Better Eyesight

The Complete Magazines of William H. Bates

Better Eyesight

The Complete Magazines of William H. Bates

EDITED BY

Thomas R. Quackenbush

North Atlantic Books
Berkeley, California

This book is solely educational and informational in nature. The reader of this book agrees that the reader, author, and publisher have not formed a professional, or any other, relationship. The reader assumes full responsibility for any changes or lack of changes experienced due to the reading of this book. The reader also assumes full responsibility for choosing to do any of the activities mentioned in this book. The author and publisher are not liable for any use or misuse of the information contained herein.

The educational information in this book is not intended for diagnosis, prescription, determination of function, or treatment of any eye conditions or diseases or any health disorder whatsoever. Readers and students of the Bates Method are advised to have an eye doctor monitor their eyesight. The information in this book should not be used as a replacement for proper medical or optometric care.

Any person with a history of disease, pathologies, or accidents involving the eyes should be under the care of an eye doctor, and consult with the eye doctor before doing any activity in this book.

Better Eyesight: The Complete Magazines of William H. Bates

Published by
North Atlantic Books
P.O. Box 12327
Berkeley, California 94712

Cover design by Catherine Campaigne
Book design by Paula Morrison
Printed in the United States of America

Better Eyesight: The Complete Magazines of William H. Bates is sponsored by the Society for the Study of Native Arts and Sciences, a nonprofit educational corporation whose goals are to develop an educational and crosscultural perspective linking various scientific, social, and artistic fields; to nurture a holistic view of arts, sciences, humanities, and healing; and to publish and distribute literature on the relationship of mind, body, and nature.

Library of Congress Cataloging-in-Publication Data

Quackenbush, Thomas R., 1952–
Better eyesight : the complete magazines of William H. Bates / Thomas R. Quackenbush.
p. cm.
Includes index.
ISBN 1-55643-351-4 (alk. paper)
1. Orthoptics—Miscellanea. 2. Eye—Care and hygiene—Miscellanea. I. Title.
RE992.07 Q32 2000
617.7—dc21
00-039450

2 3 4 5 6 7 8 9 / 06 05

DEDICATION

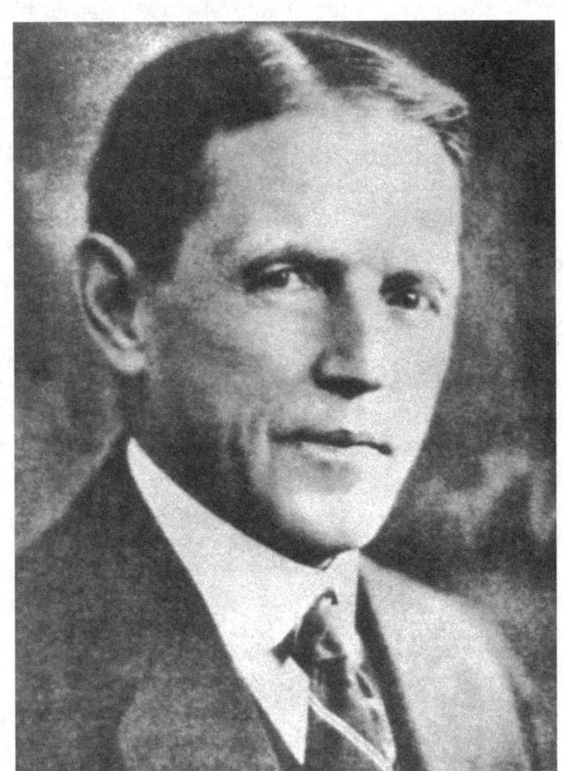

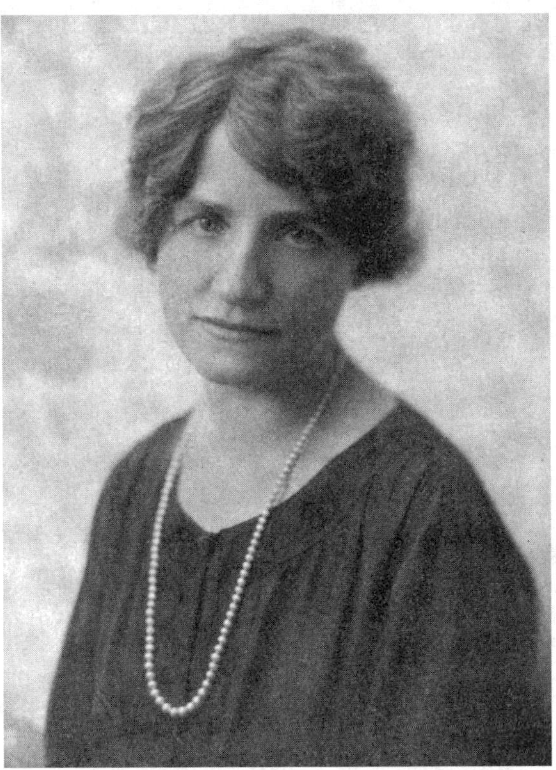

This book is dedicated to
Dr. William H. Bates, M.D.,
and
Emily A. Bates
(formerly Emily C. Lierman)

ACKNOWLEDGEMENTS

I wish to express appreciation to Kathy Glass for her expert editing, contributions, and suggestions.

I also acknowledge Paula Morrison for her book design and typesetting, Catherine Campaigne for her front cover design, Nicole George for her project management, and the staff at North Atlantic Books for their assistance in successfully completing this work. I especially appreciate Richard Grossinger's ongoing support of the Bates Method and Natural Eyesight Improvement education.

Appreciation is also expressed to my following students for their proofreading and suggestions: Dorea, Toshiyasu Abe, Barbara Cannella, Pamela Lorence Glass, Jonathan McKinnon, Robert Lichtman, Karen Pijuan, Daniela Powers, Esther van der Werf, and Timothy T. Wilson.

TABLE OF CONTENTS

LIST OF ILLUSTRATIONS AND TABLES

INTRODUCTION

If words of wisdom are gems, the collected writings of Dr. Bates constitute a treasure chest for persons serious about improving their vision by natural methods. No one before or since this "visionary" ophthalmologist has so effectively distilled the essence of the causes of faulty vision and the correct vision habits necessary for normal sight. It give me great pleasure to present this material in a modern, accessible format so others can benefit from the life's work of this brilliant yet strangely neglected eye doctor, who successfully led thousands of patients to improved vision without glasses. Dr. Bates espouses a holistic view of health and vision that was decades ahead of its time and is consistent with present-day approaches to natural health and healing. Bates' case studies and conclusions remain both powerful and inspiring to us today.

Ophthalmologist William H. Bates, M.D., is the founder of Natural Eyesight Improvement, an educational method of improving eyesight naturally. Dr. Bates self-published his landmark book *Perfect Sight Without Glasses* (a.k.a. *The Cure of Imperfect Sight by Treatment Without Glasses*) in 1920, presenting his research on the causes and solutions to many vision problems, including nearsightedness (myopia), farsightedness (hyperopia), astigmatism, strabismus (e.g. crossed eye), amblyopia ("lazy eye"), and presbyopia. Dr. Bates also reported many serious eye problems improving as a result of his educational work—including cataracts, glaucoma, retinitis pigmentosa, detached retina, conical cornea (keratoconus), iritis, atrophy of the optic nerve, and even blindness.

Dr. Bates wrote in the June 1923 issue of *Better Eyesight,* "Many people have asked me what I call my treatment. The question was a very embarrassing one because I really have no name to give it, unless I can say that my methods are the methods employed by the normal eye." The essence of the "Bates Method"—relearning correct, natural, relaxed vision habits all day long—is thoroughly presented in my textbook *Relearning to See: Improve Your Eyesight—Naturally!* More value can be derived from *Better Eyesight: The Complete Magazines of William H. Bates* if this book is read in conjunction with *Relearning to See.*

There are many references to Dr. Bates' *Perfect Sight Without Glasses* in the present book. The electronic version of *Perfect Sight Without Glasses,* including all of the illustrations, was given to the International Society for the

Enhancement of Eyesight (ISEE) by this author in 1999. At the time of the writing of the present book, *Perfect Sight Without Glasses* (with a few deletions) was on ISEE's website at http://www.i-see.org/perfect_sight/. The modern, "pop" edition of Dr. Bates' book, which was revised and abridged after Dr. Bates' death in 1931, is called *Better Eyesight Without Glasses.* Many people have found both books difficult to understand. Clarification of the Bates Method was a major motivation for writing *Relearning to See* and compiling the *Better Eyesight* magazines.

Dr. Bates wrote monthly *Better Eyesight* magazines to extend his educational outreach to the public. These writings contain outstanding elaboration of the Bates Method by Dr. Bates, his longtime assistant, nurse, and later his wife, Emily C. Lierman (Emily A. Bates), and many other Natural Eyesight Improvement teachers, including doctors. These magazines also include detailed case histories and testimonials of improved eyesight. This author considers many of the instructions and testimonials contained in these magazines of greater value than Dr. Bates' original book.

The present book is a compilation of writings from all 132 of Dr. Bates' magazines published from July 1919 to June 1930. The majority of information from each magazine is included, with only minor editing for redundancy and clarity. For example, duplicated "Questions and Answers" have been deleted. Some material, while repetitive, has been retained in this book because the variations on a particular theme are worth reading.

Some material, especially from the earlier magazines, was removed to avoid confusion. Dr. Bates changed some of his teachings in his later writings. For example, in the earlier *Better Eyesight* magazines, Dr. Bates was adamant that glasses needed to be discarded immediately and never worn again, else total success was not possible. In the later issues, he modified this position and stated that glasses could be used when necessary, although doing so would slow the progress of improving sight. Instead of removing some information, I have added editorial notes for clarification.

I am not aware of Dr. Bates suggesting the use of reduced-prescription glasses. (See Chapter 5, "Reduced Prescriptions," in *Relearning to See.)* Dr. Bates was clearly against the use of full-correction lenses. Many students have improved their eyesight by using reduced-prescription glasses when they are needed. I retained some of Dr. Bates' writings advising the immediate and permanent elimination of glasses to emphasize the importance of never wearing corrective lenses except when essential. It is not essential to completely eliminate glasses immediately to succeed; see "New Eyes for Old" by Grace Ellery Channing in the February 1920 issue, "No Glasses for Quick Results" in the October 1928 issue, and "Discarding Glasses Not Injurious" by Emily A. Bates in the September 1929 issue. In the November 1924 issue Emily C. Lierman wrote, "I was very much surprised to find that her vision had improved even though she wore her glasses. Dr. Bates and I have been surprised more than once to find a patient get well although they had worn their glasses at times." Dr. Bates writes in the October 1928 issue, "Patients who require good sight to earn a living and find it difficult to discard their glasses while under treatment have been able to make slow or rapid progress in the cure of their imperfect sight by wearing their glasses only when it was absolutely necessary."

In regard to describing lenses, e.g. "right eye, convex 3.00 D. S.; left eye, convex 3.75 D. S. with convex 0.50 D. C. 180 degrees," convex lenses are for farsightedness and presbyopia; D. S. stands for "diopters spherical"; D. C. stands for "diopter cylinder," which is a lense for astigmatism; and there is always an "axis" associated with astigmatism, which indicates the astigmatism's orientation—*not* its magnitude. Concave lenses are for nearsightedness and are also indicated by D. S. For the most part, I have standardized the nomenclature used for describing prescriptions. (For further discussion of lenses, see "Understanding Lenses and Prescriptions" in *Relearning to See.)*

A few of Bates' techniques are no longer used by modern Bates teachers and are not used in an educational setting. These techniques have been deleted.

In Dr. Bates' later writings, he taught only closed-eyelids sunning; references to his earlier versions of sunning have been removed. Never look directly into the sun with the eyelids open under any circumstances.

Many of the titles of the "Page Twos" are missing from the Table of Contents of the original *Better Eyesigh*t magazines. I have added titles to the Table of Contents of this book. "Page Two" is usually the first article of each magazine and is enclosed within a box. They are written by Dr. Bates, unless otherwise noted. Duplicate "Page Twos" have been omitted.

Most of my editorial comments are in brackets—[abc]. Sometimes I have added a short word, phrase, or comment so that a topic can be more easily located in the index.

The text blocks following "Editor's Note—" in italics are Dr. Bates' writings, not my emphasis. My emphasis is always noted as such. I do not know the author of notes in italics at the beginning of some articles (that are not preceded by "Editor's Note—"). Some may have been written by Emily A. Bates.

Starting with the February 1920 issue, there were other contributors to the *Better Eyesight* magazines. Presumably, all of the articles appearing from July 1919 to January 1920 were written by Dr. Bates and, perhaps, Emily C. Lierman.

I do not agree with all of Dr. Bates' ideas. I have

attempted to note my disagreements at their first appearances chronologically. Also, I do not use all of Dr. Bates' methods in my teaching. For example, I do not use a sun glass or the square swing.

Some of the original formatting and style has been edited in this book for easier reading. For example, where questions and answers are listed at the end of each magazine, I have numbered them for clarity and easier reference. For a few magazines, the "Questions and Answers" section title was changed by Dr. Bates to "The Question Mark"; the title has been kept in this book as "Questions and Answers" for consistency. "Shortsighted" has been standardized to "nearsighted"; "till" to "until," except in poems. "Mrs." and "Miss" have either been changed to "Ms." or deleted. While standardizing parts of these magazines, I have tried to keep as much of the original style as possible. The term "squint" has been used to describe both "strabismus" (e.g. crossed eye) and the harmful habit of narrowing of the eyelids. I have clarified this distinction in many of the earlier magazines. The context in which the term "squint" is used should make it clear to the reader which definition applies in each case. The term "squint" in reference to strabismus is no longer used today.

Volumes I-VI, from July 1919 through June 1922, contained six issues (Numbers) in each Volume. Volumes VII-XIV, from July 1922 through June 1930, contained twelve issues in each Volume.

Every August issue is a special "School Number" concerned with the eyesight of schoolchildren. Teachers and parents of schoolchildren will be especially interested in these issues. Note also the "Retardation Number" issue of April 1926. Many of the other magazines contain important information regarding schoolchildren.

A Glossary is included.

Appendix A contains a Bibliography on the Bates Method and Natural Eyesight Improvement.

Emily C. Lierman wrote a book in 1926 entitled *Stories from the Clinic*. Essentially, Emily's book is a compilation of most of the "Stories from the Clinic" articles contributed to the *Better Eyesight* magazines. All of the stories in her book are contained in the *Better Eyesight* magazines. Some of the other information contained in *Stories from the Clinic* has been included in Appendix B, "Excerpts from *Stories from the Clinic.*" I recommend reading this short Appendix before reading the *Better Eyesight* magazines. While there are 91 "Stories from the Clinic," only Stories 1-23 and 45-91 were numbered in the original *Better Eyesight* magazines. I have added the missing numbers, 24-44, and some subtitles. Emily C. Lierman's name was changed to Emily A. Bates toward the end of 1928. The middle initial "A" stands for "Ackerman." I have not been able to determine why the middle initial was changed from "C" to "A" when Emily married Dr. Bates.

Appendix C contains a "Biographical Sketch of William H. Bates, M.D."

Appendix D has information on how to contact a Natural Eyesight Improvement Teacher and other information about the Natural Vision Center of San Francisco.

Appendix E explains how to obtain information about becoming a Certified Natural Eyesight Improvement Teacher.

Appendix F, "Snellen Eyechart and Test Cards," contains reproductions of the large Snellen eyechart and many small Test Cards used by Dr. Bates and Emily Bates in their Clinic and office. Duplicates and reverse (white on black) versions of the small cards are included. You may want to assemble the Snellen Eyechart and mount it and the Test Cards on cardboard, or other suitable material, before reading the magazines, since many references are made to them.

One of the most important features of this book is the Index. There were no indexes in the original *Better Eyesight* magazines. Inclusion of the extensive Index, in conjunction with the Table of Contents, will allow the reader to find topics of interest quickly.

The power of Dr. Bates' *Better Eyesight* magazines speaks for itself. It is a mark of timeless wisdom when work such as this remains applicable long after the death of its chief proponent. The bottom line is that the Bates Method *works*, and that is the key to the longevity of these concepts among the general populace, if not within the mainstream medical community. It is my hope with this work that more people will improve their eyesight in a natural, holistic way, as many thousands of students of the Bates Method have done for more than 80 years.

Sketch (Shift), Breathe, and Blink—Always.

—TRQ
August 2000
Ashland, Oregon

EXCERPTS FROM THE INTRODUCTION TO *RELEARNING TO SEE: IMPROVE YOUR EYESIGHT—NATURALLY!*

by Thomas R. Quackenbush

Most people in this society obtain glasses or contact lenses when their eyesight becomes blurred. These crutches, or "machines of seeing," are not necessary. Nor are they natural. "Corrective" lenses do not correct the real problem. A person wearing glasses or contact lenses still has blurred vision.

Ophthalmologist Dr. William H. Bates, M.D. (1860–1931), discovered the principles and habits underlying natural eyesight. Concurrently, Bates discovered the interferences to normal sight. Bates then taught students to stop interfering with their clear vision; they were literally relearning to see.

Bates rejected contemporary theories about blurred vision because he found too much evidence in his practice as an ophthalmologist that contradicted them. Bates' decades of research on natural vision and the real causes of nearsightedness, farsightedness, astigmatism, crossed eyes, and many other vision problems went far beyond the ideas of his contemporaries. Today, most orthodox eye experts still do not understand, and do not support, his discoveries. Unfortunately, Bates was forced to leave his teaching post as instructor of ophthalmology at the New York Post-Graduate Medical School and Hospital and was ostracized from the conventional medical community because of his revolutionary discoveries.

Someone once asked Bates what technique he was using. Bates' reply was that he did not use any technique, but if it was a technique, it would be nature's technique. Bates wrote in his June 1923 *Better Eyesight* magazine, "... my methods are the methods employed by the normal eye."

Blurred vision is a message from the mind and body that a person's visual system is out of balance with nature.

Clarity is a connection; blur is a disconnection. Blur is created primarily in the mind; it is much more a disconnection from ourselves than from the world. The processes involved in improving eyesight naturally are an opportunity to reconnect with ourselves. The Bates educational method is an opportunity for internal change.

The great majority of attendees at my introductory lectures say they have seen their vision improve spontaneously. Vision fluctuates for all people. For many people in industrialized societies, sight generally becomes worse over time. Yet sometimes people see better. Most people know, either intuitively or experientially, that there is a way to improve their sight.

How is it that people accept a theory that says blurry sight is due to old age when many people—especially in non-industrialized cultures—have excellent eyesight at 40, 50, 60, 70, 80, and even 90 years of age? The idea that age and genetics determine blurry vision is also contradicted by the fact that many students have improved their sight by relearning correct vision habits. And, I have watched many children improve their vision along with their parents in my classes.

Many people experience a lowering of their sight during a period of high stress. Bates showed that when vision (excluding pathologies) lowers, it is due to acquiring incorrect vision habits. When vision improves, it is due to the person relearning relaxed vision habits. Relaxation is the key to normal, clear sight.

Broken bones heal. Burns and cuts heal. Stomach aches get better. Are we to believe that eyesight, the most important sense perception we have and one that has evolved over millions of years, is the only part of the human body that cannot heal itself? Are artificial glasses, contact lenses, drugs, and surgeries the only solutions to the functional vision problems, including nearsightedness, farsightedness, astigmatism, and strabismus? Bates concluded the answer was "no."

Personally, I had several good reasons to pursue the possibility of improving my sight: 1) I suffered physically from wearing heavy glasses and painful contact lenses every day; 2) I began to experience improvement in all parts of my health once I began receiving natural healing and education from many holistic health practitioners. Could vision improvement be the only natural healing process I investigated that did not work? 3) I experienced a dramatic improvement in my eyesight after approximately one hour while participating in a stress reduction program; this occurred before I knew about the Bates Method. So, I knew there was a way vision could improve naturally.

In the beginning, I read several eyesight improvement books. I did all of the "exercises" and "drills," but did not notice any improvement. Looking back, I realize I had almost no real understanding of the Bates Method. The processes—especially the more subtle aspects—are difficult to understand from books. I had continuing improvement of my eyesight only after receiving instructions from a Bates teacher.

Contrary to popular belief, the Bates Method is not *about* "eye exercises." Many natural eyesight improvement books present this topic in a relatively ineffective, left-hemisphere, eye exercise manner. This issue is discussed further in Chapter 19, "Brains and Vision." Since vision is primarily a right-hemisphere activity, lessons are best presented in an integrative, holistic manner, with the emphasis on the correct vision habits (or skills) to be used automatically and subconsciously our entire lifetime.

Along with improvement of clarity, many qualities of the vision system improve, e.g. color brightness and variations, contrast, spatial/depth perception, and texture awareness. There is a high correlation between memory and concentration improvement and natural eyesight improvement.

Since poor vision habits strain the neck and shoulders, no one is truly healthy who has blurred sight.

I have watched eyesight improve naturally with hundreds of students since 1983. Many of my students have freed themselves from glasses or have prevented moving into wearing glasses in the first place. If you are interested in vision re-education, study this book and other books on natural eyesight improvement to learn and apply as much as you are able; better yet, find a Bates teacher who understands and can teach you the key habits and principles of natural vision. Then, discover the joys and rewards of relearning to see—naturally. As the original jacket of Aldous Huxley's book, *The Art of Seeing,* says, this process of improving vision is "An Adventure in Re-education."

Because Dr. Bates was a medical doctor and eye surgeon (ophthalmologist), and because much of his work is discussed in this book, some terms used herein are medical. After Bates died in 1931, his wife Emily and other Natural Eyesight Improvement teachers have taught the "Bates Method" in an educational manner. The Bates Method, as presented in this book, is solely educational in nature—it is not medical or optometric.

Better Eyesight
July 1919—Vol. I, No. 1

FLASHING

Do you see imperfectly? Can you observe then that when you look at the first word or the first letter of a sentence, you do not see best where you are looking; that you see other words, or other letters, just as well as or better than the ones you are looking at? Do you observe also that the harder you try to see, the worse you see?

Now close your eyes and rest them, remembering some color, like black or white, that you can remember perfectly. Keep them closed until they feel rested, or until the feeling of strain has been completely relieved. Now open them and look at the first word or letter of a sentence for a fraction of a second. If you have been able to relax, partially or completely, you will have a flash of improved or clear vision, and the area seen best will be smaller.

After opening the eyes for this fraction of a second, close them again quickly, still remembering the color, and keep them closed until they again feel rested. Then again open them for a fraction of a second. Continue this alternate resting of the eyes and flashing of the letters for a time, and you may soon find that you can keep your eyes open longer than a fraction of a second without losing the improved vision.

If your trouble is with distant instead of near vision, use the same method with distant letters.

In this way you can demonstrate for yourself the fundamental principles of the cure of imperfect sight by treatment without glasses.

If you fail, ask someone with perfect sight to help you.

FOREWORD

When the United States entered the European war, recruits for general military service were required to have a visual acuity of 20/40 in one eye and 20/100 in the other.[1] This very low standard, although it is a matter of common knowledge that it was interpreted with great liberality, proved to be the greatest physical obstacle to the raising of an Army. Under it 21.68 percent of the registrants were rejected, 13 percent more than for any other single cause.[2]

Later the standard was lowered[3] so that men might be unconditionally accepted for general military service with a vision of 20/100 in each eye without glasses, provided one eye was correctable to 20/40. For special or limited service they might be accepted with only 20/200 in each eye without glasses, provided one was correctable to 20/40. At the same time a great many defects other than errors of refraction were admitted in both classes, such as squint not interfering with vision, slight nystagmus, and color blindness. Even total blindness in one eye was not a cause for rejection in the limited service class, provided it was not due to progressive or organic change, and the vision of the other eye was normal. Under this incredible standard, eye defects still remained one of three leading causes of rejection.

Over ten percent (10.65) of the registrants were disqualified by them, while defects of the bones and joints and of the heart and blood-vessels ran respectively one and one and a half percent higher.[4]

Most of the revelations about the physical condition of the American people that resulted from the operation of the draft law had been anticipated by persons who had been giving their attention to such matters—and whose warnings had long fallen upon deaf ears—but it is doubtful if anyone had formed an adequate conception of the truth regarding the condition of the nation's eyesight. That

1. Harvard: *Manual of Military Hygiene for the Military Services of the United States,* third revised edition 1917, p. 195.

2 "Report of the Provost Marshal General to the Secretary of War on the First Draft under the Selective Service Act," 1917.

3. "Standards of Physical Examination for the Use of Local Boards, District Boards and Medical Advisory Boards under the Selective Service Act," Form 75, issued through office of the Provost Marshal General.

4. "Second Report of the Provost Marshal General to the Secretary of War on the Operations of the Selective Service System" to December 20, 1918.

it should be impossible to raise an Army with even half normal vision in one eye, and that one man in every ten rejected for military service should have been unable, even by the aid of glasses, to attain this standard, is a situation so appalling that words fail to characterize it, so incredible that only the most unimpeachable evidence could compel belief in it. Under these circumstances it seems to me the plain duty of anyone who has found any means of controlling the evil in question to give the facts the widest possible publicity.

Most writers on ophthalmology today appear to believe that defective eyesight is part of the price we must pay for civilization. The human eye, they say, was not designed for the uses to which it is now put. Eons before there were any schools, or printing presses, electric lights, or movies, its evolution was complete. In those days it served the needs of the human animal perfectly, but it is not to be expected, we are told, that it should respond without injury to the new demands. By care it is thought that this injury may be minimized, but to eliminate it wholly is considered to be too much to hope for. Such is the depressing conclusion to which the monumental labors of a hundred years and more have led us.

I have no hesitation in stating that this conclusion is unqualifiedly wrong. Nature did not blunder when she made the human eye, but has given us in this intricate and wonderful mechanism, upon which so much of the usefulness as well as the pleasure of life depends, an organ as fully equal to the needs of civilization as to those of the stone age. *After thirty-three years of clinical and experimental work, I have demonstrated to my own satisfaction and that of others that the eye is capable of meeting the utmost demands of civilization; that the errors of refraction which have so long dogged the footsteps of progress, and which have made the raising of an Army during the recent war so difficult, are both preventable and curable; and that many other forms of imperfect sight, long held to be incurable, may be either improved or completely relieved.* [My emphasis.—TRQ]

All these discoveries have been published in the medical press, but while their reliability has never been publicly disputed, the medical profession has so far failed to make use of them. Meantime the sight of our children is being destroyed daily in the schools, and our young men and women are entering life with a defect that, if uncorrected, must be a source of continual misery and expense to them, sometimes ending in blindness or economic ruin. Admitting for the sake of argument that I may be wrong in my conclusion that these things are unnecessary, it is time I was proven to be wrong. I should not be allowed to play on the forlorn hope of a suffering world. If I am right, as I know I am, a suffering world should no longer be deprived of the benefit of my discoveries.

To give publicity to these discoveries and arouse discussion regarding them is one of the objects for which this magazine has been started. At the same time its pages are open to everyone who has any light to throw upon the problem. It has too long been the custom of ophthalmologists to disregard every fact at variance with the accepted theories. Such facts, when observed, have usually not been published, and when published they have either been ignored or explained away in some more or less plausible manner. The management of this magazine wishes to make it a medium for the publication of such facts that, it may safely be asserted, are known to every ophthalmologist of any experience, and which, if they had received proper consideration, would long ago have led us out of the blind alley in which we are now languishing.

While I think it may be truthfully said that many of my methods are new and original, other physicians, both in this country and in Europe, have cured themselves and others by treatment without glasses. Lay persons have done the same.

In *The Autocrat of the Breakfast Table,* Oliver Wendell Holmes published a very remarkable case of the cure of presbyopia.

"There is now living in New York State," he says, "an old gentleman who, perceiving his sight to fail, immediately took to exercising it on the finest print, and in this way fairly bullied nature out of her foolish habit of taking liberties at five-and-forty, or thereabouts. And now this old gentleman performs the most extraordinary feats with his pen, showing that his eyes must be a pair of microscopes. I should be afraid to say how much he writes in the compass of a half-dime, whether the Psalms or the Gospels, or the Psalms and the Gospels, I won't be positive."[5]

An officer in the American Expeditionary Forces, whose letter is published below, wrote to me about a year ago that he has cured himself of presbyopia, and after half a lifetime of misery was entirely free from eye discomfort. There must be many more of these cases, and we want to hear of them.

FUNDAMENTAL FACTS

For about seventy years it has been believed that the eye accommodates for vision at different distances by changing the curvature of the lens, and this theory has given birth to another, namely, that errors of refraction are due to a permanent organic change in the shape of the eyeball. On

5. Everyman's Library, 1908, pp. 166 and 167.

these two ideas the whole system of treating errors of refraction is based at the present time.

My experiments and clinical observations have demonstrated that both these theories are wrong.[1] They have shown:

(1) That the lens is not a factor in accommodation; [see my comments in "Presbyopia: Its Cause and Cure" in the April 1927 issue.—TRQ]

(2) That the change of focus necessary for vision at different distances is brought about by the action of the superior and inferior obliques, which, by their contraction and relaxation, change the length of the eyeball as the length of the camera is changed by the shortening and lengthening of the bellows;

(3) That errors of refraction are due to the abnormal action of these muscles and of the recti, the obliques being responsible for myopia and the recti for hypermetropia, while both may combine in the production of astigmatism;

(4) That this abnormal action of the muscles on the outside of the eyeball is always due to mental strain of some kind.

This being the case it follows that all errors of refraction can be cured by relaxation. All methods of treatment, therefore, are simply different ways of obtaining relaxation. And because it is impossible to relax the eye muscles without relaxing the mind—and the relaxation of the mind means the relaxation of the whole body—it also follows that improvement in the eyesight is always accompanied by an improvement in health and mental efficiency.

The fact that all errors of refraction are functional can often be demonstrated within five minutes. When a person with myopia, hypermetropia, or astigmatism, looks at a blank wall without trying to see, the retinoscope, with a plane mirror, at six feet, indicates, in flashes or more continuously no error of refraction. The conditions should be favorable for relaxation and the doctor should be as much at his ease as the patient.

It can also be demonstrated with the retinoscope that persons with normal sight do not have it all the time.[2] When the vision of such persons becomes imperfect at the distance it will be found that myopic refraction has been produced;[3] when it becomes imperfect at the near point it will be found that hypermetropia has been produced.

CENTRAL FIXATION

An invariable symptom of all abnormal conditions of the eyes, whether functional or organic, is the loss of central fixation. [Many modern Bates teachers have replaced this phrase with the term *centralization,* since *central fixation* could be misunderstood as a type of staring, a harmful vision habit.—TRQ] When a person with perfect vision looks at a letter on the Snellen test card he can always observe that all the other letters in his field of vision are seen less distinctly. He can also observe that when he looks at the bottom of even the smallest letter on the card, the top appears less black and less distinct than the part directly regarded, while the same is true of a letter of diamond type, or of the smallest letters that are printed. When a person with imperfect sight looks at the card, he can usually observe that when he can read a line of letters, he is able to look at one letter of a line and see it better than the others, but the letters of a line he cannot read may look all alike, or those not directly regarded may even be seen better than the one fixed.

These conditions are due to the fact that when the sight is normal the sensitiveness of the fovea is normal, but when the sight is imperfect from whatever cause, the sensitiveness of the fovea is lowered so that the eye sees equally well, or even better, with other parts of the retina. Contrary to what is generally believed, the part seen best when the sight is normal is extremely small. The textbooks say that at twenty feet an area having a diameter of a quarter of an inch can be seen with maximum vision, but anyone who tries at this distance to see every part of one of the small letters of the Snellen test card—the diameter of which is about a quarter of an inch—equally well at one time will immediately become myopic. The fact is that the nearer the point of maximum vision approaches a mathematical point, which has no area, the better the sight.

The cause of this loss of function in the center of sight is mental strain; and as all abnormal conditions of the eyes, organic as well as functional, are accompanied by mental strain, all such conditions must necessarily be accompanied by loss of central fixation. When the mind is under a strain the eye usually goes more or less blind. The center of sight goes blind first, partially or completely, according to the degree of the strain, and if the strain is great enough the whole or the greater part of the retina may be involved. When the vision of the center of sight has been suppressed, partially or completely, the patient can no longer see the point that he is looking at best, but sees objects not regarded

1. William H. Bates, "The Cure of Defective Eyesight by Treatment Without Glasses" in the *New York Medical Journal,* May 8, 1915; "A Study of Images Reflected from the Cornea, Iris, Lens and Sclera" in the *New York Medical Journal,* May 18, 1918.

2. William H. Bates, "The Imperfect Sight of the Normal Eye" in the *New York Medical Journal,* September 8, 1917.

3. *Idem:* "The Cause of Myopia" in the *New York Medical Journal,* March 16, 1912.

directly as well, or better, because the sensitiveness of the retina has now become approximately equal in every part, or is even better in the outer part than in the center. Therefore, in all cases of defective vision the patient is unable to see best where he is looking. [Since peripheral vision is incapable of perceiving sharp detail, the issue of the loss of central *clear* vision emphasized by Dr. Bates here is of great importance.—TRQ]

This condition is sometimes so extreme that the patient may look as far away from an object as it is possible to see it and yet see it just as well as when looking directly at it [albeit unclear.—TRQ] In one case it had gone so far that the patient could see only with the edge of the retina on the nasal side. In other words, she could not see her fingers in front of her face, but could see them if she held them at the outer side of her eye. She had no error of refraction, showing that while every error of refraction is accompanied by eccentric fixation, the strain that causes the one condition is different from that which produces the other. The patient had been examined by specialists in this country and Europe, who attributed her blindness to disease of the optic nerve, or brain; but the fact that vision was restored by relaxation demonstrated that the condition had been due simply to mental strain.

Eccentric fixation, even in its lesser degrees, is so unnatural that great discomfort or even pain can be produced in a few seconds by trying to see every part of an area three or four inches in extent at twenty feet, or even less, or an area of an inch or less at the near point equally well at one time, while at the same time the retinoscope will demonstrate that an error of refraction has been produced. [Some Bates teachers refer to *eccentric fixation* as *diffusion*, or *spreading the vision*.—TRQ] This strain, when it is habitual, leads to all sorts of abnormal conditions and is, in fact, at the bottom of most eye troubles, both functional and organic. The discomfort and pain may be absent, however, in the chronic condition, and it is actually an encouraging symptom when the patient begins to experience them.

[Many chronic conditions, not just with vision, are preceded by periods of discomfort and pain. As the problem continues, the pain and discomfort can disappear. It is a common experience in natural, holistic healing that when chronic health problems begin improving, the original discomfort and pain return temporarily. Some common terms given to this healing process are *healing crisis* and *aggravation phase*. See *healing crisis* in the Glossary.—TRQ]

When the eye possesses central fixation it not only possesses perfect sight, but it is perfectly at rest and can be used indefinitely without fatigue. It is open and quiet; no nervous movements are observable; and when it regards a point at the distance the visual axes are parallel. In other words, there are no muscular insufficiencies. This fact is not generally known. The textbooks state that muscular insufficiencies occur in eyes having normal sight, but I have never seen such a case. The muscles of the face and of the whole body are also at rest, and when the condition is habitual there are no wrinkles or dark circles around the eyes.

In most cases of eccentric fixation, on the contrary, the eye quickly tires and its appearance with that of the face is expressive of effort or strain. The ophthalmoscope reveals that the eyeball moves at irregular intervals, from side to side, vertically or in other directions. These movements are often so extensive as to be manifest by ordinary inspection, and are sometimes sufficiently marked to resemble nystagmus. [Not to be confused with *saccadic vibrations*.—TRQ] Nervous movements of the eyelids may also be noted, either by ordinary inspection, or by lightly touching the lid of one eye while the other regards an object either at the near point or the distance. The visual axes are never parallel, and the deviation from the normal may become so marked as to constitute the condition of squint. Redness of the conjunctiva and of the margins of the lids, wrinkles around the eyes, dark circles beneath them and excessive tearing are other symptoms of eccentric fixation.

Eccentric fixation is a symptom of strain, and is relieved by any method that relieves strain; but in some cases the patient is cured just as soon as he is able to demonstrate the facts of central fixation. When he comes to realize, through actual demonstration of the fact, that he does not see best where he is looking, and that when he looks a sufficient distance away from a point he can see it worse than when he looks directly at it, he becomes able, in some way, to reduce the distance to which he has to look in order to see worse until he can look directly at the top of a small letter and see the bottom worse, or look at the bottom and see the top worse. The smaller the letter regarded in this way, or the shorter the distance the patient has to look away from a letter in order to see the opposite part indistinctly, the greater the relaxation and the better the sight. When it becomes possible to look at the bottom of a letter and see the top worse, or to look at the top and see the bottom worse, it becomes possible to see the letter perfectly black and distinct. At first such vision may come only in flashes. The letter will come out distinctly for a moment and then disappear. But gradually, if the practice is continued, central fixation will become habitual.

Most patients can readily look at the bottom of the big "C" and see the top worse; but in some cases it is not only impossible for them to do this, but impossible for them to let go of the large letters at any distance at which they can be seen. In these extreme cases it sometimes requires considerable ingenuity, first to demonstrate to the patient that he does not see best where he is looking, and then to help him to see an object worse when he looks away from it than when he looks directly at it. The use of a strong light as one of the points of fixation, or of two lights five or ten feet apart, has been found helpful. The patient looks away from the light being able to see it less bright more readily than he can see a black letter worse when he looks away from it. It then becomes easier for him to see the letter worse when he looks away from it. This method was successful in the following case:

A patient with vision of 3/200, when she looked at a point a few feet away from the big "C," said she saw the letter better [but not clearly—TRQ] than when she looked directly at it. Her attention was called to the fact that her eyes soon became tired and that her vision soon failed when she saw things in this way. Then she was directed to look at a bright object about three feet away from the card, and this attracted her attention to such an extent that she became able to see the large letter on the test card worse, after which she was able to look back at it and see it better. It was demonstrated to her that she could do one of two things: look away and see the letter better than she did before, or look away and see it worse. She then became able to see it worse all the time when she looked three feet away from it. Next she became able to shorten the distance successively to two feet, one foot and six inches, with a constant improvement in vision; and finally she became able to look at the bottom of the letter and see the top worse, or look at the top and see the bottom worse. With practice she became able to look at the smaller letters in the same way, and finally she became able to read the 10-line at twenty feet, 20/10. By the same method also she became able to read diamond type, first at twelve inches and then at three inches. By these simple measures alone she became able, in short, to see best where she was looking, and her cure was complete.

The highest degrees of eccentric fixation occur in the high degrees of myopia, and in these cases, since the sight is best at the near point, the patient is benefited by practicing seeing worse at this point. The distance can then be gradually extended until it becomes possible to do the same thing at twenty feet. One patient with a high degree of myopia said that the farther she looked away from an electric light the better she saw it, but by alternately looking at the light at the near point and looking away from it she became able, in a short time, to see it brighter when she looked directly at it than when she looked away from it. Later she became able to do the same thing at twenty feet, and then she experienced a wonderful feeling of relief. No words, she said, could adequately describe it. Every nerve seemed to be relaxed, and a feeling of comfort and rest permeated her whole body. Afterward her progress was rapid. She soon became able to look at one part of the smallest letters on the card and see the rest worse, and then she became able to read the letters at twenty feet.

On the principle that a burnt child dreads the fire, some patients are benefited by consciously making their sight worse. When they learn, by actual demonstration of the facts, just how their visual defects are produced, they unconsciously avoid the unconscious strain that causes them. When the degree of eccentric fixation is not too extreme to be increased, therefore, it is a benefit to patients to teach them how to increase it. When a patient has consciously lowered his vision and produced discomfort and even pain by trying to see the big "C," or a whole line of letters, equally well at one time, he becomes better able to correct the unconscious effort of the eye to see all parts of a smaller area equally well at one time.

In learning to see best where she is looking, it is usually best for the patient to think of the point not directly regarded as being seen less distinctly than the point she is looking at, instead of thinking of the point fixed as being seen best, as the latter practice has a tendency, in most cases, to intensify the strain under which the eye is already laboring. One part of an object is seen best only when the mind is content to see the greater part of it indistinctly, and as the degree of relaxation increases the area of the part seen worse increases until that seen best becomes merely a point.

The limits of vision depend upon the degree of central fixation. [My emphasis.—TRQ] A person may be able to read a sign half a mile away when he sees the letters all alike, but when taught to see one letter best he will be able to read smaller letters that he didn't know were there. The remarkable vision of savages, who can see with the naked eye objects for which most civilized persons require a telescope, is a matter of central fixation. Some people can see the rings of Saturn or the moons of Jupiter with the naked eye. It is not because of any superiority in the structure of their eyes, but because they have attained a higher degree of central fixation than most civilized persons.

Not only do all errors of refraction and all functional disturbances of the eye disappear when it sees by central fixation, but many organic conditions are relieved or cured. I am unable to set any limits to its possibilities. I would not have ventured to predict that glaucoma, incipient cataract and syphilitic iritis could be cured by central fixation; but it is a fact that these conditions have disappeared when central fixation was attained. Relief was often obtained in a few minutes, and sometimes this relief was permanent. Usually, however, a permanent cure required more prolonged treatment. Inflammatory conditions of all kinds, including inflammation of the cornea, iris, conjunctiva, the various coats of the eyeball and even the optic nerve itself, have been benefited by central fixation after other methods had failed. Infections, as well as diseases caused by protein poisoning and the poisons of typhoid fever, influenza, syphilis and gonorrhea, have also been benefited by it. Even with a foreign body in the eye there is no redness and no pain so long as central fixation is retained.

Since central fixation is impossible without mental control, *central fixation of the eye means central fixation of the mind.* [My emphasis.—TRQ] It means, therefore, health in all parts of the body, for all the operations of the physical mechanism depend upon the mind. Not only the sight, but all the other senses—touch, taste, hearing and smell—are benefited by central fixation. All the vital processes—digestion, assimilation, elimination, etc.—are improved by it. The symptoms of functional and organic diseases are relieved. The efficiency of the mind is enormously increased. The benefits of central fixation already observed are, in short, so great that the subject merits further investigation.

A TEACHER'S EXPERIENCES

A teacher forty years old was first treated on March 28, 1919. She was wearing the following glasses: O. D. convex 0.75 D. S. with convex 4.00 D. C. 105 degrees; O. S. convex 0.75 D. S. with convex 3.50 D. C. 105 degrees. On June 9, 1919, she wrote:

"I will tell you about my eyes, but first let me tell you other things. You were the first to unfold your theories to me, and I found them good immediately—that is, I was favorably impressed from the start. I did not take up the cure because other people recommended it, but because I was convinced: first, that you believed in your discovery yourself; second, that your theory of the cause of eye trouble was true. I don't know how I knew these two things, but I did. After a little conversation with you, you and your discovery both seemed to me to bear the earmarks of the genuine article. As to the success of the method with myself I had a little doubt. You might cure others, but you might not be able to cure me. However, I took the plunge, and it has made a great change in me and my life.

To begin with, I enjoy my sight. I love to look at things, to examine them in a leisurely, thorough way, much as a child examines things. I never realized it at the time, but it was irksome for me to look at things when I was wearing glasses, and I did as little of it as possible. The other day, going down on the Sandy Hook boat, I enjoyed a most wonderful sky without that hateful barrier of misted glasses, and I am positive I distinguished delicate shades of color that I never would have been able to see, even with clear glasses. Things seem to me now to have more form, more reality than when I wore glasses. Looking into the mirror you see a solid representation on a flat surface, and the flat glass can't show you anything really solid. My eyeglasses, of course, never gave me this impression, but one curiously like it. I can see so clearly without them that it is like looking around corners without changing the position. I feel that I can almost do it. [3-D vision.—TRQ]

I very seldom have occasion to palm.[1] Once in a great while I feel the necessity of it. The same with remembering a period.[2] Nothing else is ever necessary. I seldom think of my eyes, but at times it is borne in upon me how much I do use and enjoy using them.

My nerves are much better. I am more equable, have more poise, am less shy. I never used to show that I was shy, or lacked confidence. I used to go ahead and do what was required, if not without hesitation, but it was hard. Now I find it easy. Glasses, or poor sight rather, made me self-conscious. It certainly is a great defect, and one people are sensitive to without realizing it. I mean the poor sight and the necessity for wearing glasses. I put on a pair of glasses the other day just for an experiment, and I found that they magnified things. My skin looked as if under a magnifying glass. Things seemed too near. The articles on my chiffonier looked so close I felt like pushing them away from me. The glasses I especially wanted to push away. They brought irritation at once. I took them off and felt peaceful. Things looked normal.

I see better in the street than I ever did with glasses. I can see what people look like across the street, can distinguish their features, etc., a thing I could not do with glasses or before I wore them. I can see better across the river and further into people's houses across the street. Not that I indulge, but I noticed an increase of power while looking out of the window in school.

Speaking of school, I corrected an immense pile of examination papers the other day, five hours at a stretch, with an occasional look off the paper and an occasional turn about the room. I felt absolutely no discomfort after it. Two weeks previous to this feat I handled two hundred designs over and over again, looking at each one dozens and dozens of times to note changes and improvement in line and color. Occasionally, while this work was going on,

1. By palming is meant the covering of the closed eyes with the palms of the hands in such a way as to exclude all the light, while remembering some color, usually black. [See: "The Palming Cure," January 1920 issue.]

2. William H. Bates, "Memory as an Aid to Vision" in the *New York Medical Journal,* May 24, 1919.

I had to palm in the mornings on rising.

I use my eyes with as much success writing, though once in a while after a lot of steady writing they are a little bit tired. I can read at night without having to get close to a light. I mention this because last summer I had to sit immediately under the light or I could not see.

From the beginning of the treatment I could use my eyes pretty well, but they used to tire. I remember making a large Liberty Loan poster two weeks after I took off my glasses and I was amazed to find I could make the whole layout almost perfectly without a ruler, just as well as with my glasses. When I came to true it up with the ruler I found only the last row of letters a bit out of line at the very end. I couldn't have done better with glasses. However this wasn't fine work. About the same time I sewed a hem at night in a black dress using a fine needle. I suffered a little for this, but not much. I used to practice my exercises at that time and palm faithfully. Now I don't have to practice or palm; I feel no discomfort, and I am absolutely unsparing in my use of my eyes. I do everything I want to with them. I shirk nothing, passing up no opportunity of using them. From the first I did all my schoolwork, read every notice, wrote all that was necessary, neglecting nothing. Everything I was called upon to do I attempted. For instance, I had to read President Wilson's 'Fourteen Points' in the assembly room without notice in a poor light—unusual wording, too—and I read it unhesitatingly. I have yet to fail to make good.

Now to sum up the school end of it, I used to get headaches at the end of the month from adding columns of figures necessary to reports, etc. Now I do not get them. I used to get flustered when people came into my room. Now I do not; I welcome them. It is a pleasant change to feel this way. And—I suppose this is most important really, though I think of it last—I teach better. I know how to get at the mind and how to make the children see things in perspective. I gave a lesson on the horizontal cylinder recently, which, you know, is not a thrillingly interesting subject, and it was a remarkable lesson in its results and in the grip it got on every girl in the room. What you have taught me makes me use the memory and imagination more, especially the latter, in teaching.

Now, to sum up the effect of being cured upon my own mind. I am more direct, more definite, less diffused, less vague. In short, I am conscious of being better centered. It is central fixation of the mind. I saw this in your latest paper, but I realized it long ago and knew what to call it."

ARMY OFFICER CURES HIMSELF

An engineer, fifty-one years old, had worn glasses since 1896, first for astigmatism, getting stronger ones every couple of years, and then for astigmatism and presbyopia. At one time he asked his oculist and several opticians if the eyes could not be strengthened by exercises, so as to make glasses unnecessary, but they said, "No. Once started on glasses you must keep to them." When the war broke out he was very nearly disqualified for service in the Expeditionary Forces by his eyes, but managed to pass the required tests, after which he was ordered abroad as an officer in the Gas Service. While there he saw in the *Literary Digest* of May 2, 1918, a reference to my method of curing defective eyesight without glasses, and on May 11 he wrote to me in part as follows:

"At the front I found glasses a horrible nuisance and they could not be worn with gas masks. After I had been about six months abroad I asked an officer of the Medical Corps about going without glasses. He said I was right in my ideas and told me to try it. The first week was awful, but I persisted and only wore glasses for reading and writing. I stopped smoking at the same time to make it easier on my nerves.

I brought to France two pairs of bow spectacles and two extra lenses for repairs. I have just removed the extra piece for near vision from these extra lenses and had them mounted as pince-nez with shur-on mounts to use for reading and writing, so that the only glasses I now use are for astigmatism, the age lens being off. Three months ago I could not read ordinary headline type in newspapers without glasses. Today, with a good light, I can read ordinary book type (18-point), held at a distance of eighteen inches from my eyes. Since the first week in February, when I discarded my glasses, I have had no headaches, stomach trouble, or dizziness, and am in good health generally. My eyes are coming back, and I believe it is due to sticking it out. I ride considerably in automobiles and trams, and somehow the idea has crept into my mind that after every trip my eyes are stronger. This, I think, is due to the rapid changing of focus in viewing scenery going by so fast.

Other men have tried this plan on my advice, but gave it up after two or three days. Yet, from what they say, I believe they were not so uncomfortable as I was for a week or ten days. I believe most people wear glasses because they 'coddle' their eyes."

Better Eyesight
August 1919—Vol. I, No. 2

SCHOOL NUMBER

HOW TO USE THE SNELLEN TEST CARD FOR THE PREVENTION AND CURE OF IMPERFECT SIGHT IN CHILDREN

The Snellen test card is placed permanently upon the wall of the classroom, and every day the children silently read the smallest letters they can see from their seats with each eye separately, the other being covered with the palm of the hand in such a way as to avoid pressure on the eyeball. This takes no appreciable amount of time and is sufficient to improve the sight of all children in one week and to cure all errors of refraction after some months, a year, or longer.

Children with markedly defective vision should be encouraged to read the card more frequently.

Records may be kept as follows:

John Smith, 10, September 15, 1918.
R. V. (vision of the right eye) 20/40.
L. V. (vision of the left eye) 20/20.

John Smith, 11, January 1, 1919.
R. V. 20/30.
L. V. 20/15.

The numerator of the fraction indicates the distance of the test card from the pupil; the denominator denotes the line read as designated by the figures printed above the middle of each line of the Snellen test card.

It is not necessary that either the inspector, the teachers, or the children should understand anything about the physiology of the eye.

A HOUSE BUILT ON SAND

That the results of the present method of treating defects of vision are far from satisfactory is something that no one would attempt to deny. It is well known that many patients wander from one specialist to another, seeking vainly for relief, while others give up in despair and either bear their visual ills as best they may without assistance, or else resort to Christian Science, mental science, osteopathy, physical culture, or some of the other healing cults to which the incompetence of orthodox medicine has given birth. The specialists themselves, having daily to handle each other's failures, are scarcely better satisfied. Privately they criticize each other with great asperity and freedom, and publicly they indulge in much speculation as to the underlying causes of this deplorable state of affairs.

At the recent meeting of the Ophthalmological Section of the American Medical Association, Dr. E. J. Gardiner of Chicago, in a paper on "The Present Status of Refraction Work,"[1] finds that ignorance is responsible for the largest quota of failure to get satisfactory results from what he calls the "rich heritage" of ophthalmic science, but that a considerable percentage must be attributed to other causes. Among these causes he enumerates a too-great dependence on measuring devices, the delegation of refraction work to assistants, and the tendency to eliminate cycloplegics [paralysis of the eye muscle responsible for accommodation.—TRQ], in deference to the prejudices of patients who have a natural objection to being incapacitated by "drops."

On the same occasion, Dr. Samuel Theobald of Johns Hopkins University noted a tendency to "minimize the importance of muscular anomalies" as an important cause of many failures to give relief to eye patients. Among cases that have come into his hands after glasses had been prescribed by other ophthalmologists he has often found that "though great pains had been taken to correct even minor faults of refraction, grave muscular errors had been entirely overlooked." From this fact and from the small number of latent muscular defects noted in the hospital reports that he has examined, the conclusion seems to him inevitable that such faults are in large measure ignored.

Dr. Walter Pyle of Philadelphia laid stress on "neces-

1. For reports of all the papers quoted, see *Journal of the American Medical Association,* June 21,1919.

sary but often neglected refinements in examination of ocular refraction." "Long practice, infinite care and attention to finer details," he said, "are imperative requisites, since a slight fault in the correction of a refractive error aggravates rather than relieves the accompanying asthenopic symptoms." This care, he says, must be exercised not only by the oculist but by the optician, and to the end that the latter may be inspired to do his part, he suggests that the oculist provide himself with the means for keeping tabs on him in the form of a mechanical lens measure, axis finder and centering machine.

Dr. Charles Emerson of the Indiana University School of Medicine suggested a closer cooperation between the ophthalmologist and the physician, as there were many patients who could not be helped by the ophthalmologist alone.

The fitting of glasses by opticians is usually condemned without qualification, but in the discussion that followed these papers, Dr. Dunbar Roy of Atlanta said that the optician, just because he does not use cycloplegics, frequently fits patients with comfortable glasses where the ophthalmologist has failed. When a patient needs glasses, said Dr. Roy, he needs them when his eyes are in their natural or normal condition and not when the muscle of accommodation is partially paralyzed. Even the heavy frames used in the adjustment of trial lenses were not forgotten in the search for possible causes of failure, Dr. Roy believing that the patient is often so annoyed by these contrivances that he does not know which is causing him the most discomfort, the frames or the glasses.

Nowhere in the whole discussion was there any suggestion that this great mass of acknowledged failure could possibly be due to any defect in fundamental principles. These are a "rich heritage," the usefulness of which is not to be questioned. If they do not produce satisfactory results, it must be due to their faulty application, and it is taken for granted that there are a select few who understand and are willing to take the trouble to use them properly.

The simple fact, however, is that the fitting of glasses can never be satisfactory. The refraction of the eye is continually changing.[2] Myopia, hypermetropia and astigmatism come and go, diminish and increase, and the same adjustment of glasses cannot suit the affected eyes at all times. One may be able, in many cases, to make the patient comfortable, to improve his sight, or to relieve nervous symptoms; but there will always be a considerable number of persons who get little or no help from glasses, while practically everyone who wears them is more or less dissatisfied. The optician may succeed in making what is considered to be a satisfactory adjustment, and the most eminent ophthalmologist may fail. I personally know of one specialist, a man of international reputation, who fitted a patient sixty times with glasses without affording him the slightest relief.

And even when the glasses do what is expected of them they do very little. Considering the nature of the superstructure built on the foundation of Donders, and the excellent work being done by leading men, Dr. Gardiner thinks the present status of refraction work might be deemed eminently satisfactory if it were not for the great amount of bad and careless work being done; but I do not consider it satisfactory when all we can do for people with imperfect sight is to give them eye crutches that do not even check the progress of the trouble, when the only help we can offer to the millions of myopic and hypermetropic and astigmatic and squinting [strabismic] children in our schools is to put spectacles on them. If this is the best that ophthalmology can do after building for three-quarters of a century upon the foundation of Donders, is it not time that we began to examine that foundation of which Dr. Gardiner boasts that "not one stone has been removed"? Instead of seeking the cause of our failure to accomplish even the little we claim to be able to do in the ignorance and carelessness of the average practitioner, great as that ignorance and carelessness often are; in the neglect of cycloplegics and the refinements of lens adjustment; in the failure to detect latent muscular anomalies; in the absence of cooperation between specialist and general practitioner: would it not be wiser to examine the foundation of our superstructure and see whether it is of stone or of sand?

2. William H. Bates, "The Imperfect Sight of the Normal Eye" in the *New York Medical Journal,* September 8, 1917.

THE PREVENTION OF MYOPIA

Methods That Failed

The publication in 1867 by Professor Hermann Cohn of Breslau of a study of the eyes of ten thousand schoolchildren first called general attention to the fact that while myopia is seldom found in the preschool age, the defect increases steadily both in percentage of cases and in degree during the educational period. Professor Cohn's investigations were repeated in all the advanced countries and his observations, with some difference in percentages, were everywhere confirmed. The conditions were unanimously attributed to the excessive use of the eyes for near work, and, as it was impossible to abandon the educational system, attempts were made to minimize the supposed evil effects of the reading, writing and other near work which it demanded. Careful and detailed rules were laid down by various authorities as to the size of type to be used in schoolbooks, the length of the lines, their distance apart, the distance at which the book should be held, the amount and arrangement of the light, the construction of the desks, the length of time the eyes might be used without a change of focus, etc. Face-rests were even devised to hold the eyes at the prescribed distance from the desk and to prevent stooping, which was supposed to cause congestion of the eyeball and thus to encourage elongation. The Germans, with characteristic thoroughness, actually used these instruments, Cohn never allowing his children to write without one, "even at the best possible desk."[1]

The results of these preventive measures were disappointing. Some observers reported a slight decrease in the percentage of myopia in schools in which the prescribed reforms had been made; but on the whole, as Risley has observed in his discussion of the subject in Norris and Oliver's *System of Diseases of the Eye,* "the injurious effects of the educational process were not noticeably arrested."

"It is a significant, though discouraging fact," he continues, "that the increase, as found by Cohn, both in the percentage and in the degree of myopia, had taken place in those schools where he had especially exerted himself to secure the introduction of hygienic reforms, and the same is true of the observations of Just, who had examined the eyes of twelve hundred and twenty-nine of the pupils of the two High Schools of Zittau, in both of which the hygienic conditions were all that could be desired. He found, nevertheless, that the excellent arrangements had not in any degree lessened the percentage of increase in myopia. It became necessary, therefore, to look beyond faulty hygienic environments for the cause of the pathological states represented by myopia."[2]

With the passage of time, further evidence to the same effect has steadily accumulated. In all investigation in London, for instance, in which the schools were carefully selected to reveal any difference that might arise from the various influences, hygienic, social and racial, to which the children were subjected, the proportion of myopia in the best lighted and ventilated school of the group was actually found to be higher than in the one where these conditions were worst.[3] It has also been found that there is just as much myopia in schools where little near work is done as in those in which the demands upon the accommodative power of the eye are greater, while in any case it is only a minority of the children in any school who become myopic, although all may be exposed to practically the same eye conditions. Dr. Adolf Steiger, in his recent book on *Spherical Refraction,* bears witness, after a comprehensive survey of the whole question, to the "absolutely negative results of school hygiene,"[4] and Dr. Sidler Huguenin reports[5] that in the thousands of cases that have come under his care he has observed no appreciable benefit from any method of treatment at his command.

Facts of this sort have led to a modification of the myopia theory, but have produced no change in methods of myopia prevention. A hereditary tendency toward the development of the defect is now assumed by most authorities; but although no one has ever been able to offer even a plausible explanation for its supposed injuriousness, and though its restriction has been proven over and over again to be useless, near work is still generally held to be a contributing cause and ophthalmologists still go on in the same old way, trying to limit the use of the eyes at the near point and encourage vision at the distance. It is incomprehensible that men calling themselves scientific, and having had at least a scientific training, can be so foolish. One might excuse a layman for such irrational conduct, but how men of scientific repute who are supposed to write authoritative textbooks can go on year after year copying each other's mistakes and ignoring all facts which are in conflict with them is a thing which reasonable people can hardly be expected to understand.

In 1912,[6] and a good many times since, I published the observation that myopia is always lessened when the subject strains to see at the near point, and always produced in the normal eye when the subject strains to see at the distance. These observations are of the greatest practical importance, for if they are correct, they prove our present methods of preventing myopia to be a monumental blunder. Yet no one, so far as I have heard, has taken the trouble to test their accuracy. I challenged the medical profession to produce a single exception to the statements I made in the 1912 publication, and that challenge has stood for seven years, although every member of the Ophthalmological Section of the American Medical Association must have had an opportunity to see it, and anyone who knows how to use a retinoscope could have made the necessary tests in a few minutes. If any did this, they failed to publish the results of their observations, and are, therefore, responsi-

1. *The Hygiene of the Eye In Schools,* English translation, edited by Turnbull, p. 127.

2. *System of Diseases of the Eye,* 1897, Vol. II, p. 361.

3. *British Medical Journal,* June 18, 1898.

4. *Die Entstehung der sphärischen Refraktionen des menschlichen Auges,* Berlin, 1913, p. 540.

5. *Archiv f. Augenhlt.,* Vol. LXXIX, 1915, translated in *Archives of Ophthalmology,* Vol. XLV, No. 6, November 1916.

6. William H. Bates, "The Cause of Myopia," in the *New York Medical Journal,* March 16, 1912.

ble for the effects of their silence. If they found that I was right and neglected to say so, they are responsible for the fact that the benefits that must ultimately result from this discovery have been delayed. If they found that I was wrong, they are responsible for any harm that may have resulted from their indifference.

THE PREVENTION AND CURE OF MYOPIA AND OTHER ERRORS OF REFRACTION

A Method That Succeeded

You cannot see anything with perfect sight unless you have seen it before. When the eye looks at an unfamiliar object it always strains more or less to see that object, and an error of refraction is always produced. When children look at unfamiliar writing or figures on the blackboard, distant maps, diagrams, or pictures, the retinoscope always shows that they are myopic, though their vision may be under other circumstances absolutely normal. The same thing happens when adults look at unfamiliar distant objects. When the eye regards a familiar object, however, the affect is quite otherwise. Not only can it be regarded without strain, but the strain of looking later at unfamiliar objects is lessened.

This fact furnishes us with a means of overcoming the mental strain to which children are subjected by the modern educational system. It is impossible to see anything perfectly when the mind is under a strain, and if children become able to relax when looking at familiar objects, they become able, sometimes in an incredibly brief space of time, to maintain their relaxation when looking at unfamiliar objects.

I discovered this fact while examining the eyes of 1,500 schoolchildren at Grand Forks, North Dakota, in 1903.[1] In many cases children who could not read all of the letters on the Snellen test card at the first test, read them at the second or third test. After a class had been examined the children who had failed would sometimes ask for a second test, and then it often happened that they would read the whole card with perfect vision. So frequent were these occurrences that there was no escaping the conclusion that in some way vision was improved by reading the Snellen test card. In one class I found a boy who at first appeared to be very myopic but who, after a little encouragement, read all the letters on the test card. The teacher asked me about this boy's vision, because she had found him to be very "nearsighted." When I said that his vision was normal she was incredulous and suggested that he might have learned the letters by heart or been prompted by another pupil. He was unable to read the writing or figures on the blackboard, she said, or to see the maps, charts, and diagrams on the walls, and did not recognize people across the street. She asked me to test his sight again, which I did very carefully under her supervision, the sources of error which she had suggested being eliminated. Again the boy read all the letters on the card. Then the teacher tested his sight. She wrote some words and figures on the blackboard and asked him to read them. He did so correctly. Then she wrote additional words and figures, which he read equally well. Finally she asked him to tell the hour by the clock twenty-five feet distant, which he did correctly. It was a dramatic situation, both the teacher and the children being intensely interested. Three other cases in the class were similar, their vision, which had previously been very defective for distant objects, becoming normal in the few moments devoted to testing their eyes. It is not surprising that after such a demonstration the teacher asked to have a Snellen test card placed permanently in the room. The children were directed to read the smallest letters they could see from their seats at least once every day with both eyes together and with each eye separately, the other being covered with the palm of the hand in such a way as to avoid pressure on the eyeball. Those whose vision was defective were encouraged to read it more frequently, and in fact needed no encouragement to do so after they found that the practice helped them to see the blackboard, and stopped the headaches or other discomfort previously resulting from the use of their eyes.

In another class of forty children, between ages six and eight, thirty of the pupils gained normal vision while their eyes were being tested. The remainder were cured later under the supervision of the teacher by exercises in distant vision with the Snellen card. This teacher had noted every year for fifteen years that at the opening of the school in the fall all the children could see the writing on the blackboard from their seats, but before school closed the following spring all of them without exception complained that they could not see it at a distance of more than ten feet. After learning of the benefits to be derived from the daily practice of distant vision with familiar objects as the points of fixation, this teacher kept a Snellen test card continually in her classroom and directed the children to read it every day. The result was that for eight years no more of the children under her care acquired defective eyesight.

This teacher had attributed the invariable deterioration in the eyesight of her charges during the school year

1. William H. Bates, "The Prevention of Myopia in Schoolchildren," *New York Medical Journal,* July 29, 1911.

to the fact that her classroom was in the basement and the light poor. But teachers with well-lighted classrooms had the same experience, and after the Snellen test card was introduced into both the well-lighted and the poorly-lighted rooms and the children read it every day, the deterioration of their eyesight not only ceased but the vision of all improved. Vision which had been below normal improved, in most cases, to normal, while children who already had normal sight, usually reckoned at 20/20, became able to read 20/15 or 20/10. And not only was myopia cured, but the vision for near objects was improved.

At the request of the superintendent of the schools of Grand Forks, Mr. J. Nelson Kelly, the system was introduced into all the schools of the city and was used continuously for eight years, during which time it reduced myopia among the children, which I found at the beginning to be about six percent, to less than one percent.

In 1911 and 1912 the same system was introduced into some of the schools of New York City[2] with an attendance of about ten thousand children. Many of the teachers neglected to use the cards, being unable to believe that such a simple method, and one so entirely at variance with previous teaching on the subject, could accomplish the desired results. Others kept the cards in a closet except when they were needed for the daily eye drill, lest the children should memorize them. Thus they not only put an unnecessary burden upon themselves, but did what they could to defeat the purpose of the system, which is to give the children daily exercise in distant vision with a familiar object as the point of fixation. A considerable number, however, used the system intelligently and persistently, and in less than a year were able to present reports showing that of three thousand children with imperfect sight over one thousand had obtained normal vision by its means. Some of these children, as in the case of the children of Grand Forks, were cured in a few minutes. Many of the teachers were also cured, some of them very quickly. In some cases the results of the system were so astonishing as to be scarcely credible.

In a class of mental defectives, where the teacher had kept records of the eyesight of the children for several years, it had been invariably found that their vision grew steadily worse as the term advanced. As soon as the Snellen test card had been introduced, however, they began to improve. Then came a doctor from the Board of Health who tested the eyes of the children and put glasses on all of them, even those whose sight was fairly good. The use of the card was then discontinued as the teacher did not consider it proper to interfere while the children were wearing glasses prescribed by a physician. Very soon, however, the children began to lose, break, or discard their glasses. Some said that the spectacles gave them headaches or that they felt better without them. In the course of a month or so most of the aids to vision which the Board of Health had supplied had disappeared. The teacher then felt herself at liberty to resume the use of the Snellen test card. Its benefits were immediate. The eyesight and the mentality of the children improved simultaneously, and soon they were all drafted into the regular classes because it was found that they were making the same progress in their studies as the other children were.

Another teacher reported an equally interesting experience. She had a class of children who did not fit into the other grades. Many of them were backward in their studies. Some were persistent truants. All of them had defective eyesight. A Snellen test card was hung in the classroom where all the children could see it, and the teacher carried out my instructions literally. At the end of six months all but two had been cured and these had improved very much, while the worst incorrigible and the worst truant had become good students. The incorrigible who had previously refused to study, because it gave him a headache to look at a book or at the blackboard, found out that the test card, in some way, did him a lot of good; and although the teacher had asked him to read it but once a day, he read it whenever he felt uncomfortable. The result was that in a few weeks his vision had become normal and his objection to study had disappeared. The truant had been in the habit of remaining away from school two or three days every week, and neither his parents nor the truant officer had been able to do anything about it. To the great surprise of his teacher he never missed a day after having begun to read the Snellen test card. When she asked for an explanation he told her that what had driven him away from school was the pain that came in his eyes whenever he tried to study or to read the writing on the blackboard. After reading the Snellen test card, he said, his eyes and head were rested and he was able to read without any discomfort.

To remove any doubts that might arise as to the cause of the improvement noted in the eyesight of the children, comparative tests were made with and without cards. In one case six pupils with defective sight were examined daily for one week without the use of the test card. No improvement took place. The card was then restored to its place and the group was instructed to read it every day. At the end of a week all had improved and five were cured. In the case of another group of defectives the results were similar. During the week that the card was not used no improvement was noted, but after a week of exercises in distant vision with the card, all showed marked improvement, and at the

2. William H. Bates, "Myopia Prevention by Teachers," *New York Medical Journal,* August 30, 1913.

end of a month all were cured. In order that there might be no question as to the reliability of the records of the teachers, some of the principals asked the Board of Health to send an inspector to test the vision of the pupils, and whenever this was done the records were found to be correct.

One day I visited the city of Rochester, and while there I called on the Superintendent of Public Schools and told him about my method of preventing myopia. He was very much interested and invited me to introduce it in one of his schools. I did so, and at the end of three months a report was sent to me showing that the vision of all the children had improved, while quite a number of them had obtained perfect sight in both eyes.

This method has been used in a number of other cities and always with the same result. The vision of all the children improved and many of them obtained perfect sight in the course of a few minutes, days, weeks or months.

It is difficult to prove a negative proposition, but since this system improved the vision of all the children who used it, it follows that none could have grown worse. It is therefore obvious that it must have prevented myopia. This cannot be said of any method of preventing myopia in schools which had previously been tried. All other methods are based on the idea that it is the excessive use of the eyes for near work that causes myopia, and all of them have admittedly failed.

It is also obvious that the method must have prevented other errors of refraction, a problem which previously had not even been seriously considered because hypermetropia is supposed to be congenital and astigmatism was until recently supposed also to be congenital in the great majority of cases. Anyone who knows how to use a retinoscope may, however, demonstrate in a few minutes that both of these conditions are acquired; for no matter how astigmatic or hypermetropic an eye may be, its vision always becomes normal when it looks at a blank surface without trying to see. It may also be demonstrated that when children are learning to read, write, draw, sew, or to do anything else that necessitates their looking at unfamiliar objects at the near point, hypermetropia, or hypermetropic astigmatism, is always produced. The same is true of adults. These facts have not been reported before, so far as I am aware, and they strongly suggest that children need, first of all, eye education. They must be able to look at strange letters or objects at the near point without strain before they can make much progress in their studies, and in every case in which the method has been tried it has proven that this end is attained by daily exercise in distant vision with the Snellen test card. When their distant vision has been improved by this means children invariably become able to use their eyes without strain at the near point.

The method succeeded best when the teacher did not wear glasses. In fact, the effect upon the children of a teacher who wears glasses is so detrimental that no such person should be allowed to be a teacher; and since errors of refraction are curable, such a ruling would work no hardship on anyone. Not only do children imitate the visual habits of a teacher who wears glasses, but the nervous strain of which the defective sight is an expression produces in them a similar condition. In classes of the same grade with the same lighting, the sight of children whose teachers did not wear glasses has always been found to be better than the sight of children whose teachers did wear them. In one case I tested the sight of children whose teacher wore glasses and found it very imperfect. The teacher went out of the room on an errand and after she had gone I tested them again. The results were very much better. When the teacher returned she asked about the sight of a particular boy, a very nervous child, and as I was proceeding to test him she stood before him and said, "Now, when the Doctor tells you to read the card, do it." The boy couldn't see anything. Then she went behind him and the effect was the same as if she had left the room. The boy read the whole card.

Still better results would be obtained if we could reorganize the educational system on a rational basis. Then we might expect a general return of that primitive acuity of vision which we marvel at so greatly when we read about it in the memoirs of travellers. But even under existing conditions it has been proven beyond the shadow of a doubt that errors of refraction are no necessary part of the price we must pay for education.

There are at least ten million children in the schools of the United States who have defective sight. This condition prevents them from taking full advantage of the educational opportunities which the State provides. It undermines their health and wastes the taxpayers' money. If allowed to continue, it will be an expense and a handicap to them throughout their lives. In many cases it will be a source of continual misery and suffering. And yet practically all of these cases could be cured and the development of new ones prevented by the daily reading of the Snellen test card.

Why should our children be compelled to suffer and wear glasses for want of this simple measure of relief? It costs practically nothing. In fact, it would not be necessary, in some cases, as in the schools of New York City, even to purchase the Snellen test cards, as they are already being used to test the eyes of the children. Not only does it place practically no additional burden upon the teachers, but, by improving the eyesight, health, disposition and mentality of their pupils, it greatly lightens their labors. Further, no one would venture to suggest that it could possibly do any harm. Why, then, should there be any delay about introducing it into the schools? If there is still thought to be need for further investigation and discussion, we can investigate and discuss just as well after the children get the cards as before, and by adopting that course we will not run the risk of needlessly condemning another generation to that curse which heretofore has always dogged the footsteps of civilization—namely, defective eyesight. I appeal to all who read these lines to use whatever influence they possess toward the attainment of this end.

THE STORY OF EMILY

The efficacy of the method of treating imperfect sight without glasses has been demonstrated in thousands of cases, not only in my own practice but in that of many persons of whom I may not even have heard; for almost all patients when they are cured proceed to cure others. At a social gathering one evening a lady told me that she had met a number of my patients; but when she mentioned their names, I found that I did not remember any of them, and said so.

"That is because you cured them by proxy," she said. "You didn't directly cure Ms. Jones or Ms. Brown, but you cured Ms. Smith and Ms. Smith cured the other ladies. You didn't treat Mr. and Ms. Simpkins, or Mr. Simpkins' mother and brother, but you may remember that you cured Mr. Simpkins' boy of a squint and he cured the rest of the family."

In schools where the Snellen test card was used to prevent and cure imperfect sight, the children, after they were cured themselves, often took to the teaching with the greatest enthusiasm and success, curing their fellow students, their parents and their friends. They made a kind of game of the treatment, and the progress of each school case was watched with the most intense interest by all the children. On a bright day, when the patients saw well, there was great rejoicing, and on a dark day there was corresponding depression. One girl cured twenty-six children in six months; another cured twelve in three months; a third developed quite a varied teaching and did things of which older and more experienced practitioners might well have been proud. Going to the school which she attended one day, I asked this girl about her sight, which had been very imperfect. She replied that it was now very good, and that her headaches were quite gone. I tested her sight and found it normal.

Then another child whose sight had also been very poor spoke up. "I can see all right, too," she said. "Emily cured me." "Indeed!" I replied. "How did she do that?" The second girl explained that Emily had had her read the card, which she could not see at all from the back of the room, at a distance of a few feet. The next day she had moved it a little farther way, and so on, until the patient was able to read it from the back of the room, just as the other children did. Emily now told her to cover the right eye and read the card with her left, and both girls were considerably upset to find that the uncovered eye was apparently blind. The school doctor was consulted and said that nothing could be done. The eye had been blind from birth and no treatment would do any good.

Undaunted, Emily undertook the treatment. She told the patient to cover her good eye and go up close to the card, and at a distance of a foot or less it was found that she could read even the small letters. The little practitioner then proceeded confidently as with the other eye, and after many months of practice the patient became the happy possessor of normal vision in both eyes. The case had, in fact, been simply one of high myopia, and the school doctor, not being a specialist, had not detected the difference between this condition and blindness.

In the same classroom, there had been a little girl with congenital cataract, but on the occasion of my visit the defect had disappeared. This too, it appeared, was Emily's doing. The school doctor had said that there was no help for this eye except through operation, and as the sight of the other eye was pretty good, he fortunately did not think it necessary to urge such a course. Emily accordingly took the matter in hand. She had the patient stand close to the card, and at that distance it was found that she could not see even the big "C." Emily now held the card between the patient and the light and moved it back and forth. At a distance of three or four feet this movement could be observed indistinctly by the patient. The card was then moved farther away, until the patient became able to see it move at ten feet and to see some of the larger letters indistinctly at a less distance. Finally, after six months, she became able to read the card with the bad eye as well as with the good one. After testing her sight and finding it normal in both eyes, I said to Emily:

"You are a splendid doctor. You beat them all. Have you done anything else?" The child blushed, and turning to another of her classmates, said, "Mamie, come here." Mamie stepped forward and I looked at her eyes. There appeared to be nothing wrong with them. "I cured her," said Emily. "What of?" I inquired. "Crossed eye," replied Emily. "How?" I asked, with growing astonishment.

Emily described a procedure very similar to that adopted in the other cases. Finding that the sight of the crossed eye was very poor, so much so, indeed, that poor

Mamie could see practically nothing with it, the obvious course of action seemed to her to be the restoration of its sight; and, never having read any medical literature, she did not know that this was impossible. So she went to it. She had Mamie cover her good eye and practice the bad one at home and at school until at last the sight became normal and the eye straight. The school doctor had wanted to have the eye operated upon, I was told, but fortunately Mamie was "scared" and would not consent. And here she was with two perfectly good, straight eyes.

"Anything else?" I inquired, when Mamie's case had been disposed of. Emily blushed again, and said, "Here's Rose. Her eyes used to hurt her all the time, and she couldn't see anything on the blackboard. Her headaches used to be so bad that she had to stay away from school every once in a while. The doctor gave her glasses, but they didn't help her and she wouldn't wear them. When you told us the card would help our eyes I got busy with her. I had her read the card close up, and then I moved it farther away, and now she can see all right, and her head doesn't ache any more. She comes to school every day, and we all thank you very much." This was a case of compound hypermetropic astigmatism.

Such stories might be multiplied indefinitely. Emily's astonishing record cannot, it is true, be duplicated, but lesser cures by cured patients have been very numerous and serve to show that the benefits of the method of preventing and curing defects of vision in the schools which is presented in this number of *Better Eyesight* would be far-reaching. Not only errors of refraction would be cured, but many more serious defects; and not only the children would be helped, but their families and friends also.

Better Eyesight
September 1919—Vol. I, No. 3

VISION AND EDUCATION

Poor sight is admitted to be one of the most fruitful causes of retardation in the schools. It is estimated[1] that it may reasonably be held responsible for a quarter of the habitual "left-backs," and it is commonly assumed that all this might be prevented by suitable glasses.

There is much more involved in defective vision, however, than mere inability to see the blackboard, or to use the eyes without pain or discomfort. Defective vision is the result of an abnormal condition of the mind, and when the mind is in an abnormal condition it is obvious that none of the processes of education can be conducted with advantage. By putting glasses upon a child we may, in some cases, neutralize the effect of this condition upon the eyes and by making the patient more comfortable may improve his mental faculties to some extent, but we do not alter fundamentally the condition of the mind and by confirming it in a bad habit we may make it worse.

It can easily be demonstrated that among the faculties of the mind which are impaired when the vision is impaired is the memory; and as a large part of the educational process consists of storing the mind with facts, and all the other mental processes depend upon one's knowledge of facts, it is easy to see how little is accomplished by merely putting glasses on a child that has "trouble with its eyes." The extraordinary memory of primitive people has been attributed to the fact that owing to the absence of any convenient means of making written records they had to depend upon their memories, which were strengthened accordingly; but in view of the known facts about the relation of memory to eyesight it is more reasonable to suppose that the retentive memory of primitive man was due to the same cause as his keen vision, namely, a mind at rest.

The primitive memory as well as primitive keenness of vision have been found among civilized people, and if the necessary tests had been made it would doubtless have been found that they always occur together, as they did in a case which recently came under my observation. The sub-

1. *School Health News,* Department of Health of New York City, February 1919.

ject was a child of ten with such marvelous eyesight that she could see the moons of Jupiter with the naked eye, a fact which was demonstrated by her drawing a diagram of these satellites which exactly corresponded to the diagrams made by persons who had used a telescope. Her memory was equally remarkable. She could recite the whole content of a book after reading it, as Lord Macaulay is said to have done, and she learned more Latin in a few days without a teacher than her sister who had six diopters of myopia had been able to do in several years. She remembered five years afterward what she ate at a restaurant, she recalled the name of the waiter, the number of the building and the street in which it stood. She also remembered what she wore on this occasion and what everyone else in the party wore. The same was true of every other event which had awakened her interest in any way, and it was a favorite amusement in her family to ask her what the menu had been and what people had worn on particular occasions.

When the sight of two persons is different it has been found that their memories differ in exactly the same degree. Two sisters, one of whom had only ordinary good vision, indicated by the formula 20/20, while the other had 20/10, found that the time it took them to learn eight verses of a poem varied in almost exactly the same ratio as their sight. The one whose vision was 20/10 learned eight verses of the poem in fifteen minutes, while the one whose vision was only 20/20 required thirty-one minutes to do the same thing. After palming, the one with ordinary vision learned eight more verses in twenty-one minutes, while the one with 20/10 was only able to reduce her time by two minutes, a variation clearly within the limits of error. In other words, the mind of the latter being already in a normal or nearly normal condition, she could not improve it appreciably by palming; while the former whose mind was under a strain was able to gain relaxation, and hence improve her memory, by this means.

When the two eyes of the same person are different, a corresponding difference in the memory has been noted according to whether both eyes were open or the better eye closed. A patient with normal vision in the right eye and half-normal vision in the left when looking at the Snellen test card with both eyes open could remember a period for twenty seconds continuously, but could remember it only ten seconds when the better eye was closed. A patient with half-normal vision in the right eye and one-quarter normal in the left could remember a period for twelve seconds with both eyes open and only six seconds with better eye closed. A third patient with normal sight in the right eye and vision of one-tenth in the left could remember a period twelve seconds with both eyes open and only two seconds when the better eye was closed. In other words, if the right eye is better than the left the memory is better when the right eye is open than when only the left eye is open.

Under the present educational system there is a constant effort to compel the children to remember. These efforts always fail. They spoil both the memory and the sight. The memory cannot be forced any more than the vision can be forced. We remember without effort, just as we see without effort; and the harder we try to remember or see, the less we are able to do so.

The sort of things we remember are the things that interest us, and the reason children have difficulty in learning their lessons is because they are bored by them. For the same reason, among others, their eyesight becomes impaired, boredom being a condition of mental strain in which it is impossible for the eye to function normally.

Some of the various kinds of compulsion now employed in the educational process may have the effect of awakening interest. Betty Smith's interest in winning a prize, for instance, or in merely getting ahead of Johnny Jones, may have the effect of rousing her interest in lessons that have hitherto bored her, and this interest may develop into a genuine interest in the acquisition of knowledge; but this cannot be said of the various fear incentives still so largely employed by teachers. These, on the contrary, have the effect, usually, of completely paralyzing minds already benumbed by lack of interest, and the effect upon the vision is equally disastrous.

The fundamental reason, both for poor memory and poor eyesight in schoolchildren, in short, is our irrational and unnatural educational system. Montessori has taught us that it is only when children are interested that they can learn. It is equally true that it is only when they are interested that they can see. This fact was strikingly illustrated in the case of one of the two pairs of sisters mentioned above. Phebe, of the keen eyes, who could recite whole books if she happened to be interested in them, disliked mathematics and anatomy extremely, and not only could not learn them, but became myopic when they were presented to her mind. She could read letters a quarter of an inch high at twenty feet in a poor light, but when asked to read figures one to two inches high in a good light at ten feet she miscalled half of them. When asked to tell how much "2" and "3" made, she said "4," before finally deciding on "5"; and all the time she was occupied with this disagreeable subject the retinoscope showed that she was myopic. When I asked her to look into my eye with the ophthalmoscope she could see nothing, although a much lower degree of visual acuity is required to note the details of the interior of the eye than to see the moons of Jupiter.

Nearsighted Isabel, on the contrary, had a passion for

mathematics and anatomy and excelled in those subjects. She learned to use the ophthalmoscope as easily as Phebe had learned Latin. Almost immediately she saw the optic nerve and noted that the center was whiter than the periphery. She saw the light-colored lines, the arteries; and the darker ones, the veins; and she saw the light streaks on the blood vessels. Some specialists never become able to do this, and no one could do it without normal vision. Isabel's vision, therefore, must have been temporarily normal when she did it. Her vision for figures, although not normal, was better than for letters.

In both these cases the ability to learn and the ability to see went hand in hand with interest. Phebe could read a photographic reduction of the Bible and recite what she had read verbatim, she could see the moons of Jupiter and draw a diagram of them afterwards because she was interested in these things; but she could not see the interior of the eye nor see figures even half as well as she saw letters because these things bored her. When, however, it was suggested to her that it would be a good joke to surprise her teachers, who were always reproaching her for her backwardness in mathematics, by taking a high mark in a coming examination, her interest in the subject awakened and she contrived to learn enough to get seventy-eight percent. In Isabel's case, letters were antagonistic. She was not interested in most of the subjects with which they dealt and, therefore, she was backward in those subjects and had become habitually myopic. But when asked to look at objects which aroused an intense interest her vision became normal.

When one is not interested, in short, one's mind is not under control, and without mental control one can neither learn nor see. Not only the memory but all other mental faculties are improved when the eyesight becomes normal. It is a common experience with patients cured of defective sight to find that their ability to do their work has improved.

The teacher whose letter was quoted in the first issue of *Better Eyesight* testified that after gaining perfect eyesight she "knew better how to get at the minds of the pupils," was "more direct, more definite, less diffused, less vague," possessed, in fact, "central fixation of the mind." In another letter she said, "The better my eyesight becomes the greater is my ambition. On the days when my sight is best I have the greatest anxiety to do things."

Another teacher reports that one of her pupils used to sit doing nothing all day long and apparently was not interested in anything. After the test card was introduced into the classroom and his sight improved, he became anxious to learn, and speedily developed into one of the best students in the class. In other words his eyes and his mind became normal together.

A bookkeeper nearly seventy years old who had worn glasses for forty years found after he had gained perfect sight without glasses that he could work more rapidly and accurately and with less fatigue than ever in his life before. During busy seasons, or when short of help, he has worked for some weeks at a time from 7 a. m. until 11 p. m., and he reports that he felt less tired at night after he was through than he did in the morning when he started. Previously, although he had done more work than any other man in the office, it always tired him very much. He also noticed an improvement in his temper. Having been so long in the office and knowing so much more about the business than his fellow employees, he was frequently appealed to for advice. These interruptions, before his sight became normal, were very annoying to him and often caused him to lose his temper. Afterward, however, they caused him no irritation whatever. In the case of another patient whose story is given elsewhere, symptoms of insanity were relieved when the vision became normal.

From all these facts it will be seen that the problems of vision are far more intimately associated with the problems of education than we had supposed, and that they can by no means be solved by putting concave, or convex, or astigmatic lenses before the eyes of the children.

THE DOCTOR'S STORY

One of the most striking cases of the relation of mind to vision that ever came to my attention was that of a physician whose mental troubles, at one time so serious that they suggested to him the idea that he might be going insane, were completely relieved when his sight became normal. He had been seen by many eye and nerve specialists before he came to me and consulted me at last, not because he had any faith in my methods, but because nothing else seemed to be left for him to do. He brought with him quite a collection of glasses prescribed by different men, no two of them being alike. He had worn glasses for many months at a time without benefit, and then he had left them off and had been apparently no worse. Outdoor life had also failed to help him. On the advice of some prominent neurologists, he had even given up his practice for a couple of years to spend the time upon a ranch, but the vacation had done him no good.

I examined his eyes and found no organic defects and no error of refraction. Yet his vision with each eye was only three-fourths of the normal, and he suffered from double vision and all sorts of unpleasant symptoms. He used to see people standing on their heads and little devils dancing on the tops of the high buildings. He also had other illusions too numerous to mention in a short paper. At night his sight was so bad that he had difficulty in finding his way about, and when walking along a country road he believed that he saw better when he turned his eyes far to one side and viewed the road with the side of the retina instead of with the center. At variable intervals, without warning and without loss of consciousness, he had attacks of blindness. These caused him great uneasiness, for he was a surgeon with a large and lucrative practice, and he feared that he might have an attack while operating.

His memory was very poor. He could not remember the color of the eyes of any member of his family, although he had seen them all daily for years. Neither could he recall the color of his house, the number of rooms on the different floors, or other details. The faces and names of patients and friends he recalled with difficulty, or not at all.

His treatment proved to be very difficult, chiefly because he had an infinite number of erroneous ideas about physiological optics in general and his own case in particular, and insisted that all these should be discussed; while these discussions were going on he received no benefit. Every day for hours at a time over a long period he talked and argued. Never have I met a person whose logic was so wonderful, so apparently unanswerable—and yet so utterly wrong.

His eccentric fixation was of such high degree that when he looked at a point forty-five degrees to one side of the big "C" on the Snellen test card, he saw the letter just as black as when he looked directly at it. The strain to do this was terrific, and produced much astigmatism; but the patient was unconscious of it, and could not be convinced that there was anything abnormal in the symptom. If he saw the letter at all, he argued, he must see it as black as it really was, because he was not color blind. Finally he became able to look away from one of the smaller letters on the card and see it worse than when he looked directly at it. It took eight or nine months to accomplish this, but when it had been done the patient said that it seemed as if a great burden had been lifted from his mind. He experienced a wonderful feeling of rest and relaxation throughout his whole body.

When asked to remember black with his eyes closed and covered he said he could not do so, and he saw every color but the black which one ought normally to see when the optic nerve is not subject to the stimulus of light. He had, however, been an enthusiastic football player at college, and he found at last that he could remember a black football. I asked him to imagine that this football had been thrown into the sea and that it was being carried outward by the tide, becoming constantly smaller but no less black. This he was able to do, and the strain floated with the football until, by the time the latter had been reduced to the size of a period in a newspaper, it was entirely gone.

The relief continued as long as he remembered the black spot, but as he could not remember it all the time, I suggested another method of gaining permanent relief. This was to make his sight voluntarily worse, a plan against which he protested with considerable emphasis. "Good heavens!" he said, "Is not my sight bad enough without making it worse."

After a week of argument, however, he consented to try the method, and the result was extremely satisfactory. After he had learned to see two or more lights where there was only one, by straining to see a point above the light while still trying to see the light as well as when looking directly at it, he became able to avoid the unconscious strain that had produced his double and multiple vision and was not troubled by these superfluous images any more. In a similar manner other illusions were prevented.

One of the last illusions to disappear was his belief that an effort was required to remember black. His logic on this point was overwhelming, but after many demonstrations he was convinced that no effort was required to let go, and when he realized this, both his vision and his mental condition immediately improved.

He finally became able to read 20/10 or more, and although more than fifty-five years old, he also read diamond type from six to twenty-four inches. His night blindness was relieved, his attacks of day blindness ceased, and he told me the color of the eyes of his wife and children. One day he said to me, "Doctor, I thank you for what you have done for my sight; but no words can express the gratitude I feel for what you have done for my mind."

Some years later he called with his heart full of gratitude, because there had been no relapse.

LYING A CAUSE OF MYOPIA

I may claim to have discovered the fact that telling lies is bad for the eyes. Whatever bearing this circumstance may have upon the universality of defects of vision, it can easily be demonstrated that it is impossible to say what is not true, even with no intent to deceive, or even to imagine a falsehood, without producing an error of refraction.

If a patient can read all the small letters on the bottom line of the test card, and either deliberately or carelessly miscalls any of them, the retinoscope will indicate an error of refraction. In numerous cases patients have been asked to state their ages incorrectly or to try to imagine that they were a year older, or a year younger, than they actually were, and in every case when they did this the retinoscope indicated an error of refraction. A patient twenty-five years old had no error of refraction when he looked at a blank wall without trying to see; but if he said he was twenty-six, or if someone else said he was twenty-six, or if he tried to imagine that he was twenty-six, he became myopic. The same thing happened when he stated or tried to imagine that he was twenty-four. When he stated or remembered the truth his vision was normal, but when he stated or imagined an error he had an error of refraction.

Two little girl patients arrived one after the other one day, and the first accused the second of having stopped at Huyler's for an ice-cream soda, which she had been instructed not to do, being somewhat too much addicted to sweets. The second denied the charge, and the first, who had used the retinoscope and knew what it did to people who told lies, said, "Do take the retinoscope and find out." I followed the suggestion, and having thrown the light into the second child's eyes, I asked, "Did you go to Huyler's?" "Yes," was the response, and the retinoscope indicated no error of refraction. "Did you have an ice cream soda?" "No," said the child; but the telltale shadow moved in a direction opposite to that of the mirror, showing that she had become myopic and was not telling the truth.

The child blushed when I told her this and acknowledged that the retinoscope was right, for she had heard of the ways of the uncanny instrument before and did not know what else it might do to her if she said anything more that was not true.

The fact is that it requires an effort to state what it not true, and this effort always results in a deviation from the normal in the refraction of the eye. So sensitive is the test that if the subject, whether his vision is ordinarily normal or not, pronounces the initials of his name correctly while looking at a blank surface without trying to see, there will be no error of refraction; but if he miscalls one initial, even without any consciousness of effort, and with full knowledge that he is deceiving no one, myopia will be produced.

CURED IN FIFTEEN MINUTES

Patients often ask how long it takes to be cured. The answer is that it takes only as long as it takes to relax. If this can be done in five minutes, the patient is cured in five minutes, no matter how great the degree of his error of refraction, or how long its duration. All persons with errors of refraction are able to relax in a few seconds under certain conditions, but to gain permanent relaxation usually requires considerable time. Some persons, however, are able to get it very quickly. These quick cures are very rare, except in the case of children under twelve; but they do occur, and I believe the time is coming when it will be possible to cure everyone quickly. It is only a question of accumulating more facts and presenting them in such a way that the patient can grasp them quickly.

A very remarkable case of a quick cure was that of a man of fifty-five who had worn glasses for thirty years for distant vision and ten years for reading, and whose distant vision at the time he consulted me was 20/200. When be looked at the Snellen test card the letters appeared gray to him instead of black. He was told that they were black, and the fact was demonstrated by bringing the card close to him. His attention was also called to the fact that the small letters were just as black as the large ones. He was then directed to close and cover his eyes with the palms of his hands, shutting out all the light. When he did this he saw a perfect black, indicating that he had secured perfect relaxation and that the optic nerve and visual centers of the brain were not disturbed. While his eyes were still closed he was asked, "Do you think that you can remember with your eyes open the perfect black that you now see?" "Yes," he answered, "I know I can."

When he opened his eyes, however, his memory of the black was imperfect, and though able to read the large letters, he could not read the small ones. A second time he was told to close and cover his eyes, and again he saw a perfect black. When he opened them he was able to retain complete control of his memory, and so was able to read the whole card. This was ten minutes after he entered the office.

Diamond type was now given him to read, but the letters looked gray to him and he could not distinguish them. Neither could he remember black when he was looking at them because in order to see them gray he had to strain, and in order to remember black he would have had to relax, and he could not do both at the same time. He was told that the letters were perfectly black, and when he looked away from them he was able to remember them black. When he looked back he still remembered them black, and was able to read them with normal vision at twelve inches. This took five minutes, making the whole time in the office fifteen minutes. The cure was permanent, the patient not only retaining what he had gained, but continuing to improve his sight, by daily reading of fine print and the Snellen test card, until it became almost telescopic.

Better Eyesight
October 1919—Vol. I, No. 4

THE SWINGING CURE

If you see a letter perfectly, you may note that it appears to pulsate or move slightly in various directions. If your sight is imperfect, the letter will appear to be stationary. The apparent movement is caused by the unconscious shifting of the eye. The lack of movement is due to the fact that the eye stares, or looks too long at one point. This is an invariable symptom of imperfect sight, and may often be relieved by the following method:

Close your eyes and cover them with the palms of the hands so as to exclude all the light, and shift mentally from one side of a black letter to the other. As you do this, the mental picture of the letter will appear to move back and forth in a direction contrary to the imagined movement of the eye, just so long as you imagine that the letter is moving, or swinging, you will find that you are able to remember it, and the shorter and more regular the swing, the blacker and more distinct the letter will appear. If you are able to imagine the letter stationary, which may be difficult, you will find that your memory of it will be much less perfect.

Now open your eyes and look first at one side and then at the other of the real letter. If it appears to move in a direction opposite to the movement of the eye, you will find that your vision has improved. If you can imagine the swing of the letter as well with your eyes open as with your eyes closed, as short, as regular, and as continuous, your vision will be normal.

SIMULTANEOUS RETINOSCOPY

Much of my information about the eye has been obtained by means of simultaneous retinoscopy.

The retinoscope is an instrument used to measure the refraction of the eye. It throws a beam of light into the pupil by reflection from a mirror, the light being either outside the instrument—above and behind the subject—or arranged within it by means of an electric battery. On looking through the sight-hole one sees a larger or smaller part of the pupil filled with light, which in normal human eyes is a reddish yellow because this is the color of the retina, but which is green in a cat's eye, and might be white if the retina were diseased. Unless the eye is exactly focused at the point from which it is being observed, one sees also a dark shadow at the edge of the pupil, and it is the behavior of this shadow when the mirror is moved in various directions which reveals the refractive condition of the eye. If the instrument is used at a distance of six feet or more and the shadow moves in a direction opposite to the movement of the mirror, the eye is myopic. If it moves in the same direction as the mirror, the eye is either hypermetropic or normal; but in the case of hypermetropia the movement is more pronounced than in that of normality, and an expert can usually tell the difference between the two states merely by the nature of the movement. In astigmatism the movement is different in different meridians. To determine the degree of the error, or to distinguish accurately between hypermetropia and normality, or between the different kinds of astigmatism, it is usually necessary to place a glass before the eye of the subject.

This exceedingly useful instrument has possibilities which have not been generally realized by the medical profession. It is commonly employed only under certain artificial conditions in a dark room; but it is possible to use it under all sorts of normal and abnormal conditions on the eyes both of human beings and of the lower animals. I have used it in the daytime and at night; when the subjects were comfortable and when they were excited; when they were trying to see and when they were not; when they were lying and when they were telling the truth. I have also used it under varying conditions on the eyes of many cats, dogs, rabbits, birds, turtles, reptiles and fish.

Most ophthalmologists depend upon the Snellen test card, supplemented by trial lenses, to determine whether the vision is normal or not, and to determine the degree of any abnormality that may exist. This is a slow, awkward and unreliable method of testing the vision, and absolutely unavailable for the study of the refraction of the lower animals and that of human beings under the conditions of life. The test card can be used only under certain favorable conditions, but the retinoscope can be used anywhere. It is a little easier to use it in a dim light than in a bright one, but it may be used in any light. It is available whether the subject is at rest or in motion, asleep or awake, or even under ether or chloroform. It is also available when the observer is in motion. It has been used successfully when the eyelids were partly closed, shutting off part of the area of the pupil; when the pupil was dilated; when it was contracted to a pinpoint; when the subject was reading fine print at six inches, or at a greater distance; and when the eye was oscillating from side to side, from above downward, or in other directions.

It takes a considerable time, varying from minutes to hours, to measure the refraction with the Snellen test card and trial lenses. With the retinoscope, however, the refraction can be determined in a fraction of a second. With the Snellen test card and trial lenses it would be impossible to get any information about the refraction of a baseball player at the moment he swings for the ball, at the moment he strikes it, and at the moment after he strikes it. With the retinoscope, however, it is quite easy to determine whether his vision is normal, or whether he is myopic, hypermetropic, or astigmatic when he does these things; and if any errors of refraction are noted, one can guess their degree pretty accurately by the rapidity of the movement of the shadow.

With the Snellen test card and trial lenses conclusions must be drawn from the patient's statements as to what he sees; but the patient often becomes so worried and confused during the examination that he does not know what he sees, or whether different glasses make his sight better or worse; and, moreover, visual acuity is not reliable evidence of the state of the refraction. One patient with two diopters of myopia may see twice as much as another with the same error of refraction. The evidence of the test card is, in fact, entirely subjective; that of the retinoscope is entirely objective, depending in no way upon the statements of the patient.

By means of simultaneous retinoscopy it has been demonstrated that the refraction of the eye is never constant; that all persons with errors of refraction have, at frequent intervals during the day and night, moments of normal vision when their myopia, hypermetropia, or astigmatism disappears completely; and that all persons, no matter how good their sight may ordinarily be, have moments of imperfect sight when they become myopic, hypermetropic, or astigmatic. It has also been demonstrated that when the eye makes an effort to see, an error of refraction is always produced, and that when it looks at objects without effort, all errors of refraction disappear no matter how great their degree or how long their duration. It has been further demonstrated that when the eye strains to see distant objects myopia is always produced in one or all meridians, and when it strains to see near objects hypermetropia is always produced in one or all meridians.

The examination of the eyes of persons while asleep, or under the influence of ether or chloroform, has shown that the eye is rarely at rest during sleep or while the subject is unconscious from any cause. Persons whose sight was normal while awake were found to have myopia, hypermetropia and astigmatism when asleep, and if these errors were present when they were awake, they were increased during sleep. This explains why so many people are unable to see as well in the morning as at other times and why people waken with headaches and pain in the eyes. Under ether or chloroform, errors of refraction are also produced or increased, and when people are sleepy they have invariably been found to have errors of refraction.

Under conditions of mental or physical discomfort, such as pain, cough, fever, discomfort from heat or cold, depression, anger, or anxiety, errors of refraction are always produced in the normal eye or increased in the eye in which they already exist. In a dim light, in a fog, or in the rain, the retinoscope may indicate no error of refraction in eyes which ordinarily have normal sight; but a pilot on a ship on a rainy night usually has an error of refraction because he is straining to see, and it is rare to find persons in positions of responsibility under unfavorable conditions with normal vision.

In order to obtain reliable results with the retinoscope it must be used at a distance of six feet or more from the subject. When used at a distance of three feet or less, as it commonly is, the subject becomes nervous and unconsciously strains, thus altering his refraction.

FLOATING SPECKS

A very common phenomenon of imperfect sight is the one known to medical science as *muscae volitantes,* or *flying flies.* These floating specks are usually dark or black, but sometimes appear like white bubbles, and in rare cases may assume all the colors of the rainbow. They move somewhat rapidly, usually in curving lines, before the eyes, and always appear to be just beyond the point of fixation. If one tries to look at them directly they seem to move a little farther away. Hence their name of *flying flies.*

The literature of the subject is full of speculations as to the origin of these appearances. Some have attributed them to the presence of floating specks—dead cells or the debris of cells—in the vitreous humor, the transparent substance that fills four-fifths of the eyeball behind the crystalline lens. [Floating specks *can* be due to debris in the eyeball. See Glossary.—TRQ] Similar specks on the surface of the cornea have also been held responsible for them. It has even been surmised that they might be caused by the passage of tears over the cornea. They are so common in myopia that they have been supposed to be one of the symptoms of this condition, although they occur also with other errors of refraction, as well as in eyes otherwise normal. They have been attributed to disturbances of the circulation, the digestion and the kidneys, and because so many insane people have them, they have been thought to be an evidence of incipient insanity. The patent-medicine business has thrived upon them, and it would be difficult to estimate the amount of mental torture they have caused, as the following cases illustrate.

A clergyman who was much annoyed by the continual appearance of floating specks before his eyes was told by his eye specialist that they were a symptom of kidney disease and that in many cases of kidney trouble, disease of the retina might be an early symptom. So at regular intervals he went to the specialist to have his eyes examined, and when at length the latter died, he looked around immediately for someone else to make the periodical examination. His family physician directed him to me.

I was by no means so well known as his previous ophthalmological adviser, but it happened that I had taught the family physician how to use the ophthalmoscope after others had failed to do so. He thought, therefore, that I must know a lot about the use of the instrument, and what the clergyman particularly wanted was someone capable of making a thorough examination of the interior of his eyes and detecting at once any signs of kidney disease that might make their appearance. So he came to me, and at least four times a year for ten years he continued to come.

Each time I made a very careful examination of his eyes, taking as much time as possible, so that he would believe that it was careful; and each time he went away happy because I could find nothing wrong.

A man returning from Europe was looking at some white clouds one day when floating specks appeared before his eyes. He consulted the ship's doctor, who told him that the symptom was very serious and might be the forerunner of blindness. It might also indicate incipient insanity, as well as other nervous or organic diseases. He advised him to consult his family physician and an eye specialist as soon as he landed, which he did. This was twenty-five years ago, but I shall never forget the terrible state of nervousness and terror into which the patient had worked himself by the time he came to me. I examined his eyes very carefully and found them absolutely normal. The vision was perfect both for the near point and the distance. The color perception, the fields and the tension were normal, and under a strong magnifying glass I could find no opacities in the vitreous. In short, there were absolutely no symptoms of any disease. I told the patient there was nothing wrong with his eyes, and I also showed him an advertisement of a quack medicine in a newspaper which gave a great deal of space to describing the dreadful things likely to follow the appearance of floating specks before the eyes, unless one began promptly to take the medicine in question at one dollar a bottle. I pointed out that the advertisement, which was appearing in all the big newspapers of the city every day, and probably in other cities, must have cost a lot of money and must, therefore, be bringing in a lot of money. Evidently there must be a great many people suffering from this symptom, and if it were as serious as was generally believed, there would be a great many more blind and insane people in the community than there were. The patient went away somewhat comforted, but at eleven o'clock—his first visit had been at nine—he was back again. He still saw the floating specks and was still worried about them. I examined his eyes again as carefully as before, and again was able to assure him that there was nothing wrong with them. In the afternoon I was not in my office, but I was told that he was there at three and at five. At seven he came again, bringing with him his family physician, an old friend of mine.

I said to the latter, "Please make this patient stay at home. I have to charge him for his visits because he is taking up so much of my time; but it is a shame to take his money when there is nothing wrong with him." What my friend said to him I don't know, but he did not come back again.

I did not know as much about *muscae volitantes* then as I know now, or I might have saved both of these patients a great deal of uneasiness. I could tell them that their eyes were normal, but I did not know how to relieve them of the symptom, which is simply an illusion resulting from mental strain. The specks are associated to a considerable extent with markedly imperfect eyesight because persons whose eyesight is imperfect always strain to see; but persons whose eyesight is ordinarily normal may see them at times because no eye has normal sight all the time. Most people can see *muscae volitantes* when they look at any uniformly bright surface, like a sheet of white paper upon which the sun is shining. This is because most people strain when they look at surfaces of this kind. The specks are never seen, in short, except when the eyes and mind are under a strain, and they always disappear when the strain is relieved. If one can remember a small letter on the Snellen test card by central fixation, the specks will immediately disappear, or cease to move; but if one tries to remember two or more letters equally well at one time, they will reappear and move. Usually the strain that causes *muscae volitantes* is very easily relieved.

[According to some writers, all people have debris floating in their eyes. A person is more likely to notice floating specks if the eyes are strained. Generally, floating specks are ignored by the mind when a person has correct vision habits.—TRQ]

CORRESPONDENCE TREATMENT

Correspondence treatment is usually regarded as quackery, and it would be manifestly impossible to treat many diseases in this way. Pneumonia and typhoid, for instance, could not possibly be treated by correspondence, even if the physician had a sure cure for these conditions and the mails were not too slow for the purpose. In the case of most diseases, in fact, there are serious objections to correspondence treatment.

But myopia, hypermetropia and astigmatism are functional conditions, not organic as the textbooks teach and as I believed myself until I learned better. Their treatment by correspondence, therefore, has not the drawbacks that exist in the case of most physical derangements.

In the case of the treatment of imperfect sight without glasses there can be even less objection to the correspondence method. It is true that in most cases progress is more rapid and the results more certain when the patient can be seen personally; but often this is impossible, and I see no reason why patients who cannot have the benefit of personal treatment should be denied such aid as can be given them by correspondence. I have been treating patients in this way for years, and often with extraordinary success.

Some years ago an English gentleman wrote to me that his glasses were very unsatisfactory. They not only did not give him good sight, but they increased instead of lessening his discomfort. He asked if I could help him, and since relaxation always relieves discomfort and improves the vision, I did not believe that I was doing him an injury in telling him how to rest his eyes. He followed my directions with such good results that in a short time he obtained perfect sight for both the distance and the near point without glasses, and was completely relieved of his pain. Five years later he wrote me that he had qualified as a sharpshooter in the Army.

After the United States entered the European war, an officer wrote to me from the deserts of Arizona that the use of his eyes at the near point caused him great discomfort which glasses did not relieve, and that the strain had produced granulation of the lids. As it was impossible for him to come to New York, I undertook to treat him by correspondence. He improved very rapidly. The inflammation of the lids was relieved almost immediately, and in about four months he wrote me that he had read one of my reprints—by no means a short one—in a dim light with no bad aftereffects; that the glare of the Arizona sun, with the thermometer registering 114°, did not annoy him, and that he could read the 10-line on the test card at fifteen feet almost perfectly, 15/10⁻, while even at twenty feet he was able to make out most of the letters, 20/10⁻.

A third case was that of a forester in the employ of the U. S. Government. He had myopic astigmatism and suffered extreme discomfort, which was not relieved either by glasses or by long summers in the mountains where he used his eyes little for close work. He was unable to come to New York for treatment and although I told him that correspondence treatment was somewhat uncertain, he said he was willing to risk it. It took three days for his letters to reach me and another three for my reply to reach him, and as letters were not always written promptly on either side he often did not hear from me more than once in three weeks. Progress under these conditions was necessarily slow, but his discomfort was relieved very quickly and in about ten months his sight had improved from 20/50 to 20/20.

In almost every case the treatment of cases coming from a distance is continued by correspondence after they return to their homes; and although the patients do not get on so well as when they are coming to the office, they usually continue to make progress until they are cured.

At the same time it is often very difficult to make patients understand what they should do when one has to communicate with them entirely by writing, and probably all would get on better if they could have some personal treatment. At the present time the number of doctors in different parts of the United States who understand the treatment of imperfect sight without glasses is altogether too few, and my efforts to interest them in the matter have not been very successful. I would consider it a privilege to treat medical men without a fee, and when cured they will be able to assist me in the treatment of patients in their various localities.

Better Eyesight
November 1919—Vol. I, No. 5

THE MEMORY CURE

When the sight is perfect, the memory is also perfect, because the mind is perfectly relaxed. Therefore the sight may be improved by any method that improves the memory. The easiest thing to remember is a small black spot of no particular size and form; but when the sight is imperfect it will be found impossible to remember it with the eyes open and looking at letters or other objects with definite outlines. It may, however, be remembered for a few seconds or longer when the eyes are closed and covered, or when looking at a blank surface where there is nothing particular to see. By cultivating the memory under these favorable conditions, it gradually becomes possible to retain it under unfavorable ones, that is, when the eyes are open and the mind conscious of the impressions of sight. By alternately remembering the period with the eyes closed and covered and then looking at the Snellen test card or other letters or objects, or by remembering it when looking away from the card where there is nothing particular to see and then looking back, the patient becomes able, in a longer or shorter time, to retain the memory when looking at the card, and thus becomes able to read the letters with normal vision. Many children have been cured very quickly by this method. Adults who have worn glasses have greater difficulty. Even under favorable conditions the period cannot be remembered for more than a few seconds, unless one shifts from one part of it to another. One can also shift from one period, or other small black object, to another.

REASON AND AUTHORITY

Someone—perhaps it was Bacon—has said, "You cannot by reasoning correct a man of ill opinion which by reasoning he never acquired." He might have gone a step farther and stated that neither by reasoning, nor by actual demonstration of the facts, can you convince some people that an opinion which they have accepted on authority is wrong.

Patients whom I have cured of various errors of refraction have frequently returned to specialists who had prescribed glasses for them, and, by reading fine print and the Snellen test card with normal vision, have demonstrated the fact that they were cured, without in any way shaking the faith of these practitioners in the doctrine that such cures are impossible.

A girl of sixteen, who had progressive myopia of such high degree that she was not allowed to read and was unable to go about on the streets without a guide, was assured by the specialist whom her family consulted that her condition was quite hopeless and that it was likely to progress until it ended in blindness. She was cured in a very short time by means of the methods advocated in this magazine, becoming able to discard her glasses and resume all the ordinary activities of life. She then returned to the specialist who had condemned her to blindness to tell him the good news; but, while he was unable to deny the fact that her vision was normal without glasses, he said it was impossible that she would have been cured of myopia, because myopia was incurable. How he reconciled this statement with his former patient's condition he was unable to make clear to her.

A lady with compound myopic astigmatism[1] suffered from almost constant headaches which were very much worse when she took her glasses off. Every week, no matter what she did, she was so prostrated by eyestrain that she had to spend a few days in bed; and if she went to a theatre, or to a social function, she had to stay there longer. She was told to take off her glasses and go to the movies; to look first at the corner of the screen, then off to the dark, then back to the screen a little nearer to the center, and so forth. She did so, and soon became able to look directly at the pictures without discomfort. After that nothing troubled her. One day she called on her former ophthalmological adviser, in the company of a friend who wanted to have her glasses changed, and told him of her cure. The facts seemed to make no impression on him whatever. He only laughed and said, "I guess Dr. Bates is more popular with you than I am."

In some cases patients themselves, after they are cured, allow themselves to be convinced that it was impossible that such a thing could have happened and go back to their glasses.

1. A condition in which the eye is nearsighted in all meridians, but more so in one than in the others.

A clergyman and writer, age forty-seven, who had worn glasses for years for distance and reading, had what I should have considered the good fortune to be very quickly cured. By the aid of his imagination he was able to relax in less than five minutes, and to stay relaxed. When he looked at fine print it appeared gray to him, and he could not read it. I asked him if he had ever seen printer's ink. He replied, of course, that he had. I then told him that the paragraph of printed matter which he held in his hand was printed in printer's ink, and that it was black and not gray. I asked him if he did not know and believe that it was black, or if he could not at least imagine that it was black. "Yes," he said, "I can do that"; and immediately he read the print. It took him only about a minute to do this, and he was not more than five minutes in the office. The cure was permanent and he was very grateful—for a time. Then he began to talk to eye specialists whom he knew, and thereupon grew skeptical as to the value of what I had done for him. One day I met him at the home of a mutual friend, and in the presence of a number of other people he accused me of having hypnotized him, adding that to hypnotize a patient without his knowledge or consent was to do him a grievous wrong. Some of the listeners protested that whether I had hypnotized him or not, I had not only done him no harm, but had greatly benefited him and he ought to forgive me. He was unable, however, to take this view of the matter. Later he called on a prominent eye specialist who told him that the presbyopia (old-age sight) and astigmatism from which he had suffered were incurable and that if he persisted in going without his glasses he might do himself great harm. The fact that his sight was perfect for the distance and the near point had no effect upon the specialist, and the patient allowed himself to be frightened into disregarding it also. He went back to his glasses and, so far as I know, has been wearing them ever since. The story obtained wide publicity, for the man had a large circle of friends and acquaintances; and if I had destroyed his sight I could scarcely have suffered more than I did for curing him.

Fifteen or twenty years ago the specialist mentioned in the foregoing story read a paper on cataract at a meeting of the Ophthalmological Section of the American Medical Association in Atlantic City, and asserted that anyone who said that cataract could be cured without the knife was a quack. At that time I was assistant surgeon at the New York Eye and Ear Infirmary, and it happened that I had been collecting statistics of the spontaneous cure of cataract at the request of the executive surgeon of this institution, Dr. Henry D. Noyes, Professor of Ophthalmology at the Bellevue Hospital Medical School. As a result of my inquiry I had secured records of a large number of cases which had recovered, not only without the knife, but without any treatment at all. I also had records of cases which I had sent to Dr. James E. Kelly of New York and which he had cured, largely by hygienic methods. Dr. Kelly is not a quack, and at that time was Professor of Anatomy in the New York Post Graduate Medical School and Hospital and attending surgeon to a large city hospital. In the five minutes allotted to those who wished to discuss the paper, I was able to tell the audience enough about these cases to make them want to hear more. My time was, therefore, extended, first to half an hour and then to an hour. Later both Dr. Kelly and myself received many letters from men in different parts of the country who had tried his treatment with success. The man who wrote the paper had blundered, but he did not lose any prestige because of my attack with facts upon his theories. He is still a prominent and honored ophthalmologist and in his latest book he gives no hint of having ever heard of any successful method of treating cataract other than by operation. He was not convinced by my record of spontaneous cures, nor by Dr. Kelly's record of cures by treatment; and while a few men were sufficiently impressed to try the treatment recommended, and while they obtained satisfactory results, the facts made no impression upon the profession as a whole and did not modify the teaching of the schools. That spontaneous cures of cataract do sometimes occur cannot be denied; but they are supposed to be very rare and anyone who suggests that the condition can be cured by treatment still exposes himself to the suspicion of being a quack.

Between 1886 and 1891 I was a lecturer at the Post Graduate Hospital and Medical School. The head of the institution was Dr. D. B. St. John Roosa. He was the author of many books and was honored and respected by the whole medical profession. At the school they had the habit of putting glasses on the nearsighted doctors, and I had the habit of curing them without glasses. It was naturally annoying to a man who had put glasses on a student to have the student appear at a lecture without them and say that Dr. Bates had cured him. Dr. Roosa found it particularly annoying and the trouble reached a climax one evening at the annual banquet of the faculty when, in the presence of one hundred and fifty doctors, he suddenly poured out the vials of his wrath upon my head. He said that I was injuring the reputation of the Post Graduate by claiming to cure myopia. Everyone knew that Donders said it was incurable, and I had no right to claim that I knew more than Donders. I reminded him that some of the men I had cured had been fitted with glasses by himself. He replied that if he had said they had myopia he had made a mistake. I suggested further investigation. "Fit some more doctors with glasses for myopia," I said, "and I will cure them. It is easy for you to examine them afterwards and see if the cure is genuine."

This method did not appeal to him, however. He repeated that it was impossible to cure myopia, and to prove that it was impossible he expelled me from the Post Graduate, even the privilege of resignation being denied to me.

The fact is that, except in rare cases, man is not a reasoning being. He is dominated by authority, and when the facts are not in accord with the view imposed by authority, so much the worse for the facts. They may and indeed must win in the long run; but in the meantime the world gropes needlessly in darkness and endures much suffering that might have been avoided.

THE EFFECT OF LIGHT UPON THE EYES

Although the eyes were made to react to the light, a very general fear of the effect of this element upon the organs of vision is entertained both by the medical profession and by the laity. Extraordinary precautions are taken in our homes, offices and schools to temper the light, whether natural or artificial, and to insure that it shall not shine directly into the eyes; smoked and amber glasses, eye-shades, broad-brimmed hats and parasols are commonly used to protect the organs of vision from what is considered an excess of light; and when actual disease is present, it is no uncommon thing for patients to be kept for weeks, months and years in dark rooms, or with bandages over their eyes.

The evidence on which this universal fear of the light has been based is of the slightest. In the voluminous literature of the subject one finds such a lack of information that in 1910, Dr. J. Herbert Parsons of the Royal Ophthalmic Hospital of London, addressing a meeting of the Ophthalmological Section of the American Medical Association, felt justified in saying that ophthalmologists, if they were honest with themselves, "must confess to a lamentable ignorance of the conditions which render bright light injurious to the eyes."[1] Since then, Verhoeff and Bell have reported[2] an exhaustive series of experiments carried on at the Pathological Laboratory of the Massachusetts Charitable Eye and Ear Infirmary, which indicate that the danger of injury to the eye from light radiation as such has been "very greatly exaggerated." That brilliant sources of light sometimes produce unpleasant temporary symptoms cannot, of course, be denied; but as regards definite pathological effects, or permanent impairment of vision from exposure to light alone, Drs. Verhoeff and Bell were unable to find, either clinically or experimentally, anything of a positive nature.

The results of these experiments are in complete accord with my own observations as to the effect of strong light upon the eyes. In my experience such light has never been permanently injurious.

A strong electric light may lower the vision temporarily, but never does any permanent harm. In those exceptional cases in which the patient can become accustomed to the light, it is beneficial. After looking at a strong electric light some patients have been able to read the Snellen test card better.

It is not light but darkness that is dangerous to the eye.[3] Prolonged exclusion from the light always lowers the vision, and may produce serious inflammatory conditions. Among young children living in tenements this is a somewhat frequent cause of ulcers upon the cornea, which ultimately destroy the sight. The children, finding their eyes sensitive to light, bury them in the pillows and thus shut out the light entirely.

The universal fear of reading or doing fine work in a dim light is, however, unfounded. So long as the light is sufficient so that one can see without discomfort, this practice is not only harmless, but may be beneficial.

Sudden contrasts of light are supposed to be particularly harmful to the eye. The theory on which this idea is based is summed up as follows by Fletcher B. Dresslar, specialist in school hygiene and sanitation of the United States Bureau of Education:

"The muscles of the iris are automatic in their movements, but rather slow. Sudden strong light and weak illumination are painful and likewise harmful to the retina. For example, if the eye adjusted to a dim light is suddenly turned toward a brilliantly lighted object, the retina will receive too much light, and will be shocked before the muscles controlling the iris can react to shut out the superabundance of light. If contrasts are not strong, but are frequently made, that is, if the eye is called upon to function where frequent adjustments in this way are necessary, the muscles controlling the iris become fatigued, respond more slowly and less perfectly. As a result, eyestrain in the ciliary muscles is produced and the retina is over-stimulated. This is one cause of headaches and tired eyes."[4]

There is no evidence whatever to support these statements. Sudden fluctuations of light undoubtedly cause discomfort to many persons, but far from being injurious I

1. *Journal of the American Medical Association,* December 10, 1910, p. 2028.

2. *Proceedings of the American Academy of Arts and Sciences,* July 1916, Vol. 51, No. 13.

[3. Reference: Jacob Liberman, *Light: Medicine of the Future* (Santa Fe, New Mexico: Bear & Company, 1991).—TRQ]

4. *School Hygiene, Brief Course Series in Education,* edited by Paul Monroe, 1916, pp. 235–236.

have found them in all cases observed to be actually beneficial. The pupil of the normal eye, when it has normal sight, does not change appreciably under the influence of changes of illumination; and persons with normal vision are not inconvenienced by such changes.

When the eye has imperfect sight, the pupil usually contracts in the light and expands in the dark, but it has been observed to contract to the size of a pinhole in the dark. Whether the contraction takes place under the influence of light or darkness, the cause is the same, namely, strain. Persons with imperfect sight suffer great inconvenience, resulting in lowered vision, from changes in the intensity of the light; but the lowered vision is always temporary, and if the eye is persistently exposed to these conditions, the sight is benefited. Such practices as reading alternately in a bright and a dim light, or going from a dark room to a well-lighted one, and vice versa, are to be recommended. [Some Bates teachers educate students to alternate between closed-eyelid sunning and palming.—TRQ] Even such rapid and violent fluctuations of light as those involved in the production of movies are, in the long run, beneficial to all eyes. I always advise patients under treatment for the cure of defective vision to go to the movies frequently and practice central fixation. They soon become accustomed to the flickering light, and afterward other lights and reflections cause less annoyance.

TWO POINTS OF VIEW

Being anxious to know what my colleagues think of *Better Eyesight,* I lately sent notes to a number of them asking for their opinion. The following replies were so interesting that I think the readers of the magazine have a right to see them.

Dear Doctor:

As long as you ask for my opinion of your new magazine entitled *Better Eyesight,* permit me to give it to you in all frankness. It is what we call in the vernacular, "PUNK."

Meaning no personal offense, I am, Your colleague,—.

Dear Doctor:

Your little note was received this morning and am glad to have the opportunity to tell you what I think of *Better Eyesight.*

It is all that you claim for it, and I am always glad to receive it as I know that I am going to get something beneficial for myself as well as something for the good of my patients.

If the medical bigots had *Better Eyesight* on their desks, and would put into practice what you give in each number, it would be a great blessing to the people who are putting eye crutches on their eyes. I first tried central fixation on myself and had marvelous results. I threw away my glasses and can now see better than I have ever done. I read very fine type (smaller than newspaper type) at a distance of six inches from the eyes, and can run it out at full arm's length and still read it without blurring the type.

I have instructed some of my patients in your methods, and all are getting results. One case who has a partial cataract of the left eye could not see anything on the Snellen test card at twenty feet, and could see the letters only faintly at ten feet. Now she can read 20/10 with both eyes together and also with each eye separately, but the left eye seems, as she says, to be looking through a little fog. I could cite many other cases that have been benefited by central fixation, but this one is the most interesting to me.

Kindly send me more of the subscription slips, as I want to hand them out to my patients.

Yours very truly, —.

Better Eyesight
December 1919—Vol. I, No. 6

THE IMAGINATION CURE

When the imagination is perfect the mind is always perfectly relaxed, and as it is impossible to relax and imagine a letter perfectly and at the same time strain and see it imperfectly, it follows that when one imagines that one sees a letter perfectly one actually does see it, as demonstrated by the retinoscope, no matter how great an error of refraction the eye may previously have had. The sight, therefore, may often be improved very quickly by the aid of the imagination. To use this method the patient may proceed as follows:

Look at a letter at the distance at which it is seen best. Close and cover the eyes so as to exclude all the light and remember it. Do this alternately until the memory is nearly equal to the sight. Next, after remembering the letter with the eyes closed and covered, and while still holding the mental picture of it, look at a blank surface a foot or more to the side of it at the distance at which you wish to see it. Again close and cover the eyes and remember the letter, and on opening them look a little nearer to it. Gradually reduce the distance between the point of central fixation and the letter, until able to look directly at it and imagine it as well as it is remembered with the eyes closed and covered. The letter will then be seen perfectly and other letters in its neighborhood will come out. If unable to remember the whole letter, you may be able to imagine a black period as forming part of it. If you can do this, the letter will also be seen perfectly.

THE MENACE OF LARGE PRINT

If you look at the big "C" on the Snellen test card (or any other large letter of the same size) at ten, fifteen, or twenty feet, and try to see it all alike, you may note a feeling of strain and the letter may not appear perfectly black and distinct. If you now look at only one part of the letter and see the rest of it worse, you will note that the part seen best appears blacker than the whole letter when seen all alike, and you may also note a relief of strain. If you look at the small "C" on the bottom line of the test card, you may be able to note that it seems blacker than the big "C." If not, imagine it as forming part of the area of the big "C." If you are able to see this part blacker than the rest of the letter, the imagined letter will, of course, appear blacker also. If your sight is normal, you may now go a step further and note that when you look at one part of the small "C" this part looks blacker than the whole letter, and that it is easier to see the letter in this way than to see it all alike.

If you look at a line of the smaller letters that you can read readily, and try to see them all alike—all equally black and equally distinct in outline—you will probably find it to be impossible, and the effort will produce discomfort and perhaps pain. You may, however, succeed seeing two or more of them alike. This too may cause much discomfort, and if continued long enough will produce pain. If you now look at only the first letter of the line seeing the adjoining ones worse, the strain will at once be relieved and the letter will appear blacker and more distinct than when it was seen equally well with the others. If your sight is normal at the near point, you can repeat these experiments with a letter seen at this point, with the same results. A number of letters seen equally well at one time will appear less black and less distinct than a single letter seen best, and a large letter will seem less black and distinct than a small one; while in the case of both the large letter and the several letters seen all alike, a feeling of strain may be produced in the eye. You may also be able to note that the reading of very fine print, when it can be done perfectly, is markedly restful to the eye.

The smaller the point of maximum vision, in short, the better the sight and the less the strain upon the eye. This fact can usually be demonstrated in a few minutes by any one whose sight is not markedly imperfect; and in view of some of our educational methods, is very interesting and instructive.

Probably every man who has written a book upon the eye for the last hundred years has issued a warning against fine print in schoolbooks, and recommended particularly large print for small children. This advice has been followed so assiduously that one could probably not find a lesson book for small children anywhere printed in ordinary reading type, while alphabets are often printed in characters one and two inches high. The British Association for the Advancement of Science does not wish to see children read books at all before they are seven years old, and would conduct their education previous to that age by means of large printed wall-sheets, blackboards, pictures, and oral teaching. If they must read, however, it wants them to have 24- and 30-point type, with capitals about a quarter of an inch in height. This is carefully graded down, a size smaller each year, until at the age of twelve the children are permitted to have the same kind of type as their elders. Bijou editions of Bible, prayer-book and hymnals are forbidden, however, to children of all ages.[1]

In the London myope classes, which have become the model for many others of the same kind, books are eliminated entirely and only the older children are allowed to print their lessons in one- and two-inch types.[2]

Yet it has just been shown that large print is a strain upon the eyes [if a person diffuses—TRQ], while the retinoscope demonstrates that a strain to see at the near point always produces hypermetropia[3] (commonly but erroneously called "farsight"). We should naturally expect, therefore, to find hypermetropia very common among small children, and it is. Of children eight and a half years old in the public schools of Philadelphia, Risley found[4] that more than eighty-eight percent were hypermetropic, and similar figures may be found in all statistics of the subject. The percentage declines as the children become older, but hypermetropia, or hypermetropic astigmatism, remains at all ages the most common of all errors of refraction. Hypermetropia is, in fact, a much more serious problem than myopia, or nearsightedness. Yet we have heard very little about it, for the specialists have concluded from its prevalence and its tendency to pass away or become less pronounced with the growth of the body, that it is the normal state of the immature human eye and therefore beyond the reach of preventive measures. It is true that many young children are not hypermetropic, but this fact is easily disposed of by the theory that the ciliary muscle alters the shape of the lens in such cases sufficiently to compensate for the shortness of the eyeball.

The baselessness of this theory, as well as the relation of large print to the production of hypermetropia, may be demonstrated by the fact that the condition can be relieved, and has been relieved in numerous cases, by the reading of fine print combined with rest of the eyes. A child of eight was cured in a few visits by this means. Yet according to the British Association she should not, at this age, have been allowed to read any type larger than 12-point, with capitals more than an eighth of an inch in height. Many grown people have been cured of hypermetropia in the same way, and in all forms of functional imperfect sight the reading of fine print, when it can be done with comfort, has been found to be a benefit to the eyes.

1. *Report on the Influence of School-Books upon Eyesight,* second revised edition, 1913.

2. Pollock, "The Education of the Semi-Blind," *Glasgow Medical Journal,* December 1915.

3. William H. Bates, "The Cause of Myopia," *New York Medical Journal,* March 10, 1912.

4. *School Hygiene, in System of Diseases of the Eye,* edited by Norris and Oliver, Vol. II, p. 353.

SHIFTING AND SWINGING

When the eye with normal vision regards a letter either at the near point or at the distance, the letter may appear to pulsate, or move in various directions, from side to side, up and down, or obliquely. When it looks from one letter to another on the Snellen test card, or from one side of a letter to another, not only the letters, but the whole line of letters and the whole card, may appear to move from side to side. This apparent movement is due to the shifting of the eye, and is always in a direction contrary to its movement. [This is called *oppositional movement.*—TRQ] If one looks at the top of a letter, the letter is below the line of vision and therefore appears to move downward. If one looks at the bottom, the letter is above the line of vision and appears to move upward. If one looks to the left of the letter, it is to the right of the line of vision and appears to move to the right. If one looks to the right, it is to the left of the line of vision and appears to move to the left. [Note the combination of the key principles of movement and centralization in this example.—TRQ]

Persons with normal vision are rarely conscious of this illusion and may have difficulty in demonstrating it; but in every case that has come under my observation they have always become able, in a longer or shorter time, to do so. When the sight is imperfect the letters may remain stationary or even move in the same direction as the eye.

It is impossible for the eye to fix on a point longer than a fraction of a second. If it tries to do so, it begins to strain and the vision is lowered. This can readily be demonstrated by trying to hold one part of a letter for an appreciable length of time. No matter how good the sight, it will begin to blur or even disappear very quickly, and sometimes the effort to hold it will produce pain. In the case of a few exceptional people a point may appear to be held for a considerable length of time; the subjects themselves may think that they are holding it; but this is only because the eye shifts unconsciously, the movements being so rapid that objects seem to be seen all alike simultaneously.

The shifting of the eye with normal vision is usually not conspicuous, but by direct examination with the ophthalmoscope[1] it can always be demonstrated. If one eye is examined with this instrument while the other is regarding a small area straight ahead, the eye being examined, which follows the movements of the other, is seen to move in various directions, from side to side, up and down, in an orbit which is usually variable. If the vision is normal, these movements are extremely rapid and unaccompanied by any appearance of effort. The shifting of the eye with imperfect sight, on the contrary, is slower; its excursions are wider, and the movements are jerky and made with apparent effort.

It can also be demonstrated that the eye is capable of shifting with a rapidity which the ophthalmoscope cannot measure. The normal eye can read fourteen letters on the bottom line of a Snellen test card at a distance of ten or fifteen feet in a dim light so rapidly that they seem to be seen all at once. Yet it can be demonstrated that in order to recognize the letters under these conditions it is necessary to make about four shifts to each letter. At the near point, even though one part of the letter is seen best, the rest may be seen well enough to be recognized; but in the distance it is impossible to recognize the letters unless one shifts from the top to the bottom and from side to side. One must also shift from one letter to another, making about seventy shifts in a fraction of a second. [These are called *saccadic vibrations*.—TRQ]

A line of small letters on the Snellen test card may be less than a foot long by a quarter of an inch in height; and if it requires seventy shifts to a fraction of a second to see it apparently all at once, it must require many thousands to see an area of the size of movie screen, with all its detail of people, animals, houses, or trees, while to see sixteen such areas to a second, as is done in viewing movies, must require a rapidity of shifting that can scarcely be realized. Yet it is admitted that the present rate of taking and projecting movies is too slow. The results would be more satisfactory, authorities say, if the rate were raised to twenty, twenty-two, or twenty-four a second.

The human eye and mind are not only capable of this rapidity of action, and that without effort or strain, but it is only when the eye is able to shift thus rapidly that eye and mind are at rest, and the efficiency of both at their maximum. It is true that every motion of the eye produces an error of refraction; but when the movement is short, this is very slight, and usually the shifts are so rapid that the error does not last long enough to be detected by the retinoscope, its existence being demonstrable only by reducing the rapidity of the movements to less than four or five a second. The period during which the eye is at rest is much longer than that during which an error of refraction is produced. Hence, when the eye shifts normally no error of refraction is manifest. The more rapid the unconscious shifting of the eye, the better the vision; but if one tries to be conscious of a too rapid shift, a strain will be produced.

Perfect sight is impossible without continual shifting, and such shifting is a striking illustration of the mental control necessary for normal vision. It requires perfect mental control to think of thousands of things in a fraction of a second; and each point of fixation has to be thought of separately, because it is impossible to think of two things, or of two parts of one thing, perfectly at the same time. The eye with imperfect sight tries to accomplish the impossible by looking fixedly at one point for an appreciable length of time; that is, by staring. When it looks at a strange letter and does not see it, it keeps on looking at it in an effort to see it better. Such efforts always fail and are an important factor in the production of imperfect sight.

One of the best methods of improving the sight, therefore, is to imitate consciously the unconscious shifting of normal vision, and to realize the apparent motion produced by such shifting. Whether one has imperfect or normal sight, conscious shifting and swinging are a great help and advantage to the eye; for not only may imperfect sight be improved in this way, but normal sight may be improved also.

OPTIMUMS AND PESSIMUMS

In nearly all cases of imperfect sight due to errors of refraction there is some object, or objects, which can be regarded with normal vision. Such objects I have called *optimums*. On the other hand, there are some objects which persons with normal eyes and ordinarily normal sight always see imperfectly; an error of refraction being produced when they are regarded, as demonstrated by the retinoscope. Such objects I have called *pessimums*. An object becomes an optimum or a pessimum according to the effect it produces upon the mind, and in some cases this effect is easily accounted for.

For many children their mother's face is an optimum, and the face of a stranger a pessimum. A dressmaker was always able to thread a No. 10 needle with a fine thread of

1. An instrument for viewing the interior of the eye. When the optic nerve is observed with the ophthalmoscope, movements can be noted that are not apparent when only the exterior of the eye is regarded.

silk without glasses, although she had to put on glasses to sew on buttons because she could not see the holes. She was a teacher of dressmaking and thought the children stupid because they could not tell the difference between two different shades of black. She could match colors without comparing the samples. Yet she could not see a black line in a photographic copy of the Bible which was no finer than a thread of silk, and she could not remember a black period. An employee in a cooperage factory, who had been engaged for years in picking out defective barrels as they went rapidly past him on an inclined plane, was able to continue his work after his sight for most other objects had become very defective, while persons with much better sight for the Snellen test card were unable to detect the defective barrels. The familiarity of these various objects made it possible for the subjects to look at them without strain—that is, without trying to seem them. Therefore the barrels were to the cooper optimums; while the needle's eye and the colors of silk and fabrics were optimums to the dressmaker. Unfamiliar objects, on the contrary, are always pessimums.

In other cases there is no accounting for the idiosyncrasy of the mind which makes one object a pessimum and another an optimum. It is also impossible to account for the fact that an object may be an optimum for one eye and not for the other, or an optimum at one time and at one distance and not at others. Among these unaccountable optimums one often finds a particular letter on the Snellen test card. One patient, for instance, was able to see the letter "K" on the 40-, 15-, and 10-lines, but could see none of the other letters on these lines, although most patients would see some of them, on account of the simplicity of their outlines, better than they would such a letter as "K."

Pessimums may be as curious and unaccountable as optimums. The letter "V" is so simple in its outlines that many people can see it when they cannot see others on the same line. Yet some people are unable to distinguish it at any distance, although able to read other letters in the same word or on the same line of the Snellen test card. Some people again will not only be unable to recognize the letter "V" in a word, but also unable to read any word that contains it, the pessimum lowering their sight not only for itself but for other objects. Some letters or objects become pessimums only in particular situations. A letter, for instance, may be a pessimum when located at the end or at the beginning of a line or sentence, and not in other places. When the attention of the patient is called to the fact that a letter seen in one location ought logically to be seen equally well in others, the letter often ceases to be a pessimum in any situation.

A pessimum, like an optimum, may be lost and later become manifest. It may vary according to the light and distance. An object which is a pessimum in a moderate light may not be so when the light is increased or diminished. A pessimum at twenty feet may not be one at two feet or thirty feet.

For most people the Snellen test card is a pessimum. If you can see the Snellen test card with normal vision, you can see almost anything else in the world. Patients who cannot see the letters on the Snellen test card can often see other objects of the same size and at the same distance with normal sight. When letters which are seen imperfectly, or even letters which cannot be seen at all, or which the patient is not conscious of seeing, are regarded, the error of refraction is increased. The patient may regard a blank white card without any error of refraction; but if he regards the lower part of a Snellen test card, which appears to him to be just as blank as the blank card, an error of refraction can always be demonstrated, and if the visible letters of the card are covered the result is the same. The pessimum may, in short, be letters or objects which the patient is not conscious of seeing. This phenomenon is very common. When the card is seen in the eccentric field it may have the effect of lowering the vision for the point directly regarded. For instance, a patient may regard an area of green wallpaper at the distance and see the color as well as at the near point; but if a Snellen test card on which the letters are either seen imperfectly, or not seen at all, is placed in the neighborhood of the area being regarded, the retinoscope may indicate an error of refraction. When the vision improves, the number of letters on the card which are pessimums diminishes and the number of optimums increases, until the whole card becomes an optimum.

A pessimum, like an optimum, is a manifestation of the mind. It is something associated with a strain to see, just as an optimum is something which has no such association. It is not caused by the error of refraction, but always produces an error of refraction; and when the strain has been relieved it ceases to be a pessimum and becomes an optimum.

HOME TREATMENT

It is not always possible for patients to go to a competent physician for relief. As the method of treating eye defects presented in this magazine is new, it may be impossible to find a physician in the neighborhood who understands it; and the patient may not be able to afford the expense of a long journey, or to take the time for treatment away from home. To such persons I wish to say that it is possible for a large number of people to be cured of defective eyesight without the aid either of a physician or of anyone else. They can cure themselves, and for this purpose it is not necessary that they should understand all that has been written in this magazine, or anywhere else. All that is necessary is to follow a few simple directions.

Place a Snellen test card on the wall at a distance of ten, fourteen, or twenty feet, and devote half a minute a day, or longer, to reading the smallest letters you can see, with each eye separately, covering the other with the palm of the hand in such a way as to avoid touching the eyeball.

Keep a record of the progress made, with the dates. The simplest way to do this is by the method used by oculists, who record the vision in the form of a fraction, with the distance at which the letter is read as the numerator and the distance at which it ought to be read as the denominator. As already explained, the figures above the lines of letters on the test card indicate the distance at which these letters should be read by persons with normal eyesight. Thus a vision of 10/200 would mean that the big "C," which ought to be read at 200 feet, cannot be seen at a greater distance than ten feet. A vision of 20/10 would mean that the 10-line, which the normal eye is not ordinarily expected to read at a greater distance than ten feet, is seen at double that distance. This is a standard commonly attained by persons who have practiced my methods.

Children under twelve years who have not worn glasses are usually cured of defective eyesight by the above method in three months, six months, or a year. Adults who have never worn glasses are benefited in a very short time—a week or two—and if the trouble is not very bad, may be cured in the course of from three to six months. Children or adults who have worn glasses, however, are more difficult to relieve, and will usually have to practice the various methods of gaining relaxation which have been presented from month to month in this magazine and will be described in more detail in my forthcoming book, *The Cure of Imperfect Sight by Treatment without Glasses*.

Children and adults who have worn glasses will have to devote an hour or longer every day to practice with the test card, and the balance of their time to practice on other objects. It will be well for such patients to have two test cards, one to be used at the near point, where it can be seen best, and the other at ten or twenty feet. The patient will find it a great help to shift from the near card to the distant one, as the unconscious memory of the letters seen at the near point helps to bring out those seen at the distance.

If the patient can secure the aid of some person with normal sight, it will be a great advantage. In fact, persons whose cases are obstinate will find it very difficult, if not impossible, to cure themselves without the aid of a teacher. The teacher, if he is to benefit the patient must himself be able to derive benefit from the various methods recommended.

Parents who wish to preserve and improve the eyesight of their children should encourage them to read the Snellen test card every day. There should, in fact, be a Snellen test card in every family; for when properly used it always prevents myopia and other errors of refraction, always improves the vision, even when this is already normal, and always benefits functional nervous troubles. Parents should improve their own eyesight to normal, so that their children may not imitate wrong methods of using the eyes and will not be subject to the influence of an atmosphere of strain.

Better Eyesight
January 1920—Vol. II, No. 1

THE PALMING CURE

One of the most efficacious methods of relieving eyestrain, and hence of improving the sight, is palming. By this is meant the covering of the closed eyes with the palms of the hands in such a way as to exclude all the light, while avoiding pressure upon the eyeballs. In this way most patients are able to secure some degree of relaxation in a few minutes, and when they open their eyes find their vision temporarily improved.

When relaxation is complete the patient sees, when palming, black so deep that it is impossible to remember or imagine anything blacker, and such relaxation is always followed by a complete and permanent cure of all errors of refraction (nearsightedness, farsightedness, astigmatism, and even old-age sight [presbyopia]), as well as by the relief or cure of many other abnormal conditions. In rare cases patients become able to see a perfect black very quickly, even in five, ten or fifteen minutes; but usually this cannot be done without considerable practice, and some never become able to do it until they have been cured by other means. When the patient becomes able after a few trials to see an approximate black, it is worthwhile to continue with the method; otherwise something else should be tried.

Most patients are helped by the memory of some color, preferably black, and as it is impossible to remember an unchanging object for more than a few seconds, they usually find it necessary to shift consciously from one mental picture to another, or from one part of such a picture to another. In some cases, however, the shifting may be done unconsciously, and the black object may appear to be remembered all alike continuously.

THE VARIABILITY OF THE REFRACTION OF THE EYE

The theory that errors of refraction are due to permanent deformations of the eyeball leads naturally to the conclusion, not only that errors of refraction are permanent states, but that normal refraction is also a continuous condition. As this theory is almost universally accepted as a fact, therefore, it is not surprising to find that the normal eye is generally regarded as a perfect machine which is always in good working order. No matter whether the object regarded is strange or familiar, whether the light is good or imperfect, whether the surroundings are pleasant or disagreeable, even under conditions of nerve strain or bodily disease, the normal eye is expected to have normal refraction and normal sight all the time. It is true that the facts do not harmonize with this view, but they are conveniently attributed to the perversity of the ciliary muscle. This muscle is believed to control the shape of the lens, and is credited with a capacity for interfering with the refraction in some very curious ways. In hypermetropia (farsightedness), it is believed to alter the shape of the lens sufficiently to compensate, in whole or in part, for the shortness of the eyeball. In myopia, or nearsightedness, on the contrary, we are told that it actually goes out of its way to produce the condition, or to make an existing condition worse. In other words, the muscle is believed to get into a more or less continuous state of contraction, thus keeping the lens continuously in a state of convexity, which, according to accepted theories, it ought to assume only for vision at the near point. This theory serves the purpose of explaining to the satisfaction of most eye specialists why persons who at times appear to have myopia, or hypermetropia, appear at other times not to have them. After people have reached the age at which the lens is not supposed to change, this theory does not work so well, while in astigmatism it is available only to a limited extent even at the earlier ages; but these facts are quietly ignored.

When we understand how the shape of the eyeball is controlled by the external muscles, and how it responds instantaneously to their action, it is easy to see that no refractive state, whether it is normal or abnormal, can be permanent. This conclusion is confirmed by the retinoscope, and I had observed the facts long before my experiments upon the eye muscles of animals, reported in 1915[1] (to be described again in my forthcoming book) had offered a satisfactory explanation for them. During thirty years devoted to the study of refraction, I have found few people who could maintain perfect sight for more than a few minutes at a time, even under the most favorable conditions; and often I have seen the refraction change half a dozen times or more in a second, the variations ranging all the way from twenty diopters of myopia to normal.

Similarly I have found no eyes with continuous or unchanging errors of refraction, all persons with errors of refraction having, at frequent intervals during the day and night, moments of normal vision when their myopia, hypermetropia, or astigmatism wholly disappears. The form of the error also changes, myopia even changing into hypermetropia and one form of astigmatism into another.

Of twenty thousand schoolchildren examined in one year, more than half had normal eyes with sight which was perfect at times, but not one of them had perfect sight in each eye at all times of the day. Their sight might be good in the morning and imperfect in the afternoon, or imperfect in the morning and perfect in the afternoon. Many children could read one Snellen test card with perfect sight, while unable to see a different one perfectly. Many could also read some letters of the alphabet perfectly, while unable to distinguish other letters of the same size under similar conditions. The degree of this imperfect sight varied within wide limits, from one-third to one-tenth, or less. Its duration was also variable. Under some conditions it might continue for only a few minutes, or less; under others it might prevent the subject from seeing the blackboard for days, weeks, or even longer. Frequently all the pupils in a classroom were affected to this extent.

Among babies a similar condition was noted. Most investigators have found babies hypermetropic. A few have found them myopic. My own observations indicate that the refraction of infants is continually changing. One child was examined under atropine on four successive days, beginning two hours after birth. A three percent solution of atropine was instilled into both eyes, the pupil was dilated to the maximum, and other physiological symptoms of the use of atropine were noted. The first examination showed a condition of mixed astigmatism. On the second day there was compound hypermetropic astigmatism, and on the third, compound myopic astigmatism.[2] On the fourth, one eye was normal and the other showed simple myopia. Similar variations were noted in many other cases.

What is true of children and infants is equally true of adults of all ages. Persons over seventy years old have suffered losses of vision of variable degree and intensity, and in such cases the retinoscope always indicated an error of refraction. A man eighty years old, with normal eyes and ordinarily normal sight, had periods of imperfect sight which would last from a few minutes to half an hour or longer. Retinoscopy at such times always indicated myopia of four diopters or more.

During sleep the refractive condition of the eye is rarely, if ever, normal. Persons whose refraction is normal when they are awake will produce myopia, hypermetropia and astigmatism when they are asleep, or, if they have errors of refraction when they are awake, they will be increased during sleep. This is why people waken in the morning with eyes more tired than at any other time, or even with severe headaches. When the subject is under ether or chloroform, or unconscious from any other cause, errors of refraction are also produced or increased.

When the eye regards an unfamiliar object an error of refraction is always produced. Hence the proverbial fatigue caused by viewing pictures, or other objects, in a museum. Children with normal eyes who can read perfectly small letters a quarter of an inch high at ten feet always have trouble in reading strange writing on the blackboard, although the letters may be two inches high. A strange map, or any map, has the same effect. I have never seen a child or a teacher who could look at a map at the distance without becoming nearsighted. German type has been accused of being responsible for much of the poor sight once supposed to be peculiarly a German malady; but if a German child attempts to read Roman print, she will at once become temporarily myopic. German print, or Greek or Chinese characters, will have the same effect on a child, or other person, accustomed to Roman letters. Cohn repudiated the idea that German lettering was trying to the eyes.[3] On the contrary, he always found it "pleasant, after a long reading of the monotonous Roman print to return to 'our beloved German'." Because the German characters were more familiar to him than any others, he found them restful to his eyes. "Use," as he truly observed, "has much to do with the matter." Children learning to read, write, draw, or sew always suffer from defective vision because of the unfamiliarity of

1. William H. Bates, "The Cure of Defective Eyesight by Treatment Without Glasses," *New York Medical Journal,* May 5, 1915.

2. In astigmatism the eye is lopsided. In simple hypermetropic astigmatism one principal meridian is normal, and the other, at right angles to it, is flatter; hence the eye is farsighted in one curvature and normal in another. In simple myopic astigmatism the contrary is the case, one principal meridian is normal and the other, at right angles to it, more convex, making the refraction normal in one curvature and nearsighted in another. In mixed astigmatism one principal meridian is too flat, the other too convex. In compound hypermetropic astigmatism, both principal meridians are flatter than normal, one more so than the other. In compound myopic astigmatism both are more convex than normal, one more so than the other.

3. "Eyes and School-Books," *Popular Science Monthly,* May 1881, translated from *Deutsche Rundschau.*

the lines or objects with which they are working.

A sudden exposure to strong light, or rapid or sudden changes of light, are likely to produce imperfect sight in the normal eye, continuing in some cases for weeks and months.

Noise is also a frequent cause of defective vision in the normal eye. All persons see imperfectly when they hear an unexpected loud noise. Familiar sounds do not lower the vision, but unfamiliar ones always do. Country children from quiet schools may suffer from defective vision for a long time after moving to a noisy city. In school they cannot do well with their work, because their sight is impaired. It is, of course, a gross injustice for teachers and others to scold, punish, or humiliate such children.

Under conditions of mental or physical discomfort, such as pain, cough, fever, discomfort from heat or cold, depression, anger, or anxiety, errors of refraction are always produced in the normal eye, or increased in the eye in which they already exist.

The variability of the refraction of the eye is responsible for many otherwise unaccountable accidents. When people are struck down in the street by automobiles or trolley cars, it is often due to the fact that they were suffering from temporary loss of sight. Collisions on railroads or at sea, disasters in military operations, aviation accidents, etc., often occur because some responsible person suffered temporary loss of sight.

HOW LONG WILL IT TAKE?

This question is asked so constantly by persons who wish to be cured of imperfect sight that it seems worthwhile to devote a little space to its consideration. It is impossible, of course, to answer the question definitely. Cure is a question of the mind, and people's minds are different.

While patients who have worn glasses are usually harder to cure than those who have not, elderly persons who have worn them for the better part of a lifetime are sometimes cured as quickly as children under twelve who have never worn them. These cases are very rare, but they do occur. Some patients can look at the letters on the test card, or in a paragraph of fine print, and imagine them at once to be perfectly black, with the result that they immediately become able to read them. Some patients are able to palm almost perfectly from the start, and nearly all can do it well enough to improve their sight; some never become able to do it until their sight has been improved by other means.

Most patients, when they look from one side of a large letter to another, or from one side of the card to another, can imagine that the letter or the card is moving in a direction opposite to the movement of the eye. Others, whose condition may be no worse, take a week or a month or longer to do the same thing. A patient recently treated was able to do almost everything I asked her to at the first visit. I began, as I always do, by directing her to close and rest her eyes, and, as in the case of most other patients, she was able to improve her sight materially by this method. Then she went on to do a lot of other things, some of which very few patients can do at the first visit, while no one but herself, so far as I can remember, was ever able to do all of them. She was able to stare at a letter and make her sight worse, and she was able to look from one side of it to another and imagine that it was moving in a direction opposite to the movement of the eye. If the letter was seen perfectly, the movement was short, rhythmical and easy; if it was seen imperfectly, it was longer and irregular. She could not imagine a letter stationary, and if she tried to imagine it so, it blurred. When she looked at a line of letters that she could read, she realized at once that one letter was seen best and the adjoining ones worse; and when she looked at a line that she could not read, she noted that they were seen all alike. She demonstrated at once—which was very remarkable—that a perfect memory is quick and easy, and an imperfect memory slow, difficult and even impossible; that the first relieves fatigue and the second induces discomfort. She also demonstrated that while it was easy to imagine that a letter remembered perfectly was swinging, she either could not imagine such a swing in the case of an imperfectly remembered letter, or else the swing was longer and irregular. It is hardly necessary to say that this patient became able at once to read the whole card, even in a dim light. It was only when she came to fine print that she failed. She could not imagine that the letters of diamond type were swinging. She could imagine the universal swing[1] when she looked two inches away from the letters, but she could not imagine it when she looked between the lines.

These peculiarities of the mind cannot be known in advance, and therefore it is seldom possible, in any given case, to make predictions as to the length of time that will be required for a cure. This much can be stated, however: that marked improvement is always obtained in a few weeks, and that all patients obtain some benefit at the first visit. If there are any exceptions to this rule, they are so rare that I do not remember them.

As more facts are accumulated and better ways of pre-

1. When the patient becomes able to imagine that the letters on the test I card are swinging, everything else thought of also seems to be swinging. This is the universal swing.

senting things are learned, it becomes possible to cure people more quickly. I can cure people more quickly today than I did a year ago, and I expect to cure them next year more quickly than I do today. In the last three months, seven or eight patients have been cured in one visit, with a little additional help over the telephone.

When patients can give considerable time to the treatment they naturally get on faster than those who cannot or will not do this. When they follow instructions and do not waste time in discussion, or in carrying out theories of their own, they also get on faster. One of the advantages that children have over adults is that their heads are not so full of erroneous ideas, and that they are accustomed to doing as they are told.

The chief cause of delay seems to be that people will not believe the truth after it is demonstrated to them. You can demonstrate to anyone in a few minutes that rest improves the vision; but the idea that everything worthwhile must be gained by effort is so deeply ingrained in the average mind that you may not in a year be able to get it out, and so long as the patient believes that his sight can be improved by effort, he will make little progress.

In most cases it is necessary, in order to retain what has been gained, to continue the treatment for a few minutes every day. When a cure is complete it is always permanent. The patient need never think of the matter again, and may even forget how he was cured. But complete cures, which mean the attainment not of what is ordinarily called normal sight, but of a measure of telescopic and microscopic vision, are very rare; and even in these cases the treatment may be continued with benefit, for it is impossible to set limits to the visual powers of man, and no matter how good the sight, it is always possible to improve it.

RELIEF AFTER TWENTY-FIVE YEARS

While many persons are benefited by the accepted methods of treating defects of vision, there is a minority of cases, known to every eye specialist, which gets little or no help from them. These patients sometimes give up the search for relief in despair, and sometimes continue it with surprising pertinacity, never being able to abandon the belief, in spite of the testimony of experience, that somewhere in the world there must be someone with sufficient skill to fit them with the right glasses. The rapidity with which these patients respond to treatment by relaxation is often very dramatic, and affords a startling illustration of the superiority of this method to treatment by glasses and muscle-cutting. In the following case relaxation did in twenty-four hours what the old methods, as practiced by a succession of eminent specialists, had not been able to do in twenty-five years.

The patient was a man of forty-nine, and his imperfect sight was accompanied by continual pain and misery, culminating twenty years before I saw him, in a complete nervous breakdown. As he was a writer, dependent upon his pen for a living, his condition was a serious economic handicap, and he consulted many specialists in the vain hope of obtaining relief. Glasses did little, either to improve his sight or to relieve his discomfort, and the eye specialists talked vaguely about disease of the optic nerve and brain as a possible cause of his troubles. The nerve specialists, however, were unable to do anything to relieve him. One specialist diagnosed his case as muscular, and gave him prisms which helped him a little. Later, the same specialist, finding that all of the apparent muscular trouble was not corrected by glasses, cut the external muscles of both eyes. This also brought some relief, but not much. At the age of twenty-nine the patient suffered the nervous breakdown already mentioned. For this he was treated unsuccessfully by various specialists, and for nine years he was compelled to live out of doors. This life, although it benefited him, failed to restore his health and when he came to me on September 13, 1919 he was still suffering from neurasthenia. His distant vision was less than 20/40 and could not be improved by glasses. He was able to read with glasses, but could not do so without discomfort. I could find no symptom of disease of the brain or of the interior of the eye. When he tried to palm he saw gray and yellow instead of black; but he was able to rest his eyes simply by closing them, and by this means alone he became able, in twenty-four hours, to read diamond type and to make out most of the letters on the 20-line of the test card at twenty feet. At the same time his discomfort was materially relieved.

He was under treatment for about six weeks and then he left the city. On October 25 he wrote as following:

"I saw you last on October 6, and at the end of the week, the 11th, I started off on a ten-day motor trip as one of the officials of the Cavalry Endurance Test for horses. The last touch of eyestrain which affected me nervously at all I experienced on the 8th and 9th. On the trip, though I averaged but five hours sleep, rode all day in an open motor without goggles, and wrote reports at night by bad lights, I had no trouble. After the third day the universal slow swing seemed to establish itself, and I have never had a moment's discomfort since. I stood fatigue and excitement better than I have ever done and went with less sleep. My practicing on the trip was necessarily somewhat curtailed, yet there was noticeable improvement in my vision. Since returning

I have spent a couple of hours a day in practice, and have at the same time done a lot of writing.

Yesterday, the 24th, I made a test with diamond type, and found that after twenty minutes practice I could get the lines distinct and make out the capital letters and bits of the text at a scant three inches. At seven I could read it readily, though I could not see it perfectly. This was by an average daylight—no sun. In a good daylight I can read the newspaper almost perfectly at a normal reading distance—say fifteen inches. I seem able now to read ordinary print at a little distance from my eyes without straining; but I practice bringing it so close that it is not quite clear, and after closing and opening my eyes and thinking of the text as clear and black, or of a perfect black letter, it clears up. I am confident now that in a few weeks I shall be able to read the fine print at three inches. Now that the swing has established itself so well I seem to get the best results on close work by consciously relaxing as much as I can, avoiding all conscious effort to see better, and imagining words or letters perfectly clear and black. All soreness has gone from the eyeballs, but there are little muscle twitches that catch me when consciously opening or closing the lids. The last few days these almost ceased at the end of twenty minutes practice and my sight was better.

I feel now that I am really out of the woods. I have done night work without suffering for it, a thing I have not done in twenty-five years, and I have worked steadily for more hours than I have been able to work at a time since my breakdown in 1899, all without sense of strain or nervous fatigue. You can imagine my gratitude to you. Not only for my own sake, but for yours, I shall leave no stone unturned to make the cure complete and get back the child eyes which seem perfectly possible in the light of progress I have made in the eight weeks since I first went to you.

I have just been trying the big card for distance in the out-of-door light of an overcast day at two in the afternoon. At twenty feet I get all the bottom line, but the '5' and '6.' The 'B' also is black. But I think I have done a little better than this. The halos[1] begin to come out spontaneously both on the fine print and on the big card at a distance. I am sure that I only have to keep on to win."

1. When the sight is normal, the margins and openings of letters appear whiter than the rest of the background, and the lines of fine print seem to be separated by white streaks.

FACTS VERSUS THEORIES

Reading fine print is commonly supposed to be an extremely dangerous practice, and reading print of any kind upon a moving vehicle is thought to be even worse. Looking away to the distance, however, and not seeing anything in particular is believed to be very beneficial to the eyes. In the light of these superstitions the facts contained in the following letter are particularly interesting:

"On reaching home Monday morning I was surprised and pleased at the comments of my family regarding the appearance of my eyes. They all thought they looked so much brighter and rested, and *that* after two days of railroading. I didn't spare my eyes in the least on the way home. I read magazines and newspapers, looked at the scenery; in fact, I used my eyes all the time. My sight for the near point is splendid. Can read for hours without tiring my eyes. I went downtown today and my eyes were very tired when I got home. The fine print on the card (diamond type) helps me so. I would like to have your little Bible (a photographic reduction of the Bible with type much smaller than diamond.) I'm sure the very fine print has a soothing effect on one's eyes, regardless of what my previous ideas on the subject were."

It will be observed that the eyes of this patient were not tired by her two days railroad journey, during which she read constantly; they were not tired by hours of reading after her return; they were rested by reading extremely fine print; but they were very much tired by a trip downtown during which they were not called upon to focus upon small objects. Later a leaf from the Bible was sent to her, and she wrote:

"The effect even of the first effort to read it was wonderful. If you will believe it, I haven't been troubled having my eyes feel 'crossed' since. . . ."

Better Eyesight
February 1920—Vol. II, No. 2

HALOS

When the eye with normal sight looks at the large letters on the Snellen test card at any distance from twenty feet to six inches or less, it sees, at the inner and outer edges and in the openings of the round letters, a white more intense than the margin of the card. Similarly, when such an eye reads fine print, the spaces between the lines and the letters and the openings of the letters appear whiter than the margin of the page, while streaks of an even more intense white may be seen along the edges of the lines of letters. These "halos" are sometimes seen so vividly that in order to convince people that they are illusions it is often necessary to cover the letters, when they at once disappear. Patients with imperfect sight also see the halos, though less perfectly, and when they understand that they are imagined, they often become able to imagine them where they had not been seen before, or to increase their vividness, in which case the sight always improves. This can be done by imagining the appearances first with the eyes closed, and then looking at the card or at fine print and imagining them there. By alternating these two acts of imagination the sight is often improved rapidly. It is best to begin the practice at the point at which the halos are seen, or can be imagined best. Nearsighted patients are usually able to see them at the near point, sometimes very vividly. Farsighted people may also see them best at this point, although their sight for form may be best at the distance.

[Dr. Bates states that the halos around letters and between sentences appear whiter than the "margin" of the page. Many people have noticed a thin, glowing white line that appears along the edges of a white page. This thin white border can also appear to be whiter than other areas of the page. See also the subsection "The Thin White Line" in the May 1926 issue.—TRQ]

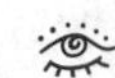

NEW EYES FOR OLD

By Grace Ellery Channing

Editor's Note—*We are constantly hearing of patients who have been able to improve their sight by the aid of information contained in this magazine, or in other publications on the same subject, without personal assistance. The following is a very remarkable example of these cases, as the improvement was made while the patient was handicapped by having to wear her glasses a great part of the time.*

There was once a gentleman who attempted to sell new lamps for old ones. And another who tried to exchange, on Waterloo Bridge, perfectly good new shillings for sixpence. In both cases the wares were as advertised, but both fell under suspicion. It is perhaps, then, not to be wondered at that an offer of new eyes for old should meet with a similar fate at the hands of a public early trained to suspect the worst—in a world where few things are as represented and nothing is to be had for nothing.

In no other way, at least, can I account for the fact that so much of the world is still in glasses, after a brief experience of my own. This is the story:

Something over a year ago, in one of those periodic fits of dejection common to those who abuse their eyes and then wonder at their failure, I chanced to take up a copy of the *New York Tribune,* open exactly at an article on eyes, in the column devoted to scientifico-medical truth.

I may as well confess at once that I read this column chiefly to scoff—a privilege reserved to those born in doctors' families. Moreover the condition of my own eyes at that moment, after years of oculists and opticians, was one to make me particularly skeptical towards anything calling itself a new "cure." Still—I ran through the article.

It was brief, a mere review of another which had appeared in the *Scientific American,* and I grasped but a fragment of the principle—that defects of vision were not necessarily integral, but might result from defectively controlled muscles distorting the eyeball, pulling it out of shape. Hence nearsightedness, farsightedness, astigmatism, etc., might be curable through muscle-control. The treatment consisted in relaxation and re-education, intelligently applied.

As I grasped it, not being hampered by scientific prepossessions, the thing appeared so simple that I exclaimed to myself, "How sensible!"—hastily qualifying it with, "How much too good to be true!" For here was something rational—something you could do for yourself, without either being cut up or poisoned. The article mentioned that patients went home and taught their families—it was so simple. There was nothing to prevent one from at least trying it on oneself.

The only detail of treatment set forth—or which I grasped—was that the eyes could be relaxed most conveniently by looking at black, and that by covering the eyes with the palms of the hands ("palming") black could be retained as a mental vision, or memory, during which the eye was at rest. By practice, one could learn to "remember black" with the eyes opened, at will, and when it was not there. Thus muscular control could be re-established.

It was at least worth trying, and I tried. (Here it is interesting to remark that the moment you look at a black thing, you realize it isn't. A really black object is hard to find, but not necessary to success; the approximate will serve. Later I discovered that a black period—of printer's ink—was sufficient, but I am giving by preference the tale of my first blundering efforts.)

My first discovery was one which anyone may make for himself; it contains the crux of the whole. This is, that after looking at black, "palming," and seeing black with the eyes shut (at first one may see gray or red), and then opening the eyes, there is an appreciable instant of clear vision in which letters or images previously blurred and hazy come out sharp and definite. For that brief instant I could read clearly; then immediately the old habit of muscular strain set in again and vision lapsed. But *that instant was enough.* For, if for any fraction of time at all vision could be reconquered, clearly the organ of vision was intact; the trouble was extraneous, functional, and might be removable. All that was needed was *to make that instant permanent,* and that, evidently, was a mere matter of re-educating the exterior muscles of the eye and fixing a habit.

So far as I was concerned that first experiment was final. I was as convinced then as I am convinced now that I, or anyone else in my case, can recover vision virtually whole, with time, patience and training. The demonstration was, for me, complete. Nobody had proved it to me, I had proven it to myself. Relaxed, eyes could return to the normal and see without glasses.

How to take advantage of my discovery was another matter. My days are largely spent in typing; my nights (too largely) in reading, both in glasses, which of course are framed to perpetuate the errors they confirm, so that every pair of glasses has to be farther from the normal than the one before. With a war on, I could neither stop working nor reading newspapers. Yet the first requisite for the new cure I assumed to be the abandonment of the glasses. (I have since heard of cases cured even while in glasses.)

I postponed, then, all hope of my own cure to some date "after Peace." But I was too interested and fascinated to quite let the matter drop. Accordingly I began to play with the small fragment of theory I had assimilated (very inaccurately, I now realize), in the scant leisure of my daily outings. I practiced "seeing black" on the coat-backs of pedestrians, and "central fixation" (which means seeing best what you look at *where* you look at it, and not its edges instead), on the street signs and advertising billboards. My companions began to recognize my "seeing black" expression. As a skeptic, I am something of a trial to them and they enjoyed, perhaps, seeing the biter bit. But I was getting results—undoubling the long-doubled stars, making one moon grow where the proverbial two had grown before. Blurred letters of fantastic height I was reducing to neat, clear rows half as high; I who had not read a headline—with just *eyes*—for years, was reading them all. Thence I passed to the higher literature; probably nobody has ever been so stirred by the genius of Mr. Shonts as I, when first I could untangle his lines. Next came the gems of verse in streetcar advertisements. Now I read them all alike indifferently, negligently, as being no great thing, down to the quite fine ones, if the vehicle is moderately light.

The first really startling intimation of gain, however, came to me one hurried morning when, taking my mail from the box, I read my letters one after another on the way to the bus, and only realized later as I was rolling downtown that I had read them all without glasses—and without noticing it. It was fully ten years since I had been able to read a line of a letter without glasses, frequently to my extreme inconvenience.

This is as far as I have gone—except that I am still going. Month by month I recover a little and a little more of my ability to see normally, and meanwhile, as a most important by-product of the gain, I lose the old fatigue and ache which, with its accompanying depression, made my hours without glasses periods of strain. Here I should explain that my eyes are always under a two-fold strain—for I listen with them. Only the partly deaf will fully understand this, but it makes the importance of this new treatment for them incalculable. And the deaf are as the sands of the sea.

Now, if gains so real and so appreciable can be made in quarter-hour and casual applications of a partially grasped theory, and while with both hands one is engaged in undoing for the remainder of the hours what one has done in the quarters, is it not fair to believe that a proper, steadfast, continuous application of the theory would work miracles for those multitudes of mankind who suffer every form of disability and handicap now covered by the term "eyestrain"? We are told that pretty much everything from flat feet to baldness can proceed from eyestrain, and for my part I believe it; I know what earstrain can do. We are also assured that children in our schools suffer by tens of thousands from defective vision, and are turned into truants, invalids and criminals. Almost the largest percentage of physical disqualifications in our Army were optical—and that under an incredibly low standard. Eyes, then, are not an academic but a vital issue. How is it possible that we fail to investigate to the last point any and every possible means of relief from an evil well-nigh universal?

This is the question I have naturally been asking, north, south, east and west, for a year past. It seems time now to ask it out loud—in print. Of course I have found excellent people to tell me that my discovery "isn't so," and other excellent people to tell me that "everybody has always known it" anyway, which does not explain to me why "everybody" is still wearing glasses. I was sufficiently interested myself to go and talk with a few of the cured enthusiasts; their attitude is about what mine would be in their case—that of those who were present at the Pool Bethesda and *saw* the miracle effected. I also had the curiosity to go and talk with the author of the revolutionary theory that eyes can be cured without glasses, himself—Dr. Wm. H. Bates.

I went to Dr. Bates through streets filled with people wearing glasses, and punctuated at intervals by the signs of oculists, opticians, and makers of optical devices for the near-blind. My own oculist's and optician's offices are usually thronged with a waiting list; it occurred to me that I might find cordons of troops keeping order about Dr. Bates'. I found neither the cordon nor the crowds. Why?

Here is a man who is either an absolute benefactor of humanity, or who makes an unfounded claim. He should be given, not for his own sake but for ours, the widest opportunity and the heartiest encouragement to prove or disprove his theory, past all possibility of question. It is indeed so extraordinary that he has not been forcibly summoned to do this before now by an impatient public, that it can only be accounted for by that ancient disability of the human mind to accept new things if strange—new lamps for old, real shillings sold for sixpence, or truth that is as simple as a lie. Yet, actually, of course, Truth is always simple—the only simple thing there is.

New eyes for old, ladies and gentlemen!

STORIES FROM THE CLINIC

No. 1: Joey and Patsy

By Emily C. Lierman

Editor's Note—*Ms. Lierman wore glasses for thirteen years. She was cured six years ago, and has since acted as a very enthusiastic assistant in the laboratory and Clinic of the editor. She is not a physician, but obtains results, having never failed to improve the sight of any patient whom she has treated—a wonderful record.*

Joey is a little boy who was struck on the head a few months ago in an automobile accident, and injured in such a way that he became almost totally blind in the left eye. Patsy is Joey's brother, and from him it was learned that when the accident occurred Joey was at the head of his troops, conducting a strategic retreat after a fierce conflict in which he had been obliged to yield to adverse fortune. His face was to the foe and the automobile was behind him. Hence the catastrophe.

A week later he was brought to the Clinic of the Harlem Hospital by his aunt. Dr. Bates examined him and found that he was suffering from optic neuritis and retinal hemorrhages of the left eye, as a result of which the vision of this eye had been reduced to mere light perception.

The child was now brought to me for treatment, and never have I seen a more forlorn little specimen of humanity. I did not know then that a gang of street boys had once looked up to him as their leader, and I never should have suspected it. There was not the shadow of a smile upon his face, and he had not a word to say. Both his face and his clothes were dirty. The latter were also ragged, while his shoes were full of holes. His teeth were wonderful, however, and beneath the grime on his small countenance one could catch glimpses of the complexion of perfect health. I told him to rest his eyes by closing and covering with the palms of his hands, and after a few minutes he was able to see the largest letter on the test card with his blind eye. I told him to do this six times a day for five minutes at a time and to come back on the next Clinic day.

The next time I saw him, he not only had made no progress, but was as blind as he had been at the beginning. His aunt said, "You scold him. Tell him you will keep him here because he will not palm or do anything he is told to do at home." I answered, "You do not wish me to lie to him, do you?" Joey looked up into my face, so sad and worried, waiting for me to defend him again as his aunt replied, "Well, I will leave him here and not take him home again."

"All right," I said. "I live in the country, and perhaps Joey would like to go home with me and play in the fields, and watch the birds build their nests, and learn how to smile as little boys should."

Well now, you should have seen that dirty little face flush up with excitement and pleasure. "Joey," I said, "you are going to love me a whole lot, because I love you already; but you must mind what I say because if you don't you will go blind."

Joey then consented to palm for a few minutes, and his sight improved so that he was able to see the large letter of the test card three feet away. He now made an effort to see the next line of two letters, but not only did he fail to do so, but he also lost the large letter. The strain had made him blind again.

How I wish I had more time to spend on a case like this! But the room was full of patients, and more were coming continually. I had to attend to them. So I asked Joey, very gently, to palm and not take his hands from his eyes until I came back. After ten minutes I returned and asked what he could see. To my surprise he read five lines of the test card with the blind eye. Much encouraged I sent him home and he promised to palm six times a day. He stayed away almost a week and I worried about him for I knew he would forget what I had told him to do. Then one day he turned up with his brother Patsy, who, I believe, is twelve years old. My, how Patsy did talk! Joey had not a word to say, and did not smile until I asked him to. Patsy said that Joey did not practice and that his father hit him on the head and threatened him with all sorts of things to make him do so. It was quite evident that he had not practiced. When I asked him to read the card, all he could see was the big letter at the top at three feet.

Poor little Joey! I gathered him in my arms, patted his dirty face, and told him that if he would count six fingers for me and practice palming as many times a day, I was sure Santa Claus would have some toys for him at Christmas time. Joey was all smiles, and stood with his eyes covered for a long time. When he again looked at the card he read the 5-line. Meantime Patsy was telling me all about the accident in which Joey had been injured, and also all about the rest of the family. His big brother was going to be married, he said, but not until another brother, eighteen years old, was out of prison. Patsy talked like a man and his voice sounded like a foghorn; but I saw that he had a gentle nature and I enlisted him as my little assistant. I asked him if he would not try to get Joey to palm more and told him that he must always speak kindly to him. I also asked him to ask his father not to hit Joey on the head again because that made the hemorrhages worse and Joey would go blind. Bless Patsy's heart. He promised to help me all he could, and I am sure he deserves much of the credit for what I was afterward able to do for Joey.

After this Joey's progress was steady. He responded to kindness as a flower responds to the sun. But if I ever forgot myself and spoke to him without the utmost gentleness—if I even raised my voice a little—he would at once become nervous and begin to strain. One day I remonstrated with him because he had not done what I had told him and a few moments later, when I asked him to read the test card with his left eye, he said, "I can only see the large letter." I began to pet him, telling him what a great man he might be some day and how important it was for him to see with both eyes. He smiled and palmed, and in a short time he again read five lines of the card.

At a recent visit he was very conspicuous because he had had his face washed. I could see that he wanted me to notice this, which of course I did, giving him high praise for his improved appearance. He smiled and started to palm without being told to, and his sight improved more rapidly than at any previous visit. His last visit was a happy one. He saw all of the bottom line at ten feet without palming.

One day Patsy appeared at the Clinic wearing spectacles. "Patsy, for heaven's sake, what are you wearing those things for?" I asked. "The nurse in school said I needed glasses and my father paid four dollars for them—but I can see without them." His vision without glasses was 20/100. After palming five minutes it improved considerably. "Do you want to be cured without glasses?" he was asked. "Sure, I don't want to wear them." "Well, you ask father's permission and I will cure you."

Fortunately his father had no objection and now Patsy sees much better without glasses than he ever did with them. He says that the blackboard looks blacker than it used to and that his lessons do not seem so hard. His vision is not normal yet, but after he has rested his eyes for part of a minute, simply by closing them, he can read the bottom line of the test card easily at ten feet.

SEEKING A MYOPIA CURE

By L. Mehler

When the Lusitania was sunk I knew that the United States was going to get into trouble, and I wanted to be in a position to join the Army. But I was suffering from a high degree of myopia and I knew they wouldn't take me with glasses. Later on they took almost anyone who wasn't blind, but at that time I couldn't possibly have measured up to the standard. So I began to look about for a cure. I tried osteopathy, but didn't go very far with it. I asked the optician who had been fitting me with glasses for advice, but he said that myopia was incurable. I dismissed the matter for a time, but I didn't stop thinking about it. I am a farmer, and I knew from the experience of outdoor life that health is the normal condition of living beings. I knew that when health is lost it can often be regained. I could remember a time when I was not myopic, and it seemed to me that if a normal eye could become myopic, it ought to be possible for a myopic eye to regain normality. After a while I went back to the optician and told him that I was convinced that there must be some cure for my condition. He replied that this was quite impossible, as everyone knew that myopia was incurable. The assurance with which he made this statement had an effect upon me quite the opposite of what he intended, for when he said that the cure of myopia was impossible I knew that it was not, and I resolved never to give up the search for a cure until I found it. Shortly after I had the good fortune to hear of the editor of this magazine and lost no time in going to see him. At the first visit I was able, just by closing and resting my eyes, to improve my sight considerably for the Snellen test card, and in a short time I was able to make out most of the letters on the bottom line at ten feet. I am still improving, and when I can see a little better I mean to go back to that optician and tell him what I think of his ophthalmological learning.

MENTAL EFFECTS OF CENTRAL FIXATION

A man of forty-four who had worn glasses since the age of twenty was first seen on October 8, 1917, when he was suffering, not only from very imperfect sight, but from headache and discomfort. He was wearing for the right eye, concave 5.00 D. S. with concave 0.50 D. C. 180 degrees; left eye, concave 2.50 D. S. with concave 1.50 D. C. 180 degrees. As his visits were not very frequent and he often went back to his glasses, his progress was slow. But his pain and discomfort were relieved very quickly, and almost from the beginning he had flashes of greatly improved and even of normal vision. This encouraged him to continue, and his progress, though slow, was steady. He has now gone without his glasses entirely for some months. His wife was particularly impressed with the effect of the treatment upon his nerves, and in December 1919, she wrote:

"I have become very much interested in the thought of renewing my youth by becoming like a little child. The idea of the mental transition is not unfamiliar, but that this mental, or I should say spiritual, transition should produce a physical effect which would lead to seeing clearly is a sort of miracle very possible indeed, I should suppose, to those who have faith.

In my husband's case, certainly some such miracle was wrought, for not only was he able to lay aside his spectacles after many years of constant use, and to see to read in almost any light, but I particularly noticed his serenity of mind after treatments. In this serenity he seemed able to do a great deal of work efficiently, and not under the high nervous pressure whose aftereffect is the devastating scattering of forces.

It did not occur to me for a long time that perhaps your treatment was quieting his nerves. But I think now that the quiet periods of relaxation, two or three times a day, during which he practiced with the letter card, must have had a very beneficial effect. He is so enthusiastic by nature, and his nerves are so easily stimulated, that for years he used to overdo periodically. Of course, his greatly improved eyesight and the relief from the former strain must have been a large factor in this improvement. But I am inclined to think that the intervals of quiet and peace were wonderfully beneficial, and why shouldn't they be? We are living on stimulants, physical stimulants, mental stimulants of all kinds. The minute these stop we feel we are merely existing, and yet if we retain any of the normality of our youth, do you not think that we respond very happily to natural simple things?"

Better Eyesight
March 1920—Vol. II, No. 3

PROGRESSIVE MYOPIA RELIEVED

By E. E. Agranove

Editor's Note—*The writer of this article, a young man of twenty, was wearing when first seen the following glasses prescribed three years earlier: both eyes, concave 6.50 D. S. with concave 3.00 D. C. 180 degrees. He also brought with him a later prescription—right eye, concave 9.00 D. S. with 4.50 D. C. 180 degrees; left eye, concave 8.00 D. S. with concave 3.00 D. C.—which indicated that there had been a very rapid advance in his myopia. The progress he made in the brief period of six weeks was very unusual.*

I was only eight years old when the teacher told me that I couldn't come to school if I didn't get glasses. So, of course, I had to get them and, of course, I hated them. They kept me out of all the games that a boy really likes, such as baseball, and they made me terribly self-conscious.

Every little while I had to get new and stronger glasses. They were changed eight times in the course of the next nine years, by the end of which time I had what the specialists pronounced to be a very bad case of progressive myopia. After that I refused to make any more changes, for I had lost faith in glasses and wasn't interested in trying new ones.

Although my eyes kept getting worse all the time, and the specialists said there wasn't a chance of a cure, I always felt sure that sometime I would find a cure, and I tried and investigated everything that seemed to offer any hope of relief. One specialist said that while I couldn't be cured, it would help me to live out of doors. So I gave up my job as a telegrapher, went West and got work in the open air. It didn't do me a bit of good. Then I went in for physical culture; but, while this improved my general health, it didn't help my eyes. I tried osteopathy and chiropractic, but they didn't help either. I read all the literature on the subject that I could find, and the invariable assertion of the authorities that my condition was hopeless did not shake my conviction to the contrary. I even made a trip to Rochester, Minnesota, for the sake of visiting the famous Mayo Clinic, where I expected to find all medical wisdom concentrated. All I got was a prescription for a stronger pair of glasses and a confirmation of the statements of my previous medical advisors and of the medical books—that myopia was incurable. I remained unconvinced, however.

I now happened to run across an article in the *Literary Digest* about a method of curing nearsightedness by squeezing the eyeball, said to have been used successfully in Paris. I wrote for further information but was told that the article was merely a reprint from *La Nature* and that the office knew nothing more about it. The editor suggested, however, that I write to Dr. Bates who was making a special study of this problem. I had already heard of Dr. Bates through another source and I lost no time in following this advice. He assured me that my condition was curable, and as I did not want to go to the expense of going to New York, I asked him if he could treat me by correspondence. He replied that while he had cured many patients by correspondence, such treatment was slow and a little uncertain, and in a case as serious as mine had better not be relied upon. As soon as I was able, therefore, I gathered together all the money that I had and went to New York, in spite of a tremendous amount of opposition and no encouragement whatever. Every doctor and every layman to whom I mentioned my purpose said I was crazy to suppose that nearsightedness could be cured when all the books said it was incurable. My brother, who is an optician, was so strong in his opposition that I don't think I should ever have got to New York if I hadn't pretended that I was going for some purpose other than the real one—and even after I got there and was able to write to him that my sight was improving, he kept urging me to come home telling me that any man who pretended to cure nearsightedness must be a quack, and that if I imagined I was getting any benefit it was because I had been hypnotized.

I arrived in New York on December 17, 1919, and went at once to Dr. Bates. When my eyes were tested with the Snellen test card, I found that at twenty feet I could see only the large letter at the top. I could read large print at five and a half inches, but could not read it any nearer or any farther, and could not see diamond type distinctly at any point.

I put in six hours a day at the office, practicing constantly with the Snellen test card, and at first found it rather discouraging and tiresome. When I tried to palm I saw all the colors of the rainbow instead of black. As I could not see anything perfectly, either at the near point or the distance, I could not remember anything I saw perfectly. Even my own signature I was unable to visualize. Neither could I imagine that the letters on the card were moving when I shifted from one side to another, or from one side of a letter to another.

At the end of a week, however, I succeeded in getting

the swing, becoming able to imagine not only that the letters on the card were swinging, but that my body and everything that I thought of was swinging also. This universal swing soon established itself so thoroughly that I was unable to stop it and the Doctor had to tell me how. I did it by staring at a letter of fine print for a few seconds. After this things began to go better. As long as I imagined the universal swing I could see black when I palmed and remember it with my eyes open. When I imagined it on the street it was as if a fog had lifted or the sun had come out from behind a cloud. My sight improved rapidly and I began to find the practice extremely interesting. I never got bored or sleepy and, in fact, never had such a good time in my life.

Besides improving my sight the swing did many other things for me. I had never done any running before coming to New York, but I now began to experiment with that form of exercise, not expecting in the least to distinguish myself. In a week, however, I was able to run eleven miles without fatigue or loss of breath, and without even feeling sore or stiff afterward. This I attributed to the swing, which I kept up all the time I was running. When I did not do this, I quickly became tired. One day I had to visit a chiropodist to have an ingrown nail treated. The first touch was excruciatingly painful. Then the chiropodist turned away to get an instrument, and I began to swing. When he resumed work I felt no pain, and the operation was finished painlessly. Even loneliness seemed to flee before this imaginary rhythmical movement, and it has now become so necessary to my existence, that I would even be willing to go back to the hated glasses rather than be without it.

When I left New York on December 31, I was able to make out some of the letters on the bottom line of the test card at twenty feet and to read diamond type from four to eighteen inches, while my eyes, which had previously been inflamed and partly closed, were clear and wide open. Incidentally, my memory, which had previously been so poor as to cause me great inconvenience and for which I had taken several memory courses in vain, had improved as much as my eyesight.

STORIES FROM THE CLINIC

No. 2: A Case of Cataract

By Emily C. Lierman

One day as I entered the Clinic I found a little white-haired woman waiting patiently to be treated. I had not seen her before and did not know what her trouble was. The usual crowd of patients was waiting for Dr. Bates and myself, so when he said to me, "See what you can do for this woman," I did not ask any questions, for I knew that whatever the condition of her eyes, relaxation would help her.

I placed her four feet from the test card, at which distance she read the 40-line (read by the eye with normal vision at forty feet), and told her how to rest her eyes by palming and how to avoid staring by shifting from one side of a letter to another. These practices helped her so much that before she left she was able to read the 30-line.

Later I learned that she had first seen Dr. Bates in March 1919 and that she had incipient cataract of both eyes. In October 1916, she had visited another dispensary where an operation was advised when the cataracts were ripe. I also learned that in spite of her seventy-three years she worked hard every day for her living, being employed in an orphan asylum where she mended the children's clothes. The fact that she was very deaf I saw for myself, of course, at the first interview, for I had to scream to make her hear. Her courage and cheerfulness under circumstances that might have daunted the bravest spirit were amazing. Her face was always radiant with smiles, and she was so witty and appreciative of everything that was done for her that each one of her visits to the Clinic was a pleasure to me.

"I have so much to be thankful for," she said one day. "I know I will see all right again. They are waiting to operate at the other dispensary, and I am waiting to fool them."

Most patients frown when they cannot see a letter, but my little cataract patient smiles instead, and remarks cheerfully, "That's the time you got me." One day she did not do as well as usual, and I found that the people in the place where she worked had been saying unpleasant things. I told her she must try not to let things of this sort disturb her, because that made her strain and made the cataracts worse. "Well," she said, "it is mighty hard not to worry; but I'll try not to."

At a recent visit she explained that she wouldn't be able to do very well because she hadn't had time to practice. "Never mind," I said. "Just do as well as you can." Without her knowing it I placed her two feet farther from the card than usual. Then I told her to palm, and after a short time I pointed to a small letter on the bottom line and asked her if she could see it. She recognized it immediately. Then I pointed to another, but she was so eager to see it that she tried too hard and failed. She closed her eyes for a few minutes without palming, and when she opened them she read the whole line. I then told her that she was two feet farther away from the card than she usually was. She was very happy about this and said, "That's the time you fooled me."

She has since become able to read the bottom line at ten feet, and one day she read it at eleven feet without knowing it and without having done any practicing at home.

On sunshiny days she can read the "W. H. Bates, M.D." on Dr. Bates' card, and for over a month she has done all her sewing without glasses. There is no doubt that she is going to fool them at the other dispensary.

Along with the improvement in her eyes has been a considerable improvement in her hearing. Noises in her ears which she describes as a "ringing and a singing" are promptly relieved by palming, and she says that the relief, which at first was only temporary, is now becoming more constant. She also says that she hears conversations better than she used to.

[See "Stories from the Clinic, No. 60: Two Cases of Cataract" in the February 1925 issue for a follow-up to this case.—TRQ]

HOW I WAS CURED

By Victoria Coolidge

Editor's Note—*This is the first of a series of articles by the same author. Next month she will tell how she cured other people. Owing to her high degree of hypermetropia, her own cure is particularly interesting.*

When I went to see Dr. Bates, I had been wearing glasses for twenty-six years. A prescription for glasses given to me in 1899 read: right eye, convex 5.00 D. S. with convex 0.50 D. C. 180 degrees; left eye, convex 5.00 D. S. with convex 1.00 D. C. 180 degrees. Another given to me in 1917 read nearly the same. I had consulted five different eye specialists, some of them several times, and they all told me the same thing—very poor sight is caused by malformation of the eyeball and no possibility of cure.

Fortunately, I was only a child when I first put on glasses and these statements, instead of discouraging me, made me feel that I was very important and should be the envy of all my schoolmates. As I grew older, however, I began to have headaches; so I had my glasses changed and my home study was reduced to one hour. As the changing of my glasses meant, at that time, a trip out of town, both parts of the treatment were very pleasant—more pleasant than effective, for the headaches continued.

Each time the eye specialist gave me stronger glasses, and gradually my vision for distant objects became worse and worse. When I went to the theatre I could not see the faces of the actors distinctly unless I sat as near as the fifth or sixth row from the stage; and when I discussed the play with the persons who accompanied me, the accuracy with which they could describe the features and expressions of the actors, without the aid of eyeglasses or opera-glasses, seemed unbelievable. The feeling of depression which I experienced on these occasions, however, was only momentary, and on the whole I was resigned to my fate.

But resignation was not so complete as to dull entirely my sense of ocular deformity; and, especially when I had had some fresh reminder of it in the shape of a headache or inability to finish a book because of tired eyes, I searched the magazines eagerly for discoveries about the eye. I felt sure that science had not said the last word about that subject. In January 1918, my attention was called to an article entitled "New Light Upon Our Eyes," in the *Scientific American,* and I lost no time, in reading it. You may be sure the article stated that Dr. Bates, who was already well known to the scientific world as the discoverer of adrenalin, had made a series of experiments on animals, the results of which struck at the very foundations of the present method of treating errors of refraction. They indicated, in short, that the lens is not a factor in accommodation, and that the deviations from the normal in the shape of the eyeball which produce errors of refraction are caused by a strain of the extrinsic muscles. As soon as the strain is removed, by perfect relaxation, the eyeball resumes its normal shape and there is no error of refraction. The remedy, therefore, was not to put glasses before the eyes, but to remove the strain which caused the abnormal action of the outside muscles.

The morning after reading the article I took off my glasses and tried to knit, but put them on more quickly than I had taken them off, for my sight was so poor without them that I made several mistakes and experienced a feeling of nausea. I believe that I had never until that moment realized how very poor my sight had become. I began to leave off my glasses whenever I had no close work to do, in spite of the fact that I had been warned by one eye specialist never to let them leave my nose during waking hours, and I determined to see Dr. Bates the very next time I came to New York.

The following August I called on Dr. Bates. I was prepared to make any sacrifice or to spend any amount of time—five years, ten years—it didn't matter, if my eyes were only getting better all the time instead of worse. The only thing that troubled me was the fear that he might tell me that my case was hopeless. This thought was so prominent in my mind, in fact, that I told him at once that I was afraid he could do nothing for me. I wanted him to know that I was prepared, so that if I must hear my doom I might hear it without delay.

After making a careful examination of my eyes, Dr. Bates asked me what was the lowest line that I could read on the test card. I found that I could read the 30-line at a distance of fourteen feet. Then he asked me if I could see anything on the line below. I said I could see the hollow square. Then he directed me to close my eyes, remembering how the square looked. I was able to do that, and he next directed me to look at the blank wall, still remembering the square; while I was doing so he examined my eyes again with a retinoscope and found them normal. When the strain was removed from my eyes by remembering the square perfectly and looking at the blank wall without trying to see anything, my vision became normal. The impossible had evidently been accomplished. For a few moments, at least, the lopsided eyeballs with their consequent errors of refraction had been miraculously rounded out. Dr. Bates now asked me to close my eyes, and then left me for about fifteen minutes. When he returned, he handed me one of his professional cards, and asked me if I could read anything on it. It seemed to me, I remember, a very foolish question, because I had previously told him that I could read nothing without glasses. A newspaper looked like a big gray blur, and the harder I tried to see it, the more blurred it became. However, I took the card and tried to read it, but, as I expected, without success. So he asked me to close my eyes again, this time covering them with the palms of my hands, and thinking of the blackest thing I could remember, which happened to be black paint. I did this for perhaps twenty minutes. After this he gave me the same card again, and directed me to hold it close to my eyes, about six inches, and to look alternately at the top and bottom of the letters. Much to my amazement and joy, a "B" came out clearly enough for me to recognize it. I kept on in this way, occasionally closing my eyes, until I could see "Bates," "Dr. W. H. Bates," and finally the telephone numbers printed in small type. I felt as if I were in a dream, or, as if I must be someone else. I lived in the clouds for the rest of the day, but somehow managed to get in some palming and some practice with the Snellen card.

The next day I did better, and I have kept on improving ever since. The best of it is that every gain is permanent. Dr. Bates told me that I would never have to wear glasses again, but I kept them near me for two or three weeks in case of emergency, just as Dr. Manette, in Dickens' *Tale of Two Cities,* used to keep his shoemaking tools and bench at hand in the event of his relapsing into his disordered state of mind. I never had to use them, however, and about six months ago I sold them for old gold. My vision is now 20/20 in a good light and 20/30 in any light and I can read diamond type at six inches.

AFTER GLASSES FAILED

By Florence Miller

I began to wear glasses when I was fifteen years old and wore them unchanged for seven years. Then I went to another specialist who gave me new ones—stronger, I suppose. I wore these for a year and then, not feeling quite comfortable in them, I consulted a third specialist who changed them again. These lenses I wore for four years, by the end of which time I had begun to have constant though not severe headaches. I went back to the third specialist a second time, but he said he could not improve upon the lenses I was wearing, and I went on having the headaches, which gradually became worse until sometimes I had to go to bed with them.

One day my son, ten years old, came home and said that the teacher had told him that he needed glasses. Naturally I did not wish to see him wearing spectacles if there was any way of avoiding it, and as my husband, who is a physician, had recently heard Dr. Bates read a paper at a medical society on his method of curing errors of refraction without glasses, I took my boy to see him. Dr. Bates not only assured me that the child could be cured, but improved his sight markedly at the first visit.

Then he turned to me and said, "I can cure you, too." "But I couldn't possibly go without glasses," I said; "I get such awful headaches when I do." "Do you want to be cured very much?" he asked. "I would do anything in this world," I said, "to be cured." "If so," he answered, "I can cure you, and you will be able to go without your glasses without getting headaches." "What do you want me to do?" I asked. "I want you to take off your glasses," he said, "and come and see me every day for a while."

I took the glasses off and have never worn or wanted them since; just what became of them I don't know. My impression is that I gave them to the Doctor and that he put them in a cabinet where he deposits treasures of that kind. He says he told me to throw them in the ashcan and that I afterwards said I had done so. At any rate I am sure that I never put them or any other glasses before my eyes since that day.

This was on July 14, 1914, and my vision, as tested by the Snellen test card without glasses, was 20/200 in each eye. The Doctor said I had compound myopic astigmatism, and that my glasses were concave 0.50 D. S. with concave 1.50 D. C. 180 degrees.

It was troublesome and tedious learning to see. For two months I went to see Dr. Bates nearly every day and he spent half an hour or more with me. For another two months I went twice a week. Since then I have continued to practice more or less regularly with the test card. But the results have been worth all the trouble.

Most of the practice time I spent simply resting my eyes by closing them, or by covering them with the palms of my hands, then looking at the test card for a moment and resting again. The Doctor told me that when I looked at a letter on the test card and did not see one part of it better than the rest I was immediately to look away and rest my eyes. He also recommended me to imagine that I saw one part of a letter best with the eyes open and closed alternately. In this way I finally became able to look at each and every letter on the card and see one part of it best when my vision became normal, and even double what is ordinarily considered normal.

On July 20, less than a week after I began to take the treatment, I was able to read most of the letters on the bottom line of the test card at twenty feet, and in two weeks I could read all of them, 20/10. At first I was able to do this only temporarily, but gradually I became able to hold the letters longer. On August 12, I was able to report that for the first time in years I had not had a headache for a whole week. By September 2, I was able to read and sew as much as I liked without any discomfort in my eyes. When I wore glasses the theatre and movies had always hurt my eyes terribly, but instead of advising me to stay away from these places, Dr. Bates urged me to go to the movies and look at them just as I did at the test card—that is, by alternating vision with rest. I was to look first at the corner of the screen, then off to the dark, then a little nearer the center, and so forth. In this way I soon became able to look directly at the pictures without discomfort.

For the last five years my sight has steadily improved. My form of astigmatism was such as to positively obliterate all horizontal lines. To see such lines at all I had to turn my head or the object. Lines of music would hold only a minute or less. I have gradually become able to hold these lines longer and longer, and now I never lose them unless very tired. As for headaches I have had none at all during these years that could not be accounted for by indigestion or neuralgia, and very few even of these.

Last spring I went to see Dr. Bates about an ulcer on my cornea. He tested my sight and found it, even under these conditions, better than normal.

Better Eyesight
April 1920—Vol. II, No. 4

REST

All methods of curing errors of refraction are simply different ways of obtaining rest.

Different persons do this in different ways. Some patients are able to rest their eyes simply by closing them, and complete cures have been obtained by this means, the closing of the eyes for a longer or shorter period being alternated with looking at the test card for a moment. In other cases patients have strained more when their eyes were shut than when they were open. Some can rest their eyes when all light is excluded from them by covering with the palms of the hands; others cannot, and have to be helped by other means before they can palm. Some become able at once to remember or imagine that the letters they wish to see are perfectly black, and with the accompanying relaxation their vision immediately becomes normal. Others become able to do this only after a considerable time. Shifting is a very simple method of relieving strain, and most patients soon become able to shift from one letter to another, or from one side of a letter to another in such a way that these forms seem to move in a direction opposite to the movement of the eye. A few are unable to do this, but can do it with a mental picture of a letter, after which they become able to do it visually.

Patients who do not succeed with any particular method of obtaining rest for their eyes should abandon it and try something else. The cause of the failure is strain, and it does no good to go on straining.

HOW I HELPED OTHERS

By Victoria Coolidge

When I had become able to read without glasses, and my headaches had become less and less frequent, and less severe each time, I was so enthusiastic over my experience that I was anxious to help others. My brother was my first patient. He was so much interested in what had been done for me that he wanted to try it himself; but I never dreamed of being able to help him, because his eyes were almost as bad as my own had been, his glasses being: right eye, convex 3.25 D. S.; left eye, convex 3.75 D. S. with 0.50 D. C. 180 degrees. However, I knew the treatment could do no harm, so I decided that I would try to show him as nearly as I could what Dr. Bates had done for me. Imagine my surprise when I found that he too, by holding the fine print six inches from his eyes and looking alternately at the top and bottom of the letters, became able to read it just as I had become able to do so. He proved to be a model pupil as soon as he had demonstrated to his own satisfaction that he must leave off his glasses all the time if he wanted to make any appreciable progress. He has now done without them for about a year and has made remarkable progress in that time, the secret of his success being a great desire to be cured, an intelligent grasp of the idea of central fixation, and perseverance in practicing central fixation at every possible opportunity.

The next person I was able to help was a friend who, while visiting me, happened to notice the Snellen test card hanging on the wall. She asked me what I was doing with it, and I explained, adding that she was very fortunate in having normal vision. "I thought I had," she said, "but I have had so many headaches that I consulted an eye specialist the other day and he gave me glasses." She was so displeased to think she had to wear them and had found it so difficult to get used to seeing with them that I asked her if she would like to try Dr. Bates' treatment without glasses. She said that she would jump at the chance. I told her to read the card every day at ten, fifteen, and twenty feet, and to palm whenever she had a headache. That was in August. On December 19 she telephoned that she had practiced reading the card every day, that she had had no trouble with headaches, and that she was reading 20/10 easily with the better eye and fairly well with the other. Shortly after she began the treatment herself, she was able to improve the vision of a child nine years old from 20/50 to 20/20.

It has been many times pointed out in this magazine that children under twelve years old who have never worn glasses are easily cured; and so for the past month I have been trying to see what I could do for such children, and for some who were older—including two who had worn glasses, one some time previously and the other up to the time I began to treat her. I have worked with six and they have all improved. One girl, fifteen, who had worn glasses a few years ago for imperfect sight in one eye but who had discarded them, improved in a half-hour from 20/70 to 20/50 by alternating palming, or sometimes just closing her eyes and then reading the Snellen test card. This improvement was permanent.

Another girl, sixteen, had worn glasses for a year, chiefly for headache, she said, although her vision in both eyes was but 20/200. As she could read without her glasses without much difficulty, she was only too glad to take them off, as most girls of that age are, but she was afraid of the headaches. I asked her to try it, and she has done so for about three weeks during which time her vision improved to 20/70 and she had no headaches.

The following is the record of four little girls who have improved by reading the Snellen test card daily, and palming:

Name	Age	Vision Sept. 1919 Phys. Rec. Card	Dec. 11	Dec. 31
Catherine	10	R.20/50	20/40	20/40
		L.20/50	20/40	20/40
Blanche	10	R. 4/50	6/40	6/30
		L. 4/50	6/40	6/30
Vinnie	9	R.20/50	20/40	absent
		L.20/40	20/30	
Sylvia	10	R.20/40	20/15	20/10
		L.20/40	20/15	20/10

Catherine's vision afterwards (January 22) improved to 20/20. The case of Sylvia was so interesting that it will be treated in more detail next month.

STORIES FROM THE CLINIC

No. 3: Retinitis Pigmentosa

By Emily C. Lierman

I am not a physician and I know very little about the disease of the eyes known as retinitis pigmentosa except how to relieve it. I have been told that in this condition spots of black pigment are deposited in the retina, that parts of the retina are destroyed, and that the nerve of sight is diseased. Eye books which describe the disease say that it usually begins in childhood, and progresses very slowly until it ends in complete blindness. The field of vision is contracted and, because they cannot see objects on either side of them, patients frequently stumble against such objects. In most cases the vision is much worse at night than in the daytime. The books say further that no treatment is known which helps these cases. Nevertheless, Dr. Bates reported in the *New York Medical Journal* of February 3, 1917, a case of retinitis pigmentosa which had been materially benefited through treatment by relaxation, and by the use of the same methods I have been able to greatly improve the sight in several cases of the same kind.

My first case of retinitis pigmentosa was Pauline, a little girl of twelve who came to the Clinic in October 1917. At five feet from the card she could read only the 70-line, and her eyes vibrated continually from side to side, a condition known as nystagmus. She was very shy and extremely nervous, and appealed to me pathetically for glasses so that she could see the blackboard and the teacher would not think her stupid and make fun of her. I have noticed that eye patients often suffer from extreme nervousness; but this poor child had the worst case of nerves I ever saw, and the slightest agitation made her sight worse. If in asking her to read a line on the test card I raised my voice and spoke a little peremptorily, her face would flush and she would say, "I cannot see anything now." But just as soon as I lowered my voice and took pains to speak gently, her sight cleared up.

I began her treatment by telling her to cover her eyes with the palms of her hands and remember the letters she had seen on the card. This improved her sight so much that before she left she was able to see all of the 50-line at five feet, and—what thrilled me most of all—the dreadful movement of her eyes had stopped. She came quite steadily to the Clinic, and every time she came I was able to improve her sight so that at last she became able to read the writing on the blackboard at school.

Then I did not see her again for six months. When she came back she told me that she had been working in a laundry during the summer because she hated school. She had also been ill during the summer and her mother had taken her to a hospital for treatment. While she was there an eye specialist had looked at her eyes, and this made her so nervous that they had started to vibrate from side to side.

He said to her, "You ought to have your eyes treated; they are very bad." "I am having them treated at the Harlem Hospital Clinic," she answered. "I know how to stop that vibration." Then she palmed for a while and when she uncovered and opened her eyes the doctor looked at them again. "Why they seem all right now," he said. "You had better go to that Doctor until you are cured. He can do more for you than I can."

I was very much pleased to find that in spite of having stayed away so long, she had not forgotten what I had told her and was able to stop her nystagmus. I tested her sight and found that it was no worse than when I had last seen her. In fact, in some ways, it was better. She was not so nervous, and she said that her family and friends noticed that her eyes looked better. She herself was now very enthusiastic and anxious to have me help her. I told her to palm as usual, and left her to treat other patients. Five minutes later she read the 30-line at thirteen feet. I now told her to look first to the right of the card and then to the left, and to note that it appeared to move in a direction opposite to the movement of her eyes; then to close her eyes and remember this movement. She did this, and when she opened her eyes she read two letters on the 20-line. At a later visit she read the whole of the 20-line at thirteen feet.

The last patient I treated for this dreadful disease was an old man of seventy. He came to the Clinic on January 14, 1920, and when I first saw him, he was standing with many others, waiting patiently for Dr. Bates to speak to him. Our work has to be done very rapidly because of the very short time we have to treat so many patients, and I very seldom have time to observe individuals as I would like to do. But because of his unusual appearance, I at once singled this dear old man out from the crowd. Most men of his age who come to our Clinic are unkempt, dirty and ragged. But this man was well groomed. His clothes, though worn and old, were well-brushed, his shoes were polished, his collar clean, his tie neatly adjusted. He had a great abundance of snow-white hair, neatly parted and brushed, and his skin was like a baby's, "pink and white."

Dr. Bates asked me to treat him with the usual remark, "See what you can do for this man," and I placed him four feet from the card, asking him to read what he could. "I'm afraid I can't see so well, ma'am," he said, "my eyes bother me a good deal." "I'm going to show you how to rest your eyes so that they won't bother you," I answered.

The best he could do at this distance was to read the 50-line. I told him to palm, and in less than five minutes he saw a number of letters on the 40-line. The next time he came I put him nine feet from the card, and at this distance he read all the letters on the 30-line. He was so happy and excited over this that I became excited too. I forgot that I had other patients waiting for me and encouraged him to talk, a thing which I am seldom able to do with the patients. I was glad afterward that I did so, for he had a wonderful story to tell.

"Do you know, ma'am," he said, "for two nights I palmed and rested my eyes for a long time before I went to bed and what do you think?—I slept all the night through without waking up once. Now I think that is great, ma'am, because for years I have had insomnia. I would sleep only a little while; then I would get up and smoke my pipe to pass the time."

At a later visit I put him twelve feet from the card, and at this distance also he was able to read the 30-line. When I told him what he had done he was again greatly pleased and excited. "You know I'm so much better"' he said, "that I didn't even notice that I was farther away than usual. Thank you, ma'am. God bless you, ma'am."

During the practice, when he failed to see a letter I was pointing to, I said, "Close your eyes and tell me the color of your grandchild's eyes." "Blue, ma'am." he said. "Keep your eyes covered, keep remembering the color of baby's eyes." He did this, and after a few minutes his sight cleared up and he saw the letter. After we had finished the practice I again encouraged him to talk, and he told me more about his insomnia.

"Do you know, ma'am," he said, "after I had had two night's sleep without waking up, I didn't dare tell any of my family about it, for fear that it wouldn't last and I would only disappoint them. So I waited. Now, do you know, ma'am, it is just two weeks that I have slept the night through without waking up once, and so I told my wife about it. She is so happy, ma'am, I just can't tell you, for it has been many years since I was able to do that."

I wish I could have a picture of his face when he is telling of the improvement in his eyesight and general health. It would be a picture of gentleness, love, kindness and gratitude. Recently he looked up into my face and said, "I am seeing you better now, ma'am. You look younger."

In two months his vision improved from 10/200 to 10/30. As he made but eight visits in this time, I feel that this record is remarkable. I also feel that the statements in the books about the impossibility of doing anything for patients with retinitis pigmentosa are in need of modification.

PERFECT SIGHT WITHOUT GLASSES

By Evelyn Cushing Campbell

Editor's Note—*The author of the following article is engaged in literary work which compels her to use her eyes constantly for reading and writing. When first seen she was wearing the following glasses: right eye, convex 1.50 D. S.; left eye, convex 1.25 D. C.*

One of several problems which long disturbed my mind, both consciously and subconsciously, was whether the distressing condition of my eyes was caused by bodily ailments, or my general state of ever-present weariness was due to trouble with the eyes. Without glasses, my eyes felt blurred and strained; after wearing them for a time, the immediate relief was succeeded by increased weariness and a desire to throw them far away. Often I thought, "How happy would I be if I never again had to put on my glasses!"

My problem has now been solved. The haunting spectre of anxiety which stalked ever at my side has vanished, and I have entered upon a state of beatific bliss and satisfaction with life in general. I have acquired perfect vision without glasses, and at the same time a relaxed state of once over-strained nerves which gives me a glimpse of what heaven may hold in store for world-weary mortals.

A visit to Dr. Bates wrought this seeming miracle, so far beyond any hope or expectations in which I had ever dared to indulge that I now confess, as an article of faith, that hereafter I shall always believe that everything is possible.

The first treatment occupied not more than half an hour, but in that brief time I passed from the inability to read type of medium size, except at arm's length, to reading type less than half the size at a proximity to the eye which formerly had made the letters absolutely illegible.

My recollections of the entire treatment are by no means consecutive nor complete, but the results were more than conclusive that the basic principle must be sound.

After some preliminary tests with charts, Dr. Bates informed me that there was nothing wrong with my eyes. This in itself was a tremendous relief, as it immediately suggested the possibility of benefit by means other than the wearing of nerve-racking eyeglasses.

"Close your eyes and rest them," I was told. The closing was at once accomplished, but the resting process proved to be more elusive. Almost at once the eyelids began to twitch so constantly that only with great difficulty was I able to keep the eyes closed at all. Upon opening them, the letters on the test card were very much blurred and suggestive of little dancing figures.

Instructions followed to close the eyes again and, first, to remember the white of starch; then the black of coal. When the eyes were reopened from the blackness, they felt distinctly rested and it was possible to read lines upon the card which previously had been very unclear.

"Now close your eyes and remember an agreeable color—the green of trees, of grass, the color of flowers." This I did, seeing the green leaves of oak trees with sunlight upon them, the blue of a river glimmering beyond; brighter green of grass on a hillside; yellow flowers with fine-fringed petals upon which had alighted a butterfly of deeper yellow; reddish-yellow tiger-lilies; pink roses, red roses, yellow roses; blue sky with cumulus cloud masses.

Upon opening my eyes, the first line of printing on a card which had been much blurred at a distance of, say nine inches, could now be read with ease. The card was then brought three inches nearer, with the result that the printing once more became indistinct.

Directions now followed to close the eyes and again remember a color. After some hesitation I brought to my mind yellow, but the eyes did not feel rested as on the former occasion. This I thought might be due to the effort to concentrate upon an object of that color—a yellow curtain hanging in my apartment. My comment to this effect met the response that I must not make any effort, that all effort was bad for the eyes.

Another instruction was to close the eyes, covering them with the cupped palm, fingers crossed lightly upon the brow with no pressure upon the eye itself, and to remember black. This is called *palming*. The blackness at first was filled with swirling, grayish, elongated globules, and the eyelids twitched. No other color was visible and the swirling particles gradually became less apparent.

"Now remember a black point, or period, and imagine it swinging like a pendulum." My first attempt was a failure, but I finally succeeded and, to my amazement, found upon opening the eyes that I was able to read diamond type on a small card held at a distance of six inches from the eyes. This really surpassed everything else, for formerly the person who held anything before my eyes at this close range had inflicted positive suffering upon me, and was usually greeted with an expression of ill-suppressed irritation, for the attempt to focus the eyes at this point produced at once a feeling of nausea.

A peep into the mirror showed my eyes much clearer and less filled with weariness than I had been accustomed to see them after hours of sleep. Completely convinced of the uselessness of wearing aids to eyes that did not aid but only irritated, I went home to consign the hated glasses to the darkest and deepest corner of my "Botany Bay" trunk. They have lain there undisturbed for over a year. I have never since that day felt the need of them, and my eyes have performed without fatigue tasks which would have been quite beyond them in the days when I depended on eye-crutches. One day recently, when I had to finish a piece of work in a limited time, I worked at my typewriter from nine in the morning until four the following morning, only stopping for meals, and my eyes were just as fresh when I finished as when I began.

BETTER EYESIGHT APPRECIATED

Editor's Note—*The testimony of the following letter to the value of the experiences of patients recently published in this magazine is very interesting. The statements about the effect of central fixation upon the desire for sleep are also significant, and the facts have been duplicated in many other cases.*

I am keenly interested in this medium through which your discoveries and the experiences of your patients are made known to the public. My eyesight is improving steadily, and I find that I am grasping and applying the principles set forth in your magazine more intelligently every day.

I have improved physically and mentally since I started. Ever since I can remember, I have had the greatest difficulty in rousing myself from a very heavy sleep in the morning into which I seem to fall after a night of constant dreaming. As a result, I feel heavy with fatigue and positively stupid mentally. One doctor whom I consulted said that these nocturnal disturbances were due to indigestion, or a bad conscience! I told him I guessed it was both! As soon as I awaken in the morning, I start my exercises and after palming, flashing and swinging, I feel as if a fog had lifted and as if I were suddenly released from a weight that had held me down. I start the day with a clear mind and a buoyant energy that enables me to accomplish twice as much as I used to. This has been a very interesting experience to me, and a very curious one. I suppose some mental scientists would say that I forget my fatigue because I focus my attention and interest on something else, which may be true to a certain extent, but not wholly, because it does not explain the sudden clear vision and physical freedom of which I immediately become conscious.

Better Eyesight
May 1920—Vol. II, No. 5

Seven Truths of Normal Sight

1. Normal Sight can always be demonstrated in the normal eye, but only under favorable conditions.
2. Central Fixation: The letter or part of the letter regarded is always seen best.
3. Shifting: The point regarded changes rapidly and continuously.
4. Swinging: When the Shifting is slow, the letters appear to move from side to side, or in other directions, with a pendulum-like motion.
5. Memory is perfect. The color and background of the letters, or other objects seen, are remembered perfectly, instantaneously and continuously.
6. Imagination is good. One may even see the white part of letters whiter than it really is, while the black is not altered by distance, illumination, size, or form of the letters.
7. Rest or relaxation of the eye and mind is perfect and can always be demonstrated.

When one of these seven fundamentals is perfect, all are perfect.

FINE PRINT A BENEFIT TO THE EYE
Its Effect the Exact Contrary of What Has Been Supposed

It is impossible to read fine print without relaxing. Therefore the reading of such print, contrary to what is generally believed, is a great benefit to the eyes. Persons who can read perfectly fine print, like the above specimen are relieved of pain and fatigue while they are doing it, and this relief is often permanent. Persons who cannot read it are benefited by observing its blackness, and remembering it with the eyes open and closed alternately. By bringing the print so near to the eyes that it cannot be read, pain is sometimes relieved instantly because when the patient realizes that there is no possibility of reading it, the eyes do not try to do so. Persons who can read fine print perfectly, imagine that they see between the lines streaks of white whiter than the margin of the page; persons who cannot read it also see these streaks, but not as well. When the patient becomes able to increase the vividness of these appearances (see "Halos" in *Better Eyesight,* February 1920) the sight always improves.

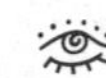

MY HEADACHES
By R. Ruiz Arnau, M.D.

From my childhood until about three years ago—I am now forty-six—I suffered from headaches, periods of intense supraorbital pain lasting from twenty-four to thirty-six hours unless relieved by repeated doses of some derivative of antipyrin. A notable feature of these attacks was their regularity; every six days—seven at the most—I would awake with a feeling of discomfort near the right temple, the forerunner of immediate torment. Unless relieved by the use of a sedative, varying according to the time and also the results or lack of results obtained from previous doses, the painful paroxysm, with all its train of nausea, eructation, polyuria, excessive sensitiveness to light and noise, and complete incapacity for physical or mental activity, would run its course producing a condition truly unbearable for one or two days. In the intervals between the attacks I was absolutely normal, and even accomplished more, perhaps, than the ordinary person, thus compensating for the time lost by headache. Under these conditions I went through my studies at the high school and took my medical course. Thereafter, for a period of about twenty years, I followed the profession of an active general practitioner, wrote many articles and several books, always subject to the terrible prospect of the period of migraine which unfailingly appeared with invariable regularity.

As I enjoyed, or thought I enjoyed, perfect vision, I lived to the age of thirty-three accepting the idea of hereditary rheumatic migraine; my mother suffered from similar headaches all her life, and so also did my sisters. I had been told that if the headaches were due to such a cause, they would be modified or disappear after thirty years old, some other indisposition, perhaps, taking their place. With that hope I almost wished the years to pass quickly so that I might not only be free from an excessively painful malady, but be able to devote myself to the intense mental labor to which my vocation and tastes had always inclined me. My thirtieth birthday came and went, however, with no cessation of the headaches and no diminution in their severity.

With the passing of the years, too, came a desire to cultivate a specialty requiring deep, constant and careful theoretical and practical work. For this purpose it was necessary for me to read a number of books printed in small type, and as my professional work, then very arduous, left me but little free time, I had to read them at all hours and in all places, often in moving vehicles. In the space of a few months, my age being then thirty-four, I found my sight ruined, constituting a new factor in my (supposedly) inherited disorders. Immediately on beginning to read I would experience ocular fatigue and a feeling of discomfort in the eyeballs, and this aggravated the headaches, although I was now in the fourth decade of my life, the period at which I had hoped for relief.

I had recourse, naturally, to an oculist, a friend of mine to whom I was accustomed to send special cases, and with whose aptness and efficiency I had always been satisfied. He examined my eyes with great care, and concluded that I had a slight hypermetropic error in both, with a slight degree of astigmatism in one. He prescribed lenses to correct only half my defect, as is customary in such cases, and after several changes, owing to the difficulty of fitting the astigmatic eye, I secured a pair of glasses which I was able to endure for a year.

Their use convinced me that the head troubles from which I had suffered during my whole life, in spite of their mathematical regularity and their supposedly rheumatic origin, had never been anything but an eloquent expression of what Anglo-Saxons term *eyestrain*. As soon as I began to wear the glasses all the features of the old pains were radically modified. Their regularity ceased and they were converted into painful disturbances of irregular occurrence, connected with work requiring use of the eyes at the near point and completely independent of other causes. If I did not read, I would be all right indefinitely; if I used my eyes for close work for even a short time, I knew that I would suffer for it, some hours later, with a period of ocular pain or headache. In a word, the trouble became a necessary consequence of visual activity and lost its old appearance of a syndrome that was established, recurrent, classical, only remotely connected with the use of the eyes.

But the fact remained that the wearing of glasses had not cured my malady. I had, it is true, got rid of the old periodical migraine, but I was left with perpetual attacks of ocular and supraorbital pain, almost continuous, though never very intense. This change I almost regretted, for when I suffered from periodical headaches I had had five good consecutive days, during which it was possible for me to do sustained intellectual work. Now prolonged application was impossible and I feared that an ailment resulting in almost continuous pain would, in time, lead to a serious state of neurasthenia.

At thirty-eight years old my trouble began to be complicated with presbyopia; and here began, if I may say so, the second Odyssey of my ocular problem. In order to read I had to increase the strength of my glasses, and this involved the use of hideous bifocals. With three different pairs of glasses in my pocket and one on my nose—one for distance, one for reading, a tinted pair to moderate the intense sunlight of the tropics where I lived, and bifocals for special occasions—I found my troubles daily increasing. I could not escape from the optician who was continually changing the refractive power of the lenses, as none of them ever suited me, and I did not cease to annoy my good friend, the oculist who, with singular patience, listened to my complaints and tried to help me.

Once during this time I had occasion to visit New York and while there I consulted a famous eye specialist. In no way was he able to mitigate my sufferings, and I returned more confused than ever to my country, Puerto Rico, and almost decided, in view of the increasing difficulty of keeping up the struggle, to give up professional life and devote myself to some work of a rural nature which would not require of my poor eyes the insupportable effort of reading the small print of periodicals and medical books.

I must add that at this time I suffered from several attacks of swelling of the upper eyelid of one or the other eye, lasting for four or five days and having no appreciable cause; that on two occasions I had an inflammation of the margins of the lids, followed the second time by a combined inflammation of both eyes and lids; while the last condition left after it a little ulcer of the right cornea, near the pupil, which required more than two months treatment on the part of my patient and capable oculist.

Another detail which I do not wish to forget is that during the whole time that I wore glasses, about nine years, and even for some months after discarding them, I frequently noticed the phenomenon known as "floating specks." These I never noticed before wearing glasses.

I had reached a state bordering on desperation when, in September 1916, professional work took me again to New York, accompanying one of my patients to whom I had recommended x-ray treatment by a well-known specialist of the great city. On the occasion of our visits the old doctor and I used to discuss the latest advances in electrotherapy, and he called my attention to some notable cases of cure brought about by this means. One day it occurred to me to say to him, "Well, friend doctor, all that is very fine, but the wonder that is to cure my particular ill has not yet been discovered." "What do you mean? What is the matter with you?" I recounted at great length the history of my eyes. The doctor laughed, left his office for a few minutes, and on returning said to me, "Why, yes, it has been discovered. Read this pamphlet, take my card, and go to see the author."

It was an article by Dr. William H. Bates of New York published a few months previously in the *New York Medical Journal,* and entitled, "The Cure of Defective Sight by

Treatment Without Glasses, or Radical Cure of Errors of Refraction by Means of Central Fixation." The reader can understand the eagerness with which I read this pamphlet, but I must confess that it caused me both surprise and disappointment. The author affirmed, as the readers of this magazine already know, that errors of refraction—myopia, hypermetropia, and astigmatism—so far from being permanent conditions due to deformities of the eyeball, congenital or acquired, and only to be corrected by glasses, are caused by a vicious contraction of the outside muscles of the ocular globe and may be cured by treatment leading to the relaxation of these muscles. In a word, the eyeball is not inextensible and the lens is not a factor in accommodation. Thus two fundamental dogmas of the doctrine established by Helmholtz and others fall to the ground. This, I reflected, could only be the work of an unbalanced mind or of a genius, and unbalanced minds are so abundant and geniuses so rare nowadays, that the latter did not seem probable. Imbued, like all doctors, with the idea that accommodation is brought about by a change in the curvature of the crystalline lens, I felt, as I read, the tremendous influence of the old school of physiological optics, with all the authority of its founders, and all the weight of things long established, accepted by the great majority and sustained by the immense mass of vested interests developed under their shadow; and I said to myself, "All this seems to me anatomically impossible."

And yet it inspired me with hope. After all, I thought, why should things not be accomplished in the eye as they are in the photographic camera in which, in order to obtain pictures at different distances, the distance between the lens and the sensitive plate is shortened or lengthened. If, in a photograph, one were to imitate that which, according to the accepted theory, occurs in the eye, it would be necessary to put in a new lens every time one desired to change the focus since there is no known device that can modify the power of a lens. Leaving the accepted theories out of consideration for the moment, it seemed to me more logical to conceive of accommodation as Bates described it than as it had appeared to Helmholtz. After some hesitation, therefore, I decided to consult the author of the revolutionary pamphlet.

I gave him a detailed account of my ailment, begging him, on finishing the tale, to tell me frankly if he considered it incurable, as in that case I would give up my career definitely and live in the country. I expected that my case, which I supposed to be exceptional, would present to him a most difficult clinical problem, and I was astonished when he said: "Is that all?" "What! You don't think that is much, Dr. Bates?" I replied, somewhat provoked, as I remembered my long years of suffering. "You will be cured, and soon," was his reply; a reply firm, decided, categorical, which for the moment increased my confusion.

Dr. Bates then explained to me that my eyes were in no way abnormal, except for having lost the power of central fixation many years before. Mental strain had brought with it ocular strain. I had contracted the muscles of the eyeball abnormally in doing close work, and with the commencement of the presbyopic age the trouble had been considerably accentuated.

It required only a few treatments by means of rest, practice with the Snellen test card, and the cultivation of the memory of a black period with the eyes alternately closed and open (glasses having, of course, been discarded), to convince me of the truth of this diagnosis and, naturally, of its logical basis. By a continuation of the same treatment my headaches were soon cured and, after many months of practice, my lost power of central fixation was restored and I regained the normal vision I have since enjoyed. I can now read diamond type at six inches, and can devote to reading or writing as much time as I wish. The intense rays of electric light, which formerly were unbearable to me, no longer cause me any inconvenience and I even enjoy looking at them for long periods.

I have, in short, learned to look at things without staring, so that every object seen seems to have a slight movement caused by the unconscious shifting of the eye, a phenomenon discovered by Bates and by virtue of which the point regarded changes rapidly and continuously.

I have been able to demonstrate in myself the "Seven Truths of Normal Sight," formulated by Bates; truths in light of which the old ideas of the refraction of the eye crumble irremediably; truths completely verifiable by every truly impartial and scientific mind which is emancipated from the tendency to persist in error solely because it is supported by authority, even such an authority as the immortal Helmholtz; truths demonstrated by careful, repeated and varied observations—by scientific experiments upon animals, and above all by the study of images obtained, after much labor and many failures, from the lens, cornea, iris and sclera. The powerful electric light employed for the latter purpose is evidently more adequate than the candle used by Purkinje for the study of the celebrated images to which his name has been given, and it suffices to compare—with an open mind—two photographs of images upon the lens obtained with the eye focused, respectively, at the distance and the near point, to become convinced that accommodation is accomplished by the lengthening of the eyeball—through the unmistakable action of the oblique muscles—and that we have here one of the most beautiful and significant achievements of the century.

And not only have I demonstrated these truths in

myself, but I have cured some patients and improved many others. Among the former was the very notable case of a young printer who, although only slightly hypermetropic, was easily fatigued by the close work demanded by his calling. Half an hour of such work brought on a severe frontal headache, growing in intensity up to midday, when he was obliged to suspend his labors. After only three weeks of treatment by the methods described, his troubles completely disappeared. Today he not only works all day without inconvenience, but even works overtime with great economic advantage to himself.

Another case was that of a lady, a lawyer, who had been told that the sight of one eye was almost lost, and who could practically do no continuous work without severe headaches. She wore a pair of large dark-tinted lenses constantly in order to protect her eyes from the tropical sunlight, and these were so disfiguring that they made her very conspicuous and, naturally, caused her much annoyance. Treatment by relaxation soon cured her headaches and other ailments, and she became able to fulfill her duties efficiently as secretary to a high judicial officer in Puerto Rico. At present she occupies an important position as a lecturer in one of the YWCA's of the United States, and according to recent advice her sight and general health continue very satisfactory.

Many of my friends who witnessed and sympathized with my sufferings and saw me wear numerous spectacles are now for the most part presbyopic and use glasses for reading. Overcome by the evidence of my case, they only await a period of leisure in order to take the treatment in which they believe, but which they erroneously suppose to demand effort and time. They find their problems solved temporarily by glasses and continue to wear them. But the patients who never find a pair of lenses satisfactory and who pass half their lives in the optician's office, who suffer from troublesome ailments of various kinds resulting from their eye troubles, these have no choice but to have recourse to the new truth and the new methods which are certain to solve their problems—not temporarily, but permanently. It is they, above all, who will publish the glad tidings they and the schoolchildren under twelve, who having, as a rule, not accustomed their eyes to glasses, and being free from the misconceptions that handicap older patients, respond with incredible rapidity to the new methods—methods as simple as they are effective, and both preventative and curative of visual defects.

In spite of indifference, in spite of the coldness with which new truths are received—the great majority not deigning even to discuss them—I have absolute confidence in the early acceptance of this wonderful discovery, so simple and, in its practical application, so fruitful. There will not be lacking dispassionate and impartial minds to verify and propagate it. The number of the cured, constantly increasing, will become at last like a tidal wave, overwhelming all opposition. Truth must conquer in the end, removing the mountains of error and prejudice.

THE STORY OF SYLVIA

By Victoria Coolidge

Sylvia is a little girl, ten years old, in the fourth grade in school. She has a good brain and is an energetic worker, but until she learned to see with central fixation, she was handicapped by defective eyesight. According to her physical record card, her vision in September 1919, was 20/40 in each eye. On November 4, 1919, I tested her eyes and found that 20/40 was the best that she could see with either eye at that time.

On this day I gave her the first lesson in central fixation. By alternately reading the Snellen card and closing her eyes to rest them, she improved to 20/30. When she had demonstrated what an improvement she could make by resting her eyes in this way, I showed her how she could rest them even more by palming, that is, covering her eyes with the palms of her hands laid gently over them, excluding all light but not pressing on the eyeballs. I asked her to do this as many times as she could during the day, five minutes at a time, and I gave her a piece of paper on which to write her name, the date, and the number of times she palmed each day for a week.

The next week I went to visit Sylvia's school and she showed me her paper. She had palmed about eight times each day, except Saturday and Sunday, when she had palmed fourteen times. I could see by the expression on her face that she had a surprise in store for me, but I was not prepared for such a surprise as followed. I had her stand six feet from the Snellen card, and she read every letter on it perfectly. Then she stood ten feet away and read it just as well. "Now stand back here," I said, pointing to a line twenty feet from the card. Nothing daunted, and with the triumphant expression still lighting up her face, she walked to the twenty-foot mark and read every letter correctly through the 15-line and some letters on the 10-line. I looked at Sylvia and then at her teacher. "Is this Sylvia?" I asked, thinking I had been teaching the wrong child. The teacher assured me that it was. Still skeptical, I looked up her physical record card and my own record to be sure that I had read the figures correctly. There they were, 20/40 on both.

At my next visit, December 18, Sylvia scorned to stand

at ten feet, and instead walked immediately to the twenty-foot mark with all the confidence in the world. This time she was able to read all the letters so quickly and so confidently that her teacher began to suspect that she had memorized them, and I must confess that I began to think so, too. Therefore, I hung up the Snellen card which belonged to the school and which had entirely different letters. Sylvia had not seen this card since September when her eyes were tested. She read the 20-line, which happened to be the last line on the card, at twenty, twenty-six, and thirty-two feet. Another day I took her out into the hall and she read the 20-line on the same card at forty feet, in a dim light, with only two errors. In addition to this, she read diamond type, first at nine inches, the nearest distance at which she could see it clearly, and at fifteen inches, the farthest; and later at six and at twenty inches. She also read writing on the blackboard from the back of the room without any difficulty.

To sum up Sylvia's case then, she was able in two weeks' time to improve her vision from 20/40, which is only half what is ordinarily considered normal, to 20/10, which is double this standard. In five weeks she was able to read a card having unfamiliar letters with a vision of 40/20, and to read diamond type clearly at six inches and also at twenty inches. This remarkable cure had been accomplished through resting the eyes by palming for five minutes at a time about nine times a day, by reading the Snellen test card every day from her seat in the schoolroom and from a point twenty feet from the card.

Sylvia, now looking for more worlds to conquer, has undertaken, with characteristic energy, the cure of one of her schoolmates. She has already succeeded in improving this child's vision from 20/30 to 20/20.

Better Eyesight
June 1920—Vol. II, No. 6

LIGHT

Light is necessary to the health of the eye, and darkness is injurious to it. Eye-shades, dark glasses, and darkened rooms weaken the sight and sooner or later produce inflammations. In all abnormal conditions of the eyes, light is beneficial. It is rarely sufficient to cure, but is a great help in gaining relaxation by other methods.

A LESSON FROM THE GREEKS

By W. H. Bates, M.D.

The failure of the muscles of the eyes to function normally under the conditions of civilization is not an isolated phenomenon. As Diana Watts, in her remarkable book, *The Renaissance of the Greek Ideal,* points out, the entire muscular system of modern civilized peoples works under such a condition of jar and strain that all muscular labor is accomplished with a maximum of effort. So far, indeed, have we drifted from our normal physical possibilities that the positions of the ancient statues seem impossible to us, and we have been forced to attribute many descriptions of the feats of heroes in the *Iliad* and *Odyssey* to poetic license. Ms. Watts, by reproducing the positions of these statues and doing other things that are beyond the power of even the strongest gymnasts and dancers trained under present methods, has fairly established her claim to have discovered the secret of Greek physical supremacy.

Greek athletics, according to Ms. Watts, was very far from being a matter of mere muscle development. Its aim was to produce a condition in which all the muscles worked harmoniously together and responded instantly to the mind's desire—thus securing a maximum of activity with a minimum expenditure of energy.

The secret she found to be very simple. It consists in such a perfect balancing of the body that, whether it is at rest or in motion, its centre of gravity is always kept exactly over its base. This perfect equilibrium involves in turn a condition of the muscles in which they are transformed from a dead weight to a living force. In this condition there is said to be a complete connection of all the muscles with the center of gravity; independent motions and independent reactions are eliminated, and a combined force is instantly brought to bear upon whatever work is required. The spine is perfectly straight, the waist muscles firm, and the weight in the standing posture is supported upon the balls of the feet. Extraordinary precision and beauty of movement results, and all sense of fatigue is said to be abolished.

To attain this equilibrium in its perfection requires much study and practice, but it can be approximated simply by keeping the spine straight and the weight over the balls of the feet, or upon the thighs if seated. By this means a large degree of relaxation is often obtained, and the effect upon the eyesight has, in several cases, been most marked.

A patient suffering from retinitis pigmentosa found that when he straightened his spine in walking or sitting, his field at once became normal, remaining so as long as the erect position was maintained. His field had already improved considerably by other methods but was still very far from normal. In the evening the position had the further effect of relieving his night blindness.

Another patient who had been under treatment for some time for a high degree of myopia without having become able to read the bottom line of the test card, read it for the first time when her body was in the position described. She was able, moreover, to maintain the position for a considerable length of time, whereas ordinarily she was extremely restless and could not remain still for more than a moment. A third patient, who could not rest her eyes by closing them or by palming, was relieved at once by this means, as was shown not only by her own feelings but by the expression of her face.

Sleeping with a straight spine has also been found to be a very effective method of improving the vision and relieving fatigue. The patient with retinitis pigmentosa, whose case has just been referred to, suffered continual relapses in the morning. No matter how well he saw in the afternoon or in the evening, he would wake up unable to distinguish the big "C" and with his memory so impaired that it would take him the whole morning to get it back. After sleeping on his back, with his lower limbs completely extended and his arms lying straight by his sides, he was able to see the 50-line at ten feet when he woke and his memory was much better than usual at that time. Further improvement resulted from further sleeping in this posture. The patient with myopia had been in the habit of waking up tired after ten or twelve hours' sleep. One night she shared her bed with a guest, and in order not to disturb the latter she tried to keep her body straight. Although she had stayed up until a very late hour talking, she awoke feeling perfectly refreshed. Another myopic patient, who had been at a standstill for six months, gained two lines after sleeping on his back for one night.

SAVED FROM BLINDNESS

By Patricia Palmer

It is very hard for an active young girl to suddenly learn that in a short time she may lose her eyesight. I had always felt a great deal of pity for blind people, but I never stopped to realize how many beautiful things they missed until I knew that I was going blind myself. I only wore glasses for three years, but in that short time I developed a very bad case of progressive myopia. In the summer of 1918 my sight became so poor that I had to stop reading altogether and even a moderately bright day hurt my eyes so much that I kept them bandaged a great part of the time. Finally, I had to put on a dark Krux lense, and the goggle-like glasses that I wore shut out all light. In the fall I started school, but as I could not see to read I was working under great difficulties. Then, through an article published some months before in the *Scientific American,* we learned of Dr. Bates' work and it seemed the last possible hope. I declared that there was no use in taking the trip to New York, because I knew he could do nothing for me; but in the end I went.

The first time I looked at the test card I could not see the big "C" until I stood within four feet of it; but in two hours I was able to flash all the letters of the third line and part of the fourth at ten feet. In four weeks I had 10/10 vision and my hearing, which had been bad, was normal.

Some weeks after I returned home a friend, who was calling, complained of a bad headache. I persuaded him to take off his glasses and showed him how to palm and swing the letters on the chart. A short time later he discovered, to his surprise, that his headache was entirely gone.

This incident made me realize that if I showed others what Dr. Bates had shown me, I could relieve, if not cure, their troubles. The next person that I worked with was a little girl with progressive myopia that had not become very serious. She worked very conscientiously, and about a month after we started, when she visited Dr. Bates, her sight was nearly perfect.

I have helped a number of people, some successfully, others not so successfully. One of my most interesting cases was a chauffeur who thought that he was unusually farsighted, but who could not see to read the paper. When I tested his eyes I found that he had only 10/20 vision. In a short time, however, he attained normal sight by palming and swinging the letters. I then told him to close his eyes and count ten, then open them for a fraction of a second. I held a book in front of him and in a short time, by closing his eyes and then glancing at it, he read parts of it. He practices on signboards, automobile licenses, or anything that he sees, and now he reads the entire paper every evening. He has noticed, too, that he is not blinded by bright lights at night as he used to be.

As to the value of swinging the little black period I am very decided. I find it my best friend, especially in a test. One time in a French examination, in the excitement of the moment, I could not think of a certain word that I knew well enough and that was very important to me. I closed my eyes and palmed for a second and remembered the period. In a flash my self-control returned to me, and with it, the word. I have tried this several times since usually with success.

I often wonder now how I could possibly have managed without my eyes, even with glasses. It is such a joy to be able to read from morning to night if I want to. Reading music is supposed to be a terrible thing for the eyes, but I do an endless amount of it and never know the difference. I find, too, that since my eyes have been well I memorize remarkably quickly, and that when I study I can grasp the contents of the text more easily than before. In the old days of glasses I had to read my history assignment two or three times before I knew what it was about, while now once is quite enough.

My greatest regret is that so few people know how to prevent eye troubles, or how to care for them after they develop. Perhaps, however, if the movement to establish Snellen test cards in the schools grows, thousands of children may be saved the agony which I and many others suffered with headaches as well as being freed from the inconvenience of glasses.

STORIES FROM THE CLINIC

No. 4: Three of a Kind

By Emily C. Lierman

George, Gladys and Charlie are three children who came to the Eye Clinic of the Harlem Hospital at about the same time. They were all of the same age, nine years; they were all suffering from about the same degree of defective sight; they all had headaches; and they got into a very interesting three-cornered contest in which each one tried to beat the others at getting cured.

George was the first of the trio to visit us. He had been sent from his school to get glasses because of his headaches, and it was easy to see from his half-shut eyes and the expression of his face that he was in continual misery. My first impulse was to try to make him smile, but my efforts in that direction did not meet with much success.

"Won't you let me help you?" I asked. "Maybe you can and maybe you can't," was his discouraging reply. "But you are going to let me try, aren't you?" I persisted, stroking his woolly head.

He refused to unbend, but did consent to let me test his vision, which I found to be 20/70, and to show him how to palm and rest his eyes. He also continued to come to the Clinic, but for three weeks I never saw him smile, and he complained constantly of the pain in his head.

Then came Gladys, accompanied by her mother who gave me a history of her case very similar to that of George. Her vision was 20/100 and in a very short time I improved it to 20/40. At her next visit it became temporarily normal, and this fact made a great impression upon George. I saw him roll his black eyes and watch Gladys while I was treating her, and later, when he thought I was not looking, I saw him walk over to her, and heard him say, "You ain't going to get ahead of me. I came before you. I wanna get cured first. See?"

I separated the two children very quickly, for I foresaw trouble; but all the time I was very grateful to Gladys for having, however unintentionally, stirred George up.

Next week Charlie came. He looked very sad, and his mother, who came with him, was sad also. His headaches were worse than those of the other children had been, and were actually preventing him from going on with his studies. Promotion time was near, and both mother and child were very anxious for fear the latter would be left behind. They hoped that by the aid of glasses this tragedy would be averted. Of course I explained to the mother that we never gave glasses at this Clinic, but cured people so they did not need them.

Then I tested Charlie's sight, and found it to be 20/100. Next I told him to close his eyes and remember a letter perfectly black, just as he saw it on the test card. He shook his head in dismay, and said, "I can't remember anything, the pain is so bad." "Close your eyes for part of a minute," I said, "then open them just a second and look at the letter I am pointing at; then quickly, close them again. Do this for a few minutes and see what happens." What happened was that in a few minutes Charlie began to smile and said, "The pain is gone."

I now showed him how to palm and left him for a while.

When I came back his sight had improved to 20/70. I was very happy about this and so was Charlie's mother. She was also very happy to think that he did not have to wear glasses.

Charlie continued to come regularly and was an apt pupil. One day he told me that he had been out sleigh-riding with the boys, and that the sun had been shining so brightly upon the snow that he couldn't open his eyes, and his head ached so much that he had to go home and go to bed.

"Why didn't you palm for a while and remember one of those letters on the card?" I asked. "That's right," he said. "I wonder why I didn't think of it." The next time he came there had been another snowstorm and he could hardly wait to tell me what had happened.

"I went sleigh-riding some more with the boys," he said, as soon as he could get my ear, "and the pain came back while I was having fun. But this time I didn't go home and go to bed. I remembered what you said, covered my eyes with the palms of my hands right in the street, and in a little while the pain all went away. I could look right at the snow with the sun shining on it, and I didn't mind it a bit."

From the start, George and Gladys were greatly interested in Charlie, and thinking that a little more of the competition that had proved so effective in George's case would do no harm, I said, "See who beats." They needed no urging from me, however. Every Clinic day, an hour before the appointed time, the trio was at the hospital door. If there was a crowd there, the children forced their way through without much ceremony, and then started on a dead run for the eye room. There they practiced diligently until Dr. Bates and I arrived and, I fear, they also squabbled considerably. There was no lack of smiles now in the case of any of the children, and as for George, he had a grin on his face all the time.

Charlie was the first to be cured. In just a month from the time of his first visit his vision had improved to 20/10. Usually patients do not come back after they are cured, but this boy kept on with the practice at home and returned to show me, and incidentally his two rivals, what progress he had made. We had a visiting physician at the Clinic that day, and I rather suspected Charlie of trying to show off when he walked to the very end of the room, a distance of thirty feet from the card. To my astonishment, and the great annoyance of George and Gladys, he read all the letters on the bottom line correctly. The colored children made haste to suggest that he had probably memorized the letters; so I hung up a card with pothooks on it such as we use for the illiterate patients, and asked him to tell me the direction in which those of the bottom line were turned. He did not make a single mistake. There seemed no room for doubt that his vision had actually improved to 30/10—three times the accepted standard of normality. Not more than one other patient at the Clinic has ever become able to read the card at this distance. Charlie returned several times after this, not from the best of motives, I fear, and I took great pleasure in exhibiting his powers to the visitors.

George and Gladys were cured very soon after Charlie, both of them becoming able to read 20/10. I was sorry that they could not have done as well as Charlie, but since their vision is now twice what is ordinarily considered normal, I think they ought to be satisfied.

A CASE OF CATARACT

By Victoria Coolidge

After I had made one visit to Dr. Bates, I was so much encouraged that I asked him if he could do anything for my father, eighty-one years old, who had cataract in each eye. He said he could, provided the patient had all his faculties and would follow directions. I replied that he was not only in full possession of his faculties but that he was blessed with vigorous health besides, and I felt sure that he would be willing to do anything to restore his sight.

When I went home, I told my father what Dr. Bates had said, but the treatment seemed so simple for such a difficult case, and his mind was so thoroughly imbued with the idea that nothing but an operation would help him, he did not make up his mind to see Dr. Bates until four months later.

He remembered having had remarkably keen vision as a young man, and in 1862 passed as normal the Army eye test, which was very strict at the beginning of the Civil War.

When he was about fifty years old, however, he began to have trouble in reading and other near work, so he put on glasses to correct this difficulty and seems to have had the same experience that so many people have—the glasses were nearly, but not quite right. He went from one doctor to another, but the result was always the same. Finally, in 1907, he consulted a well-known specialist in Albany, who, in 1919, at his request, sent him the following record of his case as it was at the time of that visit:

R. V.—20/200 corrected by glasses to 20/50

L. V.—20/50 corrected by glasses to 20/30

Ophthalmoscopic examination showed in each eye incipient cataractous changes, which were more marked in the right eye. Otherwise the interior of the eye appeared normal. Nothing was said to him personally regarding this condition, for frequently it remains unchanged for years.

He was well pleased with the glasses obtained at this

time, and for a few years had more comfort with them than with any he had ever worn; but after a while he began to have trouble with his right eye again. In 1917 he noticed that there seemed to be hard deposits in his eyes. He consulted a prominent specialist in his own locality and learned from him that he had a fairly well-developed cataract in the left eye, and an incipient cataract in the other. The doctor prescribed glasses for him and asked him to visit him once a month so that he might watch the progress of the cataracts. He said that nothing but an operation would help the left eye, but he would advise an operation only in the event of a loss of sight in both eyes, as would be the case if the cataract in the right eye should also progress, because unless both eyes were operated on at approximately the same time they would not focus together. He called on the doctor faithfully every month for about a year and a half, when he finally became tired of hearing the same discouraging story: the left cataract was rapidly developing, but the doctor would not operate unless both cataracts were ripe. And so he discontinued his visits.

It was about six or seven months after his last visit to this doctor that he called on Dr. Bates. The sight in the left eye had become so dim by this time that he could not recognize the members of his family across the table. He could see that there were people there, but he could not distinguish them. Dr. Bates made the following report of his condition at the time of his first visit:

January 1, 1918: R. V.—20/100; L. V.—Perception of light—unable to count his fingers.

At subsequent visits the following records were made:

January 2: R. V.—20/200, artificial light; L. V.—Counted fingers at six inches. Improved by shifting, swing, rest, palming (best).

January 4: R. V.—14/30; L. V.—14/200. Reads large print.

January 8: R. V.—14/15; L. V.—14/200+. Reads some words fine print continuously.

January 13: R. V.—14/10; L. V.—14/40. He reads in flashes the fine print with the right eye and some larger print with the left. His improved sight helps his hearing at times.

January 18: R. V.—14/10; L. V.—14/20 in more continuous flashes. He is reading large print more continuously with the left eye.

April 30: Obtains flashes of the fine print with the left eye better than with the right.

The treatment prescribed was as follows: Palming six times a day, a half-hour or longer at a time; reading the Snellen test card at five, ten and twenty feet; reading fine print at six inches, five minutes at a time, especially soon after rising in the morning and just before retiring at night; and reading books and newspapers. Besides this, he was to [do sunning; see Sun Treatment in Glossary.—TRQ], drink twelve glasses of water a day, walk five miles a day, and later, when he was in better training, to run half a mile or so every day.

The results of this treatment have been most gratifying. Not only have his eyes improved steadily, but his general health has been so much benefited that at eighty-two he looks, acts and feels better and younger than he did at eighty-one.

Better Eyesight
July 1920—Vol. III, No. 1

SEE THINGS MOVING
When the Sight is Normal All Objects Regarded have an Apparent Motion

When the sight is perfect the subject is able to observe that all objects regarded appear to be moving. A letter seen at the near point or at the distance appears to move slightly in various directions. The pavement moves toward a person while walking, and the houses appear to move in a direction opposite to one's own movement. In reading, the page appears to move in a direction opposite to that of the eyes and head movement. [Oppositional movement.—TRQ] If one tries to imagine things stationary, the vision is at once lowered and discomfort and pain may be produced, not only in the eyes and head, but in other parts of the body.

This movement is usually so slight that it is seldom noticed until the attention is called to it, but it may be so conspicuous as to be plainly observable even to persons with markedly imperfect sight. If such persons, for instance, hold the hand within six inches of the face and turn the head and eyes rapidly from side to side, the hand will be seen to move in a direction opposite to that of the head and eyes. If it does not move, it will be found that the patient is straining to see it in the eccentric field. By observing this movement it becomes possible to see or imagine a less conspicuous movement, and thus the patient may gradually become able to observe a slight movement in every object regarded. Some persons with imperfect sight have been cured simply by imagining that they see things moving all day long.

The world moves. Let it move. All objects move if you let them. Do not interfere with this movement, or try to stop it. This cannot be done without an effort which impairs the efficiency of the eye and mind.

THE MISSION OF *BETTER EYESIGHT*

With this number *Better Eyesight* enters upon its second year. It was started in July 1919, for the purpose of diffusing a knowledge of the truth about central fixation, and it has accomplished all that was hoped for. It has carried the message that errors of refraction are curable to thousands of people, and many of these people have been able to cure these conditions in themselves and others solely by means of the information which it has contained.

The magazine is modest in its appearance. One can get many times the amount of reading matter which it contains at any newsstand for the same money, but the value of truth cannot be estimated by the number of words required to state it, and it is the object of the editor to give the public the truth about central fixation as briefly and simply as possible. The truth can usually be stated briefly and simply. It is error which is hard to understand and which requires a multitude of words for its presentation.

The editor believes that no one who values his or her eyesight can afford to be without this magazine. It has a message not only for those whose sight is imperfect, but for those whose sight is normal. No one, however good his sight may ordinarily be, has perfect sight all the time. No one has as good sight as he might have. Therefore everyone can benefit by practicing the principles presented in this magazine. While persons with imperfect sight may thus gain normal vision, persons with so-called normal sight can always improve it and may even double the accepted standard of normality, or gain a measure of telescopic or microscopic vision. It is not a good thing to be satisfied with just normal sight. Not only is keen sight a great convenience, but it reflects a condition of mind which reacts favorably upon all the other senses, upon the general health and upon the mental faculties.

Even the blind can get some help from *Better Eyesight*. Not all blind persons are curable, but the editor believes that an increasing number of blind persons may expect help from central fixation, for already it has been found possible to relieve or cure such conditions as cataract, glaucoma, conical cornea, retinitis pigmentosa, cyclitis, opacities of the cornea, and atrophy of the optic nerve.

The magazine will continue to publish during the coming year, as it has in the past, the latest discoveries of the editor, the experiences of cured patients which have proven to be very valuable, and practical instructions for the improvement of the eyesight. On page 2 of each issue we will continue to give specific directions for self-treatment, in language as simple as possible, so that persons who are not physicians can understand it. We have had much testimony to the value of this page and the editor strongly urges every subscriber, no matter what the condition of his or her eyesight, to demonstrate these truths as they appear.

Better Eyesight stands for a revolution in the treatment of eye troubles, and has had to meet the difficulties that always beset the path of the revolutionist. For seventy-five years we have believed that errors of refraction—by which is meant the inability of the eye to focus light rays accurately upon the retina—were due to organic and irremediable causes. The editor of *Better Eyesight* has proved that these troubles are functional and curable, that the elongated eyeball of myopia (nearsightedness) the flattened eyeball of hypermetropia (farsightedness), and the lopsided eyeball of astigmatism, can be made to resume their normal shape, temporarily in a few minutes, and more continuously by further treatment. The world has been slow to receive this message. The editor is practically alone in advocating central fixation. A small number of physicians, including a few eye specialists, who have been cured or seen members of their families cured of eye troubles—without glasses, operations, or medication—have been convinced that the old theories about the eye and the treatment of defects of vision are wrong; but very few have had courage to endorse the new treatment publicly.

This is not to be wondered at, and is not a cause for discouragement. The editor now wonders at his own slowness in seeing the truth. The facts conquered his conservatism at last only because they were irresistible, and for the same reason they must ultimately conquer all conservatism. Physicians and others who refuse to accept them, or even to investigate them, will be swept aside to make room for those of more open mind.

In the meantime, *Better Eyesight* needs friends, it needs encouragement, it needs subscribers. The editor appeals to present subscribers to continue their support, and to advertise whenever and wherever they have an opportunity the good news that the eye is not a blunder of nature, as the textbooks teach, but an instrument as perfectly adapted to the needs of civilized man as to those of the savage. Persons who have cured themselves should utilize every opportunity to improve the sight of relatives and friends. All parents should be told that they have it in their power to prevent and cure defects of vision in their children and at the same time to improve their health and increase their mental efficiency. The same message should be carried to teachers and school boards. The blind should be told of this new hope for the sightless, and societies for the blind should be urged to investigate it. If everyone who has demonstrated the truth of central fixation does his or her duty in the matter, defective eyesight will soon cease to be, as it has so long been, the curse of civilization.

STORIES FROM THE CLINIC

No. 5: The Jewish Woman

By Emily C. Lierman

Just before the war a Jewish woman, sixty-three years old, came to the Clinic and begged me to help her just a little. "Please don't bother trying to cure me," she said. "That is too much to expect, and anyhow I am an old lady so what does it matter?"

Her eyes were half shut because the light bothered her and she felt more comfortable with the lids lowered. She told me that she was suffering great pain both in her eyes and head, and when I had her look at the test card at ten feet it was all a blur to her. I showed her how to palm, but the position tired her, and she said she was not accustomed to praying so long.

As she weighed over two hundred pounds and was sick in both mind and body, I asked her how much she ate every day. "Oh, I don't eat much—nothing to speak of at all," she said. "In the morning I eat eggs, or something like that, and rolls and butter and coffee. Then about ten I have a few slices of bread with more butter and more coffee. At noon I have soup, bread and butter and more coffee. For supper I have bread, butter, meat, vegetables and more coffee. That's all."

She took more food in one day than I did in three, and when I told her she ate too much, it appeared to frighten her, for she stayed away for two weeks. Eating, no doubt, was one of the few pleasures she had in life, and she did not wish to be deprived of it.

When she returned I had her palm again, and this improved her sight from 20/100 to 20/50. It also relieved her pain markedly, and when I told her that she would get still more help, both for her eyes and her body generally, if she would eat less, she agreed to do so.

In spite of her pain and misery, my patient had always been full of humor, and her witty remarks had been a source of much amusement to me; but one day, just after the declaration of war, I found her in a corner weeping. When I asked her to read the test card for me, she said with tears, "Please, nurse, I can't see anything today. My two sons have enlisted—one as a Marine, and the other as an aviator, and they are never coming back, I am afraid. I cannot sleep. I am suffering great pain all over my body. My heart is breaking."

From the beginning I had felt that she had been a devoted mother, and as I am always drawn to good mothers, I now felt a great pity for her grief. In order to get her mind off her pain, I encouraged her to talk about her boys.

"How proud you must be to have two sons to fight for your country, and for you!" I said. "I wish I had ten sons; I would give them all for my country." These remarks were not very consoling, I admit, in the presence of a sorrow like this, and the stricken mother refused to be comforted. But when I said, "You wouldn't be proud of them if they were cowards, and Uncle Sam wouldn't want them if they were criminals in a jail," she straightened up and said, "You are right. They are brave boys all right, and I am proud of them." I now tested her sight with the card and I found it better than ever before.

"You have the right medicine" she said, "I am coming again. I do not understand why I can see so well after being so blind a few minutes ago." I squeezed her arm above the elbow and asked, "Do you feel that?" "Yes," she replied. "Well, that is just what you are doing to the muscles of your eyes, and the strain blinded you. When you relaxed, the pressure was relieved and your sight improved. It was the pressure that lowered the vision."

At a later visit she brought a package for me, explaining that she had no money and wanted to express her gratitude. I took the package home and when I opened it I found a loaf of delicious real bread. My neighbors were very envious of me, because the only bread they could obtain had a flavor like that of sawdust. At the time I appreciated that bread more than a five-dollar bill.

Every time the patient came to the Clinic we talked about her boys for a few minutes, and it certainly had a good effect upon her eyesight. When the war ended and the boys came home, everyone who would listen heard of the great things they had done "over there." One would have thought one was attending an annual convention of some sort instead of an eye Clinic.

During the war and up to about six months ago, the patient came more or less regularly to the Clinic. Palming always helped her, but as she complained that it made her arms ache to hold her hands over her eyes, I had her simply close her eyes without palming. This also helped her. One day I placed her two feet farther from the card than usual and asked her how much she could see. She replied, "Now, you know I am an old woman, and I guess my eyes are getting old, too; I cannot see so far."

I told her to close her eyes and rest them, forget that she had eyes, and think of black velvet or her black hat. Ten minutes later she read 10/20 and her eyes had a natural appearance. She became very much excited and asked me what I did to her.

Dieting also helped her eyesight and nerves very much, but she could not always bring herself to forego the pleasure of eating what she wanted. She forgot most of the things I told her to do at home, but I don't think she ever forgot a meal, nor did she realize the quantity of food she consumed when she gave free rein to her appetite. If she had always done as she was told, I am sure she would have been completely cured long ago. As it was, her improvement was very remarkable. Not only did she become able to read 10/20, but at the time she stopped coming to the Clinic she said that the pain and discomfort in her eyes had entirely ceased. She was sleeping better and her general physical condition was greatly improved.

Her case made me realize more clearly than ever the relation of mental strain to defective vision. I could not help her until I found out what she had on her heart, and when, by means of a little sympathy—I could give her nothing else—I was able to get her mind off her trouble, or make it seem less to her, her nerves always relaxed. It was very remarkable the way a pleasant conversation, without further treatment, would improve her sight. The experience was afterward a great help to me in treating other patients. In the rush of work at the dispensary it has often seemed that I could not take the time to talk to the patients, to get acquainted with them, to let them tell me about their troubles. I know now that this is not a waste of time, but a very necessary part of the treatment.

WHAT GLASSES DO TO US

By W. H. Bates, M.D.

On a tomb in the Church of Santa Maria Maggiore in Florence was found the following inscription—"Here lies Salvino degli Armati, Inventor of Spectacles. May God pardon him his sins."[1]

The Florentines were doubtless mistaken in supposing their fellow citizen was the inventor of the lenses now so commonly worn to correct errors of refraction. There has been much discussion as to the origin of these devices, but they are generally believed to have been known at a period much earlier than that of Salvino degli Armati. The Romans at least must have known something of the art of supplementing the powers of the eye, for Pliny tells us that Nero

1. *Nuova Enciclopedia Italiana,* sixth edition.

used to watch the games in the Colosseum through a concave gem set in a ring for that purpose. If, however, his contemporaries believed that Salvino delgi Armati was the first to produce these aids to vision, they might well have prayed for the pardon of his sins; for while it is true that eyeglasses have brought to some people improved vision and relief from pain and discomfort, they have been to others simply an added torture, they always do more or less harm, and at their best they never improve the vision to normal.

That glasses cannot improve the sight to normal can be very simply demonstrated by looking at any color through a strong convex or concave glass. It will be noted that the color is always less intense than when seen with the naked eye; and since the perception of form depends upon the perception of color, it follows that both color and form must be less distinctly seen with glasses than without them. Even plane glass lowers the vision both for color and form, as everyone knows who has ever looked out of a window.

That glasses must injure the eye is evident from the fact that one cannot see through them unless one produces the degree of refractive error which they are designed to correct. But refractive errors, in the eye which is left to itself, are never constant.[2] If one secures good vision by the aid of concave, convex, or astigmatic lenses, therefore, it means that one is maintaining constantly a degree of refractive error which otherwise would not be maintained constantly. It is only to be expected that this should make the conditions worse, and it is a matter of common experience that it does. After people once begin to wear glasses, their strength, in most cases, has to be steadily increased in order to maintain the degree of visual acuity secured by the aid of the first pair.

That the human eye resents glasses is a fact which no one would attempt to deny. Every oculist knows that patients have to "get used" to them, and that sometimes they never succeed in doing so. Patients with high degrees of myopia and hypermetropia have great difficulty in accustoming themselves to the full correction, and often are never able to do so. The strong concave glasses required by myopes of high degree make all objects seem much smaller than they really are, while convex glasses enlarge them. These are unpleasantnesses that cannot be overcome. Patients with high degrees of astigmatism suffer some very disagreeable sensations when they first put on glasses, for which reason they are warned by one of the *Conservation of Vision* leaflets published by the Council on Health and Public Instruction of the American Medical Association to "get used to them at home before venturing where a misstep might cause a serious accident."[3]

All glasses contract the field of vision to a greater or lesser degree. Even with very weak glasses patients are unable to see distinctly unless they look through the center of the lenses, with the frames at right angles to the line of vision; and not only is their vision lowered if they fail to do this, but annoying nervous symptoms, such as dizziness and headache, are sometimes produced. Therefore, they are unable to turn their eyes freely in different directions. It is true that glasses are now ground in such a way that it is theoretically possible to look through them at any angle, but practically they seldom accomplish the desired result.

The difficulty of keeping the glass clear is one of the minor discomforts of glasses, but nevertheless a most annoying one. On damp and rainy days the atmosphere clouds them. On hot days the perspiration from the body may have a similar effect. On cold days they are often clouded by the moisture of the breath. Every day they are so subject to contamination by dust and moisture and the touch of the fingers incident to unavoidable handling that it is seldom they afford an absolutely unobstructed view of the objects regarded.

Reflections of strong light from eyeglasses are often very annoying, and in the street may be very dangerous.

Soldiers, sailors, athletes, workmen and children have great difficulty with glasses because of the activity of their lives, which not only leads to the breaking of the lenses, but often throws them out of focus, particularly in the case of eyeglasses worn for astigmatism.

The fact that glasses are very disfiguring may seem a matter unworthy of consideration in a medical publication; but mental discomfort does not improve either the general health or the vision, and while we have gone so far toward making a virtue of what we conceive to be necessity that some of us have actually come to consider glasses becoming, huge round lenses in ugly tortoise-shelf frames being positively fashionable at the present time, there are still some unperverted minds to which the wearing of glasses is mental torture and the sight of them upon others far from agreeable. As for putting glasses upon a child it is enough to make the angels weep.

Up to about a generation ago glasses were used only as an aid to defective sight, but they are now prescribed for large numbers of persons who can see as well or better without them. The hypermetropic eye is believed to be capable of correcting its own difficulties to some extent by altering the curvature of the lens through the activity of the ciliary muscle. The eye with simple myopia is not credited with this capacity, because an increase in the convexity of the lens, which is supposed to be all that is accomplished by accom-

2. William H. Bates, "Imperfect Sight of the Normal Eye," *New York Medical Journal,* September 8, 1917.

3. Lancaster, *Wearing Glasses,* p. 15.

modative effort, would only increase the difficulty, and this, it is believed, can be overcome, in part, by alterations in the curvature of the lens. Thus we are led by the theory to the conclusion that an eye in which any error of refraction exists is practically never free, while open, from abnormal accommodative efforts. In other words, it is assumed that the supposed muscle of accommodation has to bear, not only the normal burden of changing the focus of the eye for vision at different distances, but the additional burden of compensating for refractive errors. Such adjustments, if they actually took place, would naturally impose a severe strain upon the nervous system, and it is to relieve this strain—which is believed to be the cause of a host of functional nervous troubles—quite as much as to improve the sight, that glasses are prescribed.

It has been demonstrated, however, that the lens is not a factor either in the production of accommodation or in the correction of errors of refraction. Therefore under no circumstances can there be a strain of the ciliary muscle to be relieved. It has also been demonstrated that when the vision is normal, no error of refraction is present and the extrinsic muscles of the eyeball are at rest. Therefore there can be no strain of the extrinsic muscles to be relieved in these cases. When a strain of these muscles does exist, glasses may correct its effects upon the refraction, *but the strain itself they cannot relieve*. [My emphasis. This is also true of contact lenses, ortho-keratology, corneal refractive surgeries, and all other *artificial* methods of eyesight improvement.—TRQ] On the contrary, it has been shown they must make it worse. Nevertheless persons with normal vision who wear glasses for the relief of a supposed muscular strain are often benefited by them. This is a striking illustration of the effect of mental suggestion, and plane glass, if it could inspire the same faith, would produce the same result. In fact, many patients have told me that they had been relieved of various discomforts by glasses which I found to be simply plane glass. One of these patients was an optician who had fitted the glasses himself and was under no illusions whatever about them; yet he assured me that when he didn't wear them, he got headaches.

When glasses do not relieve headaches and other nervous symptoms it is assumed to be because they were not properly fitted, and some practitioners and their patients exhibit an astounding degree of patience and perseverance in their joint attempts to arrive at the proper prescription.

A patient who suffered from severe pains in the base of his brain was fitted sixty times by one specialist alone and had, besides, visited many other eye and nerve specialists in this country and in Europe. He was relieved of the pain in five minutes by the methods recommended by this magazine, while his vision at the same time became temporarily normal.

As refractive abnormalities are continually changing, not only from day to day and from hour to hour, but from minute to minute, even under the influence of atropine, the accurate fitting of glasses is, of course, impossible. In some cases these fluctuations are so extreme, or the patient so unresponsive to mental suggestion, that no relief whatever is obtained from correcting lenses, which necessarily become, under such circumstances, an added discomfort. At their best it cannot be maintained that glasses are anything more than a very unsatisfactory substitute for normal vision.

Better Eyesight
August 1920—Vol. III, No. 2

SCHOOL NUMBER

THE CURE OF IMPERFECT SIGHT IN SCHOOLCHILDREN

While reading the Snellen test card every day will, in time, cure imperfect sight in all children under twelve who have never worn glasses, the following simple, practices will insure more rapid progress:

1. Let the children rest their eyes by closing for a few minutes or longer, and then look at the test card for a few moments only, then rest again, and so on alternately. This cures many children very promptly.

2. Let them close and cover their eyes with the palms of their hands in such a way as to exclude all the light while avoiding pressure on the eyeballs (palming), and proceed as above. This is usually more effective than mere closing.

3. Let them demonstrate that all effort lowers the vision by looking fixedly at a letter on the test card or at the near point, and noting that it blurs or disappears in less than a minute. They thus become able, in some way, to avoid unconscious effort.

The method succeeds best when the teachers do not wear glasses.

At least once a year some person whose sight is normal without glasses and who understands the method should visit the classrooms for the purpose of answering questions, testing the sight of the children, and making a report to the proper authorities.

The Snellen test card is a chart showing letters of graduated sizes, with numbers indicating the distance in feet at which each line should be read by the normal eye. Originally designed by Snellen for the purpose of testing the eye, it is admirably adapted for use in eye education.

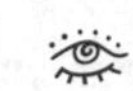

SAVE THE CHILDREN'S EYES

Editorial

With this issue of *Better Eyesight* we are again urging measures to prevent and cure imperfect sight in schoolchildren. A very simple method by which this can be done was discovered by the editor while studying the vision of the schoolchildren of Grand Forks, North Dakota, and tested over a period of eight years in the schools of this city. It consists merely, as has been frequently stated in this magazine, of exposing a Snellen test card in each classroom, and having the children read the lowest line they can see from their seats once a day or more often.

Six or seven years ago this system was tried in some of the public schools of New York City with the most gratifying results. In every case in which the card was used properly the vision of the children improved, regardless of whether the classroom was well or poorly lighted; and in every case in which it was not used the vision declined, being worse at the end of the year than it was at the beginning, regardless also of the lighting of the room. Not only was myopia (nearsightedness) prevented and cured by this method, but hypermetropia (farsightedness), a much greater curse than myopia and one the prevention of which had not previously been seriously considered, was also prevented and cured. So also was astigmatism, while the sight of those children whose sight had been normal to begin with was improved. Headaches and fatigue were relieved. The mentality of the children improved. Truants and incorrigibles were reformed. The teachers were enthusiastic about the results. So also were the children.

But unfortunately the method was contrary to the teachings of a hundred years, and hence was condemned without trial by every eye specialist consulted by the Board of Education. And thus the children, not only of New York, but of the whole country, have been deprived for years of the blessing of perfect sight. If New York had led the way, the whole country would have followed.

Through the efforts of this magazine, however, a few schools here and there have introduced the system, and we hope that before another year has elapsed there will be many more of them. An interesting report from one of these schools appears below.

IMPERFECT SIGHT CONTAGIOUS

By W. H. Bates, M.D.

The question of whether or not errors of refraction are hereditary is one about which the medical profession has exercised itself greatly. An immense amount of work has been done for the purpose of throwing light upon it, and all the time the very plain fact that these conditions are contagious has escaped observation. For an error of refraction is simply a nervous condition; and there is nothing more contagious than nervousness. A person with myopia, hypermetropia, or astigmatism is a person under a strain. This strain shows in his voice, his walk, his manner, and makes the people with whom he comes in contact nervous. These people then develop errors of refraction, temporarily if the influence is temporary, and permanently if the influence is permanent, as in the case of children who cannot escape from their nervous teachers and parents. Endless illustrations of this fact could be given. A few must suffice.

A very nervous woman wearing glasses for astigmatism brought me her very nervous child who had been wearing glasses for six months, also for astigmatism, three diopters in one eye and three and a half in the other. The child's eyes were red, strained, and partly closed, and it was quite evident that the glasses did not make her comfortable. I talked to her pleasantly for a while so as to disarm any fears of the Doctor that she might entertain, and then told her to close her eyes and rest them for fifteen minutes. When she opened them she had perfect sight for the Snellen test card in both eyes, and she read diamond type from six to eighteen inches.

I said to the mother, "There is nothing wrong with your child's eyes. When they were tested she must have been nervous." The mother answered that this was true. The child had been trying to play a duet with her sister, and got so nervous that she could not see the notes. The family was so alarmed at this sudden failure of sight that she was taken immediately to an oculist, and the result was glasses for astigmatism. As children have an astonishing power of adapting their eyes to different kinds of lenses, she had adapted her eyes to these very strong glasses sufficiently so that she could see through them, but was not able to be comfortable in them, nor in any of the others that were subsequently given to her.

Mother and child left the office in a very happy frame of mind, but a few days later the mother returned, very much discouraged and somewhat incensed. The child was just as bad as ever, she said. She couldn't read half the card.

"The reason she can't read the card," I said, "is because you test her. Let her younger sister test her and you will find that she will read it perfectly. The strain in your eyes is reflected in your voice and walk, in everything about you; you make the child nervous, and when you try to test her sight she becomes astigmatic. If you want her to get cured and stay cured, you should get cured yourself." She took my advice and is now under treatment.

In my studies of the eyesight of schoolchildren this experience was frequently repeated. When I went into a classroom where the teacher wore glasses I knew I would always find a large percentage of imperfect sight. When the teacher did not wear glasses I knew the percentage would be below the average. When the teacher tested the sight of a child it was often found to be very imperfect, but when I tested it, it might be perfect.

In one case a teacher wearing glasses told me that a certain boy was very nearsighted. He could not read writing on the blackboard, he could not tell the time by the clock, and he could not recognize people across the street. I tested his sight and found it normal. The teacher was incredulous and suggested that he must have memorized the letters. Then I wrote letters and words on the blackboard which he read just as well as he had read the letters on the card.

One day my own children came home from school with a note to the effect that they could not read the writing on the blackboard and needed glasses, and later a nurse called to reinforce the message. I tested their sight and found it normal. Then I called on the principal, told him that I was an eye specialist, and after testing the sight of the children I could find nothing wrong with it. I asked if there would be any objection to their having a test card in their classrooms so that they could read it frequently. He said he could see no reason why this should not be done, and it was. But soon after, the younger child, a little girl, came home from school in tears. The teacher and the nurse and the other children had made fun of the card and said it was absurd to suppose that such a simple thing as reading it every day could keep one from having trouble with one's eyes. Of course I knew it would do her no good to read the card under these conditions, and so I had her read it at home. The sight of both children has remained perfect, but I have no doubt that if the circumstances had been different they would have been wearing glasses today.

Children are very sensitive to nervous influences, these influences often produce temporary imperfect sight, and unfortunately they are often, in these states, fitted with glasses. Fortunately most children hate to wear glasses, and after trying them for a while frequently discard them. They also break and lose them. Thus they are saved much injury. But if the teacher or parent is conscientious and insists on the wearing of the glasses and on their renewal when lost or broken, the temporary error of refraction becomes a permanent one.

The atmosphere of the average schoolroom is extremely irritating. It makes the children nearsighted, farsighted and astigmatic. But if they have a familiar Snellen test card which they can read every day, they are always able to overcome this adverse influence. When they can read the letters on the test card which they know by heart, they are also able to read the writing on the blackboard and see other strange objects at the distance or the near point with normal sight.

STORIES FROM THE CLINIC

No. 6: The Schoolchildren

By Emily C. Lierman

A great many children visit our Clinic. Some are sent by their teachers, or the school nurse. Others hear from their friends that we cure people without glasses and come of their own accord. They are a most interesting class of patients, for they respond so quickly to treatment that one's work becomes a succession of thrills, and as a rule they are very grateful for what we do for them.

Grown people are often annoyed when they find that we do not prescribe glasses, but the children, with rare exceptions, are delighted, for they usually hate to wear glasses. Only occasionally do they insist that they must have them, because the teacher or the nurse said so. Before they leave the Clinic, however, they are always convinced that whoever told them they needed glasses made a mistake.

One day a girl tried to work me for a pair of glasses. Dr. Bates, after examining her eyes, turned her over to me with the remark that she would be an easy case. I placed her at ten feet from the card and asked her to read what she could. She said she could not read anything. I brought her to within one foot of it, and she still insisted that she could not see a letter. It occurred to me that perhaps she did not know the letters, but she said she did. I told her to palm for a while and then I tried her again at ten feet. She looked very mournful, and said, "I can't see." Then I realized at last what was the matter with her.

"Well, if you want glasses," I said, "you will have to go elsewhere, we do not give glasses here." I never saw a patient's sight improve as quickly as hers did now. She started at once to read the test card, and went right down to the bottom, missing only two letters on the last line.

In most cases the children, after they are cured, prove to be enthusiastic missionaries in the cause of better eyesight. On the same day that I cured the case just mentioned, another girl, ten years old, who was as anxious to be cured as the other one had been to avoid it, came to the Clinic. The school nurse had sent her to get glasses, but she said, "I just hate glasses and I won't wear them."

I improved her sight in ten minutes from 15/70 to 15/30, and the next Clinic day she brought with her fourteen other children and the school nurse. That was a thrilling day at the Clinic. The nurse was thrilled and I was thrilled, for in an hour's time I improved the sight of every one of those children from about 15/50 to 15/20.

The first child I treated was very cross, and did not wish to be annoyed by palming or anything else. The nurse explained to me that she was a very nervous child and never still a minute. "That doesn't matter," I said; "I'm not going to make her nervous."

I then asked the child what her name was, and she told me it was Helen. "Now Helen," I said, "the first thing you are going to do for me is to smile," which she did. "Now I wonder if you can read that test card for me?" I asked. "Oh, sure," she replied, "I'm not a baby!" She read 15/50. "Be a nice girl now and cover your closed eyes with your palms," and I showed her how to do it. She followed my instructions, and by alternately flashing the letters and palming, her vision rapidly improved to 15/20.

The next girl had closely watched Helen, and from the look on her face I could see that she would be more ready to do as I wished her to do than Helen had been. Her name was Clarice, and her vision was about the same as Helen's, namely 15/50. I told her to palm, and while she was doing this I went to the next patient, a girl who reminded me of Topsy in *Uncle Tom's Cabin,* for her head was just covered with pigtails. After I had started her palming, I went back to Clarice, and found that she could now read 15/20. And so it went through the whole fourteen. The nurse asked me a great many questions about the treatment and said she would treat the children the same way at school. At a later date she came to me again for more instructions, and said that so far she had been getting such good results that she had not found it necessary to send any more of her charges to the Clinic. She studied *Better Eyesight* very carefully and found that it enabled her to give the treatment correctly. Clarice and Helen also came back, not because it was necessary, since they and the other children were doing so well under the instructions of the nurse, but because they liked to come. After palming for a short time both of them became able to read 15/10.

The influence of the school in producing imperfect sight is sometimes startlingly illustrated by these child patients. A dear little blue-eyed girl of twelve who came to us because she had severe headaches seemed to be suffering mainly from fear of her teacher. In the morning before school she felt perfectly well; after playing in the street with the other children she also felt well; but when she went into her classroom and began work her head began to ache. It also ached when she was doing her homework, but not so badly. I asked her to read the test card at twelve feet, and unconsciously I raised my voice a little. Immediately I saw her start as if someone had scared the very life out of her. I guessed at once just what was the matter, and lowering my voice I told her as gently as possible that there was nothing to be frightened about. "What you are not able to read on that card today, you will read next time," I said.

Then I showed her how to palm and left her for a time, as there were many other children waiting to be treated. Coming back in fifteen minutes I told her to take her hands down and tell me what she could read, and I made my voice as low as I could, not much above a whisper. At once, with each eye she read 15/10, more than normal vision, and she said she had no pain. I asked her if she could guess how many children there were in her class. "Yes, about sixty," she replied. "My," I said, "if your poor mother had sixty children, wouldn't she be nervous and worried! And wouldn't you want to help her all you could! Suppose you make believe the teacher is your mother, and try to help her all you can."

This had a great effect on her. The next time she came her attitude toward her teacher seemed to have completely changed, and at every subsequent visit she always had something to say about her wonderful teacher. I feel sure that her fear of her teacher had been unnecessary, and also that it had had much to do with her condition. She had little trouble with the headaches after her first visit for when she felt one coming on, as sometimes happened when she had a hard example to do, she was able to get quick relief simply by closing her eyes.

While the work with the children is always thrilling, we sometimes have a case that is so wonderful that it stands out from all the others. A boy of ten came to us one day in a very bad condition. He did not want to look at anyone, and did not even want to raise his head because the light bothered him so. After testing his sight and finding it to be about 15/70, I placed him on a stool which, by the way, is a very precious piece of furniture in the Clinic. All our patients have to stand while they palm and practice with the test card. There are no comfortable chairs for them. But most of them are willing to do anything so that they may not need glasses, and they do not complain. For this boy, however, I was able to find a stool on which he could sit while he palmed. I told him not to open his eyes for a moment, and after I had attended to a few patients, I came back and asked him to take his hands from his eyes. What happened then seemed like a miracle. He didn't look like the same boy. His formerly half-shut eyes were wide open, and without any trouble he read the bottom line of the test card at fifteen feet. When I praised him for what he had done he smiled and said, "When shall I come again?" At the next visit he read 20/10 with both eyes, and he told me that when the light bothered him he closed his eyes and covered them with the palms of his hands, and in a few minutes he was all right.

This boy brought a friend, age twelve, who had been wearing glasses for two years or more. When he came into the room he did not wait for his turn (I guess he never thought about it in his eagerness), but placed himself right in front of me, took off his glasses and said, "You cured Jimmie's eyes. Will you cure me, too?" "Surely," I said, "if you wait your turn," and as soon as I could I tested his sight.

I found that he could see just as well without his glasses as with them—15/20. So, I asked Dr. Bates to examine him and his glasses, and it turned out that he was wearing farsighted glasses for nearsightedness. I told him to palm, and before he left the Clinic that day he saw distinctly some of the letters on the bottom line at fifteen feet. This was an even more remarkable cure than Jimmie's, for patients who have worn glasses are usually much harder to cure than those who have never worn them.

Sometimes the mothers come with the children and then I try to enlist them as my assistants, and if the mothers wear glasses I try to persuade them to cure themselves so that the children will not copy their bad visual habits, and will not be subjected to the influence of people who strain. Not long ago a mother who had trouble with her eyes brought a child for treatment and said that she would help the latter at home. I said that would be fine, and then I asked the child to help me cure her mother.

"After mother has given you a treatment," I said, "tell her to close her eyes and cover them with the palms of her hands, and to stay so until everything is black. Be very quiet so that she will not be disturbed, and when she opens her eyes you will surely find that she can see better."

Both mother and child made rapid progress. At the first visit the child's vision, which had been 15/50, improved to 15/30, and in six weeks it became 20/15. The mother now exhibits to her friends, with much pride, her ability to thread a needle without glasses.

Only one thing about this work with the children makes me sad, and that is we can do so little of it. Many children come from other districts and are, of course, turned away by the dispensary clerk. But even if the hospital rules did not require the clerk to do this, we could not admit all who come. There is a limit to the number we can treat, and there is so little space in our little eye room that already we are obliged to treat the overflow in the outside general waiting room. I wish that there could be such clinics in every hospital, and that the teachers and the nurses in the schools could be instructed in the very simple art of preserving the eyesight of the coming generation.

THE SNELLEN TEST CARD IN NEWTON

By U. G. Wheeler
Superintendent School Department,
Newton, Massachusetts

Editor's Note—*We are greatly indebted to Superintendent Wheeler for sending us the following report of the use of the Snellen test card in one of the public schools of Newton, and we hope that the success which attended his experiment will encourage other schools to try this method of preventing and curing imperfect sight in schoolchildren.*

Last fall we purchased several copies of the school number of *Better Eyesight*, and have been trying the suggested method for the prevention and cure of imperfect sight in one building in the city. The following is a copy of the report I received at the end of the school year from the principal of that school regarding the result of this trial:

In the fourth grade the teacher began using the Snellen eye chart last October. There was one case where the child tested very low in one eye. One of the children in the grade worked with her four times a day as was suggested in the booklet. The child lost the fear of using her eye, and after some time could read the card fifteen feet away. At that time her mother requested that we do no more work with her, as the oculist was afraid that she might strain her eyes. The class as a whole used the card for months. Their eyes seem to be strengthened by the constant use of it.

In the fifth grade the teacher used the card with her class and gained definite results. One interesting case was that of a girl who had trouble with her eyes. It seemed to be hereditary, as the father had the same trouble. The girl used the Snellen test card and finally was able to read it across the room. If she neglected to practice for a few days, she found it necessary to begin all over again. There was no chance for memorizing the card, as the teacher cut letters from newspapers and used them while testing her and found that she had been helped a great deal. It is thought the children's eyes were really strengthened.

In the other grades—I, II, VI, VII and VIII—the card was used, and in some cases it helped; in others cases the eye defects were too serious. However, the teachers believe that if the card is put to the right use, wonderful results may be reaped.

Better Eyesight
September 1920—Vol. III, No. 3

MAKE YOUR SIGHT WORSE

This is an excellent method of improving it

Strange as it may seem, there is no better way of improving the sight than by making it worse. To see things worse when one is already seeing them badly requires mental control of a degree greater than that required to improve the sight. The importance of these facts is very great. When patients become able to lower their vision by conscious staring, they become better able to avoid unconscious staring. When they demonstrate by increasing their eccentric fixation that trying to see objects not regarded [clearly] lowers the vision, they may stop trying to do the same thing unconsciously.

What is true of the sight is also true of the imagination and memory. If one's memory and imagination are imperfect, they can be improved by consciously making them worse than they are. Persons with imperfect sight never remember or imagine the letters on the test card as perfectly black and distinct, but to imagine them as gray and cloudy is very difficult or even impossible, and when a patient has done it or tried to do it, he may become able to avoid the unconscious strain which has prevented him from forming mental pictures as black and distinct as the reality.

To make imperfect sight worse is always more difficult than to lower normal vision. In other words, to make a letter which already appears gray and indistinct noticeably more cloudy is harder than to blur a letter seen distinctly. To make an imperfect mental picture worse is harder than to blur a perfect one. Both practices require much effort, much hard disagreeable work; but they always, when successful, improve the memory, imagination and vision.

EXPERIENCES WITH CENTRAL FIXATION

By M. H. Stuart, M.D.

Editor's Note—*We are greatly indebted to [ophthalmologist] Dr. Stuart for sending in this remarkable story of his own cure and that of his patients, all of which was accomplished without personal assistance by means of the information presented in this magazine.*

Some sixteen years ago, when working as a stenographer, I developed indigestion and became extremely nervous, one of my symptoms being a tension in the spinal cord between the shoulder blades which was extremely uncomfortable. In the late afternoon and evening I would become so nervous that I could scarcely sit still, and I have walked five miles into the country and back again to get relief. I tried dieting for the indigestion, but after two months failed to get any relief. A medical student then suggested that the trouble might be due to my eyes. I went to an oculist, who fitted me with glasses, and all my troubles ceased.

The glasses given to me were convex 0.25, axis 90. A few years later, when I was in New York doing post-graduate work at the Polyclinic, they were changed to concave 0.25, axis 180, my refraction having changed from hypermetropia to myopia. In succeeding years the myopic astigmatism increased to concave 0.75, axis 180, and finally, after I had worn glasses for some fourteen years, to concave 1.00, axis 180. The last correction I had worn for about two years when I discarded glasses for good.

Slight as my error of refraction was, I was not able to leave off my glasses for more than an hour or two without suffering from nervousness and the feeling of tenseness in the spinal cord alluded to above. At other times I was perfectly comfortable except for the last year or two, during which I had so much to do that I suffered at times from the old nervous trouble. I had no pain in my head or eyes, but the trouble in my back was so bad last fall that I had to have the services of a masseur in order to do my work.

Five years ago I first read about Dr. Bates' experiments upon the eye muscles of animals. While interested I was not prepared to abandon the accepted teachings on the subject, and I waited to hear more. Recently I read, in the May 1920 number of *Better Eyesight,* Dr. Arnau's story of how his headaches were cured, and I was so impressed by it that I determined to try the relaxation method upon myself. I palmed for five minutes and then read the test card three times with each eye as far as I could without effort. I did this six times a day for five days, and at the end of this time I had gained a very decided degree of relaxation. I had, of course, discarded glasses, and although this caused me a little discomfort at first, I was able, about a week later, to perform without them three tonsillectomies and one operation for cataract, and to remove two blind eyes.

At the same time I went through my daily routine of treating ten to thirty patients, examining eyes, ears, noses and throats, much of which work requires extra good vision. At noon I lay down to rest as usual and read the Atlanta paper. At night I read the Moultrie daily paper and anything else that I wanted to.

After the first five days of systematic relaxation I have never done anything in a routine way for myself, but if I feel nervous, or my eyes feel drawn, I swing twenty times and palm. In this way I am always able to get relief. Another method of gaining relaxation that I have resorted to is to look at an imaginary period in any dark, distant object. In this pinewoods district there are thousands of stumps, many of which have been burned and blackened. The third day after I discarded my glasses I had to drive about twenty-eight miles, and whenever my eyes felt drawn I would look in an easy relaxed way at a small point on one of these stumps and always got relaxation.

Nearly every afternoon at half past four I go out for a game of golf, and often I palm before going as I find it gives me better control of my nervous system and enables me to play a more consistent game.

I was so pleased with the results of the new treatment in my own case that I have since taught central fixation to about forty of my patients, and in only about two did I fail to improve the vision at the first sitting.

The following are some of my more notable cases.

Mr. S., an automobile mechanic, had been mentally deranged for two weeks, following an attack of flu, after which he gradually became rational, only to find that he saw double and his vision was imperfect in each eye. At the first examination he read with his right 20/120, and with the left 20/60. I suggested that he palm at least six times a day for five minutes, and on the second day he was greatly improved, reading with the right eye 20/80, left 20/40. On the third day he read with the right eye 20/40, left 20/30, an increase of vision in the right eye of 200 percent, and in the left of 100 percent. He is now at work, and when, occasionally, he had to lay off, it is not on account of any trouble with his eyes, but because of weakness in his knees.

A year ago a Mr. B. consulted me about the sight of his right eye, the left having been blind for years. His vision was 10/40, and could not be improved by any lens. I advised him to have the left eye removed, since it was a menace to the other eye. He would not consent to this and I did not see him again until May 5 of this year, when he came to my office practically blind in his right eye from sympathetic ophthalmia. At one foot he could only count fingers. I advised the immediate removal of the blind eye and of a few teeth that had pus about them, but I could not promise that his vision would be saved. That afternoon I removed the eye, and the following day I was gratified to find that he could count fingers at three feet. I sent him home with some large letters to use for the practice of central fixation, and by the fifteenth he was able to count fingers at five feet. I then told him how to practice the universal swing, and on the twenty-second he could count fingers at seven feet. On the twenty-ninth he could read the small type on the 20-line of the test card at four inches, whereas he had been entirely unable to see them previously. He states that he can now see the small chickens running about near his feet and can see small cotton plants seven feet away. I am confident that in a year or so, he will have sufficient vision to attend to the necessary work of his farm.

I have treated three cases of squint, all of them with success. One of them, Delia S., age twelve, came to me on May 15, with her right eye turned in to such a degree that the cornea was partly hidden. The sight of this eye was so imperfect that at three feet she could only count fingers. With her left eye she could read 20/30. She was told to palm, and when she returned on May 24 she was able, with the squinting eye, to count fingers at six feet, twice as far as at her first visit, and the eye was straighter. On June 5 she came again, and counted fingers at eight feet, an increase of vision since the beginning of 700 percent. On July 3, while I was writing this report, she came in, and I found that her right eye had improved to 20/60, one-third of normal, while her left had become entirely normal, 20/20. Her right eye was entirely straight at times, and I feel sure that in a few months this condition will have become permanent.

Another case of squint was that of a young girl of fourteen with rather large, pretty eyes, one of which, the right, was slightly crossed inwardly. Her sight was very imperfect—half normal in the right eye and one-third normal in the left—while like most crossed eye people, she was troubled with double vision. I asked her to palm at least six times a day, and she came back with her eyes straighter and able to read 20/30 with both. The next week showed normal vision, the eyes being at times perfectly straight.

I was particularly pleased to be able to relieve these little girls of a disfigurement which means so much more to them than it would mean to a boy, and I was much interested to note how much prettier their eyes were, apart from the disappearance of the squint, after a few treatments. They were wide open, softer-looking—in short, relaxed.

HOW I IMPROVED MY EYESIGHT

By Pamela Speyer

Editor's Note—*When first seen this patient was wearing the following glasses: each eye, concave 5.00 D. S. combined with concave 1.00 D. C. A number of competent men had said that her myopia was progressive, and that her vision was certain to become very imperfect even with glasses. They all insisted that she must wear glasses constantly. Yet after she had discarded them her vision improved in two days from 6/200 to 20/100.*

I have always been nearsighted. When I was six year old, my father took me to a famous oculist in London, and he prescribed and fitted me with my first glasses. With these lenses I was able to distinguish things at a distance which before I had not been able to see. I found that I could read or see objects at close range just as well without the glasses. The only difference that they made to my sight in this case was that print appeared smaller and less black.

Every year stronger lenses were given to me, and I visited several oculists in England and America in the hope of improvement. When I was fifteen an oculist told me that my eyesight, instead of improving each year as I had hoped, would gradually become worse. By this time I was wearing glasses all the time.

Then, quite by chance, my father heard of Dr. Bates through a friend whose eyesight had been cured by him. I was taken there at once. The first thing Dr. Bates did was to take away my glasses. I sat down in a chair, opposite which was a Snellen test card, fifteen feet away. I could not see the largest letter, a "C" about four inches by three, which people with normal vision are supposed to read at two hundred feet. He brought the card five feet nearer and then I read the "C." It appeared very blurred and indistinct. The smaller letters were so blurred that I could not see them at all.

The most helpful thing I learned was how to "palm." This I did by closing my eyes and then covering them with the palms of my hands so that I saw black and remembered it perfectly. This perfect black rested my eyes a great deal. After doing this for some ten or fifteen minutes, I looked at the card and found that I could read the two letters on the next line.

After I had learned to "palm," I learned to "swing." The reason I strained my eyes so when looking at the card was that I stared at one place. So by imagining the letter was swinging like a pendulum, I moved my eyes instead of staring as I had done before. At first the swing was a long one, but after practicing for some weeks, I began getting it shorter until it was only half an inch on each side of the letter. The short swing was more difficult to do than the long one, but it helped more in the end.

Then I learned to "flash." I looked at a small letter at fifteen feet distance and could not read it. The longer I looked the worse it grew. So by closing my eyes and remembering the swing for a few seconds, I just glanced at the letter and closing my eyes at once, I saw the letter in a flash.

All these things must be practiced every day, and even now I have to "palm" every morning and night. Palming, swinging and flashing were the three fundamentals. As soon as they were mastered, only practice remained. I have now been going to Dr. Bates for over a year and my eyesight is almost cured. I often have flashes of perfect sight. Dr. Bates has certainly helped me in a remarkable degree, more indeed than I ever thought possible when I first went to him wearing strong glasses.

SLEEPINESS AND EYESTRAIN

By W. H. Bates, M.D.

How much sleep is necessary to maintain health? This is a question which has never been satisfactorily answered. Theoretically, mental or physical work should increase the need for sleep, but it is a matter of common knowledge that many inactive persons seem to need just as much sleep as those who work, or even more.

Much time has been devoted to the investigation of the symptoms of fatigue. Analyses have been made of the blood of fatigued subjects; the action of the muscles, nerves and brain; the changes in the structure of the cells, under the influence of fatigue, the changes following sleep, have all been carefully studied. But so far very little light has been thrown upon the nature of either fatigue or sleep.

This is a fact, however, that eyestrain has always been demonstrated when fatigue was present, and that fatigue has always been relieved when eyestrain was relieved. Perfect sight is perfect rest, and cannot coexist with fatigue. Even the memory or imagination of fatigue is accompanied by the production of eyestrain and imperfect sight, while the memory of perfect sight will relieve both eyestrain and fatigue. Sleepiness is a common symptom of habitual eyestrain, and when the sight improves the need for sleep is often markedly reduced.

One patient reports that after gaining normal sight without glasses she was able to get on comfortably with seven hours sleep, whereas she had formerly not been able to avoid continual sleepiness and yawning even on nine and ten hours. The inclination to yawn on all occasions had been so overpowering, she stated, that it often subjected her to great embarrassment. On one occasion she yawned so incessantly during a call made in the early evening that the visitor concluded, not unnaturally, that her presence was a burden and departed in high dudgeon, no explanations sufficing to convince her that the yawning was not the result of boredom. The patient was made very unhappy by this condition, but finally became reconciled to it in a measure, thinking that what could not be cured must be endured. Great was her surprise and delight, therefore, when, after discarding her glasses and beginning to practice central fixation, she found herself sleeping less and not yawning so much. She made no conscious effort, she said, to check the yawning, and had indeed almost forgotten about it. She now gets sleepy only at bedtime.

Another patient, although he never had any desire to sleep in the daytime, found it very difficult to keep awake in the evening. At the opera or theatre, at lectures and social gatherings, and at church, he was always sleepy and often went to sleep. It was naturally more difficult for him to keep awake when he was not interested, but whether he was interested or not he was sure to become more or less sleepy. He never went to a lecture without going to sleep, and the world's most famous songbirds were not always able to keep him awake at the opera. In the case of dull papers or sermons, it did no good to think of something else, for the sound of the speaker's voice acted like an opiate. When he learned how to relax by the aid of the memory, imagination, shifting, swinging and palming, the trouble gradually became less, and now he can stay awake at all times and in all places where people are supposed to stay awake.

STORIES FROM THE CLINIC

No. 7: The Woman with Asthma

By Emily C. Lierman

When eyestrain is relieved all other strain is relieved, and therefore patients relieved of eyestrain are often relieved of many other symptoms. Asthma belongs to a large class of diseases with symptoms which may result from nervous disturbances instead of from organic changes. They have been called functional neuroses. It was not strange, therefore, that this patient should note an immediate improvement in her breathing after palming, and that this treatment, its combination with hygienic measures, should have permanently relieved the trouble. Many similar cases could be reported, and even when organic disease has been present, the subjective symptoms have been relieved.

One day during the summer of 1919, a woman suffering from asthma came to the Clinic. She was only forty years old, but looked fifty, and it was evident, from the wrinkles in her forehead and her half-shut eyes, that her vision was very poor. She told me that she suffered from continual pain, and I could see that she had great difficulty in breathing but her spirit was unbroken, and her exuberance was something of a problem to me. She talked continually as long as she could find anyone to listen to her, and in order to preserve any order in the Clinic I had to keep her as much as possible by herself. I was sorry to do this because her good humor was contagious and made the patients forget their pain and other troubles, but I could not have the work brought to a standstill even for such a desirable end as this.

The state of her eyesight did not seem to trouble her. It was her asthma about which she was concerned. When I asked her to read the test card she said, "Please ma'am, help me to breathe first; never mind my eyes." "You are in the wrong room for asthma," I replied, "just let me do something for your eyes, and then I will send you to another room where a good doctor will treat you for the asthma."

She smiled, evidently pleased that I had not sent her away, and proceeded to read the card as I had asked her to do. Her vision was 20/30 in each eye. I told her to palm and on no account to remove her hands from her eyes until I came back. It was fully half an hour before I was able to do this, and when I told her to uncover her eyes, she asked, "What makes me breathe so easy?" "The palming has helped you," I replied.

Her vision was now 15/20, and she said the pain in her chest and back had gone. I gave her some advice about her diet, told her to drink plenty of water, and asked her to come to the Clinic three days a week.

On the next Clinic day, to my great disappointment, I did not see her. I concluded that she did not care to bother about her eyes, and was not willing to give up the foods and drinks I had told her not to take, including meats, pastry, strong tea and other liquids much stronger than tea. Other patients were continually coming in, however, so the poor woman with asthma went completely out of my mind until two months later when she rushed into the Clinic like a cyclone. Most of these poor people do not think about waiting for their turn, and are so anxious to tell me about their relief from eyestrain and other troubles that I have to forgive them when they break the rules. This woman not only did not wait her turn but did not think it necessary to wait until I had finished with the patient I was attending to.

As soon as she saw me she yelled in a loud excited voice, "Please, ma'am, I didn't forget you. I didn't forget myself either. It felt so good after you treated me, I just palmed and palmed, and I began to breathe so much better I went out and got a job right away. During the day, my madam allowed me to rest my eyes, and I ate very sparingly. Sure, ma'am, it was no joke either, for I just love to eat good and lots of it; but I remembered what you said, and so I behaved myself. I must have starved the asthma all away."

"I am very glad to hear all this," I said. "Now let me see what the palming did for your eyes." Her vision had improved to 15/10. And it had all happened in two months. She did it and not I. When I told her this and praised her for it, she replied, "God bless you! You don't know how happy I am. I am working and supporting myself now for the first time in four years. But what surprises me the most is that I have not been drowned by this time with all the water I have been drinking."

QUESTIONS AND ANSWERS

The editor has received so many questions from the readers of *Better Eyesight* that he feels it sufficiently important to open a new department which will start next month.

Better Eyesight
October 1920—Vol. III, No. 4

GO TO THE MOVIES

They can help you to improve your sight

Cinematograph pictures are commonly supposed to be very injurious to the eyes, and it is a fact that they often cause much discomfort and lowering of vision. They can, however, be made a means of improving the sight. When they hurt the eyes it is because the subject strains to see them.

If this tendency to strain can be overcome, the vision is always improved, and, if the practice of viewing the pictures is continued long enough, nearsightedness, astigmatism and other troubles are cured.

If your sight is imperfect, therefore, you will find it an advantage to go to the movies frequently and learn to look at the pictures without strain. If they hurt your eyes, look away to the dark for a while, then look at a corner of the picture; look away again, and then look a little nearer to the center; and so on. In this way you may soon become able to look directly at the picture without discomfort. If this does not help, try palming for five minutes or longer; dodge the pain, in short, and prevent the eyestrain by constant shifting or by palming.

If you become able to look at the movies without discomfort, nothing else will bother you.

THE PROBLEM OF IMPERFECT SIGHT

By W. H. Bates, M.D.

The problem of imperfect sight is such a tremendous one that few, even of those who specialize in such matters, realize its proportions, while outside this circle there is not the remotest conception of what it means.

The literature of the subject is very confusing and contradictory; but from the facts available there can be no doubt that the great majority of schoolchildren suffer from some degree of imperfect sight, while among adults normal vision is a rare exception.

The very careful investigation of Risley showed that in the public schools of Philadelphia, among children between eight and a half and seventeen and a half, the proportion of imperfect sight was about ninety percent;[1] other investigators report lower figures, but in many cases this simply means a lower standard. The findings of Risley agree with those obtained by myself in a study of 100,000 children made under all sorts of conditions in both city and country schools.

As to the sight of the adult population the operation of the draft law has supplied us with some unimpeachable data. It was found impossible to raise an Army with even half normal vision in one eye, and in order to get the number of soldiers required it was necessary to accept for general service, men whose vision could be brought up to half normal with glasses.[2]

Such figures as the foregoing, terrible as they are, by no means exhaust the subject. In fact they are only the beginning.

Errors of refraction are so common that we have learned to take them lightly. They are usually reckoned among minor physical defects, and the average lay person has no idea of their real character. It is well known, of course, that they sometimes produce very serious nervous conditions, but the fact that they also lead to all sorts of eye diseases is known only to specialists, and not fully appreciated even by them. The complications of myopia (nearsight) constitute a large and melancholy chapter in the science of the eye, but most eye specialists say that no organic changes occur in hypermetropia (farsightedness). That this is very far from being the case was proven by Risley in the investigation alluded to above, and it is strange that his report on the subject has attracted so little attention. His studies also showed that these organic changes, occurring in all states of refraction, are very common among children and have often progressed to an extent that would be expected only after long years of eyestrain.

In the case of myopic astigmatism the percentage of diseased eyes among all the children examined ran as high as eighty-seven percent, and in the secondary schools not a single myopic eye was found with a healthy eyeground.

The condition known as *conus,* in which the choroid, or

1. *School Hygiene, System of Diseases of the Eye,* edited by Norris and Oliver.

2. "Report of the Provost Marshal General to the Secretary of War on the First Draft under the Selective Service Act," 1917. "Second Report of the Provost Marshall General to the Secretary of War on the Operations of the Selective Service System" to December 20, 1916.

middle coat of the eye, is destroyed in the neighborhood of the optic nerve exposing the white outer coat (sclera) and forming first a crescent and later even a complete circle, is commonly regarded as one of the symptoms of myopia and attributed to the tension resulting from the lengthening of the globe, but Risley's statistics show that while it is somewhat more common in this state of refraction than in hypermetropia it is by no means peculiar to it. In hypermetropia, conus was found in twenty percent of the cases, and in hypermetropic astigmatism in forty-five percent. In simple myopia it was present in forty-one percent of the cases, and in myopic astigmatism it reached sixty percent. It is a terrible thing to think that the eyes of our children should show a symptom of this character in such a large proportion of cases.

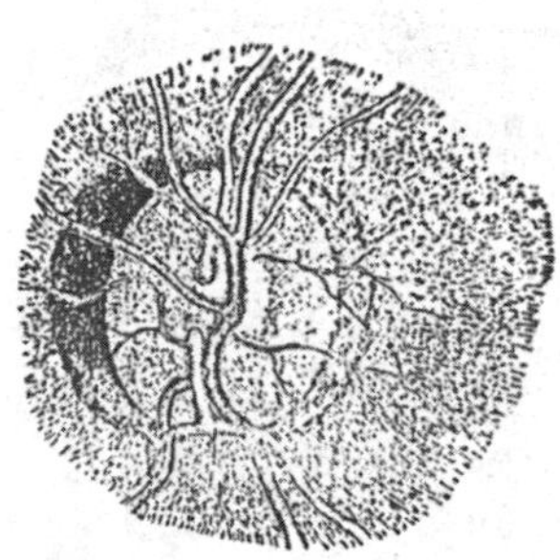

CONUS IN HYPERMETROPIA

The eyegrounds of a brother and sister age respectively ten and twelve years. Both had hypermetropic astigmatism. "The conditions here represented," says Risley, "were repeated in scores of their fellows at school."

My own experience is that errors of refraction are always accompanied by some organic change. It may be only a slight congestion, but this may be sufficient to lower the vision.

By wearing glasses, avoiding poor lights and limiting the use of the eyes for near work, it is supposed that we can do something to prevent the development of these organic diseases and to check their progress; but for none of the traditional methods of treatment is it even claimed that they can be depended upon to preserve the sight as long as it may be needed, and, Sidler Huguenin, in a paper several times referred to in this magazine, has stated that in the thousands of cases of myopia that have come under his observation they never were of any material benefit.[3]

That imperfect sight is a fruitful cause of retardation in school is well known. According to the New York City Board of Health it is responsible for a quarter of the habitually left backs.[4] But that this condition cannot be remedied by glasses has not been generally observed. By making the patient more comfortable, glasses do often improve his mental condition, *but since they cannot relieve the mental strain that underlies the visual one, they cannot improve it to normal, and by confirming it in a bad habit they may make it worse.* [My emphasis.—TRQ]

From the foregoing facts it will be seen that in the condition of the eyesight of our people we have a health problem, an educational problem, and a military problem, of the first magnitude, and one would think that if any method of either prevention or cure that was even tolerably successful had been found it would immediately be put into general use.

STORIES FROM THE CLINIC

No. 8: Atrophy of the Optic Nerve

By Emily C. Lierman

About twenty-five years ago a patient came to the New York Eye Infirmary with well-marked atrophy of the optic nerve. According to all that we know of the laws of pathology he should have been totally blind; yet his vision was normal. The case was considered so remarkable that it was exhibited before a number of medical societies, but it was by no means an isolated one. On February 8, 1917, the editor published in the New York Medical Journal, *under the title, "Blindness Relieved By a New Method of Treatment," a report of a case in which the vision was improved from perception of light to normal. He has had quite a number of such cases.*

Some time ago a woman was led into the Clinic by a friend. She had heard of Dr. Bates and had come to him in the hope that he might be able to restore her sight. The Doctor examined her eyes and found that she had atrophy of the optic nerve complicated with other troubles. She could not count her fingers, nor had she any perception of light whatever. The Doctor turned her over to me saying, "Help her, will you?"

She was very good-natured and motherly. She greeted me with a smile and said, "May the good Lord bless you, ma'am, if you can give me again the light of day." The words came from a very humble heart and were very hopeful. When I heard them I can tell you that I lost some of my courage. It might turn out that I could do nothing for her,

3. *School Health News,* February 1919.

4. *Archiv. f. Augenh.* Vol. IXXIX, 1915, translated in *Arch. Ophth.,* Vol. XLV, November 1916.

and I dreaded to disappoint her. My work is not always easy; yet I like the hard cases to come my way, because when I can help them I feel that I have done something worthwhile.

"Won't you tell me how long you have been blind?" I asked. "Yes, ma'am," she replied. "I haven't seen nothing for two years. I have been in the hospital all that time and the doctors say that maybe I will never see again. Some friend of mine said to me, 'You just go to the Harlem Hospital Clinic. There you find the Doctor that makes you see.' So I just came; that's all."

I told her to cover her eyes with the palms of her hands and asked if she could remember anything black. She replied, "Yes, ma'am, I remember stove polish black, all right." "That's fine," I said. "Now, keep remembering the black stove polish, and that will stop the strain in your eyes. When your eyes first began to trouble you, you strained to see, and every time you did that your eyes became worse. Now let us see what will happen when you stop the strain."

I stood her against the wall to make things easier for her, for we have few chairs at the Clinic, and left her to treat other patients, telling her not to open her eyes, nor to remove her palms from them, not for a moment, until I came back. Presently I became aware of a strange sound, a sort of mumbling. I was greatly puzzled, but tried not to show it for fear I would disturb the patients. All of a sudden, as I approached my blind patient, I discovered where the sound came from. She was saying in a low tone, "Black polish, black polish," just as fast as she could. Now I held a test card covered with "E's" of various sizes turned in different directions a foot away from her eyes, and told her to take her hands down and look at it. The Doctor, the other patients and myself were quite scared at the outburst that followed.

"Ma'am, that's an 'E'; that's a sure enough 'E.' I am sure that's a black 'E' on some white paper." This was a large letter on the first line, read by the normal eye at two hundred feet.

But the next moment it faded from her eyes. That was my fault. I was not quick enough. What I should have done was to have her close her eyes and palm again the moment she saw the "E." But I was greatly encouraged, not only because the patient had had a flash of vision, but because Dr. Bates had said he was sure I would help her to see again. I again told her to palm and remember black and when, in a few moments, I asked her to take down her hands and look at the card, she again saw the "E," and blacker than the first time. I now told her to close her eyes for a minute and open them for just a second, alternately, remembering the stove polish as she did so. She did this for a time and was able to see the "E" each time she opened her eyes.

"Now," I said, as I raised my hand and held it one foot from her eyes, "how many fingers can you see?" "Three," she replied, which was correct.

I told her to rest her eyes by palming many times a day, and to come and see me three times a week. I also gave her some advice about her diet and told her that enemas were quite necessary to relieve her constipation.

Next Clinic day she saw the 70-line of letters at one foot, and they did not fade away as did the "E" the first time she saw it. I told her to palm some more, and in a few minutes she counted my fingers correctly every time I asked her to, with only one exception.

"If this here seeing keeps up, ma'am," she remarked, "I sure will be able to earn my living again. The Lord bless you ma'am."

She continued to come and made slow but sure progress for a time. Then came a time when she stayed away for several months. As I was very anxious to cure her, I worried about her considerably during this time. Then one day she turned up again. She seemed to be very much frightened about something, but her eyes looked much better. I was so glad to see her, and she seemed so much upset that I refrained from scolding her as I felt like doing, and in course of time I discovered the reason for her absence. She had been under treatment for some other troubles, and some doctor or nurse had scared her into discontinuing her visits to our Clinic. She had, however, continued to palm several hours a day with most gratifying results.

"Do you know, ma'am," she said, "I can see every house number as I go visiting, and I go out to a day's work once in a while."

She continued to come quite regularly and her improvement continued. Sometimes I would find that she did not see as well as at her previous visit, but immediate improvement always followed palming. Her gratitude was pathetic, and every little while she would bring a bundle, saying, "This here is for you, ma'am. You saved me from blindness. Yes, you did, and I am mighty grateful." These bundles contained gifts of various kinds—a coconut from the West Indies at one time, grapefruit and cucumbers at another, and a third a necklace made of tropical beans of various colors.

The greatest day of her life came a few weeks ago when she washed a full set of Dresden china for her employer, without breaking a single piece, and earned four dollars and twenty cents by her day's work. If she continues to practice the palming, which she now forgets sometimes, I have no doubt that she will, in time, obtain normal vision. She now sees the largest letter on the card twenty feet away and reads the headlines in the newspapers. Recently Dr. Bates examined her eyes with the ophthalmoscope and found the appearance of the optic nerve very much improved, more blood-vessels being visible in the papilla, or head of the nerve.

[For a follow-up on this case, see the end of Emily's article "Stories from the Clinic, No. 13: Relief of Blindness at the Clinic" in the March 1921 issue.—TRQ]

HOW I LEARNED TO SEE

By Irma Meyers

This patient was fourteen years old when first seen, and was wearing the following glasses: right eye, concave 3.12 D. S. with concave 0.75 D. C. 90 degrees; left eye, concave 3.25 D. S. with concave 0.50 D. C. 90 degrees. At the second treatment her sight had improved temporarily to 20/20, and at the third she had a flash of perfect sight.

The time had come for me to consult an oculist again. I had been wearing glasses for over a year and they had always been a torment to my parents.

We were discussing the question of oculists at the table. My father contended that if there were physicians who could correct defective sight with glasses, there must be those who could cure such defects so that glasses would not be necessary. He had heard of a Dr. Bates who had cured people so that they no longer had to wear glasses.

So instead of going to an eye specialist who would probably have prescribed new glasses, father and I went to see Dr. Bates. While waiting for admission to his private office, a number of questions came to my mind. Could he cure me? Would I be able to get along without glasses for the rest of my life? It seemed too good to be true. My eyesight had been so poor that I had given up hope of ever leaving off my glasses.

Finally we were ushered into Dr. Bates' office. He examined my eyes. I could just barely read the second line of letters on the Snellen chart—which shows how defective my eyesight was. The Doctor impressed upon me that to improve my sight depended largely upon myself, and I determined to follow his directions conscientiously. I must never wear my glasses again, I was told, and that day, in the Doctor's office, was the last time I did wear those hated glasses.

Then the Doctor told me to palm—that is, to put my hands over my eyes in such a way as to exclude all the light from them. In this way my eyes became rested. I was not looking at anything, and therefore my eyes were not undergoing any strain. Next the Doctor showed me some fine print on a card and called my attention to the fact that while these letters looked perfectly black to me, those on the Snellen chart, at a distance of ten feet, were gray. The difference was due to my imagination, he said, and proved that my eyesight was not normal because the letters on the test card were just as black as those on the small card in my hand. Then he told me how to improve my imagination. In reading letters like "O," "D," and "S," which had open spaces in them, I was to imagine the white openings (the card is white, the letters are black) whiter than the margin of the card, which is the way the normal eye sees them. When I became able to do this the black letters stood out more clearly.

Besides my imagination I had also to exercise my memory. This was accomplished in this way: I looked at a certain letter on the chart. Then I closed my eyes and remembered it better than I saw it. I could not do this very well at first, but my memory improved with practice.

These and many other methods of improving the sight I learned from Dr. Bates. I visited him three times each week, and soon began to read much more on the chart than I had at my first visit. At the same time I noticed that stores, signs, houses, cars, all material objects, began to come out more clearly than before. I discovered, too, that I was not so shaky on my feet as I had been when I first discarded my eyeglasses. I felt then as if I would fall at every step I took. In school I did not have to go up to the blackboard to read what was on it, and did not have to sit as near the front as I formerly did.

After six or seven months I began to enjoy the movies. I no longer had to sit and view a picture that I could not see. (I never, as I said before, used my glasses after my first visit to Dr. Bates.) I began to enjoy the pictures as much as the people around me who had never worn glasses. In school I could sit in the last rows and read the blackboard without any trouble.

I have now been under treatment about a year, with some interruptions, and my eyesight is considered normal. At a recent test by the visiting physician at school I stood second among forty pupils. The girl who was first read just one letter more than I did, and I am sure that if I had had an opportunity to palm I would have been able to do better than she did.

I cannot express in words what I owe to Dr. Bates. I shall always be grateful to him, and I wish I could show my appreciation for his work.

At a recent visit Dr. Bates told me that my cure was not yet permanent, but I shall continue to follow his instructions and teachings implicitly until it is permanent. I sincerely hope that I shall never go back to wearing glasses, and that this recital of my experiences may help others similarly afflicted.

QUESTIONS AND ANSWERS

Editor's Note—*All readers of this magazine are invited to send questions to the editor regarding any difficulties they may experience in using the various methods of treatment which it recommends.*

Q–1a. When objects at a distance clear up, they are double. Can you suggest a remedy for this double vision? 1b. When I open my eyes after palming my sight gradually clears, but an intense pain often comes in my eyes so that they close. The pain always starts with very clear vision. Is this eyestrain?

A–1a. If the objects are double when they clear up, relaxation is not complete, and the only remedy is to secure a greater degree of relaxation. This may be done in many ways. Use the method you have found most effective. [The temporary experience of multiple images, in contrast to true double vision caused by squint (strabismus), is common when students improve their sight.—TRQ] 1b. Yes. Your sight should be best when you open your eyes. If it clears up afterward, it is because you are making an initial effort to see. This produces the pain.

Q–2a. How long should one palm and how often? 2b. How young a patient can you treat by this method, and up to what age can you expect results? How would you handle a child that did not know its letters? 2c. Is astigmatism curable by this method? 2d. How long has the method [been used]?

A–2a. As often and as long as possible. 2b. The age is immaterial. It is a matter of intelligence. Patients as old as eighty-two have been relieved. Children can be treated as soon as they are able to talk. Any small object can be used for eye training, and in the case of children who do not know their letters, kindergarten and Montessori equipment is often useful. 2c. Yes. 2d. Its evolution began thirty-five years ago. It has improved as experience was gained, and is still improving.

Better Eyesight
November 1920—Vol. III, No. 5

SQUINT [STRABISMUS] NUMBER

MAKE YOUR SQUINT WORSE
This will help you to cure it

There is no better way of curing squint than by making it worse, or by producing other kinds of squint. This can be done as follows:

To produce convergent squint, strain to see a point about three inches from the eyes, such as the end of the nose.

To produce divergent squint, fix a point at the distance to one side of any object, and strain to see it as well as when directly regarded.

To produce a vertical squint, look at a point below an object at the distance, and at the same time strain to see the latter.

To produce an oblique divergent squint, look at a point below and to one side of an object at the distance while straining to see the latter.

When successful, two images will be seen arranged horizontally, vertically, or obliquely, according to the direction of the strain.

The production of convergent squint is usually easier than that of the other varieties, and most patients succeed better with a light as the object of vision than with a letter or other non-luminous object.

SQUINT AND AMBLYOPIA: THEIR CURE
By W. H. Bates, M.D.

Squint, or strabismus, is that condition of the eyes in which both are not directed to the same point at the same time. One eye may turn out more or less persistently while the other is normal (divergent squint), or it may turn in (convergent squint), or it may look too high or too low while deviating at the same time in an outward or inward direction (vertical squint). Sometimes these conditions change from one eye to another (alternating squint), and sometimes the character of the squint changes in the same eye, divergent squint becoming convergent and vice versa. Sometimes the patient is conscious of seeing two images of the object regarded, and sometimes he is not. Usually there is a lowering of vision in the deviating eye which cannot be improved by glasses, and for which no apparent or sufficient cause can be found. This condition is known as *amblyopia,* literally *dimsightedness,* and is supposed to be incurable after a very early age, even though the squint may be corrected.

Operations, which are now seldom advised, are admitted to be a gamble. According to Fuchs,[1] "their results are as a rule simply cosmetic. The sight of the squinting eye is not influenced by the operation, and only in a few instances is even binocular vision restored." This is an understatement rather than the reverse, for a desirable cosmetic effect cannot be counted upon, and in many cases the condition is made worse. Sometimes the affected eye becomes straight and remains straight permanently, but often, after it has remained straight for a shorter or a longer time, it suddenly turns in the opposite direction.

I myself have had both failures and successes from operations. In one case the eyes not only became straight, but binocular single vision—that is, the power of fusing the two visual images into one—was restored, and when I last saw the patient, thirty years after the operation, there had been no change in these conditions. Yet when I reported to the Ophthalmological Section of the New York Academy of Medicine that I had cut away a quarter of an inch from the tendon of the internal rectus of each eye, the members were unanimous in their opinion that the eyes would certainly turn in the opposite direction in a very short time. In other cases the eyes, after remaining straight for a time, have reverted to their old condition or turned in the opposite direction. The latter happened once after an apparently perfect result, including the restoration of binocular single vision, which had been permanent for five years. The consequent deformity was terrible. Sometimes I tried to undo the harm resulting from operations, my own and those of others, but invariably I failed.

Glasses, prescribed on the theory that the existence of errors of refraction is responsible for the failure of the two eyes to act together, sometimes appear to do good; but exceptions are numerous, and in many cases they fail even to prevent the condition from becoming steadily worse.

The fusion training of Worth is not believed to be of much use after the age of five or six, and often fails even then, in which case Worth recommends operations.

Fortunately for the victims of this distressing condition, their eyes often become straight spontaneously, regardless of what is or is not done to them. More rarely the vision of the squinting eye is restored. If the sight of the good eye is destroyed, the amblyopic eye is very likely to recover normal vision, often in an incredibly short space of time. In spite of the fact that the textbooks agree in assuring us that amblyopia is incurable, many cases of the latter class are on record.

The fact is that both squint and amblyopia, like errors of refraction, are functional troubles, originating entirely in the mind. Both can be produced in normal eyes by a strain to see, and both are immediately relieved when the patient looks at a blank surface and remembers something perfectly. A permanent cure is a mere matter of making this temporary relaxation permanent.

Permanent relaxation can be obtained by any of the methods used in the cure of errors of refraction, but in the case of young children who do not know their letters these methods have to be modified. Such children can be cured by encouraging them to use their eyes on any small objects that interest them. There are many ways in which this can be done, and it is important to devise a variety of exercises so that the child will not weary of them. For the same reason the presence of other children is at times desirable. There must be no compulsion and no harshness, for as soon as any exercise ceases to be pleasant it ceases to be beneficial.

The needle, the brush, the pencil, kindergarten and Montessori material, picture books, playing cards, etc., may all be utilized for purposes of eye training. At first it will be necessary to use rather large objects and forms, but as the sight improves the size must be reduced. A child may begin to sew, for instance, with a coarse needle and thread, and will naturally take large stitches. As her sight improves, a finer needle should be provided and the stitches will naturally be smaller. Painting the openings of letters in different colors is an excellent practice, and as the sight improves the size of the letters can be reduced. Map drawing and the study of maps is a good thing, and can be easily adapted to the state of the vision. With a map of the United States a child can begin by picking out all the states of a particular color, and as the sight improves she can pick out the rivers and cities. In drawing maps the child can proceed in the same way, beginning with the outlines of countries or states, and with improved vision putting in the details. A paper covered with spots in various colors is another useful thing, as the child gets much amusement and benefit from picking out all the spots of the same color. With improved vision the size of the spots can be reduced and their number increased.

1. *Text-Book of Ophthalmology,* authorized translation from the twelfth German edition by Duane, p. 795.

Many interesting games can be devised with playing cards. "Slap Jack" is a good one, as it awakens intense interest and great quickness of vision is required to slap the Jack with the hand the moment its face appears on the table.

These ideas are only suggestions, and any intelligent parent will be able to add to them.

Both children and adults are greatly benefited by making their squint worse or producing new kinds of squint (see above). The voluntary production of squint is a favorite amusement with children, and if they show an inclination to indulge in it, they should be encouraged. Most parents fear that the temporary squint will become permanent, but the fact is just the contrary. Anyone who can squint voluntarily will never squint involuntarily.

HOW I CURED MY CHILD OF SQUINT

By Ms. B. F. Glienke

Editor's Note—*The following remarkable story is published in the hope that it may help other parents in the treatment of squinting children. The patient was first seen on April 24, 1920, her age being four. When her sight was tested with pothooks her eyes were straight and her vision normal. When tested with the letters of the Snellen test card which she could not read, or with figures which she did not know, her eyes turned and the retinoscope showed that she had compound myopic astigmatism. When she looked at a blank wall without trying to see, her eyes were again straight and her vision normal.*

When my little daughter was quite young I noticed that her eyes were crossed at times, while at others they were perfectly straight. Later the squint became more continuous, and when she was four years old she was taken to Dr. Bates. He said the trouble was entirely a nervous one, and called my attention to the fact that when the child was comfortable and happy her eyes were straight, and when she was nervous they turned. He said that she should be encouraged to use her eyes as much as possible on objects that interested her, and that she must never be scolded or punished. He also recommended a cold sponge bath and massage first thing in the morning for the purpose of quieting and strengthening her nerves and improving her general health. As I had been a teacher of drawing before my marriage and understood something of kindergarten methods, I did not find it difficult to follow his instructions. I drew pictures of animals and asked Marie to tell me if they were running, walking, or standing still, whether they were looking at her, or facing in some other direction, whether they had four legs or two. I showed her a picture of the moon, and asked her to tell me whether the horns were pointing upward, downward, or sideways. We played that the moon was full of water and had to be held right side up so that the water would not run out. She became very much interested in these pictures, and as long as the interest lasted, her eyes were straight. When they ceased to interest her the squint returned.

Sometimes I would ask her to look at the windows and tell me whether they were open at the top or bottom, whether the shades were partly down, or all the way down. Then we would look at the windows across the street and do the same thing. We also watched the passing cars, and I asked her to tell me how many people there were in them and whether these people were men, women or children. We studied the patterns of the wallpaper, and when visitors came I asked her after they had gone to tell me what kind of clothes they had on. I taught her to sew and paint, to match colors, and braid mats, to thread beads, and do things with building blocks. Her father, who is a printer, showed her specimens of diamond type, and of minion which is even smaller than diamond. She enjoyed picking out the smallest letters, and when she did so her eyes were straight.

Threading beads was the most beneficial work undertaken, its tediousness being overcome by the fact that the child's doll and all her stuffed animals, Teddy bear, bunny, dog, etc., each received its own particular necklace of beads. The cold baths and massage were also a great help.

The combined results of the treatment were wonderful. Her eyes began to be straight all the time. Her nervous condition and her appetite improved, and she slept better. Then we had some setbacks. First she had an attack of grippe with cough, headaches and fever. The squint came back and stayed with her for several weeks, until she was well. Then her eyes became straight again.

Later on when she was playing with her little brother they disagreed about something, and Marie got so nervous that her eyes became worse than on any previous occasion since she had been under treatment. The squint alternated from one eye to the other, the left eye being the worse, and the next day we were very much worried when we found that the left eye was practically blind. But we went on encouraging her to use her eyes, and in ten days she was as well as ever.

STORIES FROM THE CLINIC

No. 9: Three Cases of Squint

By Emily C. Lierman

One day as I entered the Clinic I saw two mothers standing side by side, each holding a little boy by the hand. The children were both about the same age, five years, and both were crossed eyed; but there the resemblance ceased. One seemed happy and contented, and it was quite evident that he was much loved and well cared for. The clothes of both mother and child were clean and neat, and often the boy would look at the mother for a smile, which was always there. The other boy was plainly unhappy and neglected. I could read the mind of the mother, who was anything but clean, as she stood there grasping his hand a little too tightly; and even without her frequent whispered threats of dire things to happen if the child did not keep still, I would have known that she considered him a nuisance, and not a precious possession as the first boy plainly was to his mother.

I was at a loss to know which child to treat first, but decided upon Nathan, the clean one, and tried to keep the other interested while he waited. Nathan had beautiful black curls, and should have been pretty but for the convergent squint of his right eye, which gave him a very peculiar appearance. His vision was very poor. With both eyes together he could read at ten feet only the 50-line of the test card, and with the squinting eye he read only the 70-line. I showed him how to palm, and while he was doing so I had time to talk to his mother. She said that his right eye had turned in since he was two years old and that all the doctors she had taken him to had prescribed glasses. These, however, had not helped him. I now asked Nathan to read the card again and was delighted to find that the vision of the worse eye had become equal to that of the good one, namely 10/50. I had difficulty in keeping his head straight while I was testing him, for like most children with squint he tried to improve his sight by looking at the object of vision from all sorts of angles. After he had palmed for a sufficient length of time, however, he became able to correct this habit. The extraordinary sympathy which existed between mother and child came out again during the treatment, for no matter what I said or did, the child would not smile until the mother did.

Nathan came to the Clinic very regularly for a year, and for the first six months he always wore a black patch over his better eye, the left, while atropine was also used in this eye to prevent its use in case the patch was not worn constantly. Nathan did not like the patch, and his mother had to promise all sorts of things to keep it on. After it was removed the atropine was continued. Dr. Bates had told me what to expect when the patch was removed, and so I was not shocked to see the eye turn in. I knew the condition would be temporary, and that in time both eyes would be straight. Treatment was continued for six months, and now the boy reads at times 10/15 with both eyes, and always with a smile.

The dirty boy, to whom we must now go back, was called George, and his condition was worse than that of Nathan, for he had squint in both eyes. At ten feet he read the 50-line, but complained that he saw double. I showed him how to palm, and while he was doing so his mother told me how very bad he was, adding that I must spank him if he did not mind me.

"I think he gets enough of that already," I said, but I was careful to say it with a smile, fearing that she might lose her temper and say more than I would like.

George had now been palming five minutes, and I asked him to uncover his eyes and look at the card. He was much surprised to find that he could read the 40-line without seeing the letters double. I asked his mother very quietly to be a little patient with him and help him at home, and I gave her a test card for him to practice with.

"Madam," she replied, "I am the mother of six, and I haven't time to fuss with him." "No wonder the kiddy is crossed eye," I thought, and seeing I could get no help in that quarter, I appealed to George.

When I revealed to him the possibility of a Christmas present if he came to the Clinic regularly and did what I told him he became interested. I did not know how much could be done for his eyes in the eight weeks that remained before the holidays, but I felt sure that with his cooperation we could at least make a good start. This he gave me in full measure. Never did I have a more enthusiastic patient. He came to the Clinic regularly three days a week, and often when I came late I would find him waiting for me on the hospital steps and yelling, "Here she is. I saw her first."

After he had been practicing faithfully for two weeks palming—six times a day, and perhaps more, according to his own report—he was able to keep his eyes straight while he read the test card at twelve feet. After he had done this I asked him to spell a word with five letters, and instantly his eyes turned. I had him palm again, and then I asked him to count up to twenty, his eyes remained straight, because he could do this without strain.

Two days before Christmas I brought my bundle of presents for the children. George was there bright and early, and with him had come three of his brothers to get their share too, "if there was any," as George explained. Fortunately a little fairy had prepared me for this, and I had gifts for everyone. That day George was able to keep his eyes straight both before and after his treatment, and to read 15/10 with each eye separately. I have never seen him since, and can only hope that he kept up the treatment until permanently cured.

When little Ruth, age three, first came to us Dr. Bates suggested to her mother, who was nearsighted, that she should have her own eyes cured because her condition had a bad effect on the child. She consented and now has nearly normal vision. Ruth had squint and was so tiny that I had to put her on a table to treat her. As she could not read the letters on the test card, I held before her a card covered with "E's" of various sizes turned in different directions. Her mother was quite positive that she couldn't understand what I wanted her to do, but Ruth, as often happens in such cases, had more intelligence than her mother gave her credit for. I asked her to tell me whether a certain "E" pointed upward, or to the right or left, by merely indicating the direction with her finger, and it did not take an instant for her to show her mother how bright she was. I showed her how to palm, and in a little while she indicated correctly the direction of the letters on several lines. When the letters became indistinct as I moved the card farther away, she became excited and wanted to cry, and her left eye turned in markedly. She palmed again, and while she was doing so I asked her all about her dolly, whether her eyes were blue or some other color, what kind of clothes she wore and so on. When she removed her hands from her eyes both were straight. Her mother was instructed to practice with her many times a day at short intervals, so that she would not tire of it, and in three months her eyes were straight every time I tested her sight. I was much interested to learn from her mother that if Ruth's daddy raised his voice in the slightest degree when he spoke to her, her eyes were sure to turn in. This merely confirmed my own experience that it is necessary to treat children who have defects of vision with the utmost gentleness if one wants to cure them. Ruth is not cured yet, but she hopes to be before Christmas because Santa Claus is sure to visit Room 6, Harlem Hospital Clinic, and he does not like to see children with squint.

QUESTIONS AND ANSWERS

Q–1. Can opacity of the cornea be cured?

A–1. Yes. A patient with opacity of the cornea came to the eye Clinic of the Harlem Hospital with a vision of 20/70, and in half an hour became able to read 20/40. Later his vision became normal, much to my surprise. Other cases have also been cured.

Q–2. Is retinitis pigmentosa curable?

A–2. Yes. See *Better Eyesight*, April 1920.

Q–3. My eyes are weak and cannot stand the light. Can anything be done for them?

A–3. Yes. Stop wearing dark glasses, and go out into the bright sunshine. Let the sun shine on the closed eyelids. See *Better Eyesight,* November 1919.

Q–4. Is it possible to regain the ability to read without glasses when it fails after the age of forty, the sight at the distance being perfect? If so, how can this be done?

A–4. The failure of the sight at the near point after forty is due to the same cause as its failure at any other point and at any other age, namely strain. The sight can be restored by practicing at the near point the same methods used to improve the vision at the distance—palming, shifting, swinging, etc. The sight is never perfect at the distance when imperfect at the near point, but will become so when the sight at the near point has become normal.

Better Eyesight
December 1920—Vol. III, No. 6

GLAUCOMA NUMBER

GLAUCOMA: ITS CAUSE AND CURE

By W. H. Bates, M.D.

Glaucoma is a condition in which the eyeball becomes abnormally hard, and theories as to its cause are endless. The hardness is supposed to be due to a rise in intraocular pressure, and the other glaucoma symptoms, chief among which is an excavation of the optic nerve, forming in advanced cases a deep cup with overhanging edges, are supposed to be the results of this pressure. Yet all the symptoms commonly associated with increased tension have been found in eyes in which the tension was normal.

The increased tension is supposed to be due to an excess of fluid in the eyeball, and this is commonly attributed to an impeded outflow. The aqueous humor, which is secreted very rapidly [by the ciliary process—TRQ], is supposed to escape at the angle formed by the junction of the iris with the cornea, and in glaucoma it is believed that the iris adheres to the cornea so that the angle is obstructed. Yet it is a well-known fact that in many cases no such obstruction can be found.

For more than fifty years iridectomy held the field as the only treatment which gave any hope of relief in glaucoma.

The operation, which means the removal of a piece of the iris, was introduced by von Graefe, and often gives relief for a longer or shorter time. If the patient lives long enough, however, the condition always returns. I have seen this happen after the tension had been normal for fifteen years. It is a fact mentioned by all the textbooks, moreover, that it often fails to give even temporary relief, and sometimes the condition is made worse than it was before.

The beneficial results of the operation, when it does succeed, have never been satisfactorily explained, but the accepted opinion at the present time is that they are due to the formation of a scar which is more pervious to the fluids of the eye than the normal tissue, and the object of modern operations is to obtain such a scar. For this reason sclerotomy, usually performed by the method of Elliott has gained great vogue. A piece of the entire thickness of the sclera is removed, and thus a permanent fistula covered only by the conjunctiva is formed. Through this the fluids of the interior escape. Like iridectomy this operation sometimes succeeds temporarily, but, according to Elliott himself, it may fail to check the optic atrophy and decline of vision even when the relief of tension is complete.

Although it is the consensus of medical opinion that a glaucomatous eye must eventually be operated upon and that the sooner this is done the better, some men have attempted to hold the process at bay by the use of myotics. These drugs, by contracting the pupil and thus stretching the iris, are believed to draw the latter away from the "filtration angle" and allow the excess of fluid to escape. They are commonly employed for the purpose of giving temporary relief, but some specialists advise their continuous use. Posey claimed that such treatment gives a larger proportion of successes than iridectomy.

Until a few years ago I always treated glaucoma by the old methods, not knowing anything better to do; but I never used the Elliott operation, having early learned that it is very dangerous to allow the fluids of the eyeball to escape, and having seen glaucoma produced by fistula of the cornea. I would not have ventured to predict that the condition could be relieved by relaxation, and only learned by accident that it was amenable to such treatment.

On May 9, 1915, a patient (mentioned in "Blindness Relieved by a New Method," *New York Medical Journal,* February 3, 1917) came to me with a complication of diseases which had reduced the vision of the right eye to light perception and that of the left to 20/100 (the field being also contracted). She was fifty-four years old, and had been wearing since 1910 the following glasses: both eyes, convex 2.00 D. S. with convex 1.50 D. C. 90 degrees. As her pupils were much contracted, I prescribed atropine to dilate them, two grains to an ounce of normal salt solution, one drop three times a day.

On the afternoon of May 10, she had an attack of acute glaucoma in the left or better eye. As atropine and other mydriactics are thought sometimes to produce glaucoma, the fact that the disease attacked only one eye and, at that, the better of the two, is interesting. The condition got worse as the day advanced, and during the night the pain was so intense that the patient vomited repeatedly. The next morning she came to the office, and I noted that there was blood in the anterior chamber. The vision had been reduced to light perception, and the pain again produced vomiting. I prescribed eserine—two grains to the ounce, one drop three times a day. Afterward I visited her three or four times a day in her home, and as there had been no improvement, I increased the strength of the eserine solution to four grains to the ounce and alternated it with a three percent solution of pilocarpine, both of these drugs being myotics. Still there was no improvement, and after a few days I decided upon an operation. It was performed on May 15, and was accompanied by considerable hemorrhage. Mild hemorrhages also occurred at different times during the following week. When the blood cleared away, an opaque mass was left covering the pupil. On May 23, the tension was normal and there was no pain; but, owing to the opaque matter covering the pupil, there had been no improvement in the vision.

After the operation the patient resumed the relaxation treatment. Under its influence the vision of the right eye improved, and when a few weeks after the operation there was an increase of tension in this eye, it was at once relieved by palming. For some months the vision of the left eye remained unchanged, owing to the opacity of the pupil. Then the obstruction began to clear away and the vision improved. In a year there was normal vision in both eyes. From time to time during this period and up to the present time, the patient had attacks of increased tension in both eyes; but they were always relieved in a few minutes by palming.

Since then I have used the same treatment in many cases, and I have never seen one in which the pain and tension could not be relieved in a few minutes by palming, while permanent relief was obtained by more prolonged treatment.

One of the worst cases of glaucoma I ever met with came to me on February 2, 1920. The patient was sixty years old, and his vision in the right eye or better eye was only 20/100, with marked contraction of the field on the nasal side. In the left he had only light perception. The eyeballs felt as hard as the glass shell of an artificial eye which, technically, is tension plus 3. The glaucomatous excavation of the optic nerve was so marked that it seemed as if the whole nerve had been pushed backward. The patient had been under treatment a long time, but had received no benefit.

On March 2, after swinging and palming, the vision of the right eye was 20/20—while that of the left was 20/100 in the eccentric field. On March 4, the field of the left eye had improved, and by alternating the universal swing with palming he became able, for short periods, to read diamond type with the right eye at six inches. This was twelve days after he had begun the treatment. On March 7, he flashed 20/40 with the left eye, and by the aid of the universal swing read fine print at five inches with the right, while the field of both eyes was normal. For the first time in several years he became able to see the food on his plate. Previously he had had to be fed, which was very humiliating to him. He also became able to go about without an attendant, to attend to his correspondence at the office, and to read his letters without glasses. At this point he stopped the treatment against my advice, and I have not seen him since. He was greatly helped by the universal swing, which he practiced all day.

The truth about glaucoma is that it is a functional neurosis caused by strain, and as such is curable. You can produce hardness in a normal eye by having the patient strain to see and you can soften a glaucomatous eyeball by relief of strain. These changes are so rapid that no change in the contents of the eyeball could account for them. I therefore concluded, before I had any experimental evidence of the fact, that they were due to muscular action. Later I was able to produce glaucoma in a rabbit's eye by operations upon the muscles. I shortened the superior rectus by tucking, and thereby produced a tension of plus 1. I repeated the operation upon the superior oblique, and the tension increased to plus 2. I did the same to the inferior oblique, and the tension increased to the maximum, plus 3. All this time the tension of the other eyeball remained normal.

GETTING CURED OF GLAUCOMA

By F. T. Stewart

Editor's Note—*This patient when first seen was able to read 20/50 with each eye, but the right eye was absolutely blind on the nasal side, a vertical line dividing the seeing from the blind area. The tension of the right eye was usually greater than that of the left, but at times the reverse was the case, and for short periods the tension of both eyes was normal. He had been using myotics (drops which contract the pupil) for some time, but had obtained no benefit from them. His age was fifty-eight, and he was wearing the following glasses: distance, both eyes, convex 2.75 D. S.; reading, both eyes, convex 5.00 D. S. The improvement in his field since he has been under treatment has been very remarkable, as the accepted methods of treatment, even when the results are most favorable, are not expected to enlarge the field or even to prevent a further loss.*

In the summer of 1917 I had the first symptoms of glaucoma in the form of an attack of rainbow vision. I did not know what the symptoms meant, and was not alarmed; but I went to an optician and had my glasses changed, thinking the trouble was the consequence of eyestrain. The symptoms continued, however, and I went to another optician and had the glasses changed again. Still I was no better. Then I went to a succession of oculists, some six or seven, all of them being men of considerable eminence in the profession. The first two put drops in my eyes and examined my field, but did not tell me that I had glaucoma. It was only from the third, about a year and a half after the first symptoms appeared, that I learned what was the matter with me. The last began to talk operation, but I let him talk. I think I may claim to be as game as anyone about operations. When the doctors told me that they wanted to take my stomach out and put it back again, I said, "Go ahead." If they had told me that they wanted to take off my leg, I would probably have said the same thing. But when it came to letting anyone cut into my eye it was a different matter. About the first of last July the oculist, in whose care I then was, told me that my field was getting less. He asked me to come back in October, and said if the field continued to contract he would talk operation again.

Sometime previous to this an acquaintance who said that Dr. Bates had cured him of glaucoma gave me a copy of *Better Eyesight.* I did not become seriously interested at the time, but later I asked the man for details. He told me something about Dr. Bates' methods and said he not only had great faith in Dr. Bates, but that he was the only eye specialist in whom he did have any faith.

Finally, on September 11 of this year, I went to Dr. Bates.

He told me to stop the eyedrops and take off my glasses, which I did. Having worn the latter for twenty-five years, I had considerable difficulty at first in getting on without them; but after three or four days things began to go better, and before the end of the month I read the address on the Doctor's card without artificial aid. I could not have done this when I took off my glasses if a hundred million dollars had been at stake. I can now, six weeks after the beginning of the treatment, read ordinary print at twelve inches, and under favorable conditions can read diamond type at six inches or less. There has also been a considerable improvement in my field.

My progress has been slow, but it is sure, and I see no reason why it should not continue until I get a complete cure. I have spent many hours a day palming, and this, when it is successful, softens the eyeball and improves the sight very materially. I am also able to soften the eyeball simply by a thought—that is, by the memory of some object or incident. A white cloud, the blue sky, some incident of my boyhood or of a more recent period—anything, so long as it is remembered perfectly—has this extraordinary effect. Often when I wake in the morning my eyeballs are hard, but by the aid of my memory I am always able to soften them. One morning I woke at two o'clock and went to the bathroom. There, in accordance with a habit of mine, I washed my face in cold water. As I touched my eyeballs I was shocked to find how hard they were. They were like two rocks. Immediately I paid a mental visit to Van Cortland Park and began to examine the trees, noticing the texture of the bark, the gum oozing out of it, the outlines of the leaves, etc., and before I had reached the second tree the eyeballs were soft. Often since then I have resorted to the same expedient, and always with the same result. Fortunately I know the different kinds of trees very well, and my visits to the park are interesting as well as profitable.

On the streets and elsewhere I try to imagine that everything is moving, and as long as I am able to do this the eyeballs remain soft. Since I have been under treatment I have been trying to learn to sleep on my back, as the Doctor says that the body is always under a strain unless the spine is straight. When I am able to do this I waken without pain or hardness in the eyeballs.

Recently I sent one of Dr. Bates' reprints to the specialist who wanted to operate on me, and he said he was much interested.

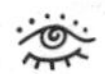

STORIES FROM THE CLINIC

No. 10: Absolute Glaucoma

By Emily C. Lierman

Editor's Note—*In absolute glaucoma there is no perception of light, and the condition is considered to be incurable. It may or may not be accompanied by pain, and in the latter case the only remedy is believed to be enucleation, or removal of the eye. So far as the editor is aware there is no case of absolute glaucoma on record in which the pain has been relieved, or any measure of sight restored, by any method except the one described below.*

A few months ago there came to the Clinic a woman of seventy-nine. At first glance one could see that she was a lady, and I guessed that at one time she had been very well off. As she stood apart from the rest of the patients waiting to be attended to she took not the slightest notice of what was going on around her, and occasionally I heard her moan with pain.

When at last Dr. Bates was able to examine her he found that she had glaucoma in both eyes, and that the right was stone-blind, possessing not even light perception. He turned her over to me, asking me to do what I could to help her and stop her pain. Fortunately I was able to find a stool for her, a rare thing at the Clinic, and placing it before a table upon which she could rest her elbows I showed her how to palm, which she did very readily. After a few minutes the pain ceased and the eyeballs became soft. I now told her to take down her hands, but she still kept her eyes shut. I thought this was because I had not told her to open them, but when I told her she might do so she asked, "Are you sure the pain will not come back if I open them. For many days I have suffered such constant pain that I cannot sleep at night, and now I feel such a sense of relief that I would really like to keep my eyes closed." "I don't think the pain will come back," I said, "and if it does you can palm again."

I now held a test card about two feet from her eyes and told her to cover her better eye and look at the card with the blind one. We had several visiting doctors at the Clinic that day, and Dr. Bates had told them about this case of absolute glaucoma. They were all standing by with Dr. Bates himself when I asked the patient to look at the card, and the excitement was intense when she said that she saw the large letter at the top.

"Oh, Doctor," I said, "she sees it!"

"Yes, I see it, I really see it," added the patient, scarcely able to credit her senses.

After a little more treatment I told her she must keep her eyes shut as much as possible when she was at home, and palm every minute she could get. I also told her never to look at any point more than a second, but to keep constantly shifting. She went away very happy and grateful for the pain had not come back.

The next time she came Dr. Bates treated her and was able to improve the vision of the right eye to 9/200, while that of the left eye improved to 9/40. He then turned her over to me I again. She was very happy and wanted to talk, which I let her do. She said she was living in a furnished room and that I hadn't any idea how worried she had been about going blind, because she had no one to look after her.

"But now," she added, "I have all sorts of hopes for the relief of my trouble, because you and Dr. Bates have done so much for me. Palming helps me so much that I am now able to sleep at night. I like to do it for hours at a time because it takes the terrible pain away."

I now told her to use her imagination to improve her sight and relieve the pain. Most of the Clinic patients become confused when I ask them to do this, but this dear old lady did not find it a bit difficult. I told her to palm, and then imagine a florist's window filled with flowers. Next I told her to imagine that she had entered the shop and was observing the flowers, and I called to her mind the red rose and the white rose, the carnation, the violet and other blossoms. Then I asked her if she could imagine the green fields in the country where the daisies grow, and she said, "Yes, and I can imagine that I am picking the daisies also."

I now told her to remove her hands from her eyes, and Dr. Bates was thrilled when she saw the "T" on the 30-line at ten feet. The patient herself laughed out loud and said, "I cannot believe it."

She came to the Clinic regularly, three days a week, for quite a while, and always happy because she was steadily improving. I was not prepared, therefore, to find her one day looking very much depressed. The trouble was that she had had a visitor who talked to her—or at her, I should say—for two long hours; this had upset her nerves so much that the pain had returned and her vision had been lowered; I pictured to myself what it must mean to listen to a steady stream of gossip for two hours, and my sight at once became imperfect. I told her what a dangerous thing it was for her to allow herself to be tortured in this way, and said that if her friends insisted upon talking to her for such a length of time she must keep her eyes closed as much as possible. Otherwise the strain would cause her to go blind. For a time she got along nicely. Then I left the city for a much-needed vacation, and while I was away I got word that she was getting worse. I came back to town and, as she was not able to come to the Clinic, I called upon her.

"Oh, nurse," she said as soon as she saw me, "my right eye pains me so that I think of nothing but death." Her thin face was lined with pain, and I could see that she was in agony. I began to talk to her about the days when she did not suffer, and how she had stopped the pain by remembering the daisies. She began to palm without my telling her to, and became able to imagine the daisy waving in the breeze. I asked her to imagine that her body was swinging with the flower. She did this, and in a few minutes her pain left her and she smiled.

"Now, isn't it strange," she remarked, "but I forgot all about using my imagination." She said that I had worked a miracle; but I explained that when she used her imagination she had to relax enough to relieve the strain in her eyes, and that had stopped the pain.

We often hear the remark, "This person makes me sick," or "That person makes me nervous," but it remained for my glaucoma patient to make me realize that these observations are literal statements of fact. All about the walls of her little room, which was very clean and sunshiny, were photographs of her children and their families. With great pride she named each one in turn, but when she came to the picture of a man and woman hanging a little apart from the rest, her tone changed.

"This is my daughter," she said of the woman, and I could see that she was very fond of her, but when she pointed to the man she said, "I cannot bear him. He makes me nervous and sick because he is not a good man."

She began to strain at once, and had to do some palming before I left to relieve her pain. Evidently it is important, if we want to avoid eyestrain, that we should keep away from the people we dislike, and think of them as little as possible.

I called on her a few times more, and by resting her eyes between each line of letters she became able to read 10/20 with the once blind eye and 10/10 with the other. The last time I saw her she was happy and comfortable.

Better Eyesight
January 1921—Vol. IV, No. 1

CATARACT NUMBER

CATARACT: ITS CAUSE AND CURE

By W. H. Bates, M.D.

Cataract is a condition in which the lens becomes opaque. It is commonly associated with advancing years, but may occur at any age. It may also be congenital (present at birth). The opacities take many different forms, and may occur in a hard or a soft lens. According to the orthodox teaching the condition is incurable except by the removal of the lens, although in the earlier stages it is sometimes ameliorated by means of drops that expand the pupil and by glasses. The textbooks are full of statements to this effect.

Yet it is perfectly well known that cataract does sometimes recover spontaneously. Many such cases are on record, and probably most ophthalmologists who have been practicing for any length of time have seen them. Fifteen or twenty years.ago, when I was assistant surgeon at the New York Eye and Ear Infirmary, I collected, at the request of the executive surgeon, Dr. Henry D. Noyes, a large number of records of such cases.

The removal of the lens, when it is soft, is usually accomplished by the operation of needling, whereby the tissues are broken up so that they may be absorbed. A hard lens is extracted through an opening at the margin of the cornea, and the best results are believed to be obtained when the opacity has become complete. Otherwise, part of the lens substance is liable to be left behind and cause trouble. Thus the patient may be kept for years in a condition of semi-blindness.

The results of the operation are not always as satisfactory as might be desired. A considerable proportion of patients regain what is considered to be normal acuteness of vision with very strong glasses, and the results are considered good when they become able to read large print at the near point and 20/50 at the distance. The patient is obliged usually to have two sets of glasses, one for distant vision to replace the focusing power of the lost lens, and the other for reading to compensate for the impairment of the accommodative power which usually follows the operation.

This impairment of accommodative power is not due to the removal of the lens, which has nothing to do with accommodation, but to the fact that the patient strains so to see that the muscles that control the shape of the eyeball fail to act properly. In some cases it is regained after the patient becomes accustomed to the new situation, without treatment, and in rare cases patients have become able to do without glasses entirely because the eyeball elongated sufficiently to compensate for the loss of the lens.

I began to treat cataract by the operative method because I did not know anything better to do. Then I learned from Dr. James E. Kelly of New York that incipient cases would yield to hygienic treatment. My first inkling of the value of central fixation in such conditions came to me through a patient who had incipient cataract in one eye and hypermetropia (farsightedness) in the other. By the time the error of refraction had been relieved the cataract had disappeared.

After this I had many similar experiences, but it did not occur to me that a ripe cataract, or a congenital cataract, could be cured by this or any other treatment.

In 1912, however, a young girl of seventeen came to my Clinic with the left eye enucleated and a congenital cataract in the right. The left had been operated upon for the same condition and, having become infected, was taken out to save the better eye. The latter having recently become worse, the patient had come to have it operated upon. Before performing the operation I thought it best to treat her by the method of relaxation, for the purpose of improving the condition of the eye as much as possible so that the operation might have a better chance of success. To my surprise the vision improved and kept on improving, until in three months it was normal and the cataract had disappeared.

One day, some half a dozen years later, a lady, fifty-five years old, came to me to be cured of presbyopia (old-age sight). Her distant vision in the right eye was 20/20, and in the left she had only light perception. This was due to the presence, in this eye, of a mature cataract. I began to treat her by the aid of the memory and imagination for presbyopia and, in order to prove to her the relation between these mental faculties and the state of the vision, I asked her to cover her right eye and note that she could not remember or imagine a black period as well as when it was open. She replied that she could, and I said it was impossible. She insisted that, nevertheless, she did it. Thinking that at the near point she would realize the imperfection of the sight of the left eye more clearly than at the distance, I brought the card closer and said, "You cannot remember the period while looking at this card with your good eye covered." She replied, "I can; and what is more, I can read the card," which she did, both at two feet and at twenty.

This was naturally a shock to me. It did not seem to me possible that a mature cataract could melt away in such a short time, but the ophthalmoscope confirmed the statements of the patient. When she remembered a period perfectly I could see the optic nerve and other details of the eyeground. Since then I have cured a great many similar cases, one of the most remarkable having been reported in *Better Eyesight,* June 1920.

I had another shock when a few months ago a traumatic cataract began to melt away under the influence of relaxation treatment. The patient came to my Clinic with an eye which had been completely blind for four years from traumatic cataract complicated with detachment of the retina. The opacity completely covered the pupil, and with the ophthalmoscope no red reflex (light reflected from the retina) could be seen. After a few treatments the patient became able to see the movements of his hand on the temporal side. Later he became able to see the hand in all parts of the field. Now he is beginning to read.

Another case of the cure of traumatic cataract is reported in the following article.

These cures are very remarkable. A traumatic cataract is one which follows an injury (trauma) to the lens, the opacity being due largely to the formation of connective tissue in the pupil and, in advance of the event, I should have pronounced the cure of such a condition impossible, although I had previously demonstrated that when patients practice central fixation connective tissue is absorbed in the optic nerve, retina and cornea. In the retina and optic nerve the circulation can be seen to improve as the connective tissue disappears, and I can only assume that this is the cause of its disappearance.

Equally remarkable is the cure of diabetic cataract without relief of the disease. A patient with such a cataract came to me on April 29, 1918, her vision being 10/200 in the right eye and 20/30 in the left. She had been seen a year and a half previously by a well-known ophthalmologist who had advised several operations, but, fortunately, she had not submitted to them. By the aid of palming, swinging, imagination and memory, her vision improved rapidly. On May 15 that of the left eye was 20/70, while later it became normal. On May 22 the vision of the right became normal temporarily. Since then she has had slight relapses in the right eye, but few or none in the left. The general diabetic condition has not changed, and it is remarkable that when it is at its worst there is very little lowering of the vision.

It is quite evident from the foregoing facts that the cause of cataract (other than traumatic) is strain, and I have found much other evidence, both clinical and experimental, to the same effect. I have not been able to produce cataract in a normal eye by strain, but in a cataractous eye I have seen the opacity come and go according as the mind of the patient was relaxed or under a strain. In one of these cases the opacity was so dense that no red reflex could be seen. Another doctor who was present looked at the eye and made the same observation. I asked the patient to remember a swinging "O" perfectly black, with a perfectly white center. This meant perfect relaxation, and when she did it I saw some of the details of the retina and the optic nerve, while the other doctor again confirmed my observation. I then asked her to think of the "O" as stationary, with gray outlines and a clouded center. This meant a great strain, and while she did it neither I nor my colleague could see the red reflex. In experimental animals I have produced cataract by operating upon the external eye muscles in such a way as to increase their pressure, and have then relieved it by cutting these muscles.

TRAUMATIC CATARACT DISAPPEARS

By Margaret Downie

Editor's Note—*This patient was first seen on October 18, 1920, when her vision in the right eye was 20/100 and in the left 14/200. She had compound myopic astigmatism in the right eye, and the pupil of the left eye was covered by a traumatic cataract which prevented ophthalmoscopic examination of the eyeground. On December 6, the cataract had been absorbed except for a spot about the size of a pinhead, and I was able to see the optic nerve and the retina clearly. With a glass to replace the focusing power of the lens—convex 7.00 D. S. with convex 3.00 D. C. 75 degrees—she was able with this eye to read 20/40, and on the same day, after palming and swinging, she obtained temporary normal vision in both eyes, the left eyeball having elongated sufficiently to compensate for the loss of the lens. The fact that astigmatism should have developed in the right eye after the injury to the left is interesting, as astigmatism has been supposed, until recently, to be congenital.*

When I was thirteen years old a bullet from an airgun, rebounding from a tree, struck my left eye and injured the lens. This resulted in the formation of a cataract which was operated upon three times. After the third operation about one-third of the cataract remained, but the doctor was afraid to operate again. I was now able with this eye to distinguish, with the aid of a strong glass, only the outlines of nearby objects.

Previous to the accident my eyes had been straight, and the vision of both normal, so far as I was aware. After the last operation, however, I found myself unable to read writing on the blackboard at school. I went to the specialist who had performed the operations, and he was astounded to find that I had a bad case of astigmatism in the good eye. He gave me the following glass: convex 3.00 D. C. 105 degrees with concave 2.50 D. C. 15 degrees. Later my left eye began to turn out.

I wore my glasses constantly, putting them on the first thing in the morning and taking them off the last thing at night. I went swimming with them, and if they were lost or broken I remained in my room until they were found or repaired. My condition caused me much unhappiness and I was particularly disturbed about the squint. I wrote to every medical journal that I knew about and to many other publications, asking if there was any cure for squint; but none of them was able to suggest anything but an operation. A few months ago I happened to hear about Dr. Bates, and I resolved to see him as soon as an opportunity offered. At the beginning of the season I came to New York from my home in Texas to study music, but with Dr. Bates in the background of my mind. Nevertheless I did not look him up immediately.

One day in the elevator of a department store my glasses were swept from my face, disappearing as completely as if they had never existed. I went to the Lost Property Office, but after waiting there a long time failed to recover them. It was a horrible experience, and the realization of my helplessness without glasses depressed me terribly. However, as it resulted in my looking up Dr. Bates immediately, it was a good thing.

I went to him with the hope that he might be able to cure my squint and astigmatism, but I never dreamed that he could cure the cataract also. When he told me he could do so I hardly knew what to think, but I resolved to do everything I could to help him cure me. I carried out the swinging treatment so vigorously that I used to get dizzy and fall over on my bed. Of course I wasn't doing it right, but the Doctor had told me to swing and I was determined to do so. I was positively terrified when he told me to palm and remember all sorts of strange things, such as the letter "F" on a piece of white starch, because I thought he was trying to hypnotize me, but I did my best, nevertheless, to carry out his instructions. Later I bought and read all the back numbers of the magazine, and learned the scientific principles on which the treatment is based.

My eyesight is now steadily improving, and I intend to keep up the treatment until I have normal vision. I have given up the music for the time being—my eyes are more important, ten times more important—and the ridicule of my friends does not disturb me. As long as that old cataract continues to melt away nothing else matters.

In addition to the improvement in my eyesight I have noticed an improvement in my memory. My memory for the things I learned out of books at school was always poor, while my memory for music has always been exceptionally good. I suppose the difference was due to the fact that one set of impressions reached me through my eyes, and the other through my ears. Now that my vision is improving I can remember the things that I see better.

I wish everyone could know of this remarkable method of curing defects of vision. I know in the end it must surmount all opposition, but meantime how many persons as afflicted as I once was will remain unhelped! It is right that we should be dubious of the new, but to hang so tightly to tradition as the medical profession seems to do makes progress unnecessarily hard.

INCIPIENT CATARACT RELIEVED

By C. L. Steenson, M.D., New York

Editor's Note—*This patient when first seen had a vision of 20/200 in each eye, and was wearing for distant vision the following glasses: right eye, concave 6.00 D. S. with 1.00 D. C. 90 degrees; left eye, 10.00 D. S. with 1.00 D. C. 60 degrees. Owing to the presence of incipient cataract in each eye these lenses improved his vision only 20/50 in the right eye and 20/100 in the left. For reading, his glasses were three diopters weaker. He now has flashes of normal vision. He was helped most by the use of his imagination.*

Since boyhood—I am now sixty-five—I have had myopia and astigmatism, for the correction of which I have worn glasses and spectacles. About two years ago cataract developed in my right eye, and a few months later in my left eye. Both were in mild degree, but still bad enough to seriously obscure the field of vision. I had previously been annoyed by vitreous opacities which made little black spots dance in the field of vision [floating specks—TRQ]. I also suffered from frequent severe headaches. My glasses were often changed without much relief.

About November 1 of this year (1920) I consulted Dr. Bates, of whom I had heard much and favorably. His methods of treatment seemed exceedingly rational, and he gave me great hopes of getting rid of my eye troubles. First of all he made me discard my glasses which, at first, seemed rather hard, but to which I have gradually become reconciled. Through what I would call a system of progressive education of sight, I have now almost got rid of the myopia, the vitreous opacities do not bother me any more, and apparently the cataracts are disappearing by degrees. The headaches have also disappeared. I have resumed, to a great extent, the literary and research work on which I have been engaged since my retirement from active practice, and I have no doubt that, ultimately, I shall be in possession of full visual power. Upon my future progress I will report at a later date.

STORIES FROM THE CLINIC
No. 11: A Case of Cataract
By Emily C. Lierman

One day last July a man of forty came to the Clinic suffering from cataract and a complication of other troubles. As I approached him he was palming. This was an unusual thing for a stranger to do, but he evidently thought that if covering the eyes with the palms was good for others it might help him also. I stood before him and said, "Can I help you?"

He paid no attention to me whatever and I soon discovered that he was deaf, so deaf that one had almost to scream into his left or better ear to make him hear. When I had at last succeeded in making him understand me he asked, "Is it possible that you will be able to do anything for me?" I answered, "I am going to try, with your help." Then I said I wanted to know something about the history of his case, and this is what he told me:

At the age of six he fell down a flight of stairs and struck his forehead on a newel post, severing an artery in the head. Later, when it was noted that his sight was deficient, physicians attributed the condition to this fall. During the thirty-four subsequent years he had been treated by many New York physicians, both at their offices and clinics. During that period he had been blind three times, and surgical treatment had been repeatedly necessary. As a boy he could never see a blackboard at school, and could read but little. Between his twenty-first and his thirty-fifth year he had enjoyed the best vision of his life; but for the past five years his sight had been steadily declining, and several doctors had told him that this would continue until he became completely blind. He was now practically blind in one eye so far as useful vision was concerned. I tested his sight and found that he could count his fingers at about three feet with the right eye, and with the left could see only the movements of his hand. Dr. Bates had previously examined him and had found that he had an inflammatory cataract in the left eye, together with other inflammatory conditions.

I told him to palm again and he complained that he saw all sorts of bright colors, and that these disturbed him very much. I then told him to remove his hands from his eyes and look at the large letter on the test card, which I held a foot away from him. After he had tried a few times he was able to remember the letter with his eyes closed; then the bright colors faded away, and after palming for fifteen minutes his vision improved from 1/200 to 1/50 in the right eye, while in the left he became able to count my fingers at three feet. Next Clinic day he became able to read 3/30 with the right eye and 1/10 with the left, while at the end of two weeks the vision of the right eye had improved to 3/10 and of the left to 3/70. At the same time his general health had improved so much that he asked me if I had time to let him tell me about it. I told him that I would be very glad to hear the story, and what he had to say interested me so much that I thought the readers of *Better Eyesight* might be interested also.

"For many years," he related, "I have suffered from insomnia, and in recent months it has been nothing unusual for me to remain awake the entire night. Frequently I stay up all night, realizing the futility of trying to induce sleep. A short time ago I did this twice in a single week. When I do sleep, my slumber has been very light and disturbed by the wildest imaginable dreaming—fires, murders, hair-breadth escapes, etc. As a result of the insomnia and eye-strain I had frequently splitting headaches, sometimes every day, and sometimes even twice a day. From these I could secure relief only by the use of what I knew to be harmful medicines. Since I came to you I have been sleeping very much better, the dreams have become much less disturbing, and the headaches have practically ceased."

Hearing this, I was encouraged to try to do even more for him; so I handed him a test card, and asked him to look at a small letter, close his eyes and remember it, and then imagine it blacker and clearer than he saw it. He was able to do this, and the constant twitching of his eyelids ceased. For a moment I forgot that he was deaf and said in an even voice, "How do your eyes feel now?" He heard me, and answered, "They feel so rested just now, I do not feel that I have eyes at all, but am seeing without them."

He came three days every week for three months, and then as he improved he came less frequently. When I last saw him he was able, with his left eye, to read 3/10 at times, and with his right 5/10, while his hearing had improved so much that I was able to talk into his better ear without raising my voice much above my ordinary conversational tone. At the same time he had been relieved of head noises, including a drumming in the ears which, he said, had often continued from three to ten days. When he first came he could not go about alone, and always walked like an intoxicated person, for which he was frequently taken. When he first left the Clinic I noticed that he bumped against the benches and he told me that the condition had been attributed by physicians whom he had consulted to incipient locomotor ataxia. After his first visit, however, he never bumped into the furniture, and before he left us his walk was almost normal.

Better Eyesight
February 1921—Vol. IV, No. 2

PAIN NUMBER

THE PREVENTION AND CONTROL OF PAIN BY THE MIND

Anyone who has normal vision can demonstrate in a few moments that when the memory is perfect no pain is felt, and can produce pain by an attempt to keep the attention fixed on a point. To do this proceed as follows:

Look at a black letter, close the eyes and remember it. Look at the letter again and again, closing the eyes and remembering it. Repeat until the memory is equal to the sight. Now press the nail of one finger against the tip of another. If the letter is remembered perfectly no pain will be felt. With practice it may become possible to remember the letter with the eyes open.

Remember the letter imperfectly, with blurred edges and clouded openings, and again press the nail of one finger against the tip of another. In this case it will be found impossible to continue the pressure for more than a moment on account of the pain.

Try to remember one point of a letter continuously. It will be found impossible to do so, and if the effort is continued long enough pain will be produced.

Try to look continuously at one point of a letter or other object. If the effort is continued long enough, pain will be produced.

PAIN: ITS CAUSE AND CURE

By W. H. Bates, M.D.

Pain is supposed to be a beneficent provision on the part of nature for advising us of injurious processes going on in the body, but, like many of nature's arrangements, it is a very clumsy one. Many of our most serious diseases are quite painless in their early stage (the only time when the warning of pain would be of any use), while a physiological process like childbirth is accompanied by such severe pain that the pangs of the woman in travail have become proverbial. Pain also occurs with no local cause whatever, being purely a creation of the mind, and it has a very destructive effect upon the body, not infrequently causing death and more often handicapping the organism in its attempts to recover from the condition that caused it. Nature's protective mechanism is, in fact, a two-edged sword striking both ways, and its control is one of the most serious problems that the medical profession has to deal with.

There has been much discussion as to the nature of pain and the mode by which it is produced, one school holding that there are special nerves for its transmission and another that it is merely the expression of a certain grade of irritation. Whatever may be said in favor of either of these points of view, it can be demonstrated that pain occurs only when the mind is under a strain and is immediately relieved when the strain is relieved. This strain may be due to a local cause, or it may occur without any local cause whatever.

That pain can be produced voluntarily by the mind has long been known. When I was a student at the College of Physicians and Surgeons, Dr. T. Gaillard Thomas used to tell us that pain could be produced in the little finger, or any other part of the body, simply by concentrating the mind upon it. Since then I have repeatedly demonstrated that pain can be produced by such a simple thing as imagining a letter or object imperfectly, or trying to look at a point for an appreciable length of time. I never knew these experiments to fail when patients could be induced to make them; but they are so uncomfortable that few are willing to do so. A physician under treatment for imperfect sight boasted that he had never had a headache or pain in his eyes in his life. I told him that I could easily show him how to produce such a pain, and that it would do him good to have one. After a week of talk he consented to make the experiment, and in a few minutes he had acquired a headache that was more interesting than pleasant. He did it by trying to look fixedly at a point. This effect was purely mental. It was not the physical strain of looking at a point that produced the pain, because there was no physical strain, the eye being incapable of looking at a point. It was the mental effort of trying to do what was impossible.

As pain can be produced by the mind without any local cause, so it can be prevented or relieved by the mind, no matter how great the local irritation may be. In other words pain is a mental interpretation of certain stimuli, and under certain circumstances such stimuli are not interpreted as pain. This, too, has long been known, there being cases on record in which individuals have possessed the power of preventing pain to an extraordinary extent. I may claim to have discovered, however, that everyone may become the possessor of this power.

It is only when the mind is in an abnormal condition that pain can be felt, or even imagined, and irritations of the nerves are followed by pain only when such irritations produce mental strain. If the mind is not disturbed by them, there is no pain, and therefore, by learning to avoid this disturbance pain can be prevented or relieved.

As the mind is always at rest when the memory is perfect, the mental condition necessary for the prevention and relief of pain can be obtained by the use of the memory. One of the simplest things to remember is a small black spot or period, and under certain circumstances anyone may become able to remember such an object. This cannot be done, it is true, at the actual moment of suffering, but, fortunately, pain is never continuous. One can see, or hear, or smell continuously; but one cannot feel pain continuously. There are always moments of freedom, and during these intermissions one can get control of the memory. In this way the pain of glaucoma, one of the most terrible conditions known to medical science, has been repeatedly relieved (see *Better Eyesight,* December 1920.) Many cases of trigeminal neuralgia have been cured after various operations commonly resorted to for the relief of this condition had failed, and the pain of childbirth and of operations has been prevented.

Persons with perfect sight never have any difficulty in preventing pain by the aid of the memory. Persons whose sight is not normal have more difficulty because imperfect sight is the result of mental strain, and it is sometimes very difficult to relieve this strain. With the help of a person who has normal sight and understands the use of the memory for this purpose, however, it can always be done.

RELIEF OF TIC DOULOUREUX

By Evelyn M. Thomson

I do not remember a time when I was able to see comfortably. At fifteen, following an attack of grippe, I began to have so much trouble with my eyes that I was taken out of school, and the late Dr. Henry D. Noyes gave me my first glasses. From that time on I wore glasses constantly, with many changes ordered by many different specialists, until I came to Dr. Bates. Sometimes they helped me; but I never was able to do any near work without discomfort, and I could not play tennis because it hurt my eyes to follow the ball.

When I was eighteen a polyp in the right middle ear broke through the drum, and a great quantity of pus poured out. This was the beginning of a long series of treatment and operations, during which I suffered increasing pain on the right side of my head, and which left me with no bones in the middle ear and an opening in the drum. After the last operation I was ill for nine months, and for a much longer time there was weakness and loss of sensibility on the left side of the body.

In 1905 I had trouble with the antrum on the left side of the face, and in order to release the pus which had collected there, a wisdom tooth was extracted, the wound being kept open for three months. A second tooth was then extracted, and one by one all the teeth on the left side of the upper jaw were taken out. Then the dentist declined to extract any more, saying that it was only increasing the trouble, instead of relieving it.

From the beginning of this condition I had a continual pain in the left side of the face, and this developed into what is known as *tic douloureux,* a painful contraction of the facial muscles, which continued for fifteen years. Everything possible was resorted to for the relief of this trouble except drugs which I refused to take, and nerve-cutting which I refused to submit to. Spinal treatment gave me more help than anything else.

From 1914 to 1918, in spite of the discomfort resulting from the use of my eyes at the near point, I read aloud for many hours every day. At the end of this time my eyes went to pieces completely. All winter I went every week to a specialist for treatment, but received no benefit. Then I went to another specialist. He gave me new glasses, but these seemed only to make the condition worse. I could not read without pain in my eyes and a contraction of the nerves and muscles on the left side of my face. At night the lid of the left eye became partially paralyzed, so that I had to force the eye open when I wakened and was afraid the time might come when I would not be able to keep it open. On the street the muscles on the left side of the face contracted all around the eye, across the bridge of the nose, and toward the temple. This I attributed to the increase of eyestrain by the wind and light.

On April 22 of last year I went to Dr. Bates in despair. My eyesight was getting worse from month to month, and the facial condition seemed also to be getting worse. In addition I suffered from noises in my left ear so loud and continuous that it seemed at times as if the top of my head would blow off.

Palming was the first thing Dr. Bates told me to do. At first I saw all sorts of lights. Then I saw gray, and at last I became sufficiently relaxed to see black. I found the use of the imagination and memory a great aid in palming. I visualized the out-of-doors and the things I had seen in my travels. This produced relaxation, and I forgot the pain and the noise in my ear. I also found it a help to be read to while palming. The universal swing relieved the tension which I had always experienced on the street.

For some months my eyes did not seem to respond to the treatment. The first intimation of gain was the natural opening of my left eye at night. Next my right eye, which had been very numb and blurred, began to have a feeling of life. Later I experienced an increase of pain in the center of both eyes. Strange to say, this encouraged me, for the new pain was quite different from the dull ache I had had before, and made me feel that life was returning to my eyes.

One day, when the pulling of the facial muscles was very severe, Dr. Bates asked me to flash a little card which he held close to my nose. This was very unpleasant at first; but suddenly the muscles relaxed, the pain in my face and eyes ceased, and I saw things at the distance clearly. It was only a flash; but after that I seemed to understand better the goal toward which I was working. Since then I have often obtained relief in this way. These glimpses of paradise are what has sustained me through months of treatment which would otherwise have been unbearably monotonous.

My vision has improved slowly, but the progress has been a constant source of excitement to me. When I first saw the faces of my friends clearly I rejoiced, and I cannot describe the feeling of relief that came to me when the dishes on the table ceased to hurt me, as all near objects had previously done. The light and the color I now see are a revelation to me. I had been told that printer's ink was black, but until I went to Dr. Bates I never saw it so. Neither did I ever see anything like the white I see now. I have a delightful time reading the signs in the subway and enjoying their colors. Not only in color, but in form, things look different to me. Instead of being flat, as they once were, they seem to have a fourth dimension. [3-D vision.—TRQ] Distant objects appear surprisingly near. Sitting in the balcony at a concert one afternoon, the orchestra seemed to be almost in my lap. In the dress circle at the opera I seemed to be almost on the stage. When I wore glasses the stage was always miles away. My vision is not normal yet; I cannot read print with comfort. But after such marvelous improvement I feel sure that this will soon come. As for the facial pain and contraction, they are practically cured. When the trouble returns, as it sometime does, I know how to relieve it.

I am very glad to have an opportunity to tell this story, and I wish I knew how to make it known to all who are suffering from the pain of defective eyesight, or of facial neuralgia, that these conditions can be cured by relaxation, and that the dreadful operations which are resorted to in the case of the neuralgia are unnecessary.

STORIES FROM THE CLINIC
No. 12: The Relief of Pain
By Emily C. Lierman

In March 1919, an Austrian woman, thirty-seven years old, came to the Clinic. She was suffering from myopia with great pain in her eyes and head, and looked so sad that one could not imagine her smiling. At the age of two she had become totally blind after a fever, and had remained so for a year and a half, during all of which time she suffered continual pain in her eyes. When her sight returned, strong glasses were given to her, but they did not relieve her pain. Neither did the glasses given to her later by various physicians. Finally an optician, finding that the glasses he had given her did not help her, suggested that she should try Dr. Bates and our Clinic.

At her first visit her pain was relieved by palming, and her vision improved from 5/70 to 5/40. She was so pleased that she smiled and kissed my hands. The pain had made her sick at her stomach most of the time, she said, so that she was often unable to retain her food, and no day was she ever free from it.

I told her to continue the palming at home, and to keep it up for an hour at a time whenever possible. For a while she got on very nicely. Her vision improved to 10/40, and whenever she felt the pain coming on she palmed, invariably obtaining relief.

Then came a day when I found her with tears in her eyes. She had had a sleepless night, she explained, and had suffered so intensely that her family was frightened. Her eyes felt as though sand was pouring out of them onto the pillow. I asked her if her eyes were still paining her, and she answered tearfully, "Yes."

I placed her comfortably on a stool, and while her eyes were covered I began to talk to her about her children. She soon forgot her pain in telling me what beautiful eyes her baby had, how thrilled the family had been when the first tooth appeared, and so on. When she uncovered her eyes the most remarkable change had come over her face. All traces of pain had disappeared, and she smiled.

One day after she had been coming to the Clinic for a year or more she was arranging to send some money to Austria and trying to fill out the necessary papers. As she was about to write her mother's name everything before her became a blank, and she experienced an intense pain accompanied by a burning sensation in her eyes. She was so frightened that she wanted to cry, but suddenly she thought about the Clinic and how her pain had been relieved by the palming. She covered her eyes with the palms of her hands for a little while, and then the pain became less and the questions on the blank began to clear up. When she tried to write, however, everything became a blank once more. Again she palmed, and this time her sister, who was with her, reminded her that she must palm for a longer time if she wanted to get results. She then palmed for fifteen minutes, her sister encouraging her as she did so. When she removed her hands from her eyes the print before her appeared perfectly distinct, she wrote the necessary answers without any difficulty, and had no more trouble with her eyes that day. She was extremely happy when she told me this. To think that she had been able to improve her sight and relieve her pain without assistance thrilled her.

When I last saw her, six months ago, her vision was 10/10 without glasses, and she had no pain.

BACKACHE CURED BY CENTRAL FIXATION

By Bessie T. Brown

Editor's Note—*The editor is much pleased to be able to publish Ms. Brown's report of the simultaneous relief of her astigmatism and the backache from which she had suffered so long. It was from her he learned the value of central fixation in relieving pain in parts of the body other than the head and eyes, and he takes great pleasure in giving her credit for the discovery.*

It is about six, or perhaps seven, years ago that I first consulted Dr. Bates concerning my eyes. I had been wearing glasses to correct astigmatism for five years. During those years of "correction" my eyes seldom gave me a comfortable day. I spared them in every way, using them as little as possible. My sight was not noticeably impaired, but I will cite a few of the many discomforts from which I suffered.

A smarting sensation in the eyes was nearly always present; also a general lassitude and a dull ache in the back. The last mentioned was never attributed to eyestrain, but to many other causes, and was treated accordingly by a physician, but without results. I was obliged to retire early every night in order to forget my pains in sleep, only to wake in the morning with eyes which felt as though a cinder from every chimney in New York City had dropped into them. This was because we strain our eyes during our sleep as well as during waking hours. To watch a stage or movie was torture; and when driving or riding on railroad trains I would keep my eyes closed, only taking occasional peeps at the passing landscape. I could not endure the glare of the sunlight on the beach or pavements, and artificial lights on the streets, in the shops or theatre, were an abomination.

My first glasses were prescribed by an optometrist, and I received no relief while wearing them. Friends advised me to consult an eye specialist of high standing in New York. I did so. He said after examination that he was not surprised that I had received no benefit from the glasses which I was wearing, and proceeded to fit me with what he considered to be the correct lenses. I was supremely happy for a few days, in the anticipation of enjoying perfect comfort as soon as I should become accustomed to the new lenses.

But alas! My happiness was short-lived. The glasses prescribed by the eminent physician gave no more satisfaction than those from the optometrist.

I returned to see the doctor after a few weeks and complained that his glasses had not helped me. He made another examination and said that he could make a slight change in the lenses, but it would not be worthwhile to do so. He also said that my eyes were not working together properly, but this condition would improve with my general health. However my health did not improve under his treatment. I felt that I was doomed to a life of suffering and tried to become reconciled to my fate.

Hope was revived a few months later when I heard of Dr. Bates and his cure of eyestrain without glasses. Dr. Bates took possession of my glasses upon my first visit to him, and I have not worn them since.

He told me to do [sunning—TRQ].

The glare of sunlight on the ground ceased to worry me and became as delightful as the pale moonlight. When the sun failed to shine, or was not convenient, I practiced at a large incandescent electric light, and very soon the artificial lights troubled me no more than the stars which twinkle in the heavens at night; and that reminds me that Dr. Bates told me that the apparent twinkle of the stars is only in the eye of the beholder.

After a few weeks of treatment I forgot to spare my eyes, as had been my habit for years. I could read or sew until midnight if I wished, and began to go out evenings and enjoy life like a normal human being. As I write tonight, the clock is striking eleven and my eyes are feeling fine and dandy, although I have been using them constantly all day sewing and embroidering.

My animation and efficiency have greatly increased. Friends have remarked that I am a new woman and continue to congratulate me upon my youthful appearance.

An acquaintance of mine, whom I had not met since I stopped wearing glasses, failed to recognize me a few days ago at the house of a mutual friend. "Why," she exclaimed, "the Ms. Brown whom I used to know was an extremely pale and worn-looking creature." Through relaxation the expression of eyes and face have become greatly changed.

I had been under treatment with Dr. Bates about three months when suddenly one day I noticed that my old and constant companion, the backache, was no longer with me, and it has never returned.

At the present time when I feel the strain coming into my eyes, I rest them by palming and remembering or recalling different familiar objects—the colors of my frocks, recalled one at a time, or the forms and shapes of pieces of china which are in constant use in my home, or the color of the eyes of members of the family. It seems marvelous to be able to go about in the shops for a good part of the day and then keep my eyes open and enjoy to the fullest extent a performance or social affair in the evening. Also, what a delight to ride through the country and feast my eyes with comfort upon the beauty of the passing landscape.

Better Eyesight
March 1921—Vol. IV, No. 3

BLINDNESS NUMBER

HOW TO OBTAIN PERCEPTION OF LIGHT IN BLINDNESS

Two things have always brought perception of light to blind patients. One is palming, and the other is the swing.

In palming, the patient should remember that this does not bring relief unless mental relaxation is obtained, as evidenced by the disappearance of the white, gray and other colors which most blind people see at first with their eyes closed and covered.

The swing may take two forms:

1. Let the patient stand with feet apart, and sway the body, including the head and eyes from side to side, while shifting the weight from one foot to the other.

2. Let him move his hand from one side to the other in front of his face, all the time trying to imagine that he sees it moving. As soon as he becomes able to do this it can be demonstrated that he really does see the movement.

Simple as these measures are, they have always, either singly or together, brought relaxation and with it perception of light from fifteen minutes or less to half an hour.

BLINDNESS: ITS CAUSE AND CURE

By W. H. Bates, M.D.

As ordinarily used, the word blindness signifies a degree of defective sight which unfits the patient for any occupation requiring the use of the eyes. Scientifically it means a state in which there is no perception of light. Speaking of this condition in his *Cause and Prevention of Blindness,* Fuchs tells us that except in extraordinarily rare cases it is incurable, and this is the accepted opinion of ophthalmology today.

The facts that have come to me during thirty-five years of ophthalmological practice have convinced me that the above statement should be reversed, and made to read, "Except in extraordinarily rare cases blindness is curable." In fact, unless the eyeball has been removed from the head, I should be unwilling to set any limits whatever to the possibility of relieving this greatest of human ills, for I have never seen a case of injury or disease of the eye which was sufficient to prevent improvement of vision. In all cases of blindness, whatever their cause, a mental strain has been demonstrated, and when this strain has been relieved perception of light has always been obtained.

Even when the eyeball has been so shrunken that the patient scarcely seemed to have an eye, sight has been restored. In one such case the cornea of the left eye had shrunk to an eighth of an inch in diameter and only a suggestion of the sclera was visible, while the right eye was reduced to a quarter of its normal size and showed only a hazy cornea and a blurred piece of iris with no pupil. The patient was ten years old and the condition of her right eye was congenital; that of the left was due to an inflammation which she suffered when she was a year old. From that time, she had had no perception of light; but in fifteen minutes she became able to see the furniture of the room indistinctly and to imagine that it was swinging. In spite of this remarkable demonstration of what could be accomplished by relaxation, her parents did not bring her again.

Atrophy of the optic nerve is one of a considerable number of diseases, like detachment of the retina, irido-cyclitis and absolute glaucoma, which have been placed beyond the pale of hope by the science of ophthalmology. Yet persons with atrophy of the optic nerve sometimes have normal vision, and persons blind from this cause sometimes recover spontaneously. At the New York Eye and Ear Infirmary thirty years ago, a patient was exhibited who had all the symptoms of atrophy of the optic nerve, but who nevertheless possessed perfect sight. The case was exhibited later at the Manhattan Eye and Ear Hospital, the New York Ophthalmological Society, and the Ophthalmological Section of the New York Academy of Medicine. Later I saw several similar cases; but when a colored woman came to my Clinic a few years ago with atrophy of the optic nerve, it did not occur to me that it would be possible to help her. Not knowing what to do, I asked her to sit down while I attended to some other patients; meanwhile my assistant, Ms. Lierman, who tells the rest of the story in a later article, got hold of her and made her see. Later many cases were relieved. A few obtained normal vision, but most of them did not have the courage to continue the treatment long enough for this purpose.

A few weeks ago a patient came to me completely blind in both eyes from atrophy of the optic nerve. Before he left the office he had become able, by the aid of the swing, to see the light with both eyes. He went away greatly encouraged, and promised to come again as soon as he returned from a neighboring city. Later he sent me a statement, signed by an oculist and witnessed by a notary public, to the effect that he was completely and incurably blind from primary optic atrophy. I have not seen him since.

The following remarkable story of a spontaneous cure was told me recently by a patient: A commercial traveler, a friend of the man who told me the story, was treated for two years in a Chicago hospital for total blindness from atrophy of the optic nerve. Although the doctors told him that his case was quite hopeless, he refused to believe it.

He talked much of a gray cloud that he had seen before his eyes at the time he became blind, and said that if he could only remember how it looked he was sure it would help him. One day he had a perfect mental picture of that gray cloud, and at once he found that he could see. He is now back in his old position, doing his usual amount of work, attending to his correspondence, and reading as well as he ever did. Doctors who have examined his eyes since say he still has atrophy of the optic nerve and ought still to be blind.

Irido-cyclitis, a combined inflammation of the iris and ciliary body, is a frequent cause of blindness. Often it results from an injury to the adjoining eye, and in that case is known as sympathetic ophthalmia. In severe cases it is believed to lead inevitably to blindness, which is, of course, thought to be incurable. Yet in all cases in which blindness has resulted from this disease I have seen perception of light, and even normal vision, restored.

One day a young girl came to my Clinic with one eye as soft as mush from irido-cyclitis (the other having been removed four years before). The iris and pupil were covered by a white scar and she had no perception of light. After palming, swinging and using her imagination for about fifteen minutes, the scar cleared up sufficiently for me to see the iris and pupil indistinctly, and two visiting doctors also saw them, while the patient saw the light. Later she became able to see people on the street and to see the pavement and imagine that it was swinging. At that point she ceased coming to the Clinic.

A case of practical blindness from this cause was cured within a month by the use of the imagination. When the patient looked at the large letter at the top of the card at one foot and was told what it was, he was able to imagine that he saw it, and thus he became able to see it actually. Then he did the same thing at ten feet. Next he imagined that he saw the first letter of the second line at ten feet, and became able to recognize the second letter. The same method was used with all the other lines until he became able to imagine the first letter of the bottom line, and then go on and read the other letters.

When his eye was examined with the ophthalmoscope the vitreous was so opaque that one could not distinguish the optic nerve and retina. He said that the light bothered him, and prevented him from imagining any of the letters on the Snellen test card. With the retinoscope at six feet, however, he stated that the light did not bother him so much, and he was able to imagine, while it was being used, that he saw a letter on the bottom line perfectly. The refraction was then normal, and a clear red reflex (light reflected from the retina) was obtained, indicating that the vitreous was now quite clear. When he failed to imagine that he saw the letter, the reflex was much blurred, indicating cloudiness of the vitreous. These are facts. I cannot offer any explanation for them.

Of detachment of the retina Fuchs says, "It is generally possible in recent and not too excessive cases of separation of the retina to obtain an improvement of the sight by a partial attachment, and in especially favorable cases even to cause the detachment to disappear completely. Unfortunately it is only in the rarest cases that these good results are lasting. As a rule, after some time, the separation develops anew, and ultimately, in spite of all our therapeutic endeavors, becomes total. In inveterate cases of total detachment it is better to abstain from any treatment." Compare this statement with the results obtained by central fixation, as told in the following article. In many other such cases useful vision has been obtained.

The incurability of blindness resulting from glaucoma is taken so completely for granted that Nettleship defines absolute glaucoma as "glaucoma that has gone on to permanent blindness." Yet in the December 1920 issue of *Better Eyesight,* and again in this issue, is reported a case in which light perception was restored in an eye stone-blind with glaucoma after a few minutes of palming. This was witnessed by several visiting doctors. Later the patient became able to read the 20-line at ten feet with this eye. As nearly half of our blind population at the present time is believed to be over sixty years old, and a great part of the blindness of later life is attributed to glaucoma, the curability of this condition is a fact of immense importance. Statistics indicate that in this country, at the present time, external injury is the most frequent cause of loss of vision between the ages of twenty and thirty-four. I believe that a great part of this blindness could be relieved, for, as I have already stated, I have never seen an eye so badly injured that its vision could not be improved. To cite only one of many similar cases, a patient injured in an automobile accident became suddenly and completely blind, either from hemorrhage into the orbit, or from injury to the optic nerve. By palming and the use of his imagination, he at once became able to count his fingers.

Perhaps the most remarkable cures of blindness are those in which the loss of vision is supposed to be due to general disease. These have frequently been relieved, partially or completely, without relief of the disease. Thirty years ago a man stone-blind with what I diagnosed to be albuminuric retinitis was led into my Clinic at the New York Eye and Ear Infirmary. This condition is so closely associated with disease of the kidneys that its existence is considered sufficient evidence of the existence of the latter. Yet the patient regained normal vision and held it up to the time of his death without any improvement in the condition of the kidneys.

On the contrary the disease of these organs became worse, and when he died a few years later the physicians who performed the autopsy wondered how he had been able to live so long. The evidence seems to me complete that the blindness was not due to the kidney trouble but to strain.

Many diseases of the eye are attributed to syphilis. Yet in every case these conditions have been relieved by rest, and often the sight has become normal without any improvement in the syphilis.

In spite of the very prompt improvement which patients obtain in these cases, they often, as the cases mentioned in the foregoing pages show, fail to continue the treatment. The weight of public and professional opinion is too much for them, and they are practically compelled to take this course. Such dogmatism is both unwise and unscientific. The causes of disease are obscure and variable, and we do not know it all. It does not seem to me that a doctor is justified in telling a patient that he is incurable just because he has never seen such a case cured, or has forgotten, because it was contrary to rule, any case that he has seen. This may cause the patient to accept as inevitable a condition which might have been cured and may even prevent nature, because of the depressing effects of discouragement, from doing what the doctor has failed to do. Still less is it justifiable for the medical profession to assume, as it now seems to do, that we have learned all there is to be known about blindness. Such an attitude throttles research and actually exposes to the suspicion of being a quack any man who tries to help these unfortunates.

RELIEF OF RETINAL DETACHMENT

By Clara E. Crandall

Twenty-five years ago Samuel D. was struck in the left eye by a nail thrown carelessly from a roof, and nineteen years later, while he was chopping wood, a stick flew up, hitting him in the face and injuring the same eye.

There were, apparently, no serious consequences from either of these accidents, but about a year after the second one the patient noted that his sight was getting dim. He consulted an oculist, thinking that he probably required glasses, and was told that he had iritis. He was given drops for this condition and had been using them for a month when, on May 12, 1916, while digging in the garden, he went suddenly and completely blind in his left eye. The cause proved to be a detached retina, and the oculist whom he consulted sent him to a hospital where he underwent a thorough examination. His teeth were x-rayed, and it was thought best to remove his tonsils. He was then kept for eight weeks motionless, flat upon his back.

At the end of this time it was found that the retina, as a result of the complete rest, had become partially reattached and the vision was, to some extent, improved. Hoping to improve it still further, the doctors operated upon the eye, but without success. Two weeks later a second operation was performed, after which the eye became totally blind again. The condition of the left eye was complicated by a traumatic cataract, and senile cataract now developed in the right. He was sent to another hospital in the autumn where he was again thoroughly examined, but the doctors decided that nothing more could be done for him.

And so, with one eye totally blind and cataract rapidly obscuring the sight of the other, Samuel went back to his work as a gardener, trying to resign himself to the dark future before him. From month to month he struggled on; but he found it increasingly difficult to do his work, and felt that the time would soon come when he would have to give it up. He suffered greatly from the strain of trying to see and complained of a constant yellow glare in the blind eye, together with many other painful and unpleasant symptoms which, he said, interfered with the sight of his right eye also.

From a time several years antedating his sudden attack of blindness Samuel has been in the employ of my family; after he became blind I went to Dr. Bates to have some eye troubles of my own treated and, hearing of the many remarkable cures that were effected by his method of treatment, it occurred to me that he might be able to do something for Samuel. It seemed to Samuel a forlorn hope, but as it was the only one, he allowed me to take him last May to Dr. Bates' Clinic in the Harlem Hospital.

At this time he was still without light perception in the left eye, and with the right was unable to make out the smaller letters on the test card when it was held a foot from his face, while even the largest letters appeared gray and blurred. Dr. Bates told him that the cataracts could be cured, and encouraged him to hope for improvement in the condition of the detached retina also. He told him to leave off the dark glasses he had been wearing, to palm as often and as long as possible, to drink twelve glasses of water a day, to imagine and flash the letters on the Snellen test card, and to imagine everything, himself included, as swinging.

Samuel followed these instructions conscientiously, and in a short time the strain and other distressing symptoms from which he had previously suffered were greatly relieved. The sight of the blind eye improved gradually. At the first visit he became able to distinguish light, and later he saw the shadowy image of a moving object, at first only when held close to the left side of his head, but afterward in all parts of his field of vision. The perception of light in the blind eye has grown steadily and the vision has so improved that now, at a distance of fourteen feet, he can see a moving object against a strong light, while at the near point he even thinks that he can sometimes catch a glimpse of the large letter on the Snellen test card.

With the right eye he can read the smallest letters on the test card at the near point, and they appear black and distinct. At fourteen feet he can flash them.

Among those who have benefited by Dr. Bates' remarkable discoveries, there is no one who owes more to them than Samuel D.; for now, instead of having to look forward to blindness and utter dependence on others, he has been enabled to take up his life with renewed courage and interest, confident that if he faithfully continues the treatment he will eventually obtain good vision in both eyes.

STORIES FROM THE CLINIC
No. 13: The Relief of Blindness

By Emily C. Lierman

Clinic day is always a happy day for me. It is true one sees at the hospital a great deal of suffering, sorrow and poverty; but it is a pleasure to be able to relieve some of the suffering, and sometimes things happen which are very amusing.

Some time ago a blind man was led into the Clinic by a friend. This was a case which really ought to have been very sad, but it turned out, instead, to be very amusing. In spite of his affliction the patient seemed to be in a happy mood and very well-pleased with himself. He was neatly dressed and his shoes, though worn, were carefully shined, while over them he wore spats. His tie was a very bright red, and his hat was a light shade of tan. A cane, which his blindness compelled him to carry, completed a costume which I am sure he considered to be that of a real swell gentleman. When I approached him he said in a very gracious manner, "Glad to see you, ma'am! Glad to see you, ma'am!"

And yet he could not see me, as I soon found out. I held my fingers before his eyes and asked him if he could see them. He answered that he could not. Further tests showed that he had no light perception whatever, and Dr. Bates said that his condition was due to atrophy of the optic nerve. I showed him how to palm, and after five minutes he pointed to an electric light in the ceiling and said, "It looks light there."

I told him at once to palm again, and when he opened his eyes he saw the shadow of my fingers moving from side to side before his face. In a few moments, however, the blindness returned. Again I told him to palm, and while he was doing so I asked him if he could remember something black, or something else that he had seen before he became blind, such as a beautiful sunset, or white clouds. He thought a while, and then remembered that in the days when he had been a housepainter he had used black paint. I told him to remember the black paint while he was palming, and then I left him to attend to other patients. When I came back to him I held two of my fingers close to his face, and asked him if he could see them.

"Ma'am," he said, "I'm not at all sure, but I think I see two fingers." I think the man must have been quite popular with the ladies, for he now remarked that one of his lady friends would be pleased if he could see her. He came quite regularly for a time, and each time I noted improvement in his vision. Sometimes this was not very marked, and then I knew that he had not been palming very much at home. He was greatly helped by the focusing of the sun's rays upon the white of his eyes with a sun glass. This had a very soothing effect. He was soon able to dispense with his guide and, when leaving the Clinic, used to use his cane to obviate collisions with the benches, nurses and patients. One day as he was leaving the room Dr. Bates called my attention to him, and I noted that instead of tapping with his cane upon the floor he was carrying it on his arm. With head erect, he walked down the long corridor, opened the door and left the hospital with apparently no more difficulty than a person with perfect sight. A little later he came without the cane. He became able at last to read the 50-line at five feet with both eyes, and then he stopped coming. Probably he thought he would be able to continue the treatment by himself.

In the October 1920 number of *Better Eyesight* I wrote about another case of blindness from atrophy of the optic nerve, the patient having no light perception. Unlike the preceding patient she was very much depressed by her condition, and begged me piteously to give her back the light of day. She had heard of our Clinic through some of the patients, and had confidence that Dr. Bates or myself would give her some relief. But I was very far from feeling this confidence. Sometimes I am a doubting Thomas. I always try, however, not to reveal this fact to the patients, but simply go ahead and do the best I can. After this woman had palmed for ten minutes or longer, all the time remembering black stove polish, she became able to see the 200-line letter a foot in front of her eyes. Since my previous article was written she has become able to read the 10-line at this distance. She is able to go out to work during the day, and to work for herself at night, and she says she sleeps better.

We have had many cases of total blindness at the Clinic, most of them due to glaucoma and atrophy of the optic nerve, a few to detachment of the retina and irido-cyclitis, and all have gained at least perception of light, while many have been more materially benefited. But most of them did not come more than a few times. It is unfortunate that the blind, as a rule, consider their condition so hopeless that it is difficult to convince them that any treatment is worthwhile, even after they have received some benefit from it.

Better Eyesight
April 1921—Vol. IV, No. 4

PRESBYOPIA NUMBER

METHODS THAT HAVE SUCCEEDED IN PRESBYOPIA

The cure of presbyopia, as of any other error of refraction, is rest, and many presbyopic patients are able to obtain this rest simply by closing the eyes. They are kept closed until the patient feels relieved, which may be in a few minutes, half an hour, or longer. Then some fine print is regarded for a few seconds. By alternately resting the eyes and looking at fine print many patients quickly become able to read it at eighteen inches, and by continued practice they are able to reduce the distance until it can be read at six inches in a dim light. At first the letters are seen only in flashes. Then they are seen for a longer time, until finally they are seen continuously.

When this method fails, palming may be tried, combined with the use of the memory, imagination and swing. Particularly good results have been obtained from the following procedure:

Close the eyes and remember the letter "o" in diamond type, with the open space as white as starch and the outline as black as possible. When the white center is at its maximum, imagine that the letter is moving and that all objects, no matter how large or small, are moving with it. Open the eyes and continue to imagine the universal swing. Alternate the imagination of the swing with the eyes open and closed.

When the imagination is just as good with the eyes open as when they are closed, the cure will be complete.

PRESBYOPIA: ITS CAUSE AND CURE

By W. H. Bates, M.D.

Presbyopia is the name given to the loss of power to use the eyes at the near point, without the aid of glasses, which usually occurs after the age of forty.

The textbooks teach that this change is a normal one; but it is a noteworthy fact that many other eye troubles often date from the time of its appearance, or develop a little later. Many cases of glaucoma start about this time, and so do many cases of cataract and inflammation of the interior of the eye. Patients with presbyopia are very likely to have conjunctivitis. They are also subject to congestion and hemorrhages of the interior of the eye. One patient developed a lot of muscular trouble and a marked degree of double vision at the time he became presbyopic, and suffered three nervous breakdowns in quick succession. He was operated on for the muscular condition and took prism exercises, but obtained very little relief. In another case a patient began to suffer—at the time she became unable to read without glasses—from a contraction of the muscles of the face, congestion of the conjunctiva and continual headaches. The strain was so great that she had to keep her eyes partly closed, and glasses did nothing to relieve her discomfort. Up to the time when her presbyopia appeared she had had none of these troubles.

The accepted explanation for the loss of near vision with advancing years is that it is due to the hardening of the lens, but it is quite impossible to reconcile the facts with this theory; for not only does presbyopia occur much below the age of forty and even in childhood, but it is often delayed beyond the age of fifty, and sometimes does not occur at all. There are also cases in which near vision is restored after having been lost. We are told that presbyopia comes early in the hypermetropic (farsighted) eye, and late in the myopic (nearsighted) eye; that premature hardening of the lens and weakness of the ciliary muscle (supposed to control the accommodation) may cause it to appear in youth; and that the swelling of the lens in incipient cataract may account for the restoration of near vision after it has been lost; but there are still many cases to which these explanations cannot be made to apply.

It is true that hypermetropia does hasten and myopia prevent or postpone the advent of presbyopia, and as myopia may exist in only one eye without the patient's being aware of it, he may think that his vision is normal both for the near point and the distance. There are cases, however, in which the vision has remained absolutely normal in both eyes long after the presbyopic age, and a considerable number of these cases have been brought to my attention. One of them, a man of sixty-five, examined in a moderate light indoors, was found to have a vision of 20/10. In other words he could see twice as far as the normal eye is expected to see. He also read diamond type at less than six inches, and at other distances, to more than eighteen inches. In reply to a query as to how he came to possess visual powers so unusual at his age or, indeed, at any age, he said that when he was about forty he began to experience difficulty, at times, in reading. He consulted an optician who advised glasses. He could not believe, however, that the glasses were necessary, because at times he could read perfectly without them. The matter interested him so much that he began to observe facts—a thing that people seldom do. He noted, first, that when he tried hard to see either at the near point or at the distance, his vision invariably became worse, and the harder he tried the worse it became. Evidently something was wrong with this method of using the eyes. Then he tried looking at things without effort, without trying to see them. He also tried resting his eyes by closing them for five minutes or longer, or by looking away from the page that he wished to read, or the distant object he wished to see. These practices always improved his sight, and by keeping them up he not only regained normal vision but retained it for twenty-five years.

"Doctor," he said, in concluding his story, "when my eyes are at rest and comfortable, my vision is always good and I forget all about them. When they do not feel comfortable I never see so well, and then I always proceed to rest them until they feel all right again."

The fact is that presbyopia is due to a strain. It is a strain similar to the one that produces hypermetropia, but differs from it in the fact that it affects chiefly vision at the near point. This can be demonstrated with the retinoscope. When a person with presbyopia tries to read, the retinoscope will show that he has hypermetropia, but when he looks at a distant object the retinoscope will show either that his eyes are normal, or that the hypermetropia is less. Simultaneous retinoscopy is difficult in the case of a reading patient, for not only is the pupil small, but in order to find the shadow it is necessary for the patient to look in one general direction all the time, and this is not easy. It is also difficult to hold a glass at one side of the eye for the measurement of the refraction in such a way that the observer can look through it while the patient does not. With a sufficient zeal for the truth, however, these difficulties can be overcome.

The strain which produces presbyopia is accompanied by a strain, more or less pronounced, of all the other nerves of the body. Hence, the many distressing symptoms from which presbyopic patients suffer. Glasses, by neutralizing the effect of the imperfect action of the muscles, may enable the patient to read, but they cannot relieve any of these strains. On the contrary, they usually make them worse, and it is a matter of common experience that the vision declines rapidly after the patient begins to wear them. When people put on glasses because they cannot read fine print, they often find that in a couple of weeks they cannot, without them, read the coarse print that was perfectly plain to them before. Occasionally, the eyes resist the artificial conditions imposed upon them by glasses to an astonishing degree, as in the case of a woman of seventy who had worn glasses for twenty years, in spite of the fact that they tired her eyes and blurred her vision, but was still able to read diamond type without them.

This, however, is very unusual. As a rule, the eyes go from bad to worse, and, if the patient lives long enough, he is almost certain to develop some serious disease which ends so frequently in blindness that nearly half of our blind population at the present time is believed to be over sixty years old. Persons with presbyopia who are satisfied with the relief given to them by glasses should bear this fact in mind.

Presbyopia is cured just as any other error of refraction is cured—by rest. But there is a great difference in the way patients respond to this treatment. Some are cured very quickly, even in as short a time as fifteen minutes; others are very slow but as a rule, relief is obtained within a reasonable time.

One of my earliest cures of presbyopia was accomplished in less than fifteen minutes by the aid of the imagination. The patient had worn glasses for reading for ten years. When I showed him a specimen of diamond type and asked him to read it without glasses he said he knew the letters were black but they looked gray.

"If you know they are black and yet see them gray," I said, "you must imagine that they are gray. Suppose you imagine that they are black. Can you do that?" "Yes," he said, "I can imagine that they are black," and immediately he proceeded to read them.

In another case a patient was cured simply by closing his eyes for half an hour. His wife was cured in the same way, and when I saw the couple six months later they had had no relapse. Both had worn reading glasses for more than five years.

While it is sometimes very difficult to cure presbyopia, it is, fortunately, very easy to prevent it. Oliver Wendell Holmes told us how to do it in *The Autocrat of the Breakfast Table.* [See the July 1919 issue.—TRQ]

Persons whose sight is beginning to fail at the near point, or who are approaching the presbyopic age, should imitate the example of this remarkable old gentleman. Get a specimen of diamond type and read it every day in artificial light, bringing it closer and closer to the eye until it can be read at six inches or less. Or get a specimen of type reduced by photography until it is much smaller than diamond type, and do the same. You will thus escape, not only the necessity of wearing glasses for reading and near work, but all of those eye troubles which now so often darken the later years of life.

HOW I WAS CURED OF PRESBYOPIA.

By Francis E. McSweeny

Editor's Note—*This patient was first seen on March 11, 1919. His right vision was 20/50 and his left vision 20/70 and, although he was fifty-one years old, he read diamond type at eight inches. He had not worn glasses for some months, and with the help of a cured patient had been able to improve his sight considerably. His last prescription for reading glasses was: right eye, convex 3.00 D. S.; left eye, convex 3.75 D. S. with convex 0.50 D. C. 180 degrees.*

I am a church organist, choir director and music teacher. Those familiar with the duties of my profession will understand what an important part good vision plays in its successful practice. I realized this and from the first, consulted the best oculists periodically in order to preserve and protect my eyesight. I was told upon reaching the "deadline" of forty-five that I had presbyopia and would henceforth be obliged to wear at least two pair of glasses, one for near and one for distant vision. I rebelled at this, but submitted for some years to the annoyance with as good grace as possible.

I knew that braces and crutches never cured weak limbs, but that exercise and use of the weak muscles, when the patient had the necessary perseverance, had often made them strong and vigorous. I began to think that glasses were like the braces and crutches, and I expected some day a method of treatment would be found that would strengthen and build up the eyes instead of weakening them. I was in this mood when Dr. Bates' treatment of imperfect sight without glasses was brought to my attention. My father and sister had received benefit from the treatment, and I believed that I could be benefited too.

When I first took off my glasses I could see nothing on the front page of the newspaper but the larger headlines. I could read down to the 30-line of the Snellen test card at 5 feet. My sister showed me how to "shift" from the top to the bottom of the letters on Dr. Bates' professional card. I read a column of the *Saturday Evening Post* that day by this method.

At first I tried to wear my glasses for close work, but after a few months I felt that this was retarding my cure and I left them off altogether. That was in January 1919. With the exception of a few Sundays at the beginning, I have done all my work without putting on my glasses even once.

It would be well for anyone who would follow my example to understand, however, that this result was not accomplished without many mistakes. I often misunderstood and lost valuable time doing things wrong. There were many discouragements, too. So many to tell me how foolish I was to try to do the impossible. I had the consolation, on the other hand, of knowing that my vision was improving all the time.

The exercises which I found most helpful were: 1. Palming—I think that nothing so relieves strain as this exercise does. 2. Flashing—This exercise helps particularly when one has been straining or using the eyes wrongly. 3. Memory practice—This has been my best exercise. One remembers a letter, picture, or other familiar object, at first with the eyes closed, then with the eyes open. If he can retain the memory of the object while looking in the direction of the test card, he will be able to read the letter easily. 4. Imagination—Imagining that the white part of a certain letter is whiter than the margin of the card. This has helped me greatly.

My present vision is: Distance (both eyes): 10/10, 15/15, some of 15/10, 20/20 and 30/30. Fine print (both eyes): best at 12 inches, some at 20 inches, can see a period at 20 inches.

I should advise anyone who contemplates taking up this treatment to first see Dr. Bates personally for diagnosis and to get right ideas in the beginning. By doing this, one would save much time and many missteps.

To those who cannot do this I should say that the first thing to do is to discard glasses altogether. Relax the mind and eye by palming. Learn to know how the eyes feel when relaxed and when doing your accustomed tasks try to keep this feeling of relaxation (lack of effort) present at all times. Do not allow the eyes to become strained. Let objects that you wish to see come to you, do not try to go to them. You will fail sometimes. If you persist, however, your failures will be less and less frequent and, as your vision improves, which it surely will, you will gain confidence. The exercises which I refer to are described in Dr. Bates' book, which contains many valuable suggestions, besides interesting matter bearing on his experiments and achievements.

STORIES FROM THE CLINIC

No. 14: Three Cases of Presbyopia

By Emily C. Lierman

As a rule, more children than adults come to the Clinic. They are sent to us by the schools, usually because they cannot see the blackboard. But during the war it was astonishing how many women came to us. Many of them were employed in factories where American flags were manufactured and could not see to do the work properly, although their sight at the distance seemed to be satisfactory. Some had trouble in threading their needles. Others complained that they saw double. One told me that she sometimes stitched her fingers to the blue field of the flag along with the stars. They all asked for glasses, of course, but were very glad to learn that they could be cured so that they could see without them.

Among these very interesting patients was a woman of about fifty who had great trouble in threading her needle, and who begged me to help her because she had her living to earn. Her distant vision was quickly improved by palming and flashing the letters on the Snellen test card. Then I suggested that she practice with fine print six inches from her eyes. Even though she did not see the letters, I told her it would help her to alternately rest her eyes by closing for a few minutes and then look at the small letters for a couple of seconds. She got immediate results from this, and was enthusiastic in her expressions of appreciation.

"Sure, ma'am, may the good angels bless you for that!" she exclaimed. "I think this very minute I would be threadin' a needle if I had one. Me old man and the young ones at home will think it fine to have meself threadin' a needle." It seemed that members of her family had been called upon to thread her needles, and had found the task somewhat irksome.

The next Clinic day she came again and, although it was afternoon, greeted me vociferously with the Irish salutation, "Top o' the mornin' to you!" "Top o' the morning to yourself!" said I, and then suggested that she should not speak so loud, as I was afraid she would disturb the other patients. I am not sure that she did any harm, however. The patients all smiled at her remark. It does me good to see these poor unfortunates smile a little, and I think it must do them good also.

She soon became able to thread her needle without any trouble, and she wanted everyone in the room to know it. The last time I saw her she said, "Sure, ma'am, me eyes are very sharp now, for the minute I set eyes on me man when he comes home at night, I can tell by the twinkle in his eye whether he has had anything stronger than water or tea."

Another woman, forty-eight years old, told me that the first time she came to the Clinic she thought she had got into the wrong place. Half a dozen people had their eyes covered with the palms of their hands to rest them, and she thought it was a prayer meeting. It was she who sewed her fingers to the flag along with the stars.

"What I need is glasses," she said, "and that's what I am here for"; but I soon convinced her that the glasses were unnecessary.

By having her alternately close and open her eyes I improved her sight for the Snellen test card from 15/40 to 15/20. Then I gave her some fine print to read, but it was only a blur to her. I now told her to palm, and imagine that she was sewing stars to the flag. When she opened her eyes her sight was worse. The very thought of those stars increased her strain and made her vision worse. This convinced her that her trouble was due to strain, and that all she needed was to get rid of the strain. I now asked her to imagine more agreeable objects at the near point. She at once became able to read the fine print, and her sight for the distance also improved. After four visits to the Clinic her vision both for the distance and the near point had become almost normal. It was quite easy for her to thread a needle and to do her work without glasses.

A woman of seventy-four, who has been coming to the Clinic for some time, works every day in an orphanage where she mends the children's clothes and does other sewing. She complained that her glasses did not fit her and she could no longer see to sew with them. I gave her a small card with some fine print on the back. "Do you mean to tell me," she asked, "that I will ever read that?" "It is possible," I said.

Her smiling face was good to see as she tried to do as I instructed her. The print was larger on one side of the card than on the other, and I asked her to read the name printed in the larger letters. She could not do so at first. I told her to close her eyes, count ten, then open them and look at the card while she counted two; then repeat. In a few minutes she saw the name on the card and also the phone number. I then had her do the same thing with the diamond type on the reverse side, and after a while she became able to see some of the letters. At later visits she obtained further improvement, and after some months she had no difficulty in sewing the buttons on the children's clothes without her glasses, although as she said, there were a lot of them and they kept her busy.

Once during the treatment I asked her to remember

the daisy in the green field as she saw it in the country last summer. "There weren't any daisies but me while I was there," she answered. "I was the only daisy."

QUESTIONS AND ANSWERS

Q–1. While I can see the letters on the Snellen test card distinctly with both eyes down to the 50-line, the right eye sees double below that point. What is the reason?

A–1. While you see the letters down to the 50-line singly and well enough to recognize them, you do not see them perfectly. Otherwise you would see them perfectly below that point. The double vision of the right eye below that point is not due to its error of refraction, but to imagination. With both eyes closed, imagine the letters single. Then look at the test card for a moment. Repeat until the letters can be regarded continuously without doubling. Practice first with both eyes together, then with the right eye separately.

Q–2. I have conical cornea. Can it be cured or relieved without glasses or operation?

A–2. Yes. One such case secured normal vision in six weeks by the aid of the methods presented in this magazine. Another case was cured in two weeks. Conical cornea is simply an anterior staphyloma, or bulging of the front of the eyeball, similar to the posterior staphyloma which so often occurs in myopia. Both are curable by the same methods.

Better Eyesight

May 1921—Vol. IV, No. 5

IMAGINATION NUMBER

HOW TO IMPROVE THE SIGHT BY MEANS OF THE IMAGINATION: NO. 1

Remember the letter "o" in diamond type, with the eyes closed and covered. If you are able to do this, it will appear to have a short, slow swing, less than its own diameter.

Look at an unknown letter on the test card which you can see only as a gray spot at ten feet or more, and imagine that it has a swing of not more than a quarter of an inch.

Imagine the top of the unknown letter to be straight, still maintaining the swing. If this is in accordance with the fact, the swing will be unchanged. If it is not, the swing will become uneven, or longer, or will be lost.

If the swing is altered, try another guess. If you can't tell the difference between two guesses, it is because the swing is too long. Palm and remember the "o" with its short swing, and you may become able to shorten the swing of the larger letter.

In this way you can ascertain, without seeing the letter, whether its four sides are straight, curved, or open. You may then be able to imagine the whole letter. This is easiest with the eyes closed and covered. If the swing is modified, you will know that you have made a mistake. In that case repeat from the beginning.

When you get the right letter, imagine it alternately with the eyes closed and open, until you are able to imagine it as well when you look at it as when your eyes are closed and covered. In that case you will actually see the letter.

IMAGINATION ESSENTIAL TO SIGHT

By W. H. Bates, M.D.

It is a well-known fact that vision is a process of mental interpretation. The picture which the mind sees is not the impression on the retina, but a mental interpretation of it. To the mind, objects seen appear to be in an upright position, but the picture on the retina is upside down. When the sight is normal the margins and openings of black letters on a white card appear whiter than the rest of the card; but this, of course, is not the fact, the whole background being of the same whiteness. One may seem to see a whole letter all alike at one time, but, as a matter of fact, the eye is shifting rapidly from one part to another. The letter may also seem to move although it is stationary.

When the vision is imperfect, the imagination is also imperfect. The mind, in short, adds imperfections to the imperfect retinal image. A great part of the phenomena of imperfect sight is, therefore, imaginary and not in any way to be accounted for by the derangement of the visual apparatus. The color, size, form, position and number of objects regarded are altered, and non-existent objects may be seen. Some persons with imperfect sight literally see ghosts. A person in a dark cellar is often under such a strain that he thinks he sees sheeted figures, and one of my patients in broad daylight used to see little devils dancing on the tops of high buildings.

It is a great relief to patients to learn that these appearances are imaginary, thus helping them to bring the imagination under control. And, as it is impossible to imagine perfectly without perfect relaxation, any improvement in the interpretation of the retinal images means an improvement in the conditions which have led to a distortion of those images; for relaxation, as all regular readers of this magazine know, is the cure for most eye troubles. There is no more effective method of improving the sight, therefore, than by the aid of the imagination, and wonderful results have been obtained by this means. At times, imagination almost seems to take the place of sight, as in the case of a patient who gained a high degree of central fixation in spite of the fact that the macula (center of sight) had been destroyed, or in those cases in which patients become able to correctly imagine letters which are seen only as gray spots without knowing what they are.

How patients manage to see best where they are looking without a macula is hard to explain, but the imagination of letters which are not consciously seen is probably made possible by a certain degree of unconscious vision. When one looks at a letter on the Snellen test card which can be seen distinctly and tries to imagine the top straight or open when it is curved, or curved when it is straight or open, it will be found impossible to do so and the vision will be lowered by the effort to a greater or lesser degree. In one case the mere suggestion to a patient that he should imagine the top of the big "C" straight caused the whole card to become blank. When one looks at a letter seen indistinctly without knowing what it is and tries to imagine it to be other than it is, one is usually able to do so, but not without strain, evidenced by the fact that the letter becomes more blurred, or by the impossibility of imagining that it has a slow, easy swing of not more than a quarter of an inch. This fact makes it possible to find out what the letter is without seeing it.

The patient begins by imagining each of the four sides of the letter taken in turn to be straight, curved, or open, and observing the effect of each guess upon the swing. If the right side is straight, for instance, and she imagines it to be straight, the swing will be unchanged; but if she imagines it to be curved, the swing will be lengthened or lost, or will become less even and easy. If she is unable to tell the difference between two guesses it is because the swing is too long, and she is told to palm and remember a letter of diamond type, with its short swing, until she is able to shorten it. Having imagined each of the four sides of the letter correctly, she becomes able to imagine the whole letter, first with the eyes closed and covered, and then with the eyes open.

When one knows what the four sides of a letter are, its identification, in some cases, is a simple process of reason. A letter which is straight on top and on the left side, and open on the two other sides, cannot be anything but an "F." If, on the contrary, it is straight on the bottom and on the left side, and open on the other two, it must be an "L." Such letters can be imagined with a lower degree of relaxation than the less simple ones, like a "V," a "Y," or a "K." If the letter is not imagined correctly, the swing will be altered, and in that case the process should be repeated from the beginning.

Having imagined the letter correctly, the patient is told to imagine it first with the eyes closed and covered, and then with the eyes open and looking at the card, until he is able to imagine it as well when looking at the card as when palming. In this way it finally becomes possible for him to imagine it so vividly when looking at the card that he actually sees it.

With most patients this method of improving the sight produces results more quickly than any other. Others, for some unknown reason, do not succeed with it. Temporary improvement is often obtained in an incredibly short space of time, and by continued practice this temporary improvement becomes permanent.

The patient who describes her case in a later article looked at the Snellen test card at ten feet one day and did not see any of the letters, even as gray spots. By the method described above she became able in half an hour to read the whole card. A schoolgirl of ten could not see anything at ten feet below the large letter at the top of the card. She was told how to make out the letters by the aid of her imagination, and then left alone for half an hour. At the end of this time she had read the whole of an unfamiliar card. A child of about the same age whose left macula had been destroyed by atrophy of the choroid (middle coat of the eye) was able with the affected eye to see only the 200-line letter on the test card, and that, only when she looked to one side of the card. She was treated by means of her imagination, and after a few months, during which time she came very irregularly, she obtained normal vision in both eyes. She is still under treatment.

A schoolgirl of sixteen with such a high degree of myopic astigmatism that she could see only the large letter at ten feet became able in four or five visits, by the aid of her imagination, to read 20/20 temporarily, and at her last visit she read 20/15 temporarily. A college student twenty-five years old, with compound hypermetropic astigmatism (four diopters in each eye), could read only 20/100 with his right eye and 14/200 with his left, and had been compelled to stop his studies because of the pain and fatigue resulting from the use of his eyes at the near point. In four visits his vision was improved by the aid of his imagination to 20/30 and he became able to read diamond type at six inches without glasses and without discomfort.

These and many other cases of the same kind have demonstrated that imagination is necessary to normal sight.

STORIES FROM THE CLINIC
No. 15: Imagination Relieves Pain
By Emily C. Lierman

A few weeks ago there came to the Clinic a very tired-looking mother, with her daughter, age twelve, who was suffering intense pain in her eyes and head. Both began to talk to me at once, and the mother told me that the child kept her awake at night with her moaning. She had taken her to another doctor in the hospital, and he, failing to relieve the pain, had sent her to Dr. Bates, thinking that her eyes might need attention. Dr. Bates examined the child, and without telling me what the trouble was, said, "Here is a good case for you; cure her quick."

The poor child could scarcely open her eyes, and her forehead was a mass of wrinkles. I tested her sight, and at twelve feet she read the 50-line on the test card. While reading the card she said that her pain was not so bad. I told her to palm, and while her eyes were covered I asked her to imagine that she saw the blackboard at school and that she was writing the figure "7" upon it with white chalk. She could do this, she said, and then I asked her to remove her hands from her eyes and look at the black "7" on the test card. She saw it very distinctly, and I noticed that her eyes had opened and that the wrinkles in her forehead had disappeared. The mother noticed this too and said, "See how wide open her eyes are!" Evidently the pain had gone, for after a moment the little girl exclaimed in great excitement, "Oh, that pain is coming back!"

I told her to close her eyes at once and palm again. Noticing how much she had been helped by her imagination, I told her to imagine the black figure blacker than she had seen it with her eyes open. She did this, and when she opened her eyes in a few minutes the pain had again disappeared and her vision had improved to 12/30. After telling her mother that the cause of all the child's trouble had been eyestrain, and that if she would palm and use her imagination she would be well in two weeks, I sent her home. Imagine my surprise when two days later she came to the Clinic with her eyes wide open, grinning from ear to ear, and having a gay old time with a school friend whom she had brought with her.

She told me that only once during the first evening after she came to the Clinic had she suffered any return of the pain. Then she had closed her eyes and covered them with the palms of her hands and imagined first that she saw a figure "7," black on a white background, and then that she saw white roses, daisies with yellow centers and green fields. She went to sleep soon after and did not wake up until morning. She had had no pain at all since that night, and when I tested her sight with both eyes together and each eye separately, I found it normal. It goes without saying that I was very happy to have accomplished in two days what I expected to take two weeks. The patient was instructed to keep on practicing and to report at least once a week at the Clinic, but she did not come again.

A boy named Harry, age eleven, now being treated at the Clinic, came to us about two weeks ago with pain in both eyes. He had been sent to us from the public school for glasses. Reading made him nervous, he said, and he did not wish to read anything on the test card but the large letters. I had him stand fifteen feet from the card, and asked him to read the letters slowly and only to see one at a time. Noticing that he was extremely nervous I lowered my voice as much as possible and talked to him as I would to a child much younger. This seemed to have a soothing effect, for immediately he seemed less nervous and shy, and he was able to read the 40-line with his left eye and the 50-line with his right. I now showed him how to palm. This seemed to afford him much amusement, but he did it faithfully because he wanted to please me, not because he thought it would help his sight. When he opened his eyes he read the 20-line with the left eye, but the vision of the right had not improved and he complained that the pain in it was still as bad as ever.

I told him to palm again, and while his eyes were covered I asked him if he ever saw a large ship getting ready to sail. He said, "yes," he had seen some of our warships on the Hudson River. I asked him how much he could imagine he saw on one of these vessels. He became intensely interested and was no longer inclined to be restless.

"Why," he said, "I can imagine a rope ladder on the side of the ship and sailors walking on the deck, and I can imagine black smoke coming out of the smokestack." Before I had told him to, he uncovered his right eye and read all the letters on the 40-line and some of those on the 30-line. He said that the pain had gone and that the letters looked blacker to him and the card whiter than before. He has come to the Clinic regularly, and now reads 15/10—better than normal—with both eyes. He still complains about a little pain in the right eye, but when he palms and imagines that he is playing baseball or doing other pleasant things, his pain stops and he always leaves the Clinic smiling.

IMAGINATION IN RETINITIS PIGMENTOSA

By Mary Blake

Editor's Note—*This patient came for examination on February 9, 1921, and for treatment on March 11. Her distant vision with glasses (concave 6.00 D. S., both eyes) was 20/40 in the right eye and 20/50 in the left, and her field had been reduced to ten degrees, so that she could see nothing above, below, or to one side of her line of vision. She was treated almost entirely by means of her imagination and has thus become able, temporarily, to read the bottom line of an unfamiliar card at ten feet. By the same means her field and color perception have at times become normal. When her imagination fails, her vision fails also. Sunning and the focusing of the rays of the sun with a sun glass upon the upper part of the sclera (white of the eye) proved very effective in overcoming her extreme sensitiveness to light.*

I began to wear glasses for nearsightedness when I was fifteen, and from that time I wore them constantly until I came to Dr. Bates five weeks ago. For the last two or three years I never took them off, except for close work, until I got into bed at night; and before I got out of bed in the morning I put them on again.

In spite of these precautions my sight became steadily worse, and for the last ten years I have spent my time and money going from one specialist to another both in this country and in Europe. Three of the most famous specialists in Switzerland told me that I had retinitis pigmentosa, a condition in which pigment is deposited in the retina, and which, I was told, always ended in complete blindness if the patient lived long enough. Nothing could be done to prevent this outcome, they said, but they advised me to wear dark glasses when I went out of doors on bright days, because by exposing my eyes to strong light I was spending my capital. For the last three years (up to five weeks ago) I did this, and for the last year, on very sunny days, I often wore dark glasses in the house also, because my eyes had become so sensitive to the light that I could sometimes find relief only by going into a darkened room. Even with dark glasses and drawn blinds, there was a kind of razzle-dazzle before my eyes which was so maddening that I almost longed for the blindness with which I had been threatened, so that I might be free from such distresses. When I looked out of a window onto a sunny street and then back into the room again, everything became perfectly black for a minute. For the last two years and a half I have not been able to go out alone in the city.

In this state of utter hopelessness, with my sight rapidly getting worse, I heard of Dr. Bates through a patient whom he was treating and, in spite of what I felt to be the incredulity of my friends, although they were considerate enough not to express it, I lost no time in consulting him. The unusualness of his methods, while it excited the suspicion of others, was a recommendation to me. I knew what the old methods accomplished, or rather what they did not accomplish, and I wanted something different. It seemed to me that Dr. Bates was the very man I had been looking for.

My friends have now been converted, but, in spite of the fact that I am able to report substantial improvement in my vision, I still meet with much skepticism in other quarters.

A doctor to whom my progress was reported by a friend wrote to her that if my trouble were imaginary Dr. Bates might help me through hypnotism or mind cure, but that if there were anything really the matter with my eyes he could do nothing by his methods. Having a relative in New

York who is an eye specialist, this doctor took the trouble to write to him and ask what he knew about Dr. Bates. The reply was that Dr. Bates was the laughing stock of all the oculists in New York. This report, when it was communicated to me, disturbed me not at all. It did not matter to me how much the other eye specialists laughed at Dr. Bates so long as he was helping me, as none of them had been able to do. Other doctors were more open-minded, but were not prepared to believe that such diseases as retinitis pigmentosa could be cured by this or any other method. One who had met some of Dr. Bates' cured patients and was inclined to believe in him said, when told that I was being treated for this condition, "Good gracious, he surely doesn't pretend to cure retinitis pigmentosa! That is an organic disease."

I said that he not only pretended to cure it, but had made substantial progress in my case. The doctor said, "I think he'll help you, but I don't believe you are ever going to see without limitations."

The improvement in my vision since I have been under treatment has been indisputable. After two weeks the intangible suffering caused by light (photophobia) left me, and it has never returned. I can go out in the brightest sunlight without glasses of any kind, and, although my eyes feel weak and I squint a little, there is no real distress. I can look out of a window onto a sunny street, and when I turn back again into the room there is no blindness. When I first took off my glasses I had to bend over close to my plate when I was eating in order to see what was on it. Now I sit in an almost normal position with such a slight bend that I don't think anyone would notice it. I also operate a typewriter while sitting in a normal position.

For three years, it has been very difficult for me to read or sew, with or without glasses. Now I do both without glasses, and instead of the distress which these activities formerly caused me, I experience a delightful feeling of freedom. And not only can I read ordinary print, but I can read diamond type and photographic reductions. About a year ago I began to lose my color perception, and up to two weeks ago I was unable to distinguish the rug from the floor in the Doctor's office. Now I can see that the floor is red and the rug blue, tan and black. At the present writing I have just become able to observe that a couch cover in my apartment, which had always appeared blue to me, is green. I am still unable to see very much at the distance; but I am beginning to make out the features of the people around me and to read signs in the streets and streetcars, and when I look out of the windows on the subway I see the people on the platforms. My field is still very limited, but I am conscious that it is slowly enlarging. The other day I pinned a piece of paper three inches from the test card, and was able to see it while looking at the card. After such improvement in the brief period of five weeks, I do not feel inclined to credit the prediction of my medical friend that I am going to regain my sight only with limitations. I hope I am going to get normal vision.

Along with the improvement in my sight there has come also a remarkable improvement in my physical condition, the natural result of freedom from suffering. I used to be a very restless sleeper, and when I woke in the morning I was greatly fatigued. Now the bed is as smooth in the morning as if I had never stirred all night, and I am much more refreshed than I used to be, although not so much so as I hope to be later. Formerly I had to force myself to write a letter. Now it is a pleasure to do so, and I am clearing off all my correspondence. Previously I could not attend to my accounts. Now I have them all straightened out. If I get nothing more from the treatment than this physical comfort and increased ability to do things, it will be worthwhile.

QUESTIONS AND ANSWERS

Q–1a. I began to wear glasses for farsightedness when I was twenty-six. I began with convex 1.00 D. S. and now, at forty-two, I am wearing convex 2.50 D. S., or was until a few weeks ago when I decided to try the methods presented in this magazine. I can read and sew with ease in the daylight, but cannot read fine print even in a strong electric light for more than a few minutes without getting a dull ache at the back of my eyeballs. Do you advise the use of the test card in my case, or is it only for children? 1b. Would the swing help me, and if so will you explain it a little more clearly? 1c. Is it best to go without the glasses as much as I can, or am I injuring my eyes by so doing? 1d. Would it retard the cure to use the glasses just for evening reading? 1e. How long will it take for my eyes to become young again, if that is possible?

A–1a. The test card is for everybody. 1b. Yes, the swing would help you. The normal eye is constantly shifting, and thus an apparent movement of objects regarded is produced. By consciously imitating this unconscious shifting of the normal eye and realizing the apparent movement which it produces, imperfect sight is always improved. 1c. You should discard your glasses permanently. They are never a benefit and always an injury to the eyes. 1d. Yes. 1e. It is entirely possible for your eyes to become young again, but it is impossible to guess how long this will take because it is impossible to tell how well or intelligently you will practice central fixation.

Q–2. Why is it that when I look at an electric light half a mile away, it looks as if there were ten or a dozen rays of light going in all directions?

A–2. Because when you look at an object half a mile away you strain to see it, and under the influence of the strain you imagine rays of light going in all directions so vividly that you seem to see them.

Better Eyesight
June 1921—Vol. IV, No. 6

DEMONSTRATE: THE FUNDAMENTAL PRINCIPLE OF TREATMENT

The object of all the methods used in the treatment of imperfect sight without glasses is to secure rest or relaxation of the mind first and then of the eyes. Rest always improves the vision. Effort always lowers it. Persons who wish to improve their vision should begin by demonstrating these facts.

Close the eyes and keep them closed for fifteen minutes. Think of nothing particular, or think of something pleasant. When the eyes are opened, it will usually be found that the vision has improved temporarily. If it has not, it will be because, while the eyes were closed, the mind was not at rest.

One symptom of strain is a twitching of the eyelids which can be seen by an observer and felt by the patient with the fingers. This can usually be corrected if the period of rest is long enough.

Many persons fail to secure a temporary improvement of vision by closing their eyes because they do not keep them closed long enough. Children will seldom do this unless a grown person stands by and encourages them. Many adults also require supervision.

To demonstrate that strain lowers the vision, think of something disagreeable—some physical discomfort, or something seen imperfectly. When the eyes are opened, it will be found that the vision has been lowered. Also, stare at one part of a letter on the test card, or try to see the whole letter all alike at one time. This invariably lowers the vision and may cause the letter to disappear.

FUNDAMENTALS OF TREATMENT

By W. H. Bates, M.D.

All errors of refraction and many other eye troubles are cured by rest; but there are many ways of obtaining this rest, and all patients cannot do it in the same way. Sometimes a long succession of patients are helped by the same method, and then will come one who does not respond to it at all.

Closing the Eyes

The simplest way to rest the eyes is to close them for a longer or shorter period and think about something agreeable. This is always the first thing that I tell patients to do, and there are very few who are not benefited by it temporarily.

Palming

A still greater degree of rest can be obtained by closing and covering the eyes so as to exclude all the light. The mere exclusion of the impressions of sight is often sufficient to produce a large measure of relaxation. In other cases the strain is increased. As a rule, successful palming involves a knowledge of various other means of obtaining relaxation. The mere covering and closing of the eyes is useless unless at the same time mental rest is obtained. When a patient palms perfectly, he sees a field so black that it is impossible to remember, imagine, or see, anything blacker, and when able to do this he is cured. It should be borne in mind, however, that the patient's judgment of what is a perfect black is not to be depended upon.

Central Fixation

When the vision is normal the eye sees one part of everything it looks at best and every other part worse in proportion as it is removed from the point of maximum (central) vision. When the vision is imperfect it is invariably found that the eye is trying to see a considerable part of its field of vision equally well at one time. This is a great strain upon the eye and mind, as anyone whose sight is approximately normal can demonstrate by trying to see an appreciable area all alike at one time. At the near point the attempt to see an area even a quarter of an inch in diameter in this way will produce discomfort and pain. Anything which rests the eye tends to restore the normal power of central fixation. It can also be regained by conscious practice, and this is sometimes the quickest and easiest way to improve the sight. When the patient becomes conscious that he sees one part of his field of vision better than the rest, it usually becomes possible for him to reduce the area seen best. If he looks from the bottom of the 200-line letter to the top, for instance, and sees the part not directly regarded worse than the part regarded ("fixed"), he may become able to do the same with the next line of letters; and thus he may become able to go down the card until he can look from the top to the bottom of the letters on the bottom line and see the part not directly regarded worse. In that case he will be able to read the letters. On the principle that a burnt child dreads the fire, it is a great help to most patients to consciously increase the degree of their eccentric fixation. When they have produced discomfort or pain by consciously trying to see a large letter, or a whole line of letters, all alike at one time, they unconsciously try to avoid the lower degree of eccentric fixation which has become habitual to them. Most patients, when they become able to reduce the area of their field of maximum (central) vision, are conscious of a feeling of great relief in the eyes and head and even in the whole body. Since small objects cannot be seen without central fixation, the reading of fine print, when it can be done, is one of the best of visual activities, and the dimmer the light in which it can be read and the closer to the eye it can be held the better.

Shifting and Swinging

The eye with normal vision never regards a point for more than a fraction of a second, but shifts rapidly from one part of its field to another, thus producing a slight apparent movement, or swing, of all objects regarded. [My emphasis.—TRQ] The eye with imperfect sight always tries to hold its points of fixation, just as it tries to see with maximum vision a larger area than nature intended it to see. This habit can be corrected by consciously imitating the unconscious shifting of the normal eye and realizing the swing produced by this movement. At first a very long shift may be necessary, as from one end of a line of letters to another, in order to produce a swing; but sometimes even this is not sufficient. In such cases patients are asked to hold one hand before the face while moving the head and eyes rapidly from side to side, when they seldom fail to observe an apparent movement of the hand. Some patients are under such a strain, however, that it may be weeks before they are able to do this. After the apparent movement of the hand has been observed, patients become able to realize the swing resulting from slighter movements of the eye until they are able to look from one side to another of a letter of diamond type and observe that it seems to move in a direction contrary to the movement of the eye. A mental picture of a letter can be observed to swing precisely as can a letter on the test card and, as a rule, mental shifting and swinging are easier at first than visual. The realization of the visual swing can, therefore, be cultivated by the aid of the mental swing. It is also an advantage to have the patient try to look continually at some letter, or part of a letter, and note that it quickly becomes blurred or disappears. When he thus demonstrates that staring lowers the vision he becomes better able to avoid it. When visual or mental swinging is successful, everything one thinks of appears to have a slight swing. This I have called the *universal swing*. Most patients get the universal swing very easily. Others have great difficulty. The latter class is hard to cure.

MEMORY

When the sight is normal the mind is always perfectly at rest, and when the memory is perfect the mind is also at rest. Therefore it is possible to improve the sight by the use of the memory. Anything the patient finds is agreeable to remember is a rest to the mind, but for purposes of practice a small black object, such as a period or a letter of diamond type, is usually most convenient. The most favorable condition for the exercise of the memory is, usually, with the eyes closed and covered, but by practice it becomes possible to remember equally well with the eyes open. When patients are able, with their eyes closed and covered, to remember perfectly a letter of diamond type, it appears, just as it would if they were looking at with the bodily eyes, to have a slight movement, while the openings appear whiter than the rest of the background. If they are not able to remember it, they are told to shift consciously from one side of the letter to another and to consciously imagine the opening whiter than the rest of the background.

When they do this, the letter usually appears to move in a direction contrary to that of the imagined movement of the eye, and they are able to remember it indefinitely. If, on the contrary, they try to fix the attention on one part of the letter, or to think of two or more parts at one time, it soon disappears, demonstrating that it is impossible to think of one point continuously, or to think of two or more points perfectly at one time, just as it is impossible to look at a point continuously, or to see two points perfectly at the same time. Persons with no visual memory are always under a great strain and often suffer from pain and fatigue with no apparent cause. As soon as they become able to form mental pictures, either with the eyes closed or open, their pain and fatigue are relieved.

IMAGINATION

Imagination is closely allied to memory, for we can imagine only as well as we remember, and in the treatment of imperfect sight the two can scarcely be separated. Vision is largely a matter of imagination and memory. And since both imagination and memory are impossible without perfect relaxation, the cultivation of these faculties not only improves the interpretation of the pictures on the retina, but improves the pictures themselves. When you imagine that you see a letter on the test card, you actually do see it, because it is impossible to relax and imagine the letter perfectly and, at the same time, strain and see it imperfectly.

The following method of using the imagination has produced quick results in many cases: The patient is asked to look at the largest letter on the test card at the near point, and is usually able to observe that a small area, about a square inch, appears blacker than the rest, and that when the part of the letter seen worst is covered, part of the exposed area seems blacker than the remainder. When the part seen worst is again covered, the area at maximum blackness is still further reduced. When the part seen best has been reduced to about the size of a letter on the bottom line, the patient is asked to imagine that such a letter occupies this area and is blacker than the rest of the letter. Then he is asked to look at a letter on the bottom line and imagine that it is blacker than the largest letter. Many are able to do this and at once become able to see the letters on the bottom line.

FLASHING

Since it is effort that spoils the sight, many persons with imperfect sight are able, after a period of rest, to look at an object for a fraction of a second. If the eyes are closed before the habit of strain reasserts itself, permanent relaxation is sometimes very quickly obtained. This practice I have called *flashing,* and many persons are helped by it who are unable to improve their sight by other means. The eyes are rested for a few minutes, by closing or palming, and then a letter on the test card, or a letter of diamond type, if the trouble is with near vision, is regarded for a fraction of a second. Then the eyes are immediately closed and the process repeated.

READING FAMILIAR LETTERS

The eye always strains to see unfamiliar objects, and is always relaxed to a greater or lesser degree by looking at familiar objects. Therefore, the reading every day of small familiar letters at the greatest distance at which they can be seen, is a rest to the eye and is sufficient to cure children under twelve who have not worn glasses as well as some older children and adults with minor defects of vision.

In the treatment of imperfect sight these fundamental principles are to a great extent interdependent. They cannot be separated as in the above article. It is impossible, for instance, to produce the illusion of a swing unless one possesses a certain degree of central fixation. That is, one must be able to shift from one point to another and see the point shifted from less distinctly than the one directly regarded. Successful palming is impossible without mental shifting and swinging and the use of the memory and imagination.

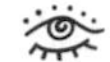

STORIES FROM THE CLINIC

No. 16: Methods That Have Succeeded

By Emily C. Lierman

The patients who come to our Clinic do wonderful things, especially the schoolchildren. We can give each one of them, as a rule, only about five minutes of our time, and yet they are able to carry out the instructions given to them at home, and to get results. This is a great tribute to their patience and intelligence.

Most of the children, and of the grown people as well, are helped by palming, and some wonderful cures have been obtained by this means alone. In my first story for this magazine I told about a little boy named Joey whose left eye had been so injured in an automobile accident that he had only light perception left. It was some time before I could get him to palm regularly, but as soon as he became willing to do it many times a day his sight began to improve rapidly, and he is now completely cured.

There are some patients, however, who cannot or will not palm. One of these was a little girl with corkscrew curls who, for all the world, looked like Topsy. She had been sent to the Clinic because she could not see the writing on the blackboard, and the school nurse told me later that she was very unruly and a great trial to her teacher. She was something of a trial to me too at first, for I could not get her to palm for a moment, and did not know what to do with her. Then I discovered that she had a wonderful memory when she chose to use it, and I resolved to treat her by the aid of this faculty. I was able to improve her sight considerably, and the very next day her teacher noticed such a change in her behavior that on the next Clinic day the school nurse came with her to see what I had done. I then asked her to remember, with closed eyes, a letter on the test card gray instead of black. She could not stand still a minute while she did so, and when she opened her eyes there was no improvement in her vision.

Then I asked her to remember the blue beads she had around her neck. She did so for five minutes, standing perfectly still all the time, and when she opened her eyes she read an extra line on the test card. I had her do this again, and again she read an extra line. The nurse was thrilled by this demonstration of the fact that perfect memory improves the sight and relieves nervousness.

Recently a poor young man called at our magazine office and asked if Dr. Bates had written a book about the treatment of the eyes. When told that there was such a book, he bought it and also subscribed for the magazine. His sister was being treated at the Clinic, he said, and he wished to take off his glasses as she had done. Later he came to the Clinic, as he lives in the hospital district. I found that he could not read newspaper print without his glasses, while his distant vision was 12/70, both eyes. This was about six months ago. He now reads diamond type, and last week his sister asked Dr. Bates if he had finer print, as her brother found the diamond type so easy that he wanted something smaller. Dr. Bates gave her a page from a photographic reduction of the Bible, and he reads this also without any trouble. The methods he used were swinging and flashing, together with palming.

The influence of this cure has been extensive and is still going on. The patient loaned the book to a myopic youth in his office, and by means of palming he was able to improve his sight so that now he dispenses with glasses for long periods. An elderly man in the same office thought the palming a very absurd practice but, having borrowed the book, he started shifting and flashing at lunch time, just to pass the time. He now does much of his work without glasses.

One mother came to the Clinic recently with her little girl, Jennie, of eight, and said the child must have glasses. The school nurse had said so. I replied that I was very sorry indeed, but that Dr. Bates did not fit glasses, and she would have to call some other day and see the doctor who did do so. She was about to leave the room when I suggested that I should test the child's sight. I felt sorry for the little girl, because she was very pretty except for her eyes, which were partly closed most of the time.

"I don't like to wear glasses," she said. "Please help me so that I won't have to wear them." The mother seemed bewildered at first, and then she said in a burst of confidence, "You know, nurse, if her glasses cost nothing, I should not worry. But all the time money, money for glasses, when all the time she breaks them."

I told the poor mother not to worry, because her child could be cured so that she would not need glasses if she would do what I told her to do. "Sure, sure," she replied. "That's all right, lady. You fix her eyes, yes? When we don't buy glasses, we got more money to buy something for her stomach, yes?"

I treated the little girl, who turned out to be a very interesting patient. We have some bright children in our Clinic and I am proud of them; but this dear little girl beat them all. She did such a wonderful thing that Dr. Bates was thrilled. Jennie had never seen the test card before, and after palming was able to read only the 30-line at fifteen feet. Below this the card was a blank to her. I asked her to follow my finger while, with very rapid movement, I pointed to the large letter at the top and so on down to the 10-line.

I now asked her to palm and, pointing to the last letter on the 10-line, which was an "F" and quite small, I asked her if she could remember some letter her teacher had written on the blackboard that way. She replied, "Yes, I can imagine I see the letter 'O,' a white 'O'." "Keep your eyes closed," I said, "and imagine that the letter I am pointing at has a curved top. Can you still imagine the 'O'?" "No," she said, "I can't imagine anything now." "Can you imagine it is open, or straight at the top?" I asked. She became excited and said, "If I imagine it has a straight top, I can still remember the white 'O'." "Fine," I said. "Can you imagine it has a straight line at the bottom?" "No," she said, "if I do that I lose the 'O.' I can imagine it's open much better." "Good," I said. "It is open. Now imagine it is open or curved to the left." "I lose the 'O'," she said, "if I imagine the left side open or curved. I think it's an 'F,' nurse."

And when she opened her eyes she saw it plainly. The fact was that, although she had been unable to see this letter consciously, she had unconsciously seen it for a fraction of a second and could not imagine it to be other than it was without a strain that caused her to lose control of her memory. And when she imagined it to be what it was she relaxed so that when she opened her eyes she was able to see it.

A little later a school nurse brought us a child who was giving her teacher a lot of trouble because she could not remember anything, and it was thought glasses might help her. She was very nervous, frowned terribly and at twelve feet the letters on the bottom line of the test card were only black spots to her. As I could not get her to palm, I asked her to look at a letter on the bottom line and with closed eyes imagine it had a straight top. She could not do this and said she could imagine it curved better. Then she found she could imagine two other sides curved and one open, and when she opened her eyes she saw the letter, a "C," distinctly, and had stopped frowning. By the same method she became able to read all the other letters on the bottom line, demonstrating that her imperfect memory had been due to eyestrain. She had unconsciously seen the letters, but the eyestrain had suppressed the memory of them. With her eyes closed the strain was relaxed, and she became able to remember, or imagine, them.

MY METHODS WITH SCHOOLCHILDREN

By a Public School Nurse

Editor's Note—Better Eyesight *considers itself fortunate to be able to publish this remarkable record of the improvement of the vision of schoolchildren by means of the methods which it advocates. The attitude of the educational authorities toward the beneficent work of this public-spirited nurse is noteworthy.*

On re-reading an article in the August 1920 issue of *Better Eyesight* I find that a nurse, after inquiry in regard to treatment of the eyes without glasses, and observations at Dr. Bates' Clinic, said she would treat the children at school in the same way. I started last fall, in a district school located in one of the suburbs of New York City, to do likewise, but, unfortunately, after having helped several children, I am advised by the school authorities to discontinue. However, I shall give some idea of the work already accomplished. In the examination for records of the children's eyesight, etc., I found several quite below normal—some with one eye more than normal and the others far below. In one case for instance, the left eye was 20/13 and the right 9/200 This child, Catherine, after having been shown how to practice, was able to help herself by cutting the letters from a newspaper and pinning them to the wall until she procured a test card. At the present time her sight is 12/50 in the right eye, a four-fold improvement. All this she has done by her own efforts and practice at home. I have helped her only once since the first examination in the latter part of March. Her mother has taken off her glasses, too, and does not suffer any more with burning of the eyes, as she did formerly. She is grateful and much pleased with her success.

Another child I brought to the Clinic, and Dr. Bates saw him after I had helped to correct a squint in the left eye, which remains straight unless he strains. The correction occurred at the beginning of the school year. The child's sight has also improved, in spite of the fact that he practices less at home than any of the others and needs constant urging.

The children come to me just before the close of the morning session, sometimes for only fifteen minutes. They palm and do the swing, either the head alone or the entire body. Lately I've found that the swing was more successful than palming alone.

When examining the children in the classroom, I found

they could read the 20-line at twenty feet after starting at 30- or 40-line, if the strain was relieved. I would point to a letter or number on the 30- or 40-line and then return to the 20-line. Almost immediately they would read 20/20.

All the children are greatly interested and pleased with their progress, and the parents fully approve. In every instance I have let the parents decide whether or not the children should be treated so that they would not need glasses. The children themselves say very emphatically that they will not wear glasses.

Better Eyesight
July 1921—Vol. V, No. 1

STOP CONCENTRATING NUMBER

HOW NOT TO CONCENTRATE

To remember the letter "o" of diamond type continuously and without effort, proceed as follows:

Imagine a little black spot (a period) on the right-hand side of the "o" blacker than the rest of the letter; then imagine a similar spot on the left-hand side. Shift the attention from the right-hand period to the left, and observe that every time that you think of the left period the "o" appears to move to the right, and every time you think of the right one it appears to move to the left. This motion, when the shifting is done properly, is very short, less than the width of the letter. Later you may become able to imagine the "o" without conscious shifting and swinging, but whenever the attention is directed to the matter these things will be noticed.

Now do the same with the "a" letter on the test card. If the shifting is normal, it will be noted that the letter can be regarded indefinitely, and that it appears to have a slight motion.

To demonstrate that the attempt to concentrate spoils the memory, or imagination, and the vision:

Try to think continuously of a period on one part of an imagined letter. The period and the whole letter will soon disappear. Or try to imagine two or more periods, or the whole letter, equally black and distinct at one time. This will be found to be even more difficult.

Do the same with a letter on the test card. The results will be the same.

THE VICE OF CONCENTRATION

By W. H. Bates, M.D.

Most patients who come to me for the cure of imperfect sight think that they have to "concentrate" in order to improve their vision. When told that they should see nothing but black when their eyes are closed and covered, they think that they can arrive at this state by "concentrating" on the black. When they look at a line of letters and see it imperfectly and all alike, they think it is because they cannot "concentrate." If they see better after closing their eyes or palming, they think it is because these things have helped them to "concentrate." It is very hard to get these ideas out of their heads, even though, after "concentrating for all they are worth," as they express it, they invariably find that their sight is worse instead of better.

By concentration they seem to mean the ability to do, see, or remember, one thing at a time, for as long a time as they want to, and to stop doing, seeing and remembering everything else; and they are quite convinced that this can be accomplished by effort. As these ideas are almost entirely erroneous, it is not strange that their sight should fail to improve under their influence.

It is physiologically impossible to see one thing at a time and exclude everything else from sight, because nature has given us a visual field of considerable range. It is true that we can see even a very small object continuously, but only if the attention shifts constantly from one part to another, because the eye is in constant motion, and any attempt to stop this motion lowers the vision and causes the object to blur or disappear. When the vision is normal the movements of the eye are short, rhythmical and easy, and each successive point fixed is seen better than any other point. In the eye with imperfect sight the movements are longer, irregular and accompanied by strain. The points fixed are not seen best, so that the object may be seen all alike at one time. In neither case is it possible to stop the motion; but the eye with imperfect sight tries unconsciously to do so and to look at each point for an appreciable length of time. This unconscious attempt to concentrate upon a point is an invariable accompaniment of imperfect sight, and is always produced by an effort to see. When, therefore, patients try to "concentrate" upon a letter, the eye attempts to stop shifting, and the vision is made worse. Even in the case of an eye with previously normal sight, such an effort will quickly cause the letters to blur or disappear.

Although the physiological reasons for it are not so plain, the mind is subject to the same law as the eye. It cannot think of one thing to the exclusion of all other things. Nor can it think continuously of an unchanging object without continuous shifting of the attention. The attempt to do these things is accompanied by a strain which is reflected in the eyes and always produces abnormal conditions there.

It is often hard to get patients to realize these facts, because the shifting of attention may be and usually is unconscious. At points where the vision is good, patients may shift normally and easily from one part of a letter to another without being aware of the fact and without noticing the swing produced by this motion. Therefore they often imagine that they can see it all alike at one time for an indefinite period. In the same way they think that they can remember or imagine a letter all alike at one time continuously. One patient looked at an "F" for the better part of an hour, seeing it all the time perfectly black and distinct and, as he thought, all alike and stationary.

He was directed to imagine with his eyes closed that a small, black spot on the upper corner of the 10-line "F" was the blackest part of the letter. Then he was told to remember a similar period on the bottom of the letter and to forget the top period. Next he was directed to shift between these two periods, remembering each one alternately as the blackest part of the letter. He did this easily and noted that every time he thought of the top period, the letter appeared to move downward; and every time he thought of the lower period, the letter appeared to move upward. When he tried to concentrate on one period, however, he immediately lost it and lost the whole letter with it. To imagine two or more periods, or the whole letter, equally black at one time was even more difficult. Having demonstrated with his eyes closed that it was impossible to think continuously of one point, or to think of two or more points equally well at the same time, but very easy to shift continuously from one point to another, he became able to realize that he could not see the letter on the test card perfectly and continuously when he saw it all alike at one time, and could not even see one point perfectly black continuously.

Most patients, when asked to remember or imagine a letter of diamond type, state that they can do it continuously and that they see it all alike at one time. When asked to concentrate on a point, or imagine one or more points equally well at one time however, they find it, as in the case just mentioned, impossible; while they have no difficulty in shifting continuously from one point to another. After having demonstrated these facts they find it impossible to remember a letter all alike at one time, and realize that when they seemed to do so they must have been unconsciously shifting and swinging.

It is strange that physiologists and psychologists have never published these facts. The normal shifting of the eye is so short and easy that it is scarcely perceptible. The apparent movement of objects regarded, produced by this motion, is also inconspicuous; yet it is sufficiently marked so that when patients are asked whether the letters they are looking at are moving or stationary they often answer that they are moving. When asked to stop the movement or imagine that the letters are stationary, they reply that they cannot, and that the attempt to do so causes discomfort or pain. One patient even noticed the phenomenon without any hint from me, and came back to me several months after I had cured her to ask for an explanation. The movement, which she noticed only when she looked at a letter continuously, not when she read a few of the letters more or less rapidly, did not trouble her, she said; in fact, when she tried to stop it she felt uncomfortable and her vision was lowered; but having never heard of it, she was afraid it might indicate something wrong with her eyes.

Psychologists tell us that it is impossible to attend continuously to an unchanging stimulus. This is true, but some of the proofs adduced in support of it are open to criticism. James says that if you try to attend steadfastly to a dot on a piece of paper, or on the wall, "you will presently find that one or the other of two things has happened: either your field of vision has become blurred so that you now see nothing distinct at all, or else you have involuntarily ceased to look at the dot in question, and are looking at something else. But if you ask yourself successive questions about the dot—how big it is, how far, of what shape, what shade of color, etc.; in other words if you turn it over, if you think of it in various ways, and along with various kinds of associations—you can keep your mind on it for a comparatively long time."[1]

It is probably true that in most cases the person who looks at a dot under the conditions in question would find his vision blurring, or his attention shifting to something else, because he would make an effort to see it. He would stare at it, or "concentrate" upon it. But a person with normal, or nearly normal vision, who looks at such a dot easily and naturally, can regard it indefinitely, because his eyes unconsciously shift from one part of it to another. Other persons, if they shift consciously and realize the apparent motion thus produced, will often find it possible to hold their attention on the dot for a considerable time, but will not see it as distinctly as persons who shift unconsciously. As for asking one's self questions about the dot, I have often tried this experiment with patients, but never found that it corrected the tendency to stare.

The idea that the attention can be forced is a very common one and is very bad for the eyes. It is greatly encouraged by popular writers, but is contrary to the teachings of more reliable psychologists who know that forced attention can only be momentary, and that it is a great strain upon the mind and the whole body. Ladd records that the subject of an experiment to determine reaction-time under concentrated attention often "though sitting quiet, sweats profusely."[2]

Since attempts to force the mind are reflected in the eyes, the popular ideas of concentration must be responsible for a great deal of that strain which is the cause of imperfect sight.

STORIES FROM THE CLINIC
No. 17: Some Results of Concentration
By Emily C. Lierman

Almost all the patients who come to us at the Clinic, especially adults, think it necessary to concentrate in order to see better. They think concentration is part of our method of treatment, and until they learn better I cannot make any progress with them.

A young girl about eighteen or nineteen years old came one day recently, holding her glasses in her hand and anxiously waiting to be treated. She told me she had worn glasses for seven years, and that she had consulted several oculists and opticians without getting any relief from the pain in her eyes. With her glasses she read 15/20, and without them 15/50, both eyes. When she closed her eyes I noticed a twitching of her eyelids. She was told to open her eyes and look at a letter on the card, then to close them and remember the blackness of the letter, thinking first of the bottom and then of the top, alternately. When a few minutes later she removed her hands from her eyes she could not see the letter which she had seen before.

I wondered why her sight did not improve, but I understood when she said, "I did what you asked me to do. You told me to remember the letter 'O,' and I held on to it and tried hard not to remember anything else. But now my pain is worse than before."

"You did not understand me," I said. "I did not ask you to hold on to the letter 'O.' I asked you to remember the blackness of it, and see or imagine one part best at a time."

She tried it again, covering her eyes with her hands, and this time I said to her, "Remember the letter 'O' as you saw it, but first remember the top best. Now what happens to

1. *Talks to Teachers,* 1915, p. 104.
2. *Elements of Physiological Psychology,* 1900, p. 543.

the bottom?" "It fades from black to gray," she said. "Now remember the bottom blacker than the top." "The same thing happens to the top," she said. "It fades to gray color." And then she added, "Please let me keep doing this for a little while, it seems to take my pain away."

After five minutes or so I had to ask her to remove her hands from her eyes, as I could not spend any more time with her, and I wanted to know if I had helped her. As she looked at the card again she saw the "O" very plainly, and also read two more lines, the 40- and the 30-lines. The twitching of her eyelids had ceased, and she was able to smile. This patient is still coming, and is now able to read most of the 10-line at fifteen feet, 15/10 minus. She is also able to read some of the letters in a paragraph of diamond type at eight inches from her eyes; but when I hold the type at six inches and ask her to fix her eyes on one corner of the card and stare at it, the whole surface becomes a blank and the pain in her head and eyes comes back.

One day an Irish mother came with her little boy of eleven, who was suffering terrible pain. Dr. Bates and I were not very busy at that moment, which was something quite unusual, and we both listened together to her story, the gist of which was, "The school nurse says he needs glasses. 'Tis trouble he's havin' with his eyes."

The boy all the while kept his eyes covered with a white cloth, and at first glance I thought he was crying because the part of his face that I was able to see was much flushed. Dr. Bates asked me to see what I could do for him, and his mother began to talk again.

"I haven't any time to be foolin' round here, ma'am," she informed me. "I got to get back to me washin.' It's glasses he needs, ma'am." When she finally stopped for want of breath, I said, "Now wouldn't it be fine and dandy to cure him so that he wouldn't need glasses?"

As I said this, down came the cloth from the boy's eyes. He was interested and returned my smile. "Just you leave him to me and I will cure him," I said to his mother. "And never mind leaving your work for him again. He can come here by himself." "Sure ma'am, is it dreamin' ye are, or is it a bit o' blarney yer given' me?" she inquired. "No," I said, "it isn't dreaming or blarney. Be a good mother and just watch your boy and see what happens."

I tested the boy's sight with the Snellen test card and found that his vision was 12/40 with each eye. Then I gave him a stool and showed him how to palm. Some minutes afterwards I told him to remove his hands from his eyes and look at the card. He stared at it as if some wild animal were after him. I discovered that his mother was threatening him, talking to him in a low tone. Evidently she thought she would please me by forcing him to do what I wished. By this time I knew that the boy was afraid of his mother, and I quietly invited her to take a nice, comfortable seat outside the room. The boy informed me that his name was Joe, and as I smoothed his hair and gave him a few pats, the most affectionate look came into his eyes. Then we got down to business again. I told him to palm and reminded him of a baseball.

"Imagine you are throwing the ball," I said. "Now imagine that you are catching it. Now look at the card."

He smiled when he saw the letters come out blacker and more distinct than before. The redness of his face, which at first I had thought was from fever, left him, and his eyes, which were Irish blue, were clear and wide open. He read the 30-line at twelve feet and part of the 20-line, which I thought was doing well for the first visit. Now it occurred to me to see what would happen if he concentrated, or stared. I told him to look at the first letter on the 40-line, a "Z," and keep his mind fixed on it no matter what happened. As he did this he began to frown, his forehead became wrinkled, and his face became red again. "I don't like to do that, nurse," he said. "All the other letters disappear and my head hurts."

I told him to palm again and remember the letter "Z," thinking first of the top, then of the bottom. When he looked at the card again he saw the letters clearly once more, and read all of the 20-line at fifteen feet. When he arrived at the 10-line, however, the first letter bothered him. He twisted his head in all directions. He stared at the letter, and finally decided to palm again. After a few moments I asked him to open his eyes, and told him that there were three of the same letters on the card, but that they were scattered here and there on the different lines. He again started to read the card, and as he saw the first letter on the 100-line, which was a "D," he said, "Now I know the first letter on the 10-line is a 'D'." Shifting his eyes from the 100-line to the 10-line letter had helped him to see it.

His last visit was a very interesting one. At the beginning of the treatment I explained to him how important it was for him to practice palming at least half a dozen times a day, but he did not feel that he could spare the time, because he earns a little money running errands for his mother. At the next to the last visit I had a talk with him about this and said, "If your eyes are cured you can earn more money during vacation time, but you cannot if they trouble you."

He promised to practice at home as many times as I wished him to, so I made him a promise. My rose garden in the country was in full bloom and I promised to bring him a bouquet the next Clinic day. Not having enough flowers for each patient, I wrapped Joe's bouquet in paper and asked Dr. Bates to carry it. Joe spied me first as we passed the long line of benches which were filled with poor people, all of them suffering from some eye trouble. His hair was combed, which was unusual, and he was spruced up generally. He was smiling, too, and his eyes were shining with great expectations. But when he saw that my hands were empty, the smile vanished, and a look of disappointment came into his eyes. I know what it means to be disappointed, so I told him at once that Dr. Bates was bringing the bouquet for him, and the sun shone for him once more. I was well repaid for those flowers, for that day Joe made wonderful progress.

He had to wait some time before I could treat him, and he never took his eyes from me. I could feel his gratitude, and my impulse was to take him in my arms and hug him tight; but I refrained, thinking he might resent the familiarity. He read the 10-line at fifteen feet, 15/10, in less than a minute, and he told me that he did not suffer any more pain in his head. He also said that his studies seemed easier to him when he remembered not to stare or think too hard of one thing.

QUESTIONS AND ANSWERS

Q–1a. After leaving off my glasses and practicing the methods advocated in your magazine for six months, I went to the oculist who gave me glasses eleven years ago to have my eyes re-examined. He said the astigmatism was exactly what it was eleven years ago, but that there had been some improvement in the nearsightedness. I am sending you the prescriptions, old and new. I apparently see better than when I took off my glasses, and there are times when I see letters measuring 3/32nds of an inch in height at a distance of ten feet. This lasts until I wink, when the letters become blurred and indistinguishable. Could there have been an improvement in the astigmatism without the oculist's observing it? 1b. What is the percentage of improvement in each eye? 1c. In your experience, when astigmatism has been cured, how does it go—all at once, or gradually? 1d. Do you think I have made enough progress to warrant my continuing, or should I go back to glasses, which always gave me comfort, and leave perfect eyesight for those more easily cured?

A–1a. Yes. During the examination you may have been under a strain. 1b. It is impossible to judge your improvement by comparing your glasses, because the refraction is continually changing. 1c. It may go in either way. 1d. Yes. Your trouble is so slight that I do not understand why it should take you so long to correct it.

Q–2. After being out in the bright sunlight everything looks intensely black to me indoors. Is this a natural consequence of the exposure of the eyes to bright light, or does the normal eye not experience it?

A–2. Many persons with imperfect sight, and also persons with ordinarily normal sight suffer in the way you describe after going indoors out of the bright sunlight, and the trouble can be relieved by any method which brings about a complete relief of strain.

Q–3. What is the quickest cure for inability to read without glasses on account of advancing years?

A–3. Close the eyes and remember a small letter of the alphabet perfectly. Open the eyes, and at twelve inches look at the corner of a card showing a specimen of diamond type, remembering the letter as well as you can. Close the eyes or palm, and remember the letter better. Alternately, remember it with the eyes open (and looking at the corner of the card) and closed, until the memory with the eyes open and closed is nearly equal. Then look between the lines and do the same thing. In this way some patients become able in half an hour to read the letters on the card. Others require days, weeks, or longer.

Q–4. Is it possible to become able to read without glasses after the extraction of cataract?

A–4. Yes. Accommodation is brought about by a lengthening of the eyeball through the action of a pair of muscles on the outside. If the patient is able to look at a printed page without effort or strain, the eyeball will lengthen sufficiently to compensate for the loss of the lens.

Better Eyesight
August 1921—Vol. V, No. 2

SCHOOL NUMBER

CHILDREN MAY IMPROVE THEIR SIGHT BY CONSCIOUSLY DOING THE WRONG THING

Children often make a great effort to see the blackboard and other distant objects in school. It helps them to overcome this habit to have them demonstrate just what the strain to see does.

Tell them to fix their attention on the smallest letter they can see from their seats, to stare at it, to concentrate on it, to partly close their eyelids—in short, to make as great an effort as possible to see it.

The letter will blur or disappear altogether and the whole card may become blurred, while discomfort or pain in the eyes or head will be produced.

Now direct them to rest their eyes by palming. The pain or discomfort will cease, the letter will come out again, and other letters that they could not see before may come out also.

After a demonstration like this children are less likely to make an effort to see the blackboard, or anything else; but some children have to repeat the experiment many times before the subconscious inclination to strain is corrected.

SIGHT-SAVING IN THE SCHOOLROOM

By Edith F. Gavin

It seemed so wonderful to me to be able to lay aside my glasses and have eye comfort after wearing them for twenty-two years with discomfort the greater part of the time! I could scarcely wait to get back home to talk to the other teachers about it and try to help a few of the children.

I began with Gertrude, who was so nearsighted that from a front seat she was unable to see very black figures one and one-half inches high printed on a white chart and hanging on the front board. Her vision on January 11, 1921, was 20/70 in both eyes, but by March 10 she had improved to 20/70 with the right eye and 20/30 with the left and could read the chart from the last seat in the row.

Matilda had complained of headaches since last September. Glasses were obtained last December, and after a two months' struggle to get used to them, she refused to wear them, saying that they made her head and eyes feel worse. I then told her how to palm and practice with the chart. She had no more headaches in school, and her mother said she didn't complain at home. Her vision also improved from 20/30 to 20/15.

I next took Walter in hand. His mother would not get glasses for him, although advised to do so by the school nurse and doctor. His vision February 18 was 20/200. Three weeks later his mother decided to get glasses for him, but his vision had improved to 20/20 in the right eye and 20/30 in the left.

Helen's teacher brought her to me, saying she was so nervous and read in such a halting manner that she felt sure that her glasses did not fit her. Her mother said that she might lay aside her glasses and Helen could hardly wait to begin. Shortly after, she was taken ill with scarlet fever and did not return, but her vision improved from 20/40 to 20/15, and her teacher said that her reading had improved noticeably.

Mollie, age six, was sent in to me February 18. She tested 20/70 in the right eye and 20/50 in the left. Her vision in May was 20/30, right, and 20/20, left.

When Rae came to my room on May 15, her vision was 20/70. Her father was very much opposed to her wearing glasses and readily gave permission for me to help her. She remained in the district only two weeks, but she had improved to 20/20 in the right eye and 20/30 in the left.

Bennie, mentally defective, required a great deal of patience, but he improved from 20/50 February 9 to 20/15 March 4.

Leo, a fifth grade pupil, was sent to me February 20 by his teacher. She said he wouldn't wear his glasses and was a poor student. He tested 20/50 in the right eye and 20/30 in the left. By March 15 his vision was 20/30, right eye, and 20/15, left, and his teacher said that he showed a marked improvement in his scholarship.

The children needing help came to me fifteen minutes before the afternoon session began. If I was busy with one, the others would work quietly by themselves, seeming to take great pride in their improvement. The chart hangs on the front wall at all times. I taught the class how to palm and often different ones would come up early to practice. Several children with apparently normal vision told me that they were able to read two or three lines more at the end of the term. To my mind there is no limit to the good that might be accomplished if this method were in general use in the schools.

MY EXPERIENCE IN TREATING MYOPIA

By Irene Kundtz

Having worn glasses constantly for seven years and then, after a week's treatment, returning to school without them, not only caused great excitement amongst my school friends, but began my experience in trying to benefit others. It was then that I really realized what a wonderful thing it was to have perfect sight and never again wear glasses.

My first patient was my chum Margaret, who roomed across the hall from me. She was now fifteen years old and had worn glasses ever since she was a small child. With her glasses off she could faintly see the large letter "C." So I immediately taught her the correct way of palming. This not only interested her but my two roommates also, for the blacker they imagined a cat or a period, the better they could read in the dim light. After palming for at least ten minutes she looked up and was greatly surprised to see the large "C" much blacker and more distinct. Then I gave her a card with diamond type and taught her to swing the little black figure "1." This was something new for all three girls, and soon I found myself treating three patients instead of one. Swinging seemed rather difficult to them until they tried moving their heads from side to side, in this way getting a short, easy swing of a quarter of an inch or less. As our time was very limited at the dormitory I was able to work with Margaret for only a half-hour, but in that short time she read three letters at a distance of fourteen feet. When her first treatment was over she promised to come again the next evening, and a little earlier if possible.

The news of Margaret being able to read three letters on the Snellen test card spread through the dormitory very rapidly, and the next morning before school I had two other girls ask if they might join the class. I was indeed glad to have them and could hardly wait until evening to resume my fascinating work.

My two new patients were both fourteen years old and had worn glasses since the second grade. As my roommates were out visiting we were able to work for forty-five minutes in peace, and each became more anxious to beat the other, for with their glasses off they could read through the 70-line. While I taught them how to palm, Margaret was practicing at swinging the figure "1" and working at the first letter in the following line, but nothing seemed to give her as much rest and benefit as palming. So after helping her she would palm again while I took care of the other two girls. At the end of forty-five minutes we had made quite a little progress, Margaret having read through the 70-line by palming alone, and the other two girls through two letters in the 50-line.

Having succeeded in helping three of my girl friends, I next began to talk to some of my teachers who had worn glasses from ten to fifteen years. But teachers as a rule are very busy correcting papers, etc.; so not being able to treat them as well, I lent them Dr. Bates' book called *Perfect Sight Without Glasses,* and found to my great delight that it worked just as well, for it not only gave them a start but interested their friends also.

Thus I continued giving treatments, sometimes for only fifteen or twenty minutes an evening, but every little bit helped and each treatment brought me more patients, and gave me more joy and courage to continue.

After treating Margaret for a week, for she was my best patient and really made the most progress, she was able to read through the 50-line, and would have continued to improve more rapidly had she been able to go to school without her glasses.

My experience in treating myopia lasted only two weeks, for at the end of that time examinations began and my evenings were occupied with studies. Helping and treating others was not only very interesting work, but was also benefiting me in continuing my daily practice.

STORIES FROM THE CLINIC

No. 18: The Schoolchildren Again

By Emily C. Lierman

We have so many interesting cases among the children sent to us from the schools to be fitted with glasses that one hardly knows where to begin when trying to tell about them. Little Agnes, eight years old, comes to my mind, not because she was more remarkable than a good many others, but because she came recently. Her mother came with her and told me that Agnes suffered from frequent headaches and that for the past year her teachers had been saying that she needed glasses, as she had great difficulty in seeing the blackboard. The mother had hesitated to take her to an oculist, however, as two of her children were already wearing glasses and she did not want to see them on a third.

I could easily see that Agnes was suffering, and when I tested her eyes with the Snellen test card I found that her vision was very poor. At fifteen feet she could not read more than the 70-line. This was so surprising in so young a child that I thought at first she did not know her letters; but when I tested her with pothooks she did no better. I now showed her how to palm, and in a few moments she read the bottom line. The mother was thrilled and said, "My goodness! When I first entered this room my hope was gone. I could think of nothing but glasses for my child. When she first read the card and I saw how bad her eyes were, I was convinced that there was no escape for her. But now that I see her vision improved so quickly I have hope indeed."

I told the mother that I was thrilled myself, and added that she could help me to cure the child if she would. "What I do for her here you can do for her at home." I said. "Encourage her to rest her eyes. Nature requires rest for the eyes, but your little girl, instead of closing her eyes when they are tired, strains to keep them open." The mother promised to do all she could, and as she was leaving she said, "God sent me here. I will send my two boys to be rid of their glasses also."

The next Clinic day Agnes brought with her brother Peter, who was wearing glasses for astigmatism and headaches. He was very attentive while I treated Agnes, who told me that she had not been having her usual headaches. Peter's vision I found to be 15/40, right eye, and 15/15, left eye. After palming only a few minutes his right eye improved to 15/15 and his left to 15/10. He was very happy when told that he did not need glasses any more, and that I could cure him during vacation. As children are cured very quickly when one helps the other at home, I expect that Agnes and Peter will soon be reading 20/10, which is twice what the normal eye is expected to do.

Another recent patient was Mary, twelve years old. She complained of such violent headaches that she could no longer attend school and stayed in bed most of the time. The school nurse had advised glasses, and she had come to get them. Mary kept her head lowered much of the time, but when I was about to treat her she tried to open one eye and look at me. The effort was so great that her face became a mass of wrinkles. As the light seemed to distress her, I decided to give her the light treatment, that is, to focus the rays of the sun on the upper part of her eyeballs with a glass. I asked her to sit on a stool where the sun could shine on her eyes. To reassure her I asked a patient who had already had the treatment to let me repeat it on her, and when Mary saw her enjoy the light bath she readily submitted to it herself. Afterward her eyes opened wide and I was able to test her sight. Her vision was 20/50, both eyes. I showed her how to palm, and when, after ten minutes, she opened her eyes, her pain was gone and her vision perfect. I was quite proud to have accomplished so much in one treatment.

Two days later Mary came again, and with her came the school nurse and a friend, both eager to hear more of the miracle that had been worked on Mary. Could it be possible, the nurse asked, that the child had been cured as quickly as she said? I was surprised myself at the change in the patient's appearance. Her eyes were still wide open, and the constant grin on her face made her almost unrecognizable as the sad creature I had seen two days before. I told the nurse what had been done for the child and how she could help the other children in her school who had eye trouble.

She came a few times more to watch our methods and told me that she was teaching all the children sent to her for examination of their eyes to palm. This always relieved them, to some extent, at once. The hard cases, however, she sent to us without delay.

A very remarkable case still under treatment is that of a girl with nystagmus, a condition in which the eyes vibrate from side to side. The child is now so much improved that ordinarily her eyes are normal, but when anything disturbs her the vibration returns. This always happens, she tells me, when the teacher asks her a question, and at the same time she loses her memory. But the teacher allows her to cover her eyes to rest them, and in a few minutes the vibration ceases and her memory improves. Before she came to the Clinic she often became hysterical and was obliged to leave the classroom. Now she is never troubled in this way.

One of the most puzzling cases I ever had was sent by the school nurse for glasses. A patient who came from the same school told me that she was stupid, and she certainly appeared to be so. I asked her if she knew her letters, and in trying to reply she stuttered painfully. I tried to reassure her by speaking as gently as I could, but without avail. I could not get her to answer intelligently. I tried having her palm, but it did not help. I held the test card close to her eyes and asked her to point out certain letters as I named them, but only in a few cases did she do this correctly. Completely baffled I appealed to Dr. Bates. He asked the child to come to him and touch a button on his coat, and she did so.

He asked her to touch another button, but she answered, "I don't see them." "Look down at your shoes," he said. "Do you see them?" "No," she answered. "Go over and put your finger on the doorknob," he said, and she immediately did so. "It is a case of hysterical blindness," the Doctor said.

The child came for some time very regularly, and now reads 15/10 with both eyes. She has stopped stuttering, and has lost her reputation for stupidity. She has become a sort of good Samaritan in her neighborhood, for every once in a while she brings with her some little companion to be cured of imperfect sight. She never has any doubts as to our capacity to do this, and so far we have never disappointed her. I hope she never brings anyone who is beyond our power to help, for I would be sorry to see that sublime faith which we have inspired in her shattered.

Two of our patients graduated in June, and after the final examinations they told me that they had been greatly helped in these tests by the memory of a swinging black period. One of them was told by the principal that if she failed to pass, it would not be because of her stupidity but because she refused to wear glasses. She gave him Dr. Bates' book, and after that, though he watched her closely, he did not say anything more about her eyes.

"I made up my mind to pass without the aid of glasses," she said, "and put one over on the principal, and you bet I never lost sight of my precious swinging period. The book has become a family treasure," she continued. "When one of us has a pain in head or eyes, out it comes. It is a natural thing to see mother palming after her work is done. She enjoys her evenings with us now because palming rests her and she does not get so sleepy."

The other graduate said, "I did not have to think of a black period when the subject was easy, but when I had to answer questions in the more difficult branches I certainly did find the period a lifesaver. I know I would have failed without it."

BETTER EYESIGHT IN NORTH BERGEN

By M. F. Husted
Superintendent Public Schools
of North Bergen, New Jersey

Editor's Note—Better Eyesight *takes great pleasure in presenting to its readers this remarkable report of the results attained in the schools of North Bergen by the use of the Snellen test card.*

[See "An Educator Offers Proof" in the September 1922 issue.—TRQ]

QUESTIONS AND ANSWERS

Q–1a. Does working by artificial light affect the eyes? I work all day by electric light—am a bookkeeper, and suffer a great deal from my eyes. I have been fitted with glasses, but cannot wear them. I feel that my eyes, instead of getting better from wearing them, get weaker. 1b. When I go out in the street after working I cannot stand the glare of the sun, and must keep my eyes half-closed; otherwise I suffer a great deal of pain. Is it so because of my eyes being accustomed to the artificial light? It is not so on Sundays. 1c. Is it advisable to wear an eye-shade while working?

A–1a. Working by artificial light should not injure the eyes. If it does, it is because you are straining them. The idea that the light is injurious may cause you to do this. If you think of it as quieting and beneficial, it may have the opposite effect. You are right in thinking that the glasses injure your eyes. 1b. The sun hurts your eyes when you go out on the street after working because you have been straining to see, not because you have been working by artificial light. Because you strain less on Sundays the sun does not hurt you. 1c. It is not advisable to wear an eye-shade while working. [Of course, safety glasses should be worn when needed.—TRQ]

Q–2. Can the blindness of squint (amblyopia) be cured?

A–2. Yes. It can be cured by the same methods that are employed to relieve strain in other cases of imperfect sight.

Better Eyesight
September 1921—Vol. V, No. 3

HOW TO IMPROVE THE SIGHT BY MEANS OF THE IMAGINATION: NO. 2

In a recent issue directions were given for improving the vision by the aid of the imagination. According to this method the patient ascertains what a letter is by imagining each of the four sides to be straight, curved, or open, and noting the effect of each guess upon the imagined swing of the letter.

Another method which has succeeded even better with many patients is to judge the correctness of the guess by observing its effect on the appearance of the letter:

Look at a letter which can be seen only as a gray spot, and imagine the top is straight. If the guess is right, the spot will probably become blacker; if it is wrong, the spot may become fainter or disappear. If no difference is apparent, rest the eyes by looking away, closing, or palming, and try again.

In many cases, when one side has been imagined correctly, the whole letter will come out. If it does not, proceed to imagine the other sides as directed above. If, when all four sides have been imagined correctly a letter does not come out, palm and repeat.

One can even bring out a letter that one cannot see at all in this way. Look at a line of letters which cannot be seen, and imagine the top of the first letter to be straight. If the guess is correct, the line may become apparent, and by continued practice the letter may come out clearly enough to be distinguished.

THE FRECKLE-FACED BOY

By W. H. Bates, M.D.

In one of the public schools of New York, some years ago, was a boy about ten years old with a very unusual amount of freckles. He had one of those smiles which some care-free boys carry around with them all the time, in all places, and under all conditions. His teacher was a very nervous person wearing glasses. Every time she spoke I was annoyed, not so much by what she said as by the disagreeable way in which she said it. As soon as I entered the room she began to find fault with me for introducing my method of curing and preventing imperfect sight in children into the school.

Pointing sternly at the freckle-faced boy she said, "That boy is very nearsighted. He holds his book too close to his eyes. He cannot read the writing on the blackboard. He is all the time looking at the Snellen test card instead of studying his lessons. He talks about it to the other children in the class and he encourages them to practice reading it. He tells them that he feels good when he reads it, makes his eyes feel better, and helps him to learn his lessons. He is impertinent because he persists brazenly in advising me, his teacher, to practice reading those fool letters which do not even spell a word and have no meaning whatever. I wish you would insist that he get glasses for his own eyes and make him stop taking glasses off the eyes of other children. Really, Doctor, it is too absurd for anything. That boy has actually persuaded the other children that they cure their headaches and improve their sight by reading that card. If it were not for the principal, I would have thrown it away long ago."

She said some other things, too, which were even more uncomplimentary. The children became restless. When she stopped for a breath I took the freckle-faced boy into a dark room and examined his eyes with the ophthalmoscope. I found them perfect, with no trace of myopia or astigmatism.

I asked him, "How is it that the teacher says you cannot read the writing on the blackboard?" He replied, still with his wonderful smile, "Because she is such a bum writer that nobody can read it; she acts often as if she couldn't read it herself." "How is it," I continued, "that you hold the book so close to your face?" He answered apologetically, "Because I get tired of the scenery." "What do you mean by that?" I asked. "Oh," he answered, "the teacher's face; I don't like it. She is always so cross; her face gives me a pain."

Then I took him back to the classroom and sent him to his seat. I asked the teacher if she could read the bottom line on the Snellen test card. She could not do so. Then I showed her an unfamiliar test card, which she saw even worse. She explained that her glasses needed to be changed. I asked the freckle-faced boy if he could read it. "Yes," he said, and promptly did so.

The teacher exploded. It was impossible, she said, that he should have read the letters; he must have found out in some other way what they were. She pointed to the clock, "What time is it?" she asked. The boy answered her correctly. Then she held up a book with very large print, which the boy also read at five feet. She was finally convinced by these and other tests that the boy's sight was better than her own.

When she was through I pointed to some very small letters which nobody could see at the distance at which the boy was sitting. He smiled, and said he could not see them. "But," I said, "you are not trying, you are making no effort to see them." At that the teacher unexpectedly struck the top of her desk with her ruler and we all jumped, with the exception of the freckle-faced boy, who had learned how to protect himself from such influences. With a rasping voice she cried, "Why don't you do what the Doctor tells you to do?" In a short time my nerves returned to something like the normal, and I turned to the boy and asked, "Why don't you try?" He replied, still smiling, "No use tryin'."

With this as my text I talked for a few moments, and told the class that the boy was right and that your sight is never perfect when you try to see. You only make yourself uncomfortable by the strain, and it never benefits you. I then proceeded to have the pupils demonstrate some facts. I directed them to keep their attention fixed on the smallest letter they could see from their seats, to stare at it, to try to see it better, to concentrate, to partly close their eyelids; in short, to do everything they could to improve their sight. I noted that the teacher, who had previously walked to the back of the room, was listening to what I was saying. The children did as I suggested, and soon found that the effort made them very uncomfortable and lowered their vision.

I now asked one pupil to tell me the smallest letter he could see. He answered, "A letter 'O' on the next to the bottom line." "When you saw it did you see it easily?" He answered, "Yes, without any trouble." Then I said to him, "When you tried to see it, when you made trouble for your eyes by an effort, by a strain, what happened?" He answered, "The letter disappeared and the whole card became blurred. I got a headache and I don't like it."

"Close your eyes," I said, "and rest them. Cover your eyes with the palms of your hands and shut out all the light. Now tell me who discovered America." "Columbus," he replied, "in 1492." "Can you spell Columbus?" I asked. "Yes," he answered, "C-o-l-u-m-b-u-s." All this time the teacher was standing with her eyes closed and covered with her hands. "You spelled it correctly," I said. "How is your headache?" "Gone," he replied, "and I feel good."

I noted that the teacher still had her eyes covered, and when the boy said his headache was relieved she nodded her head. I now directed the boy to take his hands down, open his eyes and tell me how much he could see. "Gee" he exclaimed, "I see better. The letter 'O' is all right, and I can see some of the letters on the bottom line." With that he put both his hands in the pockets of his trousers, smiled at me, and turned around and grinned at the class.

A little girl wearing glasses now timidly raised her hand, and when I told her to speak she said, "Please, sir, I have an awful headache." Her eyes looked very much strained. I told her to take off her glasses and put them on the desk, to look at the card and read what she could see. At this point, the teacher at the back of the room removed her hands from her face, took off her glasses and placed them on the desk in front of her. I asked the little girl what she could see. "I can only see the largest letter at the top of the card," she said.

She was told to close her eyes and cover them with the palms of her hands. The teacher did the same, and all the other children wearing glasses took them off, looked at the card, closed their eyes and covered them with the palms of their hands.

Then I said to the little girl who had the awful headache, "What is your first name?" "Margaret," she answered. "Can you spell it?" I asked, and she spelled it. "What is your last name?" She told me, and at my request she spelled it also. Then she smiled. "How is your headache?" "I haven't any," she answered. "Take down your hands, open your eyes and kindly read the letters for me on the card." She promptly read four lines of letters, and looked very happy when she did it.

Meanwhile the teacher and the other pupils who had been wearing glasses had been doing the same, and when they looked at the card the second time they smiled, evidently pleased with what they saw. I was surprised to observe that even the teacher smiled and when, as I was about to leave the room, she came forward and threw her glasses into the wastebasket, I was quite shocked. Turning to me she said, "Doctor, need I say anything?" "You have said it all, thank you," I replied. As I went out of the door I heard the class call out in a chorus, "Thank you, thank you."

After this the Board of Education condemned my method as "unscientific and erroneous," and forbade the use of the Snellen test card in the schools, except for the usual purpose of testing the children's sight. Thus my pleasant visits to the classrooms came to an end. Some years later, however, I called on the teacher of the freckle-faced boy to ask about him. She met me smiling and without glasses, and I noted that the Snellen test card was still on the wall. In response to my inquiry as to why it should be there after the Board of Education had forbidden its use, she replied, "The Board of Education has not the power to make me take that card down." Then I asked about the freckle-faced boy. "Graduated," she replied. As he was below the age at which children usually graduate from the public schools, I expressed some surprise. "Rapid advancement class," she said. "Got through my class in a hurry and took a lot of my other children with him to the rapid advancement class. Must be half through high school now. Bright boy."

I have written a book on *The Cure of Imperfect Sight by Treatment Without Glasses* which contains several hundred pages. The freckle-faced boy told in three words substantially what is contained in that book: "No use tryin'."

OPTIMUMS AND PESSIMUMS

A Possible Explanation

By M. E. Gore, M.D.

A lady that I was treating could not see the letter "R" on the test card, the last letter of the 50-line. It seemed strange that she was able to see the other letters on the same line, but not the "R." It occurred to me that perhaps the patient unconsciously saw this letter when she first looked at it, but, on account of some unpleasant association which it produced in her mind, she made an effort to forget it, thus causing a lowering of vision. I determined to employ an association test to find out if possible what had caused her mental distress on looking at the letter. I asked her to think of the letter "R" and tell me the first thought that came into her mind. She answered, "Red."

Now associated with red was her mother, as red had been her favorite color. Her mother had recently died, and thinking of her caused grief. I told the patient that I believed this was the cause of her lowered vision for that particular letter. To our astonishment she has since been able to see this letter without difficulty.

Another case which clearly illustrated the optimums and pessimums was a patient who was unable to see the figure "2" in a line of figures the same size and distance. On questioning her I found this number made her think of her two children which she had lost. On the other hand, she could see the letter "F" and "V" wherever they occurred. She said "F" made her think of her father whom she dearly loved, and "V" was the initial letter of his middle name.

These cases and several others of like nature have led me to the conclusion that the association of pleasant or unpleasant ideas with any of the letters is the cause of optimums and pessimums.

In most cases, by employing the association test and showing the patient the connection between the letter and the unpleasant thought, they have become able to see the letters which had been pessimums.

STORIES FROM THE CLINIC

No. 19: A Trio of Difficult Cases

By Emily C. Lierman

Myopic and farsighted patients are numerous, and I always feel confident that I can in no time improve their sight; but I suffered a case of cold feet when Dr. Bates placed in my care a young woman of twenty-seven, who came to our Clinic some time ago with a scar on her right eye almost in the center of sight. All the Doctor said to me was, "Help this patient, please," and it was my first experience with a case of that kind.

I asked the girl how long the scar had been there and also what caused it. Being a southerner, she spoke with a southern accent, and this is the way she answered me, "When I was twelve years old, mah granma was settin' by the fireplace smokin' a pet pipe, and as I was removin' a boilin' kettle of water old Granny upsets the pipe of hot ashes and done burned mah eye. Lordy, ma'am! Ah thought mah eye was burned from de socket. The doctor says I would never see again out of dat eye."

I tested her sight, and with her left eye she read 14/40, while with her right eye she could barely see my fingers one foot away. I had not the slightest idea that I could improve the right eye at all. However, I told her to stand in a comfortable position and palm for a little while. In about ten minutes or so I told her to remove her hands, and I was pleased to see that her left eye had improved to 14/15, and that with her right eye she was able to distinguish the 200-line letter at fourteen feet. Dr. Bates was dumbstruck with amazement. He said that, although he had seen opacities of the cornea resulting from constitutional disease clear up, he had never before, in his thirty-six years of experience seen any improvement in an opacity resulting from an injury, even after years of treatment. That encouraged me so much that I told the patient to palm again, and before she left the Clinic that day her right eye had improved to 14/50. She became hysterical when she found that she could see objects again with this eye. For a while she came quite regularly to the Clinic, and at her last visit her right eye improved to 20/50, while with the left she became able to read 20/10. Dr. Bates said it was a miracle. After that I never saw her again. I was sorry that she stayed away, because I was proud of what I had accomplished and wished to cure her completely.

A case of squint, which I think will interest our readers, was first seen on August 4, 1921. The patient had been wearing glasses for twelve years to correct the trouble, but without benefit. The first year her mother, who came with her, tried to console her by saying that perhaps in another year or so the squint would be cured; but instead it only got worse. Her playmates made unkind remarks about it, and when she found her sight was getting worse for reading she became utterly discouraged.

I tested her sight, and she read 12/40 with her left or better eye. When I asked her to read the card with her squinting eye she turned her head half way round to the left in trying to see. I at once showed her how to palm, and her mother and I were quite astonished when in a few minutes she opened her eyes and, with her head perfectly straight, read 12/40 with her right eye without a mistake. On August 6, two days later, she read 12/15 with each eye separately, with her right eye perfectly straight. She had followed my instructions to palm at least six times a day for as long a period as was comfortable for her. On August 9 she came to the Clinic smiling and expressed her gratitude for what had been done for her.

"I can now read a book for hours at a time," she said, "without headaches or discomfort. Just yesterday I visited another clinic where I had received treatment and asked the doctor who had treated me to let me show him what I could do. I showed him how I could palm, and then I read the test card for him with each eye separately. The doctor was thrilled, and said it seemed like a miracle, because he had told me that I could never again get along without glasses and to be sure and have them changed every year or so." That day my patient read 12/10, both eyes, and I am sure that I can cure her if she will continue to come.

Another case of squint, a little boy five years old, the most unruly youngster who ever came for treatment, was cured in less than six months. When he tried to look straight ahead his right eye turned in so far that one could hardly see the cornea. His grandmother who came with him expressed very little hope, and assured me that I would have a hard time trying to manage him or to help him. I asked him his name several times before he answered, "I ain't got no name." Later he said it was Francisco. I could see that he was straining and that he was extremely nervous. So I decided to be very patient with him, but for some time the only answers I could get from him were, "I don't wanna" and "I won't."

All sorts of apologies came from his grandmother, but I assured her that I was not discouraged with him. I made up my mind to help the little chap and in some way relieve him of that awful tension and nervous strain. I said to him, "If I had a bad eye and a good eye, I would not make my good eye do all the work. I would make the bad eye work hard so that I could see better." This interested the child for some reason, and he asked, "Have I got a bad eye?"

"Yes," I said, "and the reason it is bad is because it is lazy and you won't let it be good. All you can say when I try to tell you how to make it behave is, 'I don't wanna.' Nice boys with good eyes don't say that." Whereupon he shouted in a loud voice which startled the rest of the patients, "Make my bad eye do some work; I want good eyes like you have."

I immediately showed him a test card with pothooks pointing in different directions. I covered his left eye with the palm of my hand, and asked him to show me how the "E's" were pointing as I held the card two feet away. At that distance he was able to see the 100-line letters. He could see straight ahead with the right eye only just long enough to see those letters; then his eye turned in again. At first I could not induce him to palm, so I told him to close his eyes as though he were sleeping. He was very obedient about doing this, and his grandmother stood by in astonishment while his eyes were closed. I praised him for closing them and resting them for me, and I said if he would do this lots and lots of times every day his right eye would become straight like the left and would not be bad any more. I then told him to cover his left eye with his hand and look at the card which I had fastened on the wall five feet away. This amused him very much and he acted as though he were in for a good time. I told him to look at the 200-line letter and then quickly close his eyes; then to look at the 100-line letters and close his eyes quickly again. He was able to see these letters as well at five feet as he did at two, and this encouraged me. When he opened his eyes a third time he showed me with his hand how the next line of letter "E's" pointed.

He came regularly for a few months, and was always very obedient. Each time he came he was able to keep his eye straight, not only while practicing with the card, but also while talking to me. His grandmother bought a Snellen test card, and assisted with the treatment very faithfully at home. Now, just six months since he first came, he is able to see the 10-line of letters at ten feet away with each eye, 10/10, and has learned the alphabet by heart. Dr. Bates became very much interested in the rapid progress of the case and congratulated me frequently on the good results I had obtained. He said it was very unusual for the blindness of squint to be cured in such a short time, and that most authorities would have said it was impossible.

QUESTIONS AND ANSWERS

Q–1a. After closing my eyes tight and then opening them, I can read *Better Eyesight* at a distance of about two feet. The type stands out very black and clear. After about two or three minutes my old myopia comes back. What I want to know is whether this practice is good for the eyes and whether it will help me to see at a distance. 1b. Can you tell me what is a good thing to do to see people across the street clearly or in a meeting room at fairly close range? It is awkward not to be able to recognize people until one is close upon them.

A–1a. Yes, but I would expect you to get better results if you closed your eyes easily and naturally, instead of closing them tight. 1b. The only way to overcome this difficulty completely is to get cured, but the practice you have described sometimes helps to bring out distant objects temporarily.

Better Eyesight
October 1921—Vol. V, No. 4

HOW TO OBTAIN MENTAL PICTURES

Look at a letter on the Snellen test card.

Remember its blackness.

Shift the attention from one part of this spot of black to another. It should appear to move in a direction contrary to the imagined movement.

If it does not, try to imagine it stationary. If you succeed in doing this it will blur, or disappear. Having demonstrated that it is impossible to imagine the spot stationary, it may become possible to imagine it moving.

Having become able to form a mental picture of a black spot with the eyes closed, try to do the same with the eyes open. Alternate until the mental vision with the eyes closed and open is the same.

Having become able to imagine a black spot try to imagine the letter "o" in diamond type with the center as white as snow. Do this alternately with eyes closed and open.

If you cannot hold the picture of a letter or period, commit to memory a number of letters on the test card and recite them to yourself while imagining that the card is moving.

If some other color or object is easier to imagine than a black spot it will serve the purpose equally well.

A few exceptional people may get better results with the eyes open than when they are closed.

MENTAL PICTURES AN AID TO VISION

By W. H. Bates, M.D.

When an object is seen perfectly it is possible to form a perfect mental picture of it; when it is seen imperfectly this cannot be done. Persons with ordinarily good vision are able to form a perfect mental picture of some letter of the alphabet, especially a letter of diamond type, when looking at the Snellen test card, or at fine print; but persons with ordinarily imperfect vision can do this only under certain favorable conditions, as with their eyes closed, or when looking at a blank surface where there is nothing particular to see. They may also be able to do it when looking at objects at a distance at which their vision is fairly good, as in the case of near objects in myopia. Persons with ordinarily good vision, on the other hand, have moments when they see imperfectly, and at such times their mental pictures are imperfect.

These facts are of the greatest practical importance, because many persons easily learn how to form mental pictures, and when they become able to do so under all conditions their sight becomes perfect.

Mental vision is subject to precisely the same laws as visual perception. The mental picture must be seen or imagined by central fixation; that is, one part of it at a time must be seen best, and the attention must shift continually from one point to another. This shifting of attention produces a swing which is even more pronounced than the visual swing. Furthermore, the mind adds details that do not exist in the object remembered or imagined. If this object is a black letter on a white background, for instance, the white openings and margins will appear more intense than the reality.

It is not possible to retain a mental picture of a letter "o" of diamond type when one tries to think of one point continuously. The point may be remembered for a brief interval—a few seconds or part of a minute; then it is lost and with it the whole letter. One cannot, in short, "stare" at a point with the imagination any more than one can stare with the eye, and if one tries to do so the point disappears. If one tries to think continuously of two points of the letter, imagining them both to be equally black at the same time, the picture is lost more quickly. To think of four points or more, or to think of the whole letter perfectly black at the same time, is still more difficult.

Mental pictures cannot be retained for any length of time unless they appear to move. This movement may be so slight and easy that it is not observed until the attention is called to it, and even then it may not be realized. Some patients have told me that they could remember small letters of diamond type easily and continuously, and that they were not moving. Usually the patient can demonstrate the facts by trying to think of one part of the letter as stationary. In this case it immediately disappears. But the effort to keep the attention fixed on a point is so great that some patients cannot or will not make it. It is easier to let the attention shift naturally. In such cases I direct them to look at the letter "o" so close to their eyes, or so far away, that they are unable to see it clearly, and call their attention to the fact that now it seems to be stationary. Then I have them look at the letter at the distance at which they see it perfectly and ask them to imagine it stationary, as the letter at the preceding distance seemed to be. Usually they are able to do this, and to note that the letter blurs or disappears. After they become able to imagine that a letter which they see is stationary, they become able also to imagine that their mental picture of it is stationary, and to note that it cannot be held more than a moment under these conditions.

To imagine that other things seem to be moving helps some people to form and retain mental pictures. One patient, whose mental pictures were very poor, became able, when walking around the room and imagining things moving in the opposite direction, to imagine that a letter "o" was moving in the same direction as the furniture.

A mental picture need not be a complicated one. The perfect memory or imagination of even a small spot of color is sufficient to cure all errors of refraction—nearsightedness, farsightedness, and astigmatism—as well as many other abnormal conditions. But to form a perfect mental picture of a spot of color—say a black period—is not always easy. One may think one is imagining a black period perfectly, but when one compares one's mental picture with the reality, one usually finds that the former is several degrees paler than the latter. It is usually easier to form mental pictures with the eyes closed than with the eyes open, and by imagining a period, or other object, with the eyes closed and open alternately one can improve one's ability to imagine it under the latter condition. In a few exceptional cases, however, mental pictures are better and are more easily held with the eyes open than when they are closed.

When the sight is imperfect it is always easier to hold a mental picture when looking at nothing in particular than when looking at letters or other objects at distances at which they cannot be seen distinctly. To improve the ability to hold them under the latter conditions it is necessary, alternately, to imagine the object with the eyes closed, or looking away from the Snellen test card or printed page, and then to look back at the Snellen test card or reading matter.

Persons unable to imagine a period or letter may succeed with other objects. For example, one patient who could not imagine a white card with black letters on it which she had just seen in her hand was able, with her eyes closed, to imagine the color of her house, one part best, and the different objects—curtains, furniture, etc.—in the different rooms. She was able to see the lawn, the flowerbed, the numerous flowers, one part best, and to imagine the color of the eyes of her friends. After that she became able to imagine the white card with the black letters.

Persons who suffer from pain, fatigue, or other discomfort in their eyes, have great difficulty in forming mental pictures. Such persons, although they cannot remember a letter or other objects, are often able to remember the movement of a card held in the hand. If they cannot do this at first, they may become able to do it by alternately looking at the card and then closing their eyes and trying to recall the movement. When they become able to do this the pain stops and the sight becomes temporarily normal.

Most people are helped by learning how to fail. When they demonstrate that their sight is lowered by an imperfect mental picture, they become able to avoid such pictures. A patient with squint was cured when she learned to imagine double images. At first, with her eyes open, she could not imagine them more than two inches apart. Later, with her eyes open, she got them four feet apart, while, with her eyes closed, she could imagine one Snellen test card on one side of a bay five miles wide and another on the other. These images could be imagined either crossed or homonymous at will; that is, each eye sometimes seemed to see the image on its own side, and at other times the image seemed to be on the opposite side. When the images were homonymous the eyes turned in, and when they were crossed the eyes turned out. By means of this practice the patient gained such a degree of mental control that her eyes became almost continually straight, the slight occasional deviation not being noticeable.

AN ARTIST'S EXPERIENCE WITH CENTRAL FIXATION

By Florence Cane

Editor's Note—*This patient consulted the editor on July 20, 1921, because her vision was getting worse, and she suffered from a constant feeling of strain and fatigue in her eyes. She had worn glasses since she was seven years old for hypermetropia, commonly called farsightedness, and was now wearing convex 4.00 D. S., a rather strong lens. Yet without her glasses she was able to read fine print imperfectly, and by the aid of her memory she became able at the first visit to read it at six inches. Her discomfort was relieved at the first visit, and her distant vision, which had been imperfect, though better than her near vision, also improved.*

I have made a few observations while improving my eyesight by the methods recommended by Dr. Bates, and many thoughts and questions regarding them have suggested themselves to me.

The first thing I remember observing on leaving the Doctor's office after my first treatment was a new sense of movement and life. Never before had I seen such clear, bright color in the crowd. I walked toward the library on Fifth Avenue, and never had the sun shone so brightly, or the world looked so exciting. My heart beat faster and I felt a great elation, as if a new vision, a new power, had been given me.

The second thing I remembered was that I sat down the same evening with *The Cure of Imperfect Sight by Treatment Without Glasses,* determined to see what I could do without my glasses. I found that by shifting and palming I could read a sentence or two, later more, and after a while I could read a paragraph without stopping. I found shifting from a point above a word to one below it particularly helpful.

I went to bed at ten o'clock, but was so excited after reading there until twelve that I could not sleep much. The magnitude of the truth thrilled me. The relation of sight, memory and imagination to body, mind and soul—the use of one faculty to strengthen another—seemed to be such a wonderful conception.

Soon I observed that looking upward seemed to improve my sight. I took to practicing on high objects out of doors. I shifted on points like two apples in a tree, or on the clouds. This helped me very much, and overcame my shrinking from light. I found that I had never walked with my eyes really open before. When I told Dr. Bates about it, he said it was the light that helped me, not the height of the objects I looked at.

I have had several experiences in the application of the principles of central fixation which seem interesting enough to communicate to the readers of *Better Eyesight.* The first occurred when I had mislaid something. I had looked everywhere for it in vain. I sat down and palmed and, quietly but suddenly, I saw in my mind where I had laid it. I got up and looked, and it was there.

I burned myself at a beach fire on a piece of wood that I picked up. It had been in the fire, but it was dark and I did not notice it. I burned my thumb quite badly—enough to raise a big blister. It was very painful, and I had no remedy at hand. I remember that I had read in Dr. Bates' book about central fixation in relation to pain, and I tried remembering the small "o." After a few minutes the pain ceased until I could not tell which thumb I had burned. The same thing happened after a bee had stung me; and one night when I had a severe cold and could not sleep because of difficulty in breathing, I was greatly helped by seeing the period and making it swing. I fell asleep and continued seeing the period in my sleep.

In painting I have had the most interesting experiences of all. If I am working from the memory or imagination and it won't come the way I want, I try palming. The first time this happened, I was painting a lake with some birches at one side. I just couldn't remember how birches grew, and the trees wouldn't look right. So I closed my eyes and waited, and soon a vision came to me of myself walking in a young birch wood that I used to know; I saw how the branches grew, and felt the white glimmer of reflected light from the bark, and the tender young green of the fragile leaves, and I painted the birches with ease and joy. This use of palming may be of great value to artists, because the artist works from the image, and sometimes this image is lost. By straining and effort he cannot regain it, but by palming he may.

I have also had interesting experiences in treating others, my first pupil being my little girl. She had a great fear of the water, so that she could not let herself go, and float face down. She has a cat of which she is very fond; so I suggested that she recall her cat washing itself when she tried to float. She did this and was able to float for twelve seconds.

Another case of interest was that of a woman who was in a nervous condition, overwrought and discouraged over her problems. I began teaching her how to improve her eyesight, and at the first lesson she made such great progress that she was overcome with happiness. The magnitude of the thing she had done gave her a sense of control over herself, a new sense of power. She said, "If I can do this, why I can do anything." And it is true; she has pulled herself out of the overwrought state.

Among all the people with whom I have talked, or to whom I have tried to explain these ideas, I have met only one with a perfectly rigid mind. He was, as one would expect, a pure scientist of very high standing. He wouldn't even admit that his hand appeared to move when he swung his head from side to side with his hand eight inches before his eyes. He said it merely made him dizzy. He knew the hand was in a fixed position, so it couldn't appear to him to move. This statement showed that he only used half his functions. He used his reason but refused to allow his senses to record how things appeared.

There is one thing Dr. Bates has said that I want to question. "We can see only what we imagine, and we cannot imagine something which we have not seen or experienced." As an example, he gives our inability to imagine a foreign alphabet. Well, if that statement is true, how do we get at a new truth? I think it is from the imagination. One can conceive of new forms in art, and I should judge that a scientist must conceive a possible truth in his imagination, and then set about testing it by experiment and observation. The marriage of the two—facts and imagination—creates new truth and widens man's consciousness. This Dr. Bates has done. But he has only called imagination good. I think it is infinite, and by penetrating deeper into its mystery we are penetrating into the source of man's growth.

STORIES FROM THE CLINIC

No. 20: St. Vitus' Dance and Myopia

By Emily C. Lierman

Hyman, age ten, came to the Clinic not as a patient, but as his mother's escort. She was having her eyes treated, but her trouble was not half as bad as that of her son. His poor eyes stared painfully behind his thick glasses, and in order to see through them at all he made the most awful grimaces I ever saw. His head moved constantly in all directions, and later on I discovered that he had St. Vitus' Dance. He was an unusually bright boy, and was never satisfied unless he saw and knew everything that was going on in the Clinic. Whenever he was in the room he would stay as close to me as possible, listening eagerly to every word I said and watching every movement I made. One day I said to him, "Look here, young man, I don't mind having you watch me, but I don't think the patients like you to stare at them so much. If you want to know how I cure people, why don't you get cured yourself so that you won't have to wear glasses?" "My teacher says I must wear glasses because I cannot see the blackboard without them," he replied.

I explained to his mother that I was sure I could cure not only his eye trouble, but also the nervous twitching of his head. She did not seem to understand me, and I'm sure she doubted my ability to do anything at all for him. The boy himself seemed to be equally skeptical, but was, nevertheless, much interested. He was evidently curious to know what I would do for him, and quite willing to let me entertain him.

I tested his sight with his glasses on and found that he was able to read only 10/50, all the rest of the card being a blur. I then took the glasses off and noticed that he stared less without them. In addition his personal appearance was greatly improved, for the glasses had made him look hideous. I now told him to cover his eyes with the palms of his hands so as to exclude all the light, and to remember something perfectly. He seemed to think this was a game of hide and seek, and kept continually looking through his fingers. My patience was considerably tried, but I did not let him see this. Instead I told him that I was especially fond of little boys, and wished to help him. He squared his shoulders and made an effort to keep his head still, but failed. Finally I succeeded in making him understand that if he wanted to stop the twitching of his head, he must keep his hands over his eyes until I told him to take them down. He now became as serious as I was myself, and though I watched him while I was treating other cases, I did not once see him uncover his eyes, or peep through his fingers. No doubt the fifteen minutes that he spent in this way seemed like hours to him. When I was able to return to him, I said very gently, "Now take your hands from your eyes and look at me."

He did so, and to my delight his head was perfectly still. I now told him a story—being careful to preserve the same gentle tone of voice—about a boy who lived in the country town where I live and who stole some delicious big apples from a farmer. He ate too many of the apples, and soon began to feel that there was something wrong with his stomach. Then the farmer caught him and punished him; so he suffered both inside and out, and came to the conclusion that stealing apples was not very much fun. I took as long as I could to tell this simple tale, for my object was to keep my patient from thinking of himself, or his eyes. He seemed to find it hugely amusing. His eyes beamed with fun while he listened to me, and his head never moved once.

"Now," I said, "do some more palming for me, and then we will read the card."

When he uncovered his eyes the second time, his vision had improved to 10/30. By this time his mother's indifference had vanished. She did not know how to show her gratitude for what I had done for her boy, but promised to see that he spent a sufficient amount of time palming every day. The next Clinic day she told me that the twitching of the head had become less frequent. She was instructed to watch the boy and have him palm at once whenever she noticed the twitching. This always relieved the trouble.

Hyman was anxious to be cured before vacation began, and was quite willing to do as he was told. He came to the Clinic for two months, and at the last few visits there was no twitching, while his vision had improved to 12/10.

LET YOUR EYES ALONE

By James Hopper

I perform now and then an experiment which, I think, will interest the readers of *Better Eyesight*. It affords a striking proof of two of Dr. Bates' contentions: No. 1, that no defect of the eye is fixed, that the refraction of the eye is variable. No. 2, that the perfect refraction which means perfect sight is obtained through relaxation. Here is what I do, using first one eye, then the other:

I close the left eye, and then, taking the card with the "Seven Truths of Normal Sight" printed in diamond type, I place said card right up against the tip of my nose and, with my left eye closed, look at it with my right eye. My right eye is my bad one. It had only one-half of normal sight when I first saw Dr. Bates.

Looking at the card thus placed against my nose, I see at first nothing—or simply blurred lines. Then consciously I relax my eye, I "let it go." I can do that only gradually. I let go and let go. The best way I have found to do this is to keep my mind off the idea of reading the card, and to think of something else—a football game, a play—anything.

I can feel my eye gradually relax. There is no mistaking the process. It is one of relaxation, of letting go. And there is degree after degree of letting go. Just when I think I have reached the limit of relaxation, I feel the eye let go another notch. And then, suddenly—so suddenly it almost scares me—and clearly—so clearly it is almost weird, I see the diamond type and I read the Doctor's "Seven Truths"!

Each letter is not only black and sharp and distinct, but it is almost gigantic—two or three times the size it was when seen at six inches. There is no doubt to me that my eye has passed from a state of not seeing the type to one of seeing the type. Hence that the refraction of my eye is variable. And there is no doubt to me that the passing from the state of not seeing the type to the state of seeing the type is obtained through relaxation of the eye. And the counter proof also exists. If, while I am seeing the type perfectly and big, I set my mind deliberately to reading it—it abruptly disappears.

Working consciously, I have done something with my eye which has made it an instrument that cannot see at that distance. Working consciously, I have tightened some muscles or other, so that the eye has now the wrong shape for seeing at that distance.

Moral: Let your eyes alone, and they do the right thing. Interfere with them, butt in with your conscious will and—presto—they do the wrong thing.

Better Eyesight
November 1921—Vol. V, No. 5

THE SENSE OF TOUCH AN AID TO VISION

Just as Montessori has found that impressions gained through the sense of touch are very useful in teaching children to read and write, persons with defective sight have found them useful in educating their memory and imagination.

One patient whose visual memory was very imperfect found that if she traced an imaginary black letter on the ball of her thumb with her forefinger, she could follow the imaginary lines with her mind as they were being formed and retain a picture of the letter better than when she gained the impression of it through the sense of sight.

Another patient discovered that when he lost the swing, he could get it again by sliding his forefinger back and forth over the ball of his thumb. When he moved his fingers it seemed as if his whole body were moving.

Both these expedients have the advantage of being inconspicuous and can, therefore, be used anywhere.

The vision was improved in both cases.

THE FIRST VISIT

By W. H. Bates, M.D.

At the beginning of treatment, as well as later, it has been found to be a great benefit to have the patient demonstrate facts. It is better to avoid stating results expected, and instead let the patient discover the results for himself.

Rest Improves the Vision

The first fact to be demonstrated is that rest improves the vision. The patient is told to close his eyes and rest them, forget about them, let his mind drift, remember pleasant things. After half an hour, more or less, he is told to open his eyes and read the distant test card as well as he can. If he finds that his vision has improved the next question is, "What did you do that helped your sight?"

Obvious as the answer to this question seems to those familiar with the treatment of defective vision by relaxation, some patients find extraordinary difficulty in replying to it and one has to ask them a number of leading questions to get the proper answer, "Rest."

The amount of relief obtained from this procedure differs greatly in different cases. Some get none at all, and others very little. Others again may be cured at the first visit by this means alone. Why some people can close their eyes and rest them with so much benefit, while others fail, is not always evident; but one can often tell at the outset what the result will be. One case cured by this means rested comfortably for half an hour without any change whatever in his position. A case not benefited was very restless, moved around in his chair, got up, opened his eyes every few minutes, and was decidedly uncomfortable. For him there was no rest with his eyes closed, and his vision was not improved. Later a cure was obtained by other methods, but with much trouble.

Palming

After having rested the eyes by closing, the patient is told to cover his eyes with the palms of his hands in such a way as to exclude all the light. Usually, but not always, he is able to obtain more rest in this way than by mere closing. Those who succeed in relaxing completely see a perfect black; but this is rare, and the patient may consider himself fortunate if he is able to begin by seeing an approximate black.

Staring

Having demonstrated that rest improves the vision, the next step is to have the patient demonstrate that effort lowers it. The patient is directed to look continuously at a letter which he can see distinctly on the distant test card, and after a part of a minute the question is asked, "Do you see better or worse?" The answer is usually, "I see worse, it makes my eyes pain."

He is then directed to stare at other objects instead of letters, to make an effort to see them, concentrate on them, and to note that lowering of the vision, with fatigue, discomfort, or pain, is produced. After he has demonstrated these facts he is told that persons with imperfect sight always attempt to hold their points of fixation too long, even when the lowering of vision is caused by an injury or by a foreign body in the eye. In short, they stare, thus not only spoiling their eyesight but making themselves conspicuous and uncomfortable.

"You have your choice," I tell them. "Stare and have

poor sight and other troubles. Avoid the stare and have normal vision."

Occasionally a patient thinks that staring does improve his vision. In this case I tell him to keep on staring and improve it still more. It does not take long for him to convince himself that the improvement that results from staring is only temporary, and is followed by a lowering of the vision.

Patients who have lowered their vision and produced pain and discomfort by staring are glad to relieve the strain by closing the eyes or palming. After they have alternately stared and rested for a while it would be hard for anyone to convince them that anything is to be gained by effort when one wants to see, and they instinctively close their eyes in such a case instead of straining them.

Shifting and Swinging

Having demonstrated that staring lowers the vision, a patient is easily able to demonstrate that if he wants to see an object distinctly he must shift constantly from one part of it to another; but often he does not easily realize the apparent motion produced by this shifting. In demonstrating the facts to a new patient I usually begin by having him walk around the room and note that the furniture seems to be moving in the opposite direction. Then I have him take one step forward and one back and note that the furniture seems to move backward and forward, respectively. Next I have him hold his hand six inches in front of his face, and move his head far to the right and far to the left, alternately, without looking at the hand. Almost invariably he is able to note a very pronounced movement of the hand. After this, I have him hold a small card in his hand and note that the card appears to move with the hand. Having noticed the movement of the card in his hand, it is usually easy for him to look from one side of the test card on the wall to the other, and note that it appears to move in a direction contrary to the movement of the eye. After this, the shortening of the swing until he becomes able to look from one side to the other of a letter of diamond type and imagine that it is moving, is a mere question of practice.

Memory and Imagination

The use of the memory or imagination is an important part of the cure of imperfect sight, since a perfect memory or imagination means perfect relaxation; but I do not begin by explaining this to a patient. Instead I say, "Can you remember a small letter 'o'?"

Some patients can do this at once; others cannot. Those who can, usually think that they are remembering the letter all alike and stationary. In order to demonstrate that this is impossible, they are asked to imagine a black period on one side of the "o," to keep the attention fixed upon it, and to imagine that it is perfectly black and stationary. Generally the patient finds that he cannot do this. The period usually moves in spite of all his efforts to imagine that it is not doing so. If it does not move, it becomes gray and finally disappears. Having demonstrated that you cannot remember the period continuously unless it is moving, it usually becomes possible for the patient to realize that his attention is shifting constantly from one part of the "o" to another, and to note an apparent movement in a direction opposite to the imagined movement of the eye.

One difficulty in getting patients to make this demonstration is that the effort of remembering an unchanging object, even for a few seconds, is so great that some people cannot or will not make it. It is easier to let the attention shift naturally.

Some patients are unable to form any kind of a mental picture, and it may require much ingenuity and long practice to enable them to do it. Some become able to form mental pictures when they are able to imagine that the things they see are moving. Others are helped in remembering a black letter by imagining that it has a very white background, whiter than the card on which they saw it.

Mental pictures are formed first with the eyes closed, then with the eyes open, and as the ability to form them with the eyes open increases, the vision increases.

In every way possible the fact is impressed upon the patient that he can be cured only by rest; that he must learn to let his eyes alone; that whatever he does to improve his sight must be wrong. For home practice three general plans are recommended:

1. Practice with the Snellen test card at ten, fifteen, or twenty feet, remembering the blackness of the letters, imagining their form and their swing, and imagining the white openings and margins to be whiter than the rest of the card.
2. Reading fine print at the distance at which it is seen best, then gradually bringing it up to six inches or less and putting it off to a distance of two feet or farther.
3. Seeing things moving all day long from the time the eyes are opened in the morning until they are closed at night, and going to sleep finally with the imagination of the swing.

STORIES FROM THE CLINIC
No. 21: More Cases of Squint
By Emily C. Lierman

One day in the early part of September there came to our Clinic a very neatly dressed woman of forty-five, with her daughter, age eleven. One of the doctors from another section of the dispensary had told her of the wonderful cures wrought by Dr. Bates' methods, and convinced her that they would be effective in the case of her daughter, who was suffering from convergent squint of the left eye. I at once became more than usually interested in this case, not only because I did not want to disappoint the doctor who had sent it or cause him to lose faith in our methods, but because Selma, the patient, was a dear little girl and made a strong appeal to my sympathies. I did not notice until her eyes became straight that nature had intended her to be very pretty; but I saw her sweet smile and her absolute faith in my ability to cure her, combined with her willingness to do as she was told, was very touching.

I tested her sight with the Snellen test card, and at ten feet she was able to read, with the right eye, only the 40-line. With the left eye (the squinting one) she read only the 200-line. I showed her how to palm, and then I had a talk with the mother, who was wearing glasses, and had been wearing them for twenty-five years. I explained to her how hard it would be to cure her daughter if she continued to wear them.

"How can I possibly harm my little girl by wearing glasses?" she asked. "You are under a constant strain while you wear them," I answered, "and that affects your daughter's nerves." "But I cannot sew, read, or do other things without my glasses," she said, "so what shall I do?"

I told her to watch very closely while I was treating Selma and do just exactly what she did. She took off her glasses at once, and did not seem to doubt that she would be cured. For this I was very grateful, as mothers are not always willing to take off their glasses at their first visit, thinking, I suppose, that although I may be able to cure children, I cannot cure adults. I placed the mother where she could watch her daughter's eyes during the treatment and, as she saw them after five or ten minutes become temporarily straight, she expressed her gratitude in no uncertain terms. On leaving she invited me to her home, and every time she came after that the invitation was repeated. She bought a test card, too, for home practice, and Selma was very faithful about using it.

From that time up to the present writing, mother and daughter have come regularly three days a week. Selma now reads the 20-line with her left eye at twelve feet; and with her right eye, at the same distance, she can read the 10-line. Except when she becomes excited or overanxious, her left eye is straight most of the time. The improvement in the mother's sight seems almost equally remarkable. She reads and sews without her glasses, the lines in her face caused by strain have disappeared, and she looks so much younger that she might easily be taken for her daughter's sister. We have all become fast friends and, although I shall be glad when Selma is completely cured, I will be sorry not to see her smiling face any more at the Clinic.

At the beginning of the treatment Selma's mother could not be encouraged to discuss other treatment she had had; but when the child read the whole of the test card with both eyes straight, she began to talk.

"You don't know how grateful I am to you," she said. "It is not so long ago that I was told at another eye clinic that Selma would have to be operated on for squint. They told me that it would get worse if they didn't operate. I told them to give me time to think it over. I was a whole year thinking it over; but I could not make up my mind to the operation, as I had doubts about its curing her."

Doris, age four, has convergent squint of the right eye, and came to us also during September. It was noticed when she was two years old that the right eye was turning in and, although glasses were immediately secured for her, they did no good. When I first saw her the vision of the squinting eye was only one-quarter normal, 10/40, while that of the other eye was one-half normal, 10/20. Now the sight of both eyes is slightly above normal, 12/10.

Doris does not know the alphabet; so in treating her I have to use a card covered with letter "E's" arranged in different ways, and she tells me which way they are facing—left, right, up or down. I found it rather hard at first to get her to palm for any length of time; but one day the mother told me of a dear baby brother at home, and I told Doris to think of her brother when she closed and covered her eyes. This worked like a charm. When she thinks it is time to open her eyes, usually about a minute, she calls out, "Open them?" If I answer, "No," she keeps them closed until I say, "Ready." During the first few treatments the right eye would not keep straight for more than half a minute, but now it stays straight all the time she is reading the chart, down to the 10-line. After the treatment it turns in again, but not so badly as before; and if she is reminded to make it look straight she can do so very readily.

The child's mother has been a great help in the treatment, both at home and at the Clinic, and I think she has got a great deal of good out of it for herself. She is a most unselfish parent, absolutely devoted to her children; but this devotion causes her to get excited and nervous, so that when she arrives at the Clinic her eyes are staring almost out of her head. In a few moments she becomes relaxed, and her eyes begin to look natural.

Doris got on so nicely that her cousin Arthur, who also has a convergent squint, came for treatment. When I tested his sight I found that the vision of the squinting eye, the left one, was only 10/50, while that of the right eye was 10/20. He was a very bright boy, very obedient and lovable, and when he looked at the chart it was sad to see the left eye turn in until it was almost hidden. He made rapid progress, however, and his mother, who always comes with him, is very happy over the good results obtained in little over a month. At his first visit he was told, after reading a line of letters on the chart, to remember the last letter while he closed and covered his eyes. When he looked at the card again he was able to read another line. His vision now is almost normal, 12/15, and when he is reading the card his eyes are almost straight. His mother tells me that he gets on much better at school than he used to. He is eager to get well, and is very happy when Clinic day comes so that he may have another treatment.

I am wondering which of the trio will be cured first, and when they are I will give most of the credit to the mothers, for it is their help and the treatment given at home that has counted most.

QUESTION AND ANSWERS

Q–1a. How long should one palm at a time, and how far should one be from the test card? 1b. I do not understand shifting and swinging well enough to practice this method. Will you please explain it to me just as you would to a new patient? 1c. I am not getting the results you say one should from the treatment. For instance, I tried palming last evening, and at the beginning I could see clearly only the first three lines on the test card. After two hours work I could see and read clearly all but the last line of letters at the bottom, but when I looked at the card this morning it was just the same as when I started palming. Now, how can I get the vision to stay? Must one continue to palm every day, and if so will the improvement in time become permanent?

A–1a. The length of time you should palm depends entirely upon the results you obtain from the practice. Some patients can palm for hours with benefit; others cannot keep it up for more than a few minutes. Your distance from the test card depends somewhat on the state of your vision and somewhat on your own convenience. At whatever distance you may be—7, 10, 15, or 20 feet—practice with a line of letters which you cannot see distinctly. 1b. See "The First Visit," in this issue. 1c. We think you are doing wonderfully well and congratulate you. If you continue the palming, the improvement will in time become permanent. If you will practice shifting and swinging when not practicing with the card it will help you. (See: "The Swinging Cure" in *Better Eyesight*, October 1919.)

Q–2a. I have discarded my glasses for street use and am slowly getting used to seeing without them. However, when I go to the theatre or a movie I cannot discern the faces, expression, etc., of the actors without the aid of my glasses. When I look without them the whole proceeding is like one hazy mass before my eyes. What can I do about this? 2b. Kindly explain your terms "cupping and palming

A–2a. All you can do is to go on improving your sight. 2b. By cupping is meant cupping the hand over the eye in such a way so as to exclude the light while avoiding pressure on the eyeball. Palming cannot be explained briefly. See the January 1920 issue.

Q–3a. What is the best method to use when the patient has a dilated pupil? 3b. What special refractive condition causes white letters and dots to appear over the test card along with blurring of the letters and also without it? 3c. Is the temporary use of the reading glass as detrimental to the eyes as regular glasses?

A–3a. Any method that produces relaxation will help. Palming is particularly effective. 3b. They may occur with any error of refraction. 3c. Yes.

Q–4a. In swinging the period, should one follow it in its travel from side to side, seeing it clearly all the time? 4b. *Better Eyesight* advises sleeping on the back. Will you kindly give me explicit directions as to how to do this?

A–4a. Whether you see a period all the time you are swinging, depends upon the length of the swing. If the swing is very short, a mere pulsation, you will; if it is long, or too rapid, it will be blurred or lost altogether at times. 4b. In lying on your back the arms should be parallel with the body and the lower limbs completely extended. The height of the pillow is immaterial. The head may or may not be turned to one side. It is a good thing to go to sleep swinging or palming.

Q–5a. When I palm does it affect my eyes if I do mental work. I could palm more if it didn't matter what I am thinking about, because I could do part of my studying that way. In short, does mental work necessarily mean mental strain? 5b. Isn't there any way to cure my eyes that doesn't take so much time as palming?

A–5a. Mental work does not necessarily mean mental strain. If you can see black with your eyes closed and covered while thinking of your lessons, you are perfectly safe in doing so. 5b. The best thing for a busy person is to form a habit of constant shifting and to imagine that everything seen is moving. It is the habit of staring that spoils your sight. If you can correct this by constant shifting and the realization of the movement produced by the shift, you can get well without so much palming and you will also be able to do your schoolwork better.

Q–6. I cannot yet read or write easily without my glasses.

Can I harm my eyes by trying to do so?

A–6. You cannot harm your eyes by reading and writing without glasses if you stop often to rest them by closing or palming. Even if the use of the eyes without glasses produces pain and fatigue, the injury is less than from the wearing of the glasses.

Q–7. How can I relieve fatigue and nervousness while listening to the sermon in church?

A–7. Try swinging your thumbs over or round each other, or back and forth, and then reversing. One patient gets relief from swinging her big toe inside her shoe.

Q–8. Can a tendency to sties be relieved by relaxation?

A–8. Yes.

Q–9. Is it injurious to expose a baby's eyes to the strong sunlight while sleeping?

A–9. The strong sunlight is very beneficiary to the eyes of babies, asleep or awake. It is injurious to shade their eyes from the sun.

Better Eyesight
December 1921—Vol. V, No. 6

THINK RIGHT

"As a man thinketh in his heart, so is he," is a saying which is invariably true when the sight is concerned. When a person remembers or imagines an object of sight perfectly, the sight is perfect; when he remembers it imperfectly, the sight is imperfect. The idea that to do anything well requires effort, ruins the sight of many children and adults; for every thought of effort in the mind produces an error of refraction in the eye. The idea that large objects are easier to see than small ones results in the failure to see small objects. The fear that light will hurt the eyes actually produces sensitiveness to light. To demonstrate the truth of these statements is a great benefit.

Remember a letter or other object perfectly, and note that the sight is improved and pain and fatigue relieved; remember the object imperfectly, and note that the vision is lowered, while pain and fatigue may be produced or increased.

Rest the eyes by closing or palming, and note that the vision is improved, and pain and discomfort relieved; stare at a letter, concentrate upon it, make an effort to see it, and note that it disappears, and that a feeling of discomfort or pain is produced.

Note that a small part of a large object is seen better than the rest of it.

Accustom the eyes to strong light; note that the vision is not lowered but improved, and that the light causes less and less discomfort.

Remember your successes (things seen perfectly) forget your failures (things seen imperfectly); patients who do this are cured quickly.

THE CORRECTION OF IMPERFECT SIGHT WITHOUT GLASSES

By Dr. Etha Marion Jones

The correction of imperfect sight by central fixation, as taught by Dr. Bates, first came under my observation one year ago this September while assisting for a month in the practice of my friends, Drs. H. S. and Jennie K. Beckler of Staunton, Virginia. I was astonished at the results they were obtaining in eye cases and at once began to study the system under their supervision.

About the same time I received a letter from a sister of mine, a teacher in the Detroit Public Schools, who had worn glasses for twenty years for myopia and astigmatism. She stated in her letter that she had discarded her glasses and was taking the central fixation treatment from an osteopathic physician in Detroit who had been a student of Dr. Bates. The treatment was continued during the winter, my sister keeping right on with her schoolwork and doing extra reading at night without suffering with headaches as she had previously done. On seeing her this summer I was agreeably surprised at the change in her appearance. The strained look about the eyes and face had given place to one of relaxation, the eyes were straight, and the nervous system had lost its tension and gained a poise formerly unknown. The retinoscope showed no errors of refraction in either eye.

Encouraged by this and other cases, I decided to prepare myself to specialize in this work. After studying the anatomy, pathology and physiology of the eye all last winter, and treating several patients as best I could with my limited knowledge of the system, I decided that what I now needed most was a course of personal instruction from Dr. Bates. I went to New York for this purpose a few months ago and spent a wonderful fortnight there. The course included work in Dr. Bates' Clinic held three times a week in the Harlem Hospital. Here I had a good opportunity to study eyes by means of the retinoscope and ophthalmoscope, and I observed the changes in the refraction and pathology as the treatment progressed. I can tell of only a few of the remarkable cases which I saw, for it would take days to tell about them all.

I was especially interested in a case of squint in a girl of fourteen, who had been attending the Clinic about three months before I saw her. She had worn glasses since she was four years old to correct the trouble, but had been growing gradually worse. When her sight was first tested she read 12/40 with her left or better eye. When asked to read the card with her squinting eye, she turned her head half way around to the left in trying to see it. Ms. Lierman gave her one simple relaxing exercise to do and left her for a few minutes. At the next test she read 12/40 with the squinting eye without turning her head. Of course, that was temporary relief, as on straining again the squint would recur; but it showed what could be done by continuous treatment, and when I left New York the right eye was as straight as the left and did not change when the patient was excited or annoyed, or reading or studying. She told me she could read or study for hours at a time without headaches or discomfort, while before coming to the Clinic she could look at a book for only a few minutes at a time.

A seventy-two year old woman was responding wonderfully to treatment for cataract in the advanced stage. She had been in the Clinic for two months. At first she could not distinguish the large "C" at the top of the test card. Before I left she could read 10/40 with both eyes.

A girl of twelve was suffering from retinitis pigmentosa, a condition generally pronounced incurable, in which spots of black pigment are deposited in the retina, parts of the retina destroyed and the nerve of sight diseased. On examination by the test card, the patient could read only the 70-line at five feet. Nystagmus was one of her worst symptoms, the eyes vibrating continually from side to side. She was extremely nervous, and very sensitive in regard to her condition, the slightest annoyance making her worse. At the first treatment, the nystagmus temporarily stopped and she read the 50-line instead of the 70-line at five feet. The last day I saw her at the Clinic she could read all of the 20-line at ten feet, and the nystagmus had entirely disappeared.

After seeing these things it would seem impossible for anyone to doubt that Dr. Bates' discoveries are bound, before long, to revolutionize the practice of ophthalmology. They offer hope to millions for whom formerly there was no hope, and I am glad to have a share in the wonderful work of making them available to the world of eye sufferers.

MENTAL CONTROL IN RELATION TO VISION

By W. H. Bates, M.D.

The eye with perfect sight is always at rest. When it begins to strain, the sight becomes imperfect. The eye with imperfect sight is always straining, and when it ceases to do so the sight becomes normal. These conditions of rest and unrest are reflections of the mind. In other words, they indicate the presence or absence of mental control.

When the mind is not under control, the memory or imagination is impaired. Therefore, one cannot at the moment of seeing something imperfectly form a perfect mental picture. A person with perfect sight can remember a color, a yellow flower, a red piece of cloth, a letter of small print, a black period, a white cloud in the sky, just as well with the eyes open and looking at the Snellen test card, or reading a printed page, as with his eyes closed. A person with imperfect sight either cannot do this at all, or can do it only under certain favorable conditions, as with his eyes closed, or when looking at objects at certain distances. A nearsighted person may retain his mental control and consequent ability to form mental pictures when reading fine print at six inches, but may lose both at five inches, or when looking at certain letters on the distant Snellen test card. Some patients have a good imagination and normal sight in the daytime, but lose both by artificial light. Others have normal vision and a good imagination only when the light is dim. One patient had imperfect sight, 20/70, corrected by concave 6.00 D. S. in ordinary daylight; but when the light was dim her vision became normal, 20/20, without glasses, and her mental pictures were just as good when her eyes were open as when they were closed. She became able, by means of sunning, to remember a black period in the bright outdoor sunshine when her vision, tested with the Snellen test card, became normal in ordinary daylight.

Many cases of imperfect sight have been cured simply by having the patient demonstrate these facts. One patient had vision of 20/200 without glasses. She was nearsighted and could read fine print at a near point without trouble. She was asked to look at a small letter "o." The question was asked, "Can you see the letter easily and continuously?" "Yes," she answered.

She could also, with eyes closed, remember it without difficulty and imagine the white center much whiter than the white card on which it was printed. With some encouragement she became able to realize that she did not imagine the letters all alike; that she saw one part best, and that she did not imagine the same part best very long at a time; that her attention was constantly shifting; and that the small letter was moving slowly, easily, rhythmically, continuously, a very short distance from side to side, the movement being so inconspicuous that she would not have noted it if her attention had not been called to the fact. When she tried to keep her attention on one small part of the letter continuously for a few seconds, or part of a minute, she noted that this could not be done without effort, her mind tired, her eyes pained, although they were closed, and she lost the memory of the letter.

With her eyes open she then demonstrated that her sight was the same as her memory with her eyes closed. When she tried to keep her attention fixed on one part of the letter, the movement from side to side stopped, she experienced a sense of effort, her head began to ache, the letter blurred, all parts of it looked alike, and soon it disappeared. She was reminded that when she saw the letter distinctly, or when she imagined it perfectly, she did it easily, without effort, without strain, without any trouble or hard work whatever; but that when she saw, or imagined it imperfectly, she made a great effort.

The letters on the distant Snellen test card appeared gray and blurred to her, and all parts of each letter looked alike. Even the large letter that she could distinguish was blurred, with a gray outline, and was not as black as the small letters of the fine print which she read so easily. Her attention was called to the great difference between the size of the letters on the Snellen test card and those of the fine print, and I suggested that if she saw the larger letters on the test card gray, while the smaller letters of the fine print looked black to her, it must be because she was imagining them to be gray. I also said that if she could imagine the white openings of the small letters to be whiter than they really were, she ought to be able to do the same thing with the larger white spaces of the larger letters. Thus she was led to realize that a large part of what she saw on both the large and the small card was imaginary, and that she ought to be able to use her imagination to improve her sight when looking at the large card, as she did when looking at the small one, instead of to spoil it as she was then doing. Having demonstrated these facts she soon became able to retain her mental control when looking at distant objects, and was permanently cured.

One of the worst cases of pain and fatigue which I ever saw occurred in a young man who lived several thousand miles from New York, and came here as a last resort in the hope of being relieved of the misery he had endured as long as he could remember. The history of his treatment by numerous physicians, mostly ophthalmologists, would make an interesting story, but it is too long to be recounted here. On testing his sight I was surprised to find it good. He read the 20-line of the Snellen test card at twenty feet, and also read the finest print at various distances. At this time he had no pain. When the pain came on, however, his vision became imperfect, and as the pain was almost continuous, he said he suffered from imperfect sight most of the time. I asked him why he did not maintain his good sight continuously when he obtained so much relief from it. He replied that he was unable to do so.

He had lost his mental control to such an extent that even with his eyes closed he was unable to visualize his own signature, and when he attempted to do so and failed, the pain in his eyes and head became much worse. I had him look at a large letter on the Snellen test card and observe its white center, which he was able to see whiter than the rest of the card. I told him that the white center of the letter was not whiter than the rest of the card and that he only imagined it so. Then I asked him if he could imagine the white center as white as snow with the sun shining on it—a dazzling white. He answered, "Yes, I can imagine it as white as the snow on the top of the mountains near my home."

I told him that he had formed a mental picture of the snowcapped mountain by the aid of his memory or imagination, and that having done this with his eyes open, he ought to be able to visualize the mountain with his eyes closed. Much to my gratification he was able to do this for part of a minute, and to imagine not only the white snow on top of the mountain but also other parts of it as well. Then he demonstrated that he could imagine one part best of the snowcap, but that when he tried to imagine it all at once the mental picture disappeared and his pain increased. To see one part at a time of the snowcap was easy and his pain was relieved. To see all parts at the same time was impossible, and trying to do the impossible was a strain which produced pain. In other words, to lose his mental picture of the mountain required an effort, a very great effort which tore the nerves of his eyes and head all to pieces.

With this demonstration as a beginning, he became able to form mental pictures of other objects. The most difficult thing of all was for him to imagine printed or written letters, but this was finally accomplished, and his mental control, and consequently his mental pictures, became normal. With his eyes closed he is now able to remember or imagine large or small letters as well as he can see them with his eyes open. His pain is entirely relieved and what pleased him most—his vision has improved to 20/10, double the accepted standard of normality.

STORIES FROM THE CLINIC

No. 22: Joseph and Christmas at the Clinic

By Emily C. Lierman

Throughout the civilized world Christmas is recognized as the children's day. To hosts of boys and girls it seems the most wonderful day in the year; but there are other little folks—all too many of them—who do not know its meaning, whom Santa Claus seems to have quite forgotten.

This fact was brought home to me very forcibly during my first Christmas at the Clinic seven years ago. A boy of seven came with his sister, a little girl of five, for treatment. Both the children were thinly clad and far from clean, and seemed to feel perfectly at home near a warm radiator. There was nothing wrong with the girl's eyes, but the boy had a severe inflammation of the eyelids, along with a squint of the right eye. I was not surprised to find later that this inflammation was caused by uncleanliness. As I was about to treat him I asked him what he expected Santa Claus to give him. The time was two weeks before Christmas. He looked up and said, "Oh, he ain't never came to our house! I only sees him in the store windows." "But you have a Christmas tree on Christmas Eve, don't you?" I asked. "Nope," said he, "we never had none."

I began to think I wanted to use my influence with Santa Claus on behalf of this neglected waif, but my present business was to treat him. No, I did not begin with palming this time. I washed his eyes and face with water, and judging by the color of the towel when the operation was over I should say that he had not been washed for six months or so. I now tested his sight, and with both eyes he read the 10-line at fifteen feet. Then I covered his good eye, and with the squinting eye, the right, he read the 70-line, 15/70. I now showed him how to palm, and while his eyes were covered I told him the story of the Babe of Bethlehem. This worked like a charm, and in less than ten minutes his right eye improved to 15/30. The little fellow promised to cover his eyes to rest them many times each day; and I promised that Santa Claus would surely have a present for him at Christmas.

The progress he made was astonishing. I learned later that his father was in jail for theft, and that he had to mother his little sister and baby brother while his sickly mother went out to work; yet he found time to practice, and before Christmas he had normal vision in both eyes, though the right eye turned in at times the least little bit. As for the inflammation, it had completely disappeared under the influence of the sun treatment.

The day before Christmas I bought a Christmas tree and filled a big basket with good things to eat and a little gift for each child in the family of my little patient, and in the evening I took them to his home. The poverty I found there wrung my heart, but I had the gratification of knowing that the children at least would have a happy Christmas. The sight of the Christmas tree filled them with rapture too great for speech, and the gratitude of the mother was pathetic.

Shortly afterward the boy's visits to the Clinic ceased, and going to his home I found the scanty belongings of the family upon the sidewalk, all covered with freshly fallen snow. The next day I went again, and was told by the neighbors that the mother was in a hospital and that the children had been placed by a charitable society in an institution.

I never saw nor heard of my patient again, but he inspired me with the idea of trying to make my family at the Clinic happy at Christmas time, and incidentally I found that Santa Claus was an invaluable assistant, taking the place of baseball at other seasons. Mothers often tell me that Jimmie or Johnnie will not behave long enough for me to treat him. Well, I listen, of course, and then I begin to talk baseball or Santa Claus, according to the season of the year, and I have known the most restless of small boys to sit on a stool, or stand in a corner, for ten minutes without moving while I told of the night before Christmas, or related some incident of the baseball field. It is astonishing the interest a small boy takes in baseball. Nine times out of ten when I ask a boy to imagine something perfectly he will say, "I can imagine a baseball very well."

Santa Claus is a fair rival of baseball and appeals to girls and boys alike. I begin in September to talk about the visit he makes to the Clinic every year, and the result is magical.

Joseph, nine years old, was quite unmanageable at first and could not be enticed to palm, nor even to stand still long enough for me to test him. I finally got tired of coaxing him, and told him to wait until others had been treated. His mother, a very nervous woman, wanted to thrash him, but the little fellow didn't seem to mind that a bit. He had been sent by the school nurse for glasses, and was so sensitive to light that he could only partly open his eyes. When I was able to get back to him I said, "If you will read this card for me and do as I tell you, I will have you come here the day before Christmas when Santa Claus will give you something nice."

It worked splendidly. He read the card with both eyes together and each eye separately, getting most of the letters on the 40-line at twelve feet. He palmed when I showed him how, and before he left his sight had improved to 12/20. After he had palmed for ten minutes or so his mother remarked on how wide open his eyes were. Joseph came quite regularly after that, and was so grateful for the gift Santa Claus brought him at Christmas that, even though he was cured in a few weeks, he continued to come just to say "Hello" to the Doctor and myself.

One day, shortly before Christmas, a little girl came for treatment. Her age I cannot exactly remember, but I should imagine it was nine or ten years. Her wistful eyes looked up into mine and I guessed that she was very poor and lonely. She told me that her mother and father were both dead and that a kind neighbor who already had nine children was mothering her too. I knew just what I would like to have had Santa Claus give her, and tried to figure out just how much I could stretch my Christmas fund so that I could buy clothes and shoes for this little girl. It could not be done; but I doubt if these useful things would have made her as happy as the dolly and the necklace which I ultimately gave her, and which cost only a trifle. Like the children in the first story she was so overcome with joy that she could scarcely talk.

There was nothing seriously wrong with her eyes, but she was under a nervous strain which caused her sight to blur at times. I soon corrected this, and she was very happy when told that she didn't need glasses.

I must add that the adult patients are not forgotten at Christmas time. Each one gets a gift and an orange, and they all leave the Clinic with a smile that won't come off; all of which, I am sure, is good for their eyes. My family seems to grow each year, but somehow I always find the money for the annual distribution of Christmas joy. A good many of the patients buy Snellen test cards to practice with at home, and all this money goes into the Christmas fund; then checks come from various sources sometimes at the last moment. To all who have so generously helped me in this way I want to say, "I thank you from the bottom of my heart, and wish you all a merry Christmas and a happy New Year."

Better Eyesight
January 1922—Vol. VI, No. 1

STOP STARING

It can be demonstrated by tests with the retinoscope that all persons with imperfect sight stare, strain, or try to see.

To demonstrate this fact:

Look intently at one part of a large or small letter at the distance or near point. In a few seconds, usually, fatigue and discomfort will be produced, and the letter will blur or disappear. If the effort is continued long enough, pain may be produced.

To break the habit of staring:

(1) Shift consciously from one part to another of all objects regarded, and imagine that these objects move in a direction contrary to the movement of the eye. Do this with letters on the test card, with letters of fine print, if they can be seen, and with other objects.

(2) Close the eyes frequently for a moment or longer. When the strain is considerable, keep the eyes closed for several minutes and open them for a fraction of a second—flashing. When the stare is sufficient to keep the vision down to 2/200 or less, palm for a longer or shorter time; then look at the card for a moment. Later mere closing of the eyes may afford sufficient rest.

(3) Imagine that the white openings and margins of letters are whiter than the rest of the background. Do this with eyes closed and open alternately. It is an interesting fact that this practice prevents staring and improves the vision rapidly.

[One type of staring that the *Better Eyesight* magazines do not refer to often is the "spaced out" type. This usually occurs while a person is thinking, especially worrying, about something; the head and body are still, the breathing is shallow or almost stopped, and the eyelids are open without blinking. There is no interest in or awareness of what is around the person. This "spaced out" state is one of the worst types of staring and must be eliminated for sight to improve. There are few things worse for eyesight than to have the eye open, *and not seeing*. The common statement "You lose what you don't use" is especially true in regard to eyesight.—TRQ]

BE COMFORTABLE
By W. H. Bates, M.D.

It can be stated without fear of successful contradiction that persons with perfect sight are always comfortable, not only as to their eyes, but as to the rest of the body. As soon as they cease to be so, it can be demonstrated by examination with the retinoscope that their sight has ceased to be perfect. They become nearsighted, farsighted, or astigmatic. The art of learning to use the eyes properly is, in short, the art of learning to be comfortable. Even the memory of comfort improves the sight, while the memory of discomfort lowers it. Persons with imperfect sight often say and think that they are perfectly comfortable; but invariably such persons experience a feeling of relief when they close their eyes, demonstrating that they were not perfectly comfortable before, but had merely formed a habit of ignoring that discomfort. Persons with perfect sight, on the other hand, can immediately produce discomfort by producing imperfect sight, or even by remembering or imagining it, and persons with imperfect sight can produce a degree of discomfort that cannot be ignored by making their sight worse.

Imperfect sight cannot, in other words, be produced without effort, and this effort tears the nerves of the whole body to pieces. The same is true of an imperfect memory and imagination. To demonstrate these facts is often the best way of improving the sight.

While persons with imperfect sight may feel no discomfort when looking at letters on the test card which they do not ordinarily distinguish, they cannot blur their vision for a letter they do distinguish without great effort and discomfort. In fact, the effort and discomfort are so great that many patients cannot be induced to make the experiment. When they can be prevailed upon to do so, however, they realize that they must be unconsciously straining whenever they look at anything with imperfect sight. It is often hard to convince patients of the existence of this unconscious strain, and nothing helps more in their treatment than to have them demonstrate the facts.

What is true of the vision is true of the memory and imagination. When a letter is remembered perfectly, with the outlines clear, and the opening as white as snow or starch; when the attention shifts easily from one part of the letter to another and it appears to move in a direction opposite to that in which the attention shifts; it is remembered easily. There is no sense of effort or strain, and the individual is perfectly comfortable. When, on the other hand, a letter is remembered imperfectly, with the outline obscured by a gray cloud which is all the time changing, the mind tires so quickly that the memory of the letter is lost from time to time and has to be brought back by an effort. Discomfort is soon produced, and if the effort is continued long enough, severe pain may result. At the same time the retinoscope will show that an error of refraction has been produced, or if this condition previously existed, that its degree has increased.

Staring is uncomfortable, and lowers the vision. Shifting and the realization of the apparent movement resulting from it are comfortable and improve the vision. Let anyone try to stop the apparent movement of telegraph poles and other objects past a moving train, and discomfort, pain and carsickness result. In the same way, any effort to stop the slighter movement of stationary objects produced by the normal shifting of the eyes results in discomfort and pain, even though the individual may not previously have been conscious of the movement.

Some people are able to close their eyes and be comfortable. Such persons are easy to cure. In one case a man with presbyopia was completely relieved by keeping his eyes closed for half an hour; and the cure was permanent. Later his wife was cured by the same means. Other people cannot rest with their eyes shut, and are very difficult to cure. It is the same way with palming. Some persons, when they close and cover their eyes so as to exclude all the light, at once relax and are comfortable, and such persons are easily cured. Others strain more than ever, and are very difficult to cure.

Perfect sight, perfect memory and perfect imagination cannot, in short, coexist with the consciousness of any abnormal symptom, and all such symptoms are relieved when the sight becomes perfect, or when one is able to remember or imagine something seen perfectly.*

* Bates: "The Relief of Pain by the Aid of the Memory," *New York Medical Journal,* May 24, 1919.

MY EXPERIENCE WITH CENTRAL FIXATION

By Dr. Doris J. Bowlby

The correction of imperfect sight without the use of glasses, as taught by Dr. Bates, first came under my observation on January 1 of this year when Dr. Etha Marion Jones of St. Petersburg, Florida called my attention to the method. It appealed to me as being both simple and rational, and I began at once to study and later to practice it. Since that time I have taken glasses off about fifty patients, varying in age from ten to eighty years. Among them have been cases of squint, glaucoma, iritis, retinitis, double progressive myope and *muscae volitantes* (floating specks). Many had worn glasses for years. Yet I had great success with all of them. The following are specimens of other equally interesting cases that might be cited:

Frank, age ten, came to my office on September 1, 1921, for examination. He had been wearing glasses since he was four years old for what was supposed to be congenital myopia, and was then wearing the following:

Right eye, concave 15.75 D. S. with concave 4.00 D. C. 15 degrees; left eye, concave 15.75 D. S. with concave 4.00 D. C. 165 degrees.

With his left eye he could see only the 200-line letter at one foot, 1/200, and with his right he had only light perception. His parents hesitated about putting him in my care as it seemed incredible that he could ever be cured, but they were finally persuaded to snatch at what must have appeared to them a forlorn hope. The boy himself was unwilling to discard his glasses at first; but after the second treatment, when the vision of the left eye improved to 3/30 and that of the right to 3/40, he hesitatingly consented to go home without their aid. After his third treatment he felt safe in going anywhere without them. As he lives twenty-five miles from my office, I could see him only twice a week, but after every treatment the improvement was so marked that now, after two months, his right vision is as good as his left, both being 11/30 for the Snellen test card, while he reads diamond type at six inches and the larger type of his schoolbooks at eight inches. I feel sure that he will soon be reading 20/20. He looks and acts like a different boy and is, naturally, a very happy one. The case has attracted much attention in the village where he lives.

On September 9, a young girl of eighteen came to me because of the intense pain which she was suffering in her eyes and head. She had not been able to go to school or use her eyes in any way for over a year, and during this time had been to three specialists. Her lenses had been changed a number of times. She had dark glasses to wear whenever she went into the light, and for eight months she had spent most of her time in dark rooms. Her sight had been perfect, so far as she knew, until she had had measles four years previously. During this illness she had read and studied, and afterward her eyes were red and weak.

Two years ago she noticed that she could not see writing on the blackboard, and in a few days an eruption appeared on the eyelids and side of the face. Later she had an infected sinus and also infected tonsils, tonsillectomy and an operation upon the nose having been performed eighteen months previously. No doubt the foci of infection which had existed at least a year had something to do with her trouble. When she came to me she was suffering from conjunctival congestion, with exudation of purulent material, and there was some hardening of the eyeballs. Her left vision was 7/30 and her right vision 7/50, and she was wearing: right eye, convex 1.00 D. S. with convex 1.00 D. C. 100 degrees; left eye, convex 1.00 D. S. with convex 1.25 D. C. 80 degrees.

The patient came for treatment every day and has been very faithful in her palming and other exercises. After the third treatment all pain left her and she left her glasses with me. By October 1 she was able to return to school. She now reads the lowest line of the test card at twenty feet, 20/10, and reads diamond type at ten inches. The retinoscope shows no error of refraction in either eye, and the strained look about her eyes and in her face has given way to one of relaxation.

STORIES FROM THE CLINIC

No. 23: Congenital Blindness Relieved

By Emily C. Lierman

It is a pleasure to be able to publish the following report of the relief of congenital blindness involving not only cataract but disease of the retina. According to the accepted teachings of ophthalmology there would have been no relief for this child, and he would have been condemned to a life of blindness, a burden to himself, his family and the state.

One day about a year ago there came to our Clinic a little boy of three bearing the picturesque name of Jocky. A man and woman on the last lap of life's journey accompanied him, and I learned later they were his grandparents, his father and mother having died of influenza when he was a baby. As they held the child's hands and waited very patiently for Dr. Bates to speak to them, they both looked very sad indeed.

After the Doctor had examined the boy's eyes, he called to me and asked me to watch very carefully to see if the little fellow would follow his hand as he passed it from side to side very close to the eyes. Poor Jocky paid no attention whatever to the proceedings, for he did not see the hand at all. He could not see anything. He was blind and had been so from birth. Breathlessly the grandmother exclaimed, "Isn't there no hope at all, Doctor, please? Oh, say there is!"

Poor woman! There seemed very little room for hope. The child's pupils were filled with a white mass plainly visible to the naked eye, and Dr. Bates said that there must have occurred before birth an inflammation of the iris and the interior coats of the eyeball. This had not only caused the formation of the cataracts, but had destroyed the sensitiveness of the retina, so that the removal of the cataracts would have done no good. The Doctor did not promise anything, but carefully explained to the dear old people how necessary it was for Jocky to rest his eyes, and I then showed the grandmother how he could do this.

It was not easy for Jocky to rest. Every nerve in his body seemed to be straining. But with infinite patience his grandmother taught him to palm and encouraged him to make a game of it. "Where is Jocky now?" she would ask. Then he would cover his closed eyes with his little chubby hands, shut out all the light, and say, "Jocky gone away."

Jocky enjoyed playing this game, and the two would keep it up for hours. Even by himself, when he became tired of his other games he would cover his closed eyes with the palms of his hands and go somewhere else in his imagination. When he took his hands down he could always see better, and this naturally encouraged him to continue the game. He also enjoyed joining hands with his grandmother, or grandfather, and swinging, and the practice helped his sight very much. He did not know his letters at first, but the grandmother soon taught him with the help of the test card.

After a few months of this treatment he had made the most astonishing progress. The area occupied by the cataracts grew smaller and smaller until one pupil was half clear and the other partially so. Jocky began to go out by himself and to play with other children. At the Clinic, after he had palmed a while, his grandmother would ask him to go and find the good nurse who had been so kind to him when he first came and he would go straight to her. Then she would ask him to find Dr. Bates, and he would put his arms about the Doctor's knees and hug him affectionately. He would also go to a little girl patient suffering from crossed eyes, and the two had great fun swinging together.

Then one day the grandparents were told that Jocky

could not come to the Clinic anymore because he did not live in the district of the Harlem Hospital. We did not see or hear from him after that, and I can only hope that the grandmother kept on with the treatment and continued to get results from it.

No patient who ever came to the Clinic was more missed than Jocky when his visits ceased. As he lived quite a long way off, he did not come three days a week, like the other children, but when he did come he was like a ray of sunshine. His cunning ways endeared him to everybody, while his wonderful progress inspired confidence in the treatment and encouraged young and old to practice more industriously. He understood what we were trying to do for him and tried to help us all he could. Whenever he saw Dr. Bates coming towards him he would put his hands over his closed eyes, and say over and over again, "Jocky gone away, Doctor. See! Jocky gone away."

AFTER THIRTY YEARS

By William Murphy

Editor's Note—*This very interesting article furnishes a striking illustration of the fundamental principle of the cure of imperfect sight by treatment without glasses. All the methods used for this purpose are simply different ways of obtaining rest, and although most persons cannot obtain sufficient rest to effect a cure merely by closing their eyes, there is a minority of patients who require nothing more. The writer is mistaken in thinking that his imperfect sight was caused by excessive reading in youth. He could not have done all this reading unless he had done it without strain. And even reading under a strain would not have made him myopic. It is more likely that his trouble started with straining to see the blackboard or other distant objects in school, for it is straining to see distant objects that causes myopia.*

I was born in Ireland forty years ago, and my eyes began to fail when I was about nine or ten years old. I never knew why, but since reading *Better Eyesight* and *The Cure of Imperfect Sight by Treatment Without Glasses* I think I have found the reason.

I was an inveterate reader. I would eagerly devour every scrap of reading matter that came into my hands, and many a night I have curled up in bed all night long, reading about the hair-breadth escapes and other thrilling adventures of Buffalo Bill and Nick Carter and all the other wonderful heroes so dear to the heart of a young boy. On such nights I might get one, or maybe two, hours sleep. I would then get up and go to school. I now believe that all that reading was a very great strain on my eyes and, not having learned how to rest them, they remained under this strain for more than thirty years.

My vision grew steadily worse, but I never could bring myself to wear glasses. Several times I have been tempted to do so, but always when it came to the point I balked. One day when I was about fourteen years old, in my search for something to read, I happened upon a publication entitled *Physical Culture Magazine.* Of course I read it. It was only a pamphlet of ten or twelve pages, but it made a very strong impression upon me. Ever since then I have been a firm believer in natural methods of curing disease, and I fully expected that some day I would find a natural method that would cure my eyes. Wearing glasses was not curing them, and I simply could not get myself to put them on. Perhaps I missed something by this stubborn attitude. Perhaps there was something on the other side of the street that I did not see, but now I am sure that I gained more than I lost. If I had added the strain of glasses to my other strains, there is no knowing how much worse my eyes would have become.

Now, after waiting nearly thirty years, my long cherished hopes have been realized. I have found a way to cure my eyes by natural methods. On November 28 of last year I began the practice of central fixation, and the results have been wonderful. On that date I could read with my left eye only the 50-line at six feet. With my right eye at three feet I could barely see the great big letter at the top of the card. Eight days later my left eye had improved to 6/10 and my right eye to 6/50, and with the right eye alone, the eye that was almost blind, I read newspaper type at twelve inches.

All this I accomplished simply by closing my eyes and resting them for fifteen minutes at a time, and then looking at the card. I didn't imagine dots or swings or anything else. I just rested my eyes and looked at the card, keeping it up for about two hours.

Now I am trying something else. I noticed that whenever I attended a movie my eyes felt fine afterward. So I decided to go to a movie every day, and this is how I work it: The first day I sat up in the very first seat, close to the screen; now I am moving back a seat each day (I always go to the same theatre.) I am very careful not to strain and always close my eyes and rest them when they feel the least bit tired. In fact, this resting of my eyes is becoming quite a habit with me. The results so far have been splendid.

My greatest trouble is double vision. I have it in both eyes; but it is going away gradually, and doesn't bother me except when I look at the test card.

QUESTIONS AND ANSWERS

Q–1a. Should a house be brightly lighted by a direct electric light or a reflected white light? 1b. In many homes colored shades are used on the lights. Does that impair the sight?

A–1a. The more brightly the house is lighted the better for the sight. 1b. Yes.

Q–2a. Is it advisable to use specimens of diamond type other than the "Seven Truths of Normal Sight"? Would it be well to get a *New Testament* in diamond type? 2b. I have thus far found the flashing method the most helpful. However, after closing the eyes, I have difficulty in opening them. The lids seem to stick together, as it were. What is the cause of such stickiness and the remedy? 2c. I was trying to read the *Seven Truths* lately by the flashing method, and for about twenty minutes obtained very little results. Then, all of a sudden, upon closing my eyes, I saw the blackest object I have ever seen with closed eyes. I was startled, it seemed so real, and on opening my eyes I was surprised to find that I could read practically all of the *Seven Truths* clearly at thirteen inches without closing my eyes. I think the black object was probably the black rubber key of the electric socket in the fixture which I had unconsciously looked at from time to time during the exercise. I have not been able to do just this since. What is the probable reason for my failure? 2d. I find I see any reading matter more clearly in a bright light—sunlight or electric light—than in a dim or less bright light. Why is this? 2e. Today in trying to read the *Seven Truths* I found that I could do it at six or seven inches with few alternate closings of the eyes and flashes; but I found in accomplishing this I was partially closing my eyelids, so that I must have looked much like the Patagonians in Fig. 1 in Dr. Bates' book, said to be probably myopic when the picture was taken. I found that I could not keep my eyes thus partly closed without some strain, but I could not see the print clearly when they were wide open. Often the print would look quite blurred when I first looked at it, but it cleared perceptibly and became quite black as I continued to look. I also found myself reading today twenty pages of fairly small print at about eight or nine inches in much the same way.

A–2a. Yes, if you wish to. The *Testament* would be a good thing to have. 2b. Difficulty in closing or opening the eyes is a common symptom of strain, and may be relieved by any method that relieves strain. 2c. Such intervals of relaxation are a very common phenomenon. They will come more frequently and last longer if you continue to practice. 2d. In a bright light the contrast between black letters and their white background is more marked than in a dim light. Persons differ greatly, however, in the amount of light they require for maximum vision. Some people see better in a dim light because they think that condition a favorable one. 2e. Narrowing the eyelids (squinting) is a bad habit.

Better Eyesight
February 1922—Vol. VI, No. 2

TEST YOUR IMAGINATION!

With the eyes closed remember some letter, for example, a small letter "o." Imagine the white center to be white as snow with the sun shining on it. Now open the eyes, look at the Snellen test card and imagine the white snow as well as you can for a few moments only, without noting so much the clearness of the letters on the card as your ability to imagine the snow white center, alternating as before with the Snellen test card.

Another method: With the eyes closed, remember and imagine as well as you can the first letter, which should be known, on each line of the Snellen test card, beginning with the larger letters. Then open your eyes and imagine the same letter for a few moments only, alternating until the known letter is imagined sufficiently well that the second letter is seen without any effort on your part.

Third method: With the eyes closed remember or imagine a small black period for part of a minute or longer. Then with the eyes open, looking at no object in particular and without trying to see, imagine in your mind the black period. Should you believe that your vision is improved, dodge it and look somewhere else. This you can practice at all times, in all places, at your work as well as when sitting quietly in your room practicing with the Snellen test card. When the period is imagined perfectly with the eyes open, one cannot dodge perfect sight, which comes without any effort whatsoever.

STORIES FROM THE CLINIC
No. 24: Sixteen Schoolgirls
By Emily C. Lierman

Editor's Note—*This is the twenty-fourth of the series of "Stories from the Clinic." Can any minion of helpfulness be greater than that of Ms. Lierman's to these children of New York's crowded schools? We think not—nor do the other children of the world await any greater blessing than that which she has been fortunate enough to give to these.*

Throughout the summer of 1921 our morning and afternoon offices were filled with schoolchildren, boys and girls waiting for treatment of their eyes. They came from the Northern, Southern and Western parts of the United States. Watching them waiting patiently for their turn to see the Doctor who would take their glasses from their eyes and cure them, one could read the happy thoughts expressed in their faces. Mothers and guardians were with them to reassure them if they became impatient or the least doubtful while waiting.

To the Clinic of the same good and great Doctor in one of New York City's large hospitals, throughout the whole year, there comes a steady stream of schoolchildren, just as eager to be cured without glasses. Not always does the boy or girl have a guardian or mother to give reassurance as the different ones are waiting to be treated. Sometimes they come alone and at other times they come in pairs or with three or four other children. At the office the Doctor sees the patient for a half-hour or so, but each child at the Clinic can have only five minutes or just a little longer, for the time is short on Clinic days.

I am anxious to tell about fifteen schoolgirls, all from one class of Public School No. 90. Their ages range from nine to fourteen years. On January 5 they first appeared. That day Dr. Bates and I had to plead for admission.

Enter, the First Fifteen

There were about thirty adults, besides these schoolgirls, also waiting for treatment and all of them made a run for us when we arrived. I found that the teacher of the girls, who is very nearsighted, was at the present time being treated by Dr. Bates at his office. The progress she was making inspired her to send those of her class who were wearing glasses to the Clinic. All hands went up at once when I asked who came first.

I could see from the start that I would have my hands full. All of them had a strained expression and, because of their actions and their manner, my heart went out not just to them but to that poor nearsighted teacher!

Three out of the fifteen girls have squint and two of the three are sisters. These sisters, Helen, age 10, and Agnes, age 12, both have squint of the left eye. Helen had 14/20 with both eyes, glasses on. Glasses off she read 14/40. After palming and resting her eyes her right eye improved to 14/20, and the squinting left eye improved to 14/30 without glasses. On January 17 she read 14/15 with each eye separately. Agnes, whose squint is worse than Helen's, had 14/70 in the left eye on January 5, and on January 17 improved to 14/20. The right eye improved from 14/40 to 14/15 from January 5 to January 17.

Frieda, who also has squint of the left eye, improved from 14/40 to 14/15 in the same length of time. Her right eye has normal sight.

All the rest of the fifteen, I discovered, were nearsighted.

MARY AND MURIEL

The youngest and best behaved is nine years old. Her name is Mary. She suffered terrible pain in her eyes and head the first day she came, but after she had closed her eyes and rested them for a short time the pain went away and her sight improved from 14/40 to 14/20. The strange thing about Mary is that she did not practice at home resting her eyes as she was told to do, but nevertheless her pain never came back even though her sight did not improve any more than it had on the first day.

Muriel and another Mary had progressive myopia. Muriel became so frightened the first day she came that she ran out of the Clinic as fast as she could. She feared that the Doctor would apply drops or make her suffer in some way. Next day at school Mary told her what she had missed by running away and now, after three visits to the Clinic, Muriel is in a race with Mary and I believe she has a fair chance of being cured first.

Muriel's sight improved from 14/70 to 14/20. Palming, resting her eyes, did this for her. She practices faithfully at home. Mary's vision was 14/15 with glasses. Without them, 14/30. Now she has sight as good without her glasses as she did with them before. On January 17 her vision was 14/15. She also practices faithfully, and her father has also become interested and helps Mary at home with her chart. The remainder of the fifteen all had about the same degree of myopia and all are eager to be cured. It is encouraging to see them improve after they have rested their eyes for just a few minutes.

As I finished with these cases the Doctor called my attention to a girl from the same school who has opacity of the cornea of the left eye. She had had this trouble since she was one year old. Her age now is twelve. She had no perception of light at all in that eye when she came. On her second visit to the Clinic she could see light in that eye for the first time. Now she is beginning to see the letters on the test card.

Should children be forced to keep wearing their glasses to benefit the man who sells eyeglasses? I am willing and want to devote the rest of my life to this wonderful work, but we need help. Mothers of the children are helping; they are our assistants only in the home. Teachers who are wearing glasses and who are being cured without them are also helping, but the prejudice of some of the authorities, based on ignorance of the truth, is a stumbling block. If they would only investigate the facts we would all be better satisfied.

My girls have faithfully practiced and improved not only their eyes but in other ways. Winter storms have changed to summer breezes and they are working with a determination for better sight without glasses.

On January 14 they informed me that the school doctor said they must put on their glasses again, regardless of the fact that the sight of all of them has improved. The mothers feel quite differently about it, however, and they say that their children will not put on their glasses again no matter what the school nurse or doctor says. Since then my girls are all my willing assistants and are more determined than ever to be cured. I will be pleased to report from time to time the progress we are making.

READING WITHOUT GLASSES

By W. H. Bates, M.D.

A patient asked me how I discovered so many truths about eyesight. It may emphasize the facts and their value if I relate the events connected with the discovery of these truths.

P. T. Barnum, many years ago, wrote an essay on "How to Make Money." In the opening sentence he stated that he felt that he was able to write an essay on how to make money, because he had made money. Perhaps, similarly, as I have established medical truths I am encouraged to write how it was done.

About ten years ago I was talking to a friend of mine who showed me a letter which he desired me to read. At that time I was wearing glasses, but only for reading and on account of my age, not then knowing any means of doing without them for that purpose. My glasses were mislaid and it took me some time to find them while my friend impatiently waited. Being a friend, of course, he had the license to say things to me in a way he would not to his worst enemy.

Among other disagreeable things he said, and the tone was very emphatic, sarcastic, disagreeable, insulting, "You claim to cure people without glasses; why don't you cure yourself?" [Dr. Bates initially cured people of myopia.—TRQ] I shall never forget those words. They stimulated me to do something. I tried by all manner of means, by concentration, strain, effort, hard work, to enable myself to become able to read the newspaper at the near point.

After a few months, it dawned on me that all my efforts were useless. Previously, it had been my custom when I could not do a certain thing myself to look around and find somebody to help me, and so in the present instance I went looking for help. My old friends, the eye doctors, laughed at me and told me that I was crazy to think of the possibility of such a thing. They repeated to me the old established theories that accommodation is produced by change in the curvature of the crystalline lens. In youth the lens readily changes its form or its ability to focus. With advancing age the lens, like the bones and cartilage, becomes hard, loses its elasticity or its ability to change its shape and the eye no longer can change its focus from distant to near objects.

Hypnosis, Electricity, Neurology—and Back to Dr. Bates!

I consulted specialists of hypnotism, electricity experts, neurologists of all kinds and many others. One I called on, a physician who was an authority in psychoanalysis, was kind enough to listen to my problem. With as few words as possible I explained to him the simple method by which we diagnose nearsightedness with the retinoscope. As I looked off at the distance, he examined my eyes, and said that they were normal, but when I made an effort to see at the distance he said that my eyes were focused for the reading distance, nearsighted. Then when I looked at fine print at the reading distance and tried to read it he said that my eyes were focused for a distance of twenty feet or farther, and the harder I tried to read the farther away did I push my focus. He was convinced of the facts, namely: a strain to see at the distance produced nearsightedness, while a strain to see near produced a farsighted eye.

Then I told him what I desired, "Will you kindly suggest to me a line of investigation by which I can become able to focus my eyes for reading just as well when I am looking at the near point where I desire to see, as I am able to do when I strain to see distant objects?" He answered, "Come back in a month." At the end of three months I returned for his opinion. He said to me, "After consulting with a number of neurologists, ophthalmologists and others it is my opinion that there is only one man who can solve your problem." I eagerly asked, "Who is he?" He answered, "Dr. Bates." And so I had to go on with my work without his help.

That great truths are always simple truths, and that simplicity and humor frequently are akin, have been remarked before. But how often has one the experience of finding an appreciative and discriminating sense of humor—such as Dr. Bates'—in a scientist's reports of his experiments and discoveries?

Stumbling on the Truth

The man who finally helped me to succeed or the only man who would do anything to encourage me was an Episcopal minister living in Brooklyn. After my evening office hours I had to travel for about two hours to reach his residence. With the aid of the retinoscope, while I was making all kinds of efforts to focus my eyes at the near point, he would tell me how I was succeeding. After some weeks or months I had made no progress.

But one night I was looking at a picture on the wall which had black spots in different parts of it. They were conspicuously black. While observing them my mind imagined they were dark caves and that there were people moving around in them. My friend told me my eyes were now focused at the near point. When I tried to read he said my eyes were focused for the distance. Lying on the table in front of me was a magazine with an illustrated advertisement with black spots which were intensely black. I imagined they were openings of caves with people moving around in them. My friend told me that my eyes were focused for the near point; and when I glanced at some reading matter, I was able to read it. Then I looked at a newspaper and while doing so remembered the perfect black of my imaginary caves and was gratified to find that I was able to read imperfectly. [The end of this sentence is not clear. Dr. Bates may have meant that he was able to read the newspaper, but not with perfectly clarity. Below he clearly states that remembering the caves helped him to read. Another possibility is that "imperfectly" was a typographical error which should have been "perfectly."—TRQ]

We discussed the matter to find what brought about the benefit. Was it a strain, or what was it? I tried again to remember the black caves while looking at the newspaper and my memory failed. I could not read the newspaper at all. He asked, "Do you remember the black caves?" I answered, "No, I don't seem to be able to remember the black caves." "Well," he said, "close your eyes and remember the black caves," and when I opened my eyes I was able to read—for a few moments. When I tried to remember the black caves again I failed.

The harder I tried the less I succeeded and we were puzzled. We discussed the matter and talked of a number of things, and all of a sudden without an effort on my part I remembered the black caves, and sure enough, it helped me to read. We talked some more. Why did I fail to remember the black caves when I tried so hard? Why did I remember the black caves when I did not try or while I was thinking of other things? Here was a problem. We were both very much interested and finally it dawned on me that I could only remember these black caves when I did not strain or make an effort.

I had discovered a truth: *a perfect memory is obtained without effort and in no other way.* Also, *when the memory or imagination is perfect, sight is perfect.*

THERE SHOULD BE A BETTER EYESIGHT LEAGUE!

By Roberts Everett

I recently had the illuminating experience of an hour's intimate talk with Dr. Bates in his laboratory. It was my fortunate privilege to learn firsthand of the wonderful discoveries of Dr. Bates, his incalculable service to the poor of vision and the triumphant persistence of his methods in the face of indifference and opposition.

There was a double interest in my attention to Dr. Bates as he talked to me. There was the personal interest of my memory of a time when I had worn glasses—had *had* to wear glasses, I had been told—and of a time when, tired of much experimenting, of this lens replacing that one and this treatment following another, I had simply and determinedly discarded glasses and their ills. And successfully had done so.

But there was another interest as I listened. I realized that I was in the presence of a man and of a work that meant a definite blessing to the world. Dr. Bates, like scientists of earlier and less enlightened eras, was the discoverer and the missionary of healing methods that mankind needs. His truths of physical vision should be, by right, the property of every class and every people—as much a part of civilization's common property as the knowledge that the world is round.

And as I listened to the simple, yet for so long unaccepted, fundamentals of his discoveries and methods, it was this second, broader interest that became the overwhelming one. I felt that it became the duty of those who know of his discoveries or have been benefited by them *to spread the knowledge of them everywhere.*

The Idea of a League

So as I listened there came the idea—I believe it is a practicable idea—of a disinterested organization to carry this good word of improved vision to all who should be told of it: to the American public. An organization disinterested in all except its purpose to promulgate a healing truth, an alleviatory knowledge for the lack of which the suffering of the world today is enormously augmented.

As I learned more and more of the methods and the cures of Dr. Bates and of the needlessness of glasses, this idea became stronger and more clarified. It has been my opportunity to see certain organizations, disinterested in the larger sense but directly and enthusiastically interested in some one philanthropic or industrial truth, carry on works of education that have benefited the country or important groups or territories of it. And surely no "cause" could be more worthy of advancement, no information more worthy of promulgation, than that which will bring perfect vision and renewed faith to thousands, children and mature men and women alike.

Since that illuminating hour in Dr. Bates' laboratory I have thought much of the necessity of spreading the knowledge of the possibility of the prevention and cure of imperfect sight without the use of glasses. To those who have been benefited by the discoverer of this possibility it is a duty to so spread this knowledge, one way in which they owe it to themselves to make their lives count, in the betterment of others. So I propose to all the readers of this magazine that this work definitely be started.

How the League Can be Formed

I propose the organization of an active Better Eyesight League, devoted to the promulgation of the knowledge that the prevention and the cure of imperfect eyesight without glasses is a scientific possibility and that the man and the demonstrated methods for its achievement are at the disposal of mankind.

I propose that this Better Eyesight League be organized by readers of this magazine, by those who have been benefited by the methods of Dr. Bates, and that it be formed immediately by those who first respond to this suggestion and are the nearest in time and distance to New York.

I propose that its membership be open to all those, beyond the readers of this magazine and those who have been helped by Dr. Bates, whose pleasure and zeal it is to help their fellow men and lessen suffering.

I propose that this Better Eyesight League be formed not with the aid of Dr. Bates, if that should not be offered; but without that aid if necessary, to give the knowledge of his many cures, as well as of great discoveries, to the world. He has already within his means and to a consequently limited public told these same results and laid his knowledge of the possibilities of better eyesight open to the eyes of others. I propose that the Better Eyesight League convey this knowledge to tens and hundreds and thousands as compared to everyone that Dr. Bates has reached.

Each Reader Can Become an Organizer

To this end I suggest that every reader of this magazine the day his eye discovers this proposal write in his name and his approval of a Better Eyesight League to the office of the magazine. The envelope in the corner can be marked with the initials "B. E. L." to make sure it is read immediately. It is not necessary that Dr. Bates should ever see the letters or the names, unless that is desired. When all the letters are received there will be some means found, and word of it communicated to each name received, effectively and expeditiously to organize the League.

There should be a few weeks from now an actually functioning Better Eyesight League! Who will be first to start its organization?

QUESTIONS AND ANSWERS

Q–1. Do the rays from the Snellen Card at 20 feet enter the normal eye approximately parallel?

A–1. Yes.

Q–2. What is the function of the ciliary muscles?

A–2. I do not know.

Q–3. How do you account for this muscle and the changes in the curvature in the lens which never occur? (I have lost the page reference where you cited cases of a flattening or increase in convexity of the lens.)

A–3. I do not account for the presence of the ciliary muscle and never stated the lens changed its curvature.

Better Eyesight
March 1922—Vol. VI, No. 3

SEE THINGS MOVING

When riding in a railroad train travelling rapidly, a passenger looking out a window can imagine more or less vividly that stationary objects, trees, houses, telegraph poles, are moving past in the opposite direction. If one walks along the street, objects to either side appear to be moving.

When the eyes move from side to side a long distance, with or without the movement of the head or body, it is possible to imagine objects not directly regarded to be moving. To see things moving avoid looking directly at them while moving the eyes.

The Long Swing. No matter how great mental or other strain may be, one can, by moving the eyes a long distance from side to side with the movement of the head and body in the same direction, imagine things moving opposite over a wide area. The eyes or mind are benefited.

The Short Swing. To imagine things are moving a quarter of an inch or less, gradually shorten the long swing and decrease the speed to a rate of a second or less for each swing. Another method is to remember a small letter perfectly with the eyes closed while noting the short swing. Alternate with the eyes open and closed.

The Universal Swing. Demonstrate that when one imagines or sees one letter on a card at a distance or at a near point that the card moves with the letter, and that every other letter or object seen or imagined in turn also swings. This is the universal swing. Practice it all the time because the ability to see or to do other things is benefited.

Practice the imagination of the swing constantly. If one imagines things are stationary, the vision is always imperfect, and effort is required and one does not feel comfortable. To stare and strain takes time. To let things move is easier. One should plan to practice the swing observed by the eye with normal vision: as short at least as the width of the letter at twenty feet or six inches, as slow as a second to each movement, and all done easily, rhythmically, continuously.

READY FOR THE BETTER EYESIGHT LEAGUE!

By Roberts Everett

Editor's Note—*The cause of* Better Eyesight *is soon to come into its own through a new medium. Every reader of this article has an opportunity to become a Founder of the Better Eyesight League.*

The Better Eyesight League is to become a reality. So assured is its formation and functioning, that this article is an official call for an organization meeting in New York City, at four o'clock in the afternoon of Wednesday, March 8 at....

Last month's *Better Eyesight* carried a proposal for the forming of this League. As a result of that one article, sufficient enthusiastic support has been vouchsafed to make possible this call for an immediate organization meeting—to form a Better Eyesight League "to relieve the sufferings and discomforts of those afflicted with imperfect eyesight, to disseminate knowledge of the scientific cure and prevention of imperfect eyesight without the use of glasses, and to promote further research and investigation into the causes for imperfect eyesight and its improvement without the use of artificial lenses."

Some Letters of Approval

The February *Better Eyesight* barely had time to reach its numerous subscribers before the letters of approval of the proposal for a League began to be received. They came from New York and Missouri, from Virginia and Massachusetts, and from many other places, too. Without exception, their writers hailed the opportunity to enlist in a coordinated humanitarian movement to help alleviate a large share of the physical sufferings and discomforts of the world and to promote a general knowledge of the scientific discoveries and cures of Dr. Bates.

Says one letter from Cleveland, Ohio, "I heartily approve of any idea to band together the people who are interested in better eyesight. To assist in getting the truths that Dr. Bates has discovered to the attention of the thousands suffering from poor eyesight, it is time that we who have been benefited take a stand that will make the public recognize the possibilities of these truths."

Reads another letter, this one from Kansas City, "I wish to be a member and shall do all that I can to help such a wonderful cause."

Here is an extract from another letter, this one from New York City, "I think it would be a splendid idea to start a Better Eyesight League and will be glad if you will add my name to your list of those interested."

"My best wishes for your success. You may propose me as a member of the Better Eyesight League," writes a practicing physician from another city.

Here is still another letter, and this one, perhaps, best of all expresses the spirit animating these numerous messages of support; as if it were the world of one in the light who wishes to reach out and help those still in darkness:

"I am highly interested in your great proposition concerning a Better Eyesight League. I feel indebted to Dr. Bates who improved not only my eyesight but also my nervous condition; so I naturally wish to do my little bit to bring the life and health message to all others who are in need of it."

Pioneers in a Great Cause

A number of the writers of these letters will be present at the organization meeting in New York. At that meeting the constitution and by-laws of the League will be determined upon and adopted. Officers will be elected, disinterested men and women fired with the same zeal to promote the cause of better eyesight that is expressed in the letters quoted here. Arrangements will be made to insure publicity for the efforts of the League, so that its message of enlightenment may reach the greatest number from the start.

THE TRUTH ABOUT FATIGUE

By W. H. Bates, M.D.

This is a true explanation of fatigue. The mystery of fatigue has been one almost equal in the mind of man for ages with the mystery of death. Dr. Bates explains not merely why there is fatigue, but the lack of necessity for it!

About fifteen years ago I was ambitious to learn how to run long distances. At that time I was, it seemed to me, the poorest runner ever invented. I could not run a mile or even a quarter of a mile. To run a block brought on palpitation of the heart, and the loss of breath and fatigue was sickening. One of my dear friends told me it was impossible, that I was too old to attempt it, that it would be disastrous and that if I continued in my foolishness I would drop dead suddenly, without warning. Instead of his discouraging me, I felt an increased incentive to get busy. If I succeeded I could enjoy a conversation with my friend; but, if I failed, dropped dead, the conversation would be necessarily omitted.

At that time I belonged to a gymnasium which had a running track. The physical director promised to find out my faults. He had me run a lap and watched me closely. When I finally arrived at the starting point, all tired out, gasping for breath, he said, "Doctor, you will pardon me, I hope, when I tell you that you did not breathe naturally, but held your breath the whole distance." This knowledge was a great help; but, the strain I was under when running interfered with my breathing and was a more important factor in the cause of "fatigue" than the lack of air.

A few years ago some observations on the pulse, the heart, and the breathing before and after a race of about twenty-six miles were published. It was an interesting fact that those who finished close behind the winner had no symptoms of fatigue, loss of breath or weakened action of the heart, while the winner was in better condition at the close of the race than at the beginning. Why? Answer: At the beginning his mind was excited; and, strange to say, because he was confident of winning this great race, as he knew that he could run better than any of the men who were entered. And when he had won his mind calmed down and the action of his heart improved in consequence.

Much has been written on the cause of fatigue. A prominent physiologist, who had for many years studied the numerous theories, made the statement not long ago, "We do not know now any more about fatigue than we did many years ago."

Running Oneself Into the Ground

I determined to obtain more facts. In one race I ran about eight miles and I made all the effort possible, planning to keep running until I dropped. The experience was valuable. Before I fell I lost all sense of effort, my sight failed, the ground appeared to be rising in front of me, I lost all perception of light, and everything was midnight black. I had literally, actually, run myself into the ground. In a few minutes, I was conscious. In spite of my protests they carried me away in an automobile.

In another experiment, I entered a race of twelve miles. Just as soon as my sight failed I stopped running and walked until my vision was again normal, when I would again run some more. By alternating the walking and running I was able to finish with a sprint. A policeman invited me to sit down. Before I knew it they had me in an ambulance galloping to the hospital, with me protesting all the way. I have run in many races since, finished in good condition, and have escaped the kind attentions of the police and the ambulance service.

I now know the cause of fatigue; I know the remedy. I have cured myself. I have cured others while they in turn have relieved their friends. I can produce excessive fatigue in persons lying quietly in bed without any muscular exertion whatever. The facts are so simple they can be demonstrated by children or by adults who do not wear glasses; but the most learned eye doctors or the great scientists of the world wearing glasses cannot understand.

A Demonstration with a Period

If possible, with the eyes closed, remember a small letter "o" with a white center as white as the whitest snow. Then imagine a small black period on the right edge of the "o." Keep the attention on it, or try to see the period continuously for several seconds or for part of a minute. Note that in a few seconds it becomes more and more difficult to hold the period or a small part of the "o" stationary, the mind becomes tired, the attention wanders, the period disappears and reappears, at times the "o" is forgotten, and one demonstrates that it is impossible to keep the attention fixed on a point continuously, or to remember or imagine the letter "o" with one part stationary. Or, that it is impossible to concentrate on a point and that trying to do so or trying to do the impossible is a strain which modifies or destroys the memory or imagination, and causes discomfort and fatigue. The fatigue produced can be relieved by shifting from one part of the letter to another, when the memory or imagination of the letter again becomes normal and continuous.

Or, another demonstration: look directly at a small letter which can be seen. Keep on trying to keep the attention fixed on the letter continuously. In a short time, a few seconds, the eyes begin to tire and if the effort is made strong enough, the vision becomes imperfect, and with other disagreeable symptoms much fatigue will be experienced.

Or, still another demonstration: regard a page of fine print at a distance where it is read easily and note the restful feeling. Then hold the page farther off or at a near point where the letters are very much blurred. Make as strong an effort as possible to read the letters seen imperfectly. If the effort is strong enough one feels much fatigue. In this way one demonstrates that fatigue can be produced by eyestrain.

So many people complain that they do not have time to practice and that they have fatigue. They are less inclined to practice central fixation, the universal swing, the memory of perfect sight and other things which relieve or prevent fatigue. It should be emphasized that one has just as much time to do right as he has to do wrong and it certainly is the wrong thing to go around most of the time suffering from fatigue.

Prevention, Not Relief, for Fatigue

Theories are always wrong. As a working hypothesis the value of simply relieving fatigue is questionable.

I have a vision of the schoolchildren of this country able to do their work without discomfort or fatigue. The profession of teaching in the public schools requires much hard work and the teachers are quite properly objects of sympathy. This is all wrong because it can all be corrected. It is possible for people to do the hardest kind of work from early in the morning until late at night without any evidence of fatigue whatever. It is a puzzle for some people to explain how or why so many people are very much fatigued when they first wake up in the morning. Many society people hunt for rest and recreation. They sit in a chair and try to do nothing and wonder why they get so terribly fatigued.

I have repeatedly published that the only time the eye is at rest is when one has or imagines perfect sight. The normal eye when it is at rest is all the time moving. Fatigue is relieved by a universal swing and the relief is instantaneous, demonstrating quite decidedly that fatigue is a mental symptom. I could go on and write much more but the matter may be summed up very briefly:

(1) Fatigue is always associated with the imagination of imperfect sight.

(2) Rest or relaxation is always associated with perfect sight or the imagination of perfect sight.

STORIES FROM THE CLINIC

No. 25: What Palming did for "Pop," a Blind Man

By Emily C. Lierman

I hope and trust that our readers will forgive me for not waiting until my dear old patient could see a little better, or until I was able to accomplish a little more for him; but in this particular case I feel very much like a child, eager to tell of the most thrilling thing that ever happened in my life.

A few months ago, some time in November, this dear old man came to our Clinic, led by another man much younger. They had been told by the clerk that he could not receive treatment there because he did not live in the district. However, the nurse in charge, who is dearly loved by all the patients, did not send him away, but asked him to wait until Dr. Bates had finished with his patients and see what could be done. After our patients had been attended to, Dr. Bates had a talk with the old gentleman.

The Doctor examined him and found that he had all sorts of trouble with the nerves and muscles of his eyes. Dr. Bates then called me and asked me to look at the patient's eyes and also asked me what we could do for him. There he was, absolutely with no sight whatever, but with a smile that went straight to my heart.

A Faith That Will Not Be Denied

Before I go any further I would like all who read to know that if it had been at all possible, Dr. Bates would not have hesitated for one moment, but would have offered to treat the man himself. But it could not possibly be done because Dr. Bates labors daily, Sundays included, at the rate of sixteen hours a day. These poor people, when they hear of Dr. Bates, come from all over the United States and we do the best, the Doctor included, of course, we can for them.

As the old man held his head up toward our faces waiting to hear us say that he would be able to see again, I made up my mind to make time myself to treat him at our laboratory. Every moment of my time is taken up with our work but there was my lunch hour before Clinic on each Saturday that I could devote to his case. I had not the slightest idea that I could ever give him even perception of light or that I would have the intelligence to ever help him see like other people. One could see no iris whatever or pupil in either eye. Each eye had a thick, solid-looking white mass where the iris and pupil should be. But that day we arranged that he should come to see me each Saturday, and that I was to treat him for one hour. I made no promises to him, but said only that I would do all I could for him if he would do his part and carry out the treatment at home.

His age is seventy-four years, I learned, and he is an inmate of the Home for the Blind in Brooklyn. He said that he was first stricken with blindness in the left eye in the year 1889, and the trouble was neuralgia. In 1898 he was stricken with blindness in the right eye after suffering with chills and fever. During the year of 1898 he could see slightly with the left eye, and until 1920, when his sight gave out completely. He had been treated by noted eye specialists without success.

The first week in December he came to our laboratory, and without thinking, he said, "I am very happy to see you." And I answered very promptly, "And I am happy to see you, also." I found that he was under a terrible tension. The muscles of his arms, especially at the elbows, were so tense that I made up my mind that he would go through some sort of calisthenics with me before we started with the treatment.

Calisthenics at Seventy-four

I called him "Pop" right from the start, and he seemed to like it. Well, you should have seen the poor old fellow throw his hands over his head and try to touch the floor without bending his knees. Of course, he only got half way. Nevertheless, it was a good start. We were very serious in our exercises and, to make it appear doubly so to him, I went through the exercises with him guiding him as best I could. I taught him how to palm and to swing his body from side to side as I stood before him, holding his hands, reminding him always to loosen up at the elbows. I told him that anyone could see that he was blind because he stared so much and never seemed to close his eyes, which made his condition worse. So the next thing I taught him was to open and close his eyes often, which we call *blinking*.

The hour was over and the next time I saw him he was a very happy man. "I have so much to tell you," he said. "The other day, as I went to the washroom I did not feel for the wash basin, but I saw it and I walked over to it. But in my happiness and excitement my vision left me. Why was that, please?" I answered, "You began to strain in your excitement and caused your blindness to return." I encouraged him by saying, "Don't worry, you will be able to see more next time when you are not straining!"

Then, to my surprise, I learned that this dear old fellow has been shaving men's faces by the sense of touch. Before he became blind he was an expert barber. He loves to repeat again and again how he shaved ex-President Taft and other notable men.

Next time he came he was even more interesting. He could not wait to tell me how young he feels now and how he loves to exercise. He gave me a demonstration of how he could touch the floor with his fingertips without bending his knees, and he did it quite successfully. I was just in the act of praising him for the ability to do such a wonderful trick for a man seventy-four years young, when all of a sudden there was an accident—a button went flying to the opposite side of the room! It broke off from the back of his trousers as he touched the floor with his fingertips, and poor old "Pop" was more embarrassed than I was.

But the Treatment Goes On

However, we soon remedied the trouble and started in with our treatment. As he had no perception of light in the beginning I was quite thrilled when he pointed to both windows of our room and showed me just where the curtains were fastened. I placed him in another part of the room and I was thrilled again when he pointed with his fingers to a sunbeam shining on the rug. With this progress to encourage me, I now am striving with him to give him his greatest desire—his real eyesight. I cannot understand as yet just how he does see, but I do notice that the white mass in front of the iris is not quite as thick as formerly. The last time I saw him he told me that while he was shaving a man he suddenly saw the man's face and that he also saw another man walking past him who had entered the room quietly. He also told me that the matron of the home had entered his room, and as she passed out he asked the maid if the matron had on a bluish-gray gown and the maid, knowing that he was blind, was surprised as she answered, "Yes, it is a bluish-gray color, your sight must be coming back."

What my poor old "Pop" says now that he is most anxious about is that he may have the pleasure of seeing my face some day. There is a great deal of refinement about my dear old "Pop" and I am always anxious for the hour on Saturday to come to be with him and help him. But, of course, I merely tell him that he must not hope too seriously to see my face—for it might make him blind again! Perhaps some day I will report some further progress made in restoring of this dear old man's eyesight.

[See the May 1924 issue for more on dear old "Pop."—TRQ]

News Notes of *Better Eyesight*

Leslie's Weekly of January 21 carried an article by Herewood Carrington, Ph.D., describing the methods and possibilities of the prevention and cure of imperfect eyesight without glasses. The article was written from information supplied practically entirely by Dr. Bates, and scores of thousands of persons read it.

One evening last month, members of the Discussion Club of Grantwood, New Jersey, gathered at the home of Emma Hodkinson, listened with great interest for two hours to an exposition of Dr. Bates' methods and an account of some of his cures and experiments by Dr. Bates himself. A number of Ms. Hodkinson's guests were former patients of Dr. Bates. At the conclusion of his talk, Ms. H. Kellett Chambers proposed the formation in the future of a local branch of the proposed Better Eyesight League.

Martha Smith, who is a registered nurse in Philadelphia, is a devoted servant to the cause of better eyesight. She recently wrote to the proposed Better Eyesight League, "My interest in better eyesight has led me on to the extent of having four lending copies of Dr. Bates' book, *Cure of Imperfect Sight Without Glasses,* busy all the time, and just before the February *Better Eyesight* came I had arranged to send two copies to China. One of our nurses takes one to the North of China, and the other goes to the South portion of China. Am I eligible for membership?"

Better Eyesight
April 1922—Vol. VI, No. 4

IMPROVE YOUR SIGHT

All day long use your eyes right. You have just as much time to use your eyes right as you have to use them wrong. It is easier and more comfortable to have perfect sight than to have imperfect sight.

Practice the long swing. Notice that when your eyes move the great distance rapidly, objects in front of you move in the opposite direction so rapidly that you do not see them clearly. Do not try to see them because that stops the apparent movement.

Rest your eyes continually by blinking, which means to open and close them so rapidly that one appears to see things continuously. Whenever convenient close your eyes for a few minutes and rest them. Cover them with one or both hands to shut out the light and obtain a greater rest.

When the mind is awake it is thinking of many things. One can remember things perfectly or imagine things perfectly, which is a rest to the eyes, mind and the body generally. The memory of imperfect sight should be avoided because it is a strain and lowers the vision.

Read the Snellen test card at twenty feet with each eye, separately, twice daily or more often. Imagine white spaces in letters whiter than the rest of the card. Do this alternately with the eyes closed and opened. Plan to imagine the white spaces in letters just as white, in looking at the Snellen test card, as can be accomplished with the eyes closed.

Remember one letter of the alphabet, or a part of one letter, or a period, continuously and perfectly. [Then shift to another letter, part of one letter, or another period.—TRQ]

THE LEAGUE IS FORMED

Editor's Note—*Less than six weeks after its first proposal the Better Eyesight League had begun to function. It is to regular readers of the magazine that the League extends its first urgent invitation to membership.*

The Better Eyesight League was formally organized March 8.

Some thirty former and present patients of Dr. Bates gathered in his laboratory office that day and enthusiastically adopted a constitution and by-laws bringing into existence a permanent body for the promotion of better eyesight everywhere.

Not merely was the League definitely formed, but the spirit of devotion and eagerness which called it into being, and which is destined to give constant motive power, was crystallized into unmistakable expression. The League is not merely a paper organization—it is a living, active and determined thing.

The thirty persons actually present at the formation of the League represented three times their own number. Letters and telegrams were received before the meeting from about one hundred men and women in all parts of the country, asking for enrollment as charter members of the League. Most of these letters and telegrams conveyed the same spirit, in addition to the mere formal request for enrollment.

The constitution adopted provides for a Board of Directors of nine, from which the President, Vice President, Secretary and Treasurer are chosen, and for an Executive Committee of five, comprising these four officers and one additional member of the Board of Directors appointed by the President.

The charter members present elected Rose O'Neil, the celebrated illustrator, as the first President of the League. Roberts Everett was elected Secretary, and Emily C. Lierman, Treasurer. The constitution provides for monthly meetings.

The League has already announced in a letter to its membership that "as a true missionary of better eyesight the League will soon begin a campaign of education among the schoolchildren, physicians and general public in which you, as an active member, can greatly help."

HOW WE SEE

By W. H. Bates, M.D.

In this, and its companion article, "The Illusions of Perfect Sight," Dr. Bates recounts the mysterious part that imagination plays in vision. For this, as well as for the physiological facts recited, no one interested in the bases of perfect sight should fail to read these pages.

The theories which have been advanced by numerous writers to explain how the eye sees have all been proved to be imperfect or wrong. Mathematically and according to all the laws of optics, since every object seen is focused on the retina upside down, one ought to see things upside down. Why not? If the head is tipped to one side or at various angles objects seen are still in their proper place as before. You can stand on your head and see things right side up. According to all the laws, I believe when we see things right side up we are trifling with the exact science of optics.

It tired me exceedingly to read some of the numerous explanations offered of how we see, and they seemed all wrong. When someone found in the retina a fluid which surrounded some of the cells it was described as *visual purple*. The assumption was made that a chemical change took place in the visual purple which altered its chemical composition and produced an effect on the cells of the retina. In this way the nerve of sight was stimulated or irritated and the message carried to the brain. There has been a considerable amount of argument about this visual purple and it is difficult to find two authorities who agree on the action of the visual purple.

The eyeball has been compared to a photographic camera. When one takes a picture of an object at a near point the bellows is lengthened or a stronger lens is used, but when the camera is focused to take pictures of distant objects the bellows is shortened or a weaker lens is used. Helmholtz, a great student of the eye and a scientist of worldwide fame, sharing his studies of the eye, jokingly said that the human eye is made very imperfectly and that he believed he could make a better one by artificial means.

Physical Structure of the Eye

The eye is about one inch in diameter. It has a coat in front called the *cornea,* which is a part of the outside coat called the *sclera*. Behind the front part of the eye is a cavity containing a fluid (*aqueous humor*) resembling water in its density. The colored part of the eye, called the *iris,* is a thin vertical curtain lying at the bottom of this front cavity. In the center of the iris is an opening called the *pupil* which appears an intense black. The size of the pupil varies in different conditions. Back of the iris is a firm gelatinous body called the *lens*. Back of the lens is a larger cavity filled with a dense fluid (*vitreous humor*), and then comes the retina which is connected to the brain by the nerve fibres of the optic nerve.

In order to see, it is important or necessary that the eye should be focused properly for objects at different distances. This change in the focus has been ascribed at times either to the action of the cornea or lens. Arlt advanced the theory that the change in the focus of the eye was brought about by a change in its length, as occurs with the ordinary photographic camera. Arlt later apologized for his theory because von Graefe and public opinion were too strong for him. I have proved that Arlt was mainly right while von Graefe was all wrong in this matter.

The eye with perfect sight sees many illusions. The eye with imperfect sight sees more and different illusions. I have published a list of the illusions of perfect and imperfect sight. One cannot explain these illusions by mathematics, by chemistry, or by the anatomy or structure of the eye. A blind man will tell you, if you let him, a long list of the marvels of color, forms and objects which he often sees. I cannot escape these details; I must listen. Other doctors do not have to, but I must listen in order to keep up the hope of the patient. Hope is quite essential when you start out to cure a patient with imperfect sight. The very illusions that blind people have are a benefit in the treatment. To discourage their imagination is a crime, I now firmly believe. Why? Because the imagination when properly controlled cures blindness.

The Potency of the Imagination

Too often people look on imagination too lightly, too carelessly. They do not realize the importance of the imagination when it can be used beneficially or harmfully. One reads stories of people who have been killed by the force of their imagination, by practical jokers who made them believe that they were bleeding to death with some warm water flowing down their neck, dripping into a pail. People lying in bed not expecting to recover have at times accomplished what seemed to be impossible, and with the help of their imagination recovered completely. These facts should be investigated, studied, and realized because we can explain all the phenomena of how we see by the imagination. All the illusions of perfect sight, all the illusions of imperfect sight are imagined and not seen.

The imagination may do good or it may do harm. The imagination of perfect sight is capable of curing all errors of refraction and all diseases of the eyes. A person with a cataract who is able to imagine perfect sight with his eyes closed or with his eyes open will recover and the cataract will disappear. How, where or why I do not know. All that has been written in all the books on physiological optics on how we see is full of error because so much of it is a guess or a theory. By realizing that what we see is only what we imagine is a great help in our treatment of the various diseases of the eyes, and the more thoroughly we realize the importance of the imagination the better become our results.

The Illusions of Perfect Sight

How do we see things perfectly?

When the eye with normal vision regards a letter on the Snellen test card at twenty feet it sees the point regarded best and all other points not so well. It can see the first letter of a line blacker than the second or other letters on the same line because of central fixation, which is the ability to see best where the eye is looking.

Yet this is an illusion, because all the letters of the Snellen test card are printed equally black, equally clear. The photographic camera will take a picture of the whole card with all the letters equally black.

With normal vision it can be demonstrated that the eye sees the white part of letters or the background in the neighborhood of the letters whiter than the margin of the card or whiter than it really is. This is an illusion.

We do not see illusions; we only imagine them. If we can realize that the imagination is the principal factor of how we see and prove it to the patients, the results from treatment of imperfect sight become very satisfactory.

STORIES FROM THE CLINIC

No. 26: Operations at the Clinic

By Emily C. Lierman

So many of our office patients have asked me if Dr. Bates approves of operations on the eye or if he ever operates for cataract or other conditions. Others wish to know if there is a little Christian Science or something else mixed with our method of treatment. As I do not understand or know anything about these other things, I would like our readers to know at least that Dr. Bates always does operate on the eye when it is absolutely necessary. I have been assisting Dr. Bates for almost eight years and during that time I have helped him when he operated either at his office or at the Clinic. These operations have been done without pain or discomfort to the patient.

TO A PATIENT

By Lawrence M. Stanton, M.D.

Editor's Note—*These words of instruction and encouragement have a message not only for a single patient of Dr. Stanton's, but for the very one who seeks the better vision that true knowledge gives.*

The eyes are almost a part of the brain, and vision is more closely connected with the mind than is any one of the other special senses. Anything that effects the mind, therefore, is almost certainly reflected in the eyes and if the mind is disturbed, vision is impaired.

Importance of mental control cannot be overestimated. Perhaps this state of the mind at rest is better expressed by the word composure or equanimity than by control, as the latter somewhat suggests effort. If we could but catch these fleeting moments of clear vision, so exasperating because so elusive, and trace them to their origin I think in every case it would be found that a state of mental composure would account for them.

An unperturbed mind undoubtedly makes for clarity of physical as well as of mental vision. This is no "far-off divine event," but an effect which happens immediately and which one can demonstrate many times a day.

When you look at an object, you will see it better if you don't try to see it than you will if you try to see it. The maxim, "If at first you don't succeed try, try, try again" is never true in the sense that "try" means effort, and the futility of effort is never more convincingly shown than in our attempt to see by straining to see. If we would "venture," instead of "try," we would succeed not only eventually but often "at first."

You need not trouble about your blood pressure, but take your nerve pressure as often as you can. You can gauge your mental tension by your muscular tension; and if your muscles are taut—your arms are rigid, your hands clenched—you are mentally straining. And there are no muscles that respond more quickly to our thought than do the ocular muscles.

A patient was requested to close her eyes. She literally hanged them shut, and if she had been asked to perform the most difficult task her face could not have expressed greater strain. By our multifarious environment we are being continually bombarded, and though we must ever be ready for action, unless this action springs from self-possession it is pretty sure to misfire.

Can you perfectly recall the individual letters of the diamond type card? This is very good practice for the memory and imagination. I could not remember a small letter "t" but resolved to experiment without looking at the card. Many "t's" were at first discarded for I knew they were imperfect and not like the "t" of the card. I knew that a "t" was a long letter but whether it extended above or below the short letters of the line I could not tell. I was not sure where it was crossed in relation to the other letters in the word in which I imagined it. So poor were my mental pictures that I confounded the "t" with an "f." This, however, was a step forward, as an inverted "f" closely resembles a letter "t." I continued to experiment, knowing that if I imagined the truth I would see the letter as perfectly as when looking at it on the card. Then, suddenly, there it was, shapely and black. I still remember it clearly for "the little one does learn is unforgettable, impressed upon the mind in a different way than mere learning."

When you palm do you see a perfect black? I look out into the blackness of the darkest night and then imagine it still blacker.

Experience is only suggestive. As you are different from anyone else, so are your eyes like no others. Do your own experimenting, and prize your own successes above all things.

Better Eyesight
May 1922—Vol. VI, No. 5

RELAXATION FROM FINE PRINT

A business card, 3" x 2", with fine print on one side is held in front of the eyes as near as possible, the upper part in contact with the eyebrows, the lower part resting lightly on the nose.

The patient looks directly at the fine print without trying to see. Being so close to the eyes most people realize that it is impossible to read the fine print and do not try, in this way they obtain a measure of relaxation which is sufficient to benefit the sight very much.

The patient moves the card from side to side a short distance slowly and sees the card moving, provided the movement is not too short or too slow. The shorter the movement and the slower it is, the better.

Some patients, although the card is held very close, note that the white spaces between the lines become whiter and the black letters become blacker and clearer. In some cases one or more words of the fine print will be seen in flashes or even continuously as long as no effort is made to see or to read the fine print.

This movement of the card should be kept up to obtain the best results, for many hours every day. The hand which holds the card may soon become fatigued; one may then use the hands alternately. Some patients vary this by holding the card with both hands at the same time.

The amount of light is not important.

STORIES FROM THE CLINIC
No. 27: Some Colored Patients at the Clinic
By Emily C. Lierman

One of slavery's obscure brutalities sent a patient more than half a century later to the great metropolitan Clinic where the new science of the eye is relieving scores each week. Read this little document of human pain, and human helpfulness, and realize the wealth of fine accomplishment that the ministrations of those devoted to the cause of better eyesight have before them.

We have a colored woman who does not know where she was born. The nurse was making a record of her age, name and address and then asked her where she was born.

"I don't know where I was born. How should I know? It was so long ago—anyway, it was a very hot place, that's what I know."

Her eyes do not trouble her for reading for she does not know how to read. But she complains that her eyes burn like fire and that she cannot see at a distance. Palming helps her, and the sun treatment relieves the burning of her eyes instantly.

An old-fashioned mammy, age 72, who has been coming to us for about one year is being treated for cataract in both her eyes. When she first came she was fully convinced that we could help her so that she would not need an operation. She was employed by a former patient who was cured by Dr. Bates. At first she could just make out the 70-line at ten feet with each eye. The first treatment improved her vision to 10/40. She was told to do a great deal of palming and swinging every day and now she reads 12/20.

Incidentally, I can prove that eyestrain caused her cataracts, for one day she was sufficiently relaxed to read some of the letters on the bottom line of the card, 12/10, temporarily.

Sadness Brings Its Strain

And another day she came and I knew she was in trouble of some kind. I love to talk to her because she is so clean and neatly dressed, although very poor. Her manner is so apologetic and she is extremely grateful for the benefit she receives. This day, however, I noticed her eyes were swollen from weeping. She was eager to please me and started to read the card without success. She turned toward me and said, "Mam, I cannot read. The card is all blurred. I cannot see one letter clearly." Then she began to cry softly and told me her trouble.

"Many nights I have not slept," she said, "because my son was sent to prison. He is not bad but he did get into mischief."

She loves her boy very much but she did not tell me the nature of his trouble. But, oh, how she strained and suffered for him! I wish I could have told her boy all about it. I comforted her while she palmed and reminded her that everything might be so much worse. I observed that she was under a terrible tension all the while she palmed, but after a while, as she became more calm, I saw her relax. As she again removed her hands from her eyes to read the card, she exclaimed with relief, "My, how the letters clear up! What did you do to me? I feel so much better now." I told her that she did it all herself. The poor woman had strained so much that it made her cataracts worse.

My mind was greatly relieved because her vision had cleared up. She comes with a smile now almost every Clinic day and she is eager to read 10/10 with each eye permanently and I am striving to help her do it.

Another old mammy who remembers the Civil War very well, but does not know when she was born, also suffered from cataract in both eyes. Her condition was so bad in the beginning that she could not see anything on the test card at three feet. When she was instructed to palm she looked around the room observing several patients who were also palming and then remarked, "Good Lord, Mam, this here room looks like a prayer meetin', and believe me, ah's ready to join in too."

She had the saddest looking pair of eyes I ever saw and even as she smiled she looked sad. I found out, after we got acquainted with each other, the real reason for her look of sadness. The story she told me was almost unbelievable but I will tell the readers just what she told me.

First, I would like to say that her vision improved at the first visit so that she read 12/200 and in flashes read 12/100. This amused as well as pleased her, and she would have it that palming alone did not improve her vision but that I must have done something mysterious to her while she had her eyes closed which caused this wonderful miracle. No amount of explaining to her that day would make her understand that the eyestrain which caused the cataract was lessened by palming. Every Clinic day she was there and her vision at the present time is 12/30. She has been coming to us about one year.

Now for her story.

A Tragedy of the Past

"You know, Mam, a long time ago I had a master and he was good and kind. Then came a new master and he was bad to the help. There was twenty of us in help and we did work on the plantation. After a while I was sick and was becoming weary because a li'l stranger was on the way. The sun was hot in the fields, Mam, and my back was aching powerful bad. The old master would sure have sent me to bed but the new one he just tells me to get a move on. One day when I felt so bad and hungry I falls down on my knees. I just couldn't get up. The master beat me with a lash right before the other Negroes to teach them a lesson and said I was only lazy. When my little boy was born he did have the stripes of the lash on his back the same as was on my own back. One night I ran away with my baby and this was just before the Negroes were freed by Lincoln."

She looks very old and I should judge, as does Dr. Bates, that she is about eighty years old. It is remarkable what a good memory she has.

The strain of squint, especially in children, has a great deal to do with their disobedience. I feel quite sure of that because I know of several Clinic patients who, after they were cured, became manageable and less nervous. The change was so great in their conduct both in school and in their homes that mothers and teachers would come and tell me about it.

Some time ago in one of our back numbers of *Better Eyesight* I wrote about a little colored boy named Frisco (Francisco in the September 1921 issue) who suffered from squint in one eye. His poor mother could not live with him, he was so bad. His brothers and sisters continually punished him for the terrible tricks he played on them all. He was finally taken care of by his grandmother who did the very best she knew for his welfare.

She heard of Dr. Bates and our Clinic, so she came with him for treatment. Before I had a chance to speak to him, his grandmother told me that she was afraid he was hopeless and that I might not be able to do anything with him for he was never still a minute.

She was anxious to have his eye straightened even though he was a naughty boy. I spoke to him and the only answer he gave me was "I don't want to! I won't!" I ignored his remarks and just said, "All right, you don't need to."

Strain and Behavior

His grandmother frowned and said she was so sorry he was a bad boy. I paid no attention to him for some time and fortunately there was a little girl in the room being treated for squint, so I let him watch the little girl and me. For his benefit I said to the little girl, "You don't want a bad eye, do you? You want two good eyes, don't you? Your good eye is doing all the work; just make your bad eye do some of the work and you will soon have two good eyes instead of one."

When I was ready to treat Frisco he asked with his head and shoulders straight, "Have I got a bad eye? Won't you show me how to make the bad eye do some work?"

"Why of course I will show you," I told him. As I explained in the article I wrote about him, he became a very willing patient then and with his dear grandmother's help at home, Frisco was absolutely cured in six months.

Several months after he was cured I noticed one Clinic day a colored woman standing in line smiling pleasantly and when I asked what her trouble was she answered, "Nothing at all, nurse, I just came to tell you that Frisco has returned home to his mother. He is the best behaved of all his family and he receives the highest marks from his school teacher for his studies. He shows no more symptoms of nervousness and plays no more tricks."

This squint case was so bad that one could see only the white of the left eye. Palming, swinging and alternately opening and closing his eyes many times every day cured this boy.

THE OPTICAL SWING

By W. H. Bates, M.D.

For thousands of years mankind, both lay and professional, has overlooked a seemingly minute but vitally important phenomenon of the human system—the eye's normal inability to see a stationary object. Of the result in the science of the eye of the final observation of this vital matter, Dr. Bates tells in part in this article.

In this magazine, and in other publications, I have quite frequently written about the swing. The matter is so important that I feel that it should be described and recommended more frequently. The benefits which come from the optical swing are far-reaching and of greater importance, I find at the present time, than I realized even six months or a year ago.

When a person of normal sight regards one letter of the Snellen test card with normal vision, the letter appears to move about a quarter of an inch or less from side to side, continuously and slowly, a little more rapidly than a movement each second. This is what I call the *optical swing*.

For many thousands of years people of normal sight have regarded small and large objects which were stationary and thought that they saw them stationary. It can be demonstrated that when the normal eye imagines a letter, or a part of a letter, stationary, the letter becomes very soon imperfect. Furthermore, the letter has a jerky movement, irregular, and variable, demonstrating that it is impossible by any kind of an effort to keep or imagine a letter stationary for any length of time.

Literal Concentration Impossible

With the eyes closed most persons can remember or imagine a letter "O" with a white center, as white as they like—as white as snow. They can imagine a little black period on one edge of the "O" and keep their attention fixed on the black period for a few seconds, or part of a minute. Sooner or later, however, they note that the period moves and defies all efforts to keep it stationary, and that every once in a while the period is lost altogether.

The imagination of the period fails from the strain. Most patients also note that they lose the "O" and have to bring it back again. To concentrate on one point of the letter "O" is impossible for any length of time.

The dictionary defines *concentration* as an effort to see one thing only, or to do one thing only. I have never met any person who was able to concentrate on a point for any length of time. Concentration is impossible. Trying to do the impossible is a strain; which is the main cause of imperfect sight. For we find that all persons with imperfect sight try to concentrate—try to imagine things stationary.

It is much easier and better to let the eyes shift from one point to another than to remember or imagine imperfect sight. To stare, strain or try to concentrate is an effort which is followed by not only imperfect sight, but symptoms of discomfort, pain and fatigue.

When one can imagine the letter "O" of fine print moving from side to side, it is possible to imagine that the card on which the "O" is printed is also moving from side to side, with the same speed and in the same direction; the hand which holds the card moves; the card and everything on it, including the letter "O." When the card moves and the letter "O" moves, one can imagine the hand moves, the wrist, the arm, the whole body, in short, moving with the "O." If we imagine the "O" printed on the arm of the chair, when the "O" moves the chair moves. When the chair moves the floor moves; when the floor moves one can imagine the whole room and the objects in the room in turn to be swinging. All objects seen, remembered or imagined move with the letter "O."

The Universal Swing

This I call the *universal swing,* for one letter, or one object, cannot move without the imagination of all other objects moving at the same time. When the universal swing is imagined and one object is consciously imagined to be stationary, the universal swing stops, because it is impossible to imagine one object moving and other objects stationary when they are all connected.

A great many people have told me that they could imagine the letters on the Snellen test card to be moving and the card stationary. To do this requires a strain and, when we analyze the facts, to imagine letters moving and the card stationary, it is necessary to separate the letters from the card. There are an infinite number of ways of doing it wrong, or of imagining the swing under a strain. To imagine a letter suspended and swinging, one part more than another, requires an effort or strain. Some patients have a great facility for doing things wrong, and sometimes my ingenuity is taxed to the utmost to get them back to the right way. Some cases have required many days or weeks of conversation before they became able to practice the optical swing in the normal or proper way. It is well to repeatedly call the attention of such people to the fact that the optical swing is an evidence of relaxation, a phenomenon which is always present in normal sight, and that in all cases of imperfect sight the normal optical swing is modified or lost.

The Swing and Memory

Over and over again I have taught people to demonstrate that, when they had a perfect memory of some letter or other object, they could not retain the perfect memory if they tried to imagine things stationary. Patients who were nearsighted, myopic, who were able to read fine print at a near point with good vision, were able to demonstrate that trying to imagine letters stationary made their vision at a near point very poor. By suggesting to them the possibility of imagining the swing, at a distance or when regarding the Snellen test card, as well as they could imagine the optical swing of letters at the near point, much benefit usually followed.

About a year ago a patient was brought to me, a young girl age ten years, with considerable compound myopic astigmatism. She was unable to see the large letter on the Snellen test card more than three or four feet away with either eye. This child read fine print with normal vision. She demonstrated that she could not imagine small letters stationary and see them perfectly. When she imagined a letter was moving from side to side, not any wider than the width of the letter, her vision was continuously good, or improved. With her eyes closed the memory of the letter with its swing was not quite as good as when she regarded the letter. When she looked at the Snellen test card at fifteen feet, her memory of the letter with its optical swing was gone.

I had her practice for a while looking at the small letters with fine print at a near point, imagining one at a time with a slow, short, easy swing, and then looking at the Snellen test card for a moment only—less than a fraction of a second. This practice was followed at once by improvement and she was directed to continue the practice at her home; first to regard the same letter of fine print at the near point and imagine it moving, and to do this for a minute or longer and then look at the Snellen test card for not longer than one second.

After three days the child came in and read the whole card with normal sight with each eye. I was very much surprised and I asked the mother, "How did this happen?"

Practice Brings Cure

"Oh," she said, "the child is practicing it all the time; she is practicing it at her meals, is practicing it all day long, even when she is in bed; the first thing in the morning, as soon as she opens her eyes, she gets busy."

The optical swing was a cure; not only were her eyes cured, but the mother told me that a great many functional derangements were also relieved. The mother became interested in the cure of her child and asked for treatment of her own eyes for hypermetropia, astigmatism and presbyopia. She was as enthusiastic as the child and was cured in two visits.

NOTES FROM THE LEAGUE

The first regular monthly meeting of the Better Eyesight League was held the afternoon of April 12. Mr. Ross Varney presided in the unavoidable absence of the presiding officer.

The Secretary's report showed that the names of 500 prospective members had been sent into the League by charter members since the organization meeting held March 8.

The meeting was thrown open to suggestions regarding lines of immediate activity for the League. Many phases of activity were discussed, among them work to preserve the sight of factory and shop workers, educational work for schoolchildren, educational work among college students and among teachers, and the preparation of educational and expository publicity matter.

The members present agreed to use such educational literature in their own correspondence; and measures for acquainting prospective members of the League with its purposes and with the whole subject of the new ophthalmology were discussed in detail.

The enthusiasm and interest in the work of the League that has become manifest was strikingly shown in the volunteering of a number of those present to address noon hour meetings at factories, explaining to factory workers the menace to the eyes of too close industrial application unless the new scientific measures of prevention are understood and practiced. A number of other suggestions, all *apropos* and practical, were made and discussed.

QUESTIONS AND ANSWERS

Q–1. "When the sight is perfect the memory is also perfect because the mind is perfectly relaxed." *Better Eyesight,* November 1919. I know of a Professor of Chemistry who has remarkably fine eyes and who cannot remember the roads to drive his car home from Boston to Malden.

A–1. He does not see the roads perfectly.

Q–2. Do idiots and patients having aphasia never have perfect eyesight?

A–2. Some do.

Q–3. Am I right in thinking that you consider the reverse of this true?

A–3. Yes, with exceptions.

Better Eyesight
June 1922—Vol. VI, No. 6

DISCARD YOUR GLASSES

Easy to say, something else to do.

Patients who are really anxious to be cured can discard glasses and obtain benefit almost from the start. Wearing of glasses becomes a fixed habit. The idea of going without them is a shock. The honest determination to do all that is possible to be done for a cure makes it easy or easier to discard glasses at once. Patients tell me that after they have discarded their glasses for a few days they do not feel as uncomfortable as they expected.

It is very natural that one should hesitate to discard glasses after he has worn them for many years and obtained what seems considerable benefit. It may help to read what I have published about glasses. Most of the discomforts of the eyes are largely functional or nervous and not due to any real or organic trouble with the eyes. All the symptoms of discomfort are accompanied by a strain which produces a wrong focus of the eyes called myopia, hypermetropia, astigmatism or presbyopia. Glasses may correct the wrong focus produced by the strain, but they do not always because the eyes are not always strained to fit glasses accurately. While wearing glasses in order to see, one has to strain or, by all effort, squeeze the eyeball out of shape, and it is impossible, therefore, to obtain relaxation and see with glasses.

If one can understand what I have just stated one can realize the necessity of discarding glasses in order to obtain a cure. I feel that the facts should be emphasized and the patient made to understand the necessity of discarding glasses. This makes it easier for the patient to do without glasses.

Do not argue with yourself about the matter. When you go to a doctor you expect to take his medicine even though you may not know what it is or how it is going to act. When patients come to me for relief I say, "Discard your glasses and you can be cured."

If they are wise they do as I say without any talk.

[Many natural eyesight improvement students have successfully improved their eyesight by using reduced prescription lenses. It is not essential to completely eliminate glasses. It *is* important that corrective lenses are never used except when absolutely necessary. Generally, lenses that give clear, 20/20 or sharper acuity—at any distance—are never used. See Chapters 3–5 in *Relearning to See* for more information.—TRQ]

SOME ANIMALS' EYES

The experimental detail into which Dr. Bates has gotten in his development of the new science of ophthalmology is realized by few persons, although readers of his book, The Cure of Imperfect Sight by Treatment Without Glasses, *have some appreciation of this. This article tells some of the incidents and discoveries of his long series of experiments, some significant to science, some humorous as well.*

TURTLES

The turtle has an unusual power of changing the focus of the eye. A physician who taught in a medical college told me that every year he would remove the eye of a turtle and demonstrate that stimulating the ciliary muscle with electricity produced accommodation by altering the front surface of the lens. He had been doing this for many years.

He was a good-natured person and I asked him if he would demonstrate the facts to me, which he kindly consented to do. After removing the eye of a turtle he fastened it on a piece of cork with the help of several pins. He then told me to note that when he stimulated the eye with electricity I could see the lens change its form, with the aid of a magnifying glass. I followed his instructions carefully and told him that I did not see the lens move, but I did see a considerable agitation of the iris. With the aid of the retinoscope I found that with a strong stimulation of the eye by electricity there was no change in the focus. The doctor was able to demonstrate the same thing with my retinoscope.

During all these years the commotion produced in the iris was wrongly supposed to be associated with a change in the shape of the front part of the lens. In the other eye, having demonstrated by simultaneous retinoscopy that the lens of the turtle did not produce a change in the focus of the turtle's eye, I proceeded to demonstrate that the oblique muscle was a necessary factor in accommodation. I exposed the superior oblique muscle, which is of considerable size in the eye of the turtle. When this muscle was stimulated with electricity the doctor and I both demonstrated with the aid of the retinoscope that the eye was accommodated to a high degree.

I then cut the superior oblique muscle, when I was able to demonstrate with the retinoscope that electric stimulation of the eyeball produced no change in the focusing power of the eye. The doctor agreed with me.

Then I sewed the divided ends of the oblique muscle together again. Now the electric stimulation produced the same change in the focus as in the beginning. The eye was accommodated for the near point.

The doctor confirmed my observation. He said before he left that he was convinced that when it came to turtles Helmholtz was wrong and that all these years he had been teaching an error and would in the future omit the experiment on the eyes of turtles.

Bears

One night about ten o'clock I was testing the eyes of animals in Central Park. The watchman had kindly loaned me a lantern for my use. This lantern I placed on a stone coping which surrounded a den of bears. When possible I flashed the light from the retinoscope into their eyes and found that they were normal. When I was about to leave I started to pick up the lantern and suddenly out of the dark a bear sprang forward against the rail, poked his paw between the bars and tried to grab the light. I was so startled I jumped back in great fright. The bear seemed interested and amused; he opened his mouth and if ever a bear laughed silently he did. I am sure there was nothing wrong with his sight.

Monkeys

After examining a number of monkeys, I found by simultaneous retinoscopy some who were myopic. Usually when I examined the eyes of tigers, leopards or lions I was careful to do so at a respectful distance, but the monkeys seemed so very playful and good-natured that it did not seem necessary for me to take any precautions. While I was trying, with the help of the keeper, to get a view of the eyes of an old lady sitting up on a roost, a monkey in the adjoining cage grabbed me by the hair and produced a lot of joy among his fellows at my expense. It was so unexpected and the pull so strong that I do not believe I shall ever forget the experience, although I was more frightened than hurt. The keeper laughed louder than a lion's roar.

Wolves

A great many wolves were examined by simultaneous retinoscopy and in all cases their eyes were found to be unusually good. One night a policeman stopped me and asked in a very disagreeable tone of voice what I was doing among the animals. I explained to him that I was very much interested in finding a method of preventing myopia in schoolchildren and that facts obtained from studying the eyes of animals were a great help. Well, he softened right away and was kind enough to hold the lantern for me while I made further observations.

Leopards

It seems a safe procedure to stand in front of a cage ten or twenty feet away and flash the light of a lantern into the eyes of some wild animal, but in one case a tragedy seemed imminent. The keeper was helping me all he knew how by coaxing the animals into a position that was favorable for me to examine their eyes. He went into a cage where he thought no animal was present, in order to reach another cage that contained some leopards. Suddenly there came out from a shadow into the light another leopard, and the speed with which that keeper got out of that cage was wonderful. And he was none too soon, because the door slammed shut against the very teeth of the animal. I was able to examine the eyes of this leopard while he was annoyed and found his eyes were normal.

Other Animals, and Fish

None of the members of the cat tribe which I have examined with the retinoscope was nearsighted. One of the lions had a cataract. A hippopotamus also had a cataract. Old Jewel, an elephant I examined, was nearsighted. The distance of the eyes of the elephant from the ground may be six feet or more, and I am quite sure that this elephant did not become nearsighted from straining to see near objects. I found some buffaloes nearsighted and some other animals, also. No birds were found nearsighted. At the New York Aquarium I examined many thousands of eyes of fish and found none nearsighted. The ability of fish to focus their eyes for a very near point is wonderful. The muscles found in the eyeballs of fish are very large. Electrical stimulation produces a high degree of accommodation or focusing at the near point, except in the eyes of the shark family. These fish have no superior oblique muscle; but, when I placed a suture of strong silk thread in the place occupied by the oblique muscles in other fish, electrical stimulation produced accommodation in the eyes of all the shark family.

It is interesting to report that the cat family does not focus its eyes to see nearby. Electrical stimulation always, in my experiments, has produced near focus in the cat family, but only after a silk thread was inserted in the place usually occupied by the superior oblique muscle.

STORIES FROM THE CLINIC

No. 28: The Party

By Emily C. Lierman

Editor's Note—*If there is any pleasure keener than that of giving pleasure and comfort to a child, the great teachers and philosophers of history as well as the ordinary, man and woman has never found it out. It is the great privilege of Ms. Lierman not only to be constantly advancing the knowledge of the new science of the eye, but at the same time to be giving weekly service and comfort to many of God's children.*

In the February number of *Better Eyesight* I wrote about sixteen schoolchildren who were sent to us for treatment of their eyes. Children with imperfect sight are usually sent from the schools to us to be fitted for glasses. But all of these girls wore glasses, with the exception of two. The teacher of these children wore glasses, and they were surprised when she appeared one day without them. They all wondered how she could possibly see for she had a very high degree of nearsightedness.

In my article I wrote about the children's misbehavior and the trouble we had with them at the Clinic. As they acted wild I became more determined to cure them and began to plan very quickly in my mind just what I would like to do for them if they would only behave in the Clinic room and allow me to benefit their eyes. So a house party was promised to all whose sight improved to 20/20.

Little did I think that day in February that so many of them would obtain perfect sight so soon. But Saturday, April 22, the party was held at our afternoon downtown offices in New York City.

When schoolchildren discover that they can be cured without glasses we have very little trouble treating them because they are always anxious to be cured, with a few exceptions, of course.

The Frolic of the Thirteen

We spent an hour at the Clinic before the party and when we arrived a surprise was awaiting us. Thirteen children were all arrayed in their Sunday best and two of them presented us with bouquets of roses and carnations. They came from grateful mothers and I am certain that it meant a great sacrifice to them. The coming event must have had a good effect upon their sight for twelve of them read 20/20 with each eye separately on strange cards.

Three of the sixteen were not there. One of them stayed away because she had put her glasses on again. Her teacher informed me that she did not do so well in her studies nor with her reading on the blackboard after she had put her glasses on again. I was sorry about this because when the girl took off her glasses she was immediately benefited by the treatment and soon obtained normal sight. She became more accurate in all her studies. It was a comfort to her to see better at the distance without her glasses than she ever saw with them. I was told that previously while wearing her glasses she read figures incorrectly and usually made serious mistakes. The school nurse had visited her mother and threatened to make trouble for her if the glasses were not put on the child again. This particular girl was one of the most nervous and unruly of any girl patient I ever had. She worried her school teacher because she found it hard to be truthful. During her treatment Dr. Bates and I noticed that as her vision improved, she became less nervous and her teacher said there was a marked improvement in her conduct in school. She is coming back again for treatment as her father refuses to keep glasses on her.

After Clinic was over, two taxicabs drove the children with the Doctor and myself through the East Drive of Central Park. The flowers were budding here and there and it was like a movie show to watch the children. One of them asked me if skunk cabbage grew in the park and who feeds the squirrels in the winter time. One of my little charges has never been to the country. The party was a decided success.

Right in the midst of our fun, though, two persons called for an interview with Dr. Bates. There he was, a boy all over again, playing parlor games and laughing heartily with the children as though he had not a care in the world. I allowed the visitors who came such a long distance to see him to have only five minutes of his time, otherwise it would have been a great disappointment to him to be denied the company of the children. A game of forfeits was played and when Dr. Bates was called upon to forfeit something he gave his retinoscope. It was held over the head of the kneeling child, who was the arbiter of the fate of the owner.

"What should the owner do to redeem it?" was asked, and the answer was, "The owner must go to the next room and read the Snellen test card from top to bottom without a mistake." The Doctor promptly did this, while two of the children went with him to see that it was read correctly.

QUESTIONS AND ANSWERS

Q–1. When the memory is perfect the sight is also perfect? An eminent musician in Boston has a phenomenal memory for music but is so nearsighted that without glasses he could not see to find his way.

A–1. He sees music perfectly.

Q–2. You have said that imagining sensations of feeling, tasting, smelling, etc., are as effective as seeing in perfecting the eyesight. I know of a Professor of Psychology who is an expert in the field of smell. She has a remarkable ability to imagine odors, as I have heard her testify many times. She is so nearsighted that she has to have an attendant when she walks. I don't remember any definite statement as to her visual memory, except that I remember her remarking that when she heard a name she always by some power of association saw distinctly some color. Her memory in other respects also seems far above the average. How would you account for her nearsightedness?

A–2. Strain to see.

Q–3. "The cause of this loss of function in the center of sight is mental strain and as all abnormal conditions of the eyes, organic as well as functional, are accompanied by mental strain, all such conditions must necessarily be accompanied by loss of central fixation."—*Better Eyesight,* July 1919. Why is this necessarily true if as you say in the same magazine different strain produces eccentric fixation from that strain which produces, for example, myopia.

A–3. Imperfect sight is always accompanied by loss of central fixation.

Q–4. In visualizing a black period what background should one see?

A–4. Not important.

Q–5. How would you explain by your theory this experience? A friend of mine who has farsighted astigmatism for which she is wearing glasses, when working under pressure and with considerable nervous strain has no trouble with her eyes, but upon completely relaxing during a vacation period is troubled with smarting and aching of the eyes.

A–5. Strain, not relaxed.

Better Eyesight
July 1922—Vol. VII, No. 1

"PAGE TWO"

On page two of this magazine are printed each month specific directions for improving the sight in various ways. Too many subscribers read the magazine once and then mislay it. We feel that at least page two should be kept for reference.

When the eyes are neglected the vision may fail. It is so easy to forget how to palm successfully. The long swing always helps but it has to be done right. One may under adverse conditions suffer a tension so great that the ability to remember or imagine perfectly is modified or lost and relaxation is not obtained. The long swing is always available and always brings sufficient relief to practice the short swing, central fixation, the perfect memory and imagination with perfect relief.

Be sure and review page two frequently; not only for your special benefit but also for the benefit of individuals you desire to help.

THE STORY OF VIOLET

By W. H. Bates, M.D.

Just what, in simple words, is central fixation? If you will read this story of a ten-year-old girl who discovered it for herself you will know, not in terms of theory or in scientific phrases, but in practical simplicity.

Some years ago Violet, a young girl age 10, was brought to me for the cure of imperfect sight and squint. She was wearing quite strong glasses for relief.

The right or squinting eye, even with her strong glasses, had very poor vision. The best she could see with this eye with or without glasses was counting fingers at about three feet. Looking straight ahead of her with this squinting eye, with the other eye covered, everything was visible and perfectly dark, and what she did see at any time with this eye was off to one side. She was unable to read with this eye with or without her glasses.

With her left eye her vision was improved by glasses so that she had about one-quarter of normal vision and could read large print with more or less difficulty for short periods of time. She usually had a headache every day and at times great pain in one or both eyes.

Reading or studying her lessons was a punishment. Unlike other children she had no pleasure in reading storybooks. The trouble with her eyes interfered with her play. She spent most of her time sitting alone with no desire to talk and kept her eyes closed a good deal of the time. Without her glasses she could not read at all ordinary print.

The case to me was very interesting because of the results obtained in a short time, three weeks. When the mother asked me how long it would take, I believed and told her that if the girl received any improvement in three months she would be very fortunate. In fact she was practically cured in a week, but I was so fearful of a relapse I had her come a few weeks longer to be sure she retained what she had gained.

Glasses Off

The first thing I had her do was to discard her glasses altogether. With both eyes open her vision was 10/200. When she was able to see the large letter on the card clearly or well enough to tell what the letter was, I asked her if she saw it all alike. She said "No." She told me that she noticed that when she looked at the top of the letter she saw it best and the bottom worse. When she looked at the bottom of the letter she saw the bottom of the letter best and the top worse.

"But," I said, "the top is just as black as the bottom and one side is just as black as the other side. The letter is perfectly black in all parts." "Yes, she said, "but I do not see it that way."

I told her to try it that way. She said at once the letter blurred so that she could not tell it. When I brought the letter up close, at three feet away she saw it more distinctly than at ten feet.

"Now," I said to her, "when you try to see the letter all alike what happens?" She answered, "It blurs and if I try hard enough I cannot even tell what the letter is." I said to her, "You know the letter is perfectly black and when you see one part best you are seeing something that is not so, aren't you?" "Yes," she answered." "Now, when you see something that is not so you do not really see it—you only imagine it, don't you?" She answered, "I do not see one part best, I only imagine it."

Then I pointed to the second line, first letter. "Can you imagine the top of this letter is blacker than the bottom? Make believe it is," I told her. "Oh," she said, "I can make believe it is. I can imagine the top best."

"Can you imagine the bottom best if you want to?" "Yes, I can imagine the bottom best and the top worse. What letter is it?" she answered. "A letter 'R.' Is the letter 'R' as black as the big 'C'?" "No," she answered, "it is quite gray and all blurred on the edges." "You know it isn't gray, don't you?" "Yes, I know it isn't gray but that is the way I see it," she said.

"Isn't that an illusion? When you see gray you are seeing something that isn't true, aren't you?" "Yes, when I see it gray I am seeing something that isn't true," she answered. "Now suppose you make believe that the letter 'R' is just as black as the big 'C,' which it really is. Can you do that?" "I can make believe it is, I can imagine it is, but I have to imagine one part at a time," she said.

"All right," I said, "I can forgive you for that. Keep on imagining one part is blacker than the rest." And then she screamed with delight, "Oh goody, the whole card is getting better and I can see a thousand times more then I could before."

Better Vision Quickly

In her eagerness to prove that her sight was better, almost breathlessly, she read several lines. I said to her, "Why do you stop?" She, answered, "They all turn gray." "Oh," I said, "nonsense, they didn't all turn gray. You only made believe they did. Suppose you make believe they are black all the time, not sometimes gray, and other times black, because they are not. You know those letters are continuously black." "Yes I know it but I do not always imagine or make believe they are." "Can you make believe they are." "Oh, yes I can and can read more of them," and this she did and apologized, saying that she could not read them or imagine them perfectly black unless she made believe she saw a part of the letter best.

I was very much impressed with the fact that this child had discovered for herself what I call central fixation, or the ability to see a part of a letter better than the rest of it. She found, without any suggestion on my part, that she could not read any of the letters with maximum vision unless she did see one part best. When she came to the smaller letters she hesitated and failed to see them.

"What is the trouble?" I asked. "Oh," she said, "They are so small it seems as though I ought at least to see a small letter all alike and tell what it is."

Then I called her attention to the fact that she could not tell any of those small letters when she tried to imagine the letters all alike. I brought the card closer and encouraged her to imagine one part best of the smaller letters. At a nearer point than ten feet she was able to imagine even the letters on the bottom line, one part best, and distinguish them. She was able to demonstrate that when she saw the small letters all alike that her sight was not so good. When she looked at the card at ten feet she became able, by alternating with looking at the card nearer, to see the small letters, one part best, as well as she could at a nearer point.

Real Practice

She practiced with the card at home and did what very few of my patients are able to do—she improved her sight practicing by herself. In a few days her vision with both eyes together became normal. Then I had her cover the good eye, the left, and practice in the same way with the squinting eye, which had such very poor sight. With her eyes closed she could imagine one part best of a large letter at ten feet continuously. By flashing the large letter with the squinting eye, alternately, her ability to see one part best improved, at first in flashes and later more continuously.

When she was at home her mother said the child was spending all her time with the card. She shortened the time of her meals in order to be busy with the Snellen test card for a longer time. She even brought the card to the table and practiced with it while she was eating. It was difficult to induce her to go to sleep because she wanted to practice more. She was up in the morning soon after daylight and practiced with her card while she was dressing. She very soon had her reward, for in less than a week's time she had normal vision with each eye and the squint disappeared never to return.

It was very interesting how she improved her ability to read fine print at the near point. When I asked her, "Do you see those small letters of the diamond type one part best?" she answered "Yes." "Do you see the period of the diamond type one part best?" She answered, "Yes, but when I get started I can read it so fast that I do not have time to notice that I am seeing the letters one part best."

High Mental Efficiency

This child accomplished what I have never seen anybody else do. She could read the diamond type with each eye by central fixation so close to her eyes that the page touched her eye lashes. She could read signs farther off than any person I ever knew.

With the wonderful improvement in her sight came an increased mental efficiency. Her memory was unusual. She could read perfectly a page of history and because she saw it perfectly she was able to remember it perfectly. As a consequence her scholarship became very good indeed. Formerly she was at the foot of her class; afterwards she was at the head. She astonished her teacher with the quickness of her perceptions, her ability to understand. Formerly when her sight was poor she was a very unhappy, depressed person; later she was full of life and action and seemed to enjoy life to the utmost.

One day she met one of my patients on the street. "How are you getting along?" she asked. The patient answered gloomily, "Not as well as I would like. How are you?"

"Oh, I am all right. I am cured and I am very glad and happy over it. How much do you practice and how often do you go to see the Doctor?"

"Oh, I practice once in a while, half an hour or so a day when I think of it and I call on the Doctor about once a week."

Then Violet exclaimed, "Oh how foolish, that isn't the way I did it. I wanted to get well and I wanted to get well quick and I did just exactly what the Doctor told me to do and the more I practiced the more I improved. I found it was a good thing to do what he said, so I did it. When he told me to remember a period all day long I did it. He told me to do a whole lot of other things and some of them seemed hard, difficult, but when I found I could do them they seemed easier to do and I am glad of it."

When the patient told me of the meeting with Violet he asked me why she improved so much more than he had improved. I asked him, "Did you follow my instructions as enthusiastically as Violet did? Was there any reason, any real reason why you could not do it?" "No," he answered, "There was no reason why I should not have practiced as faithfully as Violet, but my eyes are so bad that it is difficult for me to do the right thing although you repeatedly had me demonstrate that to do the wrong thing was a strain, an effort, and required hard work and made me uncomfortable. When I did the right thing it was easier and I felt more comfortable."

This patient after his meeting and talk with Violet came to the office more frequently, practiced more continuously and made surprising progress. In a few weeks he went back to his former state of mind, and did not do so well. I have always thought if he could have had Violet with him most of the time or could have seen her daily he would have done much better. Most of my patients always do better when they have someone with perfect sight to encourage them by their example or advice.

Better Eyesight Notes

No one interested in children should fail to read "The Story of Violet" in this issue. The facts of children's vision in America today are startling. In the New York City public schools the percentage of children with imperfect vision and wearing glasses is very high. It is customary in many schools for teachers to send any child with imperfect sight promptly to a doctor to be fitted with glasses. Most such cases are of recent development and can readily be cured by the new ophthalmology.

THE MEANING OF A LEAGUER

By Ross Varney
President, Better Eyesight League

It is not a mere empty gesture to become a member of the Better Eyesight League. Those who attended its last meeting, in June, need no reminder of this: it was in the very air that night that the mission of the League is something finer than mere words, and its fulfillment to be realized by the endeavors and enthusiasm of each individual member.

The Secretary's report of work, actually begun in relation to persons known to have imperfect sight, physicians, teachers, industrial plant managers and welfare workers, gave a new idea of the scope of our activities to many of those present. So, too, was Dr. Bates' incisive, well-considered message concerning general medical practitioners and the new ophthalmology, and the many-angled discussion that followed, instructive to every person there as to actual conditions and methods to pursue in bettering them.

But if this last successful meeting and the other successful ones preceding it have made one fact predominant, it is that the cause of better eyesight rests in our individual hands! We, the members of the League, have assumed the work of propagating this tremendous, this health-and-vision revolutionizing information.

The League is concerning itself today with the problem—a most serious problem—of child vision. No worthier cause could occupy the thought and time of any person. It is a problem that can be solved by education alone—by education directed by the League and made effective largely through the individual efforts of the members of the League.

Let every member realize that the League depends upon that member—now, in this matter of school education—and in every other work that may be undertaken.

STORIES FROM THE CLINIC

No. 29: How Children Have Helped Their Parents

By Emily C. Lierman

"A little child shall lead them." is sometimes true in matters of health as well as in things spiritual. More than one suffering mother has found relief through the guidance of a child, acquainted at the Clinic with the new methods of obtaining normal vision.

One day a little girl ten years old came for treatment of her eyes.

She was alone and explained that her mother was unable to come. Her name was Mary.

She complained that she had headaches, and the pain in her eyes was so bad that at times she was put to bed for a few days. Her mother told her she was to ask for glasses. The doctor in school ordered her to get them.

At first I found it hard to make her smile. Her head and eyes pained her so much that she found it hard to look pleasant. Then, too, she did not want glasses. They frightened her, she said.

I placed her in a comfortable position and showed her how to palm. After I had treated several patients, I asked Mary to remove her hands from her eyes and to look up at me. She did so and smiled. That was encouraging. Mary smiled because the palming cured her pain.

Her sight was tested and I found her vision was normal. While she was standing I taught her how to swing her body from side to side, first on one foot, then on the other. I did the swinging motion with her to be sure she was doing it right. At first she complained of dizziness which showed that she was making an effort or trying too hard. When I told her to take it easy and swing more gracefully, the dizziness left her and she became more relaxed and enjoyed it.

"I could keep this up all day," she said. "I like it because all my pain is gone." She was instructed to keep up the palming and swinging at home and to come again the next Clinic day.

The Mother Next

When Mary came again the mother was with her. The mother was anxious to know what there was about palming and swinging that could cure eyestrain. Was it a faith cure or did we perform a miracle? She said that Mary had suffered for a long time with pain in her eyes which prevented her from attending school regularly. But for the last few days Mary, after school, had played with the children in the street instead of going to bed. She had studied her homework without being told to, after palming her eyes for ten minutes or longer.

The mother was also anxious for her to know what palming had done for her. "At first my husband and I thought Mary was joking," she said. "We did not think that such a simple thing as covering the eyes with the palms of the hands could relieve pain. Ever since my children were born I have suffered with backache and my eyes have been troubling me. Mary suggested that I should try the palming also. My eyes were rested and my backache left me. Now, won't you please tell me about the swing, too?"

I went through the motions with her until she was able to do it. The last time I saw her she told me she was not half so cross with her babies since she learned how to swing her body and see things moving. Palming helped her to read in the evenings to her husband. Mary does not complain of pain anymore, she said. She is more willing to help her mother about the house and never retires until bedtime. Relief from strain, relaxation through palming, and swinging the body from side to side cured this tired mother and Mary.

Anna's Mother

Anna, a very bright girl of twelve years, unconsciously helped her mother at a very critical time, when most expectant mothers worry and suffer, most of them silently and uncomplainingly. Anna was very nearsighted and had to have treatment for a long time before her sight improved at all. Her vision a few months ago was 10/70 in both eyes. Now she reads 15/15. Anna obtained a test card to practice with at home. This interested her mother so that she herself practiced palming.

One day her mother came to the Clinic with a tiny bundle in her arms. With a smiling face she asked me to please look at her baby boy. So proud she was as she held out her arms for me to see. "I want to tell you," she said, "that palming helped me so much just before my baby was born. I thought of you and Dr. Bates at the time, and it helped me to relax. I am so glad my daughter came to you."

This made me very happy because the mother tried the palming of her own accord. Her daughter received benefit, why shouldn't she? A great deal of credit is due her because her own good judgment was all that was necessary. Dr. Bates has records of patients who were benefited greatly in this way. Some women have told him that palming and imagination of the swing, gave them great relief and freedom from pain during childbirth.

Better Eyesight
August 1922—Vol. VII, No. 2

SCHOOL NUMBER

SCHOOLCHILDREN'S EYES

The cure and prevention of imperfect sight in schoolchildren is very simple.

A Snellen test card should be placed in the classroom where all children can see it from their seats. They should read the card at least once daily with each eye separately, covering the other eye with the palms of the hands, in such a way as to avoid pressing on the eyeball. The time required is less than a minute for both eyes. The card measures the amount of their vision. They will find from time to time that their eyesight varies. Some children are very much disturbed when they cannot see so well on account of the light being dim on a dark or rainy day, and although they usually learn the letters by heart they do not always remember or see them. It is well to encourage the children to commit the letters to memory because it is a great help for them to see them. When a child can read the Snellen test card with each eye with perfect sight, even though they do know what the letters are, it has been found by numerous observations that their eyes are also normal and not nearsighted, farsighted, nor do they have astigmatism. Many children find that when they have difficulty in reading the writing on the blackboard that they obtain material help after glancing at the Snellen test card and reading it with perfect sight.

When the eye is at rest, perfect rest, it always has perfect sight. A great many teachers and others condemn the method unwisely because they say that the children learn, and because they know what the letters are, they recite them without actually seeing them. With my instrument I have observed many thousands of schoolchildren reading the Snellen test card apparently with perfect sight, the test card that they had committed to memory, and in all cases never did I find anything wrong with their eyes.

About ten years ago I challenged a doctor, a member of the Board of Education, to prove that the children deceive themselves or others by saying that they see letters when they don't. To me it is very interesting that the most troublesome child in school, no matter how he may lie about other things with great facility and gets by with it, was never caught lying about his eyesight. I believe that every family should have a Snellen test card in the home and the children encouraged to practice reading it for a few minutes or longer a number of times every day. Some children are fond of contests and quite often a child who can demonstrate that his vision was the best of any pupil in the class had a feeling of pride and satisfaction which everyone in sporting events can understand.

COLLEGE MEN FITTED FOR ARMY

By W. H. Bates, M.D.

Nothing could have emphasized the high percentage of poor vision among students as did the war. Great numbers of young men, otherwise physically perfect, were turned down when they tried to enlist because of defective vision. Dr. Bates was able to help many of these men to pass the Army tests with perfect sight.

During the war a great many young men came to me for relief of their imperfect eyesight. They had failed to pass the eye test examination at the recruiting station. At one time, if a man failed to enlist on account of his eyesight, he was drafted and had to serve in some branch of the service which did not require good vision.

Paul had just graduated from the high school when the war broke out, and found that he could not enlist because his sight was too poor. He had about 1/5 of the normal vision. He said to me, "I consider it a disgrace to fail to pass the examination for my eyes. I want to enlist in some crack regiment; I don't want to be drafted."

He was very ambitious to join the Marine Corps. He laid his heart open to me and he was very much discouraged, very sore, and willing to do anything and everything within his power to have his eyes cured without glasses. He certainly had a strong incentive to get well. He would come to the office early in the morning, half past seven or eight, practice all the forenoon, take an hour off for his lunch, return and continue doing things to help his eyesight until nine or ten o'clock at night. He certainly was very earnest about it, and he attained a very unusual improvement in his sight in a short time, and was very happy over it, and he said to me, "Now I've almost got perfect sight and can go back home and try to enlist," and he said, "do you suppose they will take me; do you think that I am able now to pass the examination?" I said to him, "You are not entirely cured, and I doubt that you will improve when practicing by yourself." Still he was eager to enlist, went back home, applied for enlistment and failed because his vision was still too imperfect.

At once he came back and said "I am going to stick it out this time until you tell me that I am cured." And, he certainly did. In a few weeks time he became able to read 20/20 with each eye on a strange card as well as on a familiar one. I said to him, "now you palm just as much as you possibly can the day before the test and at other times during the day before you are examined, and that will make it possible for you to retain all that you have gained and pass the test of good vision successfully."

He went to his home, and afterward wrote me that he did just what I told him to and read 20/20 with each eye without any difficulty. I did not hear from him again for a year or more. He wrote me a long letter about his affairs. The following are some extracts:

"I went down to Paris Island, the Marine Training Camp, and underwent a very rigid physical examination, passing the eye test without any difficulty, 20/20. After eight weeks of severe training in the hottest part of the year, I went on the rifle range, where I made a score of 251 out of a possible 300 points. I was the second highest qualified man in my company and was awarded a sharpshooter's medal."

The Twenty-one Year Old Nineteen Year Old

A young man from Texas came to me about his eyes, which were so poor that I could not understand how he ever passed the examination. "How old are you?" I asked him. Officially I am twenty-three years old, chronologically I am nineteen. You know, Doctor, you can't enter the ranks and become an officer unless you are twenty-one years old. Can't you do something for my eyesight?"

I was able to improve his sight in a very short time so that he obtained 20/20 in each eye, which became permanent. What was interesting in his case was that he went all through the war with imperfect sight, and after the war was over he came to me to be cured.

The Twins Qualify For Service

At one time there came to the office two young men of twenty-one; twins who were quite nearsighted and who complained that they could not pass the medical examination in order to enlist. Their father, a wealthy manufacturer, came with them and enlivened the occasion by loud applause whenever one of the boys by palming swinging, memory or imagination improved his sight decidedly. We had a rollicking time whenever the father was present, and I am quite sure that his outbursts were more helpful than injurious.

One of the boys read the whole card down to next to the bottom line and then stopped. "Keep going," shouted the father, "those small letters won't do you any harm; there isn't as much to see as of the big letters," and much to my surprise the boy did read the bottom line, which meant temporary normal vision.

I really missed the old man when he ceased to visit with the boys. They came to me for several weeks after their father had returned home. They both were able to pass the examination and enter the service, for which they were grateful.

More Cures

I had a college boy, whose name is Henry, come to me some years before the war started. By persistent treatment his imperfect sight was cured, and when the war broke out he wrote me a very nice letter saying that he had passed the examination and was now in active service.

I did not hear from him for some years, when one day my attention was called to an article in a magazine in which my method was attacked and criticized for curing imperfect sight without glasses. Henry published a letter in the same magazine in which he defended my method and said it was all true, that I cured people with imperfect sight by treatment without glasses.

One day he called on me, and I asked him, "How are you getting along?" "All right." "Can you read the bottom line on the familiar card?" "Oh, yes," he answered. Then I showed him a card that he had never seen before. All the letters were strange to him. "Can you read that?" I asked. "I can," and he proceeded to read the whole card, standing as far away from it as he could get, with a vision of 18/10. I asked him if he ever had any relapses and he answered, "No." "What do you do?" "Shift," he replied. It was his constant shifting of his eyes to avoid staring and the strain that prevented him from having imperfect eyesight.

The normal eye is all the time shifting, but it is done so easily, so readily, that most people do not notice that they do it.

A young man came to me from Princeton University and said that he had been told that I cured people without glasses. He thought that glasses were a great discomfort to him; that he had just as much pain, headache and imperfect sight wearing his glasses, as he had without them and he was very anxious to be cured.

I did not think he had very much money, but he paid my fee for the first examination, and told me he would call again when he had the money. He did call again about six months later, and I said to him, "How are you?" "All right." "You must have done what I told you to do, and you must have done it thoroughly and well." "Yes, I did," he said. "You do not need any more treatment; as far as I know you are cured."

The Major was a college man, and they said he was the greatest daredevil that ever piloted an airplane. His friends said that he did not know what fear was, but when he came to me, he said, "Doctor, I am worried. There are times when I am flying my machine when my vision temporarily fails, and I can't see the compass. When I am flying high among the clouds, it is difficult for me to know whether I am flying right side up or upside down. I have heard that most deaths which occur to men who pilot airplanes are due to a temporary loss of sight. Is there anything that you can do to help me?"

What I told him to do must have been of some benefit, because he never had any more attacks of blindness, and as long as he was in the Aviation Corps, he never had any serious accidents.

I told him to take a small letter, about one-quarter of an inch in diameter, and paste it on the front part of his machine in a position where he could see it all the time. Knowing what the letter was, it was very easy for him with his wonderful vision to see that letter perfectly, and when he did, he saw everything else perfectly because one cannot remember, imagine or see one thing perfectly, without remembering, imagining or seeing everything else perfectly.

STORIES FROM THE CLINIC

No. 30: Many Schoolchildren are Helped at the Clinic

By Emily C. Lierman

"A stitch in time saves nine," says an old proverb. Similarly there is no time when detective eyesight can be cured as easily and effectively as in childhood. Hundreds of pupils from the New York public schools have had their sight restored at Dr. Bates' Clinic. Children with normal vision are always brighter mentally.

Every year toward the end of June our Clinic is a very busy place. Our room is usually filled with happy children because it is promotion time. Some of them however are not fortunate enough to be promoted, and I did not notice until a few years ago that the unfortunate children always suffered more with their eyes than the ones who were promoted to a higher class. During the winter months schoolchildren come flocking in from the district schools, all sent to us to be fitted for glasses. Since last December I have had but two cases that were not cured. This happened because in both cases the school nurse visited both mothers and threatened all sorts of things if the children did not put on their glasses again. These girls give unnecessary trouble to their teachers in school and it is all due to eyestrain. What a blessing it would be if our district nurses were given the privilege of learning how to benefit patients by our method of treatment. As they go about from home to home doing their wonderful work they could benefit mothers as well as the schoolchildren.

A middle-aged woman of the Clinic who was cured of eyestrain and who is mothering two little orphans brought one of them named Ruth to us for an examination of her eyes. Ruth is a beautiful child and smiles all the time even though she is a cripple. She has large wistful eyes but acquired a bad habit of staring which caused a constant headache. Ruth soon learned to rest her eyes by just closing them often. She was taught how to blink often which is just what the normal eye does all the time. Ruth first entered school in January 1922, and at the end of six months was promoted to 2A and 2B, advance class. Fifteen out of forty-eight children were promoted. One of the fifteen was a boy named Jerry. I remarked to Ruth that Jerry must have been very proud to be the only boy bright enough to pass. "Why no," said Ruth, "Jerry was as mad as hops because the other boys were so stupid." Jerry undoubtedly did not cherish the fact that he was the only boy among fourteen girls.

Bertha Was Soon Made Happy

Bertha, age 13, was also interesting. She came to us for the first time on June 24, 1922. I asked her how she had heard of our treatment and this is what she said: "There are so many of my schoolmates and friends who were cured by you and Dr. Bates, and so I want to be cured too. I have worn glasses for ten years and now my sight is getting worse." Bertha did not need any encouragement such as most patients do. She said she knew we could cure her and would never wear her glasses again. Her trouble was divergent squint, that is, her right eye turned out. The sight in that eye was so bad that she could only see the largest letter of the test card, which is the 200-line letter at 20 feet. With her left eye she could only read the next line which is the 100-line letters. From the first visit Bertha's sight improved so much that on July 11, which was not a full month, she now has 20/20 in both eyes. Her squint is cured but when I hold my finger close to her eyes her right eye tires and turns out the least bit. She will continue to practice the treatment so that she might be cured before school opens in the fall.

Jennie Turns Doctor

Jennie, age 10, will always be remembered by Dr. Bates and me. She is the most intelligent kiddie of her age I ever saw. She has the most to say of any kiddie I know and the joke of it is that she says something when she talks. Most talkers do not impress you, they rather tire you; but not Jennie. Her left eye had caused her a great deal of suffering and pain for a long time, so she was ready to do anything to be cured. Her vision at the beginning was 10/200 in the left eye and 10/10 in the right. Now she has temporary normal vision in both eyes. While I was ill and could not attend Clinic for a few months, Jennie came in very handy. She was so small she had to stand on a stool to reach the letters on the test card with her finger tips. Dr. Bates would ask her to point to the different letters he wanted other patients to see which was a great help to patient and Doctor.

One day a boy sixteen years old appeared for an examination. He was disagreeable and sneered because he wanted to be anywhere but the Clinic. As the room was crowded with patients Jennie took it upon herself to help. She singled out this fellow and with a voice of authority said, "Now don't be afraid little boy, the letters won't hurt you." "Tell me how much you can see." At this remark the boy laughed as loud as he could and took it all as a joke. She finally convinced him that she was serious and before he left the Clinic he had normal sight. This boy had myopia and the vision in both eyes was 15/70, and when he left the room his vision had improved to 15/10 that day. He came a few times after that but he had no more trouble in retaining normal sight.

Another day Jennie demonstrated her intelligence by treating a doctor who had come from the West to learn about the treatment. Of course she did not know she was talking to a doctor, for if she had, I fear Jennie would have lost her wonderful nerve. The doctor stood where he could observe best the patient being treated. Jennie approached him gently saying, "Now, how do your eyes trouble you?" One can imagine the doctor smiling at the little girl desiring to do so much for a big man. Without returning the smile she walked to her stool, chin up in the air as though she were a princess, and as she pointed to a letter asked the doctor if he could see it. The patients roared with laughter but that did not trouble Jennie in the least. The doctor patient said "No" he could not see the letter she was pointing at, which was the 70-line. The doctor stood 15 feet away, so he had imperfect sight. She told him to palm which he did, in jest at first, but when he saw that the little girl was really trying to help him, he did as she told him. The result was that the doctor's vision improved to 15/15 just because

Jennie taught him how to rest his eyes by palming and alternately closing and opening his eyes.

EDITORIAL

One great influence for good which the League can perform is to spread news of the cure of imperfect sight without glasses among school principals and teachers. Nothing is more pitiful than to see a little child peering out from behind heavy lensed glasses. A child with bad eyesight is slow to learn and is often nervous and unruly in school. He is hampered in his play and throughout life. Members of the League should never lose an opportunity when talking to teachers to tell about Dr. Bates' wonderful work in the public schools.

QUESTIONS AND ANSWERS

Q–1. If one's arms become tired while palming, will a black silk handkerchief covering the eyes produce the same amount of relaxation one gets from palming?

A–1. No. Palming is the best method for relaxation and improvement in vision. When tired of palming, the hands can be removed and the eyes kept closed until one feels relaxed.

Q–2. Will it still be necessary to continue practicing the methods of swinging and shifting after my eyes are cured?

A–2. When you are cured of eyestrain you will not be conscious of your eyes. However, if you strain them you will know what to do to relieve the strain.

Q–3a. Can squint be cured by treatment without glasses after an operation proved unsuccessful? 3b. Does age make any difference?

A–3a. Yes, even when it is overcorrected. 3b. No, age does not make any difference.

Better Eyesight
September 1922—Vol. VII, No. 3

COMPARISONS

In practicing with the Snellen test card, when the vision is imperfect, the blackness of the letters is modified and the white spaces inside the letters are also modified. By comparing the blackness of the large letters with the blackness of the smaller ones it can be demonstrated that the larger letters are imperfectly seen. They really have more of a blur than do the smaller letters which cannot be distinguished.

When one notes the whiteness in the center of a large letter, seen indistinctly, it is usually possible to compare the whiteness seen with the remembered whiteness of something else. By alternately comparing the whiteness in the center of a letter with the memory of a better white, as the snow on the top of a mountain, the whiteness of the letter usually improves. In the same way, comparing the shade of black of a letter with the memory of a darker shade of black of some other object may be also a benefit to the black.

Most persons with myopia are able to read fine print at a near point quite perfectly. They see the blackness and whiteness of the letters much better than they are able to see the blackness of the larger letters on the Snellen test card at 15 or 20 feet. Alternately reading the fine print and regarding the Snellen test card, comparing the black and white of the small letters with the black and white of the large letters, is oftentimes very beneficial. Some cases of myopia have been cured very promptly by this method.

All persons with imperfect sight for reading are benefited by comparing the whiteness of the spaces between the lines with the memory of objects which are whiter. Many persons can remember white snow with the eyes closed whiter than the spaces between the lines. By alternately closing the eyes for a minute or longer, remembering white snow, white starch, white paint, or a white cloud in the sky with the sun shining on it, and flashing the white spaces without trying to read, many persons have materially improved their sight and been cured.

AN EDUCATOR OFFERS PROOF

Received too late for publication in the special August School Number of Better Eyesight *is the following report by Professor Husted, Superintendent of Schools of North Bergen, New Jersey, of the astounding results in the improvement of children's vision achieved through the use of Dr. Bates' methods. The report, made independently by Professor Husted to the school commissioners of his locality, is definite, irrefutable proof, from an unquestionably neutral observer, of the efficacy of those methods.*

In the schools of North Bergen, New Jersey, are some six thousand children. They are, besides being children of a typical near-metropolitan community and a part of the coming generation of our citizens, a representative living laboratory of childhood. And in that laboratory has been performed a practical test by Professor Husted, Superintendent of Schools, the results of which are stated by him in the subjoined extract from a regular report to his school commissioners.

They are of vital significance.

Professor Husted's report says:

High Spot Normal Eye Health Crusade a Successful Three Years' Experiment

Early in October 1919, under the direction of our school nurse, Marion McNamara, a Snellen test of the eyes of all of our pupils was made. A novel health experiment was begun, a campaign for "Better Eyesight." In June a second test was made in order to verify the value of progress in this phase of health work. The June test of 1920 shows marvelous, practical, successful results. Only the skepticism of principals, teachers and pupils and lack of faithfulness in carrying out its conditions prevented the wonderful results achieved from paralleling those of an Arabian Knight's story.

Eyestrain

Swift says, "Eyestrain is so frequently the cause of headaches that the more intelligent physicians now make this the starting point in their diagnosis. It may produce loss of ambition, disinclination to study and apparent dullness. It may even develop predisposition to epilepsy and insanity. The apparently organic diseases which may be caused by uncorrected ocular defects seem to cover the entire field of pathology. Eyestrain sometimes reacts upon the moral nature and may even result in a permanently perverted disposition. Children who can focus their eyes for near objects only by constant and severe effort cannot be expected to enjoy studying."

Myopia And Other Errors Of Refraction

Bates says in *Perfect Sight Without Glasses,* "You cannot see anything with perfect sight unless you have seen it before. When the eye looks at an unfamiliar object it always strains more or less to see that object, and an error of refraction is always produced. When children look at unfamiliar writing or figures on the blackboard, distant maps, diagrams, or pictures, the retinoscope always shows that they are myopic, though their vision may be under other circumstances absolutely normal. The same thing happens when adults look at unfamiliar distant objects. When the eye regards a familiar object, however, the effect is quite otherwise. Not only can it be regarded without strain, but the strain of looking later at unfamiliar objects is lessened.

This fact furnishes us with the means of overcoming the mental strain to which children are subjected by the modern educational system. It is impossible to see anything perfectly when the mind is under a strain, and if the children become able to relax when looking at familiar objects, they become able, sometimes in an incredibly brief space of time, to maintain their relaxation when looking at unfamiliar objects."

"A Snellen test card was placed permanently in the room. The children were directed to read the smallest letters they could see from their seats at least once every day, with both eyes together and with each eye separately, the other being covered with the palm of the hand in such a way as to avoid pressure on the eyeball. Those whose vision was defective were encouraged to read it more frequently, and in fact needed no encouragement to do so after they found that the practice helped them to see the blackboard, and stopped the headaches or other discomfort previously resulting from the use of their eyes.

In 1911 and 1912 the same system was introduced into some of the schools of New York City, with an attendance of about 10,000 pupils. Many of the teachers neglected to use the cards, being unable to believe that such a simple method and one so entirely at variance with previous teaching on the subject could accomplish the desired results. Others kept the cards in a closet except when they were needed for the daily eye drill, lest the children should memorize them. Thus they not only put an unnecessary burden upon themselves, but did what they could to defeat the purpose of the system, which is to give the children daily exercise in distant vision with a familiar object as the point of fixation. A considerable number, however, used the system intelligently and persistently, and in less than a year were able to present results showing that of three thousand children with imperfect sight over one thousand had obtained normal vision by its means."—Bates, "Myopia Prevention by Teachers," *New York Medical Journal*, August 30, 1913.

The following summary shows the remarkable results of the North Bergen experiment in the use of the Bates System. The first grades are omitted because of the difficulty in making accurate tests.

Grades II to VIII

Schools	No. Tested			No. Absent 2nd Test		
	1920	1921	1922	1920	1921	1922
Grant	72	100	133	0	4	19
Robert Fulton	359	498	672	11	4	122
Franklin	341	339	418	17	3	54
Lincoln	388	585	873	21	21	135
Hamilton	211	225	204	12	1	8
Jefferson	526	542	609	33	16	41
Washington	353	543	538	11	15	67
Horace Mann	335	319	446	5	19	45
McKinley	144	157	312	17	5	36
Totals	2729	3308	4205	127	88	527

Schools	No. Below 20/20 Normal Standard			No. Below Improved			% Improved		
	1920	1921	1922	1920	1921	1922	1920	1921	1922
Grant	36	31	31	30	16	19	83.3	51.6	61.3
Robert Fulton	112	127	152	76	84	56	75.2	66.1	36.8
Franklin	103	102	100	53	53	53	61.6	51.8	53.0
Lincoln	169	131	162	103	90	71	69.4	68.6	43.8
Hamilton	78	60	42	48	40	22	72.7	66.6	52.4
Jefferson	216	181	147	109	117	86	59.5	64.6	58.5
Washington	184	134	136	107	84	80	63.4	62.6	58.8
Horace Mann	96	70	100	66	42	61	72.5	60.0	61.0
McKinley	75	38	91	55	21	52	94.8	55.2	57.1
Totals	1049	874	961	647	547	500	70.1	62.5	52.0

This is a remarkable demonstration of the priceless value of this method of treatment. That 647 or 70.1% of the 922 pupils below normal, 20/20, should have been improved in eyesight in 1920, that 547 or 62.5% should have been improved in 1921, and that 500 or 52% should have been improved in 1922 is surely a marvelous showing. The record of improvement is suggestive of what a very faithful and systematic application of these health principles may accomplish. In 1920 there were 1,049 or 38% pupils out of 2,729 tested that were below 20/20 or normal standard, while in 1921 but 874 pupils or 26% out of 3,308 were found below normal, and in 1922 only 961 pupils or 23% were below standard. This cumulative improvement is credited to our health work of 1920 and 1921. This reduction from 38% to 26% and then 23% must be due to those pupils who are benefited and remain in the North Bergen system. We have enrolled 389 new pupils from other systems this year. As the percentage of pupils below standard becomes less, (38%, 26%, 23%) the percentages of improvement has become less (70.1, 62.5, 52). This suggests that many cases remaining in our schools are less amendable to treatment and should, therefore, receive persistent and systematic attention.

Not only does this work place no additional burden upon the teachers, but, by improving the eyesight, health, disposition and mentality of their pupils, it surely lightens their labors.

THREE THINGS WHICH WILL PRODUCE BETTER EYESIGHT

By W. H. Bates, M.D.

In this article Dr. Bates offers some remarkably helpful suggestions for those who are trying to improve their sight without the use of glasses. Every reader should study the ideas offered here very carefully.

There are three things which are important or necessary for the patient to practice while under treatment.

1. Stationary Objects Should Seem to Move

The most important of all is to see things moving, or rather to be conscious that stationary objects are moving, in the opposite direction to the movement of the eyes. Unless this is done continuously one is apt to imagine stationary objects are stationary which is very injurious to the eyes. When riding in a railroad train one can imagine the telegraph poles, trees, hills, the houses and the scenery moving in the opposite direction. When one drives an automobile it is important to watch the road straight ahead, and while the car is going forward the road appears to come toward the driver and he is very apt to pay little or no attention to the movement. He does not try to imagine the road is stationary, as he knows by experience that it is impossible, and the effort makes him uncomfortable. However, the passenger in the car is interested in the scenery off to one side, and in order to see things more clearly they make an effort to imagine things are stationary. For this reason alone some people suffer from headaches, nausea or other disagreeable symptoms when riding in an automobile. They complain that moving objects make them uncomfortable. It can always be demonstrated that it is not seeing things move which is uncomfortable, but rather it is trying to stop the movement which causes the discomfort. Objects that are apparently moving rapidly are not seen clearly or perfectly. They are seen better when the car is not moving. One of the first things I have my patients demonstrate is that it is impossible to keep the attention fixed on a point and imagine it stationary for any length of time, and that the effort to do so is disagreeable and lowers the memory and imagination and sight.

Many people can remember a small letter "q" and imagine the white center as white as snow, or a white cloud in the sky, or very white starch. They can also imagine a little black period on the right edge of the "o" and imagine it perfectly black for a few seconds or longer, but the longer one tries to remember or imagine, the more difficult it becomes. The eyes and the mind become tired and the period is forgotten and the letter "q" is seen for a short time, when trying to imagine the period and the "o" stationary. It is impossible to concentrate on one point continuously. The dictionary says that concentration is an effort to keep the attention fixed on a point only and not to see anything else. To concentrate on a period on the right edge of the "o" continuously is impossible, and trying to do so is a great strain. All persons with imperfect sight consciously or unconsciously are trying constantly to do the impossible—to concentrate.

To see things moving all the time, or rather to imagine the illusion that all stationary objects are moving opposite to the movement of the eyes, is a great help in curing imperfect sight. It is well for the patient to have someone to remind them at frequent intervals of the movement of stationary objects. Many persons, when they are talking to you, feel it the proper thing to keep their eyes fixed continuously on your face, that is to say, to stare at you. Instead of moving their eyes from one eye to the other or from one side of the nose to the other, they stare at one eye continuously which lowers the vision and may cause headaches or some other discomfort. It is well to get into the habit of imagining the faces of the people are moving from side to side. In many cases when one becomes able to imagine things all day long, moving with a slow, short, easy movement from side to side, the vision becomes normal. If any other treatment, like palming or flashing or use of the memory or imagination helps the sight, the patient's ability to see things moving all day long is also benefited.

2. Snellen Test Card and Fine Print

A card with letters printed on it can be used in such a way as to obtain perfect relaxation with consequent perfect sight. The Snellen test card has letters of different sizes arranged in such a way that one can measure the amount of vision of the patient, more or less perfectly. The Snellen test card, when placed in a schoolroom and read every day with each eye separately by the pupils, always improves the sight, provided the children do not wear glasses. Most children under twelve years old are cured in a very short time, a few weeks or even less, but if they wear glasses they cannot be cured unless they stop wearing them. [See my comments in the Introduction.—TRQ] In families where the parents have poor eyesight and wear glasses it often happens that the children sooner or later appear to need glasses also. However, if they read the Snellen test card every day at 20 feet with each eye, imperfect sight is always prevented.

Children who are older than twelve and all children who have worn glasses require a longer time to obtain benefit from the use of the Snellen test card. Some of these cases may require three months, six months, or even longer. When one studies the facts it seems remarkable the amount of damage that can he done to the eyes of children from wearing glasses. Only persons who are graduates of medicine should be permitted to prescribe glasses. In some cases it is well to require a knowledge of the eye and its numerous diseases. Patients come to me wearing glasses which do not improve the sight, rather lower it, who have disease of the optic nerve, or disease of the retina of very serious nature. I have seen patients, condemned to cataract, wearing glasses which did not improve their eyesight. Patients with glaucoma, a very treacherous disease, I have observed wearing glasses that they obtained from some optician or from some ignorant so-called eye specialist.

It is a mistake to believe that even though the glasses do no good they cannot do harm. Glasses keep up the strain. A person wearing glasses for myopia has to strain all the time in order to make the eyeball elongated sufficiently to fit the glasses. It can be very readily demonstrated, as I have frequently published, that under favorable conditions all persons with myopia are temporarily normal. When they try to see they strain in such a way that the eyeball becomes nearsighted. Some days they strain more than other days, and many people tell me that they notice that, with their glasses on, their vision was extremely variable. The same is true with other errors of refraction. Reading the Snellen test card twice a day or more often, after glasses are discarded, is a great help in improving the sight. If one can memorize the letters of the Snellen test card and imagine that they can see the smallest letters on the card at 15 or 20 feet, it can be demonstrated that their eyes are normal. I believe this is a discovery worth emphasizing. Always, when a patient imagines he sees or reads the letters on the Snellen test card with perfect sight the retinoscope demonstrates that the eye is normal and he is able to read the card with normal vision. I have no exceptions. One patient who had 40 diopters in myopia, when looking at a blank wall and not trying to see the retinoscope flashing the reflection of a light on to the center of sight, demonstrated that the eye was normal for longer or shorter periods, and that when the patient regards the Snellen test card, 40 diopters of myopia can be demonstrated.

While reading the Snellen test card gives great benefit to many people it should be realized or known that there are some cases who can be cured better without reading the Snellen test card. For some persons the Snellen test card is a pessimum and the vision is lowered whenever some people regard it. I have seen a great many persons with normal sight when they regarded any ordinary objects, people's faces, houses, trees, flowers, who became highly myopic with considerable astigmatism whenever they look at the Snellen test card. One such person I cured was a champion rifle shooter. When he looked at a bull's-eye his vision was unusually good but when he looked at the Snellen test card he had compound hypermetropic astigmatism with a vision of one-quarter of the normal. Glasses in such a case would have been a crime.

3. Palming

One of the three things which patients are recommended to practice for the cure of their imperfect sight is to palm at least six times daily for five minutes or longer each time. Some persons with very poor eyesight who were anxious to recover as soon as possible have palmed nine hours daily with wonderful benefit. Palming for such long periods of time requires supervision because palming, like many other things, while it is, when done properly, a great benefit, can be used wrong. Instead of the vision improving many people have lowered their vision by palming. Instead of resting their eyes they would strain and would imagine all kinds of colors. Resting the eyes by closing and covering them with the palms of the hands improves the sight of most people. Some persons have obtained a cure by palming only. When the vision is not improved by palming do not practice it until one can learn how to palm properly. Palming has cured so many people that I always recommend it very highly to all my patients.

STORIES FROM THE CLINIC
No. 31: A Sun Treatment Cure
By Emily C. Lierman

Not long ago a girl, age 17, came to have her eyes fitted for glasses. As she stood among others waiting for treatment, I watched her as she tried in vain to keep her eyes open. She made all sorts of grimaces and her mouth was distorted as she kept trying to see things about her. One of our office patients who came to see how the work was accomplished at the Clinic was standing beside me and as she observed this girl, remarked, "Isn't she disagreeable looking? Do you suppose she will let you cure her without glasses?" My visitor was surprised when I answered, "She is in pain and cannot possibly look natural." I was eager to treat this girl because I felt that it was possible to relieve her suffering. She did not return my smile and I forgave her. I could not induce her to even glance at the test card because she said the light caused so much pain in her head and eyes. Palming seemed to relieve her so that she could open her eyes more with less pain, so she was instructed to rest her eyes by palming often during the day. Two days later she appeared again and said that palming did not always help her. I decided to try the sun treatment and see if that would help. I placed her on a stool at a window where the sun shone in and told her to look down as far as possible to be sure she would not look up at the sun during the treatment. I raised her upper lid and with our sun glass I flashed the strong rays of the sun on the sclera. This only required a part of a minute and the effect was instantaneous. What a change came over her face. For the first time she smiled and showed her pearly white teeth. All she said was, "Pain is all gone, Mam." She returned again on a sunshiny day for more sun treatment but she no longer complained of pain. The first treatment had cured her. On this same day we had another patient whom I know will interest our readers.

Eye Trouble Often Due Merely to Foreign Substances

A woman who could not speak a word of English tried very hard to tell of her suffering. Her son, age 14, was with her and he repeated to me in English what she told him in Greek. Twice she had the muscles of her left eye cut in order to relieve her pain. She was discouraged the boy said, because two operations had done her no good. I examined her eye very carefully and when I turned her upper eyelid inside out, I discovered two small eyelashes growing in. This had caused all her suffering because every time she closed her eye the end of these eyelashes rubbed the cornea of her eye. Under the supervision of Dr. Bates I promptly removed the two lashes with a pair of tweezers and immediately her trouble was over. I cannot describe my pleasure and happiness when our patients show their gratitude after their sufferings are relieved. My heart overflows with thankfulness because I am able to help.

Dr. Bates told me that day about a patient who came to him who had been treated medically by other doctors for syphilis. When he did not respond to the treatment the medicine was changed and then they gave him treatment for rheumatism. The pain still continued so he called on Dr. Bates. Dr. Bates examined his eyes and found a foreign body, a cinder lodged in his cornea. This was removed and, for the first time in weeks, the poor man was relieved entirely of pain. I could go on describing such cases but I must leave room for something perhaps more important to our readers.

Better Eyesight
October 1922—Vol. VII, No. 4

PRACTICING

A great many people have asked, "How much time should one devote to practicing the methods of central fixation in order to be cured of imperfect sight without glasses?"

The answer is—ALL THE TIME.

One should secure relaxation or rest until one is perfectly comfortable and continue feeling comfortable as long as one is awake.

The feeling of relaxation or comfort can be obtained with the memory of perfect sight. Even if one cannot remember perfect sight one can imagine it. All black objects should be imagined perfectly black. All white objects observed should be imagined perfectly white. All letters observed should be imagined perfectly and everything that is seen should be imagined perfectly.

To imagine anything imperfectly requires a strain, an effort, which is difficult. Choose the easy way. Imagine things perfectly.

If you try to imagine an object as stationary you will strain and your sight become impaired. All day long the eyes are moving from one point to another. Imagine that objects are moving opposite to the movement of the eyes. If one does not notice this, one is very apt to strain and imagine things stationary.

One can practice properly for ten minutes and be comfortable. That does not mean that all the rest of the day one can strain and tear one's eyes all to pieces without paying the penalty for breaking the law. If you are under treatment for imperfect sight be sure to keep in mind all day long from the time you awake up in the morning until you go to bed at night the feeling of comfort, of rest, of relaxation, incessantly. It is a great deal better to do that than to feel under a strain and be uncomfortable all day long.

THE MINISTER

By W. H. Bates, M.D.

Editor's Note—*The case of this minister is interesting because he found out by himself that rest is a cure or a prevention for eye troubles. He reached the same truth, partly by accident, that has been demonstrated scientifically by my experiments, research and successful practice.*

His daughter came to me for treatment of imperfect sight from myopia. After she was cured she told me that she had two brothers who also wore glasses, but that her father, a minister, 65 years old, had perfect sight in each eye for distance and for reading and had never worn glasses. I was very much interested in the father. At my request he came to the office for an interview.

His vision in average sunlight was 20/10 with each eye. An ophthalmoscopic examination revealed a normal eye with no evidence of any disease whatsoever. He read diamond type at six inches or less and as far off as he could reach, about twenty-four inches or farther. I told him that his eyes were unusually good not only for the near point but also for the distance. I asked him to tell me how he had escaped glasses for reading.

"Well Doctor, when I was about 45 years old," he informed me, "I had some trouble with my eyes after a period of hard work. As my eyes are very necessary to me in my work, I felt that I could not afford to neglect them and once consulted a well-known eye specialist. When I told him my age he was very much concerned and said that I should have had reading glasses sooner in order to prevent all strain and injury to my eyes. He gave me a prescription for glasses and insisted that I use them whenever I did any reading."

Professional Common Sense

"He talked to me at great length and explained how the focus of the eye is changed from a far point to a near one by an alteration in the shape of the focusing lens of the eye, and that with advancing years the lens became harder as the bones become harder, with increased difficulty of the lens muscle to alter its shape. On account of this fact one must wear glasses to prevent strain and injury to the eye, he said.

I obtained the glasses but did not have occasion to use

them right away and found that after a few days of rest my eyes became as comfortable as they were before I consulted the specialist. I did some reading without the glasses and without discomfort. By resting my eyes frequently I became able to read for longer and longer periods of time. And so I let matters drift and I have never felt the necessity of glasses all these years. I must admit that I am very careful not to strain them and only read when they feel comfortable."

"Closing my eyes rests them and this I do quite often and I have become so expert that I can rest them by closing them for only a few seconds at a time. Momentary closure of the eyelids for a fraction of a second is beneficial to me."

I was delighted to hear him talk and told him that he had discovered and demonstrated that my methods for treating imperfect sight are correct. When I asked him to look at one letter on the bottom line, 20/10, and asked him if he could see it continuously, he said he could. Then I asked him if he could imagine it moving from side to side, a very short, slow, easy movement. It was on the tip of his tongue to say something and then he said with an air of surprise, "Why, I verily believe I do imagine it is moving, but the movement is so slow and so short and so easy that I would not have imagined it if you had not called my attention to it."

Then I said to him, "Can you stop the movement?" He looked away. I asked him, "Why did you look away?" He answered, "Because when I tried to stop the movement it gave me a pain and I lost the letter and the whole card became blurred."

He was ready to believe me when I told him that he could demonstrate that it is impossible to imagine a letter stationary and that it could be readily demonstrated that one could only remember, imagine, or see a letter which is moving.

Effect of Painful Memories

He also demonstrated that when he saw a letter, he saw always one part best and that his eyes were continually shifting from one part of a letter to another. If he tried to see the whole letter perfectly at the same time, he felt a strain and his vision became imperfect. He was one of the very few patients who was able to demonstrate that he could not see perfectly when looking straight at a letter, and that his sight was best when he looked a very short distance to each side of a letter. Staring always lowered his vision and produced pain.

He could remember a letter "O" with a white center perfectly white with a slow, short, easy swing and remember it continuously. He could remember a number of letters, which were perfect, but if he remembered or imagined a pain, his memory became quite imperfect. The memory of fatigue, the memory of a cough, a cold, rheumatism or any other disease or the symptom of any other disease, always impaired his memory and he could not remember a letter perfectly.

I told him that a perfect memory of white, black, red, green or any other color prevented pain and he believed me. I suggested to him that being a minister he would have abundant opportunities of helping people who were sick in mind or body, that all he had to do was to teach them what he already knew about sight and he would do them a great deal of good spiritually as well as mentally.

We had a very delightful hour together and I was sorry to see him go. Before he went, I asked him, "How is it that you did not do something for your daughter and your two sons instead of recommending them to me?"

He answered, "Doctor, I am not a physician; while my treatment was a benefit to me, I did not feel that the same treatment would be a benefit to other people. Of course I could not see any harm in it, but at the same time I was timid about assuming the responsibility of practicing medicine on my family."

STORIES FROM THE CLINIC

No. 32: Iritis

By Emily C. Lierman

Two more colorful bits of human interest, from the pen of Ms. Lierman. Dr. Bates' regular clinics in the Harlem hospital are attended by many incidents replete with blended humor and pathos, and Ms. Lierman is a skillful narrator of them, indeed.

A young man came to the Clinic recently suffering terrible pain in his eyes and head. He complained that he could not stand the light. He told Dr. Bates that he had been to other clinics where they told him he had iritis. Getting no relief from eyedrops which were given him by others, he came to us to see if we could help him.

Dr. Bates examined his eyes and said that the other doctors were right. He did have iritis. I did not know what the discussion was between this young man and Dr. Bates, so while the Doctor was busy with other patients, I started to treat this case of iritis without realizing that the eye was diseased. I noticed however that the eyes were inflamed.

As I do not always ask the patient what the trouble is, on account of the short time we have to treat each patient, I go right ahead and test their sight and then work as earnestly as I know how with my patient until I have relieved the pain and improved the sight. I placed the young man fifteen feet from the test card and asked him to read as much as he was able.

He complained that the electric light near the test card caused a severe pain in his eyes. So I placed him in the sun and with my sun glass, I flashed the strong rays of the sun on the white part of his eyes after I had raised his upper eyelid and had him look down. Then I again placed him fifteen feet from the test card and this time he began to read the letters without complaining about the light until he finished reading the 40-line, when he again said the pain had returned.

I taught him how to palm and left him for a half an hour. When I returned to him I was much surprised to find that the redness of his inflamed eyes had disappeared. His vision also improved to 15/10 with each eye separate. All this time Dr. Bates was busy with other patients and was paying no attention to the young man or me. I was very happy when the Doctor told me what I had accomplished.

He said, "Did you know this man had iritis?" I said, "No." Then the Doctor proceeded to tell me what was the usual experience with the treatment of iritis, that these cases required usually three or more days before the pain in the eyes and head was relieved.

In most cases it might require two weeks of treatment before the sight could become anything near normal. Always eyedrops were prescribed to be used frequently during the day, sometimes at night, and in all cases general treatment was prescribed and this treatment was usually continued in most cases for several years. To relieve a case of iritis in the short time of one hour was very wonderful and this without local treatment and without internal medicines.

"I have never in my life seen a case of iritis so bad obtain perfect sight so quickly and acquire such wonderful relief in the condition of the eye," the Doctor said.

A Colored Mammy

A good natured old mammy came to us one day, walking very slowly with the aid of a cane. Shc was all dressed up with a faded red rose in her hat, which was gray with age. Her white apron was starched so stiff that it rustled every time she moved. When I asked her what her name was she answered, "My name is Annabelle Washington Lee." I am still wondering if George Washington and General Lee attended her christening.

Poor Mammy had squint in her left eye and I could see that she was in pain. I asked what her age was and she answered, "Now I don't know, Mam, just exactly, but maybe I am fifty and maybe I am seventy. But I do know I am crossed eyed and my head has such pain I can't sleep no how."

Dr. Bates examined her eyes and told me that she had a hemorrhage of the brain and suggested that resting her eyes would be the best treatment for her. Mammy had a strong desire to talk and before I could tell her that we had so little time to talk she said, "You know, Mam, I see you twice. Yes, Mam, I see the letters twice. Funny, but you have two heads."

Then Mammy laughed. She sat quietly with both hands covering her eyes for quite a while and I began to praise her to other patients who were not so willing to palm more than a minute or two, when all of a sudden Mammy's hands dropped to her lap and we found her fast asleep. The joke was on me all right. Mammy practiced palming faithfully at home, however, and the third time she came to the Clinic Dr. Bates examined her eyes again and said that the hemorrhage must have been cured by palming or keeping her eyes closed a great deal for the retina was all clear and there seemed to be no more trouble.

Mammy's eyes are now both straight and she does not complain about seeing double anymore. The last time I saw her she said, "Mam, the world is very different since my eyes are better and I want to smile all the time." Mammy will do anything for me but read the card. I really believe her when she says, "I am plum lazy and I just don't care about reading. I gets along very well without it."

The best she was able to do for me with the test card was 12/20 with each eye while, in the beginning, her squinting eye was 12/70 and the other eye was 12/40.

The Better Eyesight League should become a more active agency in the introduction of Dr. Bates' methods among schoolchildren.

The greatest benefits from the new ophthalmology can be offered upon the world through its children. This is true because children's eyes are more immediately responsive to proper corrective efforts, and because through the children of today a greater part of the next generation can be reached than can ever be reached of the present generation, no matter how widely the new science may be known among it.

If you who read this, as a member of the League were to call upon the principal of the nearest school tomorrow or next week, and talk with him about Dr. Bates' methods and what they have accomplished and can accomplish, it is highly probable that that principal would install the Snellen test cards and introduce the new methods in the classrooms under his direction. That would mean a true science of the eye brought home to additional hundreds of children.

Won't you make such a call on the nearest school principal before the next meeting of the League?

Is it not a fact of more than merely medical significance that patients sometimes experience the first comfort of relaxed and perfect vision under Dr. Bates' treatment, through the magic of their picturing in the imagination—and with an unconscious smile upon their lips—the blue eyes of a baby a thousand miles away, or the smile of an absent wife?

THE CURE OF IMPERFECT SIGHT REVIEWED

The Journal of the Allied Medical Associations *has recently published a page review by W. Wallace Fritz, M.D., of* The Cure of Imperfect Sight by Treatment Without Glasses, *Dr. Bates' treatise on the new science of ophthalmology. This review from an important scientific and professional publication is reprinted here.*

That all imperfect sight is caused by strain, that the removal of the strain causes a return to normal vision and that all human beings should have perfect sight without the use of glasses are points maintained by Dr. W. H. Bates in his book, *The Cure of Imperfect Sight by Treatment Without Glasses.*

Dr. Bates' statements to this effect are backed by a series of conclusive experiments which have extended over a period of more than twenty years. Four years of this time were spent in re-performing the experiments of Helmholtz, the great German ophthalmologist whose work has been accepted as the basis of all eye knowledge for years.

In this experimental work Dr. Bates proves with seeming conclusiveness that the lens of the eye is not a factor in accommodation. He shows that myopia and hypermetropia—nearsightedness and farsightedness—can be produced just as readily in eyes from which the lens has been removed as they can in eyes having a lens. On the other hand, he demonstrates through another series of experiments that accommodation depends wholly upon the exterior muscles of the eyeball.

Revolutionizes Ophthalmology

So widely do the facts presented by Dr. Bates vary from the theories which have been so long accepted as authentic as to make this work perhaps the most revolutionary statement on ophthalmology published in the last fifty years.

In presenting the experiments upon which all his conclusions are based, Dr. Bates has treated his subject with a scientific thoroughness which will command the interest and respect of every physician and which perhaps only the trained eye specialist will completely comprehend. There are illuminating and detailed chapters, for instance, on "Simultaneous Retinoscopy," "The Truth About Accommodation as Demonstrated by Experiments On the Eye Muscles of Fish, Cats, Dogs, Rabbits and Other Animals," "The Variability of the Refraction of the Eye," "The Illusions of Imperfect and Normal Sight," "Presbyopia: Its Causes and Cure," "Squint and Amblyopia: Their Causes and Their Cure," etc.

But in the description of the results obtained and of the methods of correcting imperfect sight and in the report of actual cures effected, Dr. Bates has employed a style which will both interest and instruct the lay reader as well as the physician and eye expert. It would be impossible to quote at length all of the interesting incidents and facts, and the logical deductions from many of them, with which, together with some sixty illustrations, the three hundred pages of the book are replete.

Strain is Responsible

Muscular strain is the root of all imperfect sight, says Dr. Bates, and this muscular strain is in itself caused largely by mental strain. Only through complete relaxation and a complete resting of the mind can perfect vision be obtained. The efficiency of the optic nerves, as well as of all the sensory nerves, is impaired when made the subject of effort.

Central fixation, the ability to see one part of everything looked at best, is the mode of the normal eye. The loss of this ability produces eccentric fixation, a condition of every abnormal eye which causes much discomfort and often pain. Memory and imagination are two important factors in the production of perfect eyesight.

An interesting corollary of the deductions of Dr. Bates is that it is logical to account for the keenness of practical memory of the primitive man by his exceptional keenness of vision.

Upon first reading some of Dr. Bates' statements as to what can be accomplished, it may seem to the superficially minded that surely too much is being claimed. Truly, the accepted canons of ophthalmology are flouted. The story of cure after cure said to be impossible is told. But it is in this very respect that Dr. Bates' accomplishments are accounted for, since the fundamentals of his treatments and discoveries are different fundamentals than those of Helmholtz and the host of ophthalmologists of the present school.

Cures of cataract by treatment are recorded, for instance. Revolutionary results in the treatment of squint and amblyopia and of presbyopia are cited. Myopia cures are listed.

Chapter after chapter of the book make up a fascinating, engagingly yet scientifically-told account of cure after cure of what, according to prevailing standards, was hopelessly defective and inherently incurable eyesight.

Milestone in Bibliography

An important section of the book is devoted to the prevention of myopia in schools and to home treatment for children and adults. Explicit directions for the home cure or home relief of defective vision are given.

The book is a surprisingly comprehensive, lucid, coherent and fascinating resume of a new ophthalmology which does not recognize the need of artificial lenses, founded on the experiments of Ault rather than of Helmholtz, and carried further by modern methods and equipment and by personal devotion of years—plus an equally fascinating and overwhelmingly conclusive record of the accomplishments, in actual cures of defective vision, of this new science of the eye. It is undoubtedly a milestone, and a milestone marking an abrupt and complete turn in the scientific bibliography of the eyes.

QUESTIONS AND ANSWERS

Q–1. Is reading too great a strain for the eyes?

A–1. No. Reading is good for the eyes.

Q–2. Is it an injury to read in dim light?

A–2. No. It is a benefit to the eyes.

Q–3. Is it a strain to the eyes to read while riding on a train?

A–3. No, if there is no discomfort. It is a good thing to look out of the window and see the scenery moving opposite, then continue to read.

Q–4. What causes and cures abnormal watering of the eye?

A–4. Strain produces watering of the eye. Relaxation obtained by palming and swinging will cure this trouble.

Q–5. How can one, without glasses, accustom oneself to reading by electric light?

A–5. The sun treatment, as it is explained in an article written by Emily C. Lierman in "Stories from the Clinic," September 1922 issue, is beneficial to anyone troubled by strong light of any kind. Whether it is a natural sunlight or electric light, it does not matter. The sun treatment can only be applied by an expert.

Better Eyesight
November 1922—Vol. VII, No. 5

THE VARIABLE SWING

Recently I have been impressed very much by the value of the variable swing. By the variable swing is meant the ability to imagine a near object with a longer swing than a more distant object. For example, a patient came to me with conical cornea, which is usually considered incurable. I placed a chair five feet away from her eyes, clearly on a line with the Snellen test card located 15 feet distant. When she looked at the Snellen test card and imagined the letters moving an inch or less, she could imagine the chair that she was not looking at was moving quite a distance. As is well known, the shorter the swing, the better the sight. Some persons with unusually good vision have a swing so short that they do not readily recognize it. This patient was able to imagine the chair moving an inch or less and the card on the wall moving a shorter distance. She became able to imagine the chair moving a quarter of an inch and the movement of the Snellen test card at 15 feet was so short that she could not notice it. In the beginning her vision with glasses was poor and without glasses was double, and even the larger letters on the Snellen test card were very much blurred. Now, when she imagined the chair moving a quarter of an inch and the Snellen test card moving so short a distance that she could not recognize it, the conical cornea disappeared from both eyes and her vision became normal. To me it was one of the most remarkable things I have seen in years. I know of no other treatment that has ever brought about so great a benefit in so bad a case. [See "Conical Cornea" in the May 1924 issue for the complete report.—TRQ]

The variable swing is something that most people can learn how to practice at their first visit. Some people can do it better than others. The improvement depends directly upon their skill in practicing the variable swing.

MARIAN

By W. H. Bates, M.D.

This case is reported because the child on account of her enthusiasm obtained normal vision in a short time—about a week.

The patient was ten years and six months old. She was wearing glasses constantly, concave 2.25 D. S. with convex 4.00 D. C. 90 degrees in each eye. Even with her glasses her sight was imperfect for distance. At the near point she read diamond type at six inches, the closest distance from her eyes, while she could only see it two inches farther off at eight inches without her glasses. This inability to read over a greater distance was a hindrance to comfortable reading and her eyes tired. She was taught to rest her eyes by closing them and covering them with the palms of her hands. With her eyes closed and covered she was told to think of other things than her eyesight, to remember things that were pleasant for her to remember, and she learned to do this so well that she told me that everything was dark, perfectly black all the time.

I asked her to remember a letter "O" of diamond type with a white center as white as snow. "Can you imagine it moving from side to side?" I asked her. She said, "Yes, as short a movement as the width of the letter." "Can you remember that moving letter all the time?" "Yes," she answered. Then I had her remember a little black period on the edge of the "O" and asked her to keep her attention on that period all the time. She volunteered the information that she had lost the period and could not remember the "O," that when she tried to imagine a part of the "O" or the whole of it stationary her memory failed. She was able to demonstrate that it was impossible for her to concentrate on the little black period that she imagined on the right edge of the "O" during any length of time. She said it was easier for her to alternately imagine the little black period on the left side of the "O," then the right side of the "O," and when she did that she could imagine the "O" was moving and could remember or imagine it all the time that she kept up this continuous swing. I had her read the Snellen test card as well as she could, which was almost half of normal vision. At the time I was impressed with the fact that she had unusually good vision for one who had been wearing such strong glasses for myopia and astigmatism.

She complained that the smaller letters looked gray. I asked her if she could imagine the large letters moving; she said, "The letters that I can see are moving about a quarter of an inch from side to side, but the letters that I do not see appear to be stationary. She also volunteered the information that when she looked at the letters that she could see her eyes were comfortable, but when she looked at the stationary letters that she could not see, she felt a strain—an effort—which made her uncomfortable.

I called her attention to the fact that the small letters were just as black as the large letters and, as she was not color blind, she should see them both equally black. If she saw the small letters gray her imagination of the color was imperfect. Then I had her close her eyes and remember or imagine a small letter of diamond type perfectly. I asked her if she could do it easily and she replied, "Yes." "Now, can you remember the same letter imperfectly, all blurred, gray?" I asked her. She said. "Yes, but I have to make an effort and I notice that I do not remember it all the time; it gets away from me; it is easier for me to remember it perfectly." "Well," I said, "that being true, why do you go to so much trouble; why do you make such an effort; why do you make yourself so uncomfortable; why do you make it so hard to see those smaller letters imperfectly?" That seemed to her rather startling that she had to strain and make an effort to have imperfect sight and that when she remembered or saw the letters perfectly she did it easily, without any effort, without any strain. Her sight was very much improved by resting her eyes and by imagining the letters moving and by alternately closing her eyes and remembering the letters blacker than she saw them.

It was very interesting to see how much her vision improved at the first visit. She demonstrated central fixation without much trouble. When she regarded the upper right-hand corner of the large letter on the Snellen test card she could imagine that she saw it best. If she shifted to the bottom she could see the bottom best and the top worst and could demonstrate by practicing central fixation her vision was imperfect. She said it seemed to her as though the sun came out from behind a cloud and made everything clearer when she practiced central fixation. I called her attention to the white center of a large letter "O" and had her look at it about a foot from her eyes. She said that the white center looked whiter to her than the rest of the card. Then I covered over the black part of the letter with a white card with an opening that showed the center. When the black part of the letter was covered over, the center looked, she said, the same shade of white as the margin of the card. When the whole letter was exposed the center looked much whiter than the rest of the card. I said to her, "You do not see the white center of that letter 'O' whiter than the margin. It is an illusion that you imagine," and after a little talk she soon became convinced that it was true that she did not see the white center whiter than the margin; she only thought, imagined, it so. It was a great help to her in imagining or seeing smaller letters. As she said, she could not see the white center of the letter "O" on the lower lines of the small letters, but she could imagine she did, and when she succeeded, her vision was perfect not only for the letter regarded but she was able to distinguish other letters.

For several days she practiced the methods which helped her on the first day, and her vision rapidly improved. In fact, she obtained a flash of normal sight on the second day of her treatment. Later these flashes became more frequent, more continuous, until she was able to read with normal sight more continuously. I tested her with a strange card from time to time and was pleased with the results. Her memory and imagination were very unusual. When I pointed to a small letter that she could not distinguish and asked her to imagine one side straight, she said that she could imagine it straight but she could not see it. She could also imagine it curved without being conscious of seeing the letter.

Then I said to her, "Which can you do best?" Invariably if it were a round letter she would imagine the left side curved better than she could imagine it straight or open. She could imagine the top, the bottom, and the right side curved, and knowing what the four different sides were she became able to state what the letter was. In those cases in which all four sides are the same but the letters different, like the letter "B," for example, and the letter "D," both with the left side straight, top straight, bottom straight, and the right side curved, she could imagine the letter correctly. If it were "B" she could imagine it better than "D." If the letter were "D" she could imagine it better than "B," or any other letter.

I recall numerous occasions when she would read a line of letters quite rapidly and miscall one or more letters of the line, and I said to her, "You miscalled two of those letters; which were they?" and she would tell me. "How do you know," I asked her. She answered, "Because I know I miscalled those letters because I did not see them as black or as clear as the letters I read correctly. The miscalled letters were not so black and furthermore they did not have a short, slow and as easy a swing as the letters that I saw correctly."

One day she came to the office and told me that she woke up in the morning with a severe cold in her nose and after she had palmed, as she usually did before she got out of bed, the cold left her, and when she got up and dressed it was all gone. I have seen similar cases in which palming for half an hour had relieved acute cold of the eyes, nose, throat or lungs.

On another occasion she said that she was restless and could not sleep and she said to me, "I could not sleep, so I thought I might as well spend the time in palming and the next thing I knew it was morning. Palming enabled me to go to sleep very quickly."

When it came to memory I asked her what was the best thing that she could remember and the most perfectly, and she said, "A white dress with polka dots," and sure enough when she looked at the Snellen test card and remembered that white dress with polka dots her vision became very much improved.

After she had been treated for three days I said to her mother, who was wearing glasses, "Are you willing to do all that you can to help the eyes of your child?" She answered, "Certainly." "Well," I said, "I am going to ask you to do something that may be very difficult for you to do." "Oh," she said, "I don't care what it is, I will do anything." She was wearing glasses at the time, one pair to see at a distance (which she wore constantly) and another pair which she used for reading.

"Do you know that the strain that you are under is contagious; that when you wear glasses it requires a strain on your part to squeeze your eyes all out of shape to see with the glasses." She said she had never heard of such a thing before. "Anything you want me to do I will do it," she said. I said, "Take off your glasses and never put them on again." She did this without any argument. I said, "Now practice the same thing that your daughter is practicing and you will get better. She started in right at once and I told the daughter to palm and the mother palmed, and when I told the daughter to imagine the swing the mother did the same thing. Her child improved her sight by the different methods she practiced and the mother tried to keep up with the daughter. It was very interesting to watch them. The girl would say, "I saw it first," and the mother would say, "Well, next time I will see it first."

During the week they were here, each one was trying to out-do the other. The mother was cured in about the same time as the daughter. Her vision without glasses became normal and she became able to read without glasses and to read with a great deal more comfort than she ever had when she wore glasses. I am quite sure that the cure of the mother's eyes was of great benefit to the sight of her daughter.

The interesting feature of the treatment of this young girl was that her progress was continuous and she had no relapse. It was remarkable that she obtained normal sight and was able to maintain it after so short a treatment as one week. It was still more interesting to find the mother cured in as short time as was the daughter. They had to leave town and were quite willing to practice with the

Snellen test card as long as I said it was necessary. I heard from them occasionally and then they stopped writing. One day, about a year later, I was pleased to have a visit from the mother who stopped in my office to tell me that both she and her daughter had continued to have normal sight without glasses and that they had done nothing whatever the last six months to improve their sight by way of practicing. The Snellen test card was lost and they had not taken the trouble to find it. Both of them did not know that they had eyes. Both of them read many hours a day; both of them read by artificial light; both of them used their eyes for reading while riding on railroad trains and as far as they could tell and their friends could judge, both of them had eyes as good as anyone could wish. I believe the good results obtained were entirely due to the enthusiasm of them both. I wish all my patients could be cured as quickly.

STORIES FROM THE CLINIC

No. 33: Three Cases

By Emily C. Lierman

Imperfect sight is contagious. Perfect sight is also contagious. When I am treating a patient who is suffering from eyestrain, I just swing or palm occasionally—just the same as the patient does; otherwise I begin to strain unconsciously, which makes it difficult for me to benefit the patient. Not always does the patient affect me in this way because all patients are not alike. When patients are agreeable and do what I tell them to do I can improve their sight much quicker. This thrills the patient as well as it does me. The patient becomes more and more relaxed and so do I. In the Clinic where so many poor souls come for relief, not knowing what can be done for them, we find many trying cases very hard to handle. Not long ago a friend asked me what I meant by imperfect sight being contagious. I invited her to the Clinic to observe the cases as they were being treated. Among other patients was an old-fashioned woman about 60 years old who had progressive myopia. She was so nearsighted that even with her glasses on she bumped into everything in the room as she walked. Her vision with glasses on was 5/200. With them off she could not see me or the test card at 5 feet. I removed her glasses and she complained of being dizzy so I taught her how to palm. I asked her to remember her name while she had her eyes covered and she said she couldn't. I asked her if she could remember her hat or her dress and she said, "Yes, but only for a second." After that she said there were colored lights and objects which appeared to be floating spots before her eyes. I told her to remove her hands from her eyes and to look at the large letter on the top of the test card which I held six inches from her eyes. She saw it but it was blurred. I told her to open and close her eyes alternately and look at the large letter again. This time she saw the letter clearly. Then I pointed to the 100-line letter below and she could not see anything. Instead of looking directly where I was pointing she looked to one side, about eight inches or so. The poor thing was willing enough to do as she was told but she had been doing the wrong thing for so long that it was hard for me to make her do the right thing.

My friend who was sitting quite near whispered in my ear, "Now I know what you mean by imperfect sight being contagious; I feel nervous and strained watching this case. How do you stand it, anyway?" My friend has perfect sight but just to prove that I was right I looked at her with the retinoscope and found that she was nearsighted. I proved this to her by testing her sight with the test card. This frightened her but after she had palmed her eyes for a few minutes she was relieved of her eyestrain and her vision became normal. She proved this herself by reading 15/10 with the test card. The nearsighted woman has been to see us regularly and on her sixth visit to the Clinic she reads the test card 15/200 with each eye and she can also read some words of very fine print (diamond type), six inches front her eyes by moving the card slowly from side to side and alternately closing and opening her eyes.

A young woman came to me not long ago, eager to ask questions. She was from Germany only one year ago so her English was anything but perfect. She has had tear duct trouble for some time and she wanted very much to know if Dr. Bates could cure her without an operation. Now this was the conversation between us:

"Ms. Lierman: What you call that anyhow? My eyes is running all the time. The water runs on the face instead of inside. People always say to me, 'What you cry for all der time?' Maybe sometime when I cry I wouldn't have any water left. Three times in Germany I was by the doctor and he says operation. I say no. What do you call that anyway? I go by another doctor and he did want operation but is no good. He hurt me something awful but the water is running yet."

I told her that she had trouble with her tear duct and that Dr. Bates could easily cure her by palming and swinging. When the strain was relieved the tear duct trouble would cease. She was told to call for other treatment if the palming and swinging did not help her. Evidently palming and swinging has helped her for we have not seen her since.

BETTER EYESIGHT LEAGUE

The Better Eyesight League was organized for the purpose of benefiting the vision of its members. Each one was supposed to practice improving their vision every day without glasses. After their vision became normal it was expected of them that they would help one or more persons every day.

It is a well-known fact to educators that the teacher usually learns more than the pupil. The members of the Better Eyesight League are expected to do all they can for the prevention of imperfect sight.

A large field is the schools. Imperfect sight in schoolchildren is very great. The number is not becoming less, rather it is growing. The only thing that organized medicine can recommend is glasses and glasses for schoolchildren are very objectionable, just as they are objectionable to older people.

Every teacher who has practiced our method for the prevention of imperfect sight in schoolchildren has evidence that the method always improves the sight of schoolchildren, but more than that it improves their mental efficiency. Children should practice my method for the benefit of their eyesight. Not only do they see better but their memory, their imagination, their judgment are improved. It has benefited many children who were in the habit of staying out of school. It has done much for children who were mischievous or hard to control. Many stories can be told of how individuals have been relieved of headaches and pain and dislike for school by practicing with the Snellen test card or by following the directions given in the August number of each year of *Better Eyesight*. Every family with children, every family without children, should have a Snellen test card and practice reading it for the benefit and cure of imperfect sight. All persons over 40 years old have trouble with their eyes and usually require glasses for reading. The use of the Snellen test card is a cure for adults as well as children. Of course the more chronic cases and the older the patient, other things being equal, the more time is required; but I have never seen a case yet but that the use of the Snellen test card has been of benefit. One should expect to practice reading the Snellen test card for weeks, months and years, whether sight is good or bad. If the sight is good the use of the Snellen test card would improve it even more and benefit the general nervous system to a very large extent, and it acts as a preventative of imperfect sight in middle life or older. It does not take much time and the benefits that are obtained from it are so great that I cannot urge too strongly all persons in all walks of life, young and old, to read the Snellen test card once a day.

QUESTIONS AND ANSWERS

Q–1. If I improve the vision of the poor eye will there not be a confusion of images?

A–1. Not necessarily.

Q–2. Is it possible to cure a three year old child of squint without an operation?

A–2. Yes. I have had many such cases that were cured by my method of treatment.

Better Eyesight
December 1922—Vol. VII, No. 6

THE EASY SHIFT

Some time ago a man came to me for treatment of his eyes. Without glasses his vision was about one-half of the normal. This patient could not palm without suffering an agony of pain and depression. He had pain in different parts of his body as well as in his eyes, and the pain was usually very severe. The long swing, the short swing tired him exceedingly and made his sight worse. I asked him to tell me what there was that he could remember which caused him no discomfort.

He said, "Everything that I see disturbs me if I make an effort." "I try very hard not to make an effort, but the harder I try the worse do I feel."

When he could not practice palming, swinging or memory successfully I suggested to him that he look from one side of the room to the other, paying no attention to what he saw, but to remember as well as he could a room in his home. For two hours he practiced this and was able to move his eyes from one side of the room to the other without paying any attention to the things that were moving or to the things he saw. This was a rest to him and when his vision was tested, much to my surprise, he read the Snellen test card with normal vision at twenty feet. I handed him some diamond type which he read without difficulty and without his glasses.

Since that time I have had other patients who were unable to remember or imagine things without straining and they usually obtained marked benefit by practicing the *easy shift.*

No one can obtain perfect sight without constantly shifting easily, without effort. The easy shift is easy because it is done without trying to remember, to imagine or to see. As soon as one makes an effort the shift becomes difficult and no benefit is obtained.

SOME CRITICISMS FROM A PATIENT

By W. H. Bates, M.D.

Many of my patients who were benefited by my treatment have been kind enough to speak well of my methods.

Recently I treated an elderly lady who was suffering from cataract with a considerable amount of nearsightedness. The cataract was sufficiently opaque to impair her distant vision very much, but strange to say, it did not apparently interfere at all with her ability to read fine print at a near point. She was treated twice with only temporary benefit, bought my book and returned home with instructions to write to me once a week for advice. In her first letter she said:

"Relaxation is not easy if one is part of a strenuous program of living. Here are some of the items of yesterday's hours. Before breakfast, I learned of the death by suicide of an acquaintance and of the possible loss of an item of income which has been mine for years. The mail brought me two letters, one a bill for some work done for me, one-third larger than I supposed it would be, and a request from a society in which I am interested that I would write a delicate and difficult letter. Briefly, I decided to shed all responsibility about these things."

Question—"May central fixation be illustrated by the following fact? When one reads a book, she does not read it word for word, but takes sentences, paragraphs, even pages at a glance. If there appears a word in another print, or an unfamiliar word, or a misspelled word, that word leaps out, and the rest of the text is ignored for a minute. Is not this simple and common? Central fixation seems to mean to me that when I regard any detail intently, the remainder of the object is disregarded?"

Answer—The previous paragraph is full of errors. It is impossible to read a whole word, a whole sentence, a paragraph or a page at a glance. It can be demonstrated that with perfect sight one sees one part of a letter best at a time. It is all done with incredible rapidity when one reads a page of three hundred words in a few seconds. It is not simple and it never occurs for the reader to pick unfamiliar or misspelled words without seeing each part of every letter at a time best.

Question—"I find that I can do the imaginary stunts better than the real ones; for instance, I can swing the letters better with my eyes closed or when looking at a blank wall than I can when looking at the test card. I am reminded that when I was a little girl and played with my little dishes, I could get on better with nothing in my little pitcher than I could with water to be called milk. I could imagine milk in the pitcher when I accepted the task of imagining, but when I knew it was water I would not call it milk. I know the letters do not move and I feel foolish when I allow the illusion. The most that I have gained so far is the knowledge that the eye is passive and that nothing is gained by trying to see."

Comment—This last paragraph is very encouraging. Most people can do the imaginary stunts better with the eyes closed than with the eyes open. Looking at a blank wall does not disturb the memory so much as when looking at the Snellen test card. To be able to remember a black period, a piece of white starch or white snow when looking at the Snellen test card with the eyes closed is a cure. It is alright to imagine the letters are moving because this is a physiological fact when the sight is normal because it prevents staring or trying to concentrate. The dictionary defines concentration as an effort to keep the mind focused on a point. It is unfortunate that concentration is taught or recommended so universally because it is impossible to concentrate with the mind or with the eye, and the effort to do so is always associated with imperfect sight caused by nearsightedness, astigmatism, cataract, glaucoma, disease of the optic nerve, retina or choroid.

Question—"The remarkable instances of healing in Dr. Bates' book is encouraging to anybody. But what about those who found no help?"

Answer—It is a fact that when one practices closing the eyes or palming and it is done right the vision is always temporarily improved. Too many people close their eyes without resting them or practice palming with a strain which lowers the vision instead of helping it. One can practice the long swing and produce dizziness, pain and imperfect sight by straining to see things that are moving.

The people who found no help were always people who fought me for all they were worth. I remember a physician who came to me for nine months, every day, and devoted from one to two hours trying to prove that I was wrong. Finally after numerous remonstrances I suggested to him that it did not do him any good for me just to appease him every time he called, if he desired to be cured. I advised him to try and prove that I was right. In a very short time he was cured.

The people who find no help are the people who do the wrong thing against my advice.

STORIES FROM THE CLINIC

No. 34: Christmas at the Clinic

By Emily C. Lierman

We have a very peculiar case, a girl age twelve years, at the Clinic just now. For the last two years she has been coming to us off and on. She usually turns up near Christmas time. Her vision is near normal at very rare intervals, but if I say very quickly to her, "Read the card," she stares and it is pitiable to see how distorted her mouth becomes and she says she cannot see. I do not intentionally frighten her; I forget because of the many cases we have to handle in a very short time. If I speak softly and gently and point to a large letter which she remembers easily with eyes closed, she can read every letter, 12/15, perfectly after palming a few minutes.

A PERSONAL EXPERIENCE

By James D. Dillon

At the age of six years I had a bad case of granulated eyelids, which was finally overcome by treatment, but left my eyes weak and very sensitive. From that time until I began treating my eyes according to the methods of Dr. Bates—I am now thirty-six years old—I suffered much discomfort from strain and the glare of daylight. School was more or less a burden to me because of the pain caused by reading.

I have had many prescriptions for glasses at various times but have never received real relief from them. Often I would rebel and fail to wear my glasses, always finding rest and comparative relief when doing so.

Two years ago I was fitted with the most perfect lenses I have ever had, but even these failed to relieve strain and I continued to suffer from the glare of the light. I did not suffer often from headaches but from continual smarting and irritation of the eyes, and from nervous symptoms and bad temper.

In February 1922, I began to treat myself by Dr. Bates' methods. At that time I was doing hard work with figures. In spite of misgivings at leaving off my glasses, and though I was hard pressed to persevere some days when the struggle seemed worse, I did persevere and have succeeded.

The first thing in the morning and the last thing at night,

and often during the day, I would read the Snellen test card at various distances with each eye alternately, and then with both eyes together, until I could finally read the letters clear, black and distinct. I would practice looking at a pencil point held close to the nose until it became as easy to look crossed eye as to look straight ahead. I would practice accommodation exercises by looking at near objects, then at distant objects, alternately. Palming always was a great help. Regarding very small black objects and then remembering them perfectly also helped greatly. In every way I sought to break myself of the habit of straining to see and instead to see without effort. In proportion as seeing became effortless and all fear of light vanished the vision became more perfect.

In 1920, the glare of the intense sunlight gave me much misery far into the night. Now I not only receive no harm from the light but enjoy it. In fact, I never notice the glare now; it does not disturb me. I have used many more of the exercises and ideas of Dr. Bates, as described in his book, and have much more yet to learn. I find that I greatly enjoy this method of improving my vision still more. Although I can read the 10 line of letters on the card at thirty feet easily, I wish to do better. Diamond type I read easily at four inches from my eyes. I have now practically perfect vision and have overcome all the irritation and the nervousness caused by eyestrain. During this summer, though extremely hot and trying in this desert country, I have felt better and fuller of life and vim than ever before. I know that this is due to the relief from eyestrain, which had been a great drain on my vitality.

Needless to say, I am exceedingly grateful for this relief and wish to thank the author of the book a thousand times for his great work, which has made it possible for those who suffer from eyestrain to obtain real and permanent relief even though they cannot reach him personally for treatment.

BETTER EYESIGHT LEAGUE

One member told how she helped an old blind woman by teaching her how to rest her eyes by palming. The patient reported that with its aid she had become able to take a walk unattended and visit a friend. When she became confused the patient would stop and palm for a few minutes, when her sight would at once improve for a time. The palming helped her to make the crossings successfully, to find her way and to avoid pedestrians.

There was some discussion about eyestrain during sleep. Many people suffer very much from headache, imperfect sight on first rising in the morning and the symptoms may continue for several hours.

A gentleman present related his experience. He obtained much benefit by rising at 4 a. m. with the aid of an alarm clock, when he would practice the long swing until relieved. He would then retire, sleep the rest of the night and on rising find the eyestrain much less or absent altogether.

QUESTIONS AND ANSWERS

Q–1. Has Dr. Bates' method anything to do with concentration?

A–1. No, to concentrate is to make an effort. Dr. Bates' method is rest and relaxation which cannot be obtained by concentration.

Q–2. Is auto-suggestion a benefit to the eye?

A–2. Dr. Bates has tried it and found that it is not beneficial as it does not relieve the strain.

Q–3. Can hemorrhage of the retina be cured by Dr. Bates' method of treatment?

A–3. Dr. Bates has cured many such cases.

Q–4. Can one be cured of nearsightedness without being examined personally by Dr. Bates?

A–4. Yes, we have received letters from people who have cured themselves by reading Dr. Bates' book *Perfect Sight Without Glasses.*

Q–5. Can a patient while under treatment with Dr. Bates carry on his daily work just the same?

A–5. Yes, most patients continue their work just the same without the use of their glasses even though they find it difficult at the start.

Q–6. Can the vision be improved without glasses after the lens has been removed for cataract?

A–6. Yes.

Q–7. Does Dr. Bates approve of dark glasses to protect the eyes from the glare of the sun at the sea shore?

A–7. No. Dark glasses are injurious to the eyes. The strong light of the sun is beneficial to the eyes.

Q–8. When the pupils become dilated, is that an indication of eyestrain?

A–8. No. A great many people who have dilated pupils have no trouble at all with their eyes.

Q–9. What causes sties?

A–9. Infection, which is always associated with eyestrain.

Q–10. What causes night blindness?

A–10. It is caused by a form of eyestrain which is different from the eyestrain which causes imperfect sight with other symptoms.

Better Eyesight
January 1923—Vol. VII, No. 7

BREATHING

Many patients with imperfect sight are benefited by breathing. One of the best methods is to separate the teeth while keeping the lips closed, breathe deeply as though one were yawning. When done properly one can feel the air cold as it passes through the nose and down the throat. This method of breathing secures a great amount of relaxation of the nose, throat, the body generally including the eyes and ears.

A man age sixty-five had imperfect sight for distance and was unable to read fine print without the aid of strong glasses. After practicing deep breathing in the manner described he became able at once to read diamond type quite perfectly, as close as six inches from the eyes. The benefit was temporary but by repetition the improvement became more permanent.

At one time I experimented with a number of patients, first having them hold their breath and test their vision, which was usually lower when they did not breathe. They became able to demonstrate that holding their breath was a strain and caused imperfect sight, double vision, dizziness and fatigue, while the deep breathing at once gave them relief.

There is a wrong way of breathing in which when the air is drawn into the lungs the nostrils contract. This is quite conspicuous among many cases of tuberculosis.

Some teachers of physical culture while encouraging deep breathing, close their nostrils when drawing in a long breath. This is wrong because it produces a strain and imperfect sight. By consciously doing the wrong thing, one becomes better able to practice the right way and obtain relaxation and better sight.

By the habit of practicing frequent, deep breathing, one obtains a more permanent relaxation of the eyes with more constant good vision.

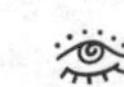

ASTIGMATISM

By W. H. Bates, M.D.

In astigmatism, the curvature of the eyeball in one principal meridian is greater than in the one at right angles to it. The eyeball is lopsided. In such an eye, rays of light are not focused. It differs from the nearsighted eye in which parallel rays of light are focused in front of the retina. In the farsighted eye, hypermetropia, parallel rays of light are focused behind the retina.

Occurrence: Astigmatism is very common and may be nearsighted astigmatism, farsighted astigmatism or it may be combined with either nearsightedness or farsightedness. Again the astigmatic eye may be farsighted in one principal meridian and nearsighted in the other. This is called mixed astigmatism. Regular astigmatism can be corrected by the use of proper glasses. Irregular astigmatism due to a malformation of the front part of the eyeball, the cornea, the lens or to the eyeball itself cannot be corrected by glasses.

In the normal eye astigmatism can always be produced by some kind of a strain. One kind of strain will produce one form of astigmatism while another kind will produce a different form. We have an instrument which measures the curvature of the front part of the eye called the ophthalmometer. With this instrument we can detect and usually measure astigmatism produced by some change in the shape of the cornea. We can observe with it the production of corneal astigmatism of varying degrees when the subject strains either unconsciously or consciously. The amount of astigmatism that can be produced by different individuals is variable. I have seen people who could consciously produce astigmatism of 3 D. By practice one can acquire the ability to consciously produce astigmatism of the cornea at different axes. This fact may explain why glasses which correct astigmatism at one time do not correct it at another time.

Many cases of normal eyes have been observed which later acquired astigmatism. In many instances patients later returned wearing glasses for the correction of astigmatism and complained that the glasses no longer suited them and when the eyes were tested no astigmatism could be found. It can be demonstrated that astigmatism may be acquired and that it may spontaneously disappear. What has been said of astigmatism caused by the malformation of the cornea is also true of the astigmatism caused by malformation of the lens or the eyeball. Many cases have been observed in which irregular astigmatism following scars on the cornea have become less or have disappeared.

Many authorities believe that most cases of astigmatism are congenital or that people are born with astigmatism. Others believe that it is usually acquired. I do not know which is correct, but I do know that whether acquired or not it can always be benefited or cured by treatment. As this always happens in my experience I believe that astigmatism is always acquired.

After the cornea or front part of the eye becomes affected with an ulcer and the ulcer heals it leaves a scar. The irregular contraction of this scar results in a malformation of various parts of the cornea. Even when the center of the cornea is clear the contraction of scar tissue at some distance away from it changes the shape of the central part of the cornea in a very irregular way. These cases of corneal opacity are usually benefited or cured by various methods employed to obtain relaxation. In general I believe that the long swing always helps and that practice of the short swing of the normal eye is usually followed by a permanent cure. In some cases of corneal astigmatism of considerable degree, 5 D or more have been cured by practice of the swing.

In the November issue of *Better Eyesight,* page two, is described the variable swing. One very remarkable case of corneal astigmatism and conical cornea with irregular astigmatism of more than 5 D was benefited in one visit by the swing and sufficiently for the patient to obtain temporary normal vision without glasses when at the beginning glasses did not succeed in obtaining normal sight. The variable swing has been a great help to many patients.

Recently a patient thirty years old, suffering from squint, nearsightedness, astigmatism in one eye, of minus 5 D with myopia and astigmatism in the other, obtained temporary normal vision with the aid of the short swing which was regulated by the feeling of the thumb and finger rubbing against each other, a quarter of an inch, from side to side. The patient obtained better vision when the body was imagined to move opposite to the direction of the moving thumb and less benefit when she imagined the body moving in the same direction as the thumb. In less than an hour she obtained normal vision for a short time. The squint became much less and at times both eyes were straight. I expect this case will obtain a permanent cure in a very short time. However, patients with a considerable amount of corneal astigmatism usually require weeks and months before they obtain a cure.

Astigmatism accompanied with a malformation of the lens is not common. Thirty years ago I treated a young girl for progressive nearsightedness. Her vision with glasses, which were very strong, concave 17 D combined with concave D. C., was only 20/100. With the ophthalmometer she had no corneal astigmatism. I removed the lens from one eye when the vision became normal, 20/20, without glasses. The case was exhibited at the Ophthalmological Section of the New York Academy of Medicine and many of the men present afterwards practiced this method of benefiting the imperfect sight of very bad cases of nearsightedness. I believe I was the first one in New York to do this operation as none of the members present recalled that anybody else had performed the same operation or published it. Many surgeons are still doing this operation for the benefit of these cases. I never did it again because my patient was not permanently benefited; the myopia or nearsightedness returned. The other eye also had 6 diopters of astigmatism with the cornea normal. For a time relaxation methods improved this eye with the astigmatism of the lens, but before she had obtained a cure she stopped treatment. I have seen other cases of astigmatism accompanied by a malformation of the lens and usually a temporary improvement in the vision can be obtained. Some of these cases have been cured. Many cataract patients have an irregular astigmatism produced by the malformation of the lens. After the cataract is cured the astigmatism disappears.

The treatment of astigmatism in my hands has been very encouraging. It is so easily produced that it seems to be just as easily relieved. It is so very common that one should realize the facts and study these cases to obtain prevention and cure. Schoolchildren acquire astigmatism very frequently and it can always be prevented by methods described in the August issue of each year of *Better Eyesight.* I am quite sure that treatment always improves or cures acquired astigmatism in schoolchildren, and that it more readily prevents it.

I cannot refrain from again repeating what I have said so often before: that the people of this country must wake up and look after the eyesight of the coming generation, and on account of the enormous number of children affected with astigmatism some radical steps should be taken for the benefit of the eyes of schoolchildren.

STORIES FROM THE CLINIC

No. 35: Staring is Bad

By Emily C. Lierman

Staring is one of the greatest evils I believe. Schoolchildren at the Clinic demonstrate it. I never make any progress in the cure of their eyes if I do not begin the treatment first, to prevent staring.

A little girl has been coming to us for a year. On her first visit, she told us that the school nurse insisted that her eyes should be examined for glasses. Her mother begged me not to put glasses on the child as she had a great dislike for them and she also believed that glasses could not possibly cure her. I was glad that I did not have to spend time convincing the mother that her little girl would not need glasses.

I tested her sight with the test card and she had 20/70 with the right and 20/100 with the left. The girl stared all the while she read the letters and I drew her mother's attention to this fact. I had instructed the child to look away in another direction after she had read one or two letters of a line; she then improved her sight with both eyes to 20/50. Her mother was a great help to me by watching very carefully when the child practiced at home. No matter what the child was doing or whenever she read a book or while studying her lessons, the mother told her not to stare. The directions for treatment at home and in school were: When she was asked to read something on the blackboard, she was not to look at the whole of a word or a sentence at once, but to look at the first letter of a word and blink her eyes, then the word would clear up and she could see the whole word without staring to see it. Then, in order to read a sentence without staring, she was to look at the first letter of the first word and then look at the last letter of the last word of the sentence; but to close her eyes frequently while doing this. How proud I was when last June she was promoted into a higher class without the aid of glasses.

I know that to the mind of our readers of *Better Eyesight* comes this thought and question. Why is she not cured by this time? It is one year now since she first came for treatment. This is my answer: The girl had normal vision with both eyes at the end of six months. Then vacation time came. Instead of our faithful patient continuing with her treatment until she could retain her normal vision, she stayed away from the Clinic and also punished her eyes in every way possible during the summer months, by straining at whatever she was doing. For the last two months she has worked with her school studies with apparently no trouble whatever, and I glory in the fact that she was never tempted to put on glasses, which I know so many of Dr. Bates' patients do, when they get discouraged and fail to get along with the treatment, without the personal instructions of the Doctor.

She was so grateful for what we accomplished that her school teacher, who had a very high degree of myopia, was encouraged through her to become a patient of Dr. Bates and is now enjoying good sight. The wonderful needle work which was done by this teacher, who by the way has become a very dear friend of mine, is most beautiful.

One of the ambulance drivers connected with the Harlem Hospital called on us not long ago. He was wearing very heavy glasses and his eyes, as they tried very hard to see, looked about the size of pinheads through his glasses. He had heard of Dr. Bates and his treatment and was eager to obtain some relief from eyestrain. Oculists told him that nothing more could possibly be done for him. His sight was gradually failing and he feared that he would soon lose his position. Dr. Bates examined his eyes and told him that he had progressive myopia, but that be could be cured if he would take the trouble.

Our room never was so crowded with patients and he had to wait some time before receiving any attention. However, while I was busy with a little boy, who enjoyed palming because it improved his sight so quickly, the ambulance driver got busy, too. Shifting and swinging also helped my little boy and he found that it was a great relief to try the different methods which helped him to relax. This interested the man very much, as the smile on his face indicated. I was very anxious to help him too and was glad when the opportunity came. He stood directly behind my little boy patient and did as well as he possibly could, just what my little patient was doing. When he first came into the room his vision was 10/200 without glasses. Before I had a chance to treat him, he had improved his sight to 10/70 all by himself. He listened while I continually repeated to the boy not to stare. When I told the boy not to look longer than a second at one letter, because if he did his sight would blur, the man followed my directions carefully, with the result that his sight improved. When I began to treat this man, he told me that he never knew he stared. He found out that when he did not close his eyes often as the normal eye does, then his vision blurred and he could not see any letter at all on the test card. I improved his sight that day to 10/40. He has not visited us again so far, but he sent in a good report, telling us that he is making steady progress improving his sight all the time.

If patients could only remember not to stare at any time, they could easily overcome their eye troubles.

A RELIEF FROM WHOOPING-COUGH

By L. L. Biddle, 2nd

My sister's children came down with the whooping-cough a little over two weeks ago. She, of course, called in for a regular physician, who said as they usually do, that it looked to him like whooping-cough and that she might as well make up her mind that they would have it for about nine weeks. I think he described it as taking three weeks to fully develop, three weeks at its most severe state and remaining three weeks to get over it. He prescribed two medicines, one of which was to give them relief when they coughed too much.

As he prophesied they continued to get worse, and the last two nights they scarcely slept at all. The youngest one, who is four, seemed to have the worse affects. He would cough for about a minute and then seem to choke or gag until finally yesterday, he spit up some blood. My sister and I got worried, however, as the medicine which the doctor prescribed to relieve the cough whenever it was at its worst, seemed to give him little relief.

Therefore, I asked Dr. Bates whether he could suggest a more satisfactory means of helping the children. He said, in his usual assuring way, "A little child about three and a half years old came to me with whooping-cough. I showed him how to palm; and every time he felt a cough coming on he would put his hands over his eyes, and by doing so lost his desire to cough."

This morning, I went into the nursery and, as usual, found them intermittently going into these terrible fits of coughing, so I explained to them as best I could how to palm. I first took the older boy, who is seven, and told him to put the palms of his hands over his eyes, making sure that he did not push the eyeballs. Then I asked him if he could imagine anything blacker and he said, "No, it is as black as anything ever saw."

I said, "As soon as you think you are going to cough put your hands over your eyes the same way again and imagine it is as dark as possible." He soon exclaimed, "I feel like coughing now." So I told him to put his hands up quickly and imagine everything was pitch black. He did so and did not cough as badly as usual. This was very encouraging, so I said, "See, that has helped you." So the next time you have the slightest idea that you want to cough, put your hands over your eyes the same way and imagine everything black." He did this and it worked magic for he did not cough at all.

The little fellow, who as I said before, is only four, had been watching very intently and as usual was trying to copy his brother, so I had little difficulty in showing him how to palm with the same results. I came back that afternoon and found the nurse in a very relieved state of mind so I asked her if she had any good news. She told me that it had worked like a charm and instead of their coughing and finally practically choking, as usual, every time either one of them felt like coughing he would put up his hands, remember something very black and prevent coughing. Moreover, the younger one became so expert that several times when he would forget to palm, the older boy would yell at him, "See black Tony, see black," and the little fellow would quickly put his hands over his eyes and the cough would stop almost instantaneously.

BETTER EYESIGHT LEAGUE

The meeting on Tuesday, December 12, was opened by the President, Mr. Varney....

An open discussion followed ... in which Mr. Varney described how he helped a friend of his. He began by asking that we, as members, should pass along our magazines and books to those who have not heard of Dr. Bates' method. He, Mr. Varney, said that an engineer friend of his had worn glasses for a number of years, and each year they had to be made stronger. This not only necessitated great trouble, but they did not improve the sight. Mr. Varney gave him his copy of *Perfect Sight Without Glasses* and explained it to his friend. The last report he had from him was that he removed his glasses (that was three months ago), and he can now do his close work without the pain and fatigue that he had while using them.

These little personal experiences pleased Dr. Bates very much, and while we were still discussing Mr. Varney's story, one lady, whose name I do not know, spoke to us in such a sincere enthusiastic way, that we could not help but catch her enthusiasm. The gist of her speech was that we all should strive with all our might to remove from the eyes of our friends, relatives, and acquaintances, the crutches that do not support, but hamper and in most cases, destroy good sight.

The thought that rankled her heart most was that now dolls are being exhibited that have miniature glasses. A woman will stroll along with a little girl, also wearing glasses, and will exclaim with ecstasies that it is the cutest thing she has seen in a blue moon, and she is going to get her little daughter just such a pair of tortoise-shelled glasses. Our speaker has discovered the fact that people are under the illusion that glasses add to one's dignity, and also look studious. This feeling is one that has to be overcome by common sense, and the application of Dr. Bates' treatment.

One of the newcomers among the members leaned forward and seemed intensely interested in all that went on. She spoke up and said that she was a teacher in Erasmus Hall High School and read the book *Perfect Sight Without Glasses,* and from it was able to lay aside her glasses, and become able to use her eyes more comfortably. Recently, she corrected more than 100 examination papers, and each time she corrected five, she palmed for a few minutes, and was benefited. After hearing the various comments from our members, she asked Dr. Bates how she could go about having the system installed in her classes. She was sure that it would promote efficiency along with better eyesight.

What really was the keynote of the meeting, though, was preserving the sight of schoolchildren. They are the innocent victims of their parents' ignorance. If we can reach them through the school authorities, it will eventually come to the notice of their parents, and in this manner it will become known, and be helpful to the present and future generation.

Better Eyesight
February 1923—Vol. VII, No. 8

THE OPTIMUM SWING

The optimum swing is the swing which gives the best results under different conditions.

Most readers of the magazine and the book know about the swing. The swing may be spontaneous, that is to say when one remembers a letter perfectly or sees a letter perfectly and continuously without any volition on the part of the patient, he is able to imagine that it has a slow, short, easy swing. The speed is about as fast as one would count orally. The width of the swing is not more than the width of the letter, and it is remembered or imagined as easily as it is possible to imagine anything without any effort whatsoever. The normal swing of normal sight brings the greatest amount of relaxation and should be imagined when one is able to succeed when it becomes the optimum swing under favorable conditions. Nearsighted persons have this normal optimum swing usually at the near point when the vision is perfect. At the distance where the vision is imperfect the optimum swing is something else. It is not spontaneous but has to be produced by a conscious movement of the eyes and head from side to side and is usually wider than the width of the letter, faster than the normal swing and not so easily produced.

When one has a headache or a pain in the eyes or in any part of the body the optimum swing is always wider and more difficult to imagine than when one has less strain of the eyes. Under unfavorable conditions the long swing is the optimum swing, but under favorable conditions when the sight is good, the normal swing of the normal eye with normal sight is the optimum swing. The long swing brings a measure of relief when done right and makes it possible to shorten it down to the normal swing of the normal eye.

EYESTRAIN WHEN SLEEPING

By W. H. Bates, M.D.

Many persons strain their eyes when sleeping. When they awake in the morning, they feel pain in their eyes with imperfect sight and often with severe headache. They may feel all tired out, not refreshed or rested by a sleep of eight hours or longer. In some cases the sleep may not have been disturbed by dreams. Dreams are not always remembered for any great length of time. There are people who can recall dreams in their early childhood twenty, thirty, forty years ago, but their recent dreams cannot be remembered longer than a few minutes or a few hours after awakening. To keep accurate records of dreams requires that they be recorded as soon as possible. Pleasant dreams do not always mean relaxation, but dreams of snakes, nightmares, fighting, crimes and horrible experiences of all sorts are usually followed by imperfect sight caused by eyestrain.

Some of my patients with a severe trouble of the eyes have told me some very awful dreams. During sleep the ticking of a clock or the outside noises in the street may be the starting point of a very exciting, disagreeable or uncomfortable dream which is due to strain.

Many patients ask, "Why do I have so much pain, discomfort, imperfect sight in the morning after a good sleep?" My answer is, "Because you strain your eyes and all the nerves of your body when you are asleep."

But for me to explain the facts further is something I cannot do. All I know is the fact that it is so. Newborn babies, half an hour after birth and later, by simultaneous retinoscopy produce a deformation of the eyeball, nearsightedness (myopia), farsightedness (hypermetropia), astigmatism of variable degree, at short intervals of a few hours. At one time, myopia will be found of the same amount in each eye; or one eye may be normal while the other eye may be myopic. At the second examination, both eyes may be normal, hypermetropic, or with any form of astigmatism. The child may produce any combination of errors of refraction by eyestrain when asleep which may persist for a longer or shorter period when awake. At times the eyes become normal when the child is awake. Squint, or strabismus, in its various forms always occurs and is also variable. The use of strong atropine, 3 1/2 percent, instilled into both eyes does not prevent the manifestations of eyestrain in newborn children when asleep.

In adults, simultaneous retinoscopy demonstrates the production of nearsightedness and other deformations of the eyeball by eyestrain during sleep but which usually become less or disappear and the eyes resume their normal shape in a few hours after awakening. Just as in babies atropine does not prevent, during sleep, the results of eyestrain.

Ether, chloroform and nitrous oxide gas are all accompanied by well-marked eyestrain during sleep produced by these agents.

Eyestrain during sleep may produce in the normal eye severe pain with hardness of the eyeball simulating the increased tension of an attack of glaucoma. In all diseases of the eyes, inflammations of the eyelids, cornea, iris, lens (cataract), retina and optic nerve eyestrain during sleep increases the severity of the symptoms with a corresponding loss of vision, temporary or more permanent. Detachment of the retina has been aggravated or produced by eyestrain during sleep.

The results of eyestrain during sleep are so disastrous that I believe proper treatment is essential.

Some patients have been benefited by palming for half an hour or longer before dropping off to sleep. "Go to sleep while palming. Palm if you wake up during the night. Practice the long or short swing before retiring," I advise.

Some people seem to sleep longer than is necessary and the eyestrain may appear increased. Some observations made of a four hour period of sleep during the night with or without a nap in the daytime seemed to show less eyestrain.

Posture during sleep has been studied. Lying on the face has generally been accompanied by an increase of eyestrain. Sleeping on the back with the arms and limbs extended with slight flexion is undoubtedly better than sleeping on the right or left side. A cramped posture is always wrong. The patient is not always conscious of his posture when asleep. In a number of cases observed by friends of the patient, one or both arms were held behind the head while asleep and strenuously denied by the patient when awake. The correction of this and other strained positions of the arms and limbs has been followed by decided benefit to the vision. Eyestrain during sleep produces or increases the symptoms of strain in various parts of the body.

Some months ago I suffered from an attack of the grippe and had a very strong cough without expectoration. This cough was spasmodic and did not bother me very much during the day, and when it did it was very easy for me to obtain sufficient relaxation to control it. But at night it was terrible, it would wake me up a few hours after I had retired and the coughing would be so severe and continuous that it was impossible for me to obtain relaxation of the eyestrain while the room was dark. I was compelled to get out of bed and light the light in order to practice the long swing which gave me relief in an incredibly short time, a few minutes or less. I would then go back to bed and sleep for a few hours or the rest of the night without being disturbed by the cough. It was interesting to me that the relief of the eyestrain was also a benefit to the bronchial or other lung tension.

For some years I had been afflicted with a chronic tuberculosis of the right elbow joint which at times caused great pain. When I became able to relax the eyestrain, to remember or imagine perfect sight, the pain in the elbow disappeared. One evening I retired as usual and slept very comfortably until one o'clock when I was awakened with an intense pain in the elbow.... I was unable to remember even my own name or any of the letters on the Snellen test card which I read every day. The doctor who was summoned gave me a hyperdermic with morphine every little while but without any appreciable relief. I kept saying, "Somebody help me to remember black," but my attendants sat around the room saying nothing and all they seemed able to do was to watch me suffer and give me morphine. This continued for four hours. During all this time I instinctively was trying to remember or imagine something that I had seen before. All of a sudden I remembered a large black "C" and the pain let up. In a few minutes I became able to remember all the letters on the Snellen test card and fell asleep. I woke up an hour later, six o'clock, apparently perfectly well without any sign of pain or soreness in the elbow. I dressed without any trouble, went downtown to the office and did a day's work without any return of the eyestrain or pain in the elbow.

STORIES FROM THE CLINIC

No. 36: Unusual Cases

By Emily C. Lierman

Not long ago a little girl, eleven years old, came to us for treatment. The school nurse was puzzled about the condition of the child's eyes and feared that the little one would be hopelessly blind within a very short time.

After Dr. Bates had examined her he said her trouble was interstitial keratitis caused by syphilis. At first, I could not do anything with her. She would not look at the test card when I asked her to, neither would she look at me. I was not annoyed at her for this because I knew that the poor child was suffering. I tried speaking softly and kindly to her and it worked like a charm. She obeyed when I told her to keep her eyes closed for a little while. Closing her eyes and resting them helped. Her eyes were a little more clear after resting them and she read 10/70 with both eyes. I told her to again close her eyes to prevent staring, and while her eyes were closed, to remember the last letter she had read on the card. The last letter of the 70-line on the Clinic test card is an "E" and when she tried to remember the whole of the letter she said her eyes began to pain her. So I told her to remember one part of the "E" at a time. This she liked to do because it was easier than to remember all of the letter at one time. I stood close to the test card pointing to the letter below the "E" and when I told her to open her eyes again she saw the letter right off. This was the 50-line. I was sorry that I had to send her home at that moment. I wished to treat her for at least a half-hour longer but others were waiting and I had so little time. She was advised to practice palming and resting her eyes regularly six times a day and to return in two days for further treatment. Her first visit began two weeks before Christmas, so each time she was treated I mentioned the possibilities of a gift for her if she would do her best, in practicing at home and doing what she could do for me at the Clinic. She is progressing very rapidly much to the surprise of Dr. Bates. He informed me that her case was so bad that he did not expect much improvement for a month or more. At the present time she reads 15/30 and her eyes look much clearer. I notice, also, that she no longer keeps her head down and she does not complain that the strong light hurts her eyes as they did before her treatments began. It is not at all easy to treat this poor little girl, because she sulks and I spend at least five minutes sometimes trying to encourage her and to make her understand that working with her eyes, while it is hard work, it is surely worth the trouble.

One day a doctor, who was a stranger both to me and to Dr. Bates, came to our room and carefully watched us as we encouraged and benefited each case. The only remark he made to me was, "Why don't you fit them with glasses and be done with it. You can get rid of these poor individuals so much quicker. They don't pay anything, so why waste your time." I was so upset when he said this, that I lost my temper.

I am anxious to tell about a mother who came a few days ago with her two children. Dr. Bates told her to wait for me and when I was ready, I would test the children's eyes. The children were sent home from school because they could not see the letters on the blackboard. The mother thought of Dr. Bates immediately so she brought her boy and girl to be treated without glasses. The trouble in both cases was eyestrain and the girl's vision improved from 15/50 to 15/15 with each eye separately by palming or just closing her eyes often to rest them. Her eyes are perfectly straight and the mother boasted about how she was cured. Dr. Bates had prescribed atropine drops to be applied every day and then to have the little girl look at distant objects as well as near objects, such as tall trees and flowers and other things. The mother would go to the park every day and have the child practice these things with each eye separately. The little boy was difficult to handle at first because he did not wish to be bothered. A perfectly normal boy would rather play ball or play a game than to sit still and fuss with his eyes. I could not win him over until I pretended to box with him. He was ready to be a prize fighter anytime he said. He very soon got tired of the game and willingly read the test card. After the test, his vision was 15/50 and after he had rested his eyes by palming his sight improved to 15/20 with the right eye and 15/30 with the left. If they obey their mother and practice at home every day, I feel sure that my two little patients will soon have normal sight.

BETTER EYESIGHT LEAGUE

By Emily A. Meder

We had a most interesting and exciting meeting in January. All formality is thrown aside when we meet, and there was a general discussion. So was the case at the January gathering. In these discussions various things relative to the League are threshed out, and the members tell what they have done during the month to promote better eyesight.

Ms. Shepard cited an experience with a friend of hers. She took this friend in hand herself, and from what she knows of Dr. Bates' treatment, being a patient herself, she proceeded to treat her friend. After removing her glasses, she could only read 10/40. She was given explicit instructions to practice palming for twenty minutes each day, and at the end of a month she could read the whole card. The pain in back of her eyes had disappeared entirely.

Ms. Shepard is one of the most energetic of our members. She does not stop at helping her friends, but tells about Dr. Bates to all her acquaintances. She introduced the method into one of the Public Schools in Orange. She will go in February to test the children's eyes, and we hope to have an interesting report in February.

Dr. Clara C. Ingham, who also practices by Dr. Bates' method, is going back to Oregon. She will have access to the orphanage, and expects to start the system there free of charge. Dr. Ingham is a true member of the League. She not only gives her time, but her valuable experience in curing defective eyesight. She is most enthusiastic and we hope to hear very favorable results of her work in Oregon, and that a Better Eyesight League is established there.

Dr. Bates spoke for a while telling of his lectures during the past month and the ones scheduled for the future. We attended his lecture at Erasmus Hall High School on Thursday evening, January 11, and were delighted at the number of people who came to hear his message. The library was full, and people were standing in the hall trying to catch what he was saying. The teachers showed great interest, and after the meeting they asked further information from some members of the League. Their interest in Dr. Bates' work was very gratifying, as they have right at hand the ones who need his help most.

MEETING AT EAST ORANGE, NEW JERSEY

By Minnie E. Marvin

A meeting of the Better Eyesight League of the Oranges was held in the Library at East Orange, New Jersey, Friday evening, January 5, at which there was an enthusiastic gathering of about two hundred. Emily C. Lierman, Dr. Bates' assistant, was the speaker.

The evening was a very enjoyable one to all, and much amusement was afforded by Ms. Lierman's little stories of humorous events and happenings at the Harlem Hospital where she and Dr. Bates are conducting their Clinic. It isn't all joy and happiness, however. There is a great deal of sorrow and pathos, too, as in the case of the old lady, seventy-six years old, having no living relatives, who is afflicted with cataracts. Then there is the old lady, seventy-nine years old, who has absolute glaucoma, and the blind girl, who was born with cataracts in both eyes, and is now beginning to actually see. There are hundreds of other cases similar to these, but Ms. Lierman cited a few of the most interesting. She has the faculty of taking these poor afflicted patients right into her heart and showing her love for them, while they in turn reciprocate by loving her and trusting her implicitly. The result is that her instructions are followed faithfully, and the patient gradually regains his or her sight.

Better Eyesight
March 1923—Vol. VII, No. 9

THE MEMORY SWING

The memory swing relieves strain and tension as well as does the long or the short swing which has been described at various times. It is done with the eyes closed while one imagines looking over first the right shoulder, then over the left shoulder, while the head is moved from side to side. The eyeballs may be seen through the closed eyelids to move from side to side in the same direction as the head is moved. When done properly it is just as efficient as the swing which is practiced with the eyes open, whether short or long. The memory swing can be shortened by remembering the swing of a small letter, a quarter of an inch or less when the eyes are closed. The memory swing has given relief in many cases of imperfect sight from myopia, astigmatism and inflammations of the outside of the eyeball as well as inflammations of the inside of the eyeball. One advantage is the fact that it can be done without attracting the attention or making oneself more or less conspicuous to others. It is much easier than the swing practiced with the eyes open and secures a greater amount of relaxation or rest than any other swing. It may be practiced incorrectly, just as any swing may be done wrong, and then no benefit will be obtained.

REST

By W. H. Bates, M.D.

The normal eye when it has normal sight is at rest. When the normal eye has imperfect sight it is not at rest. When the diseased eye is at rest it has normal sight. When the diseased eye is not at rest the sight is imperfect. There are no exceptions to these statements. In the treatment of imperfect sight without glasses it is very important that we should understand as clearly as possible what is meant by rest. The normal eye is at rest when the sight is normal or when the individual remembers or imagines normal sight. All persons with high degrees of nearsightedness have moments when the eye is normal and when the vision is normal but these moments are so short that there is not time enough to be always conscious of the normal vision.

I have a patient with myopia of 40 D measured with the retinoscope. When the patient looks at a blank wall where there is nothing much to see and does not try to see, the retinoscope demonstrates moments of longer or shorter duration when the eye is normal; but just as soon as the patient plans to read the Snellen test card or to see ordinary objects the retinoscope always demonstrates this high degree of myopia.

It can always be demonstrated that when the normal eye looks intently at one point the vision always becomes imperfect. The normal eye with normal sight does not stare, and to avoid the stare is continuously moving. When it moves from side to side the letter regarded appears to move in the opposite directions, but usually this apparent movement is so short, so slow, so easy that most people do not notice it. The eye with imperfect sight does not usually see things moving because it is usually staring. The eye with imperfect sight can be benefited by practicing seeing things moving. This can be done properly, successfully, or it can be done wrong without benefit. When done properly the eye is at rest; when done improperly the eye is under a strain and this strain can usually be felt by the patient when his attention is called to it. It is a great help to the cure of imperfect sight to have the patient demonstrate what is wrong. When you know what is the matter with you, that makes it possible to bring about relief.

In my book I describe many methods for the improvement of the vision. None of them are a benefit unless the patient by practicing them obtains rest. One can practice the swing and make the sight worse; one can close the eyes and strain them terribly. Many people are unable to rest their eyes by palming—the more they palm the more they strain. It is very difficult matter to convince some people that to have strain is a bad thing, that perfect sight can only come when the eye is at rest. Perfect sight comes to the eye when nothing is done; therefore when you do anything you are always doing something wrong. Perfect sight is passive [receptive—TRQ]. We do not see—things are seen and when things are seen with maximum vision no effort whatever is made. The eye is constantly at rest. No work is being done and the longer one uses the eye with perfect sight the more continuously is the eye at rest. Not only is the eye at rest but every nerve of the body is at rest. The body is at rest. With constant use of the eyes with perfect sight no work is done, no fatigue is felt, and one feels perfectly comfortable because the eyes are perfectly at rest.

The eye when it is at rest is very sensitive. It does not require much of an effort to destroy, to a greater or less degree, the feeling of perfect sight. If the mind remembers things perfectly the eye is at rest. When the mind remembers or imagines things imperfectly the sight is disturbed because the eye is not at rest with the memory of imperfect sight. With the eye at rest the imagination of things seen or remembered is perfect, but when the imagination of things seen or remembered is imperfect the eye is not at rest and the sight is imperfect.

It should be emphasized that when one practices any method in which the vision is improved, it is necessary that rest be secured to the eye and mind or else the vision is not improved. Nearsighted patients who have good vision at the near point can improve their sight for the distance very frequently by alternately reading the fine print with perfect sight close to their eyes and regard the letters on the distant Snellen test card in flashes.

Reading fine print with normal sight is a rest and if one can flash the distant card without effort or strain, the vision is improved as rest is maintained. However, it is possible to fail when practicing this method by doing something which prevents rest of the eyes. It is an interesting fact that when the eye is at rest one can flash letters on the Snellen test card for a short fraction of a second without interfering with the rest or relaxation of the eye.

I shall never forget the experiences that I have had with a few patients whose sight was imperfect for the distance and who were unable to read a newspaper. They were unusual in this respect that they were cured very promptly of their imperfect sight by closing their eyes and resting for a half an hour. Their vision was normal as soon as they opened their eyes and looked at the Snellen test card; they were able to read diamond type without difficulty from six to eighteen inches; the benefit was permanent. They did what very few people accomplish: they were able to obtain perfect rest by just closing their eyes.

STORIES FROM THE CLINIC

No. 37: Progressive Myopia

By Emily C. Lierman

Before I begin my story, I wish to apologize for making so many explanations throughout the article. I thought it best to do so for the benefit of those who may have the same difficulty that this poor girl had.

A girl, 23 years old, came to us in a very pitiable state. Her trouble was progressive myopia and one of the worst cases I have ever seen. The glasses she wore were so thick that her eyes seemed like very small miniature eyes when looking at her. Our book has become quite popular in Philadelphia, Pennsylvania, where her home is, and it was through a friend who has the book that she heard of Dr. Bates. She is her mother's only support which made it very hard for her to leave a good position as typist and come to our big city to see Dr. Bates, whom she was sure could cure her eyes when others had failed. Being poor, she could not afford to come to his office for treatment, so she came to the Clinic. The clerk at the desk informed her that she could not have treatment there because she did not live in the district of the hospital. She was admitted that day, however, for just one treatment and to have the privilege of an examination by Dr. Bates. After the Doctor had examined her eyes he asked me privately what on earth could be done with her in order that we could treat her there. When a severe case like this comes to us I long for a Bates Institute or something like that. My friends, some of whom were cured by Dr. Bates, have been very liberal in their support financially but so far there are not enough funds to start an institution. I asked the girl if she could establish a residence near the Clinic so that we could treat her. She said she would try. Dr. Bates then examined her eyes and said her only trouble was progressive myopia. With her glasses off she could not count my fingers at two feet from her eyes. She could see the 200-line letter, the largest letter on the test card at the same distance, but no farther. I improved her vision that day to 3/100 which was double what she had before. Her case required more time than I could give her, so she was instructed to palm her eyes for long intervals all through the day in her room and also in the evening and to come again just as soon as she could. She was told never to wear her glasses again. What a shock this was to her. As she left the room I could see how helpless she was; but before she reached the end of the corridor, on went her glasses again. She had lost her courage but I did not lose faith in her. Any girl who would leave her mother, home and position to have her eyes cured would not give up altogether, even though she was tempted to put on her glasses again. Two days later she returned and displayed her admittance card, showing that she was living in that district. She was anxious for me to know that she obtained a position as an attendant where she also had a home. Then she also wished me to know that her glasses were broken. This was the best thing that could have happened because I knew she would try all the more to be cured.

I placed the test card three feet from her eyes and all she could see was the 200-line letter. The short swing and blinking helped her and in ten minutes her vision improved to 3/100, the same as on her first visit. She comes every Clinic day and is always there ahead of time. Her progress was slow but sure and her face, which looked all the world like a stone image with slits for eyes, now has a natural appearance. She now reads 4/10 with both eyes and I am working diligently with her so that she can go back to her position and to an anxious loving mother.

She is now enjoying the movies for the first time in her life. Her sight was failing her with glasses on so she never attempted to indulge in such luxuries. She has now been under treatment two months, which seems a long time to her. She is happy because she can go along the streets and other places without fear of an accident. At a recent visit she flashed letters on the 10-line of the test card at 10 feet, 10/10. A short time ago she asked me if I go to church. The question was so unexpected. I told her I did go to church and that I was proud of the fact. I consider the Clinic my church also. Hundreds of poor souls enter our room there, just craving for a kind word or two. The Jews stand alongside of the colored folks, the Germans with the Irish. We also meet the Spanish and Italian in small numbers. Some are Catholic, others are Protestant and many other kinds of religions, but the one God is worshipped by them all. A kind word and a smile is necessary for us all and so we give it to them in abundance. The Jewish girl apologized for asking me that question. She had noticed that the kindly feeling which existed in most churches also prevailed in our Clinic.

A NEW OUTLOOK

By Mildred Shepard

If only I had known of Dr. Bates' work while I was still in school! If only I had known how to use my eyes better without glasses than with them; how to go to sleep on my back, swinging the little black "F" on my thumbnail; how to read fine print so that it would be a rest and not a strain; and how to enjoy life generally.

Looking back over the last eight or nine years, I find the remembrance of a headache long continued for days and weeks. All this time I was wearing glasses and receiving treatment from the best oculists I knew, but with no help to the headaches or to my sight, which became worse and worse. There seemed to be no cause for the headaches, and no relief except for part of a day following several consecutive nights of from ten to twelve hours sleep. Shopping or trips to town were concluded by the always to-be-expected extra heavy headache.

But now everything is different. One year ago last September Dr. Bates told me to take off the glasses that I had worn for fifteen years. It was hard for the first month or two—dreadfully hard. But the glasses were never put on again. Instead, I have been palming and swinging and shifting and flashing and imagining and remembering until now I have learned, in part, how to get better use of my eyes without glasses than I could with them. Now I am looking forward, and in fact, have begun to restfully read all those books that were put aside as being a "strain on my eyes," before I knew how.

Little by little the old "wozie feeling" in my head melted away, and now a headache is a rare thing. A few hours of restful sleep now take the place of the long hours required before I knew how to go off to sleep on my back, swinging the little black "F" on my thumbnail—a trick which I wouldn't part with. My sight has improved from 10/70 to 10/15, while I see 10/10 temporarily, which means that I will be able to keep it (normal sight) before long, I hope.

That is my one great ambition now, to be "plumb cured" so that I may go on helping other people to cure themselves. One of my friends cured herself with my help, and several others are on the way.

I say, "If only I had known of Dr. Bates and his work while I was still in school"; I might better say, "How glad I am that I know about them now!"

CRUMBS FOR BORES

By James Hopper

My trouble is eyestrain. When I first went to Dr. Bates he told me that eyestrain came nearly always of mind strain. I did not believe him. The theory seemed mystic to me, and displeasing to one asking for very tangible, physical causes.

A short time later, though, I discovered that the Doctor was right. I discovered this in a way which some will find amusing and others tragic.

In those days, every afternoon I took a walk up Fifth Avenue; and walking Fifth Avenue would practice some of the Doctor's diabolisms—such as swinging the signs and conjuring black points, I soon found that on some days these strange exercises worked perfectly—and that on other days, they wouldn't. There were days when my eyes relaxed deliciously and lost all strain, and then I walked on air. But there were days when, to the best of my efforts the eyestrain remained stubborn.

After a long search I finally found the reason for these discrepancies.

I discovered that the days when my eyestrain was stubborn and refused to yield were exactly the same days on which, in the morning mail, I had found several big bills. And the days when the swing and the black dot so easily got the best of the eyestrain were the days when, in the mail, no bills whatsoever had come.

I have not as yet discovered any absolute remedy for this state of affairs. But I will now go on to another example of mind strain causing eyestrain; one which is more pleasing in that I have in this case discovered an efficient and simple remedy, which I can recommend to all.

At the same period of my life when I walked every afternoon up Fifth Avenue, I dined every night in a certain restaurant, in Greenwich Village. This restaurant had no small individual tables, but only long tables. So you sat with friends, or acquaintances, or with people who were neither. I soon found that, dining at this restaurant, some nights my eyes were altogether relaxed and free from strain, while on other nights they strained badly in spite of all I could do. For some time I thought this was a matter of the lights. But long and close observation finally convinced me that the lighting had nothing to do with it. And finally I discovered the real reason.

It was this. When I sat with people whom I liked, and who amused me—who listened to my stories and laughed at them and did not tell too many of their own—my eyes remained nicely relaxed; I had no strain. But when I sat with bores—with people who insisted in doing all the talking and never giving me a chance—then my eyes began to strain and continued to strain.

But I found a remedy. It's crumbs.

Almost at any table where you eat, if you will look close enough you will find on the cloth—or the linoleum—a crumb. It may be a small one—but the smaller the better. I find such a crumb. I look at the right of it and see it better than the other side; I look at the left side of it and see it better than the right side. I practice on the crumb central fixation. I get it a-swinging—a short, slow swing—and feel my eyes relax, the strain leaving as if by magic.

Meanwhile the bores talk on; I let them talk. I sit there happy and at ease; I seem to be listening profoundly; they are tickled to death with themselves. But I am not listening; I am swinging my crumb. Swinging it, swinging it, and feeling my eyes, my whole being, deliciously distend.

I use this now not only at that restaurant but everywhere I go. And I go to many places now, for I have become extremely popular as a dinner guest. I am such a good listener, you see. I listen so quietly, with such profound and flattering attention.

Well, I don't. I swing crumbs.

BETTER EYESIGHT LEAGUE

By Minnie E. Marvin

Our meetings of the Better Eyesight League become more instructive and interesting every month. Some of those present came to learn about the work Dr. Bates is doing. Others came bursting with enthusiasm to make known some of the wonderful things that had been done for friends under their supervision during the past month.

One lady present told of having cured a family of five, mother, father, and three children, who had worn glasses for years. It is a peculiar fact that this lady, able to help so many as she has done, is still unable to leave off her own glasses. Dr. Bates analyzed her condition and found that though she was *preaching* central fixation she was not *practicing* it. This was the secret of her failure in her own case. Dr. Bates told her how to improve her memory, and we know that she is going to give us a favorable report of herself at the next meeting, as she did of her friends this time.

Another interesting topic was the case of a gentleman teacher in Erasmus Hall High School, Brooklyn. He told of having an "Undergraded" class of thirty-three boys and girls. These children are "sub-normal," and of course, defective sight always follows in the wake of ill-health, etc. This gentleman has cured himself and is very interested in trying to help his class. We shall be pleased to hear of his progress at our next meeting in March.

One of the "boosters" of the Better Eyesight League is a lady of about 70 years old. She has worn glasses for a great many years, and through following Dr. Bates' book, *Perfect Sight Without Glasses,* is now able to read the diamond type cards at about eight inches. She has done good work in introducing the method among her friends, and reported that they are getting fine results.

If all of our League members would pledge themselves to talk to at least one person with defective sight a week, they would have some real business to report at the next meeting. You all know what a relief you found in being able to dispense with glasses. Don't you realize how much good you will accomplish by making this relief known to others? Every day we hear someone say, "Oh! If only I had learned of this work before I became such a slave to glasses!" There are millions waiting to be told the same thing you were. We are doing our share; we trust you will do yours.

Better Eyesight
April 1923—Vol. VII, No. 10

WATCH YOUR STEP

When you know what is the matter with you, it is possible for you to correct it and bring about a cure. If you do not know what is wrong with you, the cure of your imperfect sight is delayed. Some persons have been cured quickly when they were able to demonstrate that to see imperfectly required a tremendous effort, an effort which was very difficult. Some persons are cured in one visit and they readily demonstrate that imperfect sight or failure to see is difficult. Others require weeks and months to demonstrate the facts. Perfect sight is quick, comes easy and without any effort whatever. Imperfect sight is slow and difficult. One cannot consciously make the sight worse as readily as it can be done unconsciously. There is no danger in demonstrating the facts.

Look at a small letter on the Snellen test card which can be seen clearly at ten or twenty feet, a small letter "o" for example. When the letter is seen quite perfectly it is usually seen without any apparent effort. However, by looking intently, staring at it and making an effort to improve it, the letter blurs. It can always be demonstrated that the effort to see very soon blurs the letter. Now close the eyes and rest them for a part of a minute or longer and then glance at the letter again. It will usually be as clear as it was before. Again by straining and making an effort, the letter becomes blurred. One can readily demonstrate that to make the sight worse requires an effort, a strain.

Many obstinate cases have obtained a permanent cure only after learning how to make the sight worse consciously. In my book are published "Seven Truths of Normal Sight." Prove the facts by demonstrating that the sight becomes imperfect when one or all of them is made imperfect by a strain.

AN OPPORTUNITY FOR TEACHERS

By W. H. Bates, M.D.

The future of this country is in the hands of the children. The children are in the hands of the teachers.

Parents spend relatively very little or no time with their children while the teachers supervise the lives of the children for at least six hours a day. The duties of teachers have been increased very much in recent years. There was a time when the child got all the possible education from the home, but now some children do not even get enough to eat at home and the teachers have supplied food, heat, warm clothing, fresh air, exercise and games. We ought to be very grateful to the teachers because they not only supply the necessities but also the pleasures which children need.

I am interested in the eyes of the schoolchildren. It seems to me a crime that young children should have to wear glasses; even children before they enter school, nursing babies, have occasionally been compelled to wear glasses. There was a time when I prided myself on my ability to prescribe glasses, even taught other doctors how to do it, but I never fitted young children with glasses because it was very rare to find children under six years old who could be manifestly benefited by wearing glasses. One teacher told me that the Board of Health of the City of New York not so very long ago sent a doctor to examine the eyes of her pupils. He prescribed glasses for every one of these children and even insisted that she should wear glasses. I told the teacher what to do and she very promptly became able to use her eyes without glasses and without any discomfort.

As one child after another lost their glasses, the teacher told each child who was not wearing glasses what to do to improve his sight and finally every child in her class obtained perfect sight without glasses after they stopped wearing them. Furthermore, the scholarship of her pupils improved immensely. By practicing central fixation her children had no more headaches when they looked at the blackboard or when they read their books. Surely what that teacher did was not a crime and what she did other teachers can do all over the United States. The number of children wearing glasses is steadily increasing. I have many schoolchildren brought to me wearing glasses, to be cured of their symptoms without them and I find that in a very large percentage of these cases the glasses prescribed were very weak and entirely unnecessary. By a little rest, palming and swinging, the vision became normal and the eyes perfectly comfortable without glasses.

Here is a great opportunity for all the teachers in the public and private schools to come forward and do the common sense thing for their pupils. Of the hundred and ten million people in the United States when we average five children to a family, the number of children is approximately eighty million. Of course these figures are not at all accurate but even if there were only one million schoolchildren in the United States it would be worthwhile to preserve their eyesight. The majority of people are poor; they cannot afford to pay for eyeglasses or to pay the doctor for his examination. The teachers have aided materially in supplying glasses to their pupils because they thought the glasses were necessary. Every teacher cured of imperfect sight by reading my book or practicing my treatment is able to cure every one of her pupils. There may be some exceptions to this but I have found out that so long as the child is able to see to come to school, the child can be benefited by the teacher. From time to time I have published articles on the prevention of imperfect sight in schoolchildren. From time to time I have cured teachers so that their sight became normal without glasses. Always I have urged them to do something for their pupils and many of them have, but there are a certain proportion of teachers who lack the courage of their convictions and neglect to do what they are able to do. I wish I could say something that would encourage such teachers to go ahead and benefit their pupils. They cannot do any harm to a child suffering from headaches; the child can be relieved of a headache by closing the eyes and palming. No eye specialist, no person of average intelligence would object to a child resting his eyes. Taking a rest from his studies is not a crime and most teachers can tell better than anybody else how much rest a child ought to have. Every day schoolchildren come to my office and I tell them to take off their glasses. When the children are allowed to practice my treatment they get well without glasses. I think that is much better than to condemn them to the use of glasses for the rest of their lives. My discoveries in physiological optics have demonstrated that all children wearing glasses can be cured without them.

STORIES FROM THE CLINIC

No. 38: Criminals

By Emily C. Lierman

Some years ago I was asked to go to Ossining to assist in examining the eyes of some of the prisoners. I firmly believe that if the prisoners had had no eyestrain their minds would not have turned to crime.

A foreigner who was imprisoned for arson told me in a few words how sorry he was that he set a building on fire for five dollars. He could not get work he said because he had bad sight and as a new baby was coming into his home where there were already three, he was desperate and so he did as he was bidden for a nominal sum of five dollars. Here was a foreigner who could hardly speak English who was willing to do most anything for his wife for a five dollar bill. Four years had already been spent in prison and through the kindness of Warden Osborne, who was at that time doing such wonderful work inside the prison, he was allowed to live in a cell where there was a little bit of sunshine now and then. From being in a dark cell before Osborne came, for one whole year, the sight of his right eye was practically destroyed.

There were so many patients in the room, sent there to be examined by Dr. Bates, that we had very little time to devote to each one individually; but I arranged a test card on a desk and placed him about five feet away from it and in just a few moments time I improved the sight of his good eye from 5/200 to 5/50. He was so overjoyed that he fell on his knees before me and held my two wrists very tightly, pleading with me to help him out of prison if that was possible, for he was eager to go to the new baby who arrived after his sentence. Some people might say, "Oh, yes, he told you a hard luck story," but I can understand all about it or at least enough to convince me that if conditions had been better for him when he came to this country, perhaps he might never have been there.

So many times I have found that patients who come to us at the Clinic are wearing the wrong glasses for their eyes. It is not always eyestrain which causes trouble for some patients but the mistake of the optician who commits a terrible error.

I would like to tell about a recent case, Belle, a girl eleven years old, who had myopia with glasses on and almost normal vision without them. As I do not test the strength of eyeglasses of the cases which come to me, I was not at all sure whether the child was wearing them for fun or not. The first question that came to my mind was, was she wearing her mother's glasses or someone else's, just because she enjoyed wearing glasses, so I asked Dr. Bates to test them and find out whether the child was telling the truth or not. At 15 feet I asked the child to read the test card and with glasses on she read 15/100. I took off her glasses and she just stared at the card and that was all. I told her to do the usual thing, just close her eyes to rest them for a moment or so. When she opened her eyes again and looked at the card she read without a stop from the

200-line letter down to the last letter of the 20-line. She looked at me in great surprise and smiled. The discovery that she made seemed to give her a thrill. I asked her then who fitted her for glasses.

She said that the school nurse had called to see her mother and complained that the child could not see the blackboard nor could she read the test card when her eyes were examined in school, so her mother immediately took her to an optician to be fitted for glasses. She said that the optician had charged her mother $4.50 for glasses and for the examination of her eyes. To my mind this was not only an error but a crime.

Sometimes as I go along the streets or ride in a car early in the morning to my work, I watch a policeman as he walks along his beat looking in at each store window because they are told to do so to protect the storekeeper. I wish there were policemen who understood the fitting of glasses who could invade the stores of opticians such as this one who fitted this child with the wrong glasses, and bring them to justice.

This little girl of whom I started to write is not the criminal kind. She is a wholesome kiddie, just full of life, and when I told her that it was a great mistake for her to wear those glasses she promptly put them away in the case and begged me to help her some more. I gave her perfect sight that day and she has not been to me since. Her little friend who brought her the day she came told me that Belle was not wearing glasses any more but sat in the back seat of her classroom showing off to her teacher for all she was worth reading the blackboard better than she ever did in her life. She also told me that Belle informed the teacher about our Clinic and showed the teacher how to palm. She is what I call a good League member for she is surely spreading the work in the classroom and can do more than I can because she is right there.

DR. BATES' LECTURE

By L. L. Biddle, 2nd

For the benefit of those who were unable to attend Dr. Bates' lecture, before the New York Association of Osteopaths, at the Waldorf Astoria on Saturday Evening, February 17, I decided to take down a few notes which I will now try to compile.

The chairperson introduced Dr. Bates by stating that the osteopaths take away the crutches and Dr. Bates takes away the glasses. Dr. Bates commenced by telling how he made his first discoveries and cited the opposition he had to buck against. He stated that his attitude of mind, ever since he was a little boy, was to find out all the facts possible about a subject and then work on these as a basis rather than on a guess or theory. When he commenced practicing medicine in 1885, one of the first patients who came to him had a slight degree of myopia or nearsightedness. Upon examining his eyes with the ophthalmoscope, he found that the patient was not nearsighted all of the time. When the patient was looking at a blank wall and not trying to see anything, his eyes were for short periods, normal. He persuaded this patient to go without his glasses, and his eyes finally reached a point where they stayed normal all the time.

Dr. Bates said that he then started boasting around the hospital about this cure. However, it got so on the house-surgeon's nerves that he brought up a ward patient who was nearsighted, and with him Dr. Bates managed to have equal success. Much to his surprise, instead of the rest of the doctors praising him and trying to find out how he accomplished these heretofore impossible cures, Dr. Bates suddenly became very unpopular with the rest of the staff. These successes nevertheless spurred him on in his experiments at the New York Aquarium and at the laboratory of the Columbia College for Physicians and Surgeons, and as a result he discovered that the accommodation of the eye is not brought about by a change in the shape of the lens, but by the lengthening and shortening of the eyeball itself, as the bellows of a camera.

When he explained and illustrated this to his doctor friends, it disturbed them greatly. The surgeon who had charge of the laboratory came to him and said, "Do you know that you have proven that Helmholtz is wrong, and furthermore if you wish to be accepted by scientific men you will have to show how or why he blundered?" This was quite a proposition, but Dr. Bates continued his experiments and for two years tried to prove that Helmholtz was right, but failed, and finally discovered how Helmholtz blundered; which Dr. Bates has illustrated in his book. As a reward for this, he was expelled from the University.

This was quite a handicap, but he obtained a small laboratory for himself and continued in his work. He told us of a specific case: A woman wearing very strong glasses brought her daughter to him because the little girl's eyes were getting so bad that she could not continue at school. When the woman, in her usual cross manner, told her daughter to take off her glasses and read the test card, she was only able to read the top letter. Dr. Bates then very kindly asked the child to close her eyes and rest them. After a little while he asked her to open her eyes and tell what she could see. Much to their surprise the little girl read the whole card. Her mother was very happy and said that she would see that her daughter would practice every day with the test card as Dr. Bates prescribed. In a few days, however, they returned very discouraged and the mother said that her child was only able to read the top letter on the test card. Dr. Bates said that he asked her who had tested the girl's sight, and the woman admitted that it was she. He remonstrated with her, and reminded her that he especially asked her to stay out of the room when her daughter was practicing, and to have someone with normal sight test her. He then took his little patient as before and speaking to her kindly had her rest her eyes, and she again read the whole card.

Dr. Bates stated that he cited this example to show how the strain which this woman was under from wearing very strong glasses was contagious, and harmed her daughter's sight. Moreover, he said that it showed how the child's state of mind directly affected her ability to see. For when she was spoken to kindly and her mind was relaxed, her eyes were rested and she read the whole card. He explained that when one's mind was under a strain one unconsciously tightened the muscles which encircle the eyeball, and consequently squeeze it out of shape and out of focus. But when the mind is at rest these muscles are relaxed and the eyeball is allowed to assume its proper shape and focus. He furthermore stated that all diseases of the eye can be cured by similar relaxation, which can be obtained by methods Dr. Bates has developed. He said that all children under 12 years old not wearing glasses can obtain perfect sight by reading the Snellen test card once a day, first with one eye and then with the other.

He once more reiterated his old challenge which he first gave before the New York Medical Association ten years ago, declaring that if anyone can prove one of his statements wrong, then all are wrong. He also stated that he has not found a case so bad or so blind that he could not benefit, and that he has not yet met his Waterloo.

He then returned to his seat, but was so applauded and urged to continue that he finally stated that if anyone wished to remain and ask further questions, he would be glad to answer them. This they all did, and fired questions at him until it became so late that in order to make his train, he was forced to break away.

PARENTS' AND TEACHER'S PAGE

By Emily A. Meder

We are adding this new feature to the magazine for the benefit of those who are vitally interested in the preservation of schoolchildren's eyesight.

Parents are directly responsible for the welfare of these future citizens but we find that this is lightly shifted to the shoulders of the teachers who only see the pupils one-fifth of the time that the parents do. When this great truth is brought home: THAT ALL DEFECTS OF THE EYE ARE CURABLE; THAT ALL DISEASES OF THE EYE ARE FUNCTIONAL, THEREFORE CURABLE, then we can reach the parents who are criminally placing glasses upon their children. When told in Dr. Bates' own words, it is all so logical and easy, but the difficult part of it is to convince mothers that they are doing the wrong thing.

The writer of this article has grown very fond of a little neighbor in the apartment next door. The little girl is four years old and has a very bad case of crossed eyes which is greatly exaggerated by a pair of tortoise-shell glasses. Her mother is constantly admonishing her not to run and jump with Buddy, her little brother, for fear that she might injure the precious goggles. I spoke to the mother about Dr. Bates' methods and that I knew the child could be cured; but when I suggested that she remove the glasses, the idea was met with a shudder. This woman, although having the best interest of her little daughter at heart, was doing the worst possible thing for her. She could not overcome the old set ways of doing things. She accepted as true the theories that are retarding progress and obscuring the light of newer things.

When Dr. Bates realized the value of his discoveries, he immediately took steps to have this method placed at the disposal of school officials; however, because he could not afford to pay the price to these officials for the privilege of giving away his life work, and because many obstacles were placed in his path to discourage him from removing glasses from the universe, this great work was retarded and the money and work expended, while great in itself, was only "a drop in the bucket."

The teachers and nurses of schools, however, who do not have to be financially reimbursed are doing good work. They place a test card in the classroom and have the pupils read this once every day. A record is taken of each child when he first begins and this is compared with the record taken two weeks later. The teachers are always amazed at the results.

I have in front of me a letter written to Dr. Bates from a nurse who installed this system in her school. Among other reports, is this one of great interest. She said, "The children come to me just before the close of the morning session. They palm and do the swing either with the head alone or with the entire body. Later I found that the swing was more successful than the palming, as the latter was irksome to the child." Another extract reads, "I helped correct squint in a child and his eyes remain straight unless he strains. His sight has also improved in spite of the fact that he practices less at home than any of the others and needs constant urging."

This letter speaks for itself. These are the worthwhile things and anyone who reads this page can improve the eyesight of a child with defective vision. We shall be glad to answer all questions through the magazine and give directions. Don't let your boy or girl grow up with imperfect sight. The eyes are truly the windows of the soul and if these are not normal, the whole physical outlook is altered.

If you are a teacher, look at your little charges and see if they need help. It is so easy, and means so much. If you are a mother, you will probably know now why your child does not romp with the others.

BETTER EYESIGHT LEAGUE

We noticed a greater part of those present were strangers, and people who had inquired about Dr. Bates' work, and had been advised to attend one meeting, and get some idea about his method, and how others are being helped. We were very glad indeed to see these new faces, and to have them hear the wonderful reports some of our members made. Among the most important of these reports, was that given by Dr. J. M. Watters. He is practicing Dr. Bates' method, and is keenly interested in the sight of schoolchildren. There is a sub-normal school in Orange, New Jersey, with an attendance of about forty children. Out of the forty which he examined, five had normal vision. He installed the method by explaining Dr. Bates' method to the teachers, and placing in the classroom a Snellen test card. We shall be very interested to know at the next meeting what progress has been made.

There is so much work to be done among the children, and we wish everyone who reads this magazine to have the pleasure of saying that they helped cure a child of imperfect vision. The field is so large, and the workers so few.

There were a great many who told how they improved their own vision, and how elated they were, but there were none who told if they benefited others.

QUESTIONS AND ANSWERS

Q–1. What is central fixation?

A–1. Seeing best where you are looking; that is, an object, for instance, a chair, look at the arm or the leg. The object is brought out clearer. Trying to take in the whole chair at once strains the eyes, and the object becomes blurred.

Q–2. How long does Dr. Bates' treatment take?

A–2. This depends on the seriousness and nature of your defect.

Q–3. Are cataracts curable without operation?

A–3. Yes.

Better Eyesight
May 1923—Vol. VII, No. 11

TEACH OTHERS

Many teachers have told me that when they taught arithmetic, the one who learned the most was always the teacher. Some ministers have made the remark that the one who profited mostly by the sermon was the man who delivered it.

For many years my patients who have been benefited by treatment without glasses have to a greater or less extent enjoyed the pleasure of helping others. When you think that you understand how to practice the swing with benefit, try to teach somebody else how to do it. If you find palming is beneficial, find how many of your friends who are also benefited by palming. But when you meet someone who is not benefited by what you tell them to do, you have at this time an opportunity of helping not only your friend but your own eyes as well. It seems a simple matter for you to close your eyes, rest them for a half-hour or so and find that your sight is improved by the rest. However, there are some people who are not benefited appreciably by closing their eyes and resting them. One cause of failure is the memory of imperfect sight. Many patients failed to improve because with their eyes closed they think too much of their failure to see. Patients who have improved materially usually can demonstrate that the memory of perfect sight is restful, while the memory of imperfect sight is a strain. If you have a nearsighted friend who can read ordinary print without difficulty at the near point and without glasses, you can spend an hour or two of activity in showing your friend how to demonstrate while regarding fine print that it is impossible to try to concentrate on a point without sooner or later making the sight worse, that it is impossible to remember, imagine or see stationary letters, that it is impossible to maintain normal vision with the eyes kept continuously open without blinking.

THE STORY OF BARBOUR

By W. H. Bates, M.D.

Barbour had the best imagination of anybody I ever knew in my life. I believe this is some praise because every day for many years I am teaching patients how to imagine perfectly and while doing so testing their imagination. There may be schools where the imagination is taught but I do not know where to find them and would be pleased to have someone tell me of others who teach memory and imagination. Of course I have read many books which claim to teach people how to remember better, and since memory is very important in obtaining perfect sight I have been very much interested in these books and have read them very carefully to learn what they might contain. Unfortunately I have never been able to learn anything from these books which was better than my methods.

It might interest my readers to know that some of my patients are teachers of mental science in various schools and colleges. I never found one who had a correct conception of memory and imagination. Many of them had no mental pictures at all. In fact one very prominent professor of mental science, a dean in his department in one of our well-known universities could not imagine a mental picture of his own signature or imagine a mental picture of a person's face or a mental picture of a flower or any other object. Before I could help his sight I had to teach him how to remember and how to imagine, and so when I say that Barbour had a wonderful imagination I feel that it means something.

She was eleven years old and was suffering from alternating convergent squint. She had normal vision and was wearing glasses for compound hypermetropic astigmatism which made her sight worse. When she regarded a small letter on the 10-line at twenty feet she said that she could see it when she knew what it was and this was true because when she said that she saw a letter that she knew perfectly, she was able to see other letters that she did not know. When there were two letters close together, both unknown and neither distinct, she could see both of them when she imagined she saw one after knowing what it was.

She was treated in various ways with temporary benefit for some weeks. She readily demonstrated that resting her eyes, palming, and swinging was a benefit. When she regarded a small letter at a near point, about six inches, she could see the white center of the letter "O" very white and imagine it whiter than it really was, whiter than the rest of the card. She could imagine it moving from side to side no more than its own width; but when she tried to imagine it was stationary her vision became worse and the letter "O" was not distinct. When she closed her eyes she would remember the letter "O" and imagine the white center as white as when she looked at the "O" with her eyes open. By practice she became able to demonstrate that with her eyes closed she could remember a letter "O" with its short swing and its very white center perfectly when she imagined one side of an unknown letter correctly. If the unknown letter was a "B" and she imagined the left-hand side to be straight, her memory of the "O" was perfect. If she imagined the left side was curved or open, her memory of the letter "O" was modified and sufficiently so for her to tell the difference. In the same way she was able to imagine the top was straight, the bottom was straight, and the right side was a curve. This description was also that of a letter "D." When she imagined incorrectly that the letter was a "D," her memory of the letter "O" at the same time was modified. When she imagined the truth that the letter was a "B," her memory of the letter "O" still remained perfect. In other words, when she imagined the truth of either side of an unknown letter that she had previously regarded without seeing consciously, the letter "O" remained perfect in her memory. But when she imagined an error—one or more sides of the letter incorrectly—she did not remember the letter "O" so well.

One day I held a page of diamond type, which she had never seen before, ten feet away from her eyes and directed her to look at the top, the middle, the bottom for about a half a minute. She was unable to see consciously a single letter on the page. With the retinoscope she was myopic when she tried to see the fine print, but not myopic all the time. According to simultaneous retinoscopy her eyes were normal for fractions of a second or longer. I told her mother that the distance was too great for her to read the fine print with her conscious mind, but that she saw every letter on the card perfectly with her subconscious mind; and because she saw each letter perfectly she was able, when she closed her eyes, to remember correctly where each letter was located. I asked her to tell me with the help of her imagination the first letter of the fourth word on the tenth line. This she did correctly in the same way as was just described. Then she imagined correctly the second letter of the fifth word on the fourteenth line, a small letter "c" which was similar to a capital letter "C." She was able to imagine many other letters correctly after she was told where they were located. Some letters, an "X" for example, have all four sides open, and yet in some way she became able to imagine these letters correctly better than incorrectly. The next step, made largely by her own volition, was to imagine correctly the small letters as she already had imagined capital letters. Every day her mother or I cooperated with her in imagining with her conscious mind letters which she only saw unconsciously with her subconscious mind. Her improvement proceeded rapidly until she imagined she saw one letter of a word so perfectly with so perfect a mental relaxation that she imagined she saw the whole word and many words following, one or more lines of letters as quickly as she could at times read them when looking at them at a near point.

The alternating squint disappeared, at first temporarily for a few hours, a few days or longer. She returned home and continued the daily practice of her imagination of letters seen by her subconscious mind. In one of her letters she wrote that after daily practice for forty-four days there was no return of the squint.

Her vision and squint were very much benefited by reading books printed in very fine type. The smaller the print the greater the relaxation of her eyes, and the more was her squint benefited. She became very much interested in reading fine print and was very anxious to obtain print as small as possible. So I sent her a copy of the photographic reduction of the Bible, in which the print is very small indeed. The following letter was received:

"Dear Dr. Bates: Thank you very much for the little Bible. It is the cutest thing I have ever seen. My eyes have been straight forty-four days in succession, and I'm as proud as a peacock. We only have three Christmas presents wrapped up. I hope you have a merry, merry, merry, Christmas, and a Happy, Happy, Happy New Year.

Love, Barbour."

STORIES FROM THE CLINIC

No. 39: A Case of Alternate Divergent Squint

By Emily C. Lierman

One day a young woman came to us with her little boy age nine years. Every time she looked at him it was plainly a look of disgust. The boy had the most wistful face I ever saw. He kept looking up into his mother's face and his expression was that of a deaf and dumb person. One of his eyes seemed to be looking way off to the opposite side of the room while the other eye was looking straight at her. When his other eye turned to look at her, the former would turn out in the opposite direction away from her. He had alternate divergent squint. My heart went out to James as his mother related to me the fact that her other three children had normal sight while James looked so horrible with his crooked eyes. A chill went through me when I heard her say, "I wish he had never been born." Then with more disgust in the sound of her voice she said, "I can't help it, but I hate him."

Can anyone imagine a mother disliking her own child so much? All because his eyes were crooked. Complaints came to her from the school he attended. His teacher complained that he was stupid. All this time the little fellow looked up at his mother without moving an eyelid apparently. Her question was, "What can be done with him or for him? Can you give him glasses or operate to cure his eyes?" I told the mother that glasses would never cure his squint and neither would an operation. I asked her to watch carefully and see what James was about to do for me. First, I held him very close to me and patted his woolly head. He pressed a little closer for more. He liked the beginning of his treatment. I asked him to say the alphabet for me, but he said he could not remember all of the letters. He stood ten feet from the test card. I asked him to read, starting with the largest letter at the top. He read a few letters correctly but I soon found out that he did not know many letters of the alphabet. His mother remarked then that the teacher in school thought his mind was affected because of his eyes and that there was little hope of curing him. I had my doubts about the teacher saying such a thing but I did not say so to the mother. What a pity it was to have the dear little fellow hear all this. He looked so worried and restless. Perhaps he wanted to run away somewhere because his eyes caused others so much trouble. I taught him to palm, telling him to remember a small Bible class pin I was wearing on my dress. In a few minutes I tested his sight with the "E" (pothooks) card, which is used always in cases where children do not know their letters. At ten feet he saw the 50-line. Again I told him to palm, and asked his mother not to speak to him while he was resting his eyes. In the meantime I attended to other patients. After a few moments I glanced at him and saw two big tears rolling down each cheek. He was weeping silently. His mother was just about ready to find fault with him, but I intervened and walked her gently out of the room to a bench outside the door. I whispered to James that I loved him a whole lot and if he would learn to read his letters at home and could read half of the test card correctly the next time he came, I would give him a nickel. I saw him smile, and when I was able to treat him again I found that his sight had improved to the 40-line of the "E" card. I have been wondering ever since whether it was the Bible class pin on my dress which he was asked to remember or was it a clear vision he had of that nickel I had promised him that improved his sight for the 40-line of letters. Two days later James appeared again with his mother and both were smiling. He could hardly wait to tell me that he knew his letters perfectly. His big brother taught him at home, he said, and he hoped I would be pleased as his teacher was when he read all his letters on the blackboard for her that day.

It was amusing to see James looking toward my purse which was hanging on the wall in the Clinic room. He was thinking of that nickel I promised him. I produced a strange test card which he had not seen. When he began to read the card I placed him fifteen feet away, which was five feet farther than the first day. He was so excited that his squint became worse and he could not read. Dr. Bates said his trouble was mostly nervousness. I told him to palm again and reminded him of the letter "E" with its straight line at the top and to the left, with an opening to the right. Then he became able to see the letters after a few moments' rest. I called Dr. Bates' attention to the sudden improvement in his eyes as he read one line after another until he reached the 30-line, when suddenly his eyes turned out again, but after he had rested his eyes again they became straight. I gave him the promised nickel that day, which made him very happy.

James was able to keep his eyes straight most of the time after he had been coming to the Clinic for a month. The attitude of his mother toward him was decidedly better and she promised to help him with the treatment of his eyes at home. I do not know whether James was entirely cured or not because our work at the Harlem Hospital Clinic has since been discontinued.

TEACHERS QUESTION DR. BATES

By Kathleen E. Hurty

As an interesting sequel to the January lecture given by Dr. Bates at Erasmus Hall High School in Brooklyn, there followed a most profitable evening. The January talk was to many such a revelation that some of the teachers were eager for a chance to know more of this remarkable discovery. On April 6 an opportunity was afforded to ply Dr. Bates with questions. About twenty-five teachers from the high schools and a few other friends were present. Practically everyone there had read *Perfect Sight Without Glasses* and no one needed to be convinced of the soundness of the principles involved. Therefore the discussions were largely details of technique, centering mostly about methods with children and particularly in the classroom.

Specifically, Dr. Bates recommended the following procedure:

1. That each teacher hang a Snellen test card on the classroom wall. Daily both teacher and pupils should read the smallest letters that can be seen without straining, using each eye separately. He stated that if this course be pursued faithfully over a period of time all eyes would be helped—sight improved and strain prevented.

2. That teachers do as much as possible to re-educate their pupils in the proper use of their eyes. Incorrect habits must be replaced by new correct ones, namely, pupils should be taught that any effort to see produces strain and injures the eyes. They must be taught never to look fixedly at the blackboard, teacher's face, or any object. Nor should they ever keep their eyes open for any length of time. The normal eye is always shifting and blinking. Therefore to counteract strain in a child who stares fixedly, simple exercises, such as blinking continuously for a few minutes and swinging, should be taught.

3. That children should be informed that if their eyes ache or their sight is blurred, palming is an easy means to get rest and relief.

The final impression left in the minds of those present was that teachers can do a really big work by improving sight and preventing eyestrain so that their children need never have glasses prescribed.

After the conference many stayed to ask further questions of Dr. Bates and to receive help with their own personal problems and difficulties. Some of the teachers were able to testify that they had derived immense benefit from the method. Several stated that they had already abandoned their glasses, with resulting improvement in their eyes.

HOW MY EYESTRAIN WAS RELIEVED

By Charlotte Robertson

I have had such wonderful relief by following Dr. Bates' method of treating imperfect sight and eyestrain that I should like to tell of my experience. It may be the means of giving courage to those who suffered as I did, but who hesitate to leave off their glasses. I had worn glasses but my eyes were not benefited. In fact they became worse. I went to Dr. Bates and am pleased to give some of the "exercises" advised by him which I have found very beneficial.

1. The Snellen test card I read upon arising in the morning, at noon and again in the evening, first with two eyes together and later with each eye separately.

2. Palming six times a day or more for a few minutes to half an hour, decreasing the length of time as my eyes improved.

3. I have practiced reading a little fine print daily, also some pages from Dr. Bates' book, *Perfect Sight Without Glasses,* which I have always found encouraging. At night on retiring I have used the swing together with central fixation on the small "o," and by so doing have lost the wretched strain which I have been conscious of for months, always on awakening in the morning. This exercise consists of swinging the "o" to the left and seeing the right side best, then to the right and seeing the left side best. Also swinging the black period with the "o" to the left, seeing the period on the right side of the "o" best, and to the right, seeing the period on the left side of the "o" best. First by the practice of this exercise, also with a soothing swinging motion as that of drifting in a boat in a comparatively quiet sea, I obtained relaxation when falling to sleep. My morning eyestrain had completely disappeared and in its place I awake feeling rested, refreshed and ready for the day's work.

PARENTS' AND TEACHERS' PAGE

By Emily A. Meder

It is becoming more and more gratifying to us to note the increased activity among school officials, school teachers, and last but in no wise least, among parents, in the promotion of better eyesight in children.

The slogan adopted seems to be "an ounce of prevention is worth a pound of glasses."

We are all grasping every opportunity to first, prevent defective vision, and second, to remove glasses from children who already have them.

An incident worth citing occurred in the Central Fixation office recently. A mother came to purchase a Snellen chart, and with her was a little girl about three. The youngster had a very bad case of squint and wore glasses that almost obscured the little face. We naturally surmised that the card was for the child, but learned that the mother wished it for herself. She told us she had myopia. She never dreamed that the child's eyes could be cured without operation, and was certainly elated when Ms. Lierman showed her how to treat the little one. Naturally the child was too young to read the chart, so Ms. Lierman showed her the game of seeing things swing, with the result that at times the child's eyes were perfectly straight. We are anxiously awaiting the next report from the mother, who was eager to go home and try treating the little girl herself.

A teacher from East Orange has upset a school tradition by having her pupils shift and blink while she is talking to them. She, like others, was under the impression that if her pupils stared at her and did not move this was indicative of alertness and intentness. However, upon learning of Dr. Bates' method, she has changed the old regime, and she has since informed us that she is more at ease with her class when they are relaxed.

Coinciding with this report is one received from a lady who taught her daughter, who is now ten, to look directly into the eyes of the one speaking to her. The child followed these instructions implicitly, with the result that the little girl strained her eyes so out of focus that her glasses had to be changed every few months. In desperation the mother brought her to Dr. Bates, who immediately changed the stare into a blink. They returned home within a few weeks, minus her glasses and plus perfect vision. This was mostly due to correcting the stare.

If mothers are at a loss to know where to start, let them watch the children for a short period. They will be surprised to note the prevalence among children of staring. If this is corrected, it is a good step forward.

BETTER EYESIGHT LEAGUE

By F. B. Rusk, Recording Secretary

The annual business meeting of the Better Eyesight League was held on April 10, with Ms. Hurty in the chair....

The meeting was then opened for discussion. One of Dr. Bates' patients reported a gradual but steady lessening of eyestrain by palming several times a day and swinging the "O." Another member told of the cure of a sty by palming, and Dr. Bates added other interesting cases where serious infections had been reduced by palming.

Among the most important points brought out by Dr. Bates in response to questions were the following:

Squint has never been permanently cured by operation. The only permanent cure is through relaxation of the eyes. An ingenious way of treating a young child afflicted with squint is to let him practice the foxtrot, calling his attention to the fact that the objects in the room seem to move in a direction opposite to that in which he is dancing.

GERMANY PAVES THE WAY FOR PERFECT SIGHT IN NEXT GENERATION

By Minnie E. Marvin

In every mail we have evidences of the way Dr. Bates' work is being spread all over the world. We have not only "book patients" and magazine subscribers in Europe, Asia, Africa, etc., but doctors treating imperfect sight according to Dr. Bates' method. These doctors are not among those who have studied under Dr. Bates but who have analyzed the book and with the aid of the many reprints which have appeared in the various medical journals are enabled to carry on the good work. *Apropos* of the above we have a very interesting piece of news for our readers.

About a week ago a reporter from the Universal Service Staff called at our office to learn about Dr. Bates' work. She said that Norman Hapgood, editor of *Hearst's International* who is in Europe now for the purpose of getting inside information on the political and economic situations, had cabled the Universal Service of an interesting discovery which he made incidentally. This was that while visiting the schools and soup kitchens in Germany he saw altogether only one child wearing glasses. Upon asking the reason of this he was told that the authorities are taking glasses off children all through Germany and that they were acting in this under pressure of the oculists. Mr. Hapgood was also told that this method originated in America. The reporter for the Universal News traced the origin to Dr. Bates, hence her request for further details.

Do you realize what this means? Germany, the very source from which the old theories governing our ophthalmologists originated, has at last accepted the only method of curing imperfect sight. Norman Hapgood says, "While fully accepted in Germany it is spreading slowly in America where in time it is bound to be recognized and to be universally practiced."

Why isn't the discoverer so honored by his own country?

Have You a Bible?

You all know fine print is beneficial. Do you practice reading it? Dr. Bates has proven that by reading a few lines of very fine print daily you are giving your eyes the relaxing "exercise" that will tend to prevent many common defects. We publish a Bible that is printed in microscopic type, and measures one by one and a half inches and contains the new and old Testament. Many patients past fifty have learned to read this with ease.

QUESTIONS AND ANSWERS

Q–1. Am forty-nine years old and have had to wear glasses for five years, due to gradual weakening of the eyes. Is this curable?

A–1. Old-age sight is curable, and you can discard your glasses by following the methods as outlined in the book, *Perfect Sight Without Glasses.*

Q–2. My father, eighty-three years old, has cataracts on both eyes. Can you help him?

A–2. Without personal supervision, cataracts are very hard to cure. Would advise his coming to New York. I can cure him. In the meantime, read the chapters on cataract in my book and he will get a great deal of relief.

Q–3. Why are books for small children printed in large type?

A–3. Because Boards of Education have not yet learned that it is a strain for anyone to look at big print and a relaxation to read fine print.

Q–4. Am practicing the methods in your book to cure myopia and astigmatism. Sometimes, for short periods, I see perfectly, then things fade away. Can you explain this?

A–4. This is what we call getting flashes of perfect sight. With continued practice these flashes will come more frequent and eventually will become permanent.—Then you are cured.

Better Eyesight
June 1923—Vol. VII, No. 12

TRY DANCING

There has been repeatedly published in this magazine and in my book that the imagination of stationary objects to be moving is a rest and relaxation and a benefit to the sight. Young children, when one or both eyes turn in or out, are benefited by having them swing from side to side with a regular rhythmical motion. This motion prevents the stare and the strain and improves the appearance of the eyes. It helps the sight of most children to play hide-and-seek. Children become very much excited and laugh and carry on and have a good time and it certainly is a benefit to their sight. It seems to me that these children would be benefited by going to dancing school. Many of my patients practice the long swing in the office and give strangers the impression that they are practicing steps of a dance. One patient with imperfect sight from detachment of the retina recently told me over the telephone that he went to a dance the night before and although he lost considerable sleep, his sight was very much improved on the following morning.

Dancing is certainly a great help to keep things moving or to imagine stationary objects are moving, and is always recommended. Some people have told me that the memory of the music, the constant rhythmic motion and the relaxation, have improved the vision.

COMMON SENSE

By W. H. Bates, M.D.

Many people have asked me what I call my treatment. The question was a very embarrassing one because I really have no name to give it, unless I can say that my methods are the methods employed by the normal eye. When a person has normal sight the eye is at rest, and when the eye is at rest, strange to say, it is always moving to avoid the stare. When the eye moves it is possible to imagine stationary objects are also moving. When the normal eye stares at one point of a letter or at all parts of a letter the vision always becomes imperfect. Persons with imperfect sight are always staring. Under favorable conditions all persons with near-sightedness do not stare, do not try to see, and the near-sightedness disappears for a longer or shorter time; no exceptions have been observed. In other parts of this magazine I have mentioned this fact and recorded that even patients with 40 D have moments when they are not near-sighted when they do not try to see.

The fundamental truth which should be demonstrated by all persons who desire to be cured of imperfect sight is the fact that the memory of perfect sight can only be accomplished easily and without effort. Furthermore, the memory of imperfect sight is difficult and requires time and is never continuous. Another truth of practical importance is that one cannot remember perfectly and imperfectly at the same time. What is true of the memory is also true of the imagination and of the vision.

I am in the habit of testing the vision of persons with imperfect sight at fifteen or twenty feet. Then I have them close their eyes, rest them, and if possible forget that they have eyes by remembering other things which are of interest to them. When done properly, and most people if not all are able to do it properly, the vision is always temporarily improved.

I spoke to one of my patients after this had happened and asked the question, "What did you do to improve your sight?" The patient answered, "I do not know." This seemed to me a remarkable answer. I asked a second question, "What did I tell you to do?" The patient answered, "You told me to close my eyes and rest them." "What helped you then to see better?" "I do not know," answered the patient.

Then I had to start in and talk and explain and tell the patient that it was the rest that helped the patient and not any efforts that were made. It is a matter of common sense. Most people would realize that if they rested their eyes and their sight got better that the rest must have had something to do with it; and, strange as it may appear, I have seen very few people who could realize or understand this truth.

So many people ask me how my patients are benefited. Is it Christian Science, is it auto-suggestion, is it hypnotism, psychoanalysis, psychology, or has it to do in any way with mental science? The only answer that seems to me to approach the truth is "common sense." Now when I come to review my cases and try to fit common sense to the results obtained I get all mixed up. Most people have common sense, which is ordinary intelligence or the ability to do things in a reasonable, proper way. People who are highly educated, college graduates, professional men, teachers and college professors, would be expected to have a greater amount of common sense than ordinary persons, but I am sorry to say they do not. I have very little respect for mental science because of the numerous assumptions and theories that are advanced. A theory is always something which makes me uncomfortable. I have never been able to make any progress with a working hypothesis. All my facts which were of benefit to me have no connection whatsoever with mental philosophy. I wish to confess that it gives me a great deal of unholy delight to prove and demonstrate that all the theories of physiology are wrong. This is not a popular statement to make, but I do not cure my patients by being popular. The sweetest morsel on the tip of my tongue is to say what somebody else has said before, that logic is an ingenious method of concealing the truth.

When a problem comes to me which is very difficult for me to solve, instead of starting out with a working hypothesis it is my custom to accumulate as many facts as I possibly can, to analyze these facts in various ways and by every method known to science to try to discover whether my facts are true or not; and, believe me, that is not always an easy thing to do. Someone said to me that it was impossible to scientifically prove that my method for the prevention of myopia in schoolchildren ever actually did prevent myopia or nearsightedness; in other words, that it was impossible to prove a negative proposition, or that the children did not or were not prevented from acquiring imperfect sight. It has always given me great pleasure to make the statement that every child with normal eyes who has not worn glasses, who is under twelve years old, can improve their sight by reading the Snellen test card, first with one eye and then with the other, every day. It is a benefit if the pupil learns the letters on the test chart by heart. They all improve; when I say all, I mean all, there are no exceptions. I challenged the ophthalmologists of this country to bring forward one exception to any of my statements. One exception would prove that the statement is not a truth but at best only a working hypothesis.

What is it that improves the sight of these schoolchildren? I have already stated that when the sight is normal the eyes are at rest. When the child reads a familiar card with normal sight the eyes are at rest. Common sense, just ordinary common sense, would conclude from this fact that the vision was improved by rest. Some teachers improve the sight of their children by having them close their eyes for a few minutes or less, frequently during the school session. They told me it always improves the sight when tested either with a familiar card or when tested with an unfamiliar card. When a child cannot read the blackboard his sight is usually improved by closing the eyes and resting them for part of a minute or longer.

The cure of imperfect sight without glasses is not a matter which is complicated, which can only be explained by the abstruse incomprehensible theories of the professors of mental science. The truth is that all can be explained by common sense.

One day I was testing the sight of some schoolchildren. The teacher was interested in one boy. In order to illustrate to the teacher and to the children the bad effects of staring, I asked the boy to stare at the letter "F" on the bottom line of the Snellen test card at twenty feet. This card had been permanently fastened to the wall where all the children could see it from their seats and it had been in place for some months. When I asked him to do this he sullenly said to me, "Not for me; I tried it once and it gave me a headache and spoiled my sight. I am too wise to do it again."

The boy's common sense enabled him to realize that staring was a bad thing. I told the class that if they would all profit by his experience that they would never acquire imperfect sight and need glasses.

STORIES FROM THE CLINIC
No. 40: Palming
By Emily C. Lierman

One day a mother brought her little son, Joey, nine years old, to the Clinic to be fitted for glasses. His teacher in school thought he needed them. After Dr. Bates had examined his eyes with the retinoscope, I tested his sight with the test card and then I told the mother he could be cured without glasses. This interested her greatly. She had wonderful sight herself, for she could read the smallest letters on the card at more than fifteen feet. I gave her the Doctor's diamond type card, which she read with perfect ease at four inches and also at twelve inches from her eyes. She told me her age was thirty-eight and that she was the mother of ten children. Although she was poor, her clothes were neat and clean, and Joey was just as neatly dressed as she was. She looked at him smilingly and said, "Think of it, Joey, you don't have to wear glasses." Before this little talk Joey seemed scared to death, or as though something terrible was going to happen to him, but when his mother began to show confidence in me, he smiled and looked happy, as all normal boys do. Both watched me very closely as I explained the method of palming to them. Dr. Bates found no organic trouble with Joey's eyes, but just nearsightedness. At fifteen feet he read the 50-line before palming. After palming ten minutes, Joey obtained normal sight that day. When he read the card with each eye separately his left eye seemed to be the better of the two, because he made a few mistakes in reading the 10-line letters with his right eye. He was encouraged to palm again for a few minutes, and then he became able to read 15/10 just as well with his right eye as he could with the left. His mother stood where she could see all this, and beamed with happiness as she saw her little boy's sight improve. I started to explain to her the necessity of Joey resting his eyes as soon as he wakened in the morning, because he might have strained during sleep. Also to rest his eyes again at noon, after school and before bedtime. She listened very attentively and then she said, "Maybe you think you tell me something new, but I don't think so. All the time when I nurse my babies, I put up my one hand to my eyes as I close them, and I keep quiet while my baby is nursing. Then my baby goes to sleep quicker and easier, and I am rested too." I asked her with a great deal of surprise who taught her to do this, and she answered, "Why, nobody did. I found that out myself." She was thankful, however, that Joey did not need glasses, and promised to help him every day until his eyestrain was entirely relieved.

She returned a week later with a good report of her boy. The test card I gave him for home treatment was appreciated by the whole family. Joey's mother tested the sight of all her children and found two of her little girls also had eyestrain. She taught them to palm and cured them herself. Here was a busy mother, with ten American citizens to help support and educate, and yet found time to teach them how to obtain normal sight. Surely they are worthy members of our Better Eyesight League. I saw Joey and his mother but twice, but Joey had suffered no relapse, nor has there been any complaint regarding his eyes from the school he attends.

The last time I saw Joey he was anxious for me to know that his father, who has no trouble with his eyes at all, came home from his work one evening and thought the family were all playing peek-a-boo with him. The mother had them all busy palming, which was a strange sight to him.

Most people, like myself, have not the time to palm daily. However, if I suffer from eyestrain, which sometimes happens after a strenuous day, I find the memory of palming is all that I need to obtain relaxation. The memory swing, which Dr. Bates explained so tactfully in the March 1923 *Better Eyesight* magazine, has helped a great many patients. So it is with the memory of palming, or, in other words, remember how relaxed you were and how free from strain you were the last time you were able to palm successfully, and this will help you through the day while at work, or at the theatre, or any place where it is impossible to place the palms of your hands over your eyes.

A "BOOK PATIENT'S" EXPERIENCE

By Wm. Jay Dana, B. Sc., D.C.

As result of reading Dr. Bates' book, *Perfect Sight Without Glasses,* I was enabled to discard my glasses, which I had been wearing for twenty-one years. I first heard of Dr. Bates and his book through my old partner, a doctor who had seen him personally and was able to tell me the details of the Bates Method. This doctor gave me a copy of Dr. Bates' book in March of last year, and after reading it carefully I decided to lay aside my glasses. At that time I had so much astigmatism in my right eye that anything at which I looked appeared double or blurred. For the first five days after laying aside my glasses I had considerable pain in the muscles in my right eye, but I paid little or no attention to these pains, as I knew they were due to accommodation efforts of the extrinsic muscles of the eyeball. [More likely: the release of chronically tense extrinsic muscles that create astigmatism, and/or the contraction of complementary extrinsic muscles to bring the eyeball back to its normal, round shape.—TRQ] I relaxed as much as possible during this time, used the palming quite frequently and got as much sleep as I could. By the end of three or four weeks I began to pay no attention at all to my eyes, except to shift whenever I found that my vision was not as clear as usual.

Before using these simple methods as advocated by Dr. Bates, I would have a headache in a few moments' time due to eyestrain if I read without my glasses.

I did more reading last summer in three months' time than I had done before in a year, and in spite of, or perhaps because of it, my eyesight is better than it has been since I was a boy. I found that if my eyes became fatigued I could easily rest them by reading finer print, and as my work consisted of reading many of the technical journals, I found that I could do this with benefit, as most of the technical literature is in fine print.

I take great pleasure in recommending Dr. Bates' book and his method to my friends and patients, and everyone else who is interested in having perfect sight.

Very truly yours, Wm. Jay Dana, B. Sc., D.C., Carolina State College of Agriculture and Engineering, Raleigh, North Carolina.

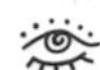

"A CHAIN IS ONLY AS STRONG AS ITS WEAKEST LINK"

By Minnie E. Marvin

In the lecture given last Monday evening before a body of chiropractic students and others numbering 200 or more, Dr. Bates demonstrated this fact very clearly in explaining his method. For the benefit of those living out of town who are unable to take advantage of these instructive talks, we will try to cover the important points discussed.

To begin with, Dr. Bates was in his finest oratorical form. His little anecdotes were genuinely appreciated, and it must be said here that in these he was not always the "hero."

It is always interesting to the new followers of Dr. Bates to learn how he came to discover the method that is revolutionizing the study of the science of the eye. This he told in his quiet, modest, matter-of-fact way, until those who knew him were almost tempted to cry out to the audience, "Let us tell you how Dr. Bates came to discover the facts he produces, and let us tell you how this scientist has been discouraged, handicapped, yes, and humiliated. Why? Because he thought for himself, and would not accept the theories that were presented to him." Our feelings notwithstanding, we did not say the things in our minds, and we venture to say, nevertheless, that everyone in the audience, be they doctor or layman, was now eager to learn more.

Dr. Bates then cited some of the theories under which the eye specialists are working today, and then, in opposition, offered his facts, which defy contradiction.

The first theory was that presented by Helmholtz, who was one of the greatest authorities on the physiology of the eye. He says that the eye changes its focus for near and distant vision by altering the curvature of the lens. Dr. Bates has shattered this theory by demonstrating on many pairs of eyes that the lens is not a factor in accommodation. In substantiation of the above, he told of an interesting experiment upon the eyes of a rabbit. The lens of the right eye was removed, each eye having been tested previously with the retinoscope and found to be normal. The wound was allowed to heal, and for a period of two years after, electrical stimulation always produced accommodation in the lensless eye precisely to the same extent as the eye having the lens. At a meeting of ophthalmologists of the American Medical Association, held in Atlantic City, Dr. Bates exhibited the subject in the anteroom, and to eye specialists from all over the world. Each one of them admitted that Dr. Bates was right, but in their subsequent articles never mentioned the fact.

Don't you see that there are exceptions to their old theories? This makes nothing more than a working hypothesis of the Orthodox Ophthalmology. Dr. Bates admits *no* exceptions. Not a single one. As he says so often, "If one exception to any statements that I have made in my lectures or in my book can be produced I will acknowledge my whole method to be wrong."

Secondly was the theory concerning presbyopia, commonly known as old-age sight. For centuries we have been led to believe that when one reaches the age of 45 or thereabouts, one was to expect an organic change to take place in the shape of the lens, which lessened the power of vision. This theory, too, was annihilated. Dr. Bates has proven that presbyopia is merely a functional derangement in the action of the extrinsic muscles and has cured thousands of this defect, including himself.

[While Dr. Bates' statements may or may not be proven, there is no *practical* difference to the thousands of people who have improved their eyesight and eliminated their need for corrective lenses by relearning correct vision habits.—TRQ]

In various experiments he has proven that age is positively no barrier to one wishing to attain perfect sight. He related the cases of the old gentleman, passed 106 years old, and the old "mammy" who lost track of her age after the 90th year. Both these were cured of old-age sight, together with other errors of refraction.

PARENTS' AND TEACHERS' PAGE

By Emily A. Meder

One of the teachers, who was attending a lecture at which Dr. Bates was expounding his treatment, explained that she was intensely interested in his method and would love to be the medium through which the children in her classes could attain better eyesight. She said, however, that inasmuch as she had no technical knowledge of the work, she was rather timid about attempting the method by herself.

For the benefit of those who are in a similar position, we want to say that no technical knowledge is necessary. If one realizes the harm done by glasses, and if one is desirous of helping those wearing them, then the good one can accomplish is unlimited.

The following instructions may be carried out either in the home or in the classroom, and while the form used is particularly applicable to teachers with large classes, it may be used in the home on a smaller scale. The installation of this method requires a little more time than is necessary for its continuation. The first step is to make a list of the children's names, together with their age and the date of the first examination. This requires about two minutes for each child. Place the Snellen test card on the wall, and have each one read as far as she can, first with one eye, and then with the other. The lines on the card are numbered. Place the child at a distance of ten feet, and if she can only see the top line which is a big "C" and line number 200, then her vision for that eye is 10/200. Her record will read as follows:

June 1, 1923	Age	Right Eye	Left Eye
Mary Anderson	12	10/200	10/100

Date of subsequent examinations: ________________

The above report indicates that Mary's sight is very defective. The line numbered 200 should be read at 200 feet by the normal eye. Here is a point to remember: when the denominator is greater than the numerator, the vision is defective.

It is not necessary to keep a daily record, but a general examination should be made every month and the improvement noted. The results will be astonishing. We have seen cases where the card was read every day in unison by the class, and was the means of raising the average 87%.

Many people question Dr. Bates as to how it is possible for the test card to make such radical improvements in children's eyesight, and he always replies that he is not certain which of the exercises are most beneficial, but seeing those black letters every day, and shifting the eyes from one letter to another breaks the stare, and tends towards complete relaxation, which is the keynote of the treatment. Concentration is the antithesis of relaxation, and if you are not relaxed, you strain. No good can be accomplished when one strains.

Another point often brought up is that a child may memorize the card. Dr. Bates says that in all the thousands of schoolchildren he has examined, many of whom have had the Snellen test card in their possession until the letters were bound to be memorized, he has never seen a case where a child would say that she could see the letter when she could not. You will find that the children are more interested in this than you would be led to believe.

Remember: *An ounce of prevention is worth a pound of glasses.*

BETTER EYESIGHT LEAGUE

By F. B. Rusk, Recording Secretary

The large room of the new headquarters of the Central Fixation Publishing Company was crowded to its utmost capacity at the May meeting of the Better Eyesight League.

Mr. M. F. Husted, Superintendent of Public Schools of North Bergen, New Jersey, was the speaker of the evening. Mr. Husted explained, with the aid of charts, the experiment he has been conducting during the past three years.

In the fall of 1919 a Snellen test of the eyes of all pupils in the North Bergen Schools was made. A Snellen test card was then placed in every classroom. Those children whose vision was defective were encouraged to read the card more frequently. In June 1920, a second examination was made in order to test the value of the methods used. The same experiment has been repeated each year since with amazing results. [See "An Educator Offers Proof" in the September 1922 issue.—TRQ]

After hearing of the remarkable benefits which accrue to children who practice central fixation, a visitor asked if there was any hope for the old folks. One of the audience volunteered that he was acquainted with a lady who had had a complete cure after wearing glasses for fifty-six years. As a result of her experience he had traveled 2,000 miles to see Dr. Bates (and attended the May meeting of the Better Eyesight League)!

In reply to the question as to whether astigmatism was curable, Dr. Bates said that if there was any one kind of astigmatism which was worse than the others, it was conical cornea—a condition with which he always had marked success.

EYES BUT THEY SEE NOT

By Emily A. Meder

The ostrich is known to be the swiftest of birds, and can outdistance the fastest horse with ease. Yet when he is attacked unexpectedly, or run into a cul-de-sac, he foolishly hides his head in the sand. He *doesn't wish to see.* Naturally his fate overtakes him, and he is doomed. His wonderful body, made especially for swift and long-distance running, his exceptional endurance, are assets which avail him nothing when he "sticks his head in the sand and will not see."

I have come in contact with people who have many desirable assets but when a thing looks a little "strange" they become dogmatic and refuse to learn. They literally stick their tails in the air and their heads in the sand. The same thing happens to them that happens to the ostrich. Their doom overtakes them. *They wear glasses.* As evidence of these "mental errors of refraction" I will tell of two instances which I noticed particularly.

In a popular magazine there appears an article each month by a very noted writer who gives beauty hints to women over forty years old. She gives very minute directions of the care of the hair, skin, teeth and figure generally, and I admit I was very surprised to see an item about the eyes. This, unfortunately, is a part of the physiognomy that is usually neglected by these Beauty Doctors. She explained that from her observations, many people received excellent relaxation by closing the eyes and forgetting that they possessed them, excluding all the light by putting the palm of the hands over the eyes very lightly, and thinking of black objects which tends to rest them more quickly. This interested me because this is part of Dr. Bates' own method. When I read on a little further, I was disagreeably astonished to read something like this—"that she had heard of a new body of oculists who say that they can cure eyes without glasses. This she says is impossible because when a woman reaches the age of forty, she simply has to fortify her eyes with glasses, as this has been done for centuries, and it does not seem possible that man has it in his power to cure the defects at this age."

This is a typical case of the ostrich again. Why doesn't this writer make herself more popular by believing this could be done, and by reading the book with an open mind. She is in a position to help thousands suffering with eye ills, and her scope is unlimited.

One more case of "mental blindness."

At a dinner given at the Hotel Astor under the auspices of the Society of Arts and Sciences, Dr. Bates was asked to speak, along with five or six other doctors, all specialists in their respective branches. Senator-elect Royal S. Copeland was Toastmaster, and a very good one he made. Everyone knows the far-reaching results of Dr. Copeland's administration when he was Commissioner of Health of the City of New York. The many improvements he made while holding that position are a credit to him. But even Dr. Copeland has a vulnerable spot that might be pierced.

Dr. Bates was the first to speak, and as he knew many others would talk after him, he limited his remarks to about ten minutes. He gave a brief synopsis of his method of treating imperfect sight, and ended by telling the audience that Germany had adopted his method, and was using it in all the schools. At the conclusion of his discourse and before the next speaker had been introduced, Senator Copeland thanked the Doctor for his remarks, and said that he was sorry that Dr. Bates did not have more time to explain his treatment but he had worn glasses so long, and besides now being a United States Senator, he was a hard man to convince.

We have no wish to "convince" anybody. If they read the book and assimilate the facts, they will convince themselves. PEOPLE WEAR GLASSES FROM HABIT, NOT BECAUSE THEY NEED THEM.

Better Eyesight
July 1923—Vol. VIII, No. 1

THE SHORT SWING

Many people with normal sight can demonstrate the short swing readily. They can demonstrate that with normal vision each small letter regarded moves from side to side about a quarter of an inch or less. By an effort they can stop this short swing, and when they are able to demonstrate that, the vision becomes imperfect almost immediately. Practicing the long swing brings a measure of relaxation and makes it possible for those with imperfect sight to see things moving with a shorter swing. It is a good thing to have the help of someone who can practice the short swing successfully. Ask some friend who has perfect sight without glasses in each eye to practice the variable swing as just described, which is a help to those with imperfect sight who have difficulty in demonstrating the short swing.

Nearsighted patients usually can demonstrate that, when the vision is perfect, with diamond type at the reading distance, one letter regarded is seen continuously with a slow, short, easy swing not wider than the diameter of the letter. By staring, the swing stops and the vision becomes imperfect. It is more difficult for a nearsighted person to stop the swing of the fine print, letter "O," than it is to let it swing. When the sight is very imperfect, it is impossible to obtain the short swing. Many people have difficulty in maintaining mental pictures of any letter or any object. They cannot demonstrate the short swing with their eyes closed until they become able to imagine mental pictures.

HENRY

By W. H. Bates, M.D.

Henry first visited me in New York about five years ago. At that time he was attending school in Connecticut. The boy was naturally of a friendly disposition. He had one virtue, which is not always found in New England or elsewhere: he asked no questions and required no explanations of anything that I might ask him to do. With him it was largely a business to be cured without glasses, and he left the solution of it entirely to me.

At his first visit his vision was less than one-half of the normal. He was wearing concave 1.50 D. S. with concave 0.25 D. C. 180 degrees. I told him that he was curable and demonstrated the fact by curing him temporarily, improving his sight to 15/10 with the aid of palming, shifting and swinging. He demonstrated that staring at one letter very soon lowered his vision, and that by shifting from one letter to another his vision improved. I asked him if he felt any different when his sight was good and when it was imperfect. He answered, "I know by the feeling in my mind, not my eyes, when I am straining and making my sight poor." This was an interesting statement and is remarkable in this way that he was the first patient I ever had who could realize that his myopia was due to a mental strain primarily. The mental strain produced the eyestrain. I asked him if he could remember mental pictures. He said that he could at times with benefit to his sight, but for some reason or other his memory was poor when he had imperfect sight. He demonstrated that when he remembered some letter of some object perfectly he did it quickly, easily and without any effort; but when he strained and tried hard to remember any mental picture he always failed. Furthermore, when he did remember the mental picture he always lost it when he strained or made any effort to remember it better. I spent a good deal of time with him all through his treatment in "Rubbing it in," as I called it. First he demonstrated that his vision was improved and became temporarily normal by resting, by not doing anything. Then, to see imperfectly, he had to strain, to work hard, and go to a lot of trouble. He was a very thoughtful person with a good deal of common sense and became able to profit from his experience.

To me his problem was not learning how to do things with his eyes, but to find out in some way how he could avoid doing anything. He repeatedly demonstrated that when his sight was normal he did not do anything, that anything he did was always wrong or always lowered his vision. He was very fond of shifting because by continually moving his eyes from one point to another, alternately closing his eyes frequently, required the ability to avoid the strain at first occasionally, later more frequently, until he became able to finally avoid the strain continuously. Many of my patients are cured by practicing one of the truths of normal sight, and he was one of them. The normal eye does not stare as long as it has normal sight; it is continually shifting to avoid the stare. He learned how to do this for a while, and then his mind would wander, and before he knew it he was staring and producing imperfect sight. He knew the proper thing to do and knew how to do it, but he often failed and lost his mental control. I said to him one time, "You have a bad habit of straining, you would be better off if you didn't have that habit." One way of getting rid of a bad habit is to acquire a beneficial habit. When you strain it makes you uncomfortable. When you shift and avoid the strain you are comfortable. Surely you should not hesitate to make the right choice. Keep shifting, enjoy yourself and be comfortable. Keep that in your mind a good deal of the time and as long as you are perfectly comfortable you know that you are not straining because the straining always makes you uncomfortable. As long as things are going all right and you are doing the right thing, then you do not need to ask yourself questions about shifting and palming and swinging; you are doing these things when you are perfectly comfortable.

Here was a boy who, like many boys, had his faults, but somehow or other they were not conspicuous. All his friends spoke well of him, and he had many. His best friend, the one who knew him the longest, was his father. Unfortunately his father was a very busy man who believed that he was doing the right thing by attending to his work and looking after his business affairs. Someone has said that the principal business of the world is children. If it were not for the children, no country would have a future. I believe this is a true statement and I believe it to the extent that I feel that the principal duty of every man, of every woman, is the business of looking after the children. Of what use is it to accumulate many dollars when your child goes around half blind wearing glasses? He is uncomfortable and not happy because of those glasses. I shall always criticize Henry's father. I do not believe I can criticize him too severely because he did not realize, and I could not make him realize, that for the best interests of his son that he should cure his own eyes for the benefit it would be to Henry. There wasn't very much the matter with his eyes, he could see perfectly at the distance without glasses, he only wore them occasionally when he had to read. Henry could have cured him of that. The father wearing glasses disturbed the mind of the son, and I have found during all these years that one of the greatest difficulties in curing children is to counteract the evil influence of the parents wearing glasses. Nearsightedness is contagious. Children are great imitators, and they consciously or unconsciously imitate the habits of their parents, even to the smallest detail. I have talked until I was all talked out trying to explain this fact to the parents of children who were wearing glasses. I have tested the sight of many thousands of children in public schools, and was very much impressed to find that in those classes presided over by teachers wearing glasses the percentage of imperfect sight in the pupils was very much increased, while in those classes where teachers did not wear glasses imperfect sight was less frequent.

Henry was an easy case to cure, as I said in the beginning; he obtained temporary perfect sight at the first visit. But why didn't he hold it; why did he have so much trouble in obtaining permanent benefit? The answer is that his father was at fault.

Henry enlisted and passed the eye tests without any difficulty. After the war was over Henry called to see me. Of course, my first question was, "How is your sight?" His laconic answer was, "Good."

As he had not been to see me in a long time, some years, I was more or less doubtful about his vision and tested him with a card that he had never seen before. I remember how he stood backed up against the opposite wall in order to get as far away as possible, and the speed with which he read the whole card with normal sight. "How did you do it?" I asked. He replied, "Shifting."

Some years later my attention was called to an article in a popular magazine which attacked my method of curing imperfect sight by treatment without glasses. In the next issue of the magazine appeared an article defending me, and signed with the initials of my dear friend, Henry.

STORIES FROM THE CLINIC

No. 41: Sarah

By Emily C. Lierman

A few years ago there came to our Clinic at the Harlem Hospital a curly-headed girl named Sarah, age twelve years. As she stood among patients who were waiting for treatment, I noticed how pretty she was. She was standing sideways with her right side toward me, and as I did not see her enter the room, I received a shock when I discovered that the left side of her face was distorted. I pretended not to notice anything wrong with her because she seemed very sensitive. However, her left eye appeared ready to pop out of its socket any moment, and both upper and lower eyelids were terribly inflamed. Dr. Bates explained the history of her case, and also the cause of her affliction, and then left her entirely in my care. She told me that at the age of four she became ill with cerebrospinal meningitis, and all of the left side of her body became paralyzed. Until she came to us she had been receiving treatment from nerve specialists, both in England, where she was born, and also in New York. Electric treatments were given without success. Money was not spared and all of her family sacrificed every penny for Sarah's medical treatment to bring about a cure. When one doctor failed, another was recommended by their friends. Finally, the family bank account dwindled to scarcely nothing and Sarah stopped treatment, believing that she could never be cured. Later, as I learned to know her better, I noticed that she was ever conscious of her trouble and would always turn the good side of her face toward me. There was one good thing about Sarah—she was never downhearted, or she never revealed it to me if she was. She was a good scholar at school and graduated at the age of 14 from the public school.

I tested her sight and she had normal vision, 10/10, in her right eye, and 10/50 with the left. I placed her in a comfortable position and showed her how to palm and told her not to remove her hands from her eyes while I was testing the sight of other patients. After a few moments I noticed while Sarah had her eyes covered that her face became terribly red and I wondered if she were comfortable or not. I spoke to her and she complained that she did not like to palm, that it made her nervous. I thought that she was not doing it right and explained to her again how easy it was to cover her eyes with the palms of her hands to obtain the relaxation which was necessary to improve the vision of her left eye. She very faithfully tried again but I noticed that she was getting more uncomfortable all the time. Her vision did not improve at all by the method of palming, so I tried her with the long swing which proved successful. I thought in time that Sarah would feel friendly toward the method of palming and that she would improve faster in that way, but I was mistaken.

For two years Sarah came to us at the Clinic quite regularly and in all that time I could not induce her to palm. She complained that it made her nervous. This was my first experience in all the years that I have been assisting Dr. Bates in that the patient could not be made comfortable by palming. The long swing was very helpful to her, holding her left forefinger in front of her or to the left side of her face, about six inches from her eyes and then slowly moving her head from shoulder to shoulder, blinking all the while she was doing this. At the first visit the vision of her left eye had improved to 10/30. Sarah was encouraged to do this long swing as many times during the day as it was possible for her to do it and she was reminded to blink her eyes very often, which she was not able to do at all with her left eye at the first visit. The upper lid of her left eye seemed stationary and she could not close this eye in sleep which gave her a strange appearance. As I never had a case like hers before, I was deeply interested and studied hard to find every possible way to help her. She was a dear bright little girl and was so willing to do everything that we wished her to do, to help in the cure of her eye. I asked Dr. Bates for permission to try helping her improve the condition of her left cheek and mouth, as well as her eye, as I thought that our method of relaxation might possibly do something for her face. The Doctor smiled his usual smile and said, "Well, you might try."

On her second visit to the Clinic her left vision had improved to 10/15 which was most encouraging to me. She told me that she had tried to palm at home just to please me, but every time she tried this it bothered her, but the long swing helped a lot. As time went on I told her to shorten the swing and move her head slowly from side to side, seeing things move opposite from the way her head was moving and this also gave her a great deal of benefit. Before she had been coming to us a month I noticed that the upper lid of her left eye was beginning to move and the inflammation which caused Sarah so much discomfort had almost entirely disappeared. Her vision stayed about the same, left 10/15, right 10/10. Always when she came, we went through the usual treatment of seeing things move opposite as she held her left forefinger to the left side or in front of her face. I sat before her, doing the treatment with her to encourage her to keep it up. During a period of eight weeks of this treatment her facial expression began to change for the better. It was more noticeable when she smiled. When I first saw her smile I noticed that her mouth would turn way over to the right side of her face.

(To be continued.)

Owing to the unusual nature of this case, and of the remarkable results obtained, Ms. Lierman is going to tell of it in detail, therefore it will be continued in the August number.

AN ENCOURAGING LETTER

By Elizabeth McKoy

I wish to tell of the results of Dr. Bates' methods of treatment on my eyes. Many times I have wished to tell of these results, but not wishing to trouble him have so far refrained.

I saw Dr. Bates first in October 1921, and since the first visit have not worn glasses. He and Ms. Lierman taught me to palm and to swing things and told me of ways to help schoolchildren. My eyes improve steadily though one of them is most of the time far from perfect as yet. I study the book and gain something from the magazine each month. As a member of the Better Eyesight League I have found that I help my own eyes most when helping others.

My brother has learned that palming and swinging will help his headaches. He came to me one day asking for some medicine for his head; I had nothing, but offered to help him. He declared he had only five minutes. I showed him how to palm and while he did it I sat beside him asking him to think of the different black objects I mentioned. I described shapes and parts of a number of familiar black objects, and he must have done his part well for at the end of the five minutes the headache was all gone much to his surprise! He has been sending his friends to me ever since. My mother's eyes are changing, second sight they call it, she palms when her eyes bother her and after palming finds she can read without her glasses.

In my home in North Carolina the past winter I have interested and helped many people. One woman who was a comparative stranger at first, I told of Dr. Bates simply because I was disturbed by her harassed look and the intense strain apparent in the eyes behind her glasses. She was willing to take off her glasses and also her daughter's glasses. She read [Bates'] book, subscribed to the magazine, and followed my instructions with much benefit. No one who asks for help fails to be interested in all I can tell them and more than half are willing to take off their glasses just on my say so. Of course those who know me well realize that whereas I was dependent on my glasses for seventeen years now I see as well or better without them. I still have difficulties, but am improving. The study becomes more and more interesting.

I am tempted to tell of some of my experiments which have especially interested me. My sight is excellent for nearby things, but I have astigmatism and cannot see so clearly in the distance. It took me months to find out for myself that I could see distant things best when I did not try to. After a good deal of practice each day I can make myself see the last line of the Snellen test card at ten feet with the worse eye. I do it best when I think of something entirely foreign to the subject or when I let people about me claim my attention as I look toward the test card. My little nephew often gets between me and the card and I find it a help instead of a hindrance when I take it calmly. Also, when I can bring up vividly to my memory attitudes and expressions of certain children or picture certain flowers in my garden, the small letters on the card will rush out at me black and distinct.

All winter in church I had time to practice a great deal. There were letters on a stained glass window above the altar. For months I could not make them out. Finally I discovered that the more closely I followed the thread of the sermon the more distinct the letters seemed, and one day as the minister was describing a scene which I could imagine vividly the letters were suddenly readable. They were gone again almost as soon; but I was able to bring them back. For this purpose one trick which succeeded admirably was to imagine that I could remove the flame-colored wings from the angel in the resurrection picture of the window and place them on the shoulders of the white-robed minister, return them to the angel and take them again and again. As soon as I could do it well, I could read the lettering. Another trick was to pick up with my eyes one of the brass vases on the altar and place it on the pulpit. There it would stand and at times be almost knocked off by the gestures of the speaker or momentarily be occupying the same position as his hand. As I look back on my childhood I remember that children are always imagining absurdities of this sort.

I practice on the streets and when no other letters are near I use moving automobile numbers for test cards. I found they generally passed too quickly for me to read. Then I discovered that I could take a glance, close my eyes quickly, then read unhurriedly with eyes shut and still have time to open my eyes and verify the numbers before they were out of sight. This pleased me as much as anything I had learned.

With children I have found that palming helped most when I read aloud to them. They all liked the swing and caught quickly on to it and also to my idea of seeing the letter best with a stolen glance.

I have enjoyed telling of Dr. Bates as much as I have enjoyed anything all winter. I have never once wished to put my glasses on again after the first visit, though for days I had many difficulties especially on the street.

Now I do not miss the glasses at all except for quite a distance and at the theatre. One most welcome result of the treatment is in connection with the severe headaches which I have always had. Always when these occurred, the pain in the eyes was acute. For the past year without glasses this eye pain has not been intense when the sick headaches came—thanks to Dr. Bates.

I do send him my sincere thanks for the results of his work with me. His book and the magazine have been of much value to me and to my friends. I have felt that the best way for me to show my appreciation was to tell of his work to as many as I saw that needed his help.

Sincerely yours, Elizabeth McKoy, Winchester, Massachusetts.

AN ENJOYABLE VACATION

By Minnie E. Marvin

Vacation time is with us again in all its glory, and most everyone is looking forward to some change in environment during the next few months. Some are pouring over "Blue Books" mapping out their trail for their auto camping trip. Others are concerned about the mode of bathing suit being used at the seashore this summer, while the rest are intent on the more dignified pastime of replenishing their wardrobes that they may more appropriately enjoy the splendors of the mountains.

Whether in the woods, at the seashore or in the mountains, we want to say to our friends and subscribers again, "Do not be tempted to wear sunglasses." Of course most of you who are familiar with Dr. Bates' book know the reason of this. He has proven again and again that the sun is very beneficial to the eye. Sometimes one experiences temporary discomfort, but this is not harmful.

This is the time of year when those wearing glasses, who have not had the good fortune to learn of Dr. Bates' method, find themselves more uncomfortable than ever. Eyeglasses are a handicap in every sport or pleasure in which one wishes to indulge, and it is for those who know how they can be dispensed with, to spread Dr. Bates' message. You will meet all cases of defective vision this summer, and when an opportunity presents itself, prove yourself a true friend, and tell those who will listen, just how the glasses can be left off and with a few moments spent in palming and swinging, the benefits will be readily manifested.

Last fall, we received quite a few testimonials from those who had learned of this work on their vacation and with the aid of the book were enabled to discard their glasses. We were also deluged with inquiries which were the result of these "vacation chats."

You will find that nine out of every ten people wearing glasses are only too pleased to learn how their eyes can be cured without them. They know that glasses do not eliminate the defects. They know that while in some cases temporary relief is afforded by the strong magnifying lenses, it stands to reason the eye is not functioning naturally since it is straining itself all out of shape to conform to the shape and strength of the glass lens.

While we are anxious for you to help as many people as possible, it is also our wish that all our friends continue to practice and help themselves during vacation. The following instance may prove of interest. A lady telephoned Dr. Bates this week asking him what she should do in regard to her son who is Dr. Bates' patient. They are going to travel through the state on a week's motor tour, and she was wondering if her son should palm while riding. Dr. Bates said that riding is extremely beneficial. The scenery, the road signs, and houses all seem to move, and this demonstrates the fact that the normal eye should never be stationary, but should continually see things moving. The boy while enjoying his trip can also practice swinging various objects. If he strains while traveling he can close his eyes and imagine the trees, the road, etc. This is equivalent to palming, and the mental relaxation is immediately apparent.

To get back to the main point at issue. When one meets a friend anxious to learn how to get rid of glasses, and all the attending discomforts, tell him all you know. We are very busy in our new office, but we shall be glad to give all the information at our command, and to explain any parts of the book that may appear ambiguous.

We are looking forward to encouraging reports from all our friends at the end of vacation time. Take your book *Perfect Sight Without Glasses* and your Snellen chart with you and you will find that your vacation is a happier one in a great many ways.

QUESTIONS AND ANSWERS

Q–1. Why is it a rest to read fine print? I should think it would be more of a strain.

A–1. Fine print is a relaxation, large print a menace. Send for the December 1919 number which explains this in detail.

Q–2. My son is taking treatment for squint. While on auto trips is it necessary for him to palm continually?

A–2. No. The finest thing he can do is to see things moving. He can do this to great advantage in a car. If his eyes burn or seem tired, he can then palm occasionally.

Q–3. I am 75 years old. Do you mean to say that you can make me see with normal vision?

A–3. We most certainly do. Old-age sight is not incurable.

Q–4. I still cannot visualize "black"; what else can I use as a substitute?

A–4. Don't try to see anything. If it is an effort to visualize black, think of something that is pleasant, for instance, a field of daisies, a sunset, etc. The result will be just as beneficial.

Q–5. Must the body be at rest before the eyes can be cured?

A–5. When the eyes are relaxed, the whole body is relaxed.

Better Eyesight
August 1923—Vol. VIII, No. 2

SCHOOL NUMBER

THE SNELLEN TEST CARD

The Snellen test card is used for testing the eyesight. It is usually placed about 20 feet away from the patient. He covers each eye alternately, and reads the card as well as he can. Each line of letters is numbered with a figure which indicates the distance that it should be read with the normal eye. When the vision is recorded, it is written in the form of a fraction. The numerator being the distance of the patient from the card, and the denominator denoting the line read. For example: If a patient at 10 feet can only read the line marked "100," the vision is written 10/100 or 1/10. If the patient at 20 feet can read the line marked "10" the vision is recorded as 20/10, which means that the sight is double that of the average eye. Reading the Snellen test card daily helps the sight. Children in a public school with normal eyes under 12 years of age who have never worn glasses were improved immediately by practicing with the Snellen test card. Children with imperfect sight also improved, and with the help of someone with perfect sight, in time the vision becomes normal without glasses. Schoolchildren oftentimes are very much interested in their eyesight and what can be accomplished with the help of the Snellen test card. They have contests among themselves to see who can read the card best in a bright light, or on a rainy day when the light is dim. Many of them find out for themselves that straining makes the sight worse, while palming and swinging improve their vision. Many of them become able to use the Snellen test card in such a way as to relieve or prevent nervousness and headaches. Many boards of educations hesitate to be responsible for any benefit that may be derived from the Snellen cards in the schools.

HYPERMETROPIA IN SCHOOLCHILDREN

By W. H. Bates, M.D.

Hypermetropia, or farsightedness, is more frequent in schoolchildren than is myopia. The statistics average in the lower grades about ten percent myopia and eighty percent or more of hypermetropia. In higher grades the percentage of myopia is increased while that of hypermetropia is decreased.

It has been generally believed for more than one hundred years that while myopia is usually acquired by schoolchildren, hypermetropia is always present at birth. Many physicians who study the eyes of schoolchildren have had more interest in hygienic methods of myopia prevention and have recommended better schools, prescribed the early use of glasses and other measures to lessen the number of children who become nearsighted after they were at school. The prevention of hypermetropia was ignored and I have never seen any article devoted to the prevention of hypermetropia in schoolchildren. In the first place it is very difficult to prove or to demonstrate the amount of hypermetropia in young children with any degree of accuracy. I spent many weary hours many years ago when I prescribed glasses, trying to measure hypermetropia with the eye under the influence of eyedrops. Twenty years ago I first introduced my method for the prevention of imperfect sight in children and kept records of the vision of the children from year to year, for eight years in one school of about two thousand pupils. In New York City I have acquired a much larger experience. The symptoms of hypermetropia were more uncomfortable and interfered much more with the mental efficiency of the children than did myopia. Most children with myopia were able to read with comfort and their imperfect sight for distance is only inconvenient at certain times, but children with hypermetropia not only have difficulty in seeing near but they also have trouble in seeing objects at a distance. Some hypermetropes have just as poor sight as children who have only myopia. Hypermetropia not only impairs the vision more than does myopia but it is associated often with a great many more uncomfortable symptoms, pain, headache, fatigue. In short, hypermetropia interferes seriously with schoolwork much more than does myopia. A great many children leave school because they cannot stand the discomfort of their eyes suffering from hypermetropia and those who continue their schoolwork suffer in many ways. They are unable to read without pain and fatigue and the memory is impaired, and they fall behind in their classes and their school life is a burden. Surely it is more important to study the problems of hypermetropia than those of myopia.

The condition of the eyes at birth has been a matter of discussion for many years. Some of the early statistics recorded considerable myopia, 90%, others found no myopia and the eyes were apparently normal. It is difficult to draw correct conclusions from most statistics.

For some years I made it a habit to test the eyes of newborn children a half-hour after birth and to examine the eyes again at regular intervals. Some children's eyes were examined every hour with the aid of the retinoscope and the eyes under the influence of eyedrops. The characteristic of them was the variability in the amount of hypermetropia. At certain hours the eyes would be apparently normal, a half-hour later they would be hypermetropic in one or both eyes; at a later period, mixed astigmatism in one eye and the other eye normal or hypermetropic. At a still later period both eyes normal. A week later both eyes might be normal or both eyes might have hypermetropia in the morning and be normal in the afternoon. Usually six months or a year later the eyes became more continuously normal. At four years old and six years old, just before they began school, the eyes of the children were usually normal. After being in school for a year or more, hypermetropia began to be manifest and increased with each succeeding year. Myopia did not appear to any great extent before the age of ten or twelve and increased while the hypermetropia appeared to diminish. I have seen some children ten years old with normal eyes, at eleven years with hypermetropia, at twelve years old myopia, at thirteen hypermetropia, at fourteen the eyes apparently normal. This variability of the eyes of young children is a matter that should be considered very seriously. Those children who practiced with the Snellen test card every day with the help of the teachers, improved. The myopia disappeared, the astigmatism disappeared, the hypermetropia disappeared and the eyes became normal. Coincident with the improvement in the sight, teachers informed me that there was a wonderful gain in the efficiency of the children. There are teachers in the city of New York still using my method for the prevention of imperfect sight in children who have obtained so much benefit from its use that they are continuing to practice it although they were ordered by the Board of Education more than ten years ago to stop using my method.

It is a great temptation to put glasses on children for the correction of hypermetropia. The glasses for the correction of hypermetropia are magnifying glasses and their effect is to enlarge the fine print of schoolbooks to such a degree as to make it much easier for the children to read.

Children who are under a strain and have imperfect sight find their vision or their ability to read improved very much by glasses, much more so than the children who wear glasses for nearsightedness. There have been many plausible theories which have encouraged eye physicians to prescribe glasses for many children who do not manifest a very high degree of hypermetropia. It is possible to put glasses on children who have normal sight, and by compelling them to wear the glasses continuously they develop hypermetropia and become able to see with the glasses. In fact there are very few people with normal sight but who can, by wearing glasses continuously, become able to see at the distance with glasses for the correction of hypermetropia when they do not have it, just as there are children who can wear nearsighted glasses and see with them although their vision may be perfectly good without the glasses.

If a child has headaches, and many children do have headaches from nervousness, from stomach trouble, conditions which often disappear by simple treatment and rest, I believe it is much better to have the children rest their eyes when they are in this condition, for a few days or a week or two because many recover without the need of glasses. Very few eye specialists realize the facts and, without even considering the possibilities that the headaches might come from something else than the eyes, have prescribed glasses whether the children needed them or not. I do not believe that any children with normal eyes, under twelve years old, ever recover or are benefited to any great extent by their use. It seems to me very much like a crime to compel children to wear glasses when their sight for distance and for near is perfectly good without them. The oculists will tell you all about latent hypermetropia, which means, in the mind of the physician, that the child is really in need of glasses although the sight is normal. They believe that the child really has hypermetropia which is concealed or corrected by a strain of a muscle inside the eyeball and that it is the strain of this muscle to correct the hypermetropia which causes the headaches, or the nervousness, or the stomach troubles or any other disease of the body generally. Some have gone to an extreme and claim that epilepsy, St. Vitus' Dance, deafness, diseases of the chest, diseases of the liver and many other diseases are caused by a strain of a muscle inside of the eyeball. This theory is wrong and the published evidence is conclusive that no muscle inside the eyeball is a factor in the focusing power of the eye.

Low degrees of farsightedness are readily curable, but in a great many cases which have convex 4, 7, or more degrees of error, the cure is for most people, or to most eye specialists, very incredible. One of my patients had convex 7 D. S. She could hardly see the large letter on the Snellen test card without her glasses. To read was impossible. After a few treatments her vision became normal at 20 feet, and she read diamond type perfectly at less than 10 inches. She wrote me a letter recently as follows, "My eyes are behaving wonderfully well. At one time it was impossible for me to read even with my glasses in a moving train. Today I read three columns of the newspaper without any trouble." Her letters are very legible and written without glasses.

STORIES FROM THE CLINIC

No. 42: Sarah (continued)

By Emily C. Lierman

Sarah seldom missed a Clinic day and she was very faithful in her treatment at home. Within a year's time she became able to smile with her mouth almost straight. I decided to try out a few ideas of my own, and suggested to her that a mirror might be of benefit in helping her to speak and smile with her mouth straight all the time. As Sarah did not like palming, I had difficulty in getting her to imagine things perfectly with her eyes closed. She had no mental pictures. Below I describe how she obtained them. The mirror would help her to watch her mouth while she was talking or studying her lessons. I told her to go into a room by herself and practice for at least an hour every day. She was to study her lessons and recite poetry out loud while looking at herself in the mirror, and to see how straight she could keep her mouth during this performance. I told her to remember, while at school, how she appeared while looking in the mirror reciting her lessons. I was amazed at the result, and so were Sarah's friends, as well as herself. This is the way she obtained the imagination of mental pictures. I always asked her to repeat the alphabet very slowly each Clinic day. After a while she became able to pronounce each letter of the alphabet with her mouth perfectly straight. She could never do this correctly unless she blinked her eyes for each letter. This may sound silly to the reader, but when Sarah did not blink before repeating a letter after me, she stared, and not only did she say the letter with her mouth crooked, but her left eye would bulge almost out of its socket. After Sarah noticed this wonderful improvement, she very often had a surprise for me when she came. One day we were late for the Clinic, but there was Sarah, sitting patiently with the rest, eager to tell me of some wonderful thing she was able to do. When her turn came, she whispered in my ear, "What do you think I can do now? I can wiggle my left ear." It sounded so funny that I wanted to laugh, but Sarah was so serious about it that I dared not. Strange to say, when I asked her to do it for me, before she did the swing, without first closing and opening her eyes, she was unable to move her ear. But when she started to move her head slowly from left to right and began to blink her eyes, she wiggled her left ear, which greatly amused the children awaiting treatment. Two years had passed and Sarah still had hopes that we could cure her, and her mother and father were very grateful because of her improved condition.

She came one day with a sty on the upper lid of the left eye. When I remarked about it, she said she had been troubled with sties for many years, and at times they were very painful. I spoke to Dr. Bates about it, and he prescribed eyedrops and salve, which gave her some relief, but the sties appeared again from time to time. At my suggestion, Sarah acquired the habit of closing her eyes frequently most of the time, day or night, while she was awake. She was permanently relieved. She believed, as I do, that rest and relaxation helped in getting rid of the sties altogether.

At school one day she passed one of her former teachers in the corridor. This teacher had not seen Sarah for a year or more. She stopped and asked if she were not a sister to Sarah. "Why, no," she answered, "I am Sarah." The teacher looked at her in astonishment and said, "I did not know you, dear; your smile is so different, and your left eye looks so much better." Sarah told her about Dr. Bates and his method of curing people without glasses. This teacher had progressive myopia for many years, and suffered greatly with her eyes. What Sarah told her did not convince her at the time, that she might also be cured, but about six months later sixteen girls from her classroom came to us at the Clinic for eye treatment. When she saw that their glasses had been removed from their eyes, and that they had improved faster in their studies, she called to see Dr. Bates at his office. In less than a year's time she herself was able to see without glasses. Every Clinic day Sarah repeated the letters of the alphabet faithfully, until she could say them with her mouth perfectly straight.

Then one day she had another surprise for me. Something she had never been able to do in all her life. She learned to whistle with her mouth straight. What a wonderful stunt that was for Sarah. This she could not do unless she first practiced the swing. Rest or relaxation always relieves tension of the body as well as the eyes. I wish to emphasize the value of rest and relaxation obtained by the swing and by blinking in curing all diseases of the eye, no matter what the cause may be.

My experience in the treatment demonstrated that many popular theories of the cause of paralysis of the motor nerves are wrong. For example, it is generally believed that when a motor nerve ceases to function properly, the recovery cannot take place until some disease or permanent organic condition is relieved. Sarah became able to close her eye quickly almost completely, after practicing the swing, which could not have occurred if the paralysis of the nerves was of a permanent nature. I am aware that cerebrospinal meningitis is caused by a germ, which is an important factor in the destruction of the nerves which control the muscles of the eye and face. I do not think that anybody will maintain that the swing had anything to do, directly or indirectly, with the germs of the disease, or with the results of the inflammation caused by the germs. My experience with the treatment of other cases of paralysis of the muscles of the eyes, caused by infection, confirms my belief that the paralysis is not due so much to local changes in the nerves as it is to mental causes. Sarah was pronounced incurable by many prominent, capable nerve specialists. I believe that one reason why local treatment did not help her was because she had no trouble with the nerves sufficient to produce the paralysis. The only treatment which helped her was mental relaxation obtained by the swing. It was the strain of her mind which produced all the symptoms of paralysis. She had no more trouble when her mind was at rest.

WHAT THE SILVER JUBILEE OMITTED

By Emily A. Meder

Civic interest was thoroughly aroused at the recent exhibition at New York's Twenty-fifth Anniversary. What old, half-forgotten memories surged through my mind as I looked once more at the obsolete horse-drawn streetcars. While gazing at these, they seemed to fade away before my sight (complete relaxation, not eccentric fixation), and I recalled the trips I used to take in these cars in the past. With a stiffly starched frock and, if I were extra stylish, a little handkerchief tucked in at the waist, I trudged beside my Dad en route to the streetcar. Upon boarding we sat peacefully for an hour and a half before we reached our destination, the Aquarium; one hour there looking at the wonders of the sea, and another two hours to get home. Practically the whole afternoon consumed for what can now be accomplished in about two hours. No wonder we swelled with pride while looking at the evolution of the various vehicles, instruments, machinery, and public conveniences. I only had one regret. Great effort, both physical and mental, was manifested in the production of such superior tools with which the humans work, but the same detailed thought was not given to devise ways for us to obtain the utmost efficiency from the greatest tool of all—

our body. I readily admit that great strides forward have been made in medicine, surgery, dentistry, and industrial appliances; but we are, in one respect, just where we started one hundred and fifty years ago. *People still wear glasses.* The Jubilee could have produced no greater thrill for me if there had been a separate showcase, with a pair of glasses carefully protected, and marked *extinct*.

There is an expression used greatly of late which, by the way, should be discarded with glasses, and that is, "Better late than never." People who apply this maxim to their daily lives are usually "fired" from their positions or are the onlookers of life, and at the tail end at that. However, to go on, Dr. Bates' work is becoming better known than ever before, and the papers are wildly clamoring for interviews, until it seems as though the public was trying to make up for lost time. We can truthfully say that it is better to come late than not at all, but looking at this from an other angle, just think of all the people who could have evaded untold misery, and even agony, if they had known of this work before.

One lady reporter had heard of Dr. Bates' cure of imperfect sight without glasses, and came for an interview about a week ago. Dr. Bates saw that she had imperfect sight, and in order to determine the trouble he applied the retinoscope, which tells at a glance the condition of the patient's eyes.

The young lady was intensely interested in this instrument as Dr. Bates explained its use to her. He also told her of one of his discoveries regarding this. Telling lies is bad for eyes. If a patient lies, the retinoscope will indicate that the shape of the eyeball has been sufficiently altered to make the focus imperfect. Defective vision is caused by strain, and to lie requires an effort or strain. Practice, of course, makes perfect, but even those accomplished in the art of "fine fabricating" have to make more of an effort than they do when telling the truth. The mental effort, therefore, produces a slight strain, which is immediately discovered by the retinoscope.

This piece of news evidently interested the reporter more than the other discoveries made by Dr. Bates, as she wrote an article dealing with the retinoscope alone. Since that time reporters have been writing about this, claiming that Dr. Bates has found a better "truth detector" than scopalamin. We know this to be true, because exceptions have been found in the use of scopalamin, whereas the retinoscope reflects the natural change in the eyeball, and this is infallible.

One of the reporters from a large city paper asked innumerable questions relative to the discovery and use of the lie-exposing qualities of the retinoscope. When these were answered to his satisfaction, I asked him why he was dwelling so much on the novel and sensational properties of this instrument, rather than the prevention and cure of imperfect sight. He answered in a way that rather dampened my good opinion of the sagacity and intelligence of the average newspaper reader. "The public is always on the lookout for something novel that will insure a thrill. Something that they can take in at a glance, which doesn't need to tax their thinking capacity. The retinoscope will supply them with a topic of conversation for a time, and they can make witty quips about installing one in the home to find out the true relation of the family budget to the dressmaker's bills." I suppose this is true, but wouldn't the public be doubly thrilled and excited if it were to be made plain to them that glasses are wrong, that they can dispense with them, and last, but not least, can cure themselves?

I hope that we all may be able to visit the next anniversary of New York City and note some of the great improvements made in the human physique, among and foremost of these being the prevalence of perfect sight and absence of glasses from all. This is coming gradually to be sure, but inevitably.

A GAME TO CURE STAGE FRIGHT

By Florian A. Shepard

"Marian is going to clap part of this piece for us before she plays it on the piano," I said to our friends at the June Recital. She wanted to because she loves to "clap" any music, and she knew she would play all the better for it.

She knew the piece perfectly, so for the sake of the audience I asked, "What time is this piece written in?" A terrified look came into her eyes, and she stared blankly. At any other time she would have answered readily and delightedly. Here was the time for our "game."

"Shut your eyes, dear," I suggested. "Can you see a picture of the piano keys?" A smile spread over her face and she nodded happily. "Now, can you see a picture of the printed music? Do you see the measure full of chords—one for each beat?" She saw them, counted them, and told us what kind of notes they were; then she remembered the time signature.

After that everything went happily and smoothly. The memory of perfect sight had helped her to forget her fear and relax while she did her part. It has helped Marian (and other pupils) many times in her lessons when she was disturbed over some mistake or supposed difficulty.

If she repeatedly makes the same mistake from a wrong habit formed at home, and fails to correct it when she tries,

I get her to close her eyes and see a "picture" of the right finger on the right note at the right time. When she opens her eyes, she usually plays the passage correctly. The memory of perfect sight helps her to relax mentally and physically, and so she gets a fresh start.

I have always asked "leading questions" when a child seemed rattled; but by helping him with "mental pictures," I have demonstrated that a pupil can think and act more naturally and efficiently. This game quiets him when he is excited or hurried, and rests him from strain.

BETTER EYESIGHT LEAGUE

Notwithstanding the fact that the New York City Silver Jubilee was at its height only one block away, and that the evening was one more conducive to a nice cool "bus" or boat ride, the meeting room of the Central Fixation Publishing Company was filled to capacity long before the meeting was called to order.

Ms. Hurty, in her very capable and business-like manner, presided, and after discussing some "old business" which has been a source of confusion to a few of the members, introduced Dr. Cornelia Brown, of East Orange, who was scheduled to be the principal speaker of the evening.

Dr. Brown is certainly a strong enthusiast for Dr. Bates' method of curing imperfect sight by treatment without glasses, and she knows whereof she speaks, for not only has she cured her own eyes, after wearing glasses for twenty years, but she has had great success in treating her patients. A year ago she started a Better Eyesight League in East Orange, and it is growing not only in size, but in popularity, ever since. She told of many experiences, and the results have been such that no one hearing her would have the slightest misgiving about their own particular case, be it ever so serious. Dr. Brown emphasized the fact that what impressed her most was the naturalness, the simplicity of this treatment. When one has imperfect sight, one has to go to a great deal of trouble to keep it imperfect. One strains, and stares continually, which is not the normal thing to do. The normal eye is forever moving, and constantly sees things move, not by making an effort, but by doing the most natural thing in the world—relaxing.

QUESTIONS AND ANSWERS

Q–1. Which is more beneficial, the short or the long swing?

A–1. The short swing, if you can maintain it.

Q–2. I find that when I imagine a period, and try to hold it, it causes discomfort. Why is this?

A–2. You are straining. Never try to hold anything. Imagine the period moving from left to right. This overcomes strain.

Q–3. I have great difficulty in seeing things move.

A–3. This is the cause of your defective vision. The normal eye sees things moving continually.

Q–4. Are the movies harmful?

A–4. No. Quite the contrary.

Better Eyesight
September 1923—Vol. VIII, No. 3

AIDS TO SWINGING

It is possible for most people to do a very simple thing—to move the fingernail of the thumb from side to side against the fingernail of one finger. This may be done when the patient is in bed or when up and walking around the house, in the street or in the presence of other people, and all without attracting attention. With the aid of the movement of the thumbnail, which can be felt and its speed regulated, one can at the same time regulate the speed of the short swing. The length of the swing can also be regulated because it can be demonstrated that when the body moves a quarter of an inch from side to side that one can move the thumb from side to side. If the long swing is too rapid it can be slowed down with the aid of the thumbnail; when it is too long it can be shortened. At times the short swing may become irregular and then it can be controlled by the movement of the thumbnail. It is very interesting to demonstrate how the short swing is always similar to the movements of the fingernail. One great advantage connected with the short swing is that after a period of time of longer or shorter duration, the swing may stop or it may lengthen. It has been found that the movement of the thumb maintains the short swing of the body, the short swing of the letters or the short swing of any objects which may be seen, remembered or imagined. A letter "O" with a white center can only be remembered continuously with the eyes closed when it has a slow, short, continuous, regular swing and all without any effort or strain. The imagination may fail at times but the movement of the thumb can be maintained for an indefinite period after a little practice. One can more readily control the movement of the thumb instead of the eye.

DODGE IT

By W. H. Bates, M.D.

Whenever your sight improves, shift quickly to something else. Dodge your improved vision. Whenever you see things imperfectly shift your eyes quickly to something else. Dodge your imperfect sight. To stare always lowers the vision. Do not stare. Dodge it. It is interesting to demonstrate the great fact that perfect sight comes so quickly that you cannot avoid seeing things perfectly. The long swing is a great benefit as long as you dodge the improvement in your sight. The short swing requires more relaxation, and to dodge the improvement in your vision is more difficult. Practice the swing which gives you the best vision, or the vision that you are able to dodge.

The eye should always be sufficiently relaxed so that you will be able to dodge. One patient was wearing very strong glasses concave 15 D. S. with which he obtained vision of only 20/70. Without his glasses he was able to remember a letter or a period perfectly as long as he did not try to see anything. With the retinoscope it was demonstrated that when his memory was perfect his eyes were normal; he had no nearsightedness. As soon as he tested his sight he lost his memory, the myopia or nearsightedness returned, and his vision became very imperfect. By practicing most of the time out of doors or in the house on ordinary objects, he became able to dodge any improvement in his sight, but not enough in the beginning, or not quickly enough, to avoid the fact that his vision in a moment became worse. He was unable to do much with the Snellen test card at first, and the temptation to stare and not dodge prevented him from shifting from one object to another quickly enough to retain his perfect memory. He finally became able to dodge any improvement in his sight before his memory failed. At the end of a week he reported one day when he came in to see me that he was cured. I tested his ability to dodge any improvement in his sight and found it as good as that of the normal eye. He could not only dodge the improvement in his sight for ordinary objects, but had at last become able to do it when he looked at the Snellen test card.

I asked him, "Can you look at the bottom line at twenty feet for so short a time that you do not lose your perfect memory?" "Yes," he answered. "Can you read any letters on the bottom line?" "I cannot help but read them."

Another patient whose vision had been equally as poor and who had nearsightedness as well was very much benefited by the memory of a short swing of her body, about one-quarter of an inch. She could maintain this swing continuously with her eyes closed, and almost as continuously when she would look at a blank wall where there was nothing to see. When she regarded the bottom edge of the card with a perfect memory of a short body swing, the letters became perfectly black but she could not at first shift her eyes, or dodge the improvement in her sight quick enough to maintain the memory of the body swing. By practicing at all times and in all places, in the house or on the street, her ability to dodge became better. It was such a shock to her to read the bottom line at six feet without glasses that she became panicky and lost her mental control, failed to dodge, and lost her improved vision. Perfect dodging of improved vision can only be done perfectly by the normal eye. The normal eye does not have normal sight continuously unless it shifts or dodges what it sees at frequent intervals.

When dodging or shifting, the shorter the shift the better provided one sees best where he is looking and sees worse all parts not regarded. One may shift to the right of the letter when the letter is to the left of the point regarded, and then shift to the left of the letter when the letter is to the right of the point regarded. Every time the eyes move to the right the letter moves to the left, every time the eyes move to the left the letter moves to the right and by doing this a few times most people become able to imagine that when the eyes move, the letter appears to move in the opposite direction. This is called The Swing, and when one is able to imagine a letter moving or swinging from side to side, the letter is not regarded directly, the stare is prevented by the shifting or dodging, and the vision is improved. When one regards a small letter of the Snellen test card at a distance where it can be seen perfectly and continuously, most people can demonstrate that they do not see the right-hand side best all the time or the left hand best all the time, but that they are shifting from one part of the letter to another, and this may all be done unconsciously. If one, however, stares at one part of the letter continuously the vision soon becomes blurred. It is necessary to keep dodging from one part of the letter to another. Every time the eyes move, one can imagine the letter moves in the opposite direction. Staring at some point of the letter continuously always blurs the sight.

Central Fixation

When the eye sees best where it is looking it is called *central fixation*. Of course when one sees one point best it must see all other parts worse. It is a great help in accomplishing central fixation to ignore or dodge all other objects or letters. To see [objects in the peripheral vision—TRQ] worse may require in a way greater rest of the mind because in central fixation a great many more things are seen worse and only one thing is seen best. It must be borne in mind that dodging may be done right or it may be done wrong like many other methods of improving the sight. Dodging is done properly when things are ignored. We do not think so much of the objects seen worse as we do of the object which is seen best. It is impossible to have perfect sight without central fixation. Central fixation is demonstrated to be a passive condition of the mind and is always accomplished without effort. It is necessary then to dodge the objects not regarded.

Blinking

It is a rest to the eyes to close them and keep them closed for a few minutes or a half-hour or longer. When the eyes are open the vision is usually improved for a moment or longer. The normal eye can look at a small letter of the Snellen test card and see it continuously but when it does so the letter is always moving and the eyes are not kept open all the time. Closing the eyes effectually dodges perfect or imperfect sight. Usually unconsciously the normal eye closes and opens quite frequently and at irregular intervals and for very short spaces of time [1/40th of a second—TRQ]. Most people can demonstrate that when they regard a letter they are able to see quite clearly, it is possible for them to consciously close their eyes and open them quick enough and see the letter continuously. This is called *blinking* and it is only another name for dodging. Dodging what? Dodging the tendency to look steadily at things all the time. All the methods which have been recommended for the improvement of the vision, central fixation, palming, swinging, blinking can all be grouped under the one word—dodging.

One of the characters in *Oliver Twist,* by Charles Dickens, was called the "Artful Dodger." Persons with good sight may not be artful but they certainly are good dodgers.

STORIES FROM THE CLINIC

No. 43: Cured in One Visit

By Emily C. Lierman

A mammy came to our Clinic complaining of great pain in the back of her eyes. She had visited a doctor before she heard of Dr. Bates and was told that her eye trouble came from indigestion and eating wrong food. After trying a diet for six months which was prescribed for her, with the result that the pain in her eyes still continued, she came to us with very little hope of being cured. After I had taken her record, name, age which she said was 32, address, and where she was born, I asked her if she had ever worn glasses.

"No Mam," said she, "And you can never make me wear them. I hate them, I do." She went off on a blue streak relating her family history. "You know, Mam, my mother had only one bad habit until she died, and thank the Lord it wasn't wearing glasses. She lived a good simple life, but my, how she did love her corn-cob pipe. But she never committed the sin of wearing glasses."

Well, this was a new one on me. I have been treating many patients for eyestrain since my work began with Dr. Bates, but this was the first one who thought that wearing glasses was committing a sin. Most people think it adds to their appearance to wear glasses and many times the Doctor was asked to prescribe plain window glass so that they could wear glasses.

I tested mammy's sight with the test card which was 10/30 with each eye. I moved the card only one foot farther away and this caused such a strain that she could only see the 40-line. Then I told her to palm and asked her to describe one of the letters she saw on the card. As she did not answer me right off I thought she had not heard me so I repeated it. She answered, "Do you know Mam, for a minute I couldn't remember a single letter." I explained to her that such was often the case; imperfect sight, imperfect memory. I pointed to the letter "E" and asked her to close her eyes and describe it. This she did by saying it had a straight line at the top, also to the left and bottom and that the right side was open. Before mammy opened her eyes I moved the card still farther away, which was now fifteen feet to be exact. Mammy had been palming about five minutes, still remembering the letter "E" of the 40-line of letters. I stood beside the card with my finger pointing to the first letter next to the bottom line, called the 15-line. Then I said, "Before you open your eyes please remember that you must not try too hard to see the letter I am pointing at. If you do not see the letter immediately, do not worry about your failure to do so but close your eyes again and remember your 'E' for a few minutes." Mammy opened her eyes and said the letter I was pointing at was an "R," which was correct. We were both very happy at the result but I had her close her eyes again and remember the "R" better than she saw it. In less than five minutes she stopped palming and read all of the 15-line correctly. I produced another card—which she had not seen, and she was able to read the same line of letters as well. This meant that she had normal vision, 15/15. Mammy thought she was all cured, but I had my doubts as to her being able to read fine print. When I held one of the Doctor's diamond type cards six inches from her eyes, one would have thought that I had intended to strike her, for she drew back her head suddenly as the little card came in view. She shook her head sadly and said, "I shall never be able to read that fine print for you. That is too much to ask." I answered, smiling at her, "No, you don't need to read it for me, read it for yourself."

She said she was willing if I would show her how to do it. I told her to move the little card slowly from side to side, flashing the white spaces between the lines of letters without trying to read. She kept this up for ten minutes or a little longer and then she screamed as the letters began to clear up, and before mammy left the Clinic she read the "Seven Truths of Normal Sight."

CATARACT CURE

By Rev. Herbert Parrish

Rector of Christ Church, New Brunswick, New Jersey

An aged member of my congregation, nearly eighty, who had been accustomed to read the Bible every day of her life and who could also read the newspaper and thread needles and sew, suddenly lost her sight early in February. She became increasingly blind and by the end of March was unable to do any reading whatever or to sew. Since there was little else that she could do, life seemed to have gone out for her, into darkness, and she was greatly distressed.

In April her daughter took her to one of the best eye specialists in this vicinity who made an examination of her eyes, said that nothing could be done at that time, charged her five dollars for the examination and handed the daughter a slip of paper as she left the office. The daughter supposed that the paper was a receipt for the five dollars, but on reaching home and opening the paper she found that it contained a single word, "Cataract." The doctor evidently hesitated to distress the old lady by telling her directly what was the matter. She had gone blind from cataracts.

Shortly after I visited the old lady at her home in order to administer the Sacrament. After the service I told her about the methods Dr. Bates used to cure cataract and I suggested that she should try palming her eyes three times a day and swinging. This she did very faithfully and before the end of the month she became able to read the larger print of the newspapers. Gradually she regained her sight and in the course of a month or two was able to resume her practice of reading the Bible daily and the ordinary print of the newspaper. She also was able again to thread needles and to sew.

She continues the palming and swinging. Her eyes have cleared up and are bright.

WHAT IS THE MONETARY VALUE OF YOUR EYES?

By Minnie E. Marvin

Did you ever stop to think of just what cash value you would place upon your eyes? Would you take a thousand or a hundred thousand dollars for your sight? To the average person this is a great deal of money. One feels that with a hundred thousand dollars one could satisfy most any ambition, be absolutely independent; but would you, without your sight?

To the artist, this money would mean a finished education among the old masters of Europe; to the physician it would mean the power enabling him to experiment along the particular lines of his endeavor for the benefit of mankind, and to the mother it would mean luxuries for her babies. But, after all, without sight these things are negligible. The greatest joy comes to the artist in beholding his finished product, and noting the glances of admiration cast upon it by an appreciative throng. The physician is rewarded by the idolatrous and grateful smiles of his patient, whom he has grasped from death's door; and is there anything more wonderful to a mother than to notice the new little charms manifested each day by her young offspring?

No, truly, there is no greater gift than sight; still some thoughtless people hold it lightly. They abuse their eyes in every conceivable way, and then, to cap the climax, cover them with a pair of glasses, and expect them to get well. A great many people spend more time hunting bargains in eyeglasses, and in getting the kind of rims adapted to their particular style of beauty, than it would take to cure their eyes by following the method outlined along the lines of common sense.

In Dr. Bates' book, *Perfect Sight Without Glasses,* is the material explained in a simple, natural way whereby every person having any form of defective vision can positively cure himself. All that is needed is a little backbone. Leave off the glasses. Allow your eyes to function naturally and see how they enjoy it. A baseball pitcher wouldn't think of binding up his pitching arm with splints weeks before a game is scheduled, would he? No, indeed; the results would certainly be disastrous to him. Neither would a marathon runner neglect his daily sprints that keep him in trim. The same principle applies to the eyes. When glasses are resorted to, the natural functioning powers of the eyes are curtailed, and as a matter of course become gradually weakened.

There has been a great deal of talk recently about some sort of organization which calls itself the Eyesight Conservation League. This League has been distributing pamphlets and circulars *anonymously* throughout the schools, byways and highways of the United States. The object of this League is to *prescribe glasses*. The reports of their representatives, submitted to headquarters at regular intervals, are merely records of the number of glasses prescribed. No mention is made of the number of children benefited.

According to their ideas, their object has been accomplished when the glasses are placed on the children, when as a matter of fact we all know that the sight will never become normal just so long as the glasses are worn. How often do you hear a person say, "Oh, my eyes are perfectly normal. Now, you see, I wore glasses for such and such a time, and the defect has been entirely cured." Have you *ever* heard it? I never have, and I doubt if anyone else has. Glasses *never* have cured defective vision.

We hope all our Better Eyesight League members and friends who know of Dr. Bates' method of curing defective sight will do all they can to put a stop to this sort of propaganda for "sight conservation." It *conserves* it, true enough; *preserves* it, might be the better word—preserves it in such a way that the normal vision is never manifested, so long as the glasses are worn.

A TALK TO THE LEAGUE

By Antoinette A. Saunders

Editor's Note—*The following is an extract taken from a talk given by Ms. Saunders before the members of the Better Eyesight League at the July Meeting, and deserves special mention.*

Plain common sense and statistics tell us that glasses have not, cannot, and never will cure errors of refraction; if they could people would wear them for a short while only, and discard them when cured. Have you ever seen a person doing so? We all know that generally the strength of the artificial lenses must be steadily increased, and in many cases it leads to cataract and blindness—and there are still people who believe that they are saving their eyesight by wearing glasses. When, oh when, will they wake up?

I dare say that errors of refraction is an imaginary disease. Dr. Bates can tell you how many patients fitted with plain glasses and even with wrong lenses, are coming to his office daily. How can they see through these ill-fitted lenses?—autosuggestion. Most of these people claim that glasses are a great comfort and they say they cannot see without them—but sometimes we catch them forgetting themselves, their eyes and glasses, and find they can read with perfect vision, an interesting article in the paper or a *lettre d'amour* just received, until they remember their glasses, and presto the perfect vision is gone. Where has it gone to? You see this is the result of autosuggestion when used in a negative way.

I have suffered long enough to know what I am talking about. From birth on I was troubled with catarrh. My eyes were frequently bloodshot, the lids swollen, inflamed and sore from a discharge. There also was a film over my eyes so that I saw everything as through a cloud. I had worn glasses for twenty-eight years. Some I lost, others I gave away to very poor people believing, at that time, that I saved somebody's eyesight. All of them were fitted by the best eye specialists here and abroad. They told me that it must be entirely my fault if I could not see with them as they were fitted most accurately and I should try to get used to them. Well, I tried hard for 28 years, but day by day in every way I got worse and worse. I was afraid to cross a street because I ran right into moving vehicles. I fell not only up and downstairs, but also over imaginary objects and was the joke of the day for my friends and acquaintances. One day I crossed Fifth Avenue at 24th Street and ran into a rope which hit me on the nose and broke the left lens. When I looked around to find out the cause of the trouble I saw the rope with my naked eye, but could not see it with my right eye, which was still covered with the lens. Then I woke up. I refused to wear glasses on the street, although the doctor warned me, prophesying that I surely would meet with a terrible accident. But after all the experiences I had had with my collection of glasses I took the responsibility on my own shoulders and stopped wearing them on the street. At work I had to use them until I met Dr. Bates, who not only improved my vision rapidly, but also cured in a couple of minutes a very severe headache of many years standing.

Today I can read fine print and some of the photographic reproduction print by good daylight. I consider myself cured—at least from the habit of wearing glasses.

I also wish to mention that my health in general has improved immensely at the same time. I have no nervous breakdowns any more. I forget what fatigue is although I am working strenuously from early morning until midnight and longer. The rheumatism which accompanied me for 35 years has vanished completely. I must admit this has one drawback, namely—I lost the ability of forecasting the weather.

In conclusion I will try to answer two questions which I know are on your mind. First: How did I improve my sight? Simply by following Dr. Bates' personal instructions and also practicing the various exercises outlined in his book. The long swing was most helpful to me.

Second: How did I overcome the difficulties of working without glasses before my vision was improved? I watched myself carefully, found out the particular way I used to strain and avoided that particular way of staring and straining. I tried to relax as well as I could and to stay relaxed during work. I gave full attention to my work and forgot my eyes. I do not ask you to kid yourselves by repeating a certain number of times, "I can see, I can see," and actually fail to see, but it is a fact whenever I thought I could see and was sure about it, I always did so without a single exception; and whenever I was uncertain and thought "maybe I can see and maybe I cannot see," sure enough I could not see a single letter of any size and at any distance. So I advise you to think, expect, remember and imagine perfect vision. We all know that our physical body is not made of one big piece of something. It consists of many trillions of tiny little cells, each tiny little cell has its own tiny little brain, it knows its work and is only too willing to perform its duty if we do not interfere with it. To illustrate this statement I will tell you about an experiment which was made in one of our many laboratories.

A scientist took one single eye-cell of a chick's embryo and transplanted it to the back of the neck. The chick was hatched out with three perfect eyes. Two in its normal place and the third on the back of its neck. Now, if a chick's eye-cell knows enough and has the power to multiply so rapidly to make up for lost time and to build up a perfect eye, although out of its normal place, then I should think we need not worry about our eyes and how they can see without glasses. The human eye must be at least just as intelligent as a chick's eye, and if so then give your eyes a chance. Have faith and confidence in yourself and in your eyes.

ANNOUNCEMENT

Although the Clinic at the Harlem Hospital has been discontinued, the records of all the interesting and peculiar cases have been kept.

Dr. Bates and Ms. Lierman visited the Clinic three days a week, the patients averaging fifty or more a day. Ms. Lierman was always able to reach the human side of these patients, some of them in agony with various diseases of the eye, some blind with cataract, and others terribly uncomfortable with minor defects. A brief synopsis of all these cases was kept, and we have pleasure in announcing that each issue of the *Magazine* will contain one of Ms. Lierman's Stories for some time to come, selected from an unlimited amount of material.

BETTER EYESIGHT LEAGUE

The speaker scheduled for the evening was Ms. Gordon, a patient of Dr. Ruiz Arnau. Being troubled with presbyopia, and severe headaches, Dr. Arnau came to Dr. Bates for relief. Upon being cured, he took the course of treatment under Dr. Bates and is practicing this method with great success. The following reports of some of his patients were received with interest:

Ms. Gordon could do nothing without her glasses, which she wore for three years. However, as they failed to improve either her vision or her sick headaches, she visited Dr. Arnau, whom, she heard, was using Dr. Bates' method. At the end of three weeks she was amazed to discover that she could not only leave off her glasses without the least discomfort, but her headaches had disappeared. She can now sew, read, thread needles and continue her work of teaching with ease. Ms. Gordon explained that if she was cured in three weeks, children ought to make rapid progress and be cured permanently in less time.

The other patients who cited their experience with Dr. Bates' method under Dr. Arnau were two little girls and a boy. The first child to speak said she had a very trying time with the doctor at school. He prescribed glasses for her, but when her parents saw she was no better they took her to Dr. Arnau. He immediately removed her glasses and had her palm for a short time in his office. When he re-examined her eyes, he saw immediate improvement. The parents were greatly gratified and sent her back to school without her glasses. However, the teacher was greatly perturbed at this breach of ancient custom, and requested the child to either resume the glasses or remain away from school entirely. The little one went home and continued the treatment under Dr. Arnau for one week. At the end of that time she was pronounced cured by him and returned to school *without her glasses*. She was again sent to the school doctor and examined. When he saw that she could read to the bottom line without discomfort, he told her to go back to her class and the subject was dropped.

The next little girl was troubled with myopia. While she could read with an effort, she could not see the little words, such as "it," "as," "an," etc. Dr. Arnau taught her how to think, see and remember black; by flashing the white spaces and remembering the little period, she was able to imagine the little words until they cleared up and she could actually see them. In a few weeks' time she could read without an effort, and if she did revert to the unconscious strain, she received immediate relief and relaxation by remembering the black period.

The young man of twelve was next to tell of his experience. He explained that the swing helped him, and he demonstrated the various swings, shifts, including the movement of the eyes from left to right to make the objects swing in a slow, easy motion.

Another member gave a brief history of her case, and concluded by saying she receives the greatest benefit from reading the test card every night before retiring. She has it always in her room and takes it with her on her vacation.

It is a curious feature of the preceding reports that each speaker claimed a different exercise helped him. The memory of black helps some most, others like the palming, and still others become nervous when palming and like the different swings. By trying each one and noting the results obtained, the most beneficial can be adapted to each individual case.

QUESTIONS AND ANSWERS

Q–1. Please state in detail why fine print is a benefit.

A–1. It requires more of an effort to accommodate the eye to large type than to small.

Q–2. Is it really possible to cure oneself by reading the book, *Perfect Sight Without Glasses?*

A–2. Yes. Follow the instructions as outlined.

Q–3. I have had good results with Dr. Bates' book, but as yet cannot leave off my glasses with comfort. May I resume them when I do close work?

A–3. No medicine is easy. Put up with the discomfort. Learn how to diminish and abolish this day by day. Leave off your glasses.

Q–4. My husband has a fully developed cataract. Can this be removed by Dr. Bates' method without operation?

A–4. Yes.

Q–5. If fine type is beneficial, why do they print children's schoolbooks in large type?

A–5. For the same reason that people wear glasses—Ignorance of the proper way.

Q–6. Trying to make things move gives me a headache. Palming gives me more relief. Why?

A–6. Making an effort to do a thing won't help you. When you are walking the street, the street should go in the opposite direction without effort on your part. Some people get more relief from palming, while swinging helps others best.

Better Eyesight
October 1923—Vol. VIII, No. 4

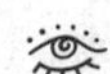

FAILURES

By W. H. Bates, M.D.

Most people with imperfect sight when they look at the Snellen test card at twenty feet believe that they see imperfectly without any effort or strain. Some people feel that to have perfect sight requires something of an effort. It is interesting to demonstrate that these two beliefs are very far from the truth. As a matter of fact it requires an effort to fail to see and *it requires no effort to have normal sight.*

In every case of imperfect sight whether due to nearsightedness or to an injury it can always be demonstrated that the nerves of the whole body are under a strain, and in every case of perfect vision it can be demonstrated that no effort whatsoever is made.

Imagine, if you are able, a small letter "o" perfectly black with a white center, to be as white as snow. When you succeed you will note that it comes easily, quickly and without any manifest effort on your part. You can choose to remember a letter "o" and you have it. This letter "o," if it is perfect, can always be demonstrated or imagined to be moving, and the movement may be so slow, so short, so easy, that you would not have imagined it without having your attention called to the letter. One can remember a perfect letter "o" or two letter "o's," as in the word "good," and at the same time remember or imagine the whole page of letters to be perfectly black, clear and distinct, although he or she is only able to see them best one at a time. Above all it can always be demonstrated that the memory of perfect sight, and the imagination and ability to see things perfectly, can only come easily, quickly and without effort.

Imagine a letter "o" again with a center as white as snow and imagine on the right edge of it a little black period. Try to keep your attention fixed on that little black period. Try to remember the blackest part of the "o"; try to imagine it stationary when not only is the period stationary but also the whole letter "o." One can hold this period black for a few seconds or a part of a minute, but, after a short time, it becomes monotonous or disagreeable or requires a strain and the period is lost and the "o" is lost momentarily, although you can get it back again. You can demonstrate quite readily that it is impossible to retain in your mind a period or a letter "o" by trying to imagine it stationary; or by trying to get your attention fixed on one point, or by staring at one point or two points or more points on the letter "o"; and trying to see them all at once and stationary is try-

MULTIPLE VISION

Persons with imperfect sight, when they regard one letter of the Snellen test card or one letter of fine print, instead of seeing just one letter, they may see two, three, six or more letters. Sometimes these letters are arranged side by side, sometimes in a vertical line one above the other, and in other cases they may be arranged oblique by any angle. Multiple vision can be produced at will by an effort. It can always be corrected by relaxation. One of the best methods is to palm, close the eyes and cover them in such a way as to exclude the light. Do this for five minutes or a half-hour or long enough to obtain normal sight. The multiple vision is then corrected.

Practice of the long swing is a great help. When the long swing is done properly the multiple images are always lessened. Do not forget that you can do the long swing in the wrong way and increase the multiple images. One great advantage of the long swing is that it helps you to obtain a slow, short, continuous swing of normal sight. When the vision is normal the letters appear to move from side to side, or in some other direction, a distance of about a quarter of an inch. The speed is about equal to the time of the moving feet of soldiers on the march. The most important part of the short swing is that it should be maintained easily. Any effort or strain modifies or stops the short swing. Then the eyes begin to stare and the multiple images return. It is a great benefit to learn how to produce multiple images at will because this requires much effort or strain, and is decidedly more difficult than normal single vision which can only be obtained easily without effort.

[Multiple images, which are often experienced with astigmatism, myopia, hyperopia, and presbyopia, should not be confused with double vision, which is often experienced with strabismus, e.g. crossed eye.—TRQ]

ing to do the impossible. You are straining and the result of the strain is that the memory, imagination and vision fail.

We have two classes of patients. One who gets well quickly in a day or at one visit. We have a second class that take their own time about getting well. They are usually under treatment for weeks and months before they recover. Why should some people get well so much quicker than others? One succeeds, the other fails. The facts are that the patient cured in one treatment does at once what he is told to do. He does not think or argue about what he is told to do, at least he does not try to explain why he is asked to do certain things, but simply goes ahead and does it and soon obtains perfect sight. It is something like the belligerent man who did not know the meaning of the word "convinced," who publicly announced in a loud voice that he was willing to be convinced, but he would like to see the man who could do it. A great many patients are like this man. They are willing to be convinced but they have their club. The club has engraved on it effort, strain, hard work.

When you have imperfect sight and look at the first letter of a line of letters on the Snellen test card which you cannot read, you can always note that you do not see the first letter or any other letter better than the rest. Usually the whole line looks pretty much the same shade of gray. Why is it? Because you are trying to see the whole line at once. You may not know it but most people can unconsciously demonstrate that they are trying to see the whole line at once. If you hold the card up close where you can readily read the same line, you will notice, or you can get somebody with good eyesight to show you that when you distinguish a letter, you do not see any of the other letters so well. To see one letter at a time is much easier than to see a whole line of letters; in fact to see a number of letters all perfectly at the same time is impossible and trying to do it is a strain. One can lift a lead pencil without any apparent effort. To lift a five pound weight requires something of an effort, but to lift ten tons of coal with one hand is impossible, and trying to do the impossible, trying to lift the ten tons of coal with one hand is an effort, a strain, and so it is with the eyesight. You can succeed oftentimes when you look at the Snellen test card without any effort to see one letter best at a time, but if you try to do the impossible, try to see the whole line of letters at once you will always fail, because you will have to make an effort. It is not an easy thing at all to fail; it is difficult; you have to try or you make an effort to do the impossible in order to fail.

This can be demonstrated by nearsighted people who can read fine print close to their eyes. When you see a line of letters, you can see one letter better than all the other letters or you can even see part of one letter best while the rest of the letter is not good.

Even persons with very good sight for the fine print close to the eyes can demonstrate that to make their sight worse or to see worse is not an easy thing to do. It requires a great effort. To prove that imperfect sight is more difficult and requires hard work, a great deal of trouble and much effort, is a great benefit.

If you close your eyes and remember a letter or word easily, perfectly, and continuously, you will find that to spoil the memory or your imagination is a difficult thing to do. Some people cannot read fine print readily, but they can read the Snellen test card at twenty feet with normal vision. To be able to look at the large letters on the card and to strain your eyes sufficiently to blot out the large letters is not an easy thing to do. It is difficult to remember, imagine or see imperfectly, to fail.

There are many patients who are convinced that they can remember or imagine with their eyes closed and oftentimes with their eyes open, letters of the Snellen test card perfectly black. Many of them can do it all right with their eyes closed, but fail to do it with their eyes open. When they are cured they become able to remember just as easily with their eyes open as they can with their eyes closed. This has suggested a method of treatment which has been highly successful. Many patients ask how long it will take to be cured. The answer is when you can remember or imagine as well with your eyes open as you are able to with your eyes closed.

STORIES FROM THE CLINIC

No. 44: The Story of Lillian

By Emily C. Lierman

At one time my work was confined to the Harlem Hospital. After awhile it was extended to other places at other times. Occasionally, when I visited a department store to make a purchase, the girl who waited on me might be suffering from the results of eyestrain, pains in the eyes or with headaches. It always gave me great pleasure to give them immediate relief with the aid of palming, swinging or in some other way. I could write many stories about the help I gave these girls and their gratitude was something worthwhile. I live in the suburbs and commute. The trainmen know me very well and always come to me to remove a cinder from their eyes, or to help them when their sight is poor, or when they are suffering in any way with their eyes. Every day during the fall, winter and spring I meet a cheerful group of girls at our station who attend high school in another town. Some of them I have known since they were babies, and while I am in their company on the train, I forget sometimes that I am grown up and join them in their fun. Several of these girls wear glasses and I offered to cure them any time they were willing to discard their glasses. We said no more about the subject until one day just before school closed for the summer, one of the girls, named Lillian, age 16, who had a higher degree of myopia than any of the rest, appealed to me to help her get rid of her glasses. I insisted that she consult her parents first and if they were willing, and would also help me with her case, I would try my best to cure her before school opened again in the fall. Lillian was very much excited about it all and begged the other girls to discard their glasses also. One girl said her mother feared that such a wonderful thing couldn't be done. Another girl thought she would wait awhile. I still feel in my heart that they did not believe in me. However, the day after school closed, Lillian called at my home with her sister, Rose, age 13. She had a decided squint of her left eye. Lillian had not spoken of Rose or that she had a sister with squint. She was afraid of imposing upon me and for that reason did not mention that her sister also had trouble with her eyes. But when Lillian came to me, Rose made up her mind that she would be cured also and so she came along with her.

I fastened a test card to an oak tree outside of our house and placed my patients ten feet from the card. I started Lillian first because I wanted, above all else, to cure her as I had planned. With glasses on she read 10/15 and with glasses off 10/70. I taught her to palm and remember something perfectly while her eyes were closed, such as a white cloud, sunset or a little flower of some kind. She did this for a few minutes and then without a stop or making a single mistake her vision improved to 10/40, both eyes. Then I tested each eye separately. Her vision fortunately was the same in each eye, which made it easy to proceed with the treatment. By closing her eyes and remembering the last letter she was able to see on the card, she became able to read another line, 10/30. When she made the slightest effort to read the smaller letters on the card the letters would disappear. I explained to her that when she stared, she made her sight worse and that was her main trouble. I told her to keep her eyes fixed on one letter without blinking her eyes and see what happened. Immediately she began to frown, her eyelids became inflamed and she complained that her eyes hurt her. She said, "Now I know why I have headaches and pain in my eyes."

On her second visit her vision improved to 10/20 after I had taught her the long swing, moving her head slowly from side to side from left to right, looking over one shoulder and then the other. She had to be reminded, as all patients do, to stop staring and to blink her eyes often, just as the normal eye does. All through the summer, Lillian practiced faithfully getting a great deal of encouragement from her sister Rose and her loving mother and father. She came to me for treatment about once a week and a few weeks before school opened we began treatment indoors with electric light instead of outdoors in the sunlight. I did this purposely because I knew that the light in school was not as bright as outdoors. Lillian became very nervous and frightened when she first read the test card by electric light. All she could see was the large "C," called the 200-line letter, at ten feet. Palming for a few moments helped her to relax enough to read several lines; then with the aid of the swing and looking at one letter and then shifting her eyes somewhere else and looking back again at the next letter, helped her to read 10/70. At each visit she improved and now reads 10/10 all the time. Before she began treatment, she had to hold a book while reading at three inches from her eyes. This was with glasses on. Since she was seven years old she had worn glasses constantly and in all that time she suffered with headaches every day. She told me that from the day I removed her glasses and started the treatment she had not had a headache or pain in her eyes. She is so grateful that I am almost swallowed up with caresses. Some friends whom she had not seen for a year called to see her folks and to enjoy a day on their farm. Lillian had worn glasses for so many years that she was not at all surprised when her friends did not know her. She stood in the doorway ready to greet them, but they thought she was a stranger. Her whole facial expression had changed. The eyelids which were swollen from eyestrain were natural looking and her large brown eyes were quite different from the tiny marble looking eyes that tried to see through the horrible thick glasses she had worn previously. When her friends finally recognized her they had to hear all about the treatment and cure.

If Lillian had not been so faithful with the treatment I could not have made such rapid progress. There were many days during the summer when she became discouraged and worried for fear she would have to put on her glasses again. Her mother was a great help to me in many ways. She was very careful to hide Lillian's glasses so that she could not possibly wear them again even if she wanted to.

Well, the first day of school came along and, of course, I was a bit anxious. I met her with the usual group of girls on the train and as she passed me by she pressed my hand and said, "Wish me luck." I asked her to telephone me that evening, which she did. This is what she said:

"When my teachers saw me they were surprised at the great change in my appearance, so I told them all about it and all you did for me. But when I asked to be placed in the last row of seats in each classroom, they were amazed!

You see, I always had to sit in a front seat near the blackboard," she said, "when I wore my glasses. I was able to read every word on the blackboard in each classroom from the last row of seats where I was sitting. I also read from my schoolbooks at eight inches from my eyes without any discomfort whatever."

I praised Lillian and said that I was glad for her. I was more than happy to have given her my evenings time, when I needed rest most of all after a day of hard but joyable work.

The interesting history of Rose, Lillian's sister, will appear in the November issue.

BETTER EYESIGHT LEAGUE

The last meeting of the Better Eyesight League was very successful, although it came in the middle of the vacation season. The large Central Fixation office was filled to capacity.

Gertrude Berdine was the speaker selected for the meeting. She told in a very interesting manner how she wore glasses for ten years and was able to discard them by practicing Dr. Bates' method under Dr. Arnau. She accomplished reading her music in two weeks' time after leaving off her glasses. She was bothered with headaches and said the swing helped her. She very rarely has a headache now.

THE POST OFFICE INCIDENT

Editor's Note—*About two months ago the Post Office noticed that we were sending an increasing number of books through the mail. They did their duty and investigated the facts by writing to a number of purchasers of the book. The following is a partial list of letters written to the postmaster, duplicates of which were submitted to us, and are printed at this time for the encouragement of those who desire good vision without glasses. We are grateful to the writers of all letters sent to the Post Office.*

1. "I was wearing spectacles for twenty-seven years. A friend of mine made me acquainted with the discovery of Dr. Bates. I bought the book, read it very carefully, and began the exercises and cured myself by following closely the directions stated in the book without consulting Dr. Bates; therefore, from the very day that I began the exercises prescribed in the book I discarded my spectacles and I never had the need of them any more. My eyes by the continual use of the spectacles had acquired a lifeless expression. They now look bright and have acquired their natural expression of my young days. I read, write and use them with remarkable comfort for anything that I must do. I recommended the same book to a friend of mine in Nassau, New York. Her children and husband, an architect by profession, were wearing spectacles, and they also cured themselves only with the knowledge of the book and the application of the exercises, in a remarkably short time.

I am living at [address deleted] for more than fifteen years and therefore my testimonial can be verified by many persons and acquaintances. I consider a blessing for the future generations the marvelous discovery of Dr. Bates, and personally I will do all that is in my power to impress on my friends the scientific and accurate importance of such valuable work done with altruistic and humanitarian spirit by Dr. Bates.

If anyone fails to have results it is only because they do not work it out accurately, continuously and conscientiously. The blame, therefore, is in their nature and not in the value of the theory. I hope my testimonial will help the future and present generations to get the just attitude and give support and value to such a remarkable discovery."

2. "I have been interested in Dr. Bates' method of treatment for the eyes for several years, and have known Dr. Bates personally for one year. From the results obtained by my patients through the use of his book and methods, I am convinced that he is right in his conclusions, and I have always found him thoroughly honest and reliable in his business methods and also in the sale and delivery of his books."

3. "I have enjoyed considerable mental comfort and, I believe, considerable practical benefit from the work in following the instructions. The 'palming' process and the mental suggestions connected with it have been followed with pleasure and profit. Dr. Bates' observation with regard to cataracts in some recorded instances having passed away was very encouraging. Believing to the fullest extent in the doctrine that what comes of its own volition should seemingly disappear either similarly or with care, I have been extracting considerable relief from the belief which amounts to a conviction.

As I have been nearly forty-seven years a practicing attorney, you can rest assured that I am neither an infant nor a neophyte, but like the man from Missouri, I must be shown and convinced. Dr. Bates has presented certain lines of thought worthy at least of investigation and consideration. I can well understand how efforts may be made to thwart him, but with me if his position is untenable it will soon be discovered and so proven. At the present time I can only speak in the most encouraging manner of the work and of his suggestions."

4. "In reference to enclosed letter, I did write for *Perfect Sight Without Glasses* and sent it on to my wife, as I thought it might interest her. I have not taken the treatment, but intend to do so the next time I vacation from business.

My wife wore glasses for 29 years. Dr. Bates told her to take them off and since that time, over a year ago, she has not worn them and can see better and longer than when she wore glasses. She is free from headaches she experienced when she wore glasses.

I believe that Dr. Bates is sincere and that he is working on really scientific lines. I believe that he has been persecuted by narrow-minded physicians who resent any change in the fundamentals of their science. I was as skeptical as could be of Dr. Bates and investigated thoroughly before I allowed my wife to take the treatment, and I am now thoroughly convinced that his method is the correct one in the majority of cases.

I should be very glad to be of any further assistance in protecting Dr. Bates or the Central Fixation Publishing Company which, I understand, is his organization, from any interference by the Government.

Please understand that I have no connection or interest in the Central Fixation Publishing Company. My only motive is that of gratitude because Dr. Bates did so much for my wife and made it possible for my little daughter to do without glasses."

5. "I have heard the optometrists and the oculists "knocking" the system and have asked each one of the known knockers if they had tried the system. Each said 'No.' They are the ones who are jealous.

I have known of very many who have been benefited beyond casual belief by Dr. Bates' system. Of course it is radical. All reforms seem radical until once adopted by the majority. As a rule, the discoverer of anything good in the healing 'art' has to be dead for about fifty years before he is given due credit for his work."

6. "I was treated for an acute condition of the left eye in the spring of 1922. I was suffering acute pain from the least ray of light, could not bandage my eye closely enough to walk on the street without agony because light would get in, and had to ride in a closed taxi cab. Dr. Bates examined my eyes for over an hour, then prescribed immediate exercises which I took in the office, remaining another forty-five minutes to do it. My eye, which had been in this inflamed painfully acute condition for five days, was relieved after fifteen minutes. I could see in twenty minutes without great pain; in forty-five minutes I could bear to look at light. I continued the exercises at home by his prescription and my eyes were normal in three or four days' time."

7. "Through your *Perfect Sight Without Glasses* I not only could throw mine away almost at once after I began to read your book last Thanksgiving, but the effects of your splendid relaxation system on my high-strung nerves is beyond words."

QUESTIONS AND ANSWERS

Q–1. What can be done for a man, blind for fifteen years who cannot tell light from darkness?

A–1. Same treatment as is used for myopia and other defects.

Q–2. How can we see things moving without making an effort?

A–2. Things only move when one is relaxed. An effort always stops things from moving.

Q–3. Why do movies hurt my eyes when they should benefit them?

A–3. Unconscious strain. Do not stare at the picture, but allow the eyes to roam over the whole picture, seeing one part best. Also keep things swinging.

Q–4. Why do some people see better by partly closing their eyes?

A–4. People with poor sight can see better by partly closing their eyes [due to the "pinhole effect"—TRQ], but when they have perfect sight squinting makes it worse. This is a good test for the vision of ordinary objects.

Q–5. When does the long swing fail to produce relaxation?

A–5. When one stares at objects moving.

Better Eyesight
November 1923—Vol. VIII, No. 5

THE BOOK: *PERFECT SIGHT WITHOUT GLASSES*

A great many people have testified that they were cured by the help that they obtained from the book. A large number, I believe, have failed to be cured with its help although most people have been able to get some benefit from it.

On the first page is described the Fundamental Principle. This should interest most people because if you can follow the directions recommended you will most certainly be cured of imperfect sight from various causes. If you have a serious injury to the eye which destroys some of its essential parts, you will find it impossible to carry out the directions. At the bottom of the page is printed: "If you fail ask some one with perfect sight to help you."

It is an interesting fact that only people with perfect sight without glasses can demonstrate the Fundamental Principle. You will read that with your eyes closed you should rest them, which is not possible if you remember things imperfectly. The book recommends that you remember some color that you can remember perfectly because it has been demonstrated that the normal eye is always at rest when it has normal sight. A perfect memory means perfect rest. Should you have perfect rest, you have perfect sight. Most people can demonstrate that they can remember some letter or other object or some color better with their eyes closed than with their eyes open. By practice some people become able to remember, imagine and see mental pictures as well with their eyes open as they can with their eyes closed. Then they are cured.

["The Fundamental Principle" from *Perfect Sight Without Glasses* is reproduced below.—TRQ]

The Fundamental Principle

Do you read imperfectly? Can you observe then that when you look at the first word, or the first letter, of a sentence you do not see best where you are looking; that you see other words, or other letters, just as well as or better than the one you are looking at? Do you observe also that the harder you try to see the worse you see?

Now close your eyes and rest them, remembering some color, like black or white, that you can remember perfectly. Keep them closed until they feel rested, or until the feeling of strain has been completely relieved. Now open them and look at the first word or letter of a sentence for a fraction of a second. If you have been able to relax, partially or completely, you will have a flash of improved or clear vision, and the area seen best will be smaller.

After opening the eyes for this fraction of a second, close them again quickly, still remembering the color, and keep them closed until they again feel rested. Then again open them for a fraction of a second. Continue this alternate resting of the eyes and flashing of the letters for a time, and you may soon find that you can keep your eyes open longer than a fraction of a second without losing the improved vision.

If your trouble is with distant instead of near vision, use the same method with distant letters.

In this way you can demonstrate for yourself the fundamental principle of the cure of imperfect sight by treatment without glasses.

If you fail, ask someone with perfect sight to help you.

THE TREATMENT OF MYOPIA

By W. H. Bates, M.D.

Myopia or nearsightedness is usually acquired by schoolchildren and others at about the age of twelve, a period when the nervous system is naturally undergoing a change.

One can demonstrate that when the normal eye stares at one part of a letter of the Snellen test card continuously at twenty feet, that it is a difficult thing to do; the eye tends to wander; and, to keep the eye fixed on one point requires an effort, a strain which lowers the vision and produces a temporary myopia. In all cases of myopia, a stare or strain or effort to see at the distance can be demonstrated. When the vision is normal, as it may be for diamond type at six inches or farther, one reads easily, readily, rapidly, and without any effort or strain whatever. It can always be demonstrated that the white spaces between the lines, words or letters are whiter than the margin of the card. By covering over the black letters, the white spaces between the lines are seen to have the same whiteness as the rest of the card or when one sees the white spaces between the lines whiter than the margin of the card one sees an illusion. An illusion is never seen, it is always imagined. We call the white spaces between the lines, when whiter than they really are, "halos," which are really never seen but only imagined. The imagination of the halos, however, may be so vivid that it is difficult for many people to realize the facts. It is most important that the patient should understand that the halos are never seen, they are always imagined.

A great many cases of myopia have been cured by demonstrating this fact. All that was necessary to bring about a cure was to encourage the patient to imagine the halos, which is more easily done than to see the letters.

Patients who are nearsighted, when they regard the letters of the Snellen test card, see the black letters a shade of gray. When their attention is called to this fact they realize that they are imagining an illusion which lowers the vision and favors the increase of myopia. In some rare instances these facts have been understood by a few patients, who said to themselves, "I do not see these gray letters, I only imagine them gray. As a matter of fact it is easier for me to imagine the letters black than it is to imagine them gray." Then they went ahead and did it and were soon cured.

No Glasses

A person who has been wearing glasses to improve the sight of myopia and has worn these glasses for a number of years is quite dependent upon them. When the glasses are removed, the vision is much less than normal and it is a curious fact that the vision without glasses does not depend directly upon the amount of myopia. A person with two diopters of myopia may have just as poor vision without glasses as one who has six or more. When a myopic patient lays aside the glasses entirely for two weeks, when the vision is again tested it is often much improved. The facts demonstrate that wearing glasses always lowers the visual acuity much below what it is when the glasses are not worn at all. It is a matter of common knowledge that when the glasses are first worn that the patient does not always obtain a minimum amount of relief. Some eye doctors, when asked to explain matters, sometime tell their patients that their eyes have to become adjusted to the glasses. It is not always easy to explain things satisfactorily, especially when some fault-finding patients complain that what they wanted was glasses to help their eyes and that they hardly expected to be called upon to adjust their eyes to fit the glasses.

Palming

One of the best methods of improving the sight of myopia is to cover the closed eyelids with one or both hands in such a way as to avoid pressure on the eyeballs. This is called palming. The patient is directed to rest his eyes and to forget them as much as possible by thinking of other things. When properly done the patient sees nothing but darkness or black. It is a failure when one sees red, blue, green, white or any other color. In such cases palming does not succeed in helping the sight. There are many cases in which palming may lower the vision, and so one must keep in mind the fact that it can be done right or it can be done wrong. The length of time necessary to palm to obtain maximum results varies with individuals. Most persons can obtain improvement in fifteen minutes while others require a longer time, a half-hour, an hour or even two or more hours of continuous palming to obtain any benefit. With improvement in the vision it usually follows that a shorter period of palming may obtain maximum results. The environment of the patient is an important factor to consider. When a patient is palming, it is well to avoid all conversation or the presence of a quantity of people. Some patients like to be read to or they enjoy conversation with their friends. These cases seldom obtain any material benefit to their sight from palming. The improved vision obtained by palming is seldom perfect. Other measures usually have to be employed to insure a lasting benefit.

Blinking

The normal eye when it has normal sight, blinks quite frequently. By blinking is meant closing the eyelids and opening them so quickly that neither the patient nor his observers notice the fact. Movies have shown that in some cases the eyes were closed and opened five times in one second. This is done unconsciously and is rather more than I can do consciously. Blinking is necessary in order to maintain normal vision continuously because if one consciously prevents blinking the vision for distance or the ability to read fine print are modified. It is interesting to me how blinking, which is so necessary for good vision, has been so universally ignored by the writers of books on diseases of the eyes. Blinking is a rest, it prevents fatigue, and very important, it improves the sight in myopia, and helps to maintain good vision more continuously.

Swinging

It has been my custom, after a nearsighted patient has palmed for half an hour or longer, to have the patient stand with the feet about twelve inches apart and sway the body from side to side, looking alternately at each side of the room without paying any particular attention to objects in front of him. By a little practice patients become able to imagine all distant objects not regarded to be moving from side to side in the opposite direction to the movement of the eyes. When the eyes move a foot or more from one side of a letter to the other side, the letter appears to move in the opposite direction, very nearly to the same extent. This movement of the letter or object is an illusion, and being an illusion, it is not seen but only imagined. A swing of an inch or more might be called the long swing, while a swing of a lesser degree might be called the short swing. When the long swing is practiced properly simultaneous retinoscopy indicates that the eyes are normal. When the short swing is practiced properly a greater improvement in vision usually follows, but the short swing stops from slight causes and the vision is then lowered. The short swing and long swing remembered with the eyes closed and remembered just as well with the eyes open, is a cure of myopia in many cases.

Memory

With the eyes closed, one may remember a small black period equally well as with the eyes open, while regarding the Snellen test card. When the period can be remembered perfectly at all times and in all places, the myopia is permanently cured.

The memory of black and the memory of white seem to be more popular with patients than the memory of other colors.

Imagination

The imagination has accomplished more in the cure of myopia than some other methods. Many people can imagine they see with their eyes open a known letter while looking at a blank wall as well as they can with their eyes closed; but when they regard the Snellen test card their ability to imagine that they see a known letter when regarding it, is not so good. Alternately imagining the known letter with the eyes open and accomplishing it better with the eyes closed has been followed by a great benefit. I have never seen patients with considerable myopia imagine an end letter of each line of the Snellen test card with a little practice as well with their eyes open as with their eyes closed. Beginning with the large letters and gradually working down to the smallest letters, they obtain normal vision entirely with the help of their imagination.

Prevention

The prevention of myopia in schoolchildren is very desirable. I recommend my published method because it always improves the vision of schoolchildren which means that automatically myopia is prevented.

The Snellen test card should be placed on the wall of the classroom where all the children can see it from their seats. Once a day the chart should be read as well as possible with each eye by the children from their seats. Every family interested in the good sight of their children should possess a Snellen test card to be read by each child at least once daily. Many adults acquire myopia. As a matter of safety and a benefit to the eyes the adults should read the card at twenty feet with each eye. They usually obtain not only benefit to the eyes but also an increased mental and physical efficiency. Some teachers have told me that palming for a few minutes occasionally during the day is followed by relaxation of the children's nerves, which is of great capital value in preserving the health of the children. Each teacher should use the Snellen test card in her classroom more or less frequently every day.

STORIES FROM THE CLINIC

No. 45: The Story of Rose

By Emily C. Lierman

Rose, age 13, is the sister of Lillian whose case was reported in the October issue of *Better Eyesight*. While I was treating Lillian, Rose was present and listened attentively to everything that was said. Rose had convergent squint of the left eye and when she became excited or tried to see at the distance, her left eye would turn in so that only the sclera or white part of her left eye was visible. At the age of three, it was noticed that her left eye turned in, and when she was four years old glasses were prescribed for her. I tested her sight with the test card and with both eyes she read 10/100. Then I told her to palm her eyes and to remember the last letter she saw on the test card. She kept her eyes closed for at least a half-hour and when she again read the card her vision had improved to 10/20. Then I tested each eye separately. She read 10/20 with the right eye, and 10/40 with the left.

I thought the improvement in the vision of her eyes was wonderful and Rose was delighted with the results of her first treatment. Her sister Lillian was thrilled as she saw that left eye straighten as the vision improved. She came to me with Lillian once every week for treatment and carried out to the letter everything I told her to do at home.

She was directed to wear a cloth patch over her good eye all day long and to do her usual duties for her mother as well as she could with her squint eye. What a faithful child she was, and how she did hate that patch. I asked her every time she came how she got along with it. "Well, Ms.

Lierman," she said, "I don't like that black patch at all. I want to take it off many times every day. I don't like to have my good eye covered, but I know I must wear it if I want to be cured; and I do want to, so I just think of you and how much better my eye looks and then I don't mind a bit."

On her second visit her left eye improved to 10/20 and her right eye became normal, 10/10. Never did I have a more enthusiastic patient. On her third visit she gave me a package sent by her mother, who tried in her kind way to show her gratitude to me. The package contained delicious homemade sweet butter, my favorite dish. Rose continued her visits and in two months her sight became normal, and her eyes were perfectly straight continuously. She practiced faithfully and the result was that, one week before school started, she was able to remove the patch permanently, without any return of the squint.

Her first day at school was very exciting to her. She said her teacher did not recognize her, but when she smiled the teacher could not mistake her then. When Rose smiles you cannot help but know and love her. Her Aunt says a miracle was performed.

She had no trouble in reading the blackboard from the last seat of her classroom where she asked to be placed, and she sees the book type much clearer than she ever did. Rose had been going to school for a week or so when her teacher noticed that a pupil, age 12, could not read the blackboard from the front seat where she was sitting. The teacher told her to have her eyes examined by an eye doctor and to be fitted for glasses. Rose heard the conversation and promptly met her schoolmate at the school door. Rose told her how she had been cured without glasses and that she would be willing to show her how to be cured also. The next day at recess, instead of joining the class outdoors for exercise, Rose and her schoolmate went back to the classroom and with the aid of a Snellen test card, which Rose had taken with her that day to school, she improved the sight of the little girl from 12/70 to 12/15 by palming, blinking and swinging. Every day the two little girls worked faithfully with great success and after less than a week, both children occupied rear seats in the back part of the room where they were able to read the writing on the blackboard without difficulty.

SEEING WITHOUT GLASSES

By Caroline Guignard

There are doubtless many men and women who have worn glasses for twelve or fifteen years, suffering annoyance and discomfort through imperfection of the substitute for normal eyesight, who feel that it would be discouraging to become personally interested in a method employed for the improvement of the eyesight of those who have used glasses a short time only or not at all. As I was one of these, but am not one of them now, I feel that I must say a word which may cause someone to read the book, *Perfect Sight Without Glasses,* who might not otherwise do so.

After reading the book, I put aside my distance glasses and began palming. At the end of three days I could look at an unshaded lamp without pain and at my fingers at a distance of six inches without pain or nausea, although I saw them very badly. I could see the hands of a watch and approximate the time without glasses. I then put away all glasses, including those I wore all the time for distance; those for reading, bifocals; for painting, and the hand glass.

I think that I began reading a little at the end of three months familiar things in clear type, *Alice Through the Looking-Glass, Aesop's Fables* and Kipling's verse, palming before each paragraph or often with each one.

Now at the end of eight months I read anything within reason in a good light, even a little diamond type, two or three chapters at a time of a Bible in pearl type [5-point], which would be pleasanter if it were not yellowed with age. I can thread a fine needle with 150 thread in a good light. Instead of paining me, my eyes feel better after using them.

I palm six half-hours or longer daily. I did not at first discover that a half-hour of palming, the last thing at night, left the vision clear the following morning.

The gesture with eyes closed of looking over one shoulder as far as possible, then over the other shoulder as far as possible, can be done for an instant or longer at almost any time.

I find a watch very useful. The one I am using has a white face one inch in diameter and the hands and figures are black. The diameter of the circle of the second hand is three-sixteenths of an inch. I glanced at the watch a great many times through the day and night as well as whenever I was awake. Almost immediately I could see which was the hour and which the minute hand and gradually began to read the figures, which slowly changed from gray to black. Now I read clearly the figures within the circle of the second hand.

Dealing cards rapidly and arranging the hands without trying to see the different cards helped me. Also reading at a glance the black and white numbers on automobiles and the black and white signboards of gas stations and wholesale districts.

Recently I rode ten days in an automobile seeing the mountains of North Carolina. Not having the Snellen test card with me, I found that reading it in my imagination at night, persisting until the figures became quite black and the card white, relaxed my eyes, as also did the swinging of the small "o" and period, recommended by Charlotte Robertson in the May magazine. After ten days of rapidly moving trees by the roadside my eyes improved.

My eyes are not yet perfect, but they are infinitely more satisfactory than they were with glasses.

A DOCTOR'S STORY

By H. W. Woodward, M.D.

About two years ago I visited New York for the purpose of investigating the claims made by Dr. Bates relative to the cure of refractive errors and the restoration of diseased eyes without the use of glasses.

I visited his Clinic at Harlem Hospital. Here I found most unusual methods practiced by the Doctor and Ms. Lierman in the treatment of disorders of the eye. I was surprised at the cheerfulness of the patients, particularly the children.

The Doctor invited me to call at his office. I did so, and again I found his methods so different from the usual oculist that I was interested at once in finding out how he did his work. The first thing that impressed me was seeing so many patients working in his waiting room. They seemed to be engaged in steadfastly regarding the letters of test cards placed upon the wall.

After I had seen the Doctor treat several patients, he turned to me and inquired about the condition of my own eyes. I replied that I had reached the age where most people require glasses for reading, but was just beginning to be annoyed by a blurring of vision when I consulted a telephone directory in a dimly lighted room. I knew that this symptom means in the almost universal experience of mankind, glasses, and more glasses, until one becomes dependent upon them. While I was contemplating this prospect, Dr. Bates explained to me that he had been through this experience, having had to wear quite strong lens for reading and that he had cured himself.

He handed me one of his professional cards. On the back of this card was printed in small diamond type seven paragraphs stating seven fundamentals of perfect sight. He requested me to hold this card about six inches from my eyes, then close my eyes and form in my imagination or memory a small letter "o" and to see it in my mind very black with a white center. After doing this for a few seconds I was to open my eyes and look at the letters on the card. I did this, and to my surprise upon opening my eyes, the letters were jet black and remarkably distinct; but for only a moment did this clear vision last. The letters soon faded away into a blur.

This experience of getting a flash of clear vision, though evanescent in character, was encouraging to me, because it suggested the possibility of conquering this tendency to blurring. In other words, if I could learn to sustain this primary normal position that my eyes relaxed into just before opening them, I would certainly achieve perfect vision. Dr. Bates instructed me to practice what I had just done twice a day. I did as he advised. At first I could not hold this flash of clear vision more than a second or two. It was too subtle. I could not get a hold on it. I continued, however, practicing night and morning for several weeks with but slight improvement. At last, however, I became able to sustain the clear vision for about thirty seconds; but if I would wink my eyes while seeing clearly, my vision would fade into a blur. In time my patience was rewarded by more improvement, for now I am often able to read the whole card without a blur.

Dr. Bates deserves much credit for the pioneer work which he is doing and for the way he keeps on doing it in spite of the hostile criticism continually directed toward him. To know him is a privilege and I am thankful to have had this experience.

BETTER EYESIGHT LEAGUE

September Meeting

On the evening of the eleventh Dr. J. M. Watters, an eye, ear, nose and throat specialist from Newark, addressed the meeting. It was an extremely impressive talk, for Dr. Watters brought with him a long and interesting list of cases for whom he had effected cures by Dr. Bates' method. He stated that when he first started this work the results actually astonished him. Eyes responded to the new treatment better than he had anticipated or dared to hope.

The histories included both old and young, men and women, with apparently all the different kinds of eye maladies. Myopia, hypermetropia, astigmatism, presbyopia and glaucoma all yielded to the eye exercises. A gentleman of 74 with cataract in both eyes, a young man who was hit in the eye with a golf ball who developed a detached retina, a patient with ruptured iris—these likewise were cured by learning and practicing the method.

Dr. Watters said that he believes best results are obtained if people practice when they feel like it. If they can enjoy it and if the exercises produce no feeling of nervousness, then the work is progressing along the right lines. There is no way of hurrying a cure and a patient must be willing to accept gradual improvement if it seems to come that way.

Dr. Bates himself gave a most valuable demonstration of the long swing. He recommended it as a help in other troubles besides eye ailments, since if done properly it produces relaxation and lack of tension throughout the whole body.

October Meeting

Perhaps no speaker has brought greater encouragement to those endeavoring to gain better eyesight than Florian Shepard of Orange, New Jersey, who spoke to our League on October ninth. The special significance of her cure lies in the fact that it has been one of the unusually slow ones.

Ms. Shepard told the history of her case and related the gradual steps in her progress. At first nothing seemed to work. Palming, swinging, everything produced strain instead of relaxation. It was only by long perseverance that she was able to arrive at any real success. Again and again Ms. Shepard spoke of the marvelous patience and understanding with which Dr. Bates helped her find a way out of all her difficulties. Her testimony proves that Dr. Bates can succeed not only with easy cases, but also with hard and unresponsive ones.

Ms. Shepard spoke of the trick of timing the swing with the thumb and finger, and Dr. Bates later discussed this point. Attention was called to the fact that the September magazine had an article on the subject.

At Dr. Bates' request Mildred Shepard gave a short account of her cure. The most interesting part of all was, perhaps, the fact that since her eyes have become normal she is much less tense and consequently less nervous in all phases of her life. She spoke of herself as having become "happy-go-lucky."

OF SPECIAL INTEREST

Throw Away Your Glasses

Doctor Bates' article in the September issue of *Hearst's International* magazine awakened more interest in his method of treatment than any previous writings. Hundreds of letters were relayed from Norman Hapgood, Editor, to Dr. Bates and contained congratulations, inquiries and appointments for treatment. A special notice of this article was placed in the *New York Times* by the editor of *Hearst's*.

In view of this fact we have had reprints made of the article and will fill orders immediately upon receipt. The title is "Throw Away Your Glasses" and it explains how this can be accomplished. Everyone interested in curing their own sight will be enlightened on many points by reading this reprint.

[This article is reproduced below in the July 1929 issue.—TRQ]

QUESTIONS AND ANSWERS

Q–1. What is the cause of cataract?

A–1. Eyestrain is the cause of cataract, but some times cataract is produced from an injury such as a blow of some kind.

Q–2. Can insomnia be cured by the method of palming?

A–2. Yes.

Q–3. Can I overdo the swing?

A–3. No, not if it is done in the right way.

Q–4. Does sunlight injure the eyes of children?

A–4. No.

Q–5. Does wearing dark glasses injure the eyes?

A–5. Yes.

Better Eyesight
December 1923—Vol. VIII, No. 6

ONE THING

By *central fixation* is meant the ability to see one letter or one object in such a way that all other letters or objects are seen worse.

Some people have been cured by practicing central fixation only, devoting little time to other methods of cure.

Swinging

When the normal eye has normal sight, the small letters of the Snellen test card are imagined to be moving from side to side, slow, continuously, not more than the width of the letter. Persons with imperfect sight have become able to imagine this illusion by alternately remembering or imagining the small letter moving from side to side continuously. With their eyes open they may be able to do it for a moment or flash it, at first occasionally, and later more continuously until they are cured.

Imagination

Imagination is very efficient in improving the vision. Some persons have told me that when they knew what a letter was, they could imagine they saw it. By closing their eyes they usually became able to imagine a known letter better than with their eyes open. By alternately imagining a known letter with the eyes open and with the eyes closed, the imagination of the letter often improves to normal when the letter was regarded. The patient who is able to do this is also able to demonstrate that when the imagination is improved for one known letter, the vision for unknown letters is also improved. By imagining the first letter of a line perfectly, the patient can tell the second letter and other letters which are not known. The imagination cure is curative when other methods of treatment have failed.

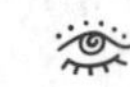

THE CADET

By W. H. Bates, M.D.

It is very important, very necessary that a soldier should have good eyesight. He cannot very well handle his opponents properly in a fight unless he can see them. Although the men at West Point are selected for their physical and mental efficiency, they are liable to acquire nearsightedness, apparently just as much as other young men. I believe that such cases should be treated before glasses are prescribed.

Mr. L., age 20, had normal sight before he entered West Point. After three years his vision began to fail. An oculist prescribed glasses. For a time the glasses gave him normal vision, but after a few months they were increased in strength. The patient did not like to wear glasses. He felt depressed over the fact that his sight was imperfect. Against his physicians' orders he laid aside his glasses most of the time and only used them for emergencies. Someone told him that it was possible for him to be cured without glasses. Full of hope he wrote to me and asked me what I could do for him. In his letter he wrote, "My trouble is myopia, brought on, I presume, by the great amount of study I had to do."

Straining to see at the distance always produces myopia in the normal eye and increases it in the myopic eye.

All persons with imperfect sight are able to demonstrate that they are staring. The normal eye, when it has normal sight, does not stare. It is a truth, that imperfect sight is always accompanied by a stare. It is a truth because there are no exceptions. When the stare can be corrected the vision always improves.

Mr. L. called October 14, 1923. His vision without glasses was less than 20/40. By palming and practicing the swing, his vision in a half-hour became normal, 20/20, in each eye. He was able to demonstrate that, when he remembered a white cloud in the sky, dazzling white with the sun shining on it and moving slowly, blown by the wind, he could imagine one letter of the alphabet perfectly. For example, he could remember or imagine he saw, with his eyes closed, a letter "O" with a white center, as white as the whitest cloud he had ever seen, but it was always moving. He could remember this and other letters perfectly black. With his eyes closed he could imagine that he put a small black period with the aid of an imaginary pen on the right edge of the "O." At my suggestion he placed another period on the left edge of the "O." When he looked to the right of the "O," the "O" was to the left of where he was looking. When he looked to the left of the "O," the "O" was to the right of where he was looking.

Every time his eyes moved to the right, the "O" moved to the left in his imagination. Every time his eyes moved to the left, the "O" moved to the right. With his eyes closed, imagining that he was looking alternately to the right and to the left, he could imagine the "O" was moving a short distance from side to side, not more than its own diameter. This he did easily, regularly and continuously.

He was asked to remember an imperfect "O," one which had no white center, a gray letter covered by a cloud which made it so obscure that it might be anything. He found this required a great effort, an effort which was tiresome. Every once in a while he lost the memory of the imperfect "O." He demonstrated that the memory or the imagination of the imperfect "O" was difficult, very difficult, while the memory of the perfect "O" was quite easy.

He was a good patient. Possibly it was the training that he had received in school which gave him the wonderful ability to do just exactly what he was told, easily, quickly and without any difficulty whatever. It certainly was a great pleasure to me to observe that he obtained his improved vision so easily. Nine-tenths of my patients have never been so obedient. Some people talk about soldiers and speak more or less lightly of their discipline. I say lightly, because my conception of discipline was materially modified after my experience with this patient. He gave me a demonstration of discipline which I had not previously read in any book.

At one time I taught some of the simpler arts of military drill as an officer in a militia student company. At that time my conception of discipline was a popular one. I can recall how it annoyed me to have my soldiers do a lot of other things besides what they were ordered to do. This interfered very much with their ability to drill properly. In my private practice, when trying to benefit my patients, I have been exceedingly annoyed by the arguments, questions and opinions indulged in by my patients when I was trying to secure perfect rest or relaxation of their minds.

STORIES FROM THE CLINIC

No. 46: Our Last Christmas at the Harlem Hospital

By Emily C. Lierman

As Christmas draws near, I keep wondering if my beloved children of the Harlem Hospital Clinic will be taken care of this year, or whether they will be neglected. I am going to miss them so much. We expect to have a tree at our new Clinic this year, distribute gifts to our Clinic patients and extend our good cheer as far as it will reach; but my heart goes out to the dear ones we had to leave behind in that other Clinic.

It is about them that I want to write, and try to give our readers a mental picture of our last Christmas with them.

First, I would like to tell of one little fellow, named Patrick, whose age was ten years. He had been coming to us for eight weeks or so before Christmas. His trouble was nearsightedness, and he had great difficulty in seeing the blackboard in school. His teacher had sent him for glasses and offered to pay for them herself. This was explained to me in a note which Patrick had with him. He was such a dear little fellow, and one of the best behaved boys in her class, she said. His family was very poor, but good people, so she wanted to pay for those glasses.

On his first visit, Dr. Bates examined his eyes, and then I started to treat him with the test card. His vision was 15/100 with both eyes, and also with each eye separately. He did not like to palm, but he kept his eyes closed as he was told, for over half an hour. His vision improved the first day to 15/20, which was very unusual. I told him to rest his eyes by closing them often every day. The second week in December, just eight weeks since his first visit, he read 15/10 on the test card.

For several years it had been our pleasure to greet Dr. Neuer in our room at the Christmas party. It was his delight to take one of the dollies and go from room to room, displaying that doll with all the joy of giving. Children suffering with tuberculosis, of whom many were cured by him, were never forgotten at Christmas time. When his eyes began to trouble him he came to Dr. Bates and was cured without glasses. He did not mind in the least standing with the rest of our Clinic patients, and when Dr. Bates invited him to his office, he said the dispensary was good enough for him.

DISCARDING GLASSES AT 60

By Dr. Adolph Selige

About a year ago a friend of mine wanted to know what I could do for one of his employees, an old man, 72 years old, who had gone nearly stone-blind, and was unable to work. I had the book and magazines of Dr. Bates and was overjoyed to put his theories to a good test, and so I told them to send the old man over.

I am happy to say that old "uncle" went back to work after the most strenuous treatment he ever had gone through in his life, and which he would never had done if it hadn't been for his niece, a woman of fair intelligence and so trained that she knew how to carry out orders. She made the old man walk the "chalk line," in regards to all the rules and regulations I laid down in regards to palming and reading the test card, and all the other stunts.

But, as I am a naturopath, and believe that diet plays a most important role in creating causes of abnormal physical conditions of all kinds, he had to live on a very strict diet too, but I had the satisfaction to see some very noticeable improvement after a few days, and was able to send him back to his employer ready to work, in less than a month's time.

I had been a victim of "Glass-o-Phobia" for something like 25 years, possibly more, for the beginning has escaped my memory entirely. My glasses were such a nuisance, my eyes smarted and pained and became sore in spite of them, and every once in a while I had to have my eyes refitted.

I was delighted with the new ray of light that filtered through the thick fog, permeating my brain in the region which is supposed to contain "good common sense in regards to eyesight," and I began to see more clearly after I had studied the book of Dr. Bates.

I resolved to apply this new knowledge to myself, and hoped to be able to get such fine success with the old uncle. There was an obstacle, however; I was a busy man, and when I was not busy with my patients, I was either reading or writing, or using my eyes in some strenuous way and, of course, I could not possibly afford the time to put my glasses away and forego the pleasure of continuing the studies I was so interested in. So I kept on postponing the event and I promised myself to do it at the very first opportunity, until one Saturday night I found myself minus glasses; I had forgotten to bring them and, instead of going back to the office, I just took the bull by the horn and decided to start "right now."

I sat and palmed and did the swing, and imagined and did all sorts of stunts and continued to do so on Sunday, nearly all day.

On Monday I just refused to be tempted to use my glasses, and put them on only in cases of the extremest emergency, such as when I had to sign my name to a letter, or when making an "Eye Diagnosis," which required effort more than a magnifying glass alone could afford me.

It was a torture for me to spend my leisure time between treatments, and my evenings and Sundays, without being able to pursue my studies, but I had resolved to stick it out and I did.

I found after a little while that my sight began to get clearer and sharper, and I did not miss my glasses so very much. I had carried them with me for emergency purposes, but used them only in very rare cases; finally I laid them away for good, when I went away on a four weeks' vacation.

During this time I took several Post Graduate Courses, made a lot of notes, and wrote under all sorts of conditions, and finally got where I did not miss them at all.

I returned to my desk three weeks ago and have not even looked for my glasses, and don't ever expect to.

It is now about three months since I began. I can read the smallest type of ill-printed newspapers at night when I have a good light to see by, but have no difficulty at all during the day time.

I can feel my sight getting better and clearer right along, and feel that eventually my eyes will see without glasses better than they ever did see with glasses on, even though I am nearing my 60th birthday.

One of the reasons why I have not many cures of eye troubles to my credit is because people are too comfortable and do not care to make any effort to regain their normal sight—they would rather wear glasses because it is less of a personal sacrifice.

As I mentioned before, I am a naturopath, and believe in the unity of disease and the unity of treatment. I should like to go into this a little deeper, as it is fundamental to health and also applies to cases of abnormal eyesight, but lack of space forbids.

I may say however, that I believe quicker and more permanent results can be secured for relieving eyestrain, and its results, when the entire body gets on a normal basis, in fact I have often found my patients to experience quite a relief for their eyes, even though I was not giving their eyes any special attention, but had merely worked towards a general adjustment of their entire physical and mental being, through diet, rest, exercise, neuropathic and other treatments, and a better mental attitude.

THE LEAGUE OF ORANGE, NEW JERSEY

The Homemakers' Association invited everyone to a meeting on the eighth, at which Ms. Lierman was to demonstrate with children how teachers and parents could prevent and cure eye troubles of children. Several informal talks were given by members who told how wonderfully their eyes had improved during the summer, and the enthusiasm of each was very marked.

THE PASSING OF MY GLASSES

By Mildred Shepard

Editor's Note—*It was at my earnest solicitation that Ms. Shepard consented, after some time, to write a brief account of the mock ceremonies which took place when she formally discarded her glasses.*

A small, but impressive, ceremony was held a short time ago, along the shore of a certain lake in Massachusetts. The occasion was the internment of "Near" and "Far," the two pairs of spectacles once worn by one now through with all glasses forever. This happy figure, posing in black robes as the bereaved, was preceded in solemn procession by similarly black-gowned attendants. Four pall bearers bore the coffin, upon which rested the remains of "Near" and "Far," now passed all use in this life—God rest their tortoise-shells. Sad, slow strains of the Funeral March, painfully drawn from a tissue-paper covered comb, mingled with those of "Mr. Gallagher and Mr. Sheehan."

With measured strides the little company moved along the lakeshore, to the famous memorial boat-landing. There were gathered the chief mourners and friends, attracted thither from the turmoil of final examinations and arriving families, not so much out of sympathy for the bereaved, we fear, as by the promise of a funeral feast of ice-cream cones.

Already the Dumb-Boatman could be seen gliding toward the stone steps. Upon his arrival the coffin was lowered upon the pillows carefully, and in great determination the bereaved climbed into the gondola and dropped upon her knees. With bated breath, the onlookers waited while the tongue-tied man swung the boat out into deep water. A great, glad smile spread over the face of the bereaved, as she laid to rest "Near" and "Far," her two steady, but now unnecessary companions of fifteen years.

UNSEEING EYES

By Emily A. Meder

We mortals have been heaped with blessings by the Divine power and, as wonderful and great as some of them are, the act of seeing is most wonderful. Sight is like a great river, with hundreds of small tributaries, and streams branching from it. One of the streams runs to the mind, another to the heart, and so on. We see something new and interesting, and immediately our mind registers this fact and causes us to speculate, surmise, and investigate. Then, if it might be a sad sight, the heart is instantly awake. There is no doubt, however, that while the sight is the greatest of God's gifts, it is also the most abused.

When one is interested in seeing glasses removed and perfect sight prevailing everywhere, incidents relative to the subject are more readily noted. Just as a person going to buy a new hat glances at all the headgear which comes to view. The same can be said of shoes and other articles of apparel. We are at that time more interested in that article, therefore more note is taken of it. This puts me in mind of a story my teacher used to tell us.

A professor desired to impress upon his young charges the value of observation, regardless of the fact that at that particular time they were not interested in the subject. He sent one-half of his class looking for a certain herb, and the other half for a particular specimen of stone. When the first half returned, they had gathered quite a bunch of the desired herb, and the second half had some of the quartz for which they were sent. The professor asked some of the members of his "herb class" if they had noticed any of the quartz while looking for the herb. They replied that they saw none at all. The same answer was given by the second half of the class when requested if they had seen any of the herbs. If the whole class had been sent for the stone and herbs together, they would probably have had good success, but not being sent for it, they did not look for it or notice it.

This brings me back to the fact that being intensely interested in people with imperfect sight who wear glasses, many unusual, and in some cases, humorous incidents are seen. One that was comical, if it had not been almost tragic, happened at Forty-second Street and Fifth Avenue, just a few days back. A party of motorists was going west, but as the car neared Fifth Avenue, the lights on the signal tower changed. The driver stopped and screwed his face into a knot to try to see the colors. I immediately saw that the man was straining dreadfully, especially as he thought he was holding traffic up, not being able to see the signals. He moved his car nearer and nearer the curb to get a better look, until he was almost on top of the light. When he finally arrived at a point of vantage where everything was visible to him, he discovered that the lights were yellow. He should have stayed where he was, as traffic was going north and south. In addition to extricating himself with difficulty, he was given a forceful opinion of himself by the angry traffic policeman.

Forty-second Street also abounds in large optical stores.

The pictures displayed in them are truly wonderful works of art. Some of them afford me great amusement, although they are worthy to be placed in an art gallery to be reviewed by the admiring public. How the artist must hate to spoil these by placing glasses on everyone of them. The most recent was a beautiful girl playing tennis. She had rosy cheeks and a happy, restful expression. In the first place, no one has that look of relaxation and happiness while wearing glasses. Secondly, it must have been a dreadful strain to look happy, and balance them while running after the ball. Somewhat like a juggler balancing a feather on his nose!

Has it ever occurred to you that children are always in danger of cars driven by people with defective vision? Just take note of the questions the traffic policeman fires at a careless chauffeur and draw your own conclusions. When they have been remonstrated for doing something wrong, the officer doesn't ask for a sample of his driving ability. The first order is "Can't you see where you're going? Are you blind?" Another question might be, "Do you see those signals? Why did you go ahead?" While the driver looks sheepish, he is politely told, "better have your eyes examined."

QUESTIONS AND ANSWERS

Q–1. Can people over fifty years old be cured without glasses?

A–1. Yes.

Q–2. Is the treatment good for nervousness?

A–2. Yes. As a general rule the long swing is the most efficient.

Q–3. Is central choroiditis curable and does it require much treatment?

A–3. Yes, choroiditis is curable and requires a great deal of treatment in some cases.

Q–4. Is conical cornea curable?

A–4. Yes, the variable swing has been a great benefit. This is described in *Better Eyesight,* November 1922.

Q–5. Why do I squint when I am out in the sun?

A–5. You are not accustomed to the strong light.

Q–6. Why do my eyes water?

A–6. Strain.

Better Eyesight
January 1924—Vol. VIII, No. 7

QUESTIONS

Asking questions is all too common with patients who have imperfect sight. There are important or necessary questions which the patient should know in order to bring about a cure. The cause of the imperfect sight should be emphasized. In all cases of imperfect sight a strain, an effort, a stare or concentration can be demonstrated. To see imperfectly requires a great deal of trouble. Even the imperfect memory or the memory or imagination of an imperfect letter is an effort. It is so great a strain that the memory or imagination fail if you keep it in mind for any length of time. Perfect sight can only be obtained without an effort, without a strain. It is impossible to remember or imagine things perfectly by an effort.

One may divide questions into (1) Proper questions; (2) Improper or useless questions.

It is a waste of time, an injury to the patient, for him to describe the infinite manifestations of imperfect sight. To know its history minutely and its variations require an effort on the part of the patient to describe these things. And this effort increases the imperfect sight. It is absolutely of no help whatever in formulating methods for its cure. Avoid asking questions about the symptoms of imperfect sight or anything connected with imperfect sight. Any question connected with perfect sight may be a good thing for the patient to know.

One may ask questions as follows: How long must one practice a perfect memory, a perfect imagination or study the latest manifestation of perfect sight? The answer to these questions are a benefit to the patient.

THE OPTICAL SWING

By W. H. Bates, M.D.

Most people when they look at stationary objects believe that they see such objects stationary; but if they observe the facts more closely, they find that when the normal eye regards a small letter of the Snellen test card with normal sight, the letter does not appear to be stationary, but seems to move from side to side, a distance about the width of the letter. This is called the *optical swing*.

During the late war, a soldier, who was rated as a sharpshooter, told me that when he regarded the bull's-eye of a target five hundred yards away or farther, that he had difficulty in aiming his gun properly because the bull's-eye seemed to move from side to side a very short distance. Both he and others who had observed it did not discuss the matter with any great interest.

The movement of a letter or other object from side to side in the optical swing is so short, so slow, that most persons with normal eyes have never noticed it. There is no reference to the optical swing in any publication which I have seen. It is a truth that in all cases of normal sight the optical swing can be demonstrated. In all cases of imperfect sight the optical swing is modified; it may be lengthened, it may become too rapid and irregular. The swing is a necessary part of perfect sight. The importance of it has not been realized. With the short optical swing the vision is good while the mental efficiency and the efficiency of the nerves and muscles is enormously increased.

The Short Swing

When the swing is short, no more than the width of the letter, the vision is normal; when the vision is normal, the swing is short. One cannot have normal vision of a letter, a normal memory or a normal imagination, without demonstrating the presence of a short optical swing.

It can be demonstrated that it is impossible to remember or imagine with the eyes closed a letter, a color, or any object without the optical swing. When the swing is stopped, an effort or strain is necessary, which may be conscious or unconscious, and the memory or imagination becomes imperfect. Normal vision is not maintained continuously without the short optical swing. It is not necessary, however, for one to be conscious of the swing in order to demonstrate normal vision.

Methods of treatment which restore the optical swing are a benefit to imperfect sight. When the short swing can be demonstrated, the vision, the memory and the imagination are normal. One cannot imagine the short swing and imperfect sight at the same time. One cannot remember or imagine pain, fatigue or any symptom of disease and the short swing at the same time. For example, the symptoms of acute indigestion have disappeared when the patient imagined the short swing of a letter or some other object. In some cases, hay fever symptoms have disappeared quickly and permanently through the use of the short swing. Bronchial troubles, the cough associated with influenza and whooping-cough, have disappeared quickly when the short swing was imagined quickly.

The Universal Swing

When you hold the Snellen test card in your hand, you can imagine a small letter "o" printed on the card to have a slow, short, easy, continuous, regular swing. Of course, when the "o" swings, the card to which it is fastened also swings; when the hand holding the card swings, the card swings and the letter "o" swings. When the letter "o" swings the card swings, the hand swings, and the wrist, the forearm, the elbow are all swinging with the "o." If the elbow rests on the arm of the chair, when the chair moves, the elbow moves; when the elbow moves, the card moves.

One can demonstrate that a letter "o" pasted on the Brooklyn Bridge moves when the bridge moves, and when the "o" moves the bridge moves. One may think of many objects, one at a time, each one in turn moving with the moving "o." This is called the *universal swing*.

The universal swing has been a wonderful benefit in improving many cases of imperfect sight, in the relief of pain, fatigue and other symptoms of disease. It can be demonstrated that when one has the universal swing the sight is perfect. If the universal swing becomes modified, the sight is imperfect. There are no exceptions. This fact has suggested successful treatment for myopia, cataract and other causes of imperfect sight.

It is well to remember that some people have difficulty in imagining the universal swing. They are very apt to separate the letter "o" from the card and imagine that either the card or the letter moves; and it is difficult for them to imagine the letter and the card fastened together and one unable to move without the other moving. Of course one can imagine the hand moving and the arm stationary, but when the hand and the arm are in a vise or fastened very closely together without any hinges, it is difficult or impossible to imagine the hand is moving without the arm moving as well. Persons who have difficulty in imaging the universal swing should consult others who can demonstrate it, explain it and help them to accomplish it.

I generally suggest to my patients that they practice the universal swing twice daily, morning and night; or better still, practice it at all times, in all places, no matter where they are or what they may be doing.

THE MEMORY SWING

With the eyes closed you can feel your eyes move under your fingers when lightly touching the eyelids. If you imagine that you are looking over your right shoulder, you can feel the eyeballs move to the right, and a long distance to the right. When you imagine that you are looking over your left shoulder, you can feel your eyeballs moving to the left, and far to the left. One can shorten the movement of the eyeballs by looking a shorter distance to the right, alternately looking to the left. With a little practice one can feel, or imagine one feels, the eyeballs are moving the shortest possible distance from side to side. The eyeballs can be seen to move under the closed eyelids. The memory swing is a good thing to practice under conditions which would not be so convenient for the other kinds of swings. One can practice the memory swing in a dark room, on a dark night, in a dark cellar, in bed, and obtain a mental relaxation or an optical relaxation or a relaxation of the nerves which is worthwhile.

THE VARIABLE SWING

Some years ago a school teacher called for treatment. She had a conical cornea, which is a very serious disease of the front part of the eye. The cornea bulges and becomes conical. The apex of the cornea becomes ulcerated, and may become perforated with loss of aqueous. Various operations have been recommended, but the results have been usually very unsatisfactory. The vision of the patient was 1/20 of the normal. She was very much benefited by the variable swing. The variable swing is shorter at twenty feet, or farther than it is at six inches. In this swing the patient holds the forefinger of one hand to one side of the temple, and while looking at the Snellen test card, the head is moved from side to side a short distance. The patient, when looking straight at the card, was able to imagine the finger moving from side to side an inch or more, while the test card moved a much shorter distance or did not appear to move at all. By shortening the movement of the head, the swing became still shorter, until the finger seemed to move no more than its own width, and the card seemed stationary. It was very remarkable how her vision improved with the improvement in the swing. At the end of about an hour of the variable swing, her vision had improved to 1/2 normal, with flashes of normal sight occasionally, which was a great deal better than the vision she obtained with her glasses.

There are some people who can practice the variable swing and obtain good results, while there are others who are not able to use it with any help or comfort. It is difficult for me to explain why or how some people obtain good results from this form of a swing, while others require supervision with a great deal of mental gymnastics from their medical adviser.

THE LONG SWING

The patient stands with the feet about twelve inches apart, facing one wall of the room. He is directed to turn his body and his shoulders to the right, and in order to do this he lifts the left heel a few inches from the floor. The whole movement is brought about by turning the body until the shoulders are square with the right-hand wall. Then the body is turned to the left, and to promote this movement the right heel is lifted a few inches from the floor. The body is turned until the shoulders are square with the left wall. It is very important that moving objects are not observed closely: do not try to see clearly objects which are moving.

This is the *long swing*, and it can be done with great benefit, because it relieves symptoms of pain when other methods do not succeed. When the patient is suffering from a severe pain, it is not easy or always possible to imagine the short swing. The long swing is the only one available under these conditions. The long swing is always a relief to some extent; and furthermore, it enables the patient very soon to obtain the short swing, which gives even greater relief from pain than the long swing. Besides relieving pain, the long swing benefits or relieves fatigue.

It is a matter of great interest that the long swing relieves pain, without necessarily correcting the cause of the pain. Pain from an injury or from a foreign body can be relieved by the long swing. The long swing does not usually give complete relief of pain, but it paves the way to the practice of the short swing, which is a greater relief.

The long swing is also a benefit to imperfect sight. The central vision is improved, and what is also unusual, the long swing improves the field of vision. It improves night blindness; it improves day blindness. The long swing has improved opacities of the cornea so dense that vision was reduced to perception of light. Yet although the opacity of the cornea was so dense in some cases that the pupil could not be seen, it would clear and the vision become normal after some weeks or months. The long swing also helps glaucoma, cataract, diseases of the optic nerve, diseases of the choroid, and detachment of the retina.

One needs a sufficient amount of light in order to practice the long swing.

THE DRIFTING SWING

One day there came to the office a patient who was among the worst that I have ever seen. In the first place, the pain that he had in his head, his eyes, his shoulders, his back, and pretty much in all parts of his body was the most severe that any of my patients has ever described. It was so severe that I have often suspected that he used a dope of some kind. Beside the pain, he complained of great depression. To hear him talk, he gave you the impression of being very miserable; and for some reason or other he could describe the condition of general misery more vividly than I have ever had the pleasure (?) of hearing it described before. His misery was mitigated to some extent, he said, when he took long walks with one or more friends and became interested in their conversation.

This case was remarkable for several reasons. With all my knowledge of various methods of resting the eyes, he failed to obtain the slightest benefit from them. In fact, he said that when he tried the treatment the pain, the depression, and his general misery were increased alarmingly, and instead of being a rest, it was actually an injury. He did not see a dark shade of black when he closed his eyes, but rather various colors—red, blue, etc.

I tried to have him practice the swing, and I exhausted my knowledge of the various kinds of swings, but was unable to have him practice successfully any swing that was of the slightest benefit: in fact, the more he tried to follow my suggestions, the worse he felt. Again I tried him with memory, encouraging him to tell me of the experiences he had had in Europe, in New York, and in his home town. He had absolutely no mental pictures, and although I had usually been able to teach people how to imagine mental pictures, in this case I failed ignominiously.

I tried many things that I knew and after I had exhausted the things that I had already practiced, I realized that I was up against it, and had to devise and have him practice with benefit something that I had never recommended before. As he could not think of anything continuously without discomfort, I suggested that he let his mind drift. As he had a very active mind and was continually thinking of a great many things, I suggested that he make no effort to keep his attention fixed on any one thing, but let his eyes keep shifting from one object to another. I asked him not to strain his eyesight to see the things about the room at all clearly, but rather to remember or specialize or think about objects in some other room. For example, when he looked at a chair in the waiting room, I asked him to remember some other chair or other object that he had seen in some other room.

It is not easy to describe what I mean by the drifting swing. Of course when he looked from right to left, the objects seen moved from left to right; when he looked up, the objects moved down, and the whole time that he spent in shifting his eyes continuously to various parts of the room, some of the objects moved opposite to the direction of his shifting. His mental pictures, if he had any, were remembered with so little responsibility on his part that he felt no discomfort. Part of the time he spent talking to some of the patients in the waiting room, and I encouraged him to take things easy, and to be as comfortable as he knew how.

In this I believe he succeeded, because when I invited him to go into another room where he could test his sight with the Snellen test card, he was smiling, a new experience for him. His vision for distance was normal, and the speed with which he read all the letters on the test card was gratifying. The rest had given him, at least temporarily, perfect sight for the distance, whereas before even with his glasses on his vision was less than one-half the normal. He was also unable to read diamond type with or without his glasses. After practicing the drifting swing he read the diamond type rapidly, perfectly and without any apparent effort at less than twelve inches.

Then he said to me, "Doctor, do you think you can help me?" I answered him, "Did you read the test card and the fine print perfectly?" "Yes," he answered and blushed. That was the first time I ever saw a man blush under such circumstances. The blush was to me an admission that he realized that I had given him a temporary cure. He sends me patients from time to time, who report that his eyes seem to be cured without glasses. All this happened some years ago, and I have been able in many other cases to obtain good results with the drifting swing when other treatment had failed.

Failures

There are some people who have great difficulty in demonstrating the illusion of stationary objects moving. Persons with imperfect sight do not ever imagine perfectly the optical swing. By practicing resting the eyes, testing the memory and imagination, they may, after some weeks, months, or a longer period, become able to imagine a short, as well as a long swing. The failure to imagine that stationary objects are moving is always due to a stare or strain. One can stare in looking straight ahead with the center of sight, and one can stare by trying to see with the sides of the retina, eccentric fixation.

The normal eye is only at rest when it is moving, and the optical swing can be demonstrated.

STORIES FROM THE CLINIC

No. 47: My Young Assistant

By Emily C. Lierman

One evening while treating some patients in my home, baby Ethel, age three, who had been living with us for over two years, came into the room and sat in a big armchair observing the treatment and listening to every word that passed between the patients and myself. She has large blue eyes, and when she is excited or interested in anything her pupils dilate and the iris seems to change color.

When I told one of the patients to palm for ten minutes, Ethel placed her hands over her eyes also. She kept perfectly still for about two minutes and then we heard a pitiful sigh. I watched and presently two little fingers of her right hand began to separate and she peeped. When she saw me smile she quickly removed her hands from her eyes and for a while she sat quietly. Presently she left the room to join other members of my family. After my patients had departed I discovered her in a room ordering the head of the household to palm. She was pointing with her little finger to an imaginary test card on the screen door. The head of the house certainly needs to do some palming and also to practice other things to improve his imperfect sight. Sometimes those whom we love are not easily persuaded to do the things that benefit them, but here was this little three-year-old very seriously giving him a treatment. Then she demanded, "Take down your hands and read the card. Do you see the 'R'? Now close your eyes and remember it," she demanded. He did so in all sincerity. "Now open your eyes and read some more." He mentioned several letters and then she said, "Swing your body, side to side, and see letters swinging opposite." He got up and swung as he was told, as all of us looked on in amazement, not daring to laugh, knowing that the little lady was very sensitive.

"Now," said she, "sit down and read some more letters." He read very faithfully, following her little finger as she touched various parts of the screen door. All of a sudden she complained, "You are staring. You shouldn't stare; that is bad." "Well," said he, "what must I do, then?" "You must blink your eyes. Just let me show you how."

She stood before him, blinking and swinging her body from side to side, looking as serious as a judge. At this moment, to our sorrow, we all laughed. I myself could not hold back a moment longer. That broke the spell, and my little three-year-old assistant began to cry. But since then her efforts have not been in vain, for I notice that her patient still keeps up the treatment. I am grateful to baby Ethel in that she was able to accomplish more for him than I could myself.

While we were sitting in our garden one day an airplane passed over our place, and as it traveled on he was able to see it miles away until it became so small to our view that it looked like a small black spot. He then closed his eyes for a while and afterward he read a newspaper for a half-hour or so. It has been a long time since he was able to read for that length of time.

When our friends called on us, baby Ethel was ever ready to show them how to palm and swing. She directed her mother to palm if her head ached or if she suffered any pain. Ethel was sincere about it all, because, as she explained it, "Dr. Bates helps big people and little people that way in his office."

She knew the Doctor very well and would talk to him about reading the test card to help children's eyes. She has perfect sight. Her eyes are never still and she blinks unconsciously all day long. If only adults would follow her example there would be less eyestrain. I am very grateful for what she accomplished for my husband. Does not the Bible say, "And a little child shall lead them."

SOME CLINIC CASES

By Dr. J. M. Watters

In the two years we have been using Dr. Bates' eye system in our offices we have discovered that our most interesting and unusual cases are to be found in the free Clinic. When this Clinic was opened last October we expected a few scattered patients to take advantage of our offer of free treatment, but great was our surprise on the first evening to find our offices and even the corridors of the building filled with men, women and children of all descriptions, each one pathetically eager to take one more chance at saving his eyesight. The variety of cases was great, ranging from simple refractive errors to various forms of squint, cataract. and glaucoma.

One very interesting case which we treated was that of a man thirty-one years old, who ten years previous had been hit in the right eye with a golf stick. He had been advised many times to have the eye removed surgically, as the eyeball was constantly inflamed. When we first examined him his vision was dim at 10/70, and his near point negative. When our Clinic closed for the summer his vision had improved to 10/15, the inflammation was no longer present, and his near point was positive.

Another interesting case was that of a young man with congenital cataracts of the zonular type in both eyes. The cataract in the right eye had apparently remained stationary, but the left had started to spread, which was his reason for coming to the Clinic. At that time the vision in the right eye was 10/30, and in the left 10/40. His near point was 12". After eight visits his vision was 10/10 in both eyes and his near point 6".

A man sixty-six years old, suffering from glaucoma, came for treatment after being told by six different specialists that only an operation could help him. We examined him and found the distance point 10/30 in both eyes, his near point negative, and a tension of 40 mm. of mercury in both eyes. At the time the Clinic closed his vision was 10/15 in both eyes, near point positive, and tension reduced to 25 mm. of Hg.

Another case of glaucoma that was of special interest was that of a man sixty years old who showed the hemorrhagic type of this disease in the right eye, with total loss of vision and a tension of 40. There was also a complicating cataract. The vision in his left eye was 10/30 and the near point was negative. When he discontinued treatment at the Clinic his left eye was normal for both the distant and the near point. In the right eye the hemorrhagic condition had entirely disappeared, the tension was reduced to 23, and the cataract was beginning to disappear. I believe that eventually the right eye will clear up entirely. The astonishing feature of this case was that an operation had been advised as the only means of relief, and one physician had even suggested removing the eyeball.

We had a number of hyperopic, presbyopic, and myopic patients, all of whom responded readily to treatment. Among the myopic type we found several patients with a vision of only 10/200 in both eyes, and in a very short time they were able to read 10/15 and 10/10. Hyperopic and presbyopic patients who were unable to read diamond type when they first came in for treatment were soon able to read fine print. Patients who complained of constant pain in their eyes, or of the inability to read or sew without discomfort, were greatly relieved and in many cases absolutely cured after a few visits.

REPORT OF THE LEAGUE MEETING

By May Secor, Recording Secretary

The November meeting of the Better Eyesight League was held on November 6. Dr. Clinton E. Achorn, an osteopathic physician of this city, was the speaker of the evening. Dr. Achorn is a former pupil of Dr. Bates and has now been practicing the Bates Method for some time.

The speaker presented a very encouraging report of the results he has obtained, correcting defective vision without the use of glasses. He emphasized the importance of the use of the memory and imagination in this work and reported a case in which the vision improved fifty percent within twenty-four hours after the patient had secured adequate use of his memory and imagination. Perfect relaxation is also essential in the correction of visual defects. Sight is impaired by strain, and fatigue follows effort.

Many cases of defective vision in children may be cured as the result of one lesson; normal use of the imagination and memory, and the facility with which the child relaxes are helpful elements in these cases. The absence of mental strain in a child is due largely to the fact that he usually forgets quickly; when his attention is called to a new object, the former object of his attention is forgotten, and so on throughout the day. The application of this principle in the correction of defective vision will prove helpful: one should see best the object or letter at which he is looking; and, proceeding to the next object or letter, he should forget the former object of his attention.

At the close of Dr. Achorn's interesting address, Dr. Bates discussed requested subjects. Dr. Bates explained the failure of hypnotism and faith in correcting defective vision as due to the presence of effort; effort precludes relaxation.

GET A GOOD START WITH SOME NEW RESOLUTIONS

By Emily A. Meder

Someone remarked recently that "promises were made to be broken." I wonder if the same train of thought is carried out with New Year's resolutions. How many of us conscientiously adhere to them throughout the year? Yet, the fact that we have made them is in our favor, for from time to time during the year they spring to life and we renew them for another week, until forgotten again.

Resolutions, however, are made for one's own benefit either financially, physically or spiritually. Begin now with the right attitude towards your eyes, and resolve that you will treat them decently. It is not necessary to pamper them; just give them half a chance and they will do the rest. Resolve that:

1. You will not overwork them by staring.
2. You will relieve them from duty by blinking constantly.
3. Palm frequently. This is relaxation to the eyes and is

what play is to the soldier. One always works better for having a little play.

4. Swing and see objects moving. This is good exercise and keeps the eyes "in trim."

5. Read small print as much as possible. This requires relaxation. You cannot read fine print very well if you strain. Large print you can read under a strain.

Let these five rules govern your eye action. They aren't difficult, and become a good habit with practice. After all, your eyes will appreciate it, and perfect sight is worth "resolving" for.

A GLAUCOMA CASE

By Dr. Harold J. Geis

Ms. Z., the mother of four children and the wife of a very wealthy farmer, was referred to me by a local physician who apparently believed what I said when I told him I felt reasonably sure that I could benefit a glaucomatous case which he had been unsuccessful in treating for several weeks. He wanted the lady to undergo an operation (an iridectomy) but she refused, thanks to the Lord and Dr. Bates.

When she called on me she felt rather skeptical, but as she said afterwards, "I was willing to take a chance inasmuch as it did not necessitate an operation."

She was unable to recognize the big "C" at six feet. In fact she could not count the fingers on my right hand at five feet. When she tried to read the card, I noted a slight tilting of the head, and I felt sure this was due to eccentric fixation. I explained to her that she made an effort to see every character on the card equally well, and that if she wanted to improve her vision and see perfectly she should see one letter best and all the other letters on the Snellen test card worse. I then had her palm for ten minutes, after which she was able to read the 70-line at ten feet. Then I told her to "flash," trying not to see the characters all equally well but just the one she was looking at should be seen best and all the other letters worse. She was enabled by this exercise to read 10/40.

After eleven treatments she can read, write, sew, and to her most important of all, go to the movies. She thinks her cure is miraculous and so do her many friends, but as I tell them, "It's all in a day's work" and simple if one understands the fundamental principle, which is muscular relaxation, of the Bates Method correctly applied.

QUESTIONS AND ANSWERS

Q–1. What causes the eyes to become bloodshot? How is it cured?

A–1. The cause is strain. It is cured by relaxation.

Q–2. Is closing the eyes and resting them during business hours as efficient as palming?

A–2. Usually not.

Q–3. Can one remember perfectly and see imperfectly?

A–3. No.

Q–4. What is the quickest cure for imperfect sight?

A–4. Imagine something perfectly. If you imagine the white Snellen test card perfectly white, you'll see the letters perfectly black. If you see them perfectly black, you can tell what they are.

Better Eyesight
February 1924—Vol. VIII, No. 8

THE TRINITY

There are three things which the normal eye practices more or less continuously, and which are necessary in order to maintain normal vision.

1. The long swing.
2. The short swing.
3. Blinking.

The long swing has been described repeatedly and most people are able to practice it successfully, especially people whose sight is good. If you have very imperfect sight you may have difficulty in demonstrating the benefit of the long swing. Some patients are indeed difficult to manage. They may be able to practice the long swing when looking out of a window with its light background. By moving the whole body, head and eyes together a long distance from side to side, one becomes able to imagine a cord of the window shade moving in the opposite direction. This makes it possible to imagine the long swing when you turn your back to the window and look at objects in the room which have a dark background. When the long swing is properly maintained, the letters of the Snellen test card become darker as long as one does not look directly at the card. Looking above the card or below it is a help in maintaining the long swing of the card when the maximum vision is obtained by the long swing. Never look directly at the card or try to read the letters when practicing the long swing.

By gradually lessening the movement of the body from side to side, the swing of the card becomes shorter and one may soon become able to flash the large letters. The swing of the card can be reduced to an inch or less.

FAIRY STORIES

By W. H. Bates, M.D.

Editor's Note—*We should read fairy stories for the benefit of our eyesight. It can be demonstrated that the imagination is a benefit to the vision and if fairy stories improve the imagination they will also improve the sight.*

The Black Fairy

Zipp, bang, again and again, the cruel boys pasted the little boy with snowballs, calling, "Four-eyes, four-eyes," at him because he could not see well and wore glasses. The snow got down his neck, inside the collar of his little jacket, it stung the skin of his face, blurred his glasses and hurt him so that he cried in pain. He could not fight them, so he ran as fast as his little legs could travel. He stumbled and fell. It seemed to the little boy that he fell down a long, long way and kept on falling, falling so long that he could not remember how long it was. He closed his eyes for a moment only it seemed, and then he stopped falling. When he opened his eyes and looked around him, he found himself lying on the grass and the grass was soft and warm, like it is in fairy land. Above him the branches of the trees were moving from a light summer breeze. Around him were bright colored flowers, with the bees buzzing to and fro. Everywhere was the bright warm sunshine. He fell asleep for awhile and awoke feeling rested. On his breast lay a little fox puppy gazing kindly at his face. He touched it with his hand and gently smoothed the top of its head. Then another little fox puppy came out from the shadow of the grass, poked its nose close to the little boy's face and licked his cheek. Then two more came romping, toddling into view, all anxious to get close to the little boy and to be petted. But suddenly he lost all interest in the puppies when the mother fox appeared with a tiny black fairy on her back. The puppies and the little boy crowded as close to her as they could. He petted the puppies while the mother fox looked on, happy and contented. A contented fox is not always or often seen. The mother fox said to the fairy, "Little black fairy, we found this boy all bruised and bloody. He is such a good little boy and he is so gentle and kind that I wish someone would make him happy. That is why I asked you to come and see him."

And then the puppies began to all talk at once. They begged the fairy to be good to the little boy, the little boy whose heart was so full of love that he even loved baby foxes. The father fox called just then and all the foxes ran away quickly, so as not to keep him waiting.

The little boy said to the black fairy, "How beautiful you are. I like to look at you. Your eyes sparkle like the diamond in my mother's ring when the sun shines on it; your teeth are white like the pearl necklace my mother wears to parties; your lips are red like my sister's ruby ring; your ears are like the fine sea shells at the seashore; your laugh sounds like the water bubbling over the pebbles in the brook, while your smile warms me inside my breast and makes me love you. Come closer to me little black fairy. Stay with me always and let me love you more than I have ever loved anybody else. When I look at you, the pain in my head leaves me, my eyes feel rested and cool, the light seems brighter, I can see everything clear, and the fog over the trees and flowers disappears."

After he spoke so nicely to the little black fairy, she giggled and laughed and blushed. She jerked her shoulders up and down, danced around on her toes, waved her hand to him, threw him many kisses and became so excited by her exertions she quite got out of breath.

After she quieted down enough so she could speak she called to him, "Oh, you dear little four-eyes," I love you for what you say. I love you so much that I want to help you as much as a fairy can help you. Let me cure your poor eyes, so that you will always have perfect sight without glasses. Love me enough and I will cure you. Never forget me. Please remember me so well that you will always see me, one tiniest part of me blacker than all the rest of me, see me on everything you look at, no matter how large or how small or how far away. Let me be your sweetheart fairy, the one little fairy you love best, and the world will be for you a heavenly place to live, with your eyes at rest with perfect sight as long as you are true to me, and never forget me."

And then she waved her hand to him and moved farther and farther away, until she appeared as small as a tiny black speck, the size of a period in the little boy's reader. But always he remembered that he loved her, and so did as she advised, and found that no matter how far away she was he was able to remember how she looked, one tiniest part of her blacker than all the rest. He loved her so much that he saw her better than everything else. The sight of her rested his eyes. And after she had disappeared from view he loved her so much better than the trees, the grass, the clouds, the flowers, that he believed he saw her better than anything else. And the better he imagined or remembered his little black fairy, or saw her in his heart better than all else, he saw more perfectly the trees, the grass, the clouds and the flowers. He was true to his love, the little black fairy, and she was true to her promise to him that he would see perfectly without glasses as long as he remembered her perfectly. When he looked at a large tree she was a good sized fairy. When he looked at a small blade of grass or a tiny flower, she was the tiniest little fairy that one could imagine.

His sight was good when he remembered how perfectly black she was; but, when she looked less black his sight was worse. He found that he had to remember his love perfectly, to be perfectly true to her in order to have perfect sight. It was all a beautiful dream; and, when you dream of fairy land, sometimes your dreams come true. You, who read this story, can you remember the blackest, blackest little black fairy, the tiniest blackest fairy that ever was? Maybe you can remember the black better with your eyes closed. Can you remember the black eyes of the black fairy when reading your book? And when you do, can you read the words better?

The next morning when his mother came into his room and wakened him with a kiss, he opened his eyes wide, with no dread of the bright sunlight which shone on his mother's face. He was all excited, laughing and talking eagerly, rapidly, of the good fortune that had come to him.

Among other things he said, "Oh, mother, I can see you without my glasses. I see the blue color of your eyes which I never saw before. The fog has gone from the pictures on the wall. I can look out the window and see the trees, the grass, the flowers, the people walking along the sidewalk, and there is father talking to a strange boy—oh no, he is the boy who lives next door. He is not a strange boy, but I see him so much clearer now without my glasses than I ever did before when I wore them. Aren't you glad? Please, I want to get dressed quickly, run down stairs and tell father all about it. I want to hurry away to school and tell the teacher I can see everything now without my glasses. And I want to tell all the boys and girls in school, the workers in the grocery store and in the market, everybody.

The White Fairy

The teacher was tired. It was very warm, and through the open windows one heard in the distance the birds calling to each other. Her head was aching, her eyes throbbing with pain. She took off her glasses to rest her eyes, and sat for awhile with her eyes closed and her head resting on her hands. And the pupils were tired, restless, and anxious to get out in the bright sunshine and play on the cool green grass in the shade of the trees. Their eyes were continually looking out the windows.

George Smith saw her first, standing on the window sill waving her hands to the children, smiling such a beautiful smile of love with her tiny rosebud of a mouth. But it was her wonderful black eyes which smiled most. They sparkled and twinkled so merrily, they were so full of life and love and happiness; they were so cheery, so encouraging, so comforting, that all were intoxicated with delight. She was only a few inches tall, but every bit of her, from the top of her head to her tiny feet, was formed with a perfection of beauty rarely seen. And how graceful she was. She found her way somehow to the top of a vacant desk; and, after delighting the children for a few moments with the most wonderful, most delightful of fairy dances, sat herself down on the top of an inkstand—but she was not quiet a moment. Her feet and hands, her whole body seemed to swing from side to side, just like the pendulum of a clock swings; and, when you looked alternately from one eye to the other they seemed to swing also. This swing was very noticeable, and the strange thing about the swing was that it was so restful and did the eyes of the children so much good. Those wearing glasses took them off and found that they could see the swinging eyes of the little white fairy as well as everything else, quite perfectly. And the teacher noted that the fog over everything she formerly saw without glasses was gone, the pain in her eyes and head was gone. She saw everything clearly, so easily that she quite forgot that she had eyes.

The teacher became interested in the eyes of her pupils. She felt that something should be done to prevent them from acquiring imperfect sight while they were attending school. As a beginning she tested the sight of all the children at twenty feet and made a record. The next day she tested them again and found that the number of cases of imperfect sight was less. This bothered her somewhat, because she could not understand how she had made any mistake. She tested them again on the third day, and was more careful and painstaking than before. Again to her surprise, she found a less number with imperfect sight. Then it dawned upon her that testing the sight of the children with the Snellen test card was a benefit. At any rate, she said to herself that she would test their sight every day for a month and note the results.

Some of the children called her attention to the fact that she had no record of the vision of her own eyes, and to please and encourage her pupils she had them test her sight every day and keep a record. Every time she read the Snellen test card it seemed to her that she read it more easily and better, and she found herself looking at the card every once in a while during the day. She acquired a certain amount of pleasure in looking at the card, and she found the pupils doing the same thing.

Standing twenty feet from the card without her glasses, at the end of the month she found that her vision with each eye was normal, and even a little better than the average normal vision. Furthermore her eyes, which formerly had bothered her more or less, although she wore glasses prescribed by a very prominent eye doctor, never gave her the relief that she now obtained without glasses by reading the Snellen test card daily.

She was very much pleased to note also that her pupils were brighter and had better memories, and studied for longer periods without becoming tired or restless. Her attendance was better than it had ever been in any one month before. One little boy told her that he no longer had headaches from studying his lessons, and that he could read what was written on the blackboard without half trying. Other teachers became interested and they obtained the same beneficial results.

STORIES FROM THE CLINIC

No. 48: Anna Bernard, the Blind Girl–Part I

By Emily C. Lierman

During the month of August 1922, while our Clinic work was still going on at the Harlem Hospital, there came one day to our office Anna Bernard, a blind girl age 25, who was led there by her younger sister.

Dr. Bates and I were extremely busy and at the time had to turn away many patients because we already had more than we could manage. As she heard me approaching her, she asked for Ms. Lierman. I said I was that person, and asked what I could do for her. She mentioned the name of a doctor's wife who had been treated successfully for cataract by Dr. Bates. A dozen or more patients were in the waiting room at the time and were listening to all she had to say, for she talked loud enough to be heard. She said, "I came with great hope that you might help me to see." She then handed me a note, written by the doctor's wife already mentioned. It read something like this:

"You have helped so many patients in your Clinic, won't you please help this girl if you can? I met her in Prospect Park, Brooklyn, as she sat beside me on a bench resting."

I am sorry to say that I frowned as I finished reading that note. I did not see how I could possibly take another case when I already had more than I could handle. She could not be treated at the Clinic because the authorities would not allow us to take cases from out of the hospital district. I was just about to say that she would have to come some other time when I was not so busy, but I caught the anxious look in her face. A look of hope, a look of faith. I could read in that face the answer she expected of me. No thought of being sent away that day without treatment had entered her mind. I solved the problem quickly and said, "I will take you this minute to our other office and see what I can do for you." At that moment, a gentleman sitting in the room gasped and sighed with relief. He smiled and said, "That was fine of you, knowing how rushed you are at present."

I disturbed Dr. Bates long enough to have him examine her eyes, and to tell me whether there was any hope of her seeing at all. Dr. Bates said she had microplithalmas in both eyes. She had no red reflex from the pupils. A white membrane was visible in both pupils and the pupils were both very small. She could distinguish light from darkness but that was all. I asked her to tell me when her sight began to fail, or how long she had been blind. What a shock it was to me to hear her say, "I was born blind; so was my mother." What chance had I, if any, to ever help that poor girl to see even just a little of this God's beautiful world? Was is possible that perhaps our Heavenly Father himself had sent her to me, and that through Him I would be guided in helping her to see? Anyhow these were my thoughts at the time, so I started right in with the treatment, just as though she had sight, and then to help her improve her sight. She had so much trouble with her poor eyes that I did not know just where to begin first. Her eyes moved rapidly from side to side, a condition called nystagmus. She also had a contraction of the throat muscles which caused a great deal of fatigue generally. Here was a big job ahead of me. I told her I would do my very best to help her if she would do exactly as I said.

Her sister, whose age was twelve, had normal vision and was called upon to assist me in the treatment. She proved later on to be a very good assistant. I asked the patient if her sense of touch was all right and she answered yes. Then I gave her an ordinary pin and told her to feel the size of it, then to feel the point and the head of it. She was told then to palm and remember the touch of the pin.

She could remember the touch of the pin very well she said, even though it was no longer in her hand. I was very much encouraged when, after a few minutes of palming, she removed her hands from her eyes and I noticed that the rapid movement of her eyes had stopped.

But when I asked her a personal question the movement of nystagmus returned. I then told her to forget the question I had asked her and to cover her eyes again with her hands to rest them. While she was doing this I told her what had been accomplished for an old blind man, who was at the present time under treatment. I related how he once had good sight and now after several years of blindness and great suffering from eye operations, he was beginning to see. I watched my patient very closely and I could see that she was interested in what I was saying, and a smile came, which was good to see. Again I told her to remove her hands from her eyes and I noticed the second time that her eyes were perfectly still. Her sister sat close by holding her breath in amazement and in an excited voice said to me, "This is wonderful. Anna has never been able to control that terrible movement of her eyes for some years. I feel sure she is going to receive benefit from your treatment and care. I want very much to help you if you will tell me how."

It has always been my greatest desire to carry on Dr. Bates' ideas and methods and to follow very closely his directions in all cases. I remembered something he said to me at one time. "If you have a pain, find out what causes it and cure the cause." So I felt with this case, that perhaps if I can cure the nystagmus and the nervous contraction of her throat, I might be better able to do more for her vision. Her sense of touch was good and her memory of the prick of the pin had helped while she rested her eyes. Now I would try the swing and see if that would help her throat. I told her to put up her forefinger and to hold it about six inches from her eyes. Then to turn her head slowly from side to side toward the right shoulder and then toward the left. I explained to her that even though she could not see her finger, she could imagine she saw it. She answered me just as I wanted her to. She said, "Oh, I can imagine the size of my finger, and when I turn my head to the right my finger seems to move to the left and vice versa."

I encouraged her to keep on moving her head from side to side and to blink her eyes to prevent staring, which had been a habit since birth. I noticed after a few minutes or so that she settled herself in a more relaxed position as she sat in her chair. Then I called her sister's attention to the fact that the contraction of her throat muscles quieted down until they stopped.

(To be continued.)

"HOW JOE COOK LEARNED TO SHIFT"

In the January number of the *American Magazine,* Joe Cook, famous eccentric comedian, says he never has seen a juggler who had to wear glasses. He himself has remarkable eyesight, and this is the way he accounts for it:

"In my work," he says, "I have to be constantly changing the focus of my eyes; adjusting it to different distances and different directions. In juggling several balls, for instance, I look up, down, to right, and to left; so quickly, of course, that even I am hardly conscious of moving my eyes. But I do move them. I am always practicing, and this exercises the muscles of the eye. I believe this keeps them strong, active and, you might say, young."

"Oculists will tell you that this is true. Exercise your eyes by looking around you, at objects that are at various distances and in different directions. If your regular job is at close work, stop once in a while and look at things farther off. Practice changing the focus of your eyes. Get several small balls and try to juggle them. It will help to keep your eyes young."

THE USE OF EYESIGHT IN A PRINTING PLANT

By Bendix T. Minden

Sight is well held to be the highest and most perfect of all the senses, whereby we are able to recognize the form, size, color, and distance of thousands of different objects in nature. Indeed, it is wonderful to behold a balloon leave the earth and watch it until it becomes a black speck in the sky. But in a printing plant, this sense is so woven into the countless acts of our occupation that we scarcely appreciate this marvelous gift, so essential not only to the simplest matters of comfort, but also to the culture of the mind and the higher forms of pleasure. It seems to be the mind behind the eye that sees, for in each department of this plant, the employees perform their work rapidly and amazingly accurate.

There is a popular opinion that persons who use their eyes for much reading or fine work are more apt to have imperfect sight than others. A visit to the majority of printing plants would disprove this theory. In the plant with which the writer is connected, there are only ten people out of 60 employed who wear glasses, and one of them has had a cataract on his eye since childhood. In three other plants visited, the percentage ran from 10 to 20 percent of those who wore glasses.

It is strange to say that the continuous use of the eye in a correct manner strengthens that organ rather than spoils the vision, which is proven not only by a printing plant, but by intimate knowledge of a juggler.

A juggler's eye, the same as a printer's, is always focusing quickly on moving objects, and it is merely this constant and automatic correct use of the eye which is so valuable for the detection of mistakes in a printing plant.

We will enter the workrooms with a piece of copy, which may be either manuscript or reprint matter. This is given to the foreman, who glances through it quickly and marks the style, size of type, measure of lines, etc. He then hands this copy to the compositor. If it is handwritten, it is not a question of the compositor being able to see, but of his brain being able to decipher the hieroglyphics of the author. In this case, inadvertently the letters were badly written—"u's" looked like "n's," the "i's" were not dotted or the "t's" crossed. This caused a mental strain, and not an eyestrain, especially when a name or a word is taken from a foreign language.

When the compositor is through setting the type, the printer's devil pulls a proof. The proof and copy are then handed to the proofreader, who proceeds to read it with the help of the copyholder.

The proofreader is called upon to exercise his eye and his brain in unison. His eye is to see wrong fonts, that is, mixed type. He is to detect mistakes in spelling, punctuation, paragraphing, grammar, or other errors. He must not have any optical illusion as to what the letters really are. The letter, the word or the punctuation mark must stand out clearly—exactly as it is.

Fortunately, the light in most printing plants is well diffused. The desk of the proofreader is placed so that the daylight comes in through the window from above and behind, and over the left shoulder, which is important for the eyes as daylight seems to be a most soothing, invigorating and strengthening tonic. The eyes appear to be rested when looking from one object or color to another of a different form or color.

In going to the pressroom, we come to another department which calls upon the eyes to see and discern a new phase of sight. A pressman uses his eyes to note the equality of impression, and to bring out the different shades of a halftone or cut, so as to make it appear as near real to the object as possible. He is called upon to see both with his eye and his mind's eye the various ink colors. By mixing different inks the pressman can produce various hues, shades or tints. To produce violet he will mix 10 parts of white, 21 parts of red, and 69 parts of blue; likewise in making the color scarlet he mixes 85 parts of red with 15 parts of orange. Thus the pressman must have a good eye in order to understand and see the colors as they are. If he were "color blind" he would be unable to distinguish even red. Our pressman had occasion to mix a color which was to match the blue sky and the green color of a dollar bill. He would look up at the sky and then down at the greenback in his hand. One not familiar with what he was doing would think he was praying for greenbacks. No, he was not doing that, but was matching colors.

We now leave the pressroom to enter the bindery. The mind's eye is here centered on the fingers, and one cannot help but remark how skillfully they do their work. Folding, counting, and numbering of sheets are done quickly and accurately. They are done so cleverly that it becomes almost automatic, thus we see a person functioning only by reason of the mind. The ladies at the wire-stitching machines, without a gauge are able, very speedily, to stitch a booklet or a leaflet in the same place almost without an error. We notice a man cutting paper on a big cutting machine. It is most remarkable how the eye can be trained to do its work so nearly perfect. Should the cutter be mistaken in his measurements, he would cut the paper wrong, thereby spoiling the job.

In passing through the plant, we go to the shipping department. Eyes are even important here, for should the shipping clerk place the wrong address on the case, it could not be very easily corrected. The case may go to Kansas instead of Kentucky. This would not only delay the delivery, but would cause considerable unnecessary labor and expense.

There are innumerable more uses of the eye in a printing plant than described in this article. Best of all, one should visit a printing plant and see for himself the wonderful workings of that valuable organ—the eye.

REPORT OF THE DECEMBER MEETING

Dr. M. E. Gore of East Orange, New Jersey was the speaker at the December meeting of the Better Eyesight League. He remarked that it was a pleasure for him to address the meeting, and he hoped that he could say something that would help someone to see. He said it is the easiest thing in the world to have perfect sight, but it takes an effort to have defective vision, and an effort and strain to continue it.

Dr. Gore gave a brief synopsis of how he became interested in Dr. Bates' work after having heard him lecture. He then attended the Clinic at the Harlem Hospital, where he was amazed at the results Ms. Lierman obtained with her patients. To test the correctness of Dr. Bates' method, as he was skeptical, he began with a patient who had very bad sight, which was further hampered by a goiter. While he was improving her sight, he was astonished to notice that the goiter was slowly diminishing in size. At the end of two years she had normal vision, and the goiter was gone. He cited a great many other cases, too numerous to mention, by which he proved that Dr. Bates was not only right, but had made a wonderful discovery.

Ms. Irwin, President of the Better Eyesight League of the Oranges, was introduced by Dr. Gore, and gave a report of her own eye trouble. Hers was a difficult case, and she deserves a great deal of credit for the tenacity she showed when everyone advised her to keep her glasses on and not to try any "new-fangled" ideas. Her history, in brief, is that she had to remain home from business at least one day a week. She had frightful headaches and could not stand the light. Her bedroom was always darkened, and the sun was never allowed to shine in on her. During that period she said she only desired a little dark nook to slink into and be alone with her troubles.

One day she heard Dr. Bates talk, and was so encouraged when he told her she could be cured that she bought his book and started immediately. She went through a great many trials before her friends would believe she really intended leaving off her glasses. She palmed on the ferry, on the train, before and after work, and wherever and whenever she had a few minutes to spare. The result was that she left off her glasses, improved her work, and was no longer troubled with headaches. She goes to the movies, and above all, likes the sun. She loves to wake up in the morning and find it streaming over her bed.

On the head of this glowing report of courage and self-control, one young lady in the audience desired to know if she could be helped. She gave a detailed description of all her symptoms, much to the amusement of the meeting, and said she was very myopic. She went on to say she wanted to improve her sight in order to leave off her glasses, and also improve her looks. She was told if she followed Ms. Irwin's example she could obtain perfect sight.

Dr. Bates was kept busy for half an hour answering questions, and explaining imagination in its relation to the cure of imperfect sight. The meeting was adjourned a half-hour later than its schedule, but everyone had learned a little more about their eyes.

QUESTIONS AND ANSWERS

Q–1. Can a child three months old be cured of squint?

A–1. Yes

Q–2. Does the bright sunlight harm a baby's eyes?

A–2. No.

Q–3. Is being in a dark room with the eyes open as beneficial as palming?

A–3. No.

Q–4. Can any other color be substituted for black when palming?

A–4. Yes, if imagined consciously and intentionally.

Q–5. How often must one read fine print to obtain benefit?

A–5. Daily.

Q–6. What one method of improving the sight is best?

A–6. Swinging and blinking.

Q–7. To palm successfully, is it necessary to remember black or try to see black?

A–7. No. When one palms successfully the eyes and mind are relaxed and black is usually seen, but any effort to see black is a strain which always fails.

Better Eyesight
March 1924—Vol. VIII, No. 9

MENTAL PICTURES

Many patients with imperfect sight complain that when they close their eyes to remember a white card with black letters, they usually fail and remember instead a black card with white letters. The vision of these patients is very much improved when they become able to remember a white card white, with the black letters remembered perfectly black. Imperfect memory, imperfect imagination, and imperfect sight are all caused by strain.

One patient could not remember a white pillow, but by first regarding the pillow and seeing one corner best and all the other corners worse and shifting from one corner to another he became able, when closing his eyes, to remember one corner in turn best, and obtained a good mental picture of the whole pillow. One cannot see a pillow perfectly without central fixation. To have central fixation requires relaxation or rest. One patient, who could not remember a large letter "C" of the Snellen test card with the eyes closed, was able to remember the colors of some flowers, and then he was able to remember a letter "C." In order to remember a desired mental picture, one should remember perfectly some other things. This is a relaxation which helps to remember the mental picture desired. It is well to keep in mind that one cannot remember one thing perfectly and something else imperfectly at the same time.

In my book is described the case of a woman with imperfect sight who could remember a yellow buttercup with the eyes closed, perfectly, but with her eyes open and regarding the Snellen test card with imperfect sight, she had no memory of the yellow buttercup.

ILLUSIONS OF NORMAL SIGHT

By W. H. Bates, M.D.

An illusion is defined by the dictionary to be something which does not exist. Illusions are not seen, they are imagined. One cannot have perfect sight without illusions.

Central Fixation

When the sight is normal, one is always able to demonstrate that things regarded are seen best while those not regarded are always seen worse. With central fixation if one recognizes or sees a letter correctly, all other letters are seen worse. With the best vision that can be obtained it can be demonstrated that one cannot see a letter or any other object perfectly without seeing one part best. No matter how large or how small the letter or object may be, it is impossible to see it perfectly without central fixation. Many people believe that when they look at a small letter or a small period that they see it all at once; but, when you notice the facts, one finds that to see or to try to see a letter, or a number of letters all perfectly, the vision becomes modified or imperfect. Some persons with unusually good vision can read the Snellen test card so rapidly that they have the impression that they see all the letters perfectly at the same time. It requires, in some cases, considerable trouble to demonstrate that this is impossible. In some obstinate cases it has required not only some hours but some days to prove that this is a fact. The letters of the Snellen test card are equally black. To see one blacker than the others, or a part of a letter blacker than the rest of it, is seeing something which is not so. The large letters and the small letters are printed in the same ink and all are equally black and although one cannot read the letters unless they see them by central fixation it is still, nevertheless, an illusion. One should emphasize the fact that it is possible to have illusions or that one cannot see perfectly unless the illusion of central fixation can be demonstrated.

Swinging

When a small letter of the Snellen test card can be seen perfectly and continuously, it can be demonstrated that the letter is moving from side to side about its own width or less or that it is moving in other directions. To look fixedly at a letter and try to imagine one point of the letter is seen continuously can be demonstrated to be impossible. One cannot obtain perfect sight by staring or trying to see things or imagine things as stationary. I have never seen this truth stated in any publication. It is just as important an illusion as is central fixation in order to have perfect sight continuously. It can be demonstrated that all persons with imperfect sight stare, concentrate, or try to see letters stationary. The illusion that the letter is moving, when the sight is normal, is brought about by the normal eye to avoid the stare and the strain of seeing things imperfectly. The point of fixation changes continuously, easily.

When one looks to the right of the letter, the letter is to the left of where you are looking. If you look to the left of a letter the letter is to the right of where you are looking. Every time your eyes move to the right, the letter moves to the left. Every time your eyes move to the left the letter moves to the right, and by alternately looking from one to the other side of a letter one becomes able to imagine the illusion that the letter is moving from side to side. When reading rapidly one does not have time to demonstrate that each individual letter is moving. Here again the imagination is responsible for the illusion of the swing. The letters do not really move, we only imagine it; and, unless we can imagine a letter moving continuously, we are unable to see it with normal sight continuously. This is a truth; it has no exceptions.

It is a necessary part of normal vision, and yet it has not, to my knowledge, been published in any book or periodical. People who write works on physiological optics have much to learn. So many of my patients who have been benefited by my methods have asked me, "Why didn't Helmholtz, Donders and all those other authorities publish the truths that you have discovered?" Nearly all ophthalmologists put glasses on people because that is all they know. I can recall the time when that was all I knew. If a patient left the office without a prescription for glasses it was not my fault. Now when persons with imperfect sight, wearing glasses, become able to practice central fixation and the optical swing in the right way, their vision becomes normal without glasses.

Halos

When the sight is normal and when one regards a letter of the Snellen test card with a white center, the white part of the letter appears whiter than it really is and whiter than the rest of the card. I use the word "halos" for this illusion. This is an illusion which can be demonstrated quite readily by covering over the black part of a letter with a screen with an opening slightly smaller than the white part of the letter, which permits the center of the letter to be observed. When this is done the white center of the letter is the same shade of whiteness as the rest of the card. Some people can imagine the illusion when it is described to them. When reading fine print the spaces between the lines appear whiter than the rest of the card, but only when the vision is good. As a general rule when one can imagine these white spaces between the lines are whiter than the rest of the card, halos are noticed, the black appears more perfectly black, and the letters can be read with normal vision. halos are imagined, not seen. Imagination of the illusion of the halos is a quick cure of myopia and astigmatism, as well as other cases of imperfect sight.

All persons who have normal sight are always able to demonstrate the halos. All persons with imperfect sight are cured, temporarily or permanently, when they become able to imagine the halos.

Blinking And Resting The Eyes

By blinking is meant frequent closing of the eyes. It is usually done so rapidly that it is not conspicuous. Many persons with normal sight have the illusion that they do not blink. They believe their eyes are always at rest and that their eyes are continually open all the time. When their attention is called to the facts, it is usually readily demonstrated with persons with normal vision. In one case the patient was able to distinguish a small letter on the bottom line at twenty feet, 20/10. He was positive that he saw the letter continuously. It was found by observing the movements of his eyes that he did two things. First: He closed and opened his eyes frequently, without being conscious of the fact. Second: He looked some distance away from the letter and back again, and did it so quickly that he was not aware that he did it. The facts can also be demonstrated, perhaps more accurately, with the help of movies. In all cases where the sight was normal, blinking occurred almost every second. In some seconds the eyes were opened and closed five times. Blinking occurs more frequently with the normal eye when the light is imperfect or when the conditions are unfavorable for perfect sight. When the light is good, or the conditions most favorable for good sight, blinking occurs at less frequent intervals. Persons with imperfect sight do not rest their eyes by blinking as often as those with normal vision. When they are encouraged to blink more frequently their sight usually improves.

STORIES FROM THE CLINIC

No. 49: Anna Bernard, the Blind Girl–Part 2

By Emily C. Lierman

Last month I wrote about Anna Bernard, the blind girl becoming able to obtain relaxation of her whole body and the muscles of her throat by practicing the swing and with the blinking, which prevented the staring. When I first handed her a test card and asked her if she could see a letter on the card, she answered, "I cannot see letters; I do not know the alphabet. I can only read and write by the sense of touch with the Braille System." Here was another problem. Of course, there was the test card with large and small "E's" pointing in different directions, which could be used to test the sight, but I had other plans. I wanted Anna to learn to read and write and give up the Braille System entirely. Her sister was called upon to help me. She was directed to cut out of cardboard, letters about the size and thickness of the big "C" on the test card. Then she was to paint them black and bring them with her next time she came.

Her sister had good news for me when I saw them again. She had taught Anna some of the letters by the sense of touch. For instance, a letter "T" had a straight piece of cardboard at the top and another straight piece through the center. A letter "C" was round with an opening to the right.

We had made a good start I thought, on this, her fourth visit. I handed her a test card, blank side up. At first she could not tell whether there was print on the card or not because she was very much excited by telling me how quickly she was learning the alphabet. This made her nervous and she strained. I got her busy with palming and while she was doing this, I told her a story. I find that all patients enjoy this, especially when they visualize or follow me closely in what I am saying. I want to say right here that I am a poor story teller, but I do the best I can. If I remember a good short story from a magazine, I tell that; or I might tell about a patient treated by me who had obtained good results. After she had rested and relaxed for ten minutes, I asked her to remove her hands from her eyes and look at the card. She remarked, "It looks all white to me. There seems to be no print on the card at all." I told her she was right. I then turned the card right side out, and as she did the long swing of her body, moving her head with her shoulders from side to side and blinking her eyes with the movement of her body, she pointed to the 200-line letter on the card in her hand and said, "That's a letter 'C'." Can anyone imagine the extent of my happiness?

For twenty-five years she was blind, born that way—never had more than a slight perception of light. Her sister forgot where she was and screamed, "My sister can see!" Anna and I cried with joy. We did not talk, just held each other's hands. I whispered in her ear, "Anna, thank God with me, will you?" "Yes, you bet," says she, "I'm doing that now."

We got busy again, and this time I told her to move the card from side to side, and to imagine her body swinging opposite. She kept this up for several minutes and then she saw the "R" and "B" of the 100-line of letters.

On September 9, 1922, after one month's treatment, her vision had improved considerably for the test card. She had to hold the card about an inch from her eyes in order to see the letters. She was directed to place her finger under the letter that she tried to see, then to move her head slowly from left to right, and in this way she saw the letters of the 70-line, one at a time. Before Anna left the office that day she said she had wonderful news for me. While walking in the street with her sister she saw moving objects for the first time in her life. In Brooklyn they have Hobble Skirt trolley cars with an entrance in the center of the car. Others have an entrance on one end only. Anna was able to see the difference from the sidewalk and told her sister when a car passed by just what kind it was. She actually saw a letterbox fastened to a lamppost and walked towards it, without assistance, to place a letter in the box. Later, Anna's sister cut out cardboard figures from one to ten, and Anna learned to tell them by the sense of touch.

On September 16, 1922, she began to read the 50-line letters of the test card at one inch from her eyes. The first on that line is a figure "5." Anna puzzled over that for a while and then she said, "The first one does not look like a letter at all, it looks very much like a figure '5' my sister has made of cardboard for me."

I cannot express in writing how happy she felt when she realized that she had seen the figure "5" correctly. I placed myself in the sun and immediately she saw a beaded medallion on my gown and also remarked how my beaded necklace sparkled in the sun.

The next thing was to teach her colors. As she never had more than a slight perception of light, the difference between bright red and bright green meant nothing to her. One day while walking with her sister, Anna stopped in front of a store where electrical supplies were displayed. In one section of this shop window was an electric heater and in the center of it was shown a red light. Anna drew her sister's attention to this and remarked, "Isn't that an angry looking thing?" When she related this to me she said, "I can get a pretty good mental picture of Satan now, since I saw that angry light."

By September 30 she had learned all the letters of the alphabet and all the figures. Her sister very patiently taught her various colors, so we had many things to work with in helping Anna to restore her sight. I owe so much of our success in her treatment so far, to her dear little sister Ella.

(To be continued.)

PREVENTING IMPERFECT SIGHT IN SCHOOLCHILDREN

By Elisabet D. Hansen

Editor's Note—*The future of our country is in the hands of the children. The future of the children is in the hands of the teachers. I wish there were more teachers like Ms. Hansen. She has solved a problem in her school of the prevention of myopia in schoolchildren by my methods. How she overcame the usual prejudice of the Board of Health and the Board of Education is interesting. I recommend her methods not only to all teachers, but also to all parents. The following letter from Ms. Hansen is worthwhile:*

Dear Dr. Bates:

I knew you would be interested in the children's compositions—they are wonderful, and the children were just as alive as their compositions.

Four times a day, immediately after the opening of school in the morning, two recesses and noon, the school Victrola is rolled in, classical music by piano, violin, orchestra or the principal song from the broadcasted opera is played. The disc chosen is played all week. They were taught to palm, and why. Sometimes they are to use their imagination on the music and weave that imagination into a three-sentence paragraph. Sometimes the memory is brought into play and we have created on paper sunsets that were as impressionistic and brilliant as any of that class of painters could produce. Another time "Crack the Whip" was used. The papers were full of life and motion. Anything that they are interested in and touch with their daily activities brings the best results.

Ten or fifteen minutes at noon we wanted to see how well they could read the test card, and the few who could stand 30 to 36 feet away and read the 10-line (30/10 to 36/10) were very proud of their eagle eyes, as they called them.

We kept a record of the improvements. Their own stories tell most plainly how much they enjoyed it, and what it did for them and others. These children are now in another room and palm when they feel the need of it. The effect is wonderful.

Lena was most resentful, when she first came to the room, about palming. She would do very little work and she had severe pains in eyes and head. She would not palm because it hurt worse when she tried, but with much persuasion she *did* try. She couldn't imagine anything at all, couldn't bring to mind a story or flower or—well—nothing. I asked her what she liked to think about when she closed her eyes. A mourning veil belonging to her mother—she was morbid to the last degree. Still the feeling between us was strained. This, of course, could not go on. We had a quiet talk, when she told me that she didn't intend to give up her glasses and believed that was what I wanted her to do. After much talking she finally believed and remembered that such a thing as glasses was never spoken of except to ask the children not to wear them when palming. But the thing that gave her faith in me was when I told her that her imaginative powers in her story work were improved a 100%, and that if she would keep up the palming in school (not at home) until June, wear her glasses by all means; they were hers and she had a right to them, that I would bet her a quarter she would believe in me. The case was dropped. I just noticed that she palmed and looked happier.

In the early part of June we were at the Art Institute when she sided up to me and asked if I had noticed anything. I said, "Well, yes, you look more cheerful—you haven't your glasses—are they broken?" She took my hand and confided to me that she did not need them any more. We tested her the next day and she was right—she could see normally. What is more, she has taken two prizes for composition work. One of $2.50, a "Thrift Essay," and the other of $100.00 from the *Herald-Examiner* on the Spark Plug contest and composition.

These are the compositions of which Ms. Hansen spoke. We picked a few of the most interesting from the fifty submitted. They are copied exactly as written, and we know they will appeal to our readers the way they did to us.

Selected Essays on Palming by Schoolchildren

Palming has helped me a great deal in my studies and has given me my beautiful imaginations come to me when I am palming. If we did not have palming four times a day I would not get a hundred in numbers from our principal.

The first time Ms. Hansen told us about palming I went home and I let my mother palm for thirty minutes and she did it every day and hasn't any glasses to wear, and I sure was happy to see my mother without glasses; it was just like wearing crutches on the eyes.

———

My eyesight is as strong as electricity, I could see very far in the distance and what do you suppose did it. Palming, which my teacher taught me a year and a half ago in room seven. Palming is the best to do for your eyes so as not to wear glasses.

———

I have strengthened my imagination and vision by palming. It has helped me in many of my studies which were very hard for me to learn. I have won a prize in the Noel State Bank Compositions. It is all I owe to palming.

———

Palming has done to me a great deal. My eyes are better than they were two years ago. Ms. Hansen is the only teacher in the Carpenter School teaching palming.

———

I taught my mother to palm. One day she said, "Peter go and buy me medicine for the eyes," and I said, "You don't need any medicine. Do this: put your two hands to your eyes and shut your eyes and only see black." She did that and I went out. After one hour I came back. I saw her still palming. I said, Ma, how are your eyes? She said, "They are all right now and so I didn't buy any medicine."

———

While I was palming I was thinking how to do my English. I was wishing for my passing mark. I was willing to try my best for the next grade. We made many mistakes in our English. The Snellen test card made our brain think a little better by palming. I thank you, Dr. Bates, for the Snellen test card and the palming that the teacher taught us to do.

———

Palming has increased my eyesight every time I palm. It has made my brains stronger. Whenever I am tired or my head aches, I just have to palm and think pleasant thoughts when I am all right.

My father who is not so well is not strong. Last night my father's eyesight was so poor that he had to wear glasses even though they are his enemies. I came home and told him how to palm. He has palmed five minutes every night and now he can see plainly and is much stronger.

———

Palming is a great helper to me. When I came to room six our teacher Ms. Hansen taught me how to palm, and to this day I don't have to wear glasses anymore.

One day my uncle told me his eyesight was getting weaker every day and I told him about our teacher how she taught me how to palm. He did the same and his eyesight improved.

———

Ms. Hansen is the only teacher that gives palming in the Carpenter School. Since I have been in room six my eyes are better. Ms. Hansen tested my eyes a few times and I improved a great deal.

My mother had a headache. I told her to put her hands before her eyes and not let any light get in. She did this and she felt better. My elder sister was wearing glasses; I told her to palm for twenty-five minutes. She did this for one week. She went to the doctor and he was surprised because her eyes were cured and he said, "You don't have to wear glasses any more."

———

Palming has improved my imagination and eyesight. It also helps me clear my mind, which I call "Making my mind a file, and not a pile." What I mean is that it helps me not to forget. Before I knew anything about palming my eyesight was very poor and I had to strain if I wanted to read. From this straining I had many headaches, but now I even can read fine print and I don't know how a headache feels like.

Editor's Note—*Ms. Lierman, Dr. Bates' assistant, was so impressed with Ms. Hansen's letter and so touched to think that there were teachers who did take an interest in the schoolchildren's welfare, that she immediately sat down and wrote the following letter to Ms. Hansen:*

My dear Ms. Hansen:

When I came to my office this morning Dr. Bates told me about your wonderful letter and asked me if I would like to read it. I want you to know that I feel just as he does about that letter. It is the most wonderful letter I have ever read in my life. Perhaps you do not realize it but there are a million words in between the lines of your letter that I understand very well. They are in your heart and you are able to give what a child needs so much, your wonderful love and understanding.

Your letter reminded me of a little girl of long ago. She was a sickly little girl and while her grandmother, who loved and cared for her, was in the home, she was happy; but after the grandmother had left her home, she was a very lonely little girl. She had three brothers, one older than herself. She also had a stepfather who did not understand children at all. Her mother, while she was very tender and self-sacrificing, had to neglect her children a great deal in order to be the breadwinner of the household.

As a patient, she came to Dr. Bates and after he cured her imperfect sight and other troubles, he inspired her to help him in this wonderful work. He has been her teacher, not only in better eyesight but also to study other things as well. The little girl I started to tell you about, is myself.

How I wish I could be near you every day and watch you as you give your love and your life to the children in your charge.

You cannot understand now just what you are doing for those children, but later on in life they will think back to you and remember all the wonderful things you did for them and how you cured their imperfect sight. Is there anything more wonderful in this world than to make people see? You are not only curing the children's eyes but you are instilling in their minds more wonderful things than better sight. I cannot say too many times to you, God bless you.

When you come to New York please come right straight to me because I love you.

Sincerely yours,
Emily C. Lierman

BETTER EYESIGHT LEAGUE

By May Secor, Recording Secretary

The January meeting of the Better Eyesight League was on January eighth; a discussion of the various phases of the Bates Method was followed by the annual business meeting of the League.

Among the clinical cases reported were two of special interest. A high schoolboy who was suffering from myopia was relieved, after one treatment, to such an extent that he was able to dispense with three pairs of glasses which he had been using. An acute case of divergent squint in a high schoolgirl was noticeably relieved in consequence of two treatments. Dr. Achorn spoke of the important roles which relaxation, memory, and swinging play in restoring normal vision.

Dr. Bates suggested:

A. *Methods for the elimination of myopia in schoolchildren, without the use of glasses:*

1. In each classroom have a Snellen card hanging where it will be plainly visible to the pupils.
2. Have each pupil read the Snellen card several times daily.
3. Have the pupils palm and swing daily.
4. Since perfect sight is contagious, and imperfect sight is contagious, consider it your duty as a teacher to acquire normal eyesight without the use of glasses.

Note: *Nurses, osteopathic physicians, and medical physicians will find that the acquisition of normal eyesight without the use of glasses will render their work more effective.*

B. *Points to be considered by all readers:*

1. Imperfect sight is the result of hard work; effort produces strain; perfect sight is attained with ease; lack of effort produces relaxation.
2. Tension indicates imperfect relaxation; staring, effort, trying to see—these interfere with perfect vision.
3. Under strain one cannot imagine, remember, nor see perfectly.

C. *To read diamond print:*

1. Hold the print not more than twelve inches from the eyes; then move it closer.
2. To eliminate staring, move the head and eyes while reading; also, move the card or book.

Better Eyesight
April 1924—Vol. VIII, No. 10

DISTANCE OF THE SNELLEN TEST CARD

The distance of the Snellen test card from the patient is a matter of considerable importance. Some patients improve more rapidly when the card is placed fifteen or twenty feet away while others fail to get any benefit with the card at this distance.

In some cases the best results are obtained when the card is as close as one foot. I recall a patient with very poor sight who made no progress whatever when the card was placed at ten feet or farther, but became able to improve the vision very materially with the card at about six inches. After the vision was improved at six inches, the patient became able to improve the card at a greater distance until normal sight was obtained at twenty feet. Some cases with poor vision may not improve when the card is placed at ten feet or farther, or at one foot or less, but do much better when the card is placed at a middle distance at about eight or ten feet. Other individuals may not improve their vision at all at ten feet, but are able to improve their sight at twenty feet or at one foot. I recall one patient with 20 diopters of myopia whose vision at ten feet was peculiar. The letters at twenty feet and at one foot were apparently all the same normal size, but at ten feet they appeared to be one-fifth of the normal size. Practicing with the card at twenty feet or at one foot helped him greatly, more than practicing with the card at about ten feet. While some patients are benefited by practicing with the card daily always at the same distance, there are others who seem to be benefited when the distance of the card from the patient is changed daily.

[See also "Imagination Cures" in the October 1924 issue.—TRQ]

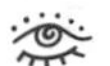

CONCENTRATION

By W. H. Bates, M.D.

The dictionary defines concentration to be an effort to keep the mind fixed on a point continuously. It can be demonstrated that this is impossible for any great length of time, a few seconds or part of a minute. All persons with imperfect sight whether due to nearsightedness, astigmatism, cataract or glaucoma try to concentrate. Since concentration is impossible, trying to do the impossible is a strain. It does a patient no good to tell him that concentration or trying to concentrate is an injury. To obtain real benefit he must prove the facts, experimenting on his own eyes.

Most people can look at the notch at the top of the letter "C" at ten or fifteen feet and try to keep their minds fixed on one point of the notch continuously. After some seconds all patients demonstrate that an effort is required and that the longer the point is fixed, the greater becomes the effort. The eyes and the mind become tired from the effort, and sooner or later the eyes move away from the notch, or the vision becomes blurred. This seems like a simple demonstration, but it may fail with individuals who have the ability to imagine erroneously that they are concentrating successfully and continuously, while unconsciously failing by closing the eyes or blinking or by shifting to some other point. These cases are difficult to manage and usually require a great deal of patience and ingenuity before the patient becomes able to demonstrate the facts.

With the eyes closed the patient may be able to remember a letter "C" with its notch, continuously, and demonstrate that the eyes are moving from one point of the "C" to another. If the patient is directed to keep the mind fixed on one point of the notch continuously and endeavor to keep the point stationary, after a few seconds or longer the notch or the point is not remembered. If one looks to the right of the notch, the notch is always to the left of where one appears to be looking with the eyes closed. Still with the eyes closed, if one imagines they are looking to the left of the notch, the notch is to the right. Every time the eyes or the mind look to the right, the notch in the "C" moves to the left. Every time the eyes or mind move to the left, the notch moves to the right; and by alternating looking from one side to another one can imagine the notch of the "C" moving from side to side in the opposite direction a short or a longer distance. This movement or swing prevents concentration, and the memory, imagination or vision usually improve.

The normal eye when it has normal sight does not try to concentrate. If one consciously tries to concentrate, the vision always becomes imperfect.

One day a professor of psychology called at the office to consult me about his eyes. His first remark was, "Doctor, I have lost the power of concentration. My eyes are very bad and so far I have not been able to obtain glasses which could help me. I am so fatigued most of the time that I find it exceedingly difficult and often impossible to deliver my lectures. I have no appetite; I do not sleep well and feel quite miserable generally."

His vision with each eye was normal, 15/10, and although only 40 years old he was not able to read the newspapers. The first thing I asked him to do was to try and keep his eyes on the left-hand side of the small letter "o," 15/15. After a part of a minute I asked him how he was getting along. He replied, "Badly. I lost the letter 'o.' The harder I try, and with all the efforts that I make, it is impossible for me to bring back that letter 'o' and, in fact, it seems to me that the harder I try the less I see."

I said to him, "When I try to concentrate on the left-hand side of that letter "o" my vision soon fails, just like yours did."

He jumped out of his chair and said, "Wait a moment, Doctor," and went out into the waiting room and brought back with him a friend who was apparently perfectly well and who had normal sight. He asked his friend to try to keep his eyes and mind concentrated on one point of the left-hand side of the small letter "o." In a few seconds the friend looked away and said to the patient, "Don't ask me to do that again." The patient asked, "Why?" The friend replied, "Because it spoiled my sight, and worse than that it gave me a pain and a headache and I don't like it." The patient smiled and motioned to his friend to retire to the waiting room again. "Pardon the confirmation," the patient said and asked this question: "If I avoid looking at a point continuously, will that help me?" I answered, "Yes, it will help you, and if you always avoid concentration you will always be relieved of your eye and nerve trouble."

I suggested that he close his eyes and demonstrate the facts that it was just as impossible for him to concentrate on the memory or a mental picture of a point on one side of the letter "o," and that when he tried to do it he lost the memory of the "o"; and the effort to concentrate, while it interfered with his memory, also made him uncomfortable.

I asked him if he had demonstrated sufficiently to be convinced that one cannot concentrate for any length of time when one looks at a point or when one remembers a point with their eyes closed.

He replied, "I am convinced. I wrote a book once on concentration and it had quite a sale. I have been teaching concentration for years and I have many friends who are also teaching it."

My answer was this, "Let me remonstrate with you and with all people who advocate concentration. In the first place, you do not know what concentration is, what you are doing, or that you are teaching people to ruin their eyesight and their general health. It is the effort, the concentration, which is always present with imperfect sight, with pain, fatigue of the eyes and the body generally. You can demonstrate that with the help of trying to concentrate, pain can be produced and other symptoms of disease. It is not possible to improve the eyesight without eliminating concentration or the stare. One cannot see, remember or imagine when concentration is practiced or an effort is made to practice concentration."

I taught the patient to shift, to keep looking from one place to another because it prevented concentration. I taught him how to imagine things moving, which also prevented concentration. Palming also helped him very much. The swing and the blinking at the same time gave him the greatest relief and I kept him practicing the long swing and the blinking for a considerable time, an hour or longer, when he declared that he felt perfectly well and not only could see the Snellen test card with normal sight continuously, but he also became able to read the newspaper without any difficulty and also diamond type at six inches or less.

What became of him? I received a letter recently from the gentleman in which he said among other things, "Thank you very much for your inquiry. I have changed my occupation and no longer teach concentration. I feel perfectly well and happy and am full of gratitude for what you did for me."

One day a lady came to see me with a child about four years old suffering from alternating squint. Sometimes the right eye turned in, at other times the left eye turned in. His mother said the child was quite nervous and had not been strong or well for some time. With the mother standing and facing me, I took hold of both her hands and had her sway in unison with me from side to side. The child was interested. I then took the child in the circle, the mother holding one hand and I the other and we all three swayed from side to side. The child was delighted and enjoyed it very much.

I said to him, "Keep looking up at the ceiling," which he did while swinging. The color came into his face; he smiled and laughed and best of all the eyes were perfectly straight. I advised the mother after her return home to encourage the child to laugh, to sing, to play, to dance and to have a good time generally and that she should spend some hours daily playing with the patient. She said, "I don't know any games."

I answered, "I will teach you a few," and I placed the mother in one corner, the little boy in another, while I stood in the third. When she tried to run from one corner to another, I ran after her and tried to get there first. The child sought another corner and got it, while I tried unsuccessfully to beat him to it. It was not very long before the child was laughing and screaming with delight. We kept this game up for quite a while, and some of the patients in the waiting room came and looked in at the open door to see what was going on. The more the child laughed, the more he screamed, the more he ran, the straighter became his eyes.

The mother said, "That is easy to do." My reply was, "I am not so sure of that. You have many duties and I am afraid you will neglect the child." She answered, "Oh, no, I promise you."

I requested her to write to me and let me know how he was getting along at the end of a week. At the end of the week instead of writing she came to the office and when the little boy saw me he ran to me, threw himself in my arms and held up his face to be kissed. I was quite willing to kiss him because his eyes were perfectly straight.

STORIES FROM THE CLINIC

No. 50: Anna Bernard, the Blind Girl–Part 3

By Emily C. Lierman

It is very easy to get into a habit, at least I find it so. I had been in the habit of calling Anna Bernard, "my blind girl, or my blind patient, but I had to get out of the habit because Anna can now see. Her vision is not normal by any means. No one could expect that. Not if they had seen Anna at the beginning of her treatment. People who have had fairly good sight and then acquired cataract and other diseases of their eyes have a fair chance or a better chance to regain normal vision. I have seen many such cases entirely cured after they had intelligently carried out our treatment. But, Anna, who was born blind with cataract and also acquired other diseases, was the greatest problem I ever had. I want to say this for Anna: If she would not have had the faith in me or in my ability to benefit her, I could not have helped her. She did as she was told and that was a great deal. For instance, Anna was caning chairs for a living. She could earn at least six dollars per week. But when I told her that she stared and strained her eyes while caning chairs and that I feared she would be wasting her time and mine if she continued to do this work while under treatment, she gave it up. It was not easy for her to make this sacrifice because she was giving up her independence. Her great desire was not to be a burden on her family. She wanted to help instead of being helpless.

Her wonderful mind helped her, however, to realize that if she could see with eyes that had always been sightless, she would be able later on to earn much more than she could at caning chairs by the sense of touch.

During the months of October and November 1922, Anna made steady progress. She could read the test card up to the 40-line at a foot or so from her eyes, but the smaller letters she read holding the card quite close to her face. She came every Saturday morning accompanied by her sister Ella as usual. She had something to tell me. Now she was going to the movies and, sitting about fifteen or twenty feet away, she could at times see the heads and faces of people on the screen. She had to keep up the body swing and also to blink constantly, otherwise everything before her became a blank. If she did not keep up the practice all the time, the staring and straining to see always lowered her vision.

One day I had three visitors in our office whom I had invited especially to see the progress Anna was making. One of my visitors was a lady who happened to be in our waiting room the day Anna appealed to me first for help. This lady was a school teacher, a delightful person with a great deal of love for others. I placed her at a desk in one corner of the office, the desk separating her from the patient. To her left I placed a young man, a relative of hers who was also troubled with imperfect sight. To her right sat another young man who was at the time under treatment by Dr. Bates. All objects seen by Anna on the street and elsewhere were seen under favorable conditions, either in the bright sunlight or under strong electric light. While at the movie theatre, all lights being out, she was able to relax enough to see objects thrown on the screen. Now, I was anxious to find out how much she could see as she entered the office, where I had purposely lessened the amount of light. As she stood in the doorway I asked her if she saw anything unfamiliar in the room. Our visitors were perfectly still and intensely interested. Anna began to blink and swing her body from side to side, which was always a benefit to her. She looked about the room and then back again to the right where the visitors were sitting. She smiled and immediately walked unassisted to the desk, and as she kept up the blinking she leaned over the desk and said the center figure was a lady with a light colored waist on. There were two gentlemen also; one on either side of her. After praising her, I placed her in a chair to palm and rest her eyes for a little while. This was always necessary because in her eagerness to read or tell what she saw, she strained unconsciously and her vision blurred.

Ten minutes later I asked her to follow me about the room and tell me what she saw. A Brazilian butterfly in an oval frame hanging on the wall attracted her, and at three feet she was able to see the color of it. As she had never seen a butterfly she tried to tell me what it might be. She remembered that at one time a butterfly was described to her, so she said it might be one although she was not sure. The memory of the form of an object explained to her helped her to really see it. She was placed before a mirror and immediately she saw what it was.

I never thought when I first saw Anna that we could accomplish so much. In her home she helps with the housework and picks up things and places them where they belong. She sees the steam from the boiling tea kettle and reads the large headlines and the next size type in the newspapers. When she first learned to write with crayon for me, she wrote something in a notebook which I hope to have photographed for my book, so that those who are interested may see what she learned to do. Perhaps not all blind patients could have accomplished what Anna did. Such an extraordinary mind as she has is very rare. Her cheerfulness, her hope of seeing helped me to help her too. Her smile was with her all the time and her gratitude to me and her faithful sister was great.

She does not come for treatment just now but her letter of February 11, 1924 reads: "My dear Ms. Lierman, It pleased me greatly to receive your letter and I appreciate your interest in me very much. I am not caning chairs anymore but am taking a commercial course. With kindest regards, I remain, Sincerely, Anna Bernard."

NANCY'S MENTAL PICTURES

By Florian A. Shepard

Last week, in her piano lesson, nine-year-old Nancy couldn't play one of her "review pieces," and her memory was all mixed up. Something needed to be smoothed out.

"Shut your eyes, Nancy," I told her. "It is easy to remember. You can see a picture of it." "I don't see any picture," she answered. "You can see a picture of the page, can't you?" "No, Ms. Shepard." "Well, perhaps you haven't looked at the music lately. See, here it is: look just at this first little black note on the lowest line. Now shut your eyes and remember it." "But I can't see a picture of it," she repeated. "You can see a picture of the piano keys, can't you?" "No, Ms. Shepard." She was trying to do what I asked, but her voice sounded baffled.

"Nancy," I suggested, "have you been making valentines lately?" "I've made some, but not this year." "Well, what have you done lately that you like to do?" "I play with my doll lots." "Your dolly! What's her name?" "Betty." "And what color are Betty's eyes?" "They're blue—dark blue." "Can you see them when you shut your eyes?" "Yes, I can see her eyes," and she smiled. "When you look at her right eye, you notice that best, don't you? Then you can notice her left eye best." She nodded. "Now look at her feet, first one foot, then the other. Now look back at her eyes. Do you see her?" "Oh, yes." "Now hold her up by the piano. Can you see the music?" "No, and I can't see her either now."

I had her think of Betty's eyes again; and when she could remember the doll, I told her about the cat that walked across his master's piano so comically that the gentleman wrote a piece about it and called it the "Cat's Fugue."

Then I asked her if Betty couldn't walk on the keys and play "fugue," too. "I can see her walking on the keys!" she cried. "And can you see the music on the rack behind her?" I suggested. "She's busy doing something else now," she explained. "She's into the sugar." Presently we brought her back to the piano keys. "I can see the piano now and the music, too," said Nancy. We both smiled. "Well, now, how did we get that picture of the music?" I asked her. "By thinking of other things first," she replied, and those are the very words that Dr. Bates has often used in helping patients to improve their memories. It took only a few moments then to get the piece nicely straightened out, and we went on easily to others.

At the end of the lesson, just for fun, I tried something else with Nancy. "Can you remember the dolly now?" I asked. "Yes, I can see a picture of her." "Look at her eyes; now look at her feet. When you look at her eyes, you don't notice her feet so well, do you? And when you look at her feet, you don't see the eyes so well. Now, can you look at the eyes and the feet at the same time and see them all just as well." "Yes, I can see them all very well." "I don't think you can, dear," I told her. "I think you are looking first at one and then the other." "Well, that's the way I do it," she replied, as a matter of course. "But now look at both eyes and feet at the same time," I directed. "What happens?" "Why, it gets dim," she exclaimed in surprise.

So she found out what happens to any of us, with eyes open or closed, when we try to look at too much at one time.

REPORT OF THE FEBRUARY LEAGUE MEETING

By May Secor, Secretary

On February 12 the Better Eyesight League held its regular monthly meeting. The meeting was well attended and proved very interesting.

Dr. William West, an osteopathic physician of this city, presented an exposition of the application of Dr. Bates' system of the alleviation of functional diseases of the mind. Dr. West uses the Bates System as a means of assisting the patient to gain control of the conscious mind. The patient is taught the various Bates exercises, and is instructed to practice them several times each day; this relieves eyestrain, and alleviates mental strain.

The patient is instructed also to practice the exercises, or to perhaps simply think of the "C" or "O," whenever he finds himself losing self-control. By giving his attention to eye work for even a short period the patient secures relaxation, the nervous strain is relieved, and self-control returns. Dr. West reported the following cases:

Woman, 28; profound neurasthenia of suicidal type. In two weeks suicidal thought quelled, and insomnia and hysteria controlled.

Man, 20; mental depression overcome in three weeks.

Woman; nervous case, lost voice. Completely cured.

Woman, 40; neuralgia of eyes. Completely cured without the use of glasses.

Lack of self-control greatly enhances symptoms of a pathological condition. By means of the Bates System Dr. West assisted two adults to regain self-control, and thereby reduce symptoms. One patient was enabled to eliminate nausea during finger therapy for tonsillitis; the second patient found that self-control thus gained greatly reduced discomfit resulting from hay fever. Other patients were enabled to control intense emotions of fear and anger.

Last month Dr. Bates reported the success of Elisabet Hansen's work in a Chicago school. Dr. Bates also called attention to the effect of eyestrain upon the work of the students. Eyestrain causes mental tension which greatly hinders the learning process; conversely, the relief of eyestrain not only renders vision normal, but relieves mental tension, and permits the neurons to function normally. Among the effects of eyestrain are: irritation of the eyelid and eyeball, "watering" of the eyes, glaucoma, and detached retina.

BATES EVENING AT THE PSYCHOLOGY CLUB

The meeting of The Psychology Club, Mr. Henry Knight Miller, president, which was held on the evening of February 28, was given over to a discussion of the Bates Method.

Dr. Clinton E. Achorn, vice-president of the Better Eyesight League, presented interesting reports on a number of cases. Dr. Achorn is a former pupil of Dr. Bates, and is meeting with marked success in the correction of visual defects without the use of glasses.

Dr. Bates discussed several phases of his method, and remained until a late hour replying to questions. Ms. Lierman reported several clinical cases.

THE TIN SOLDIER

By George M. Guild

The little boy went to sleep with the tin soldier held tight in his hand. After a little while he began to dream and he imagined that he was out in the pretty sunlight with the green trees and flowers and the cool grass; and that there were men, women and children walking around. Off in the distance were a number of targets each with a bull's-eye, a round black spot in the middle, with black and white rings surrounding it. There were soldiers and sailors, all made of tin, but with a wonderful intelligence, who walked up to the firing line, aimed their guns at the targets and blazed away. The little boy's tin soldier kept fretting, fuming and scolding, saying over and over again, "Let me at them, let me at them. I could hit the target, I could hit the bull's-eye, I could win the prize!" And so the little boy granted his request and allowed him to march up to the firing line, aim his gun and fire.

With a look of great disgust he came back to the little boy and said, "It wasn't my fault I missed the bull's-eye, but the gun kicked me and spoiled my aim." So the little boy said, "Well, try again." The little tin soldier loaded up his gun, walked up to the firing line and aimed at the bull's-eye. In a few moments he took his gun down, turned to the little boy and said, "Somebody is moving that bull's-eye from side to side, I can see it moving. How can anyone be expected to hit the bull's-eye when it is moving?" The little boy soothed him as well as he could and suggested to him that it would be better to do the best he could, even if it did move, to still blaze away.

The little tin soldier aimed his gun at the target and said, "This is outrageous. When I try to keep the bull's-eye from moving it all gets blurred and disappears just as soon as I try to imagine it stationary or try to keep it stationary."

Then the little boy advised him that if he could not see it stationary it would be better for him to see it when it was moving, since that was the only way he could see it.

And so the little tin soldier said, "Well I don't care, I will let it move and I know I can hit it." Then he raised his gun, aimed quickly, pulled the trigger and at once the signal came back, "Bull's-eye." Then the little tin soldier was so pleased that he tried to dance, which was rather difficult because his joints were all tin. He found it rather creaky and hard to move around very gracefully.

Then he fired the second time, bull's-eye number two. Then the third, the fourth and the fifth time and got a bull's-eye every trip. The people became very much excited and rushed up to the tin soldier and praised him and patted him on the back and told him he was the finest tin soldier that ever lived.

All this flattery pleased him exceedingly; and always when he aimed his gun he waited until he could see the bull's-eye moving and when the movement was slow, short and easy he pulled the trigger and got the bull's-eye, and this thing went along pretty much all the afternoon until the little boy got tired of the boasting tin soldier.

The next morning the sun came out bright and strong, and the little boy was sitting up in bed when his mother came in to give him his usual good morning greetings. With his arms around her neck he said, "Mamma dear, my little tin soldier beat them all. Oh! He hit the target over and over again while no other soldier came anywhere near hitting it. I am awfully proud of my tin soldier and I hope you will be proud of him too, because he did so well. If it hadn't been for what you told father about central fixation and seeing things move or how the normal eye sees things with normal sight, my little tin soldier would not have done so well or so much better than all the others."

IN THE OFFICE

By Emily A. Meder

The Central Fixation office is a busy one. The regular routine is continually being interrupted by telephone calls, and personal visits from people who demand firsthand information.

One of our recent visitors was a writer who wore very heavy glasses. What I first noticed was that, while I was speaking, she would stare out of the window, as though in a trance, and slowly nod her head from time to time. This was to give me the impression that she was deeply interested in what I was saying, and carefully weighing each statement.

Staring, I told her, is bad. (I had noticed her doing this so I dropped a little hint.) She broke forth in smiles and made the astonishing remark that she thought it was bad also, and that she never stared. I politely told her she did, and how.

QUESTIONS AND ANSWERS

Q–1. What is the best thing to practice when glasses are removed and eyes are terribly weak?

A–1. Palming, if it is beneficial.

Q–2. How can one improve their imagination?

A–2. By improving the memory. When the memory of a letter becomes perfect, or one can remember it with their eyes open or with their eyes closed equally well, it is possible to imagine it perfect.

Q–3. What is the difference between the wink and the blink?

A–3. Winking consists in closing one or both eyes for an appreciable length of time. Blinking the eyes is closing and opening so quickly that most people do not know they do it.

Better Eyesight
May 1924—Vol. VIII, No. 11

TIME TO PRACTICE

Many busy people complain that they have not time to practice my methods. They say that wearing glasses is quicker and much easier. Persons with normal vision or perfect sight without glasses are practicing consciously or unconsciously all the time when they are awake. When one sees a letter or an object perfectly the eyes are at rest. Any effort to improve the sight always makes it worse. The only time the eyes are perfectly at rest is when the vision is perfect. Persons with imperfect sight have to strain in order to see imperfectly. Persons with headaches, pain and other symptoms of discomfort in the eyes or in other parts of the body are under a constant strain to see, which is usually unconscious.

When a patient says he has no time to practice, he is mistaken. He has all the time there is to use his eyes in the right way, or he can use them in the wrong way. He has just as much time to use his eyes properly as he has to use them improperly. He has the choice and when patients learn the facts, to complain that they have no time to practice is an error.

Some patients object to removing their glasses on the ground that their vision is not sufficiently good for them to attend to their work, and feel that they have to put off the treatment until they have a vacation. Some of my patients have very poor vision and yet find time to practice without their glasses. Some school teachers with 15 diopters of myopia with a vision of less than 10/200 have found time to practice without interfering with their work. In fact, practicing without their glasses soon enabled them to do their work much better than before.

CONICAL CORNEA

By W. H. Bates, M.D.

Conical cornea has been considered for many years to be incurable. It is usually progressive and in advanced cases besides very imperfect sight, many patients suffer with disagreeable symptoms of pain and inflammatory troubles of the cornea. Numerous operations have been performed without any improvement in the sight. In the beginning the cornea of one eye may be the only one affected. After some years both eyes may become affected.

About ten years ago a girl, age twenty, came to me with a diagnosis of conical cornea in the right eye, the left eye being nearly normal. The vision of the right eye was 10/200, not improved by glasses. I told the patient that I did not think I could improve the conical cornea but I might be able to relieve her of the pain and discomfort in her good eye. Palming, after a half-hour or longer, relieved her discomfort temporarily and, much to my surprise, the vision of the eye with conical cornea was improved from 10/200 to 10/50. The patient felt much better at this quick relief and improvement in the sight of the eye with conical cornea, as it was the first encouragement that she had had in a long time. Under the relaxation treatment this patient's vision continued steadily to improve until it became normal after some weeks. The conical cornea disappeared. The patient had not only normal sight for distance but she was also able to read diamond type as close as six inches or less and as far off as two feet. I strongly advised her to practice the palming at least two hours daily and to return for observation at regular intervals. I have not seen her since.

A second case was that of a physician, age 40 years. He had suffered with imperfect sight and discomfort in the right eye for about fifteen years. In the beginning his vision, he said, had been improved to some extent by strong cylinders but gradually, with the increase of the conical shape of the cornea, no glasses were found which gave him the slightest improvement in his sight. He was first seen May 12, 1922. The vision of the right eye was 10/200 and the vision of the left was 20/30.

This case was very remarkable in that he obtained in about one week flashes of normal vision in the right eye by practicing relaxation methods, palming, swinging and the memory of mental pictures. His treatment was very interesting to me, especially his ability to do things wrong. He was a genius when it came to deceiving himself as well as others. I had considerable difficulty in restraining his enthusiasm to treat all my patients that he met. I told him that I was very anxious to have him treat people after he recovered because I believed that would be a help to him, but until he was cured it would be just as well for him not to talk about his treatment because he did not understand it and not only misled others but it interfered with his own recovery. He stopped treatment unfortunately before he was cured, but he felt that he had improved so much with me that he could go right along in the same way and complete his cure working by himself when he had time to spare from his practice.

The third case was referred to in the November 1922 *Better Eyesight* magazine in the article "The Variable Swing." She was a woman, age 24, a school teacher, and was first seen October 14, 1922. She had conical cornea in both eyes. The vision of the right eye was 10/200 while that of the left eye was 10/200 plus.

With strong cylinders she obtained 20/200 vision in the right eye and about 20/70 in the left eye. She could read diamond type at four inches with each eye, but much better with the left eye than she could with the right. Palming helped her, but her best vision was obtained by practicing the long swing alternating with the short swing. When she held her forefinger about one foot in front of her face and a little below the level of her eyes, by moving her head and eyes from side to side, without regarding her finger, she became able to imagine her [stationary—TRQ] forefinger was moving from side to side opposite to the movement of her eyes.

While maintaining the swing of her finger she was able to imagine that distant objects were moving opposite to the imagined movement of her finger, or [the distant objects appeared to move—TRQ] in the same direction that her eyes and head moved but much less. [This is called *double oppositional movement.*—TRQ] By increasing the amplitude of the swing of her forefinger she also increased the swing of distant objects. When she shortened the swing of her finger, distant objects she imagined had a much shorter swing or none at all. Looking at the Snellen test card with her finger in front of her was somewhat confusing. She got along better by holding her finger some inches to one side of her face, quite a distance from the Snellen test card.

This was a new method of practicing the optical swing; and, because the amplitude varied, I called it the Variable Swing. Like many other swings the benefit of it is not always the same. Some people get a great deal of improvement in their vision from it while others obtain none whatever. At the first visit, with the use of palming, the variable swing, the long swing, the short swing, and the imagination of the halos this patient obtained normal vision temporarily, and to me it seemed very remarkable that she should obtain such good vision in so short a time. On leaving she was told to never again wear her glasses, to practice at home the same methods which benefited her eyes while under my supervision, but nothing more was heard from her.

Other cases of conical cornea were treated and relieved in a short time and were kept under observation for a number of years. It was very difficult to prevent these patients from putting on their glasses from time to time without any special reason. Some told me that glasses lowered their vision for a time but that after their removal their vision slowly came back by practicing the relaxation methods. In other cases the vision did not improve at all after wearing glasses for a short time but when they came back under my supervision for treatment of their eyes the vision was again improved to the normal. The time necessary to accomplish this was variable and in some cases required treatment for a longer time than when they were first seen. Sometimes the patients would return to their former doctor who had been unable to help them, who would test them with glasses, which always produces disaster. Naturally one would not be surprised to learn that in such cases the attending physician had libeled me very strongly. When such patients returned to me they had a knowledge of physiological optics as taught in the orthodox way which was quite wonderful. No ophthalmologist of the old school has any conception of the bad mental effect on these cases of conical cornea from the glasses. Any of my patients who came to me for treatment of their eyes usually had a hard time in breaking away from the influence of the orthodox physician.

The truth is very wonderful. It is a truth that persons with normal vision have a good imagination of mental pictures, sometimes best with the eyes open and sometimes best with the eyes closed. When any patient with imperfect sight obtains a good imagination or a perfect imagination, the vision becomes normal no matter what may be the cause of the imperfect sight. A perfect imagination of a period is a cure for nearsightedness no matter how great it may be or how long it may have been present. It is a cure for farsightedness, astigmatism, cataract, glaucoma, detachment of the retina, atrophy of the optic nerve, as well as conical cornea.

STORIES FROM THE CLINIC

No. 51: More about "Pop"

By Emily C. Lierman

I promised the readers of our March 1922 *Better Eyesight* magazine that some day, if I could possibly do more for dear old "Pop," I would again write about him. As I became better acquainted with him, I encouraged him to talk. He was always cheerful when he came and tried to follow me in everything I directed him to do. He told me a little of his personal affairs, but was very careful not to arouse pity. Even though he has lived in the Home for the Blind for some time, he feels independent. He said the only sadness he ever had in his life was when his wife no longer wanted him. That was when he lost his eyesight and could not support her. After she cast him out of her home, she inherited some money and property, but before she died she lost all her earthly possessions. All he wishes for now is just enough sight to be able to work and also see the faces of his many friends.

We worked together diligently month after month hoping he would surprise me some day and actually see. I want to be very truthful and say that even today I cannot realize that he will ever see enough to get along by himself. Yet, all things are possible and I do not lose hope, even though he is 77 years old. One day he said, "I know I am going to see again, for once in a while I see my whole hand but it looks like a baby's hand. When I go out in the street I can see the brass railing attached to our front steps. I can see a man's face at times when I am shaving him, but I see his face a gray color instead of pink or a flesh color." "Pop" has always been a barber by trade.

My main point is to keep up his interest and see that he practices faithfully. In order to earn a few pennies, he caned chairs in the workshop. He stared while he was doing this work and that was a drawback. Yet I had not the courage to stop him from earning his spending money. After a day of this kind of work he complained of seeing bright colors before his eyes, which indicated that he strained while caning his chairs. For quite a few weeks he was not employed in this way, so he practiced more faithfully than ever. Then came a wonderful change in his left eye, which in the beginning looked much worse than the right eye. I believe the sun treatment helped him very much. This was given to him, if it happened to be a sunny day, every time he came to the office. He was placed in the sun, and while looking down, his upper lid was raised and the sun was focused on the sclera, or white part of the eye, with the sun glass.

The solid white mass which covered the pupil and iris gradually became less. The upper part of the iris and pupil have become visible in the left eye. The constant twitching of his eyes ceased. If I could be with him more and remind him not to stare, I know the relaxation and rest that he gets from the treatment would give him his wish and also mine—the return of his eyesight.

Week after week he kept coming with always the same

cheery greeting, "I am glad to see you Ma'am." I became acquainted well enough with him to say, "Now, you big bluffer, you know right well you don't see me." This remark would always bring a hearty "ha, ha" from him, and then we would proceed earnestly with the treatment. Dear, dear old "Pop", surely God will answer my prayers for you if it is His will that you should have your sight again. It is now the third year that he is coming to us for treatment and neither of us have given up hope yet. Only a short while ago I noticed that he was becoming more feeble and that he is not so sure of his steps as he walks along with his guide, a dear boy of fourteen years. Recently he asked me a question which was indeed hard to answer. It was this, "When do you think I will see again? Do you think in six months or so?" Before I answered I watched him and thought perhaps within six months he may be called to his Heavenly Home where there were no eye troubles; so I said, "You see, I don't know for sure, but wouldn't it be great if you will see again in six months?" It would be hard to put into print all the wonderful things he has promised me when that time comes. His favorite expression at the office, when he suddenly discovers a sunbeam on the carpet is "Gee Rusalem, that's great." Then, in all his excitement, as his vision fades away in the next moment, he asks "Why don't I keep on seeing?" There is always the same answer, for there is only one reason: strain. When he holds the test card five inches from his eyes after palming for a few minutes, he is able to see black spots on the card instead of letters. He shows me the outline of the large black letter "C" at the top of the card.

One day he said in an excited tone; "This week the Matron of our Home came into my room, and while I palmed my eyes she read something from a magazine to me. I laid down my pipe on a table before I palmed, and after the woman left my room I had forgotten all about my pipe. Later on, as I passed by the table I saw the pipe very plainly and picked it up. I called out to my friends in the next room and told them about this wonderful thing. I can shave a man's face now, not by the sense of touch always, but I can really see his face sometimes."

He calls me his "Shining Light," bless his heart. It thrills me and makes me want to do greater things and to be a better woman.

Now, up to date February 1924, the upper part of the iris and pupil of his left eye is almost clear. Dr. Bates hopes as I do for better results in the near future.

THE MIND'S EYE

By Edith McNamara

Do you enjoy your mind's movies or your mental pictures? I do. I get four times the value of a trip to the country or any place else by remembering the mental pictures of it perfectly.

I was not conscious at the time that while my physical eye was seeing everything around me, my mind's eye was making a mental picture of it to be brought back later with the help of a perfect memory. After a few experiments with perfect mental pictures, I came to the conclusion that I could only imagine what I remembered. It was impossible to imagine an object unless I could remember it perfectly. If I could not remember it perfectly it became only a jumbled up, hazy recollection of some thing.

I think it's lots of fun playing tag with the memory or mental pictures. I like to dig out of my memory all the perfect mental pictures I can—one by one—for central fixation plays a big part in mental pictures, remembering one thing best at a time.

Having once been to Canada, my favorite way of getting relaxed is to go there by mental pictures. I go along a beautiful country road, remember a lake that had impressed me, visualize it with my mind's eye and so on. Sometimes I skip a couple of towns and arrive in Canada very quickly and other times I get enough relaxation by just staying in one town for a while.

Why don't you try this? Perhaps someone will tell you a story that will remind you of an incident which happened years ago. Follow it up with the help of your memory and see how perfect a mental picture you can obtain. I am sure that you will find pleasure and relaxation in so doing. If you have to make an effort to form this mental picture let it alone for a while, and then go back to it again and start where you left off. This will benefit you in your palming.

LECTURE TO THE PSYCHOLOGY CLUB

Dr. Bates' lecture, given before the New York Psychology Club, proved to be intensely interesting. Two outstanding topics upon which Dr. Bates dwelt at great length were concentration, and the prevention and cure of imperfect sight in schoolchildren. Everyone knows of Dr. Bates' interest in helping teachers to help the children. He gave a history of the Snellen test card, the discovery of its benefits to everybody, and his efforts to have these placed in the classrooms.

Dr. Bates opened the talk by saying he was glad to speak before these psychologists, and would like to tell them a case of a professor of psychology, who was also a teacher of concentration. This case was printed in detail in the April 1924 issue of *Better Eyesight* and we refer our readers to it. It explains how one man not only spoiled his sight, but undermined his general health, by concentrating. The professor was proud of the fact that he concentrated and he believed he did it quite well. He did. So well that if he had persisted, he probably would have had to resign from his position on account of his inability to see.

This discussion of concentration brought out the fact that teachers in schools like to have their children concentrate on what they (the teachers) are saying. One teacher who is using this method with great success said that formerly if her children gazed at her in unblinking silence, without moving, she congratulated herself that she was holding their attention. She now has them palm while she describes things, and says that it "sinks in" better. She has them read the Snellen test card in the mornings and afternoons, as a sort of refreshing exercise. Reading the card, palming for a few minutes with the windows open, does away with the afternoon languor of the pupils.

For the benefit of those who had never heard of the Snellen test card, Dr. Bates exhibited one, explaining its uses, and benefits. He explained that while he did not invent the card, he did discover the many benefits derived from reading it daily.

One of the important points brought out relative to the importance of the card was the following: It was placed in the classroom of children who did not fit in any of the grades. The pupils of this class were criminally inclined, maliciously mischievous or backward in their lessons for other reasons. He explained his method to the teacher in charge and was gratified to find her an intelligent woman and interested in the experiment. She followed Dr. Bates' instructions, and when he returned some months later, she had an amazing report for him. The children not only improved in their lessons, but had overcome their abnormal tendencies. In fact a good majority of them had "skipped" a class and were promoted to a higher grade.

Dr. Bates brought his discourse to a close with the report of these cases.

Ms. Lierman was then called upon to make a few remarks. She laughingly apologized for the fact that Dr. Bates dwelt on children so much, and did not once mention any of the adult patients whom he benefited. She said that she also is anxious to help the children, but she thinks that everyone is at heart a child. Her oldest "child" is 77 years old. She calls him "Pop" and his story is continued in this month's issue. (Ms. Lierman is very fond of "Pop", and the patients are delighted every Saturday morning with the cheerful "Good morning 'Pop'" with which she greets him and his own sprightly answers.)

REPORT OF THE LEAGUE MEETINGS

By May Secor, Secretary

MARCH

The regular monthly meeting of the Better Eyesight League was held on Tuesday evening, March 11.

Dr. Achorn, vice-president of the League, called attention to the necessity of adapting the Bates exercises to the needs and temperament of each patient. The personal equation must be solved in each case.

William James has suggested that when a new theory is presented to an individual, it is well for him to inquire, "Will it work?" and "If it works, is it worthwhile?" Dr. Achorn advised prospective followers of the Bates Method to consider the method in the light of these two questions. Will the Bates Method work? An answer to this question may readily be found in Dr. Bates' book entitled *Perfect Sight Without Glasses* and in testimonials of Dr. Bates' patients. If the method works, is it worthwhile? Is it worthwhile to be freed from slavery to eyeglasses? If doubtful of the reply to this query, consult members of the League who now enjoy perfect sight without the use of glasses.

Dr. Bates discussed the personal equation, and assured those present that he has thus far been able to help all those who have presented themselves to him for treatment. Solution of the personal equation in many cases requires careful thought and much patience; however, it is a vital matter. Dr. Bates again emphasized the great assistance which imagination renders in restoring normal vision, and referred to several cures in which the imagination had played an important role.

It was stated that the elementary schools of several cities are conducting two types of classes for pupils who have defective vision:

A. "Sight Conservation Classes" which care for pupils whose sight is noticeably below normal, and

B. "Classes for the Blind" which care for children having little or no sight.

Dr. Bates urged that a definite program for the development of vision be included in the daily schedule for all classes of these types. Sight cannot be restored nor improved unless the eyes are used, and used intelligently, in such a way as to eliminate eyestrain. In no case is it advisable to adhere to large print; one may begin with large print, and then train the child to use smaller print, teaching him how to eliminate eyestrain—how to use his eyes normally. Teach the child to palm, to swing, to shift, to use his imagination, and to use his memory. Follow a definite constructive program to improve the vision of all pupils whose eyesight is below normal.

Dr. Bates stated that the continued use of large print causes acute eyestrain, and that this has been demonstrated in cities which introduced the exclusive use of large print in the lower grades of the schools; acute eyestrain and headaches became prevalent in these grades. The restoration of small print was followed by a great reduction in the number and acuteness of headaches, and cases of eyestrain.

The meeting was adjourned at the close of Dr. Bates' discussion.

April

The April meeting of the Better Eyesight League was held on April 8.

Dr. Cornelia Brown, president of the Orange Better Eyesight League, reported that the Orange League has increased its membership and scope of work. Evening classes for the correction of visual defects are being conducted in East Orange by Dr. Brown and Dr. Gore. Dr. Brown urged each patient who adheres to the Bates Method to follow the method actively and faithfully. It is by this means only that the patient may receive a maximum benefit, and that the effectiveness of the method may be demonstrated. The speaker also advised the application of Dr. Bates' "Seven Truths of Normal Sight" in the performance of one's daily tasks.

Michelangelo once stated that a man could not build a perfect cathedral unless he could imagine it moving. Dr. Bates correlated this principle with shifting. Dr. Bates also suggested palming and sun treatment as a means of securing perfect relaxation in the case of inward turning eyelashes.

Mr. George Weiss, a student of Erasmus Hall High School and son of the corresponding secretary of the League, reported several cases in which he has assisted in eliminating eyestrain and myopia.

At the close of Mr. Weiss' report the meeting was adjourned.

Teacher's Conference Scheduled for May League Meeting

The May meeting of the Better Eyesight League will be held at eight o'clock on Tuesday evening, May 13. This meeting is designed especially for teachers, and will be devoted to explanations and demonstrations of Dr. Bates' method for the cure of visual defects without the use of eyeglasses. Teachers and their friends are cordially invited to be present on the thirteenth, and to learn how Dr. Bates' methods may be applied in the classroom.

FINE PRINT

By W. H. Bates, M.D.

The photographic reduction of the fine print can be used with great benefit to patients suffering from high degrees of nearsightedness. At first it has to be held at a certain close distance from the eyes and cannot be seen so well if placed an inch farther or an inch nearer. When read easily or perfectly, the white spaces between the lines appear much whiter than they really are and the card seems to be moving from side to side or in other directions, if one takes the trouble to notice it. The eyes are blinking frequently and this is also usually an unconscious act.

More perfect rest or relaxation of the eyes is obtained by reading this fine print perfectly than by doing some other things. By alternately looking at the large letters of the Snellen test card at five or ten feet or farther and reading the fine print close to the eyes, one can obtain flashes of improved vision at the distance. By practicing, these flashes become more frequent and the letters are seen more continuously. The method is to be highly recommended because it seems to be one of the best methods of improving the distant vision.

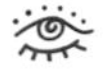

THE DE GRAFF FUND FOR THE PREVENTION OF MYOPIA IN SCHOOLCHILDREN

Mr. Jere De Graff was a patient who derived benefit from the treatment of Dr. Bates, and felt that something should be done to prevent imperfect sight in schoolchildren. He subscribed $7.50 for this fund. The money is to be for the purchase of Snellen test cards to be given to school teachers for use in the classroom. When Dr. Bates learned this he offered to subscribe double the amount of the total subscriptions, provided the teachers who receive the Snellen test card will pay ten cents each, agree to discard their glasses permanently, and render a report of the vision of the children, as well as their own, before and after treatment, at least once every six months.

Dr. Bates has also requested the Central Fixation Publishing Company to allow a special price on the Snellen test cards for teachers using them in the classrooms. The price, therefore, to schools will be twenty-five cents for the regular style and seventy-five cents for the cardboard style.

QUESTIONS AND ANSWERS

Q–1. What is the cause and cure of granulated eyelids?

A–1. The cause is strain. The cure has been accomplished by practicing the universal swing, by palming and other methods of correcting the strain.

Q–2. What can I do to help my sight when my vision blurs while reading?

A–2. Palm more frequently or imagine the white spaces between the lines are whiter than the other parts of the page.

Q–3. Does palming help nervousness?

A–3. Yes, when it is done right. It can be done wrong.

Q–4. Is glaucoma curable?

A–4. Glaucoma is curable. Some cases of blindness from glaucoma have been permanently cured by palming for long periods of time.

Q–5. Does the cataract become absorbed by relaxation treatment?

A–5. In cases which have been cured, the opacity of the lens disappeared and the lens regained its normal condition.

Better Eyesight
June 1924—Vol. VIII, No. 12

BLINKING

The normal eye when it has normal sight rests very frequently by closing the eyes for longer or shorter periods, and when practiced quickly it is called *blinking*. When the normal eye has normal sight and refrains from blinking for some seconds or part of a minute, the vision always becomes imperfect. You can demonstrate that normal vision at the near point or at the distance is impossible without frequent blinking. Most people blink so easily and for such a short period of time that things are seen continuously while the blinking is done unconsciously. In some cases one may blink five times or more in one second. The frequency of blinking depends on a number of factors.

The normal eye blinks more frequently or more continuously under adverse conditions as when the illumination is diminished, the distance is increased, or the print read is too pale, or otherwise imperfect. The distraction of conversation, noise, reflections of light, or objects so arranged as to be difficult to see—all increase the frequency of blinking of the normal eye with normal sight. If the frequency of blinking is diminished under adverse conditions or from any cause the vision soon becomes imperfect.

The imperfect eye or the eye with imperfect sight blinks less frequently than the normal eye. Staring stops the blinking. The universal optical swing, or the long or short swing when modified or stopped are always accompanied by less frequent blinking.

Blink in the early morning,
Blink when the sun sets at night;
Blink when the sun is dawning,
But be sure you do it right.

BLINDNESS

By W. H. Bates, M.D.

A great many people are blind or have vision so imperfect that they are unable to find their way about a strange place with the aid of their eyes. They are usually an object of interest to their friends and are frequently recommended to try every new form of treatment which comes out that promises any relief. They are too often disappointed.

The orthodox ophthalmologist has been guided by a certain number of rules. For example, a patient who has no perception of light is at once considered incurable, no matter what may be the condition of the eyes. The first shock that I experienced in such cases was in that of a girl who had total blindness in one eye only, the other being fairly good. She had been to many physicians, and all pronounced her incurable because she had no perception of light in the blind eye. This was a long time ago, and at that time I did not know as much as I do now and told the patient that nothing could be done to improve the blind eye. The eye itself appeared normal. There was no opacity and no organic disease which I was able to find. She told me that one doctor said she was born with something wrong with the eye center in the brain, which accounted for the blindness in the one eye. However, I treated her, planning to improve the slightly imperfect sight that she had in the good eye. Much to my surprise, the vision in the blind eye simultaneously began to get better. The first improvement the patient noticed was that she could see strong light off to the outer side of the eye, while her vision straight ahead and to her left was still dark. One of the most remarkable things about the case was the rapidity with which the blind eye obtained perception of light when the vision improved for objects and letters of the Snellen test card. After two weeks of daily treatment the vision of the right eye had improved to 10/200, and at the end of another week she had 20/20. From the results of treatment and other reasons I believe that this was just a case of blindness from squint without the squint, which is called in the textbooks *amblyopia ex anopsia.* After doing her so much good, I expected that she would return or at least send word how she was getting along. She was not heard from again. I believe if there had been any relapse, she might have returned. Sometimes these cases do relapse, and I learn the facts from friends of the patient.

About five years ago a patient was led into my office, blind from retinitis pigmentosa. The vision of the right eye was perception of light, while that of the left eye was 5/200. The pupils of both eyes were small, and in order to examine the interior of her eyes her pupils were dilated with a weak solution of atropine. It was followed very quickly by an attack of acute glaucoma. This subsided after about two weeks. The vision of the better eye was lowered to perception of light while that of the right eye, which had been practically blind for many years, had improved to 10/200. This was a great surprise because it was so unexpected. After many months of daily treatment she obtained normal vision in the right eye and almost normal vision in the left eye. She stopped treatment against my advice. The case was published in the *New York Medical Journal,* February 3, 1917.

Glaucoma is a very treacherous disease. One may have an attack and recover promptly under treatment. The same patient may have a number of attacks of temporary blindness, but sooner or later the patient will suffer an attack of glaucoma with total blindness, from which no recovery follows spontaneously. The patient goes to some competent ophthalmologist who at once tells him that there is no hope of anything being done. At one time I examined with a microscope six eyes which had been enucleated for the relief of great pain from absolute glaucoma. Not one of these eyes was imperfect in any way. Quite frequently I have seen cases of absolute glaucoma which came to me for treatment, and which were completely relieved by palming and obtained normal vision in a very few days or weeks, some in even a shorter time. One such case, about ten years ago, had pain so severe that he was unable to attend to his business and had been strongly advised to have the eye removed. He came to me as his last resort. After a half-hour of palming the pain disappeared and has not returned since in all this time. I saw the patient a few days ago and he is still full of gratitude for the benefit he received.

If my method never did anything more than to relieve the tension and pain of glaucoma, I would feel that I had done something worthwhile. Whenever I think of those glaucoma cases I relieved, it is a very difficult matter for me to refrain from boasting. There are many eye doctors of my acquaintance who do not believe that palming does much for glaucoma, although I have gone to a great deal of trouble to advertise the fact. So strongly impressed on the minds of ophthalmologists that absolute glaucoma is incurable, that I can understand how difficult it is for men of experience to imagine that any of these cases can be benefited. Some day, soon I hope, some doctor will try the palming on a hopeless case and be gratified to find that these cases can be helped. If he has the courage to publish the facts he will find that his fellow practitioners will not be as severe with him as he might expect. Some eye specialists have privately observed my work; and, although they at the time admitted that I was right and everybody else was wrong, they hesitated to endorse any of my discoveries publicly.

Many patients have said to me, "You cured me after other doctors failed. When I went back to some of them and reported the facts, they had nothing to say. What is the matter with them?"

Recently I was asked if my methods were of any benefit to the blindness of babies who have lost their sight from an infection soon after birth. I believe that these cases can be prevented by the well-known simple treatment as most doctors agree, but after the disease has caused blindness very few or no doctors believe that much can be done to restore the sight.

Some years ago I treated a girl, age fourteen, whose right eye was blind following a severe inflammation of her eyes soon after birth. She was unable to see moving objects with this blind eye, but had perception of light. I had her hold the Snellen test card in her hand, close to her face, and to move it from side to side for a half-hour or longer. In the beginning she could not imagine that the card was moving, but by appealing to her common sense she admitted that she did move the card, and furthermore that although she could not see it move, she could imagine it. The next day she practiced in the same way, and told me that she could imagine some black specks on this moving card and that the card was beginning to look more or less white. In a week's time she was able, as a result of daily use of the card, to see about half the letters with the card held close to her eyes. In another week she read the whole card. Then the card was placed gradually farther off, and at the end of about three months the opacity on the front part of her eye had almost entirely disappeared and her vision had improved to 20/20.

I wish to emphasize that many cases of so-called incurable blindness can be completely relieved. It is wrong for any doctor or group of doctors who cannot cure cataract, for example, without an operation, to insist that because they cannot cure it nobody else can.

STORIES FROM THE CLINIC

No. 52: Lewis, A Blind Boy

By Emily C. Lierman

Not long ago he came to us. Only twelve years old, but blind. His name is Lewis. If Lewis had been born blind he would not have had so many plans about the future, nor would he have been so sad.

During the month of March 1923, he was operated upon for mastoiditis. Dr. Bates found with the ophthalmoscope that the boy had atrophy of the optic nerve of both eyes. From the history of the case he believed that the cause of the trouble was probably associated with an abscess of the brain from the disease of the left ear.

After the operation for the relief of the brain abscess, a cerebral hernia appeared above and behind the left auditory canal. The hernia was about two inches long by one inch wide and projected outside the skull a distance of about one inch. For several months before the boy was seen by us, the size of the cerebral hernia, we were told by the mother, had not changed. Before the operation or before the mastoid trouble he was a perfectly normal, healthy boy, full of life and hope.

The morning of his first visit to us, a telephone message came. A teacher from the school for the blind wished Dr. Bates would see him. The appointment was made and inside of one hour the boy arrived with his mother. Her eyes were staring at the Doctor's face as he examined Lewis' eyes, straining every nerve of her body, fearing the verdict might be, "No more hope." After the examination, Dr. Bates came to my office and told me about the case and asked, "Wouldn't you like to see him? I think you could help him to see again." Oh! Wonderful faith. It is the faith Dr. Bates has in me that keeps me going. His encouragement has helped me to benefit cases that would otherwise have seemed hopeless to me.

When I entered the room where Lewis was, I saw a very forlorn looking boy sitting all huddled up in his chair, staring out of sightless eyes. His mother talked a blue streak to me, which was something like this:

"Oh, mine boy that he should be blind. Bless do you think he can once more see? One year he was blind, can see nothing. Before that he was big and healthy."

Of course the mother's heart was crying out loud for help, and it was pitiable to hear her. I tried to explain that we would do everything possible for her boy, but I could not get a word in edgeways. I just closed my eyes for a few moments and prayed for help. I then spoke to Lewis as though he could see me and placed a test card in his hands, advising him to keep his eyes closed and relax in his chair as much as possible while he was doing this. I told him it was very necessary not to worry or to think of his blindness. He could think of a sunset, he said, also a white cloud in a blue sky. With just a few minutes of this treatment he opened his eyes and saw that the card was white. I had him close his eyes again very quickly and asked him to remember the whiteness of drifted snow. He said he could remember or imagine he saw the snow, but he could imagine a white cloud much whiter. I said all right, keep remembering the white cloud, but imagine it is moving. He said he could do that easily. After a half-hour or more, Lewis opened his eyes and flashed a big black spot on the top of the card. I said, "If you will move the card slightly from side to side you will become able to see what that black spot is on the top of the card." Another half-hour had passed by, both of us doing our very best, when all of a sudden my patient said, "It is a letter 'C'!"

Then the mother screamed, "Ach Gott, mine boy sees." She threw her hands in the air, murmuring all the while that her poor boy could see. Then she became hysterical and disturbed all the patients in the treatment rooms. I placed my arm gently around her and led her into my office, and then we both cried. My heart was with this poor mother, but my thoughts were of the boy, too. We had left him all alone and I was worried. I told her to offer a little prayer of thanks to Him who had heard my plea. I said, "Your God is my God, too, so ask Him to help us." I left her to see what Lewis was doing and I found him faithfully palming his eyes.

Although weary and tired after I had worked with Lewis over two hours, I was repaid a thousandfold when he read every letter of the 70-line and 50-line as he moved the test card slowly from side to side, close to his eyes, blinking all the time. He was instructed to stand and swing his body from side to side to lessen the tension of his body; also to blink his eyes all the time to stop staring; then to practice with the test card many times a day, moving it slowly from side to side as he flashed the letters of each line on the card.

On his second visit he read the smallest letters on the card, the 10-line, but to do this he had to hold the card so close that it touched his nose. On his third visit he read the bottom line, holding the card an inch or more away from his nose. The sun treatment always helps him and he is advised to stay in the sun as much as possible. The cerebral hernia, which on his first visit was very much inflamed or red in appearance, had lost most of its redness and the size of the hernia was less.

On his last visit I placed him in front of a large mirror, and he saw it plainly. He could also see me standing behind him as he looked into the mirror. The sad look in his eyes is no longer there. His smile is wonderful to see and his mother is more than grateful because of the hope we have given her in restoring the sight of her boy.

SINBAD THE SAILOR

By George M. Guild

Why Sinbad? Of what benefit to the readers of this magazine or to people who desire a cure of imperfect sight without glasses can a reference to Sinbad be? In *Arabian Nights* tales he occupies a prominent place. In his many voyages he described many strange things which happened and which were very wonderful, although not always probable or true. Being a sailor, he used his eyes principally for distant vision. He had good eyesight, but after one of his numerous voyages he returned to his home in Baghdad and complained to his friends that his sight for distance had become poor, so poor that he was unable to recognize people ten feet away. An Egyptian astrologer sold him a pair of glasses for a price which made a big hole in his savings. For a time he was happy because his vision was decidedly improved by the glasses, but it was not long before his imperfect sight required stronger glasses, and the strength of his glasses was frequently increased. In a shipwreck he had difficulty in reaching the shore because the water clouded his glasses so that they became useless. Whenever it rained the glasses became too clouded to help him to see. In many emergencies, when he most needed his glasses, they failed him. When swimming he could not see any better than without his glasses. It embarrassed him very much when trying to reach land, because he was unable to locate it. Other sailors would throw water in his face, fog his glasses, and tease the blind man without risk to themselves. With his glasses he suffered great pain and fatigue.

While visiting a city in a foreign land and walking the streets without seeing much, a stranger handed him a parchment on which was written:

"Go where all things are moving,
Watch and think the livelong day;
The truth is always proving
Your sight will return, I say."

The words gave him some hope and he believed that in one of his voyages he would find some land or country where all things would be moving and nothing immovable or stationary. In a voyage to India he felt that in this country he would find a land where all things were moving. After a long day of traveling he entered a temple where many worshippers on their knees were alternately raising their arms and faces on high and then bowing to the ground saying, "Allah is Allah, God is Allah."

To avoid attracting attention he imitated the others while remembering that the paper of instructions told him to watch and think. He noted that when he raised his head up that things in front of him seemed to move down or in the opposite direction, and that when he bowed his head down to the ground things appeared to move up. At last he believed that he had found a place where all things were moving. By going through the motions without the prayer he found that it worked just the same. After he left the temple he was able to notice that when he walked straight ahead, things to each side of him and the ground in front of him appeared to move in the opposite direction. He was able to demonstrate then, without any effort, that the place where all things are moving was wherever he happened to be, and since he was always moving his eyes during the day, it was possible for him to see things moving opposite all day long.

Watch and think was ever in his mind. He became able to demonstrate that when he imagined the movement easily that all pain, discomfort or fatigue in his eyes and in other parts of his body were prevented or relieved. It was not long before he found that the light became brighter; and with this increased illumination, his vision improved.

When the swing was practiced with an effort, very little or no benefit followed. He discovered that the swing was a great help to his vision when practiced at night, and brought him more comfort than the same time devoted to sleep. All this time he believed that he had discovered a truth: that the cause of his imperfect sight was a strain or an effort to see, and that he was cured by rest and not by effort.

He returned to Baghdad overflowing with the wonderful news. He called on the Egyptian astrologer who had sold him his glasses, and with a happy smile on his face reported the facts.

The astrologer was furious and screamed in a loud voice:

"Out upon you, you lying knave. I believed your story of the mammoth bird, the roc, your experiences with mermaids and many others of your strange tales, but this is too much. To be cured of poor sight by rest is too absurd. You must be crazy." Then he drove Sinbad from his house, announced to the mob of people outside to shun him for a liar, a cheat, and a fool.

For many years later Sinbad held his peace, but did not neglect to help the blind until their number became sufficiently great to overwhelm the ignorant astrologer and others like him.

THE BLACK FAIRIES

By Margaret Edwards—Age 8

Editor's Note—*Margaret Edwards is a young subscriber of London, England. She was very much impressed by Dr. Bates' story, "The Black Fairy." Her story will suggest to mothers and teachers an interesting and successful way of improving the memory and the physical and mental efficiency of children.*

On the top of a grassy hill the fairies live. All kinds of fairies—flower fairies, butterfly fairies, yellow fairies, green fairies, blue fairies, red fairies, orange fairies and black fairies.

Black fairies, you will say at once? Yes, black fairies; and the black fairies are very small, but very useful.

Perhaps you would like me to tell you what their work is.

Well, early in the morning they creep to the village and hide in the bushes, waiting for the schoolboys to come. Sometimes they see things that make the tears come into their eyes—they see little boys who wear spectacles knocked about by the bigger boys. Then the black fairies come back at night, when the small boys have gone to bed. They creep in at the window, and whisper to the boys in their dreams. The black fairies ask them what they want best, and they say, "To have perfect eyesight." So the black fairies say, "Always remember us, and see us before you in everything."

Then the black fairies disappear, and you can imagine the boys' delight when they wake up in the morning and remember the black fairies, and find they can see perfectly well without their spectacles.

HELP OTHERS

By Emily A. Meder

When we help others, we help ourselves. A teacher of arithmetic learns more than any of the class. This principle so well known is valuable for persons with imperfect sight. Some eye patients have told me that they did not obtain any permanent benefit until after they tried to improve the sight of others.

The League is now two years old and is a "grandmother." There is a League in East Orange, one on its way in the Middle West, and in England. We hope to have Leagues in all the large cities before long.

One prevalent cause of defective vision is staring. This is usually unconscious, but none the less dangerous. We call your attention to this fact because it is the first thing to correct when helping your friends.

KINDERGARTEN CHILDREN BENEFITED

By Emily C. Lierman

A kindergarten teacher who attended one of our recent lectures requested me to help one of her little charges who is afflicted with squint. She informed me that the little one is very poor, so I advised her to bring her to my Clinic.

To become more acquainted with me and the way the cases are managed there, this teacher, at my cordial invitation, visited the Clinic. I would like to tell more about the teacher and what she has accomplished with her slight knowledge of our method.

She has a sunny disposition, and I can well imagine a good mental picture of the children as they greet her every day in the classroom. She loves her little pupils, and is also a great lover of nature. It is her happiness to bring the two together in her work.

She explains to her class, in her lovable, sweet way, just how the flowers grow, and makes them understand what happens before the first shoots peep their noses above the ground.

This teacher's name is Cecilia B. Eschbach and the kindergarten is connected with the Brooklyn Orphan Asylum. A short time ago I received the following letter from her which I thought would interest our readers.

"Dear Ms. Lierman:

In spite of North Wind's biting breath, the little children of the kindergarten know spring is here. Their gardens give evidence of it, for the crocuses are up, the daffodils have twelve fat buds; the hyacinths and tulips, too, have grown to quite a size. To create a situation for conversation about awakening spring, I placed eight empty flower pots in a paper bag. The one who opened the bag was called the gardener. He chose eight children and gave them each the name of a flower to go with the pots.

Every child was familiar with the following flowers and could name and identify the real ones: crocus, tulip, dandelion, daffodil, hyacinth, Easter lily, pink sweet peas, and rose. The little gardener decided to give away his flowers, but could not remember the name of the eighth one. I said, 'Palm your eyes, William.' He did so, and in a moment said, 'Pink sweet peas.'

The children have learned to palm their eyes with good results. Two who have a cast in their eyes play the swinging game and keep looking at the ceiling. Sometimes we sing it, or sway to the rhythm of the piano. They are improving.

Hoping this report will be of interest to you and thanking you for your kindness,

I am, Very truly yours, Cecilia B. Eschbach."

AT THE MOVIES

By A. L. Reed

Ms. Reed is studying this method, and is practicing at the East Orange Clinic. The following report will be helpful to those who experience discomfort at the movies.

Glasses and strain at the movies produced imperfect sight and headache; the removal of the glasses and using the eyes without strain relieved the headache and improved the vision more than with the glasses.

My patient had not been to the Clinic in several weeks and when she entered with a twinkle in her eye, I knew something was coming. After a few minutes' work she explained, "I've got to admit you are right. The last time I came you told me something that made me think you were wrong. You said the movies were good for the eyes if we looked at them right. Last week I went to the movies and in a short time I had a headache. Then I thought of what you had told me and decided to try it. First I took my glasses off and tried to relax all over; then I stopped trying to hold the pictures still, and just let them go. I looked at one thing at a time and didn't worry about the rest. After a few minutes I realized that my headache was gone, and my next surprise was when it dawned on me that I was seeing the picture clearer than I had ever seen it with my glasses on. I didn't miss much of the show either after I stopped trying to see it all at once, and straining after every little detail.

When I came out of the theatre I said to my husband, "I guess I was wrong instead of Ms. Reed, and I'll go back to the Clinic and get some more help."

I told her that she certainly had profited by the show, thanks to Dr. Bates' method.

Better Eyesight
July 1924—Vol. IX, No. 1

CURABLE CASES

Patients wearing glasses for the relief of imperfect sight may expect better vision after they are cured than they ever had before with glasses. Adults who have good distant vision but require glasses after middle life for reading are also curable without glasses. Such patients, although they may read very well with glasses, complain that, as a rule, they must hold the page at one distance in order to read with the best vision. This reading distance is usually about twelve inches. Some cases require one pair of glasses for reading books or newspapers, but cannot see clearly at a greater distance without another pair of glasses. Musicians especially find that glasses that give them good vision for reading books are useless to them for reading music or for playing the piano. To see closer than twelve inches may require still another pair of glasses. To see more distant objects may require still another pair. Some of my patients have shown me numerous pairs of glasses, each one adapted for certain specific distances. It is a great relief to such cases to be cured, because then they are able, not only to see perfectly at the distance without glasses, but they can read the fine print as well at six inches as they can farther off. The eye with normal sight is able to change its focus at will for all distances without any discomfort whatever.

Patients with cataract, glaucoma and other diseases of the eyes may not be able to see even with glasses. When they are cured by my methods they become able to see normally in all kinds of light, in a bright light or in a dim light. Pain, fatigue and other discomforts of the eyes are all relieved.

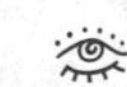

PRACTICAL SUGGESTIONS

By W. H. Bates, M.D.

Many people complain that they are so busy they do not have the time or opportunity to practice my methods with the Snellen test card for the cure of imperfect sight without glasses. While the Snellen test card can be used with benefit, there are other objects which can also be used just as well. One can obtain perfect relaxation, perfect sight, easily and continuously by the use of a perfect memory. A familiar face can often be remembered perfectly when one fails to remember letters perfectly. Stenographers tell me that they can remember the characters of shorthand better than the letters of the Snellen test card. They have in this way obtained sufficient relaxation to correct or cure their nearsightedness without glasses. Such patients can practice when riding in a car, when walking on the street or when occupied in various ways.

If one can find some object which they can remember perfectly, whether it be a hammer of a carpenter, mortar or trowel used by a bricklayer, a brush by an artist, an instrument used by a surgeon, familiar things seen frequently, a cure without glasses may be obtained without the use of the Snellen test card.

I recall a case of a musician with a high degree of nearsightedness who complained that every time he looked at the Snellen test card he was tempted to strain and his vision was lowered. It was a remarkable fact that he was unable to remember a bar of music. He could play nothing whatever from memory but he could remember a very small area of a black note of music, an area as small as a period in an ordinary newspaper. By practicing with this period and nothing else, dodging any improvement in his sight by shifting frequently, his memory of the black period improved. If he imagined his vision for a distant object was improved he was compelled to look somewhere else as quickly as possible or else lose his memory of the period. He had to be very careful in order to keep the memory of a period to avoid testing his sight. When the period was remembered perfectly, the relaxation which followed was very pleasant and he enjoyed the memory of the period at all times and in all places.

He was a very skillful pianist and played very complicated pieces on sight, and told me that the memory of the period was a great benefit to his playing. He became so interested in his period that he said at no time of the day or night when he was awake did he forget his period; and, instead of being a distraction to him, it increased his efficiency, mental and physical, enormously. He became able to walk out at night, even when it rained, find his way about the streets and return home without trouble, which was something that he had never been able to do while he was wearing his glasses. His myopia was only partially corrected by concave 16 D. In less than two weeks he read the bottom line of the Snellen test card at twenty feet, 20/10. Furthermore, there was an astonishing improvement in his memory for music. He told me that he became able to read a complicated score of music, sit down and play it right off from memory, a feat which he had never been able to do previously with the most familiar music.

One patient, a lady with myopia, came to me from a distant Western city. She was very frank and told me that she was employed as a stenographer in an office and her income was very moderate indeed. She felt that her sight was gradually leaving her because she required stronger glasses every year. She suffered much from fatigue, pain and other discomforts of her eyes. Her first words to me were, "Doctor, I will go through any operation or any form of treatment and will do anything that you say in order to get cured quickly."

I tested her statement. While she was holding her glasses in her hand I turned to leave the room, and as I walked toward the door I said to her, "Get rid of your glasses." "How?" she asked. I answered, "Smash them." Before I reached the door I heard a crash, and turned around and saw that she had taken me literally by smashing the glasses on the arm of the chair. She was cured in a few visits.

Another patient who did not have as much nearsightedness as the above asked me what she should do in order to get cured quickly. I told her that the most important thing at the start was to stop wearing her glasses and never put them on again even for any emergency. Then she started an argument and asked me all kinds of questions. What should she do when she went to the theatre when she couldn't see the stage? What should she do about her music when she couldn't see the notes without her glasses? She wanted to know, and insisted upon it, just how much time she would have to devote to practicing. She wanted to know if she would have to practice after she was cured. This was several years ago. She is still under treatment. At times she gets flashes of normal vision. Even now she will do things wrong although she knows it is wrong, apologize and promise to do better.

It is not faith that cures, but a proper use of the eyes.

Imperfect sight is not cured by a club. Ms. Lierman in her series "Stories from the Clinic" has repeatedly emphasized the value of kindness. In one case, a boy ten years old was brought to the Clinic by his mother, who was very much excited, annoyed, and indignant when the school insisted that the boy should have glasses. The mother was out of patience with the boy because he had lost his eyesight. If he had lost his hat or his shoes she could not have been more excited or upset. Her first words to the boy came with a slap in the face. "Mind what the lady says. Do as she tells you. Try as hard as you can. See those letters over there and don't cry." The boy said he could not read any of them and his mother shook him to make him see better. He complained that when he looked at the card it gave him a pain.

Ms. Lierman separated the mother and had her sit some distance away. Then she talked kindly to the little boy, asked him where he went to school and was his teacher kind to him. He replied, "She is all the time scolding me even when I don't do nothing." Then Ms. Lierman talked to him about baseball and Babe Ruth and asked him if he liked to play baseball in the summertime. He was somewhat suspicious at first, but in a little while he began to thaw. He was asked to smile, which he did with some difficulty. Ms. Lierman was gentle and very kind to him.

All of a sudden he shouted, "Oh, I can read that card over there," which he read down to the 50-line. The boy, with a little persuasion, closed his eyes and covered them with the palms of his hands, while Ms. Lierman told him fairy stories, which were very hard for him to believe. In ten minutes, after he opened his eyes he read almost all the smaller letters on the card, and by repeating the palming a few times, at brief intervals, he obtained flashes of normal vision. He left the Clinic smiling and happy, with his mother following after him in a daze.

You cannot force children to see by harshness, and what is true of children is also true of adults.

STORIES FROM THE CLINIC

No. 53: Shock Causes Blindness

By Emily C. Lierman

On July 16, 1923, there came to our office a man suffering with blindness caused by a sudden shock. As I stood before him and asked him what his trouble was, his eyes looked up toward the ceiling and immediately I noticed he could not see me. He had been sent to us in the hope that Dr. Bates would be able to restore his sight. Previous to his visit on that day I received a telephone message from a woman employed by the Compensation Bureau of the City of New York. She told me that he was blind and it was the opinion of eye specialists consulted that there was no hope of his sight ever being restored. Dr. Bates examined his eyes with the ophthalmoscope and found that he had atrophy of the optic nerve and that he was under a terrible tension.

With each eye separately he could see the 200-line letter of the test card at one foot temporarily. He could only do this in flashes, because he stared continuously, which blinded him. The variable swing improved his vision to 6/200 and his field was also improved by the swing. He came daily to the office for treatment, and on July 21 he read 9/20 after he had palmed his eyes for a long time. Sunning improved his vision also. His general depression became less and he informed me that he was feeling much better after each office visit. For a long time he did not have very much to say, but after he had become better acquainted with us all, he began to talk about his case. He had been working in the movie studios for quite a few years and apparently he felt no discomfort in his eyes. This is the story he told me:

"I was standing on the top rung of a ladder readjusting electrical parts used in the studio for taking movies. At the time there was just an ordinary light such as is used in most offices. Without my knowing it, a strong Kleig light was suddenly turned on and I received a sudden shock which caused blindness instantly. I was taken care of and then was taken home. Since then I have not been able to work. It seemed as though my troubles were multiplied when my little baby boy took sick and died. I had no money with which to bury him until my wife's parents came to our aid. Christmas came very shortly, with no hope of Christmas cheer for my other child, a little girl just three years old. We were in debt, but I had planned, when I was able to work again, to pay back the money which was used to bury my baby. My wife tried to console me and make me feel that things were not quite so bad, but I saw no hope ahead of me on account of my blindness."

We felt all the more here at the office that our patient should have all the treatment that could be given him in order to restore his sight, if possible, and we worked diligently all through the fall and winter with steady results.

During the month of May we had many rainy days with very little sun. This patient has demonstrated to us that the sun is very necessary for the eyes. During all these months of almost daily treatment he has not had such poor vision as he had in the last few weeks. His vision was lowered to 10/50 and he became very much discouraged. After the sun had shone for a day he came to the office feeling light hearted and happy. He was given the sun treatment and immediately his vision improved to almost normal, reading 10/10 at times. The Doctor questioned his ability to dodge automobiles at the crossings here in our big city. His answer was that he could get along very well on bright days when the sun was shining, but he still feared the traffic on rainy days. While this conversation was going on, the patient was looking very intently at the Doctor's face as he stood about three feet away. He did not move an eyelash, but just stared all the while he talked. He had forgotten the very thing that helped him—blinking. All of a sudden he exclaimed, "Doctor, now as I look at you, you haven't any head."

"No," the Doctor replied, "seems to me the other day somebody told me I did have a head. But you never can tell; some people don't always tell the truth." Immediately the patient apologized and hastened to say, "Oh! But Doctor, when I come close enough to you I can see that you have a head."

Dr. Bates has always advocated the movies. Whenever a patient stares he advises him to go to the movies. Dr. Bates enjoys them himself and goes as often as he is able to.

We owe a great deal to the movie artists, for a great part of their work is done under unfavorable conditions. The Kleig light, while it is powerful, is not injurious to the eyes of the actors and actresses when their eyes are properly used. Most of them work under a terrible tension, with the feeling that their eyes will be injured by the strong glare. A great many eye specialists no doubt have treated injury to the eyes apparently caused by the Kleig light. The light would be harmless if those who work in the studios could keep their minds relaxed and if they could also understand and use our method—resting the eyes all day long.

Dr. Bates discovered many years ago the benefit of strong light on the eyes and I have seen many patients cured by the sun treatment alone. Some of these cases were seriously affected because of their inability to stand even the rays of the sun. It is curious but true that this patient has been benefited mostly by a magnifying glass which focused the light on the white part of each eye as he looked down while the upper lid was raised. In the beginning of his treatment the mere mention of light would make him frown and shrink with fear. Now he enjoys sitting in the sun all day long and realizes that it gives him the greatest benefit. He is steadily improving. While he is not entirely cured, he reads the bottom line of the test card occasionally at ten feet.

He has great hopes of being cured and is so grateful for what has been done for his eyes that he insisted upon my writing to two of our most popular actresses of the screen who are interested in his case. We are striving to cure him so that we can send a note of thanks to those who are interested in him and to try and encourage others who might be troubled by the Kleig light to come to us to be benefited as he was.

NERVOUS SYMPTOM RELIEVED

By Edith T. Fisher, M.S., M.D.

About seven months ago this patient, who is a physician, forty-one years old, first came to me. He had studied his own case thoroughly and I shall present it in his words as he described it to me.

"Since I was seven years old I have worn glasses, and since then I have had attacks of nervousness, accompanied by headaches, which have become more frequent and more severe as I have grown older. My poor vision is due to astigmatism, asthenopia and hypermetropia, and I think all my nervous symptoms are the result of this condition of my eyes.

About once a week, sometimes more often, I have an excruciating headache accompanied by great weakness and nervousness. This always begins with a feeling of constriction in my eyes and spreads to my forehead, then gradually develops into a terrible headache. It continues all day and the following day I am completely exhausted.

In addition to this weekly headache I have the same feeling of constriction in my eyes and across my forehead continually. This comes on in the morning after I have been up about two hours and it makes me very nervous.

If I read ten or fifteen minutes this sensation of constriction increases and I become so weak that I have to lie down and rest; then I am able to read again for a short time. If I continue to read without resting, one of the severe headaches will develop.

At times for apparently no reason I suddenly feel an overwhelming desire to sleep. This usually occurs when I have been in a bright light or under a strain, as when we are entertaining or being entertained, and I assure you it is extremely embarrassing to fall asleep while conversing with someone. I can overcome this feeling for a short time, but gradually I become so exhausted that in spite of everything I can do, I fall asleep. Sometimes I awake in five minutes, sometimes not for fifteen, but I always feel refreshed. This invariably happens if I go anywhere, so I have given up everything and stay at home as much as possible.

My eyes are very sensitive to the light and I usually wear a pair of dark glasses over my other glasses. Last summer on bright days I wore two pairs of colored glasses so as to protect my eyes as much as possible from the sun.

I have tried many different kinds of treatment, but all without any relief.

"When I heard of Dr. Bates' method of curing imperfect sight without glasses I tried resting my eyes, but when I close them and try to relax I have a feeling of unsteadiness in the eyeball, which is almost a jerking, and this makes me more nervous. So I thought I was probably palming incorrectly.

I asked him if he had tried to imagine or remember anything while he was palming and he answered "No, I just try to relax, and the harder I try the more nervous I get."

I explained to him that by making an effort to relax he was increasing the strain. While he was talking I noticed that he had not blinked. His forehead was deeply wrinkled and there was a constant twitching of the facial muscles on the right side.

With his glasses he read 10/10; without them, 10/15; with the left eye, 10/15, and with the right, 10/50. He was unable to read the diamond type.

First I explained about blinking, but when he tried this he contracted all the facial muscles. After watching me he tried it again, but without success. Then I told him to sit in as comfortable a position as possible, close his eyes and cover them with his hand in such a way as to exclude the light without making any pressure upon the eyeballs. He said, "I've tried this, Doctor, and the unsteadiness in my eyeballs makes me very nervous."

I then asked him if he could remember the small black letter "o" that he had seen on the test card, but he could not. I asked him about many different objects, if he could remember or imagine them, but the only thing he could remember was a sunset he had seen last summer. This he could remember if he looked at the sky, then the trees, and then the grass, shifting from one to another and seeing each perfectly. After palming in this way about twenty minutes, I asked him if he could imagine a blue sky with a very white cloud moving across it. This he could do now, but for a short time only, and when he lost it he had to remember the sunset before he could imagine the blue sky and white cloud.

After palming half an hour he read 10/40 with his right eye and half of 10/10 with his left. I reminded him to blink, and though he did not contract all his facial muscles it was still a great effort for him. He said, "I don't think I ever blinked before, and this is the first time I have been able to palm without having that unsteadiness in my eyeballs." Then I explained to him that when he remembered the sunset perfectly his eyes were at rest, and when his eyes were at rest all the nerves in his body were at rest.

After palming again for half an hour he was able to imagine a small black letter "o" on the white cloud, but only for an instant. Each time that he lost it he had to imagine first the sunset, then the blue sky with the white cloud, and finally the letter "o," which he was able to imagine longer each time. He could imagine the "o" moving in the opposite direction as he looked from the right side to the left side of the "o," and in this way developed a swing, but he could keep it for a few seconds only.

The sensitiveness to light, I told him, could be overcome by sitting in the sun every day. He seemed to think he ought to wear his dark glasses until his eyes were stronger, but he promised to follow my directions. Before he left the office that day he said, "I can't remember when I have felt so relaxed."

Three days later I saw him again. He had been palming eight times a day, half an hour each time. In addition to this he had been practicing with the test card, swinging, shifting and sitting in the sun. He was very anxious to do everything that would help cure his condition.

His vision had improved to 10/30 with the right eye and 11/10 with the left. He blinked easily now, but still stared at times. He told me, "When I notice that feeling of constriction in my eyes, I know I have been staring; then I palm a few minutes and that uncomfortable sensation disappears." There was now only an occasional twitching of the facial muscles on the right side.

His vision improved slowly, and when I saw him the last time, just three months after I had first seen him, he read 10/10 with the right eye and 15/10 with the left. The diamond type he read easily. All the nervous symptoms had entirely disappeared. Before he left he said, "I have read a book in the last three days that it would have taken me at least six months to read before I discarded my glasses. Of course, I am glad to have my eyes normal, but I can't tell you how happy I am to be free from all those other symptoms."

I have heard from him several times since and he has had no relapse.

NOTES FROM PATIENTS

These paragraphs were taken from some patients' letters. We find that everyone has his own way of palming, swinging, etc. Some patients like to take drifting trips while palming. Others find more relaxation in thinking of black and remembering certain flowers. The way which is most helpful to you is the best to follow.

From a Patient Who Likes to Drift

I think by this time I have floated down every river in the world. I am not sure about those of Persia and Patagonia, but otherwise I have covered them pretty well. Geographically speaking, it has been quite interesting, for one can have at will monkeys leaping from branch to branch along the shore, or polar bears putting out a paw at one from large icebergs, and all the time being perfectly comfortable. There are really great possibilities in this method of overcoming pain and in improving the sight. I have not had a severe pain since the first trip, and the minute one starts off, I float and lose the pain.

From A Book Reader

In early spring here in this desert country the intensity of the sunlight increases with such rapidity that many people are disagreeably affected in their eyes at that time. I have been wearing a broad brimmed Stetson sombrero for its shade. But I also noted that my eyes seemed unduly sensitive to the bright light. Remembering Dr. Bates' rule that light is good for the eyes, not coddling with shade, I discarded the sombrero and now wear a cap, with the result that the over-sensitiveness to light is gone.

REPORT OF THE LEAGUE MEETINGS

A regular meeting of the Better Eyesight League was held on the evening of May 13. Anticipating a demonstration of Dr. Bates' method a large audience was in attendance. Katherine Hurty, President of the League, presented May Secor as chairperson of the meeting. The latter's experience as a teacher of various grades of the elementary school and as a member of the Speech Improvement Department of New York City's school system enabled her to speak from the teacher's standpoint.

Ms. Secor became interested in the method in an effort to find some means by which schoolchildren may be relieved of eyestrain. The stammerer who suffers from eyestrain is especially worthy of attention. Ms. Secor had worn glasses for fully fifteen years when on March 15, 1923, as a means of investigating Dr. Bates' method, she removed her bifocals and began daily practice. Upon awakening each morning she devotes twenty minutes to this work, with the result that she has eliminated entirely the use of glasses, and enjoys normal eyesight and freedom from eyestrain combined with a full daily program of work and study.

Teachers are familiar with the fact that a large percentage of pupils and teachers suffer from eyestrain; these sufferers include many who wear glasses. It is therefore incumbent upon educators to include in the daily program of the kindergarten and of each class in the elementary and high school definite exercises which will tend to relieve eyestrain; palming, reading the Snellen chart, swinging, shifting, and sunning may be used for this purpose. When the pupils have learned how to practice these exercises they may do so at odd times during the day. It will then be necessary to reserve only a short daily period for eye work; a part of the time now devoted to physical education could with profit be used in this way. Dr. Bates assures us that eyestrain is frequently produced by coming into contact with persons who are suffering from eyestrain; it is therefore extremely important that each supervisor, teacher and parent should secure normal vision without the use of glasses, thus eliminating eyestrain in his own case.

The speaker had observed that many teachers and librarians who were so fortunate as to work in rooms to which the sun's rays have access darkened their rooms in order "to save" their eyes; among these teachers and librarians were many cases of eyestrain which had not been relieved by the use of artificial lenses. As early as 1910, probably earlier, eminent oculists began to realize that the sun's rays are beneficial to the eyes; today we find that children readily appreciate the value of sun treatment.

Ms. Secor emphasized the value of palming in restoring normal vision. The meeting then assumed a clinical aspect, Dr. Bates, Dr. Achorn, Ms. Hurty, and the speaker assisting the members and visitors to palm; relaxation was secured more readily when the individual was led to assume a happy mental attitude. The speaker advised teachers to train pupils in such a manner that the eye exercises will always be accompanied by a pleasurable emotion. The use of palming by the student of music was also discussed; in many cases fatigue has been eliminated or greatly reduced by palming for a period of five minutes after each twenty minutes or half-hour of practice (vocal or instrumental.)

The speaker then called upon Ms. Hurty to discuss the use of the Snellen chart in the classroom. Ms. Hurty reported that many pupils in her "eye group" had greatly improved their vision by reading the chart each day. When difficulty is experienced in reading certain letters on the chart, one or more of the following suggestions are offered: palm, swing, and close the eyes after reading each letter; read fine print, then read the chart; close eyes, open, and look at left side of letter, report its appearance; repeat with right side of letter, then read the letter; walk up to the chart, read the letter, return to former position and read it (imagination of assistance here.) The officers of the League then assisted those present in reading the chart.

Dr. Bates was then requested to discuss the long swing. He described and demonstrated the long swing and emphasized its efficacy in securing relaxation and in relieving acute pain. The swing was then practiced by those present. Several classroom problems relative to the elimination of eyestrain were discussed. At the close of this discussion the meeting was adjourned.

QUESTIONS AND ANSWERS

Q–1. Some days I can read the Snellen test card to the 15-line, others only to the 30- or 20-line.

A–1. When the eyestrain is less, the vision is always better.

Q–2. By following instructions in the book, can cataract be benefited without consulting a physician?

A–2. Yes.

Q–3. Are memory and imagination the same? When we remember an object, do we have to visualize it?

A–3. A perfect memory cannot be obtained unless you are able to imagine that you see or visualize what you remember.

Q–4. When I try to imagine a black period, it blurs and I get all colors but black.

A–4. When you fail to remember a period with your eyes closed, open your eyes and see it, then close your eyes and remember it as well as you can for a moment; alternate.

Q–5. I am always conscious of eyestrain in church.

A–5. Eyestrain is caused by a stare or an effort to see. Close your eyes frequently and rest them.

Better Eyesight
August 1924—Vol. IX, No. 2

SCHOOL NUMBER

THE PREVENTION OF MYOPIA

The August number of *Better Eyesight* is a school number devoted almost exclusively to the problem of the cure or prevention of nearsightedness in schoolchildren. The great value of the method as a preventive is emphasized by the fact that the vision of all schoolchildren has always improved, and when the vision is improved, of course imperfect sight is prevented. It is well to remember that my method for the prevention of myopia in schoolchildren is the only one that is a success. It has been in continuous use for more than twenty years in the public schools of New York and other cities. Once daily or more often the children read the card, first with one eye and then with the other, covering each eye alternately with the palm of the hand in such a way as to shut out all the light without any pressure on the eyeball. Teachers who have studied my book or have been patients find it an advantage to have the children palm five minutes three or four times a day. They claim that palming quiets the children and gives them an improved mental efficiency which is a great help to their memory and imagination, as well as their sight. I believe other children should be taught how to palm, swing, blink and improve their vision of the Snellen test card. The method is of great value to young children in the kindergarten, children in the high schools, and should be practiced by students and teachers in colleges and universities. In the military school and naval academy the method should be employed for the prevention of imperfect sight.

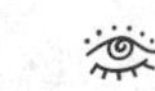

SCHOOLCHILDREN

By W. H. Bates, M.D.

Most schoolchildren when they enter school have good vision. After some months or a year, many of them acquire imperfect sight; others do not. It is interesting to compare the facts connected with children who acquire imperfect sight with the facts connected with children who do not acquire imperfect sight. It is important to consider the problem of the teachers. It is a fact that some teachers who do not wear glasses seldom have children acquire imperfect sight in their classes. Teachers who wear glasses or who have imperfect sight have a large percentage of children with acquired poor vision while under their care. It is not necessary to theorize on this matter. It is sufficient to know that teachers who have imperfect sight are under a great mental and nervous strain. This strain is contagious. After children are transferred to a room in which the teacher has normal vision, many of the pupils regain their normal sight again.

It should be emphasized that teachers wearing glasses or teachers with imperfect sight should not be allowed a license to teach. There is a school of several thousand children in New York where many of the teachers are wearing glasses.

All the children who are unmanageable, whose scholarship is so low that they can not keep up with their grade, are transferred to special classes. The teacher who was able to handle these misfits without any apparent trouble whatever had normal vision and her temperament had a quieting influence on the children. Ten years ago this teacher introduced my method for the cure and prevention of imperfect sight in schoolchildren. The results that she obtained are very important. In a few weeks all her children with imperfect sight obtained improved or normal vision. Some of the children had the truant habit. One boy was under the supervision of the Truant Officer three or four days a week. The teacher had him practice with the Snellen test card which improved his vision very much and relieved his headaches so that he became able to study his lessons without discomfort. The practice with the Snellen test card was a great relief to his nerves and gave him more benefit than running away from school. He became an enthusiastic pupil and his truant propensities were permanently cured.

Many of her children complained that they could not

read the letters on the blackboard and when they tried, it gave them a headache. After using the Snellen test card the headaches disappeared, their vision improved, and they were able to read the writing on the blackboard without discomfort. To me it was a remarkable fact that every one of her children was cured with the help of the Snellen test card and the cure of their imperfect sight was accompanied with a cure of their eye and other discomforts.

Some school teachers wearing glasses for imperfect sight were able to obtain a cure without glasses by the help obtained by reading my book. Now it is an encouraging fact that patients, soon after they are cured without glasses, have a great desire to help others, and the more they try to help others, the greater the benefit to themselves. One teacher was so enthusiastic that she not only cured all the children in her own class, but encouraged other teachers to send their children to her who had imperfect sight. Her practice increased to such an extent and produced such a favorable impression upon the principal that she was allowed four periods a week in which to devote all her time to the cure of the children.

A kindergarten teacher reported some wonderful results obtained in two cases of squint. Both of these children were wearing glasses for the benefit of their eyes, but they obtained no decided or permanent benefit. As these children did not know the letters of the alphabet, a card was used by the teacher which had printed on it large and small letters "E" which pointed in various directions. When the children had good sight they were able to tell in which direction each letter "E" was pointed: either up, down, to the right or to the left. The card was placed about fifteen feet away from the children.

Each child would stand, cover one eye with the palm of the hand and regard the chart with the other eye. If the pupil could not see the direction in which the small letters were pointing, with the open eye, this eye was covered also with the palm of the hand. In a few seconds, one hand was removed for a moment, just long enough for the pupil to determine which way the "E" pointed; but, if the child failed, the eye was again palmed for a few moments or part of a minute. This process was repeated until the pupil became able to tell in which direction the letters "E" on the bottom line pointed.

One time, the two children with squint developed measles and were sent to the hospital for two weeks where they did not wear their glasses. It is well known by physicians and others that measles is often hard on the eyes. Some children acquire imperfect sight during an attack of measles and this imperfect sight may continue during the lifetime of the patient. The teacher was very much gratified to learn that in spite of this handicap the two children with squint returned to school with their eyes no worse than before.

The teacher held the two hands of each child in turn and had the child look up and swing for a time with her. Then the teacher would look at the cheeks of the child and remark on the condition of the redness of the face following the exercise, avoiding any mention of the eyes. The children were led to believe that the exercise was not for the eyes at all, but just to see if it gave them a better color in their cheeks. This was quite important because if attention was called to the eyes of the children who had squint, the squint was very apt to become worse. When the eyes were ignored the practice of the swinging always improved the squint and these children were soon cured. The teacher was so encouraged by her results that she recommended the method very strongly to other teachers and to the parents of the children.

When a child first enters school it is well to keep in mind that children in school have a great many new and unexpected things to contend with. They are brought in contact with many other children who are new, strange and different. Their own teachers and the teachers in the other classes have an effect upon the child. Going to and from school, the child meets many strangers and these strangers have an effect upon the mind of the child. Children are great imitators. They learn to walk by watching others walk. They learn to talk and play from the influence of other children. Being great imitators they absorb many bad habits as well as new and strange ones. While it is a good thing for a child to be taught how to practice habits of decency and order, at the same time they are absorbing a great many habits which are an injury to them. If a child has a nervous teacher with imperfect sight who is constantly straining her eyes to see, the child would be very apt to imitate the eyestrain of the teacher. If, on the other hand, the teacher has good eyesight and good nerves, the child may absorb or acquire habits of great benefit. It is well to emphasize the bad effect of the strain of a teacher with imperfect sight and nerves upon the mind of the child. We may say that children in schools are exposed to influences both good and bad which are different from those in the home. Sometimes the influences in the schools are more beneficial than what the child meets with at home.

STORIES FROM THE CLINIC

No. 54: School Number

By Emily C. Lierman

While our Clinic at present is not as large as it was at the Harlem Hospital, we have very interesting cases, and some of them are schoolchildren.

One little chap, age seven years, whose name is Fredrick, is one of the brightest boys I have known. His father is one of the carpenters who helped make the partitions in our office. We were treating patients long before our present office building was completed. He therefore had the opportunity to see some of the patients as they came to our Clinic, and also saw the patients leave the office after their first treatment. One day he remarked that some cases appeared so much improved after only one treatment, that it seemed as though a miracle had been performed.

He being a poor man, I offered to help him or any of his family, if they at any time needed treatment for their eyes. "Oh!" he said, "I have two little boys, but they have nothing wrong with their eyes." But he thanked me just the same and said he would remember my offer.

On April 12, 1924, just a year after I had spoken to him, his son Fredrick, whom I have already mentioned, came with his mother. How I wish I had a son like him, or a couple of them. He was very attentive while I was talking, and his big blue eyes looked into mine. I think he was speculating whether I was all right or not. He seemed to feel very much at home with me right from the start, so I had no difficulty in improving his vision. His mother told me that the school nurse had sent him home with a note saying that he needed glasses. His father refused to get them and suggested that the mother bring him to me. As Fredrick answered my questions he looked directly at me and there was no sign of a frown or strain of any kind, but I did notice that he listened without blinking for more than two minutes or longer. As the normal eye blinks unconsciously every few seconds, I soon realized what his trouble was and that he could be cured in a short time. Dr. Bates examined him with the ophthalmoscope and said there was nothing organically wrong with his eyes, only eyestrain.

The letter test card troubled him at first, so I had him read the card with "E's" pointing in different directions. As he looked at the card, his facial expression became entirely changed. His forehead was a mass of wrinkles as he tried to see in what direction the "E's" were pointing. His vision with both eyes was 10/20. With each eye separately he read 10/20 right and 10/30 left. I left him for half an hour after I had told him to palm and to be sure not to open his eyes until I said so. When I returned to him, I tested his vision again and he read 10/10 with each eye separately and blinking after seeing each letter, with no sign of a wrinkle or change in his face whatever. His mother purchased a test card and promised to help the boy with his eyes every day at home, before and after school. She was told to bring Fredrick to the Clinic again in a few weeks. On May 3, 1924, I saw him again and he appeared very happy. His mother very proudly told me that his report card showed the highest marks in all his schoolwork. I wondered why Fredrick did not look toward his mother while she was praising him. I did not have to wait very long, however, to find out the reason. She had warned him before they arrived that she would tell me how careless he was with his stockings, and he did not wish me to know. Yes, Fredrick had only one fault. But only one, said his mother. There is not a day passes without his mother discovering holes in the knees of his stockings. Of course, I said this was a terrible crime, but putting glasses on him would have been a worse crime. Fredrick gained a point when his mother smiled on him. The school nurse who had ordered him to get glasses, noticed that Fredrick did not frown any more. He sees the blackboard at any distance now without trouble. My little patient was really cured in one visit.

Two high schoolgirls are also getting good results in the Clinic. Their teacher had trouble with her own eyes and had cured herself with the help of Dr. Bates' book. Later she became a student and took a private course of instruction from Dr. Bates just because she realized what a great help she would be to her pupils in school. She has been successful in benefiting the sight of a great many schoolchildren and feels that it is all worthwhile.

One of the two girls mentioned is named Rita. She suffered with progressive myopia and for two years her sight was steadily getting worse. The whole card seemed gray and blurred to her, the letters were indistinct. After palming for five or ten minutes at a time, her vision always improved. In six months' time she became able to read 12/30 on the test card with both eyes. She also sees the blackboard clearer and better than she has for over two years. When Rita's teacher came with her on her first visit to the Clinic, she was much surprised to see her do so well with the test card for the first time.

The other girl, named Erma, has divergent squint of her left eye. When she first came, which was six months ago, the left eye was turned decidedly to the left. When she covered her right eye, she could not read the test card very well with the left. It was difficult for Erma to keep her head straight as she tried to read the card. After she had palmed both eyes for ten or fifteen minutes, the letters of the card cleared up and now she reads some of the letters on the 10-line, eight feet away from the card. She has become able to keep her head straight when she reads with the squinting eye. Her left eye becomes perfectly straight when she covers her right eye, but it turns out again when reading with both eyes. The squint however is very much better and she is determined to keep on with the treatment until she is cured.

PALMING COMPOSITIONS

By the Pupils of Elisabet D. Hansen
Chicago, Illinois

1. Palming is one of the works that has helped me in room six. While writing a story, it would help me in my imagination. When I first came to room six, arithmetic was very hard for me to learn, but now it is as easy as punk.

2. About a month ago I told my sister Annie to start palming. She has glasses and I would not like her to have them any longer. She has started, and it looks like she will soon have eyes that will not need glasses.

3. Palming and the Snellen test card did me a great deal of good. It gave me more strength in my imagination, and I can do my work much better every day. I am not sorry in knowing how to palm, because in the beginning I did not like to put my hands over my eyes.

4. I told my mother to palm, it would help her, but she did not believe me. One day I said, "Mother, palm." She said, "All right." Finally a week later she could see clearly. She said, "I am glad I did what you told me."

5. Palming is a wonderful treatment for the eyes. It has done much during one and a half years. It has strengthened our imagination, rested our eyes, and kept them from wearing glasses.

6. We have a palming lesson four times a day. While we are palming we have a little music to think of something pleasant. It has cured many headaches from some of us. It is spreading everywhere, and we see lots of people doing it now.

7. Palming is very good for me; it settled my mind. I do not get so excited, and can add my columns easier. I can palm if I get nervous.

REPORT OF THE LEAGUE MEETINGS

By May Secor, Secretar

June Meeting

The June meeting of the Better Eyesight League was held on June 10. Many of the members had requested further practical work, and this was conducted by Dr. Bates, Ms. Hurty and the secretary. The following exercises were practiced: palming, reading the Snellen card, reading fine print, and the long swing.

Ms. Hurty offered the following suggestions for reading fine print: Look at the diamond type without trying to read the print; look at the white lines between the lines of print, and at the white spaces between the letters; move the head from right to left; select, on the Snellen card, a small letter which you can see well; close the eyes; when you remember the small letter perfectly, look at a letter on the small card; see this letter moving just the width of the letter. It is helpful, also, to hold the small diamond type card between the forefinger and thumb of each hand and, while reading it, move the card from left to right, a distance equal to the width of one letter.

Dr. Bates spoke of the difficulty that some persons experience in recalling visual images of familiar persons and objects; Dr. Bates has found the drifting swing helpful in these cases. To practice the drifting swing, imagine that you are lying comfortably on your back in a canoe, floating down a stream; float on, and on, and on. This will facilitate visualizing by inducing relaxation. Dr. Bates described the "period" as a "small, perfectly black area which has no special size or form." One does not imagine the period perfectly unless one imagines it moving. The memory of the period has been found helpful in alleviating or preventing pain and fatigue, physical or mental.

July Meeting

Cecilia Eschbach, a kindergarten teacher of the Brooklyn Orphan Asylum, presented a report of her work with Dr. Bates' method. Ms. Eschbach has relieved many cases of eyestrain, and has corrected two cases of squint. She offered the following suggestions for the daily kindergarten program:

1. Rest periods to be spent palming.
2. Swinging and palming to be combined in a swinging game in which two children join hands and swing (music).

Beneficial for all pupils. In cases of squint have children look at the ceiling while they swing.

3. Game with splints. Keep the "E" or "pothook" eye card hanging in the room. Have children sit at a table 10 or 15 feet from this eye card, and facing it. Request children to make a picture with splints of the fourth line (or any other line) of characters on the card. Train the children to palm whenever they have difficulty in seeing the characters on the card.

4. When "reading" this "E" card the child may indicate which way each "E" points by pointing the open hand in the same direction.

Elisabet D. Hansen, a Chicago teacher, also reported her eye work. She is thoroughly convinced that the Bates Method should be introduced in all schools because of its great educational value.

Dr. Achorn, vice-president of the League, spoke of the advisability of eliminating strain throughout the body, as well as in the eyes, in order to lessen fatigue. Dr. Achorn believes that permitting a reasonable amount of movement throughout the body is comparable to blinking and shifting in order to relieve eyestrain. For this reason he advises an "alert" sitting posture.

THE FAIRY CONVENTION

By George M. Guild

The fairies were holding their annual meeting in a large wood where many of them perched themselves on the branches of the trees and looked down on a large flat portion of ground covered with nice, soft, cool, green grass. The white fairy was unanimously elected to be the leader and chose for her assistant the black fairy and they both sat on a toadstool in the center of the open space where they could be seen by all. The white fairy made a speech of welcome and recommended that the first order of the evening would be a dance by all the fairies, and then they all danced in time with the white fairy. The white fairy swayed from side to side and whirled around on her toes waving her arms in all directions to all the fairies who danced with her and imitated her to the best of their ability. At first she danced slowly and then, as she became warmed up, she danced faster and faster until it made one dizzy to see her whirling around. The black fairy was able to keep up with her most of the time and the other fairies did the best they could, but there were none there who could do the things the white fairy performed. She kicked her feet higher than her head in front and smacked her shoulder blades when she kicked backwards, and every time her foot hit a shoulder blade you could hear the sound all over the place. As the dance proceeded, one by one the fairies fell to the ground completely exhausted, and in time they had all stopped. The applause was considerable, and it was not very long before the other fairies became anxious for fear the white fairy would do herself an injury by her exertions and so they called to her, they pleaded with her to stop and rest, which she finally did.

Then the white fairy called on the others to tell in turn some of the good things that they had done during the year. One told how she visited a sick child who was dying from diphtheria and when nobody was looking she danced on the chest of the sick child which stimulated the little one so much that she smiled. When she smiled she began to breathe better and in a little while, much to the surprise of the doctor, the child recovered.

Similar stories were told by many of the other fairies and then there came calls for the white fairy to tell what she had done. She told the story of a teacher who was very loving and kind and conscientious who had a hard time teaching her class. Most of the children had poor sight. Many of them had poor memories or suffered from headaches and pain and the teacher did not know what to do. One day she took a walk in the woods and rested her tired eyes looking at the green, and almost unconsciously called out, "Nobody helps me; I wonder if the fairies would help me?"

The little white fairy heard and appeared before her, dancing and moving around until the teacher, tired out, laid down and went to sleep; and all through her sleep the white fairy talked to her and told her what to do, and these are some of the things she told her to do:

"When your children are tired, common sense will suggest that they ought to rest. When they stare at the blackboard, the harder they stare, the more they strain, and the less they see. Every teacher knows that or should know it. Do not have them stare; let them look from one place to another, and keep moving."

And so the next day the teacher had the children close their eyes and cover them with the palms of their hands so as to rest them, and when she tested their sight she found that it was benefited. When the children complained of pain and headaches she would have them close their eyes and palm four times a day. Every day the children would cover their eyes with the palms of their hands for five minutes or longer while the Victrola played some popular music. The benefit was great because all the children obtained normal sight and became able to study their lessons without fatigue, headache or pain. They enjoyed going to school. When the other teachers saw the benefits of this kind of treatment they practiced it and they also got good results.

Then the white fairy appealed to the other fairies and beseeched them to help the eyes and the nerves and the minds of the little children in the public schools and in other schools. All the fairies applauded the white fairy for a long, long time, and she bowed her head, and the black fairy would bow her head and all the other fairies bowed their heads, and every time they bowed their heads down, the trees and the things they were not looking at seemed to go up. When they raised their heads upwards, the trees and everything moved down. It was such a pleasant sensation to see those trees moving up and down that they kept it up for a long, long time, and I guess some of them are doing it yet. They found that when they looked to the right, the trees seemed to move to the left. And when they looked to the left, the trees seemed to move to the right. This was also a very pleasant feeling. They kept this up also for some time. They became very happy and very enthusiastic and had a beautiful time.

THE EYE CLASS IN ERASMUS HALL

By George J. Weiss, Pupil

Aiding my fellow pupils in the eye class at Erasmus Hall High School has proved very interesting to me. There is no end to the little demonstrations that are in themselves proofs of Dr. Bates' method.

In one case, a boy who could only read at ten feet the line that is normally read at forty feet, was surprised to find that he was able to read the 10-line at ten feet. This came about in an unusual manner. The boy, whose name is Fred, was doing some chart work with me when I noticed him bending slightly forward and trying to see the letters. I knew that it would be useless for him to continue in such fashion, so I had him close his eyes after reading each letter. This eased him a great deal and he was able to read more than he expected. Fred became anxious again and tried to see all the letters on the bottom line without closing his eyes. I knew to let him go on that way would do him more injury than good. He gradually relaxed while I talked to him, and when he accidentally turned to the chart he saw all the letters on the 10-line at ten feet. This was a great revelation to him, for he not only proved the statement with his own eyes, but it taught him to stop trying to see.

Nearly everyone who comes to us has some fault which is the cause of his poor sight. This fault is sometimes discovered the first week, and usually no progress is made until the fault is found and corrected, as in the case of Fred. Many of our pupils stare, and as faults are mostly habit, so is staring.

It sometimes happens that they do not realize they are staring, and when they come to the next lesson they wonder why they have made no progress. This fault is always corrected by practicing the exercises regularly and conscientiously. We have found that the pupils who do so are always the quickest to be restored to normal sight.

REMINDERS FOR SUMMER EYE PRACTICE

By Kathleen E. Hurty

Ms. Hurty distributed these instructions to her patients for use during the summer. These are the fundamentals of Dr. Bates' method and are important to bear in mind at all seasons.

Palming. Do this at least three times a day for not less than five minutes each time. Always palm a few minutes just before going to sleep. In palming, best results are obtained when the whole body is comfortable and relaxed. While palming, let the imagination play with pleasant scenes and let your mind drift laxly.

Long Swing. Practice this as often as possible. Keep an easy, lazy, rhythmical motion. Things should appear to move in the opposite direction.

Snellen Test Card. Practice with the card at least twice daily, using the fine print, your memory of a letter, a short swing, blinking, etc., to help you see the letters on the card.

Sunning. Let the sun shine on your closed eyelids for short intervals. Choose preferably the early morning sunlight. It is the light rays which benefit the eyes rather than the heat rays. The sun loses some of its effect when it comes through glass.

Blinking. Normal eyes blink constantly. If you have unconsciously formed the habit of staring, practice frequent blinking in order to overcome this tendency. Practice it often.

General Directions. See things moving all day long. Never make an effort to focus. Let things come to you. Do not make a task of your eyes exercises. Make a game out of improving your vision. If you get a chance, teach someone else. It will help you. Never let a feeling of strain continue; stop and practice one of the methods of relaxation. Let me hear from you at least once during the summer.

Better Eyesight
September 1924—Vol. IX, No. 3

PERMANENT IMPROVEMENT

Many patients find that while it is easy for them to obtain a temporary improvement in their sight by palming a sufficient length of time or by other methods, they do not seem to hold it permanently. In this connection it is well to remember that the normal eye with normal sight can only maintain normal sight permanently by consciously or unconsciously practicing the slow, short, easy swing. When the normal eye has imperfect sight it can always be demonstrated that the swing stops from an effort. When the normal eye has normal sight, the eyes are at rest and all the nerves of the body feel comfortable. When the swing stops, one always feels more or less uncomfortable. To have perfect sight can only be obtained easily, without effort. To have imperfect sight always requires a strain or an effort which stops the swing. Nearsighted patients who have normal vision for reading at the near point become able, when their attention is called to it, to demonstrate that they are more comfortable when reading the fine print than they are when they fail to see distant objects perfectly.

One of the great benefits of the drifting swing is the comfortable, relaxed feeling it brings. The retinoscope always shows that the eye is not nearsighted when no effort is made. Persons with imperfect sight should imitate the eye with normal sight by practicing a perfect memory, a perfect imagination, a perfect swing, without effort, with perfect comfort all the time that they are awake. As I have said before many times, it is a good thing to know what is the matter with you because it makes it possible to correct.

QUICK CURES

By W. H. Bates, M.D.

Children are more easily cured of imperfect sight than are adults.

Children twelve years old or younger who have never worn glasses, who can read 20/100 or better, may obtain normal sight in two weeks or less by reading the Snellen test card four times a day after palming and practicing the swing for five minutes or longer. To obtain a permanent cure it is necessary that such children should devote at least five minutes a day to palming, swinging and reading the Snellen test card as long as they attend school. There is a great difference in the minds of children. Some have good memories and can maintain mental pictures perfectly for long periods of time. Many of these cases have been cured temporarily in one visit by palming for an hour or longer while remembering mental pictures perfectly.

Those children who were unable to remember or imagine mental pictures were not so readily cured, yet many of them were taught how to remember mental pictures at the first visit and, with the help of palming and swinging a sufficient length of time, they also obtained normal vision at the first visit.

A small child who plays baseball frequently becomes able to see, remember or imagine mental pictures connected with a game of baseball, and the better he remembers the ballgame the better becomes his vision.

Squint, which is more or less prevalent in young children, is oftentimes relieved promptly by playing games which require running. If the children enjoy the game, the strain of the eyes will be relieved and they will become straight temporarily. By repetition, the squint will become permanently corrected. The use of glasses in such cases should be condemned because they interfere with the cure without glasses.

People who have imperfect sight and do not wear glasses soon learn to find their way about the streets without much trouble. School teachers have been surprised to find how well they could get along in school without their glasses. A quick cure cannot be accomplished unless the patient stops wearing glasses. Some people who have worn them for thirty or forty years or longer have been cured in one visit. The patients who have been cured quickly make a lot of trouble for the doctor, because their friends who may apply for treatment expect as quick a cure. When such a thing is not possible their disappointment is very decided and their conversation may be very disagreeable.

Quick cures of patients over forty years old who have lost their ability to read the newspaper or any printed matter at the near point occur from time to time. One day five patients over fifty years old, who were unable to read at the near point without glasses, obtained normal vision temporarily in one visit. Each one demonstrated that the memory of imperfect sight required an effort; that it was difficult, tedious or fatiguing, and that imperfect sight could not be remembered or imagined continuously for any great length of time. They demonstrated that when they stared at one part of a large letter of the Snellen test card at twenty feet, after a few seconds an effort was required and the vision very soon became imperfect. When they looked at the diamond type at ten inches from their eyes they had the same feeling of strain and effort when they failed to distinguish the letters. They were able to demonstrate that when they stared, tried to concentrate, or tried to imagine the small letters were stationary, their vision became worse. When they rested their eyes and imagined things were moving, their memory, imagination and vision improved. Some of them soon became able to imagine that the white spaces between the lines were whiter than the margin or the rest of the card. By closing their eyes they felt a measure of relief and rest, and by keeping them closed or by palming for five minutes or longer, they became able to imagine the white spaces much whiter, the letters much blacker, and to imagine the card with a slow, short, easy swing of less than a quarter of an inch.

Some years ago, a remarkable patient came to see me. The first thing she said was that she had to catch a train which left in a few hours. She apologized by saying that she would have called to see me before, but she had only just heard of me from a lady that she recently met at a luncheon. Her eyes, she said, were a great trouble to her and all the glasses she had worn had not been satisfactory.

I asked her if she wanted to be cured quickly. She answered, "If you please." Then I said to her, "You can be cured quickly if you do just exactly what I say." She replied very solemnly, "I promise to do whatever you say." I handed her a small card on which was printed some lines of diamond type. I asked her what she could see. She said, "I see a gray card with a lot of blurred gray letters. They all seem to look alike and there are no spaces between the words or the letters and not always between the lines."

I said to her, "With your eyes closed, can you remember such a thing as a sunset, a red sun and different colored clouds?" She said, "Yes." Then I said, "With your eyes still closed, can you remember or imagine a white cloud in the sky, dazzling white with sun shining on it?" She answered, "Yes."

Then I gave her the following directions, "Close your eyes, keeping them closed until you can remember a white cloud in the sky, dazzling white with the sun shining on it, then open your eyes and glance at the fine print, still remembering your white cloud, but be sure and close your eyes before you have time to read any of the letters." I watched her do this for a few minutes and saw that she was following my directions properly, then I left her to practice by herself. After about half an hour I returned and asked her how she was getting along. Her face was a little bit flushed and in an apologetic tone she said, "I tried to do just exactly what you told me to do, Doctor, and I am sorry to say that although I only looked at the card for a second at a time, in flashes, contrary to your instructions, I read every word on the card." Then I explained to her that of course at the first visit she was not expected to do what I asked her to do exactly, but, under the circumstances, I thought that she had done very well indeed. I gave her some other fine print to practice with in the same way, but told her to hold it not more than six inches from her eyes. With her eyes closed she remembered the white cloud as before, keeping her eyes closed until her memory of the white cloud was perfect, and then she flashed the white spaces between the lines for a second.

I watched her for a while, and I said, "What is the trouble?" "Nothing," she said. "I close my eyes and remember the white cloud. I also remember it very well with my eyes open. When I do I cannot help seeing the white spaces perfectly white and the black letters perfectly black, but I am sorry to say that I cannot avoid reading the letters." Then I held out my hand to her and said, "Shake hands. I am very well pleased with you and this time I will forgive you for not avoiding reading the letters." She then departed for her train.

I tried the same method on a great many other patients, but very seldom did I find one who succeeded as well as she.

STORIES FROM THE CLINIC
No. 55: A Hospital Patient
By Emily C. Lierman

During the hot summer days while we were still treating patients at the Harlem Hospital Clinic, a little girl named Estelle, about eight years old, was brought in and placed in the children's ward of the hospital. She met with an accident which destroyed the sight of her left eye. Not being a Clinic case, another doctor took charge of her.

One day this doctor came to our room and asked Dr. Bates when he expected to take a vacation. Dr. Bates answered, "I take a vacation every day. Why do you ask?" The other doctor answered, "I am serious, Dr. Bates. When do you go away for a rest?" Dr. Bates replied, "When I am treating my patients, it rests me; so I don't have to go away. Is there anything I can do for you?" "Yes," said he. "There is a little girl in the children's ward upstairs and while I am away I would like to have you take care of her case. When I return I shall remove the injured eye, for it is in bad shape and the sight is completely destroyed."

Dr. Bates agreed to care for the little girl and asked me to help him. We called on Estelle soon after and the nurse in charge of the ward led the way to the tiny cot in a far corner of the room. The nurse stopped beside Estelle's cot, and the poor child looked very much frightened as the Doctor and I came along. We could only see part of her face as she lay there, because the whole left side was covered with a bandage. Before Dr. Bates could say a word to her, she began to cry and beg the new Doctor to please not hurt her like the other doctor did. The nurse began to remonstrate with her, but the Doctor soon quieted her when he promised in his gentle way that he would not hurt her one single bit. The Doctor very carefully directed the child to remove the adhesive plaster herself, and in this way the bandage was removed without discomfort or pain.

Estelle told us how she had been playing on the sidewalk near her home when she slipped and fell against the curbstone. A piece of a broken glass bottle lay in her path and it penetrated through her upper closed eyelid and cut the eye so badly that the sight was destroyed completely. Dr. Bates treated the eye later so that it did not have to be removed. Even though she could only see out of one eye, anyone observing her could not have guessed that the sight was destroyed in the left eye. Both Estelle and her mother were very grateful to us, and at every visit Estelle would fill the Doctor's pockets with fruit and candy which she was only too glad to share with the big Doctor who did not hurt her.

A PERSONAL EXPERIENCE

By Henrietta C. Clinton

For more than twenty years I had suffered from what the doctors call migraine headaches, with the usual digestive disturbances, which greatly interfered with my general health, both from their frequency and the medical remedies supposed to be necessary in such cases. I fortunately refused to wear glasses except for about three years of that time. At forty-six my vision was very bad for the near point and I had double vision in each eye. My headache became almost continuous, and I was very thin and nervously wrought up all the time.

One of the leading ophthalmologists of San Francisco told me that double vision meant incipient cataract. I walked the streets trying to realize blindness, because his opinion was that I should wear terrible lenses and wait until the cataract developed and got hard enough to be cut out.

Fortunately I did not give up my attempts to read. One day at the library I came across the article in an old *Scientific American* of January 12, 1918, about Dr. W. H. Bates' discoveries in regard to curing the sight without glasses. I immediately wrote to the Doctor, but it was some time afterwards before I understood anything about how to apply the principles toward a cure.

I am now fifty-one years old and my sight is almost perfect. I can read the photographic reductions readily and I can stand in the window of my office on the ninth floor of an office building downtown and read the numbers on the automobiles as they pass in the streets. The stenographer, who is in her early twenties, vies with me in seeing the most difficult things she can think of, and sometimes she beats me and sometimes the reverse.

I do not yet consider my sight perfect, because I can only see the 10-line on the test card at fifteen feet. My ambition is to see it at twenty or even thirty feet, and I have a great ambition to see Venus as a crescent.

Shortly after I purchased Dr. Bates' book, *Perfect Sight Without Glasses,* in which he says that some people see the rings of Saturn and the moons of Jupiter without glasses, I saw an article in the *Scientific American* in which the writer told of a tablet dug up in Asia Minor in which a priest made a prophecy. It said that "When the north horn of Venus was over a certain star certain things would happen, and that other things would happen when the south horn of Venus was over another star, showing," the article said, "that the Babylonians knew Venus to be a crescent," and added, "that the ancients must have had lenses, because it was not thought possible that the human eyesight could be ever acute enough to see Venus as a crescent."

That interested me greatly. At that time I had great difficulty in seeing newspaper print. I would squint and make my head swim with pain in order to read without glasses. I hated them, and I made up my mind that I should someday see Venus as a crescent.

The first thing I tried to do was palming. It was impossible because I tried to see the inner field black, and the more I tried to see it so, the more the lights would come. I tried to read the photographic reduction. It was impossible, because I would squint and strain. I got worse daily. I tried central fixation. I could not do it, because every time I looked at a thing I would outstare it until my eyes seemed to pop nearly out of my head.

I could not seem to know how to relax until I conceived the idea of using my imagination. The first time it occurred to me to use my imagination I was at the table and imagined that black ants were crawling over the tablecloth. To my delight I instantly saw the threads of the tablecloth. In two weeks I learned to relax enough to read newspaper print easily. I remembered that when I was a child and shut my eyes, they were shut, not merely the lids, but the whole paraphernalia of sight was shut. When one "sees lights" one does not shut the centers of sight. I kept imagining that I was a child sleeping in my little crib and that the black night was all around me. The first time complete blackness was all over the inner field it startled me so much that the lights came on worse than ever. I had begun again to regard the lights with my centers of sight and forgot to relax. But persistence gave me the power to disregard those bothersome lights.

The memory of a period escaped me until I imagined a spot of black molasses on the tablecloth. It was very black and some black ants ran all around the black fluid. I got so that I could disperse those ants and leave the very small spot of blackness moving slightly back and forth on the whitest surfaces. My period! Palming and going through that scene over and over again gave me such relaxation that I would open my eyes and read a line or two of the photographic reduction before the glaze of staring would come back. I do not know at what stage I lost the double vision. The headaches went while I was trying to see fine print, even staring and squinting at it before I learned to relax.

Another mental image I found relaxing was that of a black velvet cloak I once owned. I thought it had a rip and I had to take several spools of black silk and match the blackness of the cloak. One spool of silk would not be black enough, then I'd take another and another until I could get a spool as black as I could possibly conceive blackness.

I was also benefited by remembering some word of photographic reduction and have the letters rapidly change places with each other and spell different things. I find that in reading the test card at a distance, I can see them more distinctly if I imagine a black wand slowly pointing out the letters to me. I think it is the unconscious swinging that I do of the letters as the imaginary wand approaches the letters that helps me to see them more clearly and more centrally.

One thing that may interest other fifty-one-year-olds is that almost all the wrinkles which had been around my eyes have disappeared, and people meet me and tell me that I look ten years younger than I did ten years ago!

THE FAIRY SCHOOL

By George M. Guild

It was very hot. The school windows were wide open, but not a breath of air was stirring and the teacher and pupils were very uncomfortable from the heat. Freddie was only eight years old and he could not be blamed when his mind wandered from his work. In spite of all that he could do his head would nod, his eyes would close and he would drop off to sleep. Then he heard the White Fairy talking to the children while she sat on the teacher's desk, waving her hands and dancing around to the amusement of the children. Her eyes were so bright and full of sympathy, kindness and love that not one of the boys or girls could keep their eyes from her face.

She said, "Now watch me as I swing from side to side. Please, all of you stand up, with your feet slightly apart, facing me, and move your whole body, your head and your eyes from side to side while I am moving. Now sit down, close your eyes and cover them with the palms of your hands, resting your elbows on your desk. While you are doing this remember me standing up, smiling at you and loving you with all my heart." In five minutes she said, "Now open your eyes and watch me while I dance."

Freddie noticed how much more distinctly he could now see the face of the White Fairy. Then all of a sudden the White Fairy stopped dancing. At first the smiling eyes were very clear, but in a few seconds or so they began to blur and fade away. It was not long before he was unable to see her face or her tiny feet; they had become just a blur. He felt uncomfortable, and he must have looked uncomfortable because the White Fairy called out, "Freddie, swing your head from side to side." Freddie was only too glad to swing from side to side, and it was not long before he became able to see her tiny feet, her eyes and face just as clearly as before.

Then the White Fairy said, "Now, Freddie, close your eyes and remember me as well as you can. If you love me you will remember me." And Freddie closed his eyes, and I am quite sure that he remembered the face of the White Fairy, because he loved her so much.

After he had kept his eyes closed for a few minutes the White Fairy called out, "Open your eyes and tell me what you see. And when Freddie opened his eyes the schoolroom was gone. It seemed as though he was in the woods; it seemed as though he was a fairy and that all the other children were fairies, and he enjoyed being a fairy because when he imitated the look of love on the face of the White Fairy he thought of his mother and his father, his brothers and his sisters and other people that he could remember. He seemed to love all of them a great deal more than he had ever loved anybody in his life. The White Fairy invited him to dance with her. It was very strange to Freddie that he could dance for a long time without getting tired, and the more he danced the better did he feel.

Then the White Fairy told him to stop dancing, and while sitting on the grass she walked around him, touching his head with the tips of her fingers until he fell asleep. When he woke up, the teacher was petting his head and loving him. At once he called out, "Oh, teacher, the White Fairy taught me to dance, how to see, and now I feel just like studying."

When the teacher heard him say this she said, "Freddie, I am curious. Show me what the White Fairy helped you to do." And so, before the whole school Freddie showed how the White Fairy taught him to swing, shift and palm, and how she showed him how staring and straining made his sight worse, and that by moving his head and eyes from side to side his sight got better. Right away the children all did it, and after they had practiced with Freddie for a short time they were all very happy and told the teacher that they also felt a great deal better and, like Freddie, they wanted to get to work because they felt just like studying.

BETTER EYESIGHT LEAGUE

The vacation season is in full swing now and the August attendance at the *Better Eyesight* meeting was small. Owing to the small gathering, Dr. Bates informally opened the meeting and gave a lecture which lasted about an hour and a half. During this time he demonstrated the various swings and explained their value.

One visitor remarked that she is a high school teacher and interested in the results obtained in schools. She wished to help her children, but when practicing the method she failed to see things move. She emphatically said that when she looked at a chair it stood still, and no feat of her imagination could make it move.

She was a very difficult subject, inasmuch as she stared at everything instead of taking things easy and relaxing. Dr. Bates explained the principle of the swing, admitting that it was imaginary, but no more so than the moving of the telephone poles when one is riding in a train. The other members present benefited by her errors, because they were being shown the wrong way to do things and the correct method of improving the sight by the use of the swing.

Before the visitor left she saw the chairs moving by looking first over one shoulder and then over the other, glancing at the chairs as she swayed but not staring at them.

The most important fundamental principle to keep in mind is that defective vision is caused by strain and cured by relaxation. One of the greatest causes of strain, and the beginning of many unpleasant symptoms, is staring. [My emphasis.—TRQ] This is due to an unconscious effort to concentrate and to put the utmost energy into every act or movement.

The subject of seasickness was then discussed. Dr. Bates said this also is caused by strain. People who relax and allow their bodies to sway with the movement of the boat never become sick. A sailor's walk is spoken of as a "rolling gait." If he were to stand stiff, stare at the waves, and strain to resist the movement of the ship, he would never become a sailor.

CHIEF FOUR-EYES

By Emily A. Meder

A lady called at the office and introduced herself. She was one of our regular correspondents and I remembered her name because she had such a great deal of trouble with her thirteen-year-old son, Dick. She explained in her last letter that he is a normal, active boy who finds more enjoyment in playing baseball and leapfrog than doing his homework. As Dick wouldn't wear glasses she decided to see what Dr. Bates' method accomplished.

There is a vacant lot near her home, used by a band of "wild Indians," with her son as "Chief." The band, however, objected to a leader with glasses, and Dick became quite ingenious in inventing ways to wear them and still not wear them. She said she watched him continually. He walked innocently past her with the glasses gracefully perched on his nose, but in some mysterious way they disappeared before he reached the sidewalk. This became a nervous game of hide-and-seek between them. He said he would not be called "sissy," and she was equally sure that he would have to wear glasses in order to be cured.

About this time, news of Dr. Bates' work reached the mother's ears and she wrote to us for information. She bought the book and told Dick that if he did as she instructed he could leave his glasses off for two weeks. At the end of that time she found that he could not only go without his glasses but his sight had improved.

Dick enjoyed the palming, much to her surprise, and he did not have to be told to do it when his eyes felt strained. He is proud of his test card and his "Indians" try to outdo each other in reading it at the farthest distance. It has become a modern Indian rite.

"The best of it," Ms. Jamison said, "is that I can look at my boy now without suspicion, and he lost the hated nickname of 'Chief Four-Eyes'."

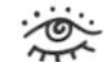

QUESTIONS AND ANSWERS

Q–1. Is there any power in the lens of dark sunglasses? Are they harmful?

A–1. Yes. Dark glasses are very injurious to the eyes.

Q–2. I improved temporarily by your method, but I am at a standstill now. What is the next step?

A–2. Practice the swinging.

Q–3. I enjoy palming, but it makes me drowsy after ten or fifteen minutes. Is this helpful?

A–3. When palming is done properly it does not make you drowsy.

Q–4. Is a case of detached retina likely to respond to treatment?

A–4. To cure detachment of the retina requires, in some cases, a year or longer.

Q–5. Could a little girl cure a cataract on her eye by blinking and swinging?

A–5. Yes, but the patient should practice many hours daily and it should be kept up for many months under the supervision of someone with perfect sight without glasses.

Better Eyesight
October 1924—Vol. IX, No. 4

THE RABBIT'S THROAT

During the past ten years, a method of breathing has been practiced which has improved the vision of many patients after other methods had failed. It consists of depressing the lower jaw with the lips closed and lowering the tongue and muscles below the chin. At the same time one breathes in through the nose and throat in a manner somewhat similar to snoring, and when done properly one can feel a coolness of the air while it passes down into the lungs. This method of breathing is accompanied with the eyelids being more widely open in a natural way without staring. The ear passages, nose, and throat dilate. The tube which goes from the throat to the middle ear becomes more widely open, with improved hearing in chronic deafness which does not respond to any other treatment. If one rests the chin with the thumb below it and the forefinger just below the lower lip, one can feel with the thumb the hardening of the muscles below the jaw accompanied with a decided swelling. By practice, the swelling and hardness increase. This suggested the title of the Rabbit's Throat because of a similar swelling below the rabbit's chin. The tension of the other muscles of the body becomes relaxed. There is a wonderful increase of muscular control.

Music teachers have told me that the singing voice becomes much better because of the relaxation of the muscles of the throat. The involuntary muscles of the digestive tract become relaxed in a striking manner with the relief of many symptoms of discomfort. Redness and inflammation of the mucous membranes of the eye, ear, nose and throat and the rest of the body are relieved in a few minutes with the aid of the Rabbit's Throat.

IMAGINATION CURES

By W. H. Bates, M.D.

The normal eye when it has normal sight imagines it sees many illusions. When the normal eye sees one small letter of the Snellen test card on the bottom line, it can be demonstrated that a swing from side to side can be imagined. If the letter does not appear to swing or if the swing is stopped, consciously or unconsciously, the vision becomes imperfect.

The white spaces between the lines of letters are always seen whiter than they really are. This is of course an illusion that the normal eye is able to imagine.

With normal vision the form of each letter is imagined correctly. For example: if the letter "O" is a perfect circle and is imagined to be an oval with the long axis vertical or horizontal, the imagination of the "O" will not be as perfect as when the "O" is imagined to be a circle. When a word is regarded, the letters are sometimes apparently transposed, and when this illusion is imagined, the vision is always imperfect.

Size: If a letter is imagined much larger than it really is, it can be demonstrated that the vision is imperfect; if the letter is imagined smaller than it really is, the vision is also lowered.

Normal vision can only be demonstrated when one sees a part of a letter best, the other parts of the letter being blurred.

The eye with imperfect sight has also an imperfect memory of a letter, its form, size or location. The white background or the spaces between the lines are less white than the margin of the card.

The stare can always be demonstrated.

The swing is also modified, being either too short, too long, too rapid, too slow, irregular and not continuous. These facts have suggested methods of treatment which have been very successful.

The best distance to practice with the Snellen test card varies widely. If no improvement is manifest in a few minutes, it is well to try practicing the vision of a letter on one card at a near point where the vision is good and to flash the more distant card alternately. [See also "Distance of the Snellen Test Card" in the April 1924 issue.—TRQ]

One patient, a girl age 18, had myopia of concave 4.00 D. S. Practicing without her glasses at fifteen feet did not improve her sight. The card was brought closer, to six feet, where her vision was 6/70. She held another card in her hand and practiced looking at the first letter of the 10-line, a letter "F," at one foot where she could see it quite perfectly with a slow, short, easy swing, and at the same time imagine her body was swinging with the "F." This she became able to do by moving her head and eyes. Later she imagined the swing of the "F" without having to move her head. She alternately regarded the "F" at the near point and imagined her body was swinging with the "F" and then flashed the first letter of each line of the Snellen test card at six feet without modifying or stopping the swing of her body. Her vision rapidly improved so that she became able to read the 10-line at six feet. The card was then placed at fifteen feet and by practicing in the same way she became able to read all the letters without stopping the body swing. She then practiced with cards that she had never seen before and was able to read the bottom line as quickly on the strange card as she could on a familiar one. When she looked at the large letters at first she unconsciously made an effort, stopped her swing, and failed to read them. By looking between the lines of letters and planning to test her swing without testing her sight, she was able to maintain the swing of the letter "F," or the swing of her body swinging with the letter "F," which improved her vision decidedly. She had more trouble in reading the larger letters than she had in reading the small letters on the bottom line.

A very interesting case called recently, a woman age 61. She complained that the doctors had repeatedly urged her to wear glasses for reading but none of the glasses gave her any benefit. When she looked at the Snellen test card at twenty feet she could read the bottom line without any trouble; and it seemed to her that the letters were always moving and that this was something wrong with her eyes. It took me about half an hour to prove that the movement of the letters was necessary and that when she tried to stop the movement, her vision always became worse. In her business she had to read very fine print most of the time. I tested her with fine print and found that she could read it perfectly as close as six inches and as far off as she could hold it.

Then I asked her, "How do your eyes trouble you?"

"They don't trouble me at all when I forget about them, but when I notice what happens when I am reading it troubles me a great deal. I found that even a small letter regarded is moving. If I try to stop it from moving it disappears and my eyes feel uncomfortable. I can usually read page after page without any trouble, but if I try to increase my speed by reading a whole sentence at a time, it causes me a great deal of discomfort."

Again it required some time to have her demonstrate that when she read with perfect comfort she read without any effort; as soon as she made an effort to see, she lowered her vision and produced headache or pain in her eyes. In various ways I emphasized the fact that when she had normal vision it came without any effort to see, but to see imperfectly required an effort and the greater the effort she made the less did she see and the more uncomfortable did she feel. I told her repeatedly that she had perfect eyes. There was no disease of the retina, there was no disease of her optic nerves and she had no sign of a cataract. The doctors also complained that her sight was too good and that she must be under a terrible strain to see so well; and, when she replied that she did not have any discomfort when her sight was normal she got into an argument which was more disagreeable than beneficial.

I think I helped this patient a great deal by just telling her the facts, that she had normal eyes and that she knew how to use them. It is interesting to know how many cases with normal vision use their eyes wrong and suffer from pain, fatigue, imperfect sight or other eye discomforts.

The imagination is a very important factor in vision. One can, by imagining a letter imperfectly, increase the hardness of the eyeball immediately, which is an important symptom of glaucoma. Conversely, the imagination of a letter seen perfectly softens the eyeball in glaucoma with great benefit to the pain and imperfect sight of this disease.

Imagination of imperfect sight has produced cloudiness of the lens or increased the opacity of the lens in cataract. In myopia the eyeball is elongated. The imagination of perfect sight is accompanied immediately by a shortening of the globe to normal and the patient obtains, temporarily at least, improved or perfect sight. One can produce myopia by the imagination of imperfect sight. In hypermetropia the eyeball is shortened. The imagination of perfect sight is followed by the lengthening of the eyeball to normal, and the patient may have normal vision temporarily. The imagination of imperfect sight for near always lessens the length of the eyeball, and produces or increases hypermetropia. All forms of astigmatism can be produced or increased by the imagination of imperfect sight. They are all cured temporarily or permanently by the imagination of perfect sight.

Wonderful cures have been accomplished, after all other methods had failed, of many eye diseases by the proper use of the imagination.

STORIES FROM THE CLINIC

No. 56: Schoolchildren

By Emily C. Lierman

Public schoolchildren come to the Clinic in great numbers throughout the whole year and are eager to be cured without glasses. Not always does the child have a guardian or mother near to encourage him while he is waiting to be treated. Sometimes they come alone, and sometimes with three or four other children.

At the office, the Doctor sees the patient for a half-hour or more, but those at the Clinic can have only five minutes or a little longer, as the time is short on Clinic days. Schoolchildren are cured quickly, however, whether it be at the office or at the Clinic. When they discover that they can be cured without glasses, we have very little trouble in treating them. They are always eager to discard their glasses, with a few exceptions, of course. Some children feel dressed up in them, because their parents wear attractive ones with gold or tortoise-shell rims. Occasionally these people come to have their glasses readjusted and the Doctor finds that these are often practically windowpane glass, without any strength whatever.

A little girl named Betty, age 13, usually found a convenient corner of our room where she could see each patient having their eyes treated. She had no trouble with her eyes, but always came with her school chum who was under treatment. She listened attentively as I encouraged the patients but never was troublesome nor asked any questions at any time. Somehow she obtained a Snellen test card and helped some of her playmates recover their vision. She brought several of them to me to be sure that they could get along without their glasses. One of them was a boy twelve years old named John, who had worn glasses for five years and was very nearsighted. At the age of seven, the school doctor ordered glasses for him. Dr. Bates examined them and discovered that the boy was wearing farsighted glasses for myopia, or nearsightedness. When they were changed one year before, the optician who sold them had made a terrible error. No wonder Johnnie was willing to have Betty help him. She told me that he could only see the 50-line of the card ten feet away without his glasses. When I tested Johnnie he placed himself fifteen feet away from the card and read every line of letters without a mistake. Then he told me how Betty spent an hour with him almost every day for three weeks until he became able to read the card at any distance Betty desired him to read it. I'm sorry she stopped coming to the Clinic. Her parents moved away and I lost a very good assistant.

Then a mother came to the Clinic with her two little girls. Marjorie, the oldest, had been to us some years previously and was cured. The youngest child was sent home by the school nurse and was told to see a doctor about her eyes. Dr. Bates told the mother to wait for me and when I was ready, I would test the children's eyes. The mother kept looking at me, smiling all the while. She asked, "Don't you remember me? Don't you remember my little girl? I brought her to you and Dr. Bates six years ago. She had alternate squint when she was three years old and Dr. Bates cured her without an operation." Marjorie's both eyes were as straight as mine, but everyone in the Clinic who would listen to the mother that day, heard how we had cured her child of crossed eyes.

Her sister Katherine, age 7, stood by, wondering what we were going to do with her. Both girls were dressed with the greatest of care and Katherine looked very much like a big French doll with her head just covered with curls. Dr. Bates examined her and said she had myopia but was not a bad case. I placed her ten feet from the test card and she read every letter correctly down to the 40-line. As I walked over to where the card was placed to assist my little patient, the mother got ahead of me, and in a soft tone of voice encouraged Katherine to palm and remember the last letter of the 40-line of the card. Katherine did so, but she had only covered her eyes for a minute when she removed her hands and opened her eyes to read again. I wanted to tell the child that she had not palmed long enough, but before I could say a word, she began to read the next line of letters as her mother pointed to each one. After each letter was read, her mother very gently told her to blink and that would help her to see the next letter without a strain.

The mother did not stop when Katherine finished reading all of the 30-line without a mistake, but kept right on to the next line, pointing to one letter and then another until she read all of the 20-line.

Then the mother advised Katherine to swing her body from side to side and to notice that everything in the room seemed to move in the opposite direction. While her mother was advising her what to do, the child did the best she could to read the card. The mother smiled when she saw how amazed I was to see her improve Katherine's eyes without my help. I asked, "Where did you learn how to do it?" She answered, "From reading your articles in the *Better Eyesight* magazine. I have been a subscriber for a number of years."

Some months later the mother called with Katherine to learn if she was cured. Her vision was 10/10 in each eye. It is interesting to report that the child was cured entirely by her mother.

THE METHOD IN ENGLAND

Editor's Note—*We have been extremely encouraged by the reports sent in from time to time by our English correspondents. No one is professionally using Dr. Bates' method in England, yet the results obtained by book patients have justified the opening of a Better Eyesight Clinic.*

Ms. Taylor's interesting letter to Dr. Bates explains the origin of the Clinic. Her firsthand information from Headquarters there is typical of the various reports sent to us.

Dear Dr. Bates:

I am so glad I got those addresses from you before I left New York. I have had the most interesting time and want to tell you about it as I am sure you and Ms. Lierman will be interested.

I found Captain Price was out of town for several weeks, but I saw his friend, Major Galloway, who is on the Council of the Better Eyesight League over here. I introduced myself as a former patient and friend of yours and Ms. Lierman's and he was just as nice as he could be, and told me all about the work they are trying to do. He said I must see K. Beswick who is Captain Price's assistant, and was the one who got him interested in the beginning. I invited Ms. Beswick to tea and she told me how everything began. It seems her mother had been blind from glaucoma for 8 years and they had tried everything including operations, without success. All she had was perception of light. Someone suggested they try osteopathy for her general health, so she took her to a well-known American here. He gave her treatment of course, but also told her about the wonderful discoveries of an American, Dr. Bates, and said he had bought your book and before he had had time to read it a patient noticed it and borrowed it. The patient had bad myopia but cured it in three weeks with the book. Ms. Beswick bought the book, went to see the woman who had cured herself, and then began on her mother. That was six months ago. I met the mother a few days ago. She took up a magazine and read the big print for me, very slowly of course. Then she told me I had on a brown dress and was dark myself. As you know my skin is dark to begin with and now I am almost black from sunburn. Then I walked down the street with her. She avoided the people all right. She could see the curb to step up but not to step down, which was exactly my trouble when I first took off my glasses. Once we came to a place where the pavement changed from dark to light and she thought it was a step down, which is natural enough.

When Ms. Beswick saw her mother's improvement she told her friend Captain Price about it. He tried it and immediately saw the wonders of it, so both of them began to practice on all their friends. When they felt more confident they opened a Clinic with three patients. That was last April and now they have forty. Captain Price is going to send you a report on the Clinic cases in a few months. They have had some wonderful successes. I asked Ms. Beswick how it was possible they could know how to treat patients with no more to go on than your book and a few letters from you.

She said the explanation, of course, was that it was the truth that you had discovered and it worked.

I will tell you a few of the cases to give you an idea of what they have done in this short time.

Some of the quick temporary cures were:

Man, myopic, has worn glasses long time. Sight very blurred 10/200. In twenty minutes read 10/40 with ease. When he went home his family persuaded him he had been hypnotized, so he has never returned.

Boy, 6 years old, bad squint in one eye, vision faint 10/200, other eye normal. In less than an hour read 10/10 with bad eye on strange card. The squint was cured temporarily for a few seconds at a time. Has had only that visit but will return after the holidays.

Ms. Beswick said Ms. Clutterbuck was the only person she had met who knew you, so she asked all about you and your work. She wanted to know if Ms. Lierman was as charming as her articles in the magazine, and I told her she was even more so.

It is wonderful what they are doing to make the method known. Captain Price is being asked to speak in some of the big cities and Ms. Beswick too.

Ms. Beswick has one or two friends who are members of Parliament. She has gotten them interested and they are working with the Ministry of Health and Education to get the system installed in the schools. She was formerly a teacher in London and she has friends who are working with the London County Council and she hopes before long to get it included in the course required at the normal schools for teachers run by the County Council. One big London high school has already installed it.

Recently a delegation was sent to England from the German Government to investigate the most modern ideas in education in England and to report with recommendations for the German schools. Ms. Beswick's friend who is in Parliament suggested that the head of the delegation see Ms. Beswick with regard to your method as applied to schoolchildren. He had several interviews with her.

Several doctors are using the method and are on the Council of the Better Eyesight League, but the medical profession as a whole have not waked up to what is going on. Ms. Beswick expects great opposition when they do. In the meantime she hopes the League will be in a strong position with titled people on the Council, etc. She has already gotten an article in a well-known magazine of the *Save the Children Fund,* which is backed by the biggest medical men in the country, and that has given the method prestige.

You mark my words it will be just like adrenalin and will come to the United States from England before the A.M.A. has finished their attacks on you. If you only live long enough I believe you will have the Nobel Prize. I am leaving London in a few days but I expect to see Ms. Beswick again. Please show this letter to Ms. Lierman.

Yours very sincerely, (Signed) Mary M. W. Taylor.

THE MAGIC CARPET

By George M. Guild

A little boy wearing a black velvet suit with a large collar which covered his shoulders was getting very restless. His nurse was trying to guide him through the crowded streets and while she held his hand and helped him along, the velvet suit with the white collar seemed perfectly willing to go with her but the large tortoise-shell rimmed eyeglasses that he was wearing over his painful eyes dragged him always in the wrong direction. The little boy with his beautiful clothes was quite frequently banging up against rough men who knocked him to one side, and every lamp post that he met welcomed him with a bang that made him cry out with pain. Finally he became so tired that he could not stand up any longer and dropped down to the curbstone and sat there for quite a while in spite of the efforts of his nurse to drag him farther. When the nurse was not looking, her attention being distracted, a nice old man with a strange hat spoke to the little boy pleasantly, sympathetically and so kindly that the little boy looked up into his face and tried to smile. The nice old man gave him a handful of candy to eat while he led him away from the nurse and sat him down on a nice green carpet in a neighboring store. The little old man came and sat down beside the little boy and told him the story about the magic carpet. When you sat on the magic carpet and said a little prayer and then called out loud some place where you would like to go, the carpet would carry you there very quickly. The little old man said to the little boy, "When you are tired of staying here, just say a little prayer that your mother taught you; call where you want to go and you will soon be there."

The little boy said his mother was a very wealthy and important person and did not have any time to teach her little boy to say his prayers. He was so disappointed that he burst into tears and cried and cried. The little old man tried to comfort him and said, "Never mind little boy. I will say a little prayer and I will say where you want to go, and then we will have a nice time going there."

Then the little old man said a little prayer and said out loud that he wanted to go to the home of the little boy in the black velvet suit. Right away the carpet rose from the floor, moved out of the doorway and up toward the sky. It all seemed so wonderful, so new, so pleasant, so agreeable;

and the louder he laughed and the more he clapped his hands, the better did he become able to see. In a very short time the carpet arrived on the lawn of a very beautiful house which was where the little boy lived. Then the little old man said to the little boy, "How is your sight?" The little boy scowled and said, "The doctor told me I must wear my glasses all the time."

The little old man removed the glasses from the little boy and said, "Wouldn't you like to see perfectly without your glasses?" This seemed a new idea to the little boy but a very pleasant one and he smiled.

The little old man then told him some nice stories about fairies and about nice little boys who grew up and became very nice big men when they learned to say a prayer at night that their mothers taught them.

The little boy was rudely shaken and he awoke and found that he was leaning against a lamp post, the little old man and the carpet were gone and the crowds were greater than ever. His nurse cried, "Where are your glasses?"

The little boy said, "I never want to wear those horrid things again because the little old man told me that I would feel a great deal happier if my eyes were cured without glasses." He looked up into his nurse's face and smiled and said, "Do you suppose I could get mother to teach me a little prayer when I go to bed at night?" The nurse was shocked and shook him some more, but she could not shake the smile from his face or the happiness from his heart because he found that he could see without his glasses a great deal better than he had ever been able to see before with them.

BATES METHOD A SUCCESS IN SCHOOLS

Editor's Note—*The following report was submitted by Mr. Husted, Superintendent of the North Bergen Schools. He is a pioneer in eye education in schools, and in spite of critical opposition and halfhearted cooperation, has had remarkable success with it.*

Early in October 1919, the Superintendent of North Bergen Schools directed our school nurse, Marion McNamara, to take a Snellen test of the eyes of all of our pupils. A novel health experiment was begun, a campaign for "Better Eyesight." In June a second test was made in order to measure the extent of progress in this phase of health work. The June test of 1920 shows marvelous, practical, successful results. Only the skepticism of principals, teachers and pupils and lack of complete faithfulness in carrying out its conditions prevented the wonderful results achieved from paralleling those of an *Arabian Nights* tale.

A Snellen test card is placed permanently in the room. The children are directed to read the smallest letter they can see from their seats at least once every day, with both eyes together and with each eye separately, the other being covered with the palm of the hand in such a way as to avoid pressure on the eyeball. Those whose vision is defective are encouraged to read it more frequently, and in fact need no encouragement to do so after they find that the practice helps them to see the blackboard, and stop the headaches or other discomfort previously resulting from the use of their eyes.

1923 Records

Special effort for exactness in records has been an aim in 1923. Out of 3,636 pupils receiving both first and final tests, 741 pupils were found below the Normal Standard of 20/20 or 19%, and of these, 565 were present at the second examination test which showed 234 of them or 52% having improved sight. As the percentage of pupils below standard becomes less, the same percentage of better sight gains become more difficult as the more serious cases carry over to the following year and are less amendable to treatment and should therefore receive special persistent and systematic attention.

Not only does this work place no additional burden upon the teachers but, by improving the eyesight, health, disposition and mentality of their pupils, it surely lightens their labors.

Curative Results and Records, 1924

A different plan for eyesight conservation was followed for 1923-1924. Every classroom in North Bergen Schools, grades II-VIII became a conservation of vision class. Each classroom was visited by the Superintendent and the values of good eyesight for pupils were dwelt upon. The method to be used in its attainment was carefully explained. Our nurses were invited to attend several of these classroom talks. Pupils with good sight volunteered to aid those with defective eyes during this special campaign to educate the eye to function without strain and thus prevent and cure defective vision. Pupils have engaged in this work with a helpful enthusiasm and teachers with a renewed interest. As this work is a physical training for the education of the eye, teachers were instructed to use some time assigned to physical training or hygiene to guide the below normal vision pupils to sufficient proper eye practice for curative effects, and the normal vision ones to sufficient practice for preventive defects.

Great care has been taken to make these reports accurate. The tests were all made by two nurses assisted by the classroom teacher and the reports were all made under nurse supervision. That 66% or 782 pupils have improved, 342 of them or 43.7% to the degree of normal vision is certainly a wonderful and worthwhile bit of health cure work and is indicative of what may be attained by this educative process under more systematic, intelligent and persistent practice.

REPORT OF THE SEPTEMBER MEETING

A regular meeting of the Better Eyesight League was held on September 9. A large attendance indicated renewed interest in the work of the League.

Ms. Hurty, president, presided. After a short business program the president discussed the aim of the League and of Dr. Bates' method. Instruction in palming was then given by the officers.

Dr. Bates emphasized the importance of the personal equation in applying his method. Palming proves most helpful in some cases, swinging in others, and the use of the imagination in others.

Mr. M. F. Husted, Superintendent of Schools in North Bergen, New Jersey, reported the result of his having used Dr. Bates' method to reduce retardation among pupils in his district. As a means to this end the method proved highly successful; furthermore, the lessening of retardation among pupils made possible a reduction in the educational budget. Last fall 4,155 children in Mr. Husted's district were examined and 1,244 cases of defective vision were recorded. During the year the pupils were merely encouraged to read the Snellen test card daily. At the close of the year 43.7% of the defective cases had attained normal vision, while 21.8% showed marked improvement. The cases of defective vision included 129 in which glasses were used; 75% of these cases were greatly improved.

Ms. Lierman discussed the work of her Clinic. Six months ago one clinical case was diagnosed as total blindness; this girl now reads the Snellen test card at two feet. Ms. Lierman reported improved vision also in a case of cataract in a woman seventy-eight years old and improved condition in a case of drooping eyelid (ptosis) in a five-year-old boy.

QUESTIONS AND ANSWERS

Q–1. I find conscious blinking a strain, because I close my eyes temporarily and seem to hold the eyeball stationary. If I shut my eyes for a longer period, would that be blinking?

A–1. No; the normal eye blinks consciously or unconsciously without effort, without strain, and quickly.

Q–2a. You mention the black period in your book. Must this be any particular size? 2b. I only imagine large round black objects like cannon balls, the center of a target, or a moving football. This is restful, but is it beneficial?

A–2a. No. 2b. Anything that is restful is beneficial.

Q–3. My little daughter has temporary perfect sight while palming, but her eyes turn in when she plays excitedly or strenuously. I thought play was relaxing.

A–3. Play may be relaxing and should be beneficial, but like other things, it can be done wrong with a great effort, without benefit.

Q–4. Please give me a simple demonstration or example of the swing. I cannot see objects moving when I know they are stationary.

A–4. When you ride in a railroad train which is traveling fast, and you look out the window, you may see the telegraph poles and other objects moving in the opposite direction.

Better Eyesight
November 1924—Vol. IX, No. 5

EYESTRAIN DURING SLEEP

Many people complain that when they first wake up in the morning they are tired, that they have headaches, and that their sight is very imperfect. Later on in the day their eyes feel better and the vision may become normal.

I have examined with the ophthalmoscope the eyes of many people during sleep and found, much to my surprise, that most people strain much more in their sleep than they ever do when they are awake. Of course, people when unconscious of their acts during sleep are not aware of this eyestrain.

The prevention of eyestrain during sleep is usually a very difficult matter. Some cases are benefited just before retiring by palming for a half-hour or longer, or until they go to sleep while palming. Others, by practicing the long swing for fifteen minutes, have found that the eyestrain becomes less. In some serious cases with imperfect sight, when the eyestrain is not prevented by palming or the swing, they are often materially benefited by shortening their hours of sleep with the help of an alarm clock. One patient had the alarm set for 3 a.m. He would then get out of bed and practice the long swing, alternating with palming for an hour or longer with the result that he slept the rest of the night very comfortably, and awoke the next morning with little or no evidence of eyestrain during sleep.

Some people have told me that they have lessened their eyestrain during sleep materially by moderate muscular exercises for a half-hour or longer. They find that they obtain the best results when the exercise is continued sufficiently long to produce muscular fatigue.

THE CURE OF MYOPIA

By W. H. Bates, M.D.

The problem of curing each case of myopia or nearsightedness requires a sufficient number of facts. Each patient has to demonstrate individually those facts which help that particular patient or which suggests successful treatment.

The cause of myopia is an effort to see at the distance. Most patients can demonstrate that when they read the Snellen test card at fifteen feet or farther, at ten feet, or nearer, staring at one point of one letter for two seconds or longer always lowers the vision. This fact is evidence that treatment which prevents the stare improves the sight.

When a nearsighted patient reads fine print with normal sight, an effort to concentrate or stare at one letter or one part of the letter seen perfectly is very soon followed by imperfect sight at the near point. All nearsighted patients can demonstrate that with the eyes closed, the memory of one letter is easy or continuous when it is imagined to be moving, and that an effort to concentrate on one part of the letter remembered requires a strain, which is soon followed by the loss of the memory of the letter.

Nearsighted patients can always demonstrate that closing the eyes and covering them with the palm of one or both hands for a half-hour or longer always improves the distant vision temporarily. It is good practice to have each patient prove over and over again by various methods that imperfect sight requires an effort, requires a strain which is disagreeable, not easy, or that with imperfect sight one has to work hard and take a lot of trouble. It is usually quite a shock to them to demonstrate more or less thoroughly that perfect sight can only be obtained easily and without effort. Even after the nearsighted patients demonstrate these facts for a time they usually keep on straining their eyes when they look at the distant Snellen test card.

All nearsighted patients are temporarily cured when their sight becomes normal at some distance, even patients with very high degrees of nearsightedness, 10 D or more, when they read with perfect sight at four inches without glasses, accommodate just the same amount as a normal eye does when it reads perfectly at four inches. They do not have an accommodation of four inches plus the amount of their myopia.

I discovered that under favorable conditions, when a nearsighted patient had a perfect memory, the myopia disappeared and the eye became normal. I also discovered that when a nearsighted patient had a perfect imagination of a mental picture of some letter or some object, the myopia disappeared and the eye became normal.

It is a fact that we remember only what we see. We imagine only what we remember. We see only what we imagine.

A nearsighted patient who reads perfectly at the near point may obtain a perfect memory by regarding one letter at the near point with perfect sight, closing the eyes and remembering it as well as he can. By alternating, the sight and the memory improve until the patient becomes able to see and remember equally well.

After this is accomplished the patient becomes able to regard a letter with normal sight at a near point and then, when looking at a distant blank wall, to remember it. By practicing, the patient becomes able to remember with the eyes open as well as he can see.

The next step is to help the patient to remember a mental picture of some letter seen perfectly at the near point just as well as when regarding the Snellen test card. The time it takes to improve the memory of mental pictures varies much with different patients. Some cases with a high degree of nearsightedness I cure in a reasonable length of time, while others with a moderate amount may require a much longer time.

The imagination is also improved by alternating with the memory. Many patients find that they can remember a letter fairly well, but when they regard it, they do not imagine they see it, then again practice helps at the near point. When a nearsighted patient regards a letter "O," for example, the white center may appear to be whiter than it really is, or whiter than the rest of the card. To prove that this is an illusion may require some trouble. It helps to cover the black part of the letter, exposing only the center which then appears to have the same shade of white as the rest of the card. When the screen is removed, exposing the black part of the letter, the white center flashes whiter. The patient, after a few trials, may become able to imagine the white center whiter than it really is.

One needs to convince the patient that this is an illusion. The white center of the letter "O" is never seen whiter than the rest of the card, it is only imagined.

After this is accomplished at the near point, it becomes possible for the nearsighted patient to imagine this illusion at a greater distance. Those patients who are thoroughly convinced that they do not see the white center of the "O" whiter than the rest of the card, but only imagine it, are soon cured, because while they find it difficult to see the letter "O" at a distance, it is easier to imagine it.

Acute myopia is usually cured by very simple treatment. Children under twelve years old who have never worn glasses are usually temporarily cured by alternately reading the Snellen test card and resting their eyes by closing them and covering them with the palms of their hands for a few minutes. Many teachers in the public schools have placed the Snellen test card permanently on one wall of the classroom in a place where all the children could see it from their seats. When the children read this card as well as they could every day, the vision usually improved without any other treatment. All the children become able to remember perfectly each letter of the Snellen test card. They not only remember what the letter is, but they also remember its blackness, the white spaces, its form, its size and its location; furthermore, they become able to imagine that they see perfectly the letters that they remember perfectly. They also discover sooner or later that a perfect imagination of one or more of the letters of the Snellen test card helps them to read the writing on the blackboard which is unfamiliar. In other words, they demonstrate that a perfect imagination of a known letter helps them to see perfectly other letters or objects that are not known. They also become convinced that a stare or strain to see the writing on the blackboard lowers the vision, just as it lowers the vision for the letters of the Snellen test card with which they are perfectly familiar. This is a fact of the greatest value in the cure and prevention of imperfect sight in schoolchildren. Every teacher should know this.

The Snellen test card, while it is of value as a test for the ability of the children to see, is of far greater usefulness as a means for improving the sight.

I have found that in schools where the Snellen test card is visible continuously, the vision of the pupils is always improved and that the children in the higher grades acquire a more perfect sight than they had when they first entered school. Most children demonstrate that the Snellen test card, while it improves the vision, is also a benefit to their nervous system. It prevents and cures headaches, lessens fatigue, encourages the children to study, and increases the mental efficiency.

STORIES FROM THE CLINIC

No. 57: Cases of Myopia

By Emily C. Lierman

I have been asked to write about myopia cases now under treatment in the Clinic. Within the last year we have had quite a number of patients who were cured of myopia in one or two visits. Some of them were not bad cases, therefore it did not take very long to cure them.

A woman of middle age who had worn glasses about

two years told me something of interest which I think our readers would like to know about. She had very little to do at the time, so to amuse herself she would stare at an object until it became distorted. She stared so wonderfully well that the object became two instead of one. Later she became able to see the object triple and she boasted about her ability to do this to anyone who would listen to her. Then one morning, after she wakened from a sound sleep, she could not see the hands of her clock. The figures were blurred. Everything in the room seemed to be covered with a veil. She tried her old stunt and stared just as hard as she could, thinking that it would help her to see things clearly. Instead, her vision became worse, so she called on an oculist. He told her that she would probably have to wear glasses for the rest of her life. He fitted her with glasses and told her never to be without them. Six months later she had to have stronger lenses. When I first saw her I thought her eyelids were stationary. I looked at her for fully three minutes without seeing her blink once. Then she told me what I have already written. I said I believed or was sure that she had brought on all this trouble herself. And she surprised me by saying, "Well, if I could make so much trouble with my eyes, surely I can undo it with your help."

[When he was a boy, a famous British actor found a book on acting stating that actors should never blink when in front of a camera. He practiced not blinking for up to twenty minutes. He got an eye infection; and he now wears thick, coke-bottle glasses.—TRQ]

She did exactly what I told her to do, and more. She practiced more often than I said, and she never talked about her eyes to anyone until she was cured. She practiced palming for an hour every morning, from six until seven o'clock. She traveled every morning and night for one hour on a railroad train and never opened her eyes the whole time she was on the train. Her friends never troubled her after she asked them not to speak about her eyes. She never used a test card but practiced whenever she had time, with a newspaper or book type. She worked with a typewriter every day, and she found that her memory helped in her work.

Sometimes she remembered a large white imitation pearl of her earring or she would remember the sparkle of a little diamond in her ring. A black period was out of the question entirely. If I just mentioned a period to her she would begin to stare.

She said it reminded her of the blurry things she saw, when her eyes first troubled her. She surely demonstrated that to remember an error is a strain.

Just six weeks after I first treated her, she was cured without glasses. She now sees things clearly at the distance, but only when she blinks, which is just what the normal eye must do to keep the vision normal. Her friends have a good time with her, when she is in the mood, for she is constantly reminding them to blink.

A young man age 23 had worn glasses steadily for ten years. With his glasses on he read 10/15 and without them 10/30. His face became a mass of wrinkles as he tried to read the letters of the test card. He complained that the white of the card was a dazzling white and gave him great pain as he tried to read the letters.

After palming for a few minutes, the wrinkles temporarily disappeared. I placed him in the sun, and as he looked down, I raised his upper eyelid. I then focused the bright rays of the sun on the white part of each eye with the sun glass. This did not take but a minute. We returned to the test card and, without a mistake, he read every letter. I told him to sit in the sun as much as possible and let it shine on his closed eyelids, and to palm every day for at least an hour altogether.

At the present time we are treating a little girl, nine years old, who was quite nearsighted and had very poor sight even with her glasses on. I was told that while her vision was poor before she had put on glasses, her eyes became much worse during the last year. She has worn them only one year, and I believe that they made her worse. The first day her vision without glasses was 7/200 with both eyes, and with each eye separately.

I told her she would have to stop wearing glasses if she wanted to be cured. The little girl was afraid to do that because her school teacher told her she should always wear them. Of course I became less enthusiastic about the cure of her eyes.

I gave her a treatment that day and improved her vision to 7/70 by having her palm for ten minutes or so, and then look at a letter on the test card that I was pointing at. I did not expect to see her again at the Clinic because she was going against my wishes by wearing her glasses, but she was there the next Clinic day, holding her glasses in her hand. She said she had worn them every day only during school hours. At other times, after her homework was finished, she practiced with the test card and palmed her eyes as much as possible.

I was very much surprised to find that her vision had improved even though she wore her glasses. Dr. Bates and I have been surprised more than once to find a patient get well although they had worn their glasses at times.

This little girl has been to us four times and she now reads 8/40. I would like to make another report of her case when she is cured. Unless she has the courage to leave off her glasses entirely, I fear it will take a long time to cure her.

THANKSGIVING FAIRIES

By George M. Guild

We have fairies in the springtime, fairies in the summer, fairies at Christmas and New Year, and also fairies at Thanksgiving.

The table was all set for a large dinner party which included not only the grandmother, the grandfather, the loving mother and the proud father, but many friends.

The Little Boy was wearing eyeglasses which were so conspicuous that they quite concealed very much of his face. He was only ten years old, but he had an appetite for everything that was good, more so than any person present. His father filled up his plate with all the good things that it would hold and, without a word to anyone, he started in to eat as he had never eaten before. Before he was half way through, he was suddenly attacked with acute indigestion which caused him such intense pain that he began to cry. His mother started to take him from the table, but he could not stand it to leave all that food behind. When he saw his mother coming, he stopped crying and begged her to leave him alone for a few minutes. All eyes were watching him, wondering what he was going to do next. After a few moments' thought, he suddenly removed his glasses, closed his eyes and covered them with his two chubby hands, with his elbows resting on the table. The color soon came back to his face, the pain left him, and in a few minutes he began to smile and was soon all right. He started in to eat again with increased energy. His father who had been watching him with a worried look on his face was very much astonished.

"What do you think of that," he said, "Where did the child find out about resting his eyes to cure his stomach-ache?"

Everybody at the table seemed dazed but had very little to say. In a little while, however, things got back to their normal state just as they were before the Little Boy became ill. He passed his plate back for more, which his father reluctantly filled again. The Little Boy began to talk, but the only words anybody could hear him say with his mouth continually stuffed with food were, "fairy," and "palming," and "teacher," and "Snellen test card." His mother could not stand it any longer. She got up, took the Little Boy in her arms and carried him to another room, held him in her lap while she asked him questions to find out what it was all about. "Oh, Mother, that was a nice dinner, and the little Thanksgiving fairy with many other fairies are dancing around on the table and they are bowing to me, they are bowing to grandpa, to grandma, and to everybody else, but principally, they seem to be paying more attention to me.

The Thanksgiving fairy, all dressed in green, is holding out her arms to me and she says, "Little Boy, don't grow up to be a four-eyed man. Take off those terrible glasses and you will have perfect sight without them, if you will only love me and never forget me. Whenever you are ill, think of me, and you can think of me best when you close your eyes and cover them with the palms of your hands."

There was a ring at the door. The Little Boy's father answered it, and ushered in the Little Boy's teacher, who had come to make a short call. When the teacher was told about the Little Boy with the attack of indigestion, and how he discarded his glasses, closed his eyes and covered them with the palms of his hands, which was followed by a very prompt and complete cure, the teacher said, "I have called to ask you to try for a time having the Little Boy do without his glasses. A great many other children have been cured of nearsightedness in a short time, and I feel that the Little Boy will also be cured so that he will get along much better without his glasses than he ever did with them."

The father's face brightened and he said to the teacher with a grateful smile, "It is so ordered."

EL USO NATURAL DE LA VISION (THE NATURAL USE OF VISION)

By R. Ruiz Arnau, M.D.

This book should appeal to Spanish-speaking people, because it contains numerous demonstrations of the truth which make it possible to cure imperfect sight by treatment without glasses. In the magazine *Better Eyesight,* of May 1920, is an article by Dr. Arnau with the title "My Headaches" in which he describes at length how he was cured of chronic headaches and imperfect sight by treatment without glasses. As a result of his cure he has become able to give relief to his patients.

The author has written a great deal about mind strain as the real and only cause of defective eyesight. He discusses the unconscious movements of the vegetative functions of the body, circulation, respiration and the constant mental shifting as entirely in accord with the new ideas of Einstein, Korbzyski and others.

The Tachorthoscope was discovered by Dr. Arnau. It is an apparatus for the treatment of patients who are not benefited promptly by other methods.

He has also investigated the use of music by which some

patients find an easy way to obtain a short swing through the auditory memory.

THE ACROBATIC "T"

By Emily A. Meder

As I look out the window the crisp air is blowing the colored leaves about like little fairy carpets. Autumn is here, with weather that delights the hiker's soul. No one but a true hiker can realize the joy of tramping in the woods or along a road, with arms swinging, eyes shifting from object to object, and the ground and trees seeming to glide slowly by as the walker passes.

This form of exercise and recreation has become very popular along with other outdoor sports. It is a good thing to call to your attention the fact that no matter what kind of sport, recreation or work you indulge in, you can rest the eyes and improve the sight while doing it. Recently while ice-skating in an indoor rink, I became dizzy going around and watching the white ice moving under my feet. I stopped for a few minutes, rested my eyes, and went on again. Instead of looking at the ice, I swung my body slowly from side to side, shifting my eyes from one skater to another. I just forgot the dizziness, and don't know whether it disappeared immediately after I palmed, or when I began to swing.

I wonder how many people find palming monotonous? One subscriber told me that he tried to palm, but found it so dull and boring, that he dropped it entirely. I asked him what he did when he palmed, what he thought of. He replied that he tried to think of black, and nothing else. Usually he saw all colors, from light gray to startling green, and he gave it up. He could not get black, so his mind returned to his business problems and other worries.

I was in sympathy with this man's state of mind, because I tried to see black, with the same results. If I let my mind drift, without charting its course, it would inevitably go over the unpleasant happenings of the day, or the work unfinished, or worse still, I would become drowsy! I was always more relaxed if I could imagine black objects, so here's the scheme I used to good advantage:

The little black "F" in the corner of the test card is a good friend of mine. I can think of it and remember it more easily than any other letter. The trouble is that it is too active and as soon as I experience benefit from its company, it hops all over the place. When I try to hold it stationary, the better to look at it, it disappears entirely. I decided to put this surplus energy to work and planned a daily dozen for Mr. "F" to do. When I palm, I summon him and he stands at attention like a soldier while I inspect him from head to foot. If he passes, he is a perfect black. Then he starts his drill. His two arms are pointed to the right when he begins. I imagine them moving to the left, and back. Then one arm is pointed to the left and one to the right, and my "F" is a "T." Both arms are then stretched up, forming a "Y." He is very versatile, and never drills twice in the same way. At one time he tried to change his straight lines to form a "C," but this was too much for even his acrobatic powers, and was painful for me to watch. He now confines himself to straight letters only, with a variation of the figures "4" and "7."

These athletic exhibitions can last fifteen minutes or longer at a time, without my becoming drowsy or bored. Try it with a letter "L" or an "O." Perhaps with training and close association it will become as dear to you as my little "F."

FINE PRINT

By W. H. Bates, M.D.

Many nearsighted patients can read fine print or diamond type at less than ten inches from their eyes, easily, perfectly, and quickly by alternately regarding the Snellen test card at different distances, from three feet up to fifteen feet or farther. The vision may be improved, at first temporarily, and later by repetition, a permanent gain usually follows.

It is a valuable fact to know that when fine print is read perfectly, the nearsightedness disappears during this period. It can only be maintained at first for a fraction of a second, and later more continuously.

Nearsighted patients and others, with the help of the fine print can usually demonstrate that staring at a small letter always lowers the vision and that the same fact is true when regarding distant letters or objects.

With the help of the fine print, the nearsighted patient can also demonstrate that one can remember perfectly only what has been seen perfectly; that one imagines perfectly only what is remembered perfectly; and that perfect sight is only a perfect imagination.

A great many people are very suspicious of the imagination and feel or believe that things imagined are never true. The more ignorant the patient, the less respect do they have for their imagination or the imagination of other people. It comes to them as a great shock, with a feeling of discomfort and annoyance, that the perfect imagination of a known letter improves the sight for unknown letters of the Snellen test card.

It is a fact that one can read fine print perfectly with a perfect relaxation, with great relief to eyestrain, pain, fatigue and discomfort, not only of the eyes, but of all other nerves of the body.

Regarding fine print, even when not read, is also of use in improving the distant vision of the Snellen test card, and the ability to read at a near point in patients whose imperfect sight is caused by astigmatism, hypermetropia (farsightedness), presbyopia and others.

REPORT OF THE OCTOBER MEETING

By May Secor, Secretary

A regular meeting of the Better Eyesight League was held on October 14. Among important facts presented were the following: The prevalence of visual defects and eyestrain is evident to anyone who gives the matter his attention. Formerly, but one course of action was open to the sufferer—to visit an oculist, have his eyes tested, receive a prescription for artificial lenses, procure them, and then endeavor to become accustomed to wearing these optical crutches.

The efficiency of the eye is variable. During an eye test the patient is able to read smaller letters on the chart at various times. When the sight is tested with the astigmatism-producing clock dial, the patient can see certain lines most clearly at one time, and others most clearly at another time. The lenses prescribed are such as "fit" the patient when his eyes register a certain number of degrees of astigmatism and myopia, for example. In order that the patient may see with the prescribed lenses it is essential that he produce the said number of degrees of astigmatism and myopia; this produces eyestrain. The need for a more efficient method for correcting visual defects is obvious.

It is here that the Bates Method functions. This method is based upon the fact that visual defects are caused by eyestrain; it therefore offers methods for the relief of eyestrain. Insomuch as the method corrects visual defects, it proves the fact to be true. Be the case one of myopia, hypermetropia, squint, or cataract, Dr. Bates removes the glasses and assists the patient to use his eyes with relaxation. This is accomplished by means of various methods: palming, reading the Snellen test card, shifting, swaying, swinging, sun treatment, and other methods involving the use of memory and imagination. These methods are described in Dr. Bates' book entitled *Perfect Sight Without Glasses.*

Dr. E. G. Kessler, M.D., expressed his gratitude for his son's cure. Dr. Kessler then discussed the importance of relaxation in securing mental rest. In this connection the doctor spoke of the use of the rocking chair, and quoted authorities who decried the "rocking habit." Dr. Bates expressed his belief that a moderate use of the rocking chair facilitates relaxation, if one "sees things moving" as he rocks; a moderate use of cradle-rocking and "swaying" was advocated for infants.

Dr. Bates demonstrated the long swing, and spoke of its helpfulness in securing relaxation. The long swing relieves eyestrain and other types of physical distress. When pain is very acute, visualization of the letters of the Snellen test card is advised also. Ms. Hurty discussed the work of A. Rollier, M.D., at his sanitarium at Leysin, Switzerland. Dr. Rollier uses sun treatment in curing tuberculosis; he finds, however, that additional results accrue, visual defects are corrected, and eyestrain relieved. This confirms Dr. Bates' claim that sunlight is effective as a cure for visual defects.

Mr. Nicholas Weiss reported several cases in which he secured relaxation by describing a horse race or a baseball inning while the patient palmed. Dr. Achorn emphasized the important role which memory plays in the Bates Method. He advised the prospective followers of the method to begin at once to practice the various methods, investigating their physiological and psychological significance as a parallel line of work. Correct use of the method will improve the vision immediately in most cases.

QUESTIONS AND ANSWERS

Q–1. If sun and light are beneficial, why do you advocate the shutting out of these two by palming?

A–1. To obtain relaxation. The sun strengthens the eyes and palming relaxes them.

Q–2. My left eye turned in and was corrected by operation. Now it turns out. What method will cure this?

A–2. You need more than one method. Complete relaxation will relieve the strain and correct the squint.

Q–3. After palming for ten minutes or longer, my eyes are rested, but I feel sleepy.

A–3. The palming is not perfect. Try imagining stationary objects to be moving when you palm.

Q–4. I was given glasses for headaches. Discarded them by your method; headaches have gone, but I strain while I sleep and my lids are swollen in the morning.

A–4. See the first article of this issue.

Q–5. Is a great amount of floating specks indicative of cataract? When I am weary these look like a flock of bees crossing my eyeballs.

A–5. No. Your particular strain produces floating specks. A different strain produces cataract.

Better Eyesight
December 1924—Vol. IX, No. 6

SUGGESTIONS

1. Imagine things are moving all the time. When riding in a railroad train, or when one looks out of the car window, telegraph poles and other objects, although they are stationary, appear to be moving. To stop the movement is impossible, and the effort to do so may be very uncomfortable. The greater the effort, the greater the discomfort, and is the cause of heart sickness, headaches and nausea. It can be demonstrated that any movement of the head and eyes produces an apparent movement of stationary objects.

2. Blink often. By blinking is meant closing and opening both eyes rapidly. When done properly, things are seen continuously and they always move with a quick jump in various directions. Regarding stationary objects without blinking is an effort, a strain which always lowers the vision.

3. Read the Snellen test card at fifteen feet as well as you can, every night and morning. Schoolchildren and others are often cured of imperfect sight by reading a familiar card, first with both eyes and then with each eye separately. It is the only method practiced which prevents myopia in schoolchildren.

4. Read fine print at six inches when possible every night and morning. If not possible, do the best you can. Just regarding the white spaces between the lines of fine print without reading the letters is a benefit.

5. Palm for five minutes, ten times daily when convenient.

PALMING

By W. H. Bates, M.D.

By palming is meant that the eyes are covered with the palms of one or both hands with the eyes closed. The object of palming is to obtain relaxation or rest of the eyes and mind. With the eyes closed and covered, the patient does not see. When properly done, the field is black and the patient does not really see anything. Most patients when they palm however, imagine they see a great many things, especially different colored lights, red, green, shades of blue and white lights in a single or multiple form, for various periods of time.

When the patient palms successfully and obtains perfect relaxation, he imagines he sees a perfect black. The number of people who can do this is small, and it can only be accomplished by individuals who have perfect sight.

While palming, one does not obtain relaxation by any kind of an effort or a strain. When nothing is done, one does not do anything. It is well to realize that palming may be done properly, or it may be done wrong.

It has been demonstrated that all persons with imperfect sight have a conscious or unconscious strain when they try to see. Palming can only accomplish relaxation when the patient does not try to see while palming. Some people realize that when their eyes are closed and covered with the palms of the hands, it is not possible to see anything, and so they do not try; but other people may strain their eyes to see while palming, although they know it is wrong. In such cases, it is very evident that mental control is lost. They do things that they do not plan to do. Some people can let their minds drift from one thing to another without much, if any, effort. Some cases become able to palm more successfully than others.

One of my patients discovered a very simple and efficient method to improve palming. While treating a friend who previously had never obtained any benefit from palming, she told him a story of a black ant. This black ant came out of the dark soil and climbed up the stem of a beautiful rose. It was slow work with the ant, but it kept on climbing, going on to the extremity of first one branch and then another, crawling to the extreme tip of every leaf until finally it located the flower. It crawled with great labor over the petals, until it found deep down in the center of the rose, a little white cup filled with honey. The patient could picture the ant carrying off some of the honey, crawling to the top of the flower, and then down back to the stem, finally meeting another ant on the ground, with whom he had a short talk with much gesticulating of heads and feet. Then the second ant started off on the same journey.

The patient, while palming, listened very attentively to this talk, which was drawn out for fifteen minutes or half an hour. He volunteered the information that at last he could see black, and when he removed his hands from his closed eyelids and opened his eyes, his vision for the Snellen test card was unusually good. Before he palmed, he was unable to see a single letter and was practically blind. After palming and visualizing the story of the ant, he was able to see his way about the room without being led, and to read some of the letters of the Snellen test card.

The story of the ant, with its successive mental pictures, suggests other stories of other things with other mental pictures. Some persons are able to let their minds drift while palming. It is normal for the mind to think of many things that come and go without any effort or strain being made. It is quite an art to let the mind drift and think of all sorts of things without any effort or without trying to see one thing in particular. As long as we are awake, it is perfectly normal to think of many things which come into the consciousness without any effort.

A school teacher who suffered from eyestrain with severe headaches, was able to obtain relief almost immediately by imagining herself in a boat which was drifting. She enjoyed drifting down some river of the north, with a scenery consisting mostly of ice and snow. For a change, she would select some tropical river with its tropical vegetation, birds and animals. She had seen a bird of paradise in captivity and enjoyed the memory of its brilliant feathers. Crocodiles seemed very interesting, and the play of the monkeys in the trees was also of interest and gave her mind much to think about. While drifting down these rivers, she became so interested in her imagination of the change in scenery that she quite forgot her eyestrain and her headaches while palming. When she noticed or thought of her palming, she found that she was seeing a perfect black, which means that she saw nothing at all with her eyes closed and covered with the palms of her hands.

One patient who had great difficulty in palming successfully was very much disturbed by seeing different colored lights. When she tried to get rid of them by an effort, they became much worse, and her discomfort was increased by the palming, instead of being relieved.

I suggested to her that she think of some enjoyable trip she had made going to Europe. She replied that she was always seasick, and the trip did her no good. The only thing that she could remember without discomfort was a walk in the woods, making note of the names of the different birds she saw. She was much interested in botany, and could tell the names of most of the wild flowers near her home.

Some people while palming can remember the branches of trees or high grass moving in the wind. The running water of a brook can be remembered with benefit, provided no effort is made. A trip to the seashore becomes restful and enjoyable when one imagines the waves flowing in and out. When riding in a rapidly moving train, the scenery observed when looking out of a window appears to be moving and is usually restful to the eyes and mind. When riding in an automobile, the driver imagines the road moving toward the car without an effort and is more relaxed than a passenger who is interested in the moving scenery and strains to see it and tries consciously or unconsciously to stop the movement.

If one makes an effort to see things stationary, a headache, eye pain or some other discomfort may be felt. Palming becomes restful and beneficial when the memory of moving objects becomes perfect or when one can remember the imaginary movement of stationary objects. By remembering stationary objects apparently moving when palming as well as they can be imagined when riding in a car, one may obtain the desired relaxation.

The memory of halos, when palming as well as they can be imagined with the eyes open is also a great benefit. Alternating is a benefit to the sight as well as to the memory, and palming becomes improved with a greater amount of relaxation.

Flashing or palming for a brief moment, alternating with the eyes open for a longer time, improves palming and the vision.

STORIES FROM THE CLINIC

No. 58: Christmas

By Emily C. Lierman

I wish everyone who is interested in our Clinic could have been with us last year at Christmas time. We had our first tree. Not only did our Clinic patients enjoy it, but our private patients as well. I fear too, that on more than one occasion, a private patient was kept waiting much longer than he cared to wait, while Dr. Bates hovered around that Christmas Tree. He never takes a vacation because he loves his work so much, but that tree needed his attention he thought, even though he was keeping his patients waiting. His orders were not to purchase anything cheap. His Clinic family is precious to him and must have the best of everything. When it came time to distribute the toys and candies to the children, I saw him peeping in at the doorway. The children all love him because he does so much for them. All this added pleasure of having a tree for them did him a world of good.

EYE EDUCATION

By Margaret Robinson

Ms. Robinson, a school teacher and patient of Dr. Bates, has been able to help a great many of her friends, although she herself is not entirely cured. Her own failures enable her to direct her pupil in the right and wrong method. We are publishing a few of her cases which she benefited.

MYOPIA

Ms. P., a school teacher, had worn glasses for fifteen years. She said she came from a nearsighted family, and her right eye was very prominent. After removing her glasses she read R.V., 10/70; L.V., 10/30. In a few weeks of practice she read R.V., 10/15; L.V., 10/10. In a little over a month she started to teach again.

A year later, Ms. P. reported that she sees 10/10 with each eye and is having no trouble with near or distant vision. The prominent right eye now looks like the other.

EXOPHTHALMIC GOITER

Ms. K. had worn glasses for six years. Her vision with both eyes was 10/10. She was discouraged with her eyes, however, because they were very prominent, with dilated pupils. One physician told her she had a goiter disturbance. She could not see the movies without her glasses, had a great dread of bright lights, and her eyes were constantly inflamed.

Ms. K. had no faith in the new method of treatment, but tried it as a last resort. She did not cooperate very well, but in six weeks she caught the trick of relaxation. Her eyes became more comfortable and she used them for all purposes. Six months later this patient reported that while she had no further trouble with her eyes, she had to practice the palming and swinging every day to keep relaxed.

SQUINT

The left eye of Darwin was injured by instruments at birth. It turned in frequently when he was a baby, and became noticeably worse when he attended school. Darwin was twelve and wore glasses for three years, but the oculist who treated him said the eye was no stronger as a result. The vision after removing glasses was Right 10/10, Left 10/200. Palming improved his sight in flashes, and the squint became less noticeable. At the end of three months he read 10/30 on a strange card. In five months he could read diamond type a little, and ordinary type slowly. His left eye tired quickly, and he didn't have the patience to practice.

The left eye is straight practically all the time and the boy's appearance is greatly improved. He can read 12/10 on the chart when using both eyes.

Darwin is so comfortable that he has lost interest in practicing further, and the parents are satisfied with the eye straight. For this reason there may be no further progress.

HEADACHES

William, ten years old, had almost constant headaches. He read 10/15 badly on the test card. Type and figures blurred so much in his schoolbooks that it was difficult for him not to make mistakes. He made little progress for about two weeks and would always report that his headaches were just as bad, and that he could read no better. Then one day he announced that he had one headache at noon for only half an hour. He also read better, then stopped coming for lessons.

William returned in four months to have his eyes tested and read 10/10 with each eye separately, with no headaches. A year later he visited me again, and his eyes looked splendid. He read 12/10 with either eye, no headaches, read as long as he wished to, and had no trouble with schoolbooks as far as seeing was concerned.

CHRISTMAS FAIRIES

By George M. Guild

Yes, he was very unhappy. The rich man with all is wealth lived alone in his big house. He sat in an easy chair suffering from a violent headache. It was Christmas Eve, but for him there was no joy, no pleasure. Then came a little white fairy who danced and smiled before him. He was puzzled because all his life long he had never seen a fairy and consequently never believed in their existence. But now he had to believe the evidence of his own eyes. She climbed to his knee and he felt her tiny feet as she finally reached his shoulder and took the glasses off his eyes. For some unaccountable reason, he felt better. The little white fairy was never still a moment. She interested him. He watched every movement she made. And then came other fairies, who danced around him on the floor, on his lap, his hands, and his head. Their eyes were full of a wonderful kindness and love.

He became more and more interested and finally asked, "What can I do for you all?" The little white fairy replied: "Come with us and see the newborn baby."

And then, guided by the fairies, he walked out on the

street, through crowds of people until he came to a tenement in a darkened street. He climbed many stairs until they reached a closed door at the top of the building. He opened the door and entered a room where poverty, dirt and sickness were very evident. On a soiled bed lay a sick woman with her newborn child. She was thin, awfully thin, with eyes full of pain and mental suffering. There were five children in the room who looked very miserable indeed; but when they saw the fairies come dancing in, they began to smile and clapped their hands with pleasure.

The rich man looked around the room for a few moments, beckoned to the white fairy and both left the room. They were not gone long, but when they returned they brought with the help of others, a Christmas Tree with all that goes with it, baskets of food, enough to feed them all for many weeks to come. And then there were dolls for the girls, toys for the boys, bedding and clothes for the mother. The men who brought the things arranged the tree with its many ornaments and candles. What a lot of laughter was there. Even the sick mother had to smile. The white fairy fixed the Star of Bethlehem at the top of the tree when all knelt for a few moments, even the rich man knelt and also the men from the stores. The rich man had never been so happy in his life. He kept swinging with the fairies. He tried to dance. It was a happy time for all.

The neighbors became interested in the proceedings. First one and then another child edged to the open door, with that look of fear so sad to see in the eyes of the children of the poor. They were invited to come in and see the fairies dance, and to see them climbing all over the Christmas Tree, arranging everything in some way better, all with a smile and a laugh. It was quite contagious.

It was impossible for the saddest person there to look sad, feel sad or have a grouch of any kind. The fairies had dissipated all the darkness, the evil, the suffering and the pain. One even forgot to notice the dirt. After the children came the grown-ups, the young wives, young mothers, old wives, old mothers with many men, pushing and shoving to get into the room where the fairies were. The festivities continued for several hours, but nobody paid any attention to the time.

After the fairies had gone and the rich man found himself in his chair without his glasses and without his headache, perfectly comfortable, with his sight better than it had ever been before in years, he acquired a lasting smile. He always says, "The fairies took off my glasses and I will never wear them again."

TENSION

By W. R. Anderson, Jr.

Editor's Note—*This patient was told he was an incurable case and needed to wear glasses for the rest of his life. We hope this report will encourage our readers to continue with their practice, even if they fail to see immediate improvement. This case is remarkable in that the patient had the perseverance to follow the instructions outlined in the book, in the face of this discouraging verdict.*

Dear Dr. Bates:

I take great pleasure in thanking you for the help which I have received from studying your methods of treating defective vision.

On March 20, 1924, a family friend, herself one of your patients, brought me a copy of your book, *Perfect Sight Without Glasses.* At that time, my eyes were in wretched shape. Since birth I had suffered from what some oculists had diagnosed as atrophy of the optic nerve, others as prenatal malnutrition of the optic nerve. There was supposed to be a small area in the center of the retina with normal vision, while the outer portions of the retina were said to be dead. I also suffered from a high degree of myopia, which glasses failed to correct. The left eye turned in [crossed eye—TRQ]. The eyeballs themselves were hard and fixed in a dull stare, and were so sunken and lifeless in appearance that many people thought I was blind.

At various times other oculists in New York and other cities fitted me to glasses, tested my fields, and said there was nothing more to do.

I had read only a short way in your book when I realized that I was trying to accomplish the impossible. Two days after I began studying your methods I discarded my glasses. I began at once to exercise my eyes by shifting them from point to point. At first this shifting required constant effort since the eyeballs had been without movement for more than twenty years (I am now twenty-six years old and had worn glasses since the age of four.) Gradually the shifting became easier, until now it calls for no effort. It is not yet so rapid as it should be. There must have been almost a paralysis of the recti muscles, and the minor pulsation of the eyeballs, which you describe as occurring in the normal eye at the rate of from seventy to several thousand per second, is still absent. I look to time to make this condition right.

There has also been some improvement in accommodation. When I discarded my glasses I could not read the largest letters on signs across the street. Now these letters and other smaller ones are clear. I believe that eyestrain, continued through many years, has caused a spastic condition of the muscles of accommodation, and that with the relief of this strain accommodation will become normal. This may take six months or a year, but it will come.

Nearsighted as I am, I am able to see more clearly without glasses than I ever did with them. I have less trouble in getting about and no longer feel confused in the midst of street traffic. While I was wearing glasses I could never play baseball or take part in other sports, so that my friends thought that I was "just naturally studious." A short time after I gave up my glasses, I started to play "catch" with a tennis ball. It was hard work at first, and I usually missed the ball. The rapidity with which I improved was amazing. When I can see the ball against a plain background, such as the sky or a blank wall, I can now catch it nearly every time when it is thrown from a distance of even fifty feet or more. You bet I get a "kick" out of it! Within a year I expect to be playing tennis.

In my case eyestrain was accompanied by a rigidity of my whole body. The muscles of my neck, especially, were contracted, and I could turn my head only with difficulty. Whether this condition resulted from or helped to cause the eyestrain I do not know. At any rate, this stiffness in my neck has worn off as my eyes have grown better. About two weeks ago my neck relaxed. Now, for the first time in my life, I can move my head without effort and am no longer conscious of my body at every step.

I shall keep you informed as to my progress. This progress I owe to your book. I hope that it will help others as much as it is helping me.

Sincerely yours, Wm. R. Anderson, Jr.

REPORT OF THE NOVEMBER MEETING

By May Secor, Secretary

A regular meeting of the Better Eyesight League was held on November 11.

Dr. J. M. Watters of Newark, New Jersey reported cases of the following visual disorders which he has successfully treated during the past year by means of the Bates Method: myopia, hypermetropia, convergent squint, corneal ulcer, simple glaucoma, atrophy of the optic nerve due to syphilis, and central scatoma.

Ms. Frederick Schaefer presented a case of myopic squint in which there had been a decided bulging of the eye. Glasses were voluntarily discarded before the first lesson. Twenty-four hours after the initial lesson the bulging was almost entirely relieved. Two weeks' practice noticeably relieved the squint and improved the vision.

Dr. Bates spoke on the use of his method with children. To cure squint in an infant, Dr. Bates advised the mother to hold the child in her arms and sway, and also to move the child up and down. If the child is older, one may have him play swinging games, and dance; these forms of exercise are usually more effective if accompanied by music.

The Doctor reported a case of central scatoma in which there was no sight in the scatoma eye; parts of the eye were destroyed by disease. Dr. Bates treated the other eye to improve the vision, and at the end of two weeks was surprised to find that sight had developed in the scatoma eye. In this case normal vision was restored in both eyes.

Dr. Bates urged those present to bear in mind that his method is one of eye education. In order that cures may be permanent, it is essential that the patient shall live up to the Bates standard of relaxation, and consequently be free from eyestrain. If the patient permits his eyes to function normally the cure will be permanent.

SUPPLEMENT TO OCTOBER REPORT

Louise Talma, age 18; New York City; pianist; wore glasses 7 years—general use; voluntarily removed glasses June 10, 1924; obtained instruction from Dr. Bates' book and from officers at League meetings; June 10—read large "C" of Snellen card at 2 feet, and music at 3 inches; October 14—reads entire chart at 12 feet, and music at 11 inches.

QUESTIONS AND ANSWERS

Q–1. When palming and remembering black, is it advisable to keep the image stationary and to keep the same image, or is it just as good to shift from one object to another?

A–1. When palming and remembering black, one should imagine everything remembered to be moving and not stationary. It is necessary to shift from one image or from one object to another.

Q–2. My little son becomes fidgety while palming. Do you prescribe something else equally beneficial?

A–2. Your little son may become able to palm for a few minutes at a time. Sometimes swaying from side to side helps.

Q–3. I am presbyopic (old-age sight.) How can I improve my vision by reading fine print, when I can not even see it?

A–3. You can improve your vision for reading fine print by alternately remembering the whiteness of snow for a second while looking at the white spaces between the lines of print, then close your eyes and remember or imagine the same white more continuously, better and more easily. By alternating, you may become able to remember the white as well when flashing the card, as you can with your eyes closed with improved vision.

Q–4. I cured myself by following the directions in your book, but cannot seem to benefit my mother. She is near-sighted and doubtful of good results in her case.

A–4. The fact that you cured yourself by following the directions in my book makes it possible to cure your mother in the same way.

Better Eyesight
January 1925—Vol. IX, No. 7

SUN TREATMENT

It is a well-known fact that the constant protection of the eyes from the sunlight, or from other kinds of light, is followed by weakness or inflammation of the eyes or eyelids. Children living in dark rooms, where the sun seldom enters, acquired an intolerance for the light. Some of them keep their eyes covered with their hands, or bury their faces in a pillow and do all they possibly can to avoid exposure of their eyes to ordinary light. I have seen many hundreds of cases of young children brought to the Clinic with ulceration of the cornea, which may become sufficient to cause blindness. Putting these children in a dark room is a blunder. My best results in the cure of these cases were obtained by encouraging the patients to spend a good deal of the time out of doors, with their faces exposed to the direct rays of the sun. In a short time these children became able to play and enjoy themselves a great deal more out of doors, exposed to the sunlight, than when they protected their eyes from the light. Not only is the sun beneficial to children with inflammation of the cornea, but it is also beneficial to adults.

When the patient looks down sufficiently, the white part of the eye can be exposed by gently lifting the upper lid, while the sun's rays strike directly upon this part of the eyeball. In most cases it is possible to focus the strong light of the sun on the white part of the eyeball with the aid of a strong convex glass, being careful to move the light from side to side quite rapidly to avoid the heat. After such a treatment, the patient almost immediately becomes able to open his eyes widely in the light.

MENTAL STRAIN

By W. H. Bates, M.D.

It can be demonstrated that all persons conscious of imperfect sight have a mental strain. To try to do the impossible is a strain. It is impossible with the eyes closed to remember or imagine a small black area continuously black and stationary. Persons with perfect sight or a perfect memory, when trying to imagine a small black period stationary, notice an effort or mental strain very quickly, in a few seconds or less, while persons with imperfect sight or an imperfect memory may strain for a longer time before they become conscious of an effort. To concentrate the attention on a point for any great length of time usually causes discomfort, fatigue, or pain, in the eyes or elsewhere.

MYOPIA, OR NEARSIGHTEDNESS

Myopia, or nearsightedness, is caused by a strain or an effort to see distant objects. It can always be produced in the normal eye temporarily, or more permanently, by trying to see distant objects. With perfect sight the eyes and mind are at rest. All the sensitive nerves of the body are passive. Myopia is never continuous. At frequent intervals, lasting for a fraction of a second or longer, the patient is conscious of flashes of better vision. To test the facts, the retinoscope is reliable. When a patient with myopia looks at a blank wall without trying to see or remembers something perfectly, the retinoscope used at the same time demonstrates that there are periods of time when the eye in normal. This fact can be demonstrated in all cases.

Even patients with 30 of 40 diopters of myopia are not myopic all the time. This fact is offered as evidence that myopia, as described by many authors, is not a permanent condition of the eyeball. It can also be demonstrated that when the mind is at rest, and there is no mental strain when the patient remembers or imagines a letter, a color, or some other object perfectly, the myopia disappears. To have imperfect sight from myopia requires much mental effort, time, and trouble to produce it. Every person with myopia has to maintain a mental strain with all its discomforts, in order to maintain a degree of myopia. These facts suggest successful methods of treatment. Since mental strain or an effort to see distant objects is the cause of myopia, mental relaxation or rest is followed by benefit. By closing the eyes for five minutes or longer, while letting the mind drift from one thought, or memory, to another, slowly, easily, and continuously, rest of the mind is obtained, and when the eyes are opened, the vision is usually improved for a short time, or for a flash.

BLINKING

Blinking, in which the eyes are opened and closed frequently, is a great help, because the eyes and mind obtain a measure of rest when the eyes are closed, even momentarily. Many patients obtain a greater amount of rest by closing the eyes and covering them with the palms of one or both hands for a few minutes, or longer. We have to consider individuals because, while there are many cases benefited by palming for a half-hour or longer, there are others who do better when they palm for a few minutes only, or for short periods of time. Mental strain is usually unconscious. It is a bad habit. When myopic patients learn that they have this unconscious bad habit of mental strain, or when they find out what is the matter with them, it helps in the cure. When patients think it is no fault of theirs that they have imperfect sight, treatment becomes more difficult. To change the unconscious bad habit of mental strain to a habit of relaxation and rest requires that the patient consciously practices relaxation and rest until the conscious practice by repetition becomes an unconscious habit.

HYPERMETROPIA, OR FARSIGHTEDNESS

Hypermetropia, or farsightedness. The length of the eyeball is shortened in hypermetropia, which is the opposite of myopia. The cause of hypermetropia is a mental strain to see near objects. When a patient reads fine print with normal sight at twelve inches, with the use of the retinoscope at the same time it can be demonstrated that the eye is accurately focused for twelve inches. But when the patient fails to read perfectly at twelve inches or nearer, he usually feels the discomfort of mental strain, and the retinoscope demonstrates at the same time that the eye is focused for a greater distance than twelve inches. In all cases examined, the mental strain to see near objects produces not myopia, but just the opposite, hypermetropia.

When hypermetropia is not great enough to prevent reading fine print perfectly at a near point, the retinoscope demonstrates that the eyes are accurately focused for that distance. As occurs under similar conditions with normal or myopic eyes, the hypermetropic eye can only read perfectly without a mental effort. If the hypermetropic eye fails to read fine print perfectly, the retinoscope always demonstrates that the eyes are focused for a greater distance. The vision of the hypermetropic eye is improved by the same methods which improve the vision of the myopic eye. Since the cause of hypermetropia is a mental effort, its cure is obtained when the mental effort disappears.

Presbyopia

When the vision for the distance remains good while the ability to read at the near point fails, the condition is called presbyopia. In most textbooks, if not all, on the eyes, the statement is made that presbyopia begins soon after the age of forty, and increases gradually until the ability to accommodate is entirely lost. Most ophthalmologists have observed that sometimes presbyopia may begin before the age of forty, or it may not appear until a much later date. I have seen patients over sixty years old who had normal sight in each eye for the distance, and the ability to read the diamond type at six inches or less with each eye. A popular belief of the cause of presbyopia is that it is due to hardening of the lens, which prevents the lens from changing its shape. I have quite frequently published facts which demonstrated that the lens was not a factor in accommodation, and that the cause of presbyopia was a mental strain when trying to see or read at a near point. Such patients, when they read the distant test card with normal vision, feel comfortable, but when they plan to read the newspaper or fine print at twelve inches or nearer, they are conscious of mental strain or effort, and the greater the mental strain, the less does the patient see. Presbyopia is cured by practicing relaxation methods. Closing the eyes and resting them for five minutes or longer may enable some patients to read fine print at twelve inches or less in flashes. Very gratifying results have followed palming for an hour, or longer, in some cases, while in others palming was a failure. Any method which secures mental relaxation is always a benefit.

Presbyopic patients are often cured quickly by a perfect imagination of the halos, which are the white spaces between the lines of letters that appear whiter than the margin of the page.

Astigmatism

Astigmatism is caused by mental strain, and is cured by relaxation of the mental strain.

STORIES FROM THE CLINIC

No. 59: Mental Strain

By Emily C. Lierman

At one time a young man, age twenty-seven, came to us suffering from severe mental strain. His large staring eyes would make anyone uncomfortable just by looking at him. I approached him in the usual way, asking him what his trouble was. He smiled and said, "Now, that's just what I am trying to find out. Nobody seems to want me. Everybody thinks I am crazy." I answered, "You are wrong. I don't think you are crazy." Just the same, this poor fellow did make me feel sort of creepy. I was just a little afraid of him, but did not dare to show it.

He had much to say, but the main thing he wanted me to know was that he was not insane. When he calmed down a bit, I said, "Now let me say something. I know that you are staring so badly that if you don't stop it, you can easily become insane or blind." I wanted him to understand that I could not help him, nor anyone else, if he continued staring his eyes out of his head.

I asked Dr. Bates to examine his eyes and to tell me what treatment was best for him. The doctor said there was nothing organically wrong with his eyes, but that he was under a terrible mental strain. I understood very well what was before me when Dr. Bates said, "I think you had better knock on my door if the patient tries you too much."

After I had taken his name and address, I asked him where he was employed. His eyes protruded and he stared without blinking, as he answered, "Didn't I tell you that no one wants me? I cannot get any work. America is at war; does Uncle Sam want me? No, I have been to all the recruiting stations here in New York, and all of them have refused me. I want to fight for my country's flag, but they won't give me a chance." He actually wept, and I could not refrain from crying too. His mind was affected, yes, but when he was calm all he could think of was Uncle Sam and how he wanted to fight for him. I was not acquainted with him a half-hour when I understood easily enough why the United States could not use him. He demonstrated to Dr. Bates and to me very clearly that one can not have normal vision with a mental strain. I placed him ten feet from the test card and told him I wanted to test his vision. He answered, "I hope you will be able to improve my sight, because I think my nervousness will also improve."

He read a few lines of the card, but when he reached the 50-line he leaned forward in his chair, wrinkled his forehead, and his eyes began to bulge. At that moment a small mirror from my purse came in very handy. I held it before him, and the expression of his face changed immediately from strain and tension to a look of amazement.

He waited for me to speak, and what I said affected him terribly. He covered his face with his hands and wept. I kept very quiet, but touched his shoulder lightly to reassure him. When he raised his head a few moments later, he said, "Maybe that is why they refused me. I guess they saw what you saw. No wonder they thought I was crazy." I feared more hysteria, so I said that if he would let me help him, no doubt the United States Army would be glad to admit him into the service. He left the office after his first visit feeling very much encouraged. I could not improve his vision beyond the 50-line that day, and I decided not to test each eye separately. All I could record was 10/50 with both eyes.

One week later he came again. Apparently he had forgotten to practice anything he was told to do. His vision was still 10/50 with both eyes. I directed him to cover his one eye, and read the card with the other. His vision with each eye separately was the same, namely 10/50.

He told me that I had encouraged him so much that he tried again to enlist. I said, "You cannot expect to win out unless you take time to practice. This you must do all day long. When you tire of palming, keep your eyes closed and imagine something perfectly." While I was telling him all this, he had his eyes covered with his hands, and was moving his body from side to side, very slowly. What he did next certainly frightened me at first.

While his eyes were still covered, he asked me in a loud voice, "Do you mind if I sing 'America' while I am reading the card?" I answered, "No, but perhaps the other patients might object. Just wait a moment and I will ask the Doctor."

Dr. Bates said if singing was his way of relaxing, by all means let him sing. That was all that was necessary. This poor fellow sang every word without a mistake. After each verse he would stop long enough to read the card. After the first verse he read two more lines, 10/30. When he finished the hymn, he also finished reading the whole card without a mistake, 10/10. He blinked his eyes as he moved his body from side to side, and there came a great change in the expression of his face. I directed him to sing "America" when he practiced reading the test card at home every day. He left us in a very happy mood and promised to practice as he was told.

We did not hear from him for a whole year. One day there came a letter from him, written in Bellevue Hospital, but mailed by a friend outside. He stated in his letter that he was all right, although he was confined. He also explained why he was sent there. It seems that when he applied at a recruiting station for enlistment, they found his vision imperfect. When he insisted that if they would only let him sing "America," his vision would at once become normal, the officers of the recruiting station considered this statement so absurd that they believed he must be crazy.

He was sent to the insane ward of Bellevue Hospital, where he was promptly admitted. While there, he wrote a play of three acts, all about the doctors, the nurses and patients. It was well written, and after he had persuaded some of the doctors to read it, they recommended his discharge.

He called to see us and I found his vision was normal, 10/10. His mental strain was relieved and did not return except temporarily, when he became excited and talked rapidly.

A TEACHER'S EXPERIMENT

By Edith Wood, Allendale, New Jersey

Editor's Note—*This is a fine example of the results that can be obtained by teachers, parents and others, who have charge of children.*

In September, while testing the eyes of my pupils, I came across Stephen Bodnar, a boy of ten, who was apparently blind in his right eye. In testing him, I brought him so close that his nose almost touched the test card, and still he said he could see nothing. I concluded there was nothing to be done. Some days later the pupils were lined in the yard, when an idea came to me. I called Stephen to one side so that we would be out from the shadow of the building. I covered his left eye with his cap, and turned his face directly toward the sun. Then I asked if he saw anything. He said, "No, it is all yellow." Next I passed my hand back and forth so that the shadow would pass over his eye. He said, "It gets light and dark." I knew then that there was sight there, so I arranged with Stephen to come to my room at one o'clock the next day.

I fixed a shield for his good eye, and when he came next day, after adjusting the shield, I took him to the window and asked him what he could see out there. He replied, "Nothing." Next I took a manila card four by seven inches. Printed on it were the figures "6A^3." I had not planned to use the printing on the card. I merely passed it back and forth so that the shadow passed over his eye. In swinging the card I began close to his face, and gradually increased the distance, requesting him to let me know when he no longer saw the shadow.

When I got about two feet away from his face, he said he could not see the shadow any more. When I held the card at four feet, he said, "I can see you. You have on a dark dress, and it has light spots on it." I immediately asked him to look out of the window, and he saw the boys and girls moving about. He could also see houses and a tree.

The next day at one o'clock he came again, and we repeated the work of the day before. After a few minutes he said, "There are letters on that card." I held the card still and asked him if he could tell me the letters. He said there was a "6" and an "A," but he could not tell the smaller number "3," although he could see it was there. I put the card down, and asked him to look at me, and tell me what he could see. I had a gold watch, suspended from my neck by a black ribbon. He said, "You have a ribbon round your neck." I closed one eye and left the other open, and he told me what I had done. While I was fixing his attention on my face with my left hand I brought my watch out. He said, "I can see your watch." I said, "Be careful, Stephen, or I'll fool you. Isn't that a large yellow button?" "No, it's a watch, for I see a ring, and a ribbon fastened to it," he answered.

Next he looked out of the window, and he could tell what the children were doing and how many windows there were in the houses. I told him about palming and the long swing, and asked him to do them morning and night, which he said he would do. I remember that he astonished me so with what he could do, that I thought he must be peeking with the other eye. I tried to prevent him from turning his head, but he would do it, so I got behind him and held his head. He read just the same as before.

I have seen very little of Stephen of late. When I last saw him he could read the whole test card at eighteen feet, and he could read from a book held at the normal reading distance.

Stephen's progress at the start was so rapid that it astonished me. After about one week's work with the shadow, I dropped that and confined the work to the test card and the book. Had any one told me this story, I'm free to say that I would have been skeptical.

SUGGESTIONS TO PATIENTS

By Emily C. Lierman

While sitting, do not look up without raising your chin. Always turn your head in the direction that you look. Blink often.

Do not make an effort to see things more clearly. If you let your eyes alone things will clear up by themselves.

Do not look at anything longer than a fraction of a second without shifting.

While reading do not think about your eyes but let your mind and imagination rule. When you are conscious of your eyes while looking at objects at any time, it causes discomfort and lessens your vision.

It is very important that you learn how to imagine stationary objects are moving without moving your head or moving your body.

Palming is a help to you, and I suggest that you palm for a few minutes many times during the day, at least ten times. At night just before retiring it is well to palm for half an hour or longer.

NEW YEAR FAIRIES

By George M. Guild

A certain man had much money. One day he gave forty million dollars to charity, and had a lot left. He invited me to spend an evening at his home. He asked me if I would like to learn how he made his money. I answered, "No." "What would you like to talk about?" was his next question. I replied, "Although you seem to be well advanced in years, your hair is not gray and your eyes seem good, because I notice that you are able to read without glasses. How have you been able to preserve your eyesight all these years?"

He smiled and answered, "I do not know unless it was due to the influence of the New Year Fairies." He stopped and waited for me to say something. All I said was, "Tell me about it."

He let his mind drift away from me and his surroundings to a time long ago when he was a poor boy living on a farm. He told me that he had many brothers and sisters, all of them now dead. Christmas, one year, had been a very sorry affair. They had very little to eat, and their poverty was extreme.

New Year's Eve, as he sat by the open fire, a small boy of ten, he felt very hungry, very despondent, and very unhappy. He watched the flames of the burning wood, watched them grow larger, grow smaller, change their color, and as he watched, a fairy appeared in the light. She had the most beautiful eyes that he had ever seen. They were so bright, clear, full of sympathy and love, that he could not look away from them. She seemed to read his mind, and spoke encouraging words to him, which made him feel better. Then another fairy, all dressed in blue, a very beautiful blue, waved her hands to him, threw him a kiss and started to dance. While she was dancing, other fairies came out of the dark and danced with her. It seemed to him that wherever there was a spot of light, there was a fairy, many fairies, all of them with the same sympathetic, loving, blue eyes of the first fairy.

The memory of these eyes has never been lost. He said that he could see them now just as clearly as he did long ago. The memory of these eyes brought with it a wonderful feeling of rest, relaxation, and comfort. It seemed to him that those fairies brought a blessing which had helped him to accomplish many things which other people believed were impossible.

After he went to bed in the dark, it seemed that he could still see the burning fire and all those fairies with their sympathetic and loving eyes. When he awoke the next morning his attitude of mind was entirely different. He ran to each member of the family, his father, his mother, each sister and brother, threw his arms around them and wished them all a Happy New Year. He tried to dance as he had seen the fairies dance; he tried to smile as he had seen them smile; he tried to be as sympathetic and as kind to everybody as the fairies had been to him. He was all eagerness to be busy. Formerly he had shirked what little work was expected from him; but now he had an uncontrollable desire to get busy, to do things. He had no feeling of fatigue no matter how hard he worked, or how much he accomplished. His mother was amazed to have him fly around the kitchen and to help her in as many ways as he possibly could. He brought in more wood for the stove than could be used in a week. He ran to the barn and started in cleaning house. It was the first time in his life that he felt a desire to do something to help the horses, the cows, and other animals. He got busy with a few tools and fixed up the chicken-coop, stopped all the cracks so that the cold air would not blow on the chickens, and all the time he was thinking of those eyes of the New Year Fairies, because the memory of their love did him so much good.

He felt a desire to go to school, and tramped through the deep snow two miles to get there. The teacher was surprised to see him and asked him what he desired. "I want to go to school. I want to learn things. I want to be a big man. I want to make people happy."

The teacher smiled, gave him a desk, some paper, a pencil, and a few pages of a primer, and told him to copy as much of it as he possibly could. He used up a great deal of paper, and before school was out he had done something very wonderful, because he had copied all the pages that had been given him.

He told me that his health was always good, and as far as his eyes were concerned, he never gave them a thought. He knew that he could see well, but he was not conscious that he had eyes most of the time. When he was forty-five he had an attack of the grippe, from which he soon recovered, but when he tried to read the newspaper, he was very much alarmed to discover that his sight was very poor. He at once consulted an eye specialist, who told him that he needed glasses because all persons in middle life, past the age of forty, needed glasses.

He had some business to attend to which occupied his time for a few days. During that time he tried to rest his eyes by not looking at the newspaper. After avoiding any use of his eyes for reading for four days, they felt quite comfortable. Later he picked up a newspaper and was surprised to find that he could read it for a short time. When his eyes tired, he rested them, and he discovered that by reading the paper and alternately resting his eyes, his vision improved to normal.

At subsequent periods in his career he had similar attacks of being unable to read, which were always relieved by rest. He felt that as long as he could improve his sight by resting the eyes, it would be perfectly safe for him not to wear glasses.

"It may sound very peculiar to you," he said, "but I find that I can obtain perfect relief immediately when I remember the sympathy and love in the eyes of those New Year Fairies."

REPORT OF THE LEAGUE MEETING

By May Secor, Secretary

A regular meeting of the Better Eyesight League was held on the evening of December 9.

Ms. Hurty gave an exposition of the Bates Method. Agnes Herrington, a teacher in Erasmus Hall High School of Brooklyn, told of the great benefit she had derived from the use of this method. Ms. Herrington wore glasses for ten years; she has now discarded them, with the exception of occasional use to read very small figures. Dr. Bates advised those who experience difficulty in reading small print to relax by means of palming and swinging; this will relieve eyestrain, and the small print will become legible. Ms. Herrington found the following most helpful: sun treatment, blinking, and imagining a white cloud upon which is placed a black dot having a period on either side.

Mr. George Weiss reported several cases which are under treatment at Erasmus Hall High School. These cases are all showing marked improvement. One case has been cured of insomnia as a result of relief from eyestrain. Mr. Norman Bernat, a member of Ms. Hurty's eye group at Erasmus Hall, reported that by means of the Bates Method he has secured normal vision. For seven years he had used artificial lenses—one set for general use, one for reading, and one for "the sun." Mr. Bernat demonstrated the long swing in an unusually pleasing and relaxed manner.

Dr. Bates reported a case in which the patient was unable to see things moving. The Doctor requested the patient to look at the upper left-hand corner of the small square of the Snellen card, to sway, and to hold the corner stationary. The patient followed instructions, and a severe headache resulted; after this experience, however, she was able to see things moving. Dr. Bates explained that it is sometimes advisable to teach a patient how to use his eyes in the wrong way in order to effect a cure. Another case had occasional attacks of complete blindness. Dr. Bates taught this man how to consciously produce complete blindness; the lesson was a difficult one. The result, however, was complete relief from attacks of blindness. After his cure, the man served overseas; when he returned to New York his vision was still normal.

Dr. Bates treated one case which had been diagnosed by neurologists as insanity. This man had double vision at times, and frequently saw imaginary figures dancing on the top of tall buildings; it sometimes appeared to him, also, that men approaching him took off their heads and carried them under their arms. In this case a correction of the visual defects removed all apparitions and the man was recognized as normal. Dr. Bates spoke also of a little girl who attained very high visual acuity by means of central fixation, seeing best a part of each letter. The Doctor stated that floating specks are the result of imperfect imagination, and are a sign of strain.

ANNOUNCEMENT

We are pleased to announce that Captain C. S. Price of London, England will visit Dr. Bates around the latter part of January. He is planning to discuss with Dr. Bates the best methods which are employed for the cure of imperfect sight without glasses. The spread of Dr. Bates' method in England is largely due to Captain Price's enthusiasm and success in helping others. There are now two clinics, and a Better Eyesight League in England, all reporting favorable results. We are hopeful that Captain Price will attend the February meeting of the League.

QUESTIONS AND ANSWERS

Q–1. What is the difference between the long and the short swing?

A–1. In the long swing, objects appear to move an inch or more. In the short swing, objects appear to move an inch or less.

Q–2. My hands become tired when I palm. Can I sit in a dark room instead of palming? Can I cover my eyes with a dark cloth?

A–2. No. I have found this to be a strain.

Q–3. While palming, is it necessary to close the eyes?

A–3. Yes.

Q–4. When I read and blink consciously, I lose my place.

A–4. This is caused by strain, which prevents one from remembering the location of letters.

Better Eyesight
February 1925—Vol. IX, No. 8

CATARACT NUMBER

THE BABY SWING

Young babies suffer very much from eyestrain. The tension of the eye muscles is always associated with the tension of all the other muscles of the body. Their restlessness can be explained by this tension. I was talking with an Italian mother in the Clinic one day about restless children, and asked her why it was that her baby was always so quiet and comfortable when she came to the Clinic, while many other babies at the same time were very restless and unhappy.

"Oh," she said, "I love my baby. I like to hold her in my arms and rock her until she smiles." "Yes, I know," I said, "but that mother over there is rocking her baby in her arms, and the child is screaming its head off." "Yes," exclaimed the Italian mother, "but see how she rocks it."

Then I noticed that the other mother threw the child from side to side in a horizontal direction with a rapid, jerky, irregular motion, and the more she jerked the child from side to side, the more restless did it become.

"Now, Doctor," said the Italian mother, "you watch me."

I did watch her. Instead of throwing the child rapidly, irregularly, intermittently from side to side, she handled her baby as though it had much value in her eyes, and moved her not in straight lines from side to side, but continuously in slow, short, easy curves. The Italian mother picked up the other mother's child, and soon quieted it by thc same swing.

I learned something that day.

CATARACT

By W. H. Bates, M.D.

Cataract is a form of imperfect sight in which the lens of the eye becomes opaque. It usually begins after the age of fifty, and may progress in the course of a year or longer to complete blindness. In most cases perception of light can be demonstrated in all parts of the field. In many cases, cataract in one or both eyes is found at birth. There are also a smaller number of cataracts which appear after an injury to the eyes. Diabetes and other general diseases are believed to be a cause of cataract. As a rule cataract is progressive.

In 1895, a well-known ophthalmologist asked me, one of his assistants, to collect the histories of all cases of cataract which recovered without treatment. There were many such cases. It seemed to me that since recovery of cataract occurred without treatment, although the majority needed an operation for the removal of the lens before they were able to see, some form of treatment might help more of these cases. I sent some of my private patients to general practitioners who at that time by various methods did benefit these patients in quite a number of instances.

Not long afterwards I attended a meeting of the Ophthalmological Section of the American Medical Association, and listened to a paper on the treatment of cataract in which the writer declared that any doctor who claimed to cure cataract without an operation was a quack or something worse. I did not think he was right, and gave a talk on my experience, which produced something of a sensation.

More than forty years ago, when I was a student in a medical college, one of the professors gave a lecture on the eye. He had a number of nucleated eyeballs from the cow. He demonstrated that when the eyeball was squeezed with the aid of his fingers, an opacity or cataract of the lens at once appeared. I could see this more than twenty feet away. When the squeeze was relieved, the lens at once became apparently perfectly clear. I have repeated this experiment on the eyes of other animals without failure.

One day I was studying the eye of a patient with partial cataract. While the patient was talking of various things of no special consequence, I could see through several openings in the cataract, areas of a red reflex, which was evidence that the lens was not completely opaque. I asked the patient how much she could see, and while she told me the letters on the Snellen test card that she could read, the opacity of the lens was incomplete. She then made an unsuccessful effort to remember some of the smaller letters, when much to my surprise, the whole lens became opaque. I repeated the observation as follows:

I asked her, "Can you remember that you saw the big 'C'?" "Yes," she answered, and then at once the lens cleared in part, and I could see the red reflex through the open spaces.

Then I asked her, "Can you remember having seen any of the smaller letters on the bottom line?" I could see that she was making a considerable effort when the lens became completely opaque. I was so interested that I had a number of friends of mine repeat the experiment, and they were just as much astonished as I was when they obtained the same result.

So many patients are depressed, or become very unhappy, when they learn that they have cataract. The prospect of an operation, with its dangers and uncertainties, is too often a punishment. When an elderly patient with loss of vision is brought to me for treatment, the friends or relatives usually request me not to tell him that he may have cataract. For many years I followed this practice and just gave the patient glasses. I felt a great responsibility which I was always anxious to be rid of. I was ashamed of my cowardice. It was a great relief to have such patients consult some other physician. At the present time this has all been changed. I welcome cataract patients now and rejoice in the fact that they have cataract, because I am always able to improve the vision at the first visit, and ultimately cure them if they continue some months, or longer, under my supervision. Cataract is more readily cured than diseases of the optic nerve or retina. I believe that I am justified in telling the patients that the cause of the imperfect sight is due to cataract, because when they know what is wrong with them, they are more likely to continue to practice methods of treatment which are helpful.

The vision of every case of cataract always improves after palming, when the patient learns how to do it right. I have seen many serious cases obtain normal vision with the disappearance of the cataract by practicing the palming and nothing else.

It was a shock to me to see a case of traumatic cataract recover with the aid of palming. Cataract, occurring in patients with diabetes, has also disappeared without treatment or cure of the diabetes.

Treatment which is a benefit to cataract has for its object relaxation of the eyes and mind.

The quickest cure of cataract is obtained by the memory or imagination of perfect sight. It can be demonstrated that when the patient remembers some letter as well with the eyes open as with the eyes closed, that the vision is improved, and when the memory is perfect with the eyes open, perfect vision is obtained at once and the cataract disappears. This startling fact has been ridiculed by people who did not test the matter properly.

When the patient stares, concentrates, or makes an effort to see, the memory, imagination, and the vision always become worse. The patient and others can feel, with the tips of the fingers lightly touching the closed upper eyelid, that the eyeball becomes harder when imperfect sight is remembered or imagined. But when perfect sight is remembered or imagined, it can always be demonstrated that the eyeball becomes as soft as is the case in the normal eye. When the patient practices the swing successfully, or practices other methods which bring about relaxation of the muscles on the outside of the eyeball, it becomes soft, and the cataract is lessened.

After an operation for the removal of cataract, a thin membrane usually forms over the pupil of the eye, which impairs the vision. This membrane is called a *secondary cataract.* Sometimes another operation, a puncture through this membrane, is beneficial. In a recent case, a man, after the removal of the lens for congenital cataract, came to me for treatment. Without glasses his vision was 15/200; with convex 15.00 D. S., the vision was improved to 15/70+.

The patient hesitated about taking treatment at this time because he had heard that I always removed the glasses. He felt that on account of his work, he had better defer the treatment until such time as it was convenient to go without his glasses. I asked him if he would go without his glasses if I improved his vision so that he could see as well, or better, without them, as he was now able to see with them. He answered that he would do as I recommended. With the aid of palming, swinging, and perfect memory and imagination, the vision very promptly improved to 15/15.

STORIES FROM THE CLINIC

No. 60: Two Cases of Cataract

By Emily C. Lierman

So many times I have been asked, "Is it really possible to cure cataract by Dr. Bates' method?" I can prove that it is. In the March 1920 number of *Better Eyesight,* I wrote about a case of cataract under treatment at the Harlem Hospital Clinic. This case was a woman seventy-three years old who was determined to be cured without an operation.

In October 1916, she had visited another dispensary where an operation was advised. The doctors there told her, however, that she must wait until the cataract was ripe before the operation could be performed. Later she heard about Dr. Bates curing cataract without an operation, and tried out the method as well as she could all by herself. In March 1919, she visited Dr. Bates in his office, and he helped her.

This woman made her living by mending clothes in an orphanage, so we were glad to treat her in the Clinic where she did not have to pay. Three days a week she came, no matter how bad the weather was.

On her first visit she read the 40-line at four feet from the test card, then her vision blurred. She knew just what to do, and I did not have to tell her to palm. Just once she peeped at me through her fingers and said, "I'll fool the other doctors yet. My eyes won't have any cataract if I keep this up." She had a way of smiling out loud, and she still has. Her disposition has not changed a bit in all the time I have known her.

Recently she came to the Clinic to see me. In the room were two school nurses and a young man who were there to observe the cases under treatment. I was not so sure that my dear old lady had retained her improved vision, because I had not seen her for a year or more. I placed the test card eight feet from her eyes and she read every letter correctly up to the 15-line without the aid of palming. At times she read 10/10 after resting her eyes with the aid of palming and blinking.

The test I made this day was the best yet, because she read a card which she had never seen before. Then I placed her in the sun and gave her the Doctor's fine print card, which she held six inches from her eyes. She looked at me in a funny way, and said, "Oh, I can read that easily." Then she proceeded to read the diamond type to the amazement of the others in the room.

Someday I am afraid the little lady will get into trouble. Whenever she sees a child in the street wearing glasses, she gets very much excited. Recently she stopped two women with a child on the street and found fault with them because the little girl, three years old, was wearing glasses. "Why don't you take that child to my Doctor; he can cure her without glasses!"

Those who know our dear old lady can very well understand her good intentions, but how about the mother and friend of this little girl? They must have thought at first that she was of unsound mind. The women treated her kindly and accepted the *Better Eyesight* magazine which she offered them.

We had another case of cataract under treatment at the Clinic, a man sixty-three years old. He had to have someone to lead him when he first came, which was less than a year ago. After his fourth visit to the Clinic he was able to travel by himself. When Dr. Bates examined him with the retinoscope on the first day, he could see no red reflex in either eye.

I gave him a test card which he held very close to his eyes, and after he had palmed for a little while and imagined he saw the test card moving opposite to the movement of his body, he could make out the big "C" of the card at two inches from his eyes, but it looked very much blurred to him. Before he left the Clinic that day he became able to read several lines of the test card, and the letters cleared up which, of course, gave him a great deal of encouragement. What helped him so quickly was that he was quite sure we could improve his sight. He did exactly as he was told. Keeping up that steady swing of his body while standing, slow and easy, without any effort, stopped the staring, or prevented it. Palming and imagining his body was moving were a rest and relaxation to him also.

After he had been coming for a month or more, he became able to read all the letters of the test card as he held the card very close to his eyes. Three months later he was able to read the large letters of the card two feet away, and the 10-line letters of the bottom line at three inches from his eyes. Always when he came, which was every Saturday morning, he had something encouraging to tell us about his eyes. The signs in the subway on his way from Brooklyn became more clear and distinct. He was able to dodge people in a crowd. At the present time, even people with normal vision have to be mighty careful to avoid injury both in the street and in the subway.

It is now about ten months since this patient first came for treatment, and on his last visit he read very fine print at three inches from his eyes, and saw the 50-line letters more than a foot away. His vision improves by practicing with print much finer than diamond type, and his jolly disposition is also a great help.

It is a great relief to be able to say to a Clinic patient when he first comes to us, "You are welcome here for treatment, no matter where you live." At the Harlem Hospital Clinic, the authorities there turned away many poor souls who needed treatment of their eyes. Each district has a free hospital, and those who lived in another district were not admitted. While it was pitiful, it had to be so, because we could not take care of them all.

Here in our office also, we have to limit the number of patients treated in the Clinic, so we can only take care of patients who have no source of income, or who are sent to us by physicians.

STRAIN

By Emily A. Meder

We are often awed by the almost uncanny wisdom of the philosophers and teachers who lived centuries ago. After extensive experiments and research work, our scientists discovered certain properties in a drug, which proved invaluable during the War. It was later found out that this property had been used as an everyday remedy in Japan for centuries. It is well known that India possesses the secret of cures for various diseases, which our scientists would be glad to know of.

Dr. Bates has made the important discovery that all cases of defective sight are caused by strain, tension or rigidity of the eye and mind. There are a great many people who refuse to accept this fact, although their imperfect sight and perhaps other troubles are due to this cause.

Read what one Chinese sage wrote about strain many, many years ago, "In love or in hate, rigidity is final; in art fatal. Elasticity means life in the plants and flowers and trees, and in the wings of a bird, as in the mind. When the sap goes from the branches, they become rigid, and the storms break them down. When the artist's mind closes against the new ideas that are the mind's strength, as the sap is the trees, the brain becomes rigid and arid, and neither philosophy, poetry nor painting can be produced thereby."

"Rigidity and death are synonymous." The eyes have perfect sight when they are relaxed. It is not difficult; when there is an absence of strain, the eyes do nothing. They don't squint, or stare, or try to see.

When the eyes are relaxed, the body is relaxed, strain disappears, and the truth of Dr. Bates' discovery is proven.

CLINIC REPORTS FROM LONDON

We have heard from several of our English correspondents praising the work done by the Better Eyesight League of Great Britain and Ireland. We are pleased to publish one of Mr. Price's reports. Notice that all cases are accepted, including those with little perception of light, which have to be led into the office. A history of the progress of these severe cases proves the usefulness and need of this work.

A Man Blind in One Eye for Many Years

This is the case of a man who has endeared himself to all of us. He is a match seller in the gutter of one of our streets and partly because of his curly hair and partly because of his sunny smile we have christened him Curly. There are occasions when his cheeriness is of great assistance to the other patients.

His vision when first tested was 10/60 with the right eye and nothing whatever with the left. He had no perception of light in the left eye and said that he had not had for many years, and was told at the hospital that it was quite gone and nothing could be done.

His vision has improved to 10/50 and the left eye is much better and has quite a good perception of light. His near sight has improved more than his distant.

(We are in hopes that Captain Price can send us a further report of Curly's progress.)

Blind for Five Years

(This case should encourage those who have only slight perception of light.)

A few weeks ago there was lead into the Clinic a man of 65 who told us he had been blind for five years and the doctors at the hospital had told him nothing more could be done for him, as his case was hopeless. On testing his sight we found the right vision 3/80 and the left vision only just perception of light.

He was eager to know if we thought he could be helped and listened attentively while he was being told how to palm and how to strengthen his eyes by splashing them with cold water. He started right away palming and was left to amuse himself in this way while other patients were attended to, and afterwards he said his eyes felt rested and much easier. He was asked what he was to do at home during the week to see if he had remembered the directions given to him, and then went home in a very hopeful frame of mind.

The following week he came along and looked rather more cheerful and was very excited to tell us that he thought he could see a little with the blind eye. Both eyes were tested, the right one was now 3/60, and with the blind eye he could see the big "C," the 200-line when the chart was held close.

Two weeks later we held the Clinic in another room and we were amazed to see him walk boldly in alone. He was looking much better and very proud of himself. He had been under the doctor's care for the last two or three months as he was generally run down, and this week he was delighted to tell us that he had caught his doctor napping. His doctor had greeted him one morning by saying how much better his eyes were looking, how much brighter and more alive. "Yes, because I am having treatment for them," said our friend. He told the doctor of the treatment, whose reply was that it was rubbish and could not possibly do any good. "Well, you said yourself how much better they were looking, and they must look very different for you to notice them and remark on them, and besides I can see more than I did."

He continues to be very much in earnest and is now able to see 3/30 with the right eye, and can read the 40-line quite easily close up to the other eye which previously had only perception of light.

A Man Who Has Worn Glasses for 60 Years

This man, without his glasses, was very helpless. He had no vision at all with the right eye, just perception of light, but very slight. The left eye was such that he could read with difficulty the 60-line at 6 inches. In three weeks the vision with both eyes was improved, so that at 6 inches he could read the 20-line comfortably and the 15-line with difficulty. The right eye is better but the improvement is not so marked as that of the left. It is a great joy to help this man; he is so grateful for the smallest thing that one does, and his childlike faith and obedience is something rarely seen. The reason he has made so much progress in so short a time is due to the fact that he cooperates willingly and with pleasure and is really interested in getting his sight.

THE ELEPHANT AND THE FAIRIES

By George M. Guild

It is a fact that few of us realize that we have never seen a fairy wearing glasses. Why shouldn't they wear glasses? Little boys and girls wear glasses. Little boys and girls like fairies, yet it is unheard of for fairies to imitate what other people do, and wear those dreadful goggles which spoil the eyes and faces of beautiful young children. Many a fairy has whispered in the ears of children that glasses are bad. Many a fairy has whispered into the ears of a mother that glasses were an injury to the eyes, with the result that mothers who enjoy the society of their children are troubled about the glasses.

One evening after everybody had gone to bed, the father of a family sat in his chair dozing after he had read the evening paper. Many fairies came and whispered in his ears that glasses were bad for his children. He tried to argue the matter with them.

"Why shouldn't they wear glasses? The doctor says it

does them good. They cost a lot of money, and my children are all the time breaking them. But if it does them good, why shouldn't they wear them?"

The fairies remonstrated with him and told him that he could not see with his eyes, he could not see with his mind, and that he was just as blind as the five men were who tried to describe an elephant which they had never seen. "Well, tell me all about it," said he. So one of the fairies perched herself on his right shoulder, and told him the story which illustrated how wrong some people can be.

Once upon a time, many centuries ago, an elephant came to a small village where no person had ever seen such a creature before. Five blind men were coaxed with some flattery to give their opinion of the elephant.

One grasped the tail and declared, "The elephant is very much like a snake." The roar of laughter from the spectators upset him very much. The second blind man leaned against the side of the elephant and said, "The elephant is very much like a high wall." The applause of the mob was tremendous. The third handled one of the elephant's legs. "Yes," he said, "The elephant is very much like a pillar." The applause which followed bothered him. The fourth grasped one of the elephant's ears, and very solemnly asserted, "The elephant is similar to a fan." More applause and laughter greeted this opinion which also disturbed the blind man. The fifth felt of the sharp pointed tusks and said, "The elephant is very much like a spear." As an encore to the applause, he corrected himself and announced, "The elephant is like two spears."

The five blind men gathered together. The vigorous arguments of each blind man, to prove that he was right and that all the others were wrong, amused the populace for some hours.

The world is full of blind people who have eyes, and minds which do not see. The world is full of Good Fairies who teach us how to see with our eyes and minds.

The next morning the father told his wife all about his experience with the fairies, and when the children appeared for breakfast wearing their large rimmed spectacles, he saw how their eyes and faces were injured by them. His wife saw the same thing, and they both exclaimed in one breath, "Take off those horrid glasses, and never wear them again."

Then the little girl took off her glasses and dropped them in the wastebasket with a smile. The little boy dropped his on the floor and, with the heel of his heavy shoe, he smashed them into little bits, and laughed.

The father was astonished, and asked, "Why did you do that?" The little boy laughed loudly and cried, "Because I have got the best of the horrid things. They never did me any good. They hurt my eyes and kept me off the baseball team. I cannot tell you how glad I am to be rid of them." The little girl also was smiling, and they soon were all smiling, and they have been smiling pretty much all the time ever since.

REPORT OF THE LEAGUE MEETING

By Dorothy Maitland

The annual business meeting of the Better Eyesight League was held Tuesday evening, January 13.

For the benefit of the visitors, Ms. Hurty briefly outlined the work of the League and the part each loyal member takes in it. This is to improve his own vision and help others to improve theirs. The work with children was emphasized as being the most essential point in the League's work. Those in charge of children were asked to cooperate with the League in order to reach those children whose defective vision can be corrected at the start.

Ms. Hurty cited a case of a boy in her class last year who suffered with severe headaches. He received no special treatment but worked out suggestions with good results. He now claims Ms. Hurty cured his eyes and relieved his headaches entirely.

Dr. Bates gave us an interesting talk on cataracts. He explained that although all imperfect sight is due to strain, each defect is caused by a different kind of strain. When one has cataracts, the eyeballs become hard. Relaxation through swinging, a perfect memory or a perfect imagination softens the eyeball and the cataract disappears. Dr. Bates claims that nearly all cases of cataract are materially benefited at the first visit. Babies with cataracts have been cured when the mothers swayed them in their arms.

Have you learned to swing by means of your thumb? If not, try it now. Place your thumb and forefinger together and rub them lightly in a circular movement. When done correctly you will feel your whole body move and everything about you will seem to move.

An instance was cited of a movie director who carried a large diamond in his vest pocket and, unless he kept moving that diamond between his thumb and forefinger, he could not direct his cast. The gentleman who related the case realized the significance of it as soon as the thumb movement was explained to him, and he was very glad to tell us about it.

Perfect sight is natural and a normal condition, and those who have bad vision sometimes instinctively do those things which help them and improve their sight.

HELPFUL HINTS FROM CORRESPONDENTS

These are extracts from letters received from book readers and others. They might suggest new ways of improving your vision.

I am proud of my ability to eliminate headaches, fatigue, and even nausea resulting from eyestrain. I formerly retired to my room when one of my severe headaches came on, and required the entire household to be absolutely quiet. Now, if my head or eyes pain, I go to my room, palm for a few minutes, swing the card, and feel rested. The headaches usually disappear when I am relaxed. Another discovery! The headaches only come when I do something wrong. The last one was caused by late shopping, rushing to put the house in order, and cooking the whole dinner myself. When I slowly did the long swing (with the broom in one hand and a duster in the other), I grew calm enough to greet my guests pleasantly."

"I was shocked to discover that I was a starer. I knew that Dr. Bates advocated blinking to prevent the stare, and thought that I blinked and shifted constantly. Upon watching myself, however, I found that I only blinked when I remembered to do it consciously. I have made it a rule now to blink my eyes at the end of each line. This compulsory rule is becoming easier, and I believe that it will become a good habit real soon."

QUESTIONS AND ANSWERS

Q–1. What is most helpful when one is dreadfully nearsighted and finds it almost impossible to see without glasses?

A–1. Practice palming as frequently as possible every day. Keeping the eyes closed whenever convenient for five minutes ten times a day is also helpful.

Q–2. I notice that my squint eye does straighten after palming, but reverts when I stop. How can I tell when and how I strain?

A–2. Avoid staring after palming and blink all the time. You can demonstrate that staring is a strain by consciously doing it for a few seconds.

Q–3a. If glasses are harmful, how do you account for the benefit the wearer receives; 3b. Also, relief from headaches?

A–3a. Eyeglasses are harmful because the benefit received is not permanent; 3b. The mental effect of glasses helps some people, but the headaches are not relieved permanently and the vision is usually made worse.

Q–4. Why is fine print beneficial?

A–4. Fine print is beneficial because it cannot be read by a strain or effort. The eyes must be relaxed.

Q–5. How can I correct the vision of my three-year-old son, who won't palm and doesn't understand it? He is farsighted.

A–5. Make a test card with black letters on white paper. The letters are to be composed of "E's" pointing in various directions. These are to be graduated in size, from about 3 1/2 inches to a quarter of an inch. Have the child read them from 10 to 20 feet away. Have him blink constantly while telling in which direction the "E's" are pointing.

Better Eyesight
March 1925—Vol. IX, No. 9

THE ELLIPTICAL SWING

The normal eye when it has normal sight is always able to imagine stationary objects to be moving from side to side about one-quarter of an inch, slowly and without effort. This is called the swing. In order that the swing may be continuous, the movement of the head and eyes should be in the orbit of an ellipse (an elongated circular direction).

A patient, age seventy-seven, with beginning cataract in both eyes had a vision of 3/200 when she looked to one side of the card. When she looked directly at the card or the letters, she complained that she could not see them so well, or at all. She was recommended to practice swaying the body from side to side. Every time she moved to the right or to the left, she stopped at the end of the movement and stared, and that prevented relaxation. With the help of the Elliptical Swing, she obtained at once very marked benefit. Her vision was improved almost immediately when she looked directly at the letters, and her vision became worse when she looked to one side of the card.

A young man, age sixteen, was treated for progressive myopia for a year or longer. His vision improved for a time, then improvement stopped. Some months later his vision had not become permanently improved. Palming and swinging no longer helped him. I noticed that when he would move his head from side to side, he stopped at the end of the swing and stared. When he practiced the Elliptical Swing, his head and eyes moved continuously, and the staring was prevented. At once there was a decided improvement in his vision and this improvement continued without any relapse.

[The modern "Infinity Swing" is more beneficial. See "The Infinity Swing" in *Relearning to See*.—TRQ]

LIMITS OF VISION

By W. H. Bates, M.D.

The textbooks on the eye which have been published during the past hundred years or more state that normal vision is limited by the anatomical structure of the retina. They describe the size of the center of sight to be so small that it is not possible for the normal eye to see the line marked "20" on the Snellen test card at a greater distance than twenty or thirty feet.

It is well known that persons can read smaller letters, or letters one-half that size, at the same distance. It can be demonstrated that the small letter "o," with a white center which can be imagined to be whiter than the margin of the card, can be seen perfectly at any distance when one can imagine the white center perfectly white. Some patients become able to imagine such a letter perfectly at thirty feet, a vision of 30/10. Others can imagine the small letter perfectly at a distance of forty feet, 40/10, at fifty feet, 50/10. The perfect imagination of the letter "O," or of other objects, is always associated with perfect sight of other letters or objects not known.

Field. In many cases of imperfect sight not only is central vision lowered, but there is also a loss of the ability to see objects off to one side. Perfect imagination is a cure for an imperfect field. In some cases of imperfect sight not only may the whole field be limited in its extent, but also small areas of the field may be absent or modified. In some cases of disease of the optic nerve or of the center of sight, the patient's vision looking straight ahead may be imperfect or absent. Some cases of no perception of light in any part of the field have been observed in which the imagination of perfect sight has been followed by a prompt recovery. It is difficult to understand in some cases of destruction of the center of sight of the retina, with total or partial loss of vision, how the use of a perfect imagination has been followed by a permanent cure.

Night Blindness. Some persons with imperfect sight see better in a bright light than they do in a dim light, and some cases are so marked that they have been described as cases of night blindness. These cases are cured at first temporarily, later more continuously, by the perfect imagination of the letter "O" or some other object, as well in a dim light as in a bright light.

Day Blindness. Day blindness also occurs quite frequently. Some patients in a good light, with correcting glasses, may read only 20/100, but after the light is dimmed, the vision may become 20/10 without glasses. These cases are quite readily cured by the intelligent use of sunning. When the patient becomes able to imagine letters in a bright light as well as in a dim light, the vision becomes normal

Color Blindness. All persons with imperfect sight have an imperfect perception of colors. They may see large letters blacker than small letters, or the white spaces in the neighborhood of large letters whiter than the white spaces of small letters. Some patients will describe the color of the large letter "C" of the 200-line as blood-red, or they may see the large or small letters a shade of blue or yellow, or purple, or any color. The perfect imagination of one letter or other object is a cure in these cases of color blindness. Even cases of color blindness associated with diseases of the retina or of the optic nerve are cured by the intelligent use of the imagination. Persons born with color blindness are also cured in the same way.

Size. The size of letters of the Snellen test card or of other objects depends entirely upon the imagination. If the imagination is perfect, one may imagine the size of known or unknown letters at the near point or at the distance correctly. If the imagination is imperfect, the size of letters or other objects will be imagined incorrectly. It is interesting to observe that artists who are familiar with the sizes of things which they draw, very seldom present a perfect drawing of one object. A portrait painted by one painter may look entirely different from a portrait of the same person by some other artist. Most artists fail to make an accurate drawing of various objects because of the variation in their imaginations from day to day, or under different conditions of light.

A drawing may be made of a plaster cast which may appear all right when first completed, but may contain many faults when studied by the same artist at other times, in other places, or under a different light.

Treatment. It can be demonstrated that we see not the image focused upon the retina, but our interpretation or our imagination of this image. Imagination, when used properly, is the most satisfactory, most accurate, most helpful method that we know to obtain perfect sight. It can be demonstrated that if our imagination for something is as good at twenty feet, forty feet, sixty feet, or farther, as it is at a nearer point where we see it perfectly, our vision is just as good as our imagination. It can be demonstrated that it is only possible to remember perfectly what has been seen perfectly. We can only imagine perfectly what we can remember perfectly. We can only see perfectly what we can imagine perfectly. These facts can be considered to be true because there are no exceptions. The difference between a theory and the truth is only a difference of fact. A theory is not destroyed by any exception, but one exception destroys the truth. The truth admits of no exception. The only reason we cannot see a star with the naked eye as well as with the telescope is our lack of imagination. To improve the imagination it is first necessary to improve the memory; to improve the memory it is first necessary to improve the sight; to improve the sight it is first necessary to improve the imagination.

Halos. For example, persons with good sight appear to see the white spaces between the lines of fine print to be whiter than the margin of the page. It can be demonstrated that this is an illusion. We do not see illusions; we only imagine them. When the white spaces between the lines appear whiter than the margin of the page, we call these white spaces halos. Most of us believe we see them, and it is very difficult for many people to realize that the halos are not seen, but only imagined. The halos might be called the connecting link between imagination and sight. To see the halos is to improve the imagination, and the vision for the letters is also improved. One can improve the vision for reading not by looking at the letters, but by improving the imagination of the halos. To look at the letters very soon brings on a strain, with imperfect sight. To look at the white spaces and to improve their whiteness, is a benefit to the imagination and to the vision. One cannot read fine print at all unless the halos are imagined. By practice one becomes able to imagine or to see the halos more perfectly—the better the imagination, the better the sight.

STORIES FROM THE CLINIC

No. 61: Two Blind Girls

By Emily C. Lierman

Rosalie

One day a doctor asked me if I would help two blind girls that he knew. I said I would be glad to see them and help them if I could. One was Eleanor, age sixteen, and the other, Rosalie, age seventeen.

Dr. Bates examined their eyes with the retinoscope, and this is what he found. Eleanor had myopia in the right eye and atrophy of the optic nerve in the left eye. This is very seldom or never cured. There was a good deal of inflammation inside of both eyes.

Rosalie had retinitis pigmentosa in both eyes, and could not count fingers in an ordinary light. This is also a very serious defect. In a very strong light she could at times count fingers if held close to her eyes. Rosalie would cure anyone of the blues because she carried a smile that was continuous. She had black curly hair and olive skin. I held a conversation with her for a few minutes purposely in order to get acquainted, and also to watch her eyes while she was talking. The first thing that I noticed was that she stared and kept both eyes open all the while she was talking. I did not see her blink at all. She had a habit of talking rapidly, and I noticed that she moved her eyes from side to side about at the same rate that she spoke. This is called nystagmus. I held the pothooks card with the letter "E" of different sizes pointing in various directions close to her eyes, and she said I was holding something white before her.

I asked, "Do you see anything else on the card?" "No," she answered.

Then I placed the palms of her hands over her closed eyelids and told her that this was palming. I told her that it was necessary to remember agreeable things, and she said she could easily remember her music. I could well believe that because she already had a good reputation as a pianist. She had won the district bronze medal, the highest reward she could obtain in her school. After she had palmed a while, ten minutes, I held the test card close to her eyes and asked her what she saw. She said the white card was covered with black spots. Quickly I told her to palm again for a short time. After about five minutes I told her to look at the card again, and this time she recognized the large "E" of the 200-line. We all rejoiced, because the rapid movement of her eyes from side to side had stopped temporarily.

Then I placed the card on my desk about a foot away from her, and told her to palm again. When she opened her eyes later she saw the 100-line letters.

The next time she came I placed her two feet away from the card. After palming a short time she read the 70-line letters. She palmed again, and this time her vision improved to 2/50.

The chaperon for the two girls did not realize that it was possible for Rosalie to read the alphabet or to read figures. She taught Rosalie at my suggestion. Her vision improved after six visits to 1/40 for the pothooks, the letter and figure cards. The nystagmus had disappeared permanently. I am sorry that she was unable to visit me until she was cured.

Eleanor

Eleanor's vision with each eye was 3/100. Her vision was improved by palming and by the long swing. She could make out figures much easier than letters, so I placed the figure test card at five feet from her eyes. While she was moving her body from left to right, she was told to glance at the figure I was pointing at. She was told not to look at the figure longer than a second, otherwise she would be tempted to stare, and her vision would be lowered. She practiced this for a few minutes and her vision with both eyes improved to 5/50. Her left eye, which had atrophy, was greatly relieved by the sun treatment.

Every time she came for treatment, which was once a week usually, her vision improved for another line of the test card. Changing cards helped to improve her vision also. After the regular "C" card was used, we tried the pothooks card. Eleanor never had anything to say, but did just as she was told. When her vision improved and she became able to read small letters and figures, she would smile and become very much excited. In one week's time her vision improved to 6/20 with both eyes. Then I gave her small type, called diamond type, and asked her to hold it six inches from her eyes. She could see black spots on the little card, she said, but nothing more. I gave her the sun treatment for a few seconds, and right away she became able to read the fine print.

Later we used a black card with white letters, which Eleanor liked very much. I placed it ten feet away from her and I noticed that she turned her head over to one side in order to read the letters. The distance of only one foot caused her to strain while trying to read the strange card. I directed her to swing and blink as she flashed the white letters I was pointing at. In less than a half-hour she read the letters one line after another with her head perfectly straight. She was given the sun treatment about six times in one hour and was encouraged to read the card after each treatment, and before she left me her vision had improved to 6/20.

I did not see her again for a few weeks, and I feared that she would not get along so well by herself. When I saw her again she surprised me by reading all the different cards she had practiced with and she was able to keep her head perfectly straight. Her vision had improved to 6/10. Eleanor plays the violin and sings. Always when I guided her in reading the card with her head straight, I reminded her of her violin and how well she could play something that she knew. This always helped to improve her vision.

Eleanor and Rosalie left the city for a time, and I did not see them again.

REPORT OF THE LEAGUE MEETING

By Mabel A. Young, Secretary

The regular meeting of the Better Eyesight League was held on Tuesday evening, February 10.

The speaker of the evening was Captain C. S. Price of London. He said that there is a Better Eyesight League of many members in England, but that they do not hold regular meetings, as is done here. Each member is doing definite work. Having no direct contact with Dr. Bates, they have gained their knowledge of his methods from an intensive study of his book. It is interesting to note that the different workers, more or less isolated, gained similar results by different methods.

The members of the English League have tried to avoid anything that would cheapen the work. They try to hold it above any idea of empiricism or quackery, and take their work where they find it near at hand. They first cured their relatives and neighbors. They worked for results, got them, and the news has spread.

Captain Price spoke more particularly of his own work, and that of his colleague, K. Beswick. He said that back of all eye troubles are mental factors. He has given much thought to the psychological side of this work. People need, first of all, to be made to realize the value of sight. Relaxation is a prime necessity, and the ways of securing it are numerous. No two patients respond to treatment in the same way. The teacher must approach them on their own ground. He would not use the same method with an artist as with a mathematician. The body must also be considered as a whole, and the eye as a part of the body. Very poor people commonly live under conditions which make relaxation impossible, and many of them visit the Clinic and ask to be allowed to merely sit there and rest. A tired person must rest before he can relax.

Thousands of poor patients are treated in the free Clinic each year, some of them having been discharged from the hospitals as incurable. Myopia is rare among them, and cataract and blindness are common. The work was first carried on in institutions, but as its unorthodox character became known, Captain Price and Ms. Beswick were debarred from working there. The patients followed them, however, and visited them in their free time at the office.

Captain Price described several cases. One man had his eye removed by an operation. The other had not been used for eighteen years, and had atrophied. After six weeks practice, the patient was able to open the lids an eighth of an inch. The eye when seen was a horrid looking mass—inflamed and sunken. It is now fully developed, has perception of light, and he can distinguish colors.

A lady who had been blind eight and a half years from glaucoma, and who had been discharged from the hospitals as incurable, now plays cards without glasses and takes her friends to see the shops.

Captain Price's talk was followed by a discussion, when he answered the members' questions. Dr. Darling, Dr. Achorn, and Mr. Husted spoke, the latter telling of his wonderful success with this method in the schools. Ms. Lierman described several interesting recent cases from her Clinic.

THE TWO PRINCES

By George M. Guild

A young prince and his brother were confined in a tall, stone tower far away from their home. The jailer had received orders to feed them very little, and if they died he would receive a big reward. Under these circumstances the two princes did not have an enjoyable prospect. Both of them were famous throughout the kingdom because they had seen fairies.

Furthermore, they had taught other young children how to see fairies. They spent a great deal of their time in the top of the tower looking for the fairies in the distant woods and in the green fields close by. This improved their sight and the improvement in their vision was followed by an improvement in their ability to remember, imagine, and to plan things to help other people as well as themselves. If you look for the fairies, sooner or later you will see them. The desire to see the fairies is a great benefit to the eyesight. They wrote many letters to their friends asking to be rescued. The fairies visited the young princes frequently, and advised them to treat the jailer very kindly and to notice the result. It was not long before the jailer, under the influence of the kind treatment recommended by the fairies, treated them better than most fathers treat their children.

One day, as they were looking out of the window high up in the walls of the tower, they saw coming towards them an army of children. It seemed that all the musicians in the country were with them. The dancing and the laughter were very considerable. When the children reached the tower, without the permission of the jailer, many of them rushed in and overflowed the place. Those who couldn't get in, stayed outside and made an awful lot of noise. Suddenly from the woods an army of fairies appeared, all dancing and singing and happy as they could be. The children welcomed them, clapped their hands and invited them to dance on the green. While the fairies were dancing and the children were trying to imitate them, the princes came down from the tower and danced with them. The jailer was so taken up by the unexpected attentions of the children that he forgot all about his prisoners.

One of the fairies said, "Let us play 'Follow the leader'." She started off to run, and all the others behind her, but there were so many that they lost the leader and found themselves just going back toward London.

About this time the jailer appeared, and in a loud voice

called out that he had something to say. So they placed him on top of a pillar where he could be seen by everybody. "My friends," he said, "I am only a poor jailer. Some wicked men in London came to me and offered me money to murder the two princes, because after they were killed their cousin would ascend the throne. But the fairies treated me so nicely and the princes treated me so nicely that instead of being their enemy, I am now their friend. Follow me to the house of those wicked men, and we will put them in a jail from which there is no escape."

All the men and women and the fairies and the children followed him to the house where the wicked people lived, and they were all dragged out and thrown into jail and placed under the care of the jailer. Then the princes and the fairies and all the people rushed up to the palace of the king and queen, and drove away the wicked soldiers who were holding them prisoners. The two princes were restored to their parents and there was great rejoicing. The king and queen felt very much indebted to the fairies because it was through their activity that things had all turned out so well. The two princes improved their sight very much by looking for the fairies; and the eyesight of the children in the kingdom was improved because they had to imitate the princes and be in the fashion.

READ FINE PRINT

All of our imperfect sight is just the result of our using our eyes wrong, and permitting bad habits to grow on us. Staring is only a bad habit, but it causes a great deal of trouble. When it is stopped and the eyes are rested by palming and blinking, the sight is immediately benefited.

Bad habit number two—The reading of large type in preference to finer print. It requires more of an effort to see a large letter than a small one, strange as it may seem. When you look at the big "C" on the Snellen test card, you don't see it all at once. You have to look at one part best, the hook on the upper right-hand corner or the curve on the left side. You cannot look at the hook, the space on the right and the curve on the left side all at once. Some people think they see it at the same time, but they do not. Their eyes shift from one point to another, unconsciously.

Fine print is a benefit because it cannot be read while the eyes are under a strain. They have to be relaxed. For instance, in reading the chapter printed below, you cannot accomplish anything by staring at the letters, or screwing your face into a knot. Do not look at the letters but at the white spaces between them, and imagine them whiter than the margin. Blink and shift constantly to avoid the stare. If your eyes feel strained, stop and palm. You will notice that where it all looked blurred before, a word will appear clear and distinct. By constant practice more words clear up, until the entire chapter can be read easily.

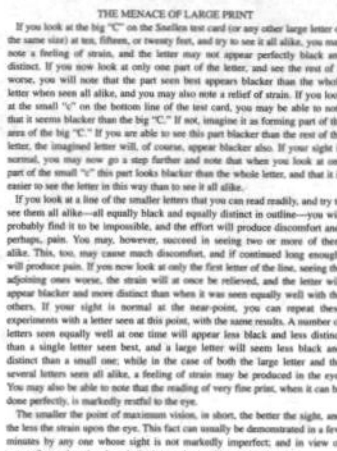

THE MENACE OF LARGE PRINT

If you look at the big "C" on the Snellen test card (or any other large letter of the same size) at ten, fifteen, or twenty feet, and try to see it all alike, you may note a feeling of strain, and the letter may not appear perfectly black and distinct. If you now look at only one part of the letter, and see the rest of it worse, you will note that the part seen best appears blacker than the whole letter when seen all alike, and you may also note a relief of strain. If you look at the small "c" on the bottom line of the test card, you may be able to note that it seems blacker than the big "C." If not, imagine it as forming part of the area of the big "C." If you are able to see this part blacker than the rest of the letter, the imagined letter will, of course, appear blacker also. If your sight is normal, you may now go a step further and note that when you look at one part of the small "c" this part looks blacker than the whole letter, and that it is easier to see the letter in this way than to see it all alike.

If you look at a line of the smaller letters that you can read readily, and try to see them all alike—all equally black and equally distinct in outline—you will probably find it to be impossible, and the effort will produce discomfort and, perhaps, pain. You may, however, succeed in seeing two or more of them alike. This, too, may cause much discomfort, and if continued long enough, will produce pain. If you now look at only the first letter of the line, seeing the adjoining ones worse, the strain will at once be relieved, and the letter will appear blacker and more distinct than when it was seen equally well with the others. If your sight is normal at the near-point, you can repeat these experiments with a letter seen at this point, with the same results. A number of letters seen equally well at one time will appear less black and less distinct than a single letter seen best, and a large letter will seem less black and distinct than a small one; while in the case of both the large letter and the several letters seen all alike, a feeling of strain may be produced in the eye. You may also be able to note that the reading of very fine print, when it can be done perfectly, is markedly restful to the eye.

The smaller the point of maximum vision, in short, the better the sight, and the less the strain upon the eye. This fact can usually be demonstrated in a few minutes by any one whose sight is not markedly imperfect; and in view of some of our educational methods, is very interesting and instructive.

[A 2-point reduction of the first part of "The Menace of Large Print" article from the December 1919 issue has been substituted for the original reduction of "St. Matthew's Beatitudes."—TRQ]

QUESTIONS AND ANSWERS

Q–1. Explain what you mean when you say "imperfect sight, imperfect memory."

A–1. If you see an object imperfectly, blurred or gray instead of black, you cannot remember it perfectly. You will remember it as you see it.

Q–2. My eyes feel fine after I palm and let my mind drift on various black objects. The period is more difficult though.

A–2. Perfect mental pictures of ordinary objects means a perfect mental picture of a period. To try to see is an effort or strain, and produces defective sight.

Q–3. By blinking do you mean shutting and opening the eyes quickly, or is done slowly, like a wink?

A–3. Blinking is done quickly, and not slowly like a wink. Watch someone with perfect sight do this unconsciously, and follow his example.

Q–4. How can one overcome the stare if it is unconscious?

A–4. Blink consciously, whenever possible, especially when reading. Never look at an object for more than a few seconds at a time. Shift your attention.

Q–5. I have noticed when I palm that my eyeballs hurt from the pressure. When I loosen this tension the light filters in.

A–5. Palming is done correctly with the fingers closed and laid gently over each eye, using the palms like a cup. If this is done properly there is no pressure and the light is shut out. [It is not essential to shut out the light completely.—TRQ]

Better Eyesight
April 1925—Vol. IX, No. 10

FLOATING SPECKS

When a patient stares or strains to see by looking at a light-colored surface he may see, or imagine he sees, floating black specks, strings of black thread or small light-colored globules resembling tears. The floating specs may be apparently a quarter of an inch or more in size and they may be of any shape.

The ability to see or imagine floating specks may occur in children or in adults of any age. Some children have been known to lie on their backs on the ground, look up at light colored clouds and amuse themselves for hours by watching what appeared to be floating specks.

Many nervous people have been made very unhappy, consciously or unconsciously imagining that they see these floating specks.

The cause of floating specks is an imperfect memory of perfect sight. Persons with normal vision who have never been conscious of floating specks can be taught how to imagine them by straining—to imagine letters, colors or other objects imperfectly.

Conversely, patients who are conscious of floating specks are unable to imagine them and perfect sight at the same time.

In the treatment of floating specks it is important to convince the patients thoroughly that they are only imagined and not seen. It helps very much to impress on the patient's mind that to see these floating specks requires a sufficient strain to lose a perfect imagination of all objects seen, remembered or imagined at all times and in all places.

Note.—Floating specks, October, 1919, *Better Eyesight*.

Muscae volitantes (floating specks), pages 176 and 236, *Perfect Sight Without Glasses*.

[I am aware of three common types of floating specks. The first type is small debris floating randomly in the eye, which some claim to be remnants of blood vessels that are in the center of the eye in the early stages of fetal development. This is likely the type of floating specks experienced by most people. Generally, the less this first type is thought of, and the better the sight, the less they are seen. The mind tends to disregard them when sight is used correctly.

The second type is larger debris, also floating randomly, which may be due to an accident to, or disease of, the eye. (See also "Retinitis Pigmentosa" in the September 1929 issue for "floating spots" in the vitreous humor.)

The third type is blood corpuscles that travel through the veins and arteries located in the top layers of the retina. In certain bluish-purple lighting situations (like certain types of sky light), these corpuscles can be seen traveling along specific paths (through the blood vessels) and can even be observed to pulse rhythmically along these paths synchronized with the pulse of your heartbeat! Since there are no blood vessels above the fovea centralis, these corpuscles are only observed in the peripheral vision. There is an exhibit at the San Francisco Exploratorium where the corpuscles can be observed flowing through these blood vessels in your retina!—TRQ]

QUICK CURES

By W. H. Bates, M.D.

Quick cures are desirable. At the same time let me hasten to state that we must use the word "cure" with great care. It means a great deal more than most physicians realize. A patient's definition of a cure is more complete, more thorough, and more lasting than he realized or remembered at his first visit.

To promise any patient a cure is unwise from a scientific standpoint. In my work I take particular pains to make the patient understand that I do not expect or guarantee a cure in any case. The most I say to them is "Yes, I have cured people much worse than you, but that is no guarantee that I can give you the slightest benefit."

This seems to eliminate a certain amount of subconscious antagonism on the part of the patient, who may consciously say that he desires to be cured, but deep down in his heart feels unconsciously, "I don't believe you can do it with my help, and I am quite sure you can't do it if I oppose you."

Like the Irishman who said, "He was willing to be convinced, but he would like to see the man who could do it."

Quick cures have their disadvantages. A patient feels that since his benefit came easily, now, with his good sight, he can go off at any time he likes and have a spree, in which he stares and strains and uses his eyes to his heart's content without any danger of a relapse. He forgets that all persons with normal vision can acquire imperfect sight at any time. The attending physician must be on his guard when referring to those patients who have been cured quickly, and not give the impression that it is an easy thing to do, because too often those patients who know about quick cure cases expect to be cured themselves in the same way as quickly and as permanently. If they are not, they are disappointed, and they have a way of expressing that disappointment which hurts. Personally I am very much upset every time a patient surprises me with a quick cure, because of the favorable criticism which may follow and which is seldom desired by the attending physician. If we could only practice quick cures in favorable cases and not have to struggle with the obstinate ones, things would get along perhaps better.

It is well to bear in mind that most quick cures happen when least expected and we do not always know what particular thing accomplished it.

One question is often asked, "What kind of cases are most quickly cured?" I do not believe that we have sufficient facts to answer this question at all intelligently, because mild cases of imperfect sight may require long periods of time—years before recovery, or a permanent recovery, occurs. I have a number of patients whose amount of imperfect sight is very small, indeed, and yet after some years of more or less continuous treatment they are still not permanently relieved. In other cases a large amount of nearsightedness or farsightedness, without any special reason, practicing the same method of treatment, would obtain a permanent cure at one visit. I wish I knew why.

Quite a number of patients with imperfect sight for the distance, and also unable to read the newspaper at a near point, have been permanently cured after a half-hour or more of palming. Other cases have practiced palming apparently just as faithfully without much if any relief after many months. It would be perhaps a good thing to know why palming was so very beneficial in some cases, while in others the benefit was imperfect.

One patient, 60 years old with imperfect sight from cataract, whose vision was not improved at all by glasses, obtained normal vision without glasses at the first visit. The cataract and all the other troubles disappeared almost immediately after palming. It was interesting to learn that this patient had worn quite strong glasses for nearly fifty years. During this time even with his glasses he suffered pain, fatigue and other discomforts. He told me that all he wanted or that he would be satisfied with, was the cure of the cataract so that possibly, with glasses, he could do his work. The very thought of it made his face brighten, but when after palming he obtained not only a cure of his imperfect sight but of every other symptom he could remember, he certainly was grateful and he showed it in his face.

Another patient said he was 106 years old. His vision for distance was poor and he was unable to read fine print with or without glasses. He had cataract in both eyes, so opaque that no red reflex could be seen in any part of the pupil with an ophthalmoscope. He was placed in a dark room and told to close his eyes and keep them closed. At the end of a half-hour his vision was improved to 10/10 and he read diamond type at six inches without glasses. He was told to repeat this treatment frequently during the day in order to avoid a relapse. He came back at the end of a week with his vision still further improved. As he went out of the office without an attendant to guide him, he stopped and spoke the only words I ever heard him say, "Doctor, you did me good." I wish I knew what I did or did not do. It would be a great satisfaction to me to find out how the patient by closing his eyes for a half-hour improved his sight so much and so quickly. A large number of other patients have been told the same thing; the same words were used as were spoken to him, but the results were seldom repeated.

It is well to emphasize that under the most favorable conditions quick cures are exceedingly rare. They generally occur when least expected, but when they do occur the definition of the word "cure" includes a great many more benefits than the patients expect.

One of the quickest cures I ever had was in the case of a very ignorant man who was suffering from sympathetic ophthalmia. At school, he told me, he could never understand fractions, and yet I found that he had the most wonderful imagination in my experience. Although he could not tell the big "C" at ten feet, when I brought it up close to him he said that he could imagine it and could imagine it perfectly. Knowing that it was a big "C," he was able to imagine it perfectly at ten feet, and when I told him that the first letter on the line below was an "R," he became able almost immediately to imagine it so perfectly that he could imagine he saw a letter "B" on the same line, and a letter "T," the first letter on the line below. He kept insisting that he did not see any of these letters. He only imagined them.

When I pointed to the first letter on the bottom line he said it all looked black. When I told him that the first letter was an "F," at once he said he could imagine it perfectly, and much to my surprise, after the perfect imagination of that letter "F," he became able to imagine in turn the other letters on the bottom line which he did not know. He kept insisting that he did not see these letters—that he only imagined them. But always when he imagined perfectly one letter on the Snellen test card, the whole card became clearer and perfectly distinct and he could see or distinguish neighboring letters which he did not know. His imagination improved his sight to normal. To walk around the room without running into the furniture and to see surrounding objects, all he had to do was to imagine one letter of the alphabet perfectly.

Many of my patients have been teachers in the various universities, have the highest intelligence and are authorities in their fields, yet whose imagination of mental pictures was very poor.

STORIES FROM THE CLINIC

No. 62: Quick Cures

By Emily C. Lierman

Patients who are cured quickly of imperfect sight are those who become able to improve their memory and their imagination quickly and without effort. A little girl named Madeline, age ten years, came with her mother, who was very anxious to have her child cured without glasses. The mother had been notified by Madeline's school teacher that her little girl could not read correctly what was written on the blackboard from her seat, which was about ten feet away. She was one of the daintiest little girls I have ever seen. I can imagine her as one of the white fairies written about in our little magazine, which I believe a great many children enjoy. I feel sure that there are many mothers among our subscribers and that they realize the relaxation and rest which is given to the child-mind as the mother reads about the good fairies just before the sandman comes.

This is how Madeline was cured in one visit. She was placed ten feet from the test card and she read all the letters correctly down to the 20-line, 10/20, but the letters were not clear and black to her. She was told to palm for ten minutes or so. Then she read the card again, and this time the letters appeared clear and black. The mother was told to notice how she stared when trying to see one of the smaller letters of the 15-line. I told Madeline she must blink her eyes all the time to prevent staring, which always lowered the vision. As she glanced at the letters each time she moved to the left and then to the right, not forgetting to blink her eyes, her vision improved to 10/10. She was placed in another room, fifteen feet from another card, which she had not seen, and without a stop she read all the letters of the card. Now, I wanted to find out if I could improve her vision further with the aid of her memory. I told her to close her eyes and palm and remember something she had seen without effort or strain. She answered, "I cannot think of anything just now, and the more I try the less am I able to do as you ask me." I asked her then to tell me what lesson she liked best at school. "Oh! I just love arithmetic," she said. I asked her if she would add up some figures for me while she was palming and she answered, "Yes." I started with easy figures at first, like nine, three and eight. She added as quickly as I announced the figures. Then I made the lesson more difficult, but she did not once make a mistake. All this time she was smiling and enjoying the whole thing. We kept this up for about fifteen minutes, and then while her eyes were still closed, I moved the test card as far away as I could place it, which was eighteen feet. Madeline was told to remove her hands from her eyes and stand and swing as she did before. She read every letter on the card correctly. Her vision had improved to 18/10 by the aid of her memory for figures.

Madeline was cured quickly because she was able to remember figures perfectly. Her mental pictures of them were perfect. Her mind was relaxed, and by the aid of the swing and remembering to blink often, as the normal eye does, she had no more eyestrain.

A little boy, age seven, was brought to me not long ago. His nurse, who was extremely fond of him, did not want glasses put on the little fellow. He told me very emphatically that he just would not wear them. No one would dare put them on him, he said.

His little forehead was a mass of wrinkles as he tried to read even the largest letters of the test card at ten feet. I asked the nurse to sit where she could watch him at the start and then see the change that I was sure would come to his face after he was taught to read without effort or strain. With each eye separately he read 10/50. As he tried to read further he wriggled and twisted his little body around in the big armchair where I had placed him.

"Now," I said, "little man, just close your eyes and place your hands over them and shut out all the light. Sit still, if you like." "Oh," said he, "I like sitting still if I keep my eyes covered, but I don't like doing it too long." I said, "All right, keep them covered for a little while and I will read you a fairy story that tells something about the elephant, too."

That was all that was necessary. My patient sat perfectly still as I read the whole fairy tale. The nurse remarked that for a long while he had not been able to sit still for more than five minutes at one time.

After the fairy story was read, I told the little chap to stand, feet apart, with eyes still closed, and I guided him in moving his body from right to left until he became able to do it gently by himself. Then he was told to open his eyes and keep moving or swinging his body to the right and then to the left. He was directed to blink his eyes while doing this. He exclaimed, with great surprise, "My, the card and letters seem to be moving opposite." I said, "That's right, my boy; now follow my finger as I point to the letters." He did, and to our surprise he read the whole card without a mistake, 10/10. The wrinkles in his forehead were gone. I told the nurse to help him many times every day with the test card just as I did. She promised also to bring him back to me if he had any relapse. So far I have not heard from her. I do believe my little boy was cured in one visit.

HUNGRY FAIRIES

By George M. Guild

Once upon a time, a young man, a reporter, found himself in a Southern city without a cent of money. He desired to take passage on a steamboat for New York. As the time came for the boat to sail, and not having met anyone he knew, he finally plucked up sufficient courage to talk to the Captain about it. The Captain listened in sympathetic interest, being one of those jovial, happy kind of people who are often interested in somebody else besides themselves, and interrupted the reporter and asked him, "What paper do you write for in New York? Do you suppose that you could write a story about our line of steamers which would be a good advertisement for our boats?"

The reporter being very anxious to get back in some way to his home town answered the Captain as best he could. The Captain then took out a ticket from his pocket, handed it to the reporter and told him that if he would promise to write a good advertisement of his boat which would encourage an increased number of people to travel by his line that he would be satisfied.

The reporter took the ticket and in his gratitude promised whatever the Captain desired. The reporter had the ticket, which insured his passage home, but he did not know what he could do for food as he had no money to purchase it. The steamer left the dock and headed for New York. Lunch time came and in order not to make himself conspicuous, he sought an unusual part of the boat where there were no people who might ask embarrassing questions.

He sat down on a steamer chair, closed his eyes and tried to forget that he had a stomach and that he was hungry. As he sat there resting, a fairy came dancing along the deck, came close up to him, patted him on the back and invited him to get up and dance with her. As there was no one around he accepted the fairy's invitation, and so they danced forward and back, sideways and round and round. And as they danced other fairies appeared and danced with him. He enjoyed the dance very much and was sorry when some of the passengers appeared and the fairies vanished.

After a while he began to feel hungry again, and at the same time he remembered how the fairies, when they danced side to side and other directions, swung their bodies as they danced. Being small fairies the swing was very short, and when he remembered the swing of the fairies he became able to remember the swing just as short. As he swung or imagined he was swinging, the hunger left him and he smiled and was pleased.

The afternoon passed and supper time arrived and again he sought an unoccupied part of the boat. Again he found a steamer chair and occupied it as previously, and while there the fairies again appeared and persuaded him to dance with them as he had done before.

The more he danced the better he felt, and as the dance went on and he practiced the swinging, side to side and other directions, he quite forgot his hunger, and when he did that the fairies smiled and encouraged him to keep on with the swing.

The next morning at breakfast time his hunger had become worse than it was the day before. Again the fairies appeared and told him that they were very hungry, that they were very anxious to be carried by the steamer to their home in New York. From there they expected to go to some of the parks and obtain some food, being fairies they did not need very much food. What they wanted was quality more than quantity. The reporter told them that, for him, he was willing to pass up the quality of the food provided he obtained sufficient quantity.

They all laughed at this and began to dance more rapidly than ever before, and in order to forget his hunger the reporter danced with them just as fast as he could.

And so the days passed for him quite rapidly. At times he found it difficult to explain why he missed so many of his meals. The help of the fairies made it possible for him to forget his hunger at all times provided he remembered or imagined the swing of the hungry fairies.

In due time the steamer reached New York. When the gang plank connected the steamer with the dock, our reporter started to leave the vessel with the other passengers. When he came to the man who takes the tickets he handed out his ticket and started to walk away. But the ticket man stopped him and looked at the ticket in a puzzled way. He said to the reporter, "How is this? Your ticket gives you three meals a day on the boat and you haven't had a single meal punched. What's the matter. Wasn't the food good enough for you?"

The reporter answered, "Yes, but you see I am under a diet and did not have to take my meals regularly," and then ran down the gang plank and disappeared in the crowd with a feeling of something which he could not describe.

The memory of the hungry fairies, however, was a pleasant memory. He walked along practicing the swing until he met a friend who saw to it that he got a good square meal. The reporter told his friend the story of the fairies and how they had helped him to endure the hunger and made his trip a pleasant one with their sympathy, kindness and the swing.

His friend laughed so long and so heartily that the reporter was quite annoyed. It amused his friend very much to hear that he carefully avoided the dining room, and was ravenously hungry for a whole week—with a paid meal ticket in his pocket!

CONCENTRATION AND RELAXATION

By Lawrence M. Stanton, M.D.

I know of no writer who has so clarified the murky philosophy of concentration and relaxation as has Dr. Bates, and yet the final word has not been said, as he himself would undoubtedly avow.

Therefore, but with humblest intention, I offer a few thoughts upon the subject which is of the utmost importance to those who are striving for better eyesight.

To my patients I have forbidden the practice of concentration, saying that the very word suggests strain, or else I bid them modify the dictionary's definition. I have reasoned that if by concentration you mean, as Dr. Bates says, doing or seeing one thing better than anything else, you may speak of concentration; but if by concentration you mean, as the dictionary says, doing one thing continuously to the exclusion of all other things, then you must abandon the practice as an impossibility.

Concentration, however, cannot psychologically be ignored, and recent psychology, I believe, has given us a new interpretation which is worthy of our consideration.

Attention underlies concentration, as that word is commonly used, and Ribot's[1] statement of attention is very enlightening. Ribot says "that the state of attention which seems continuous is in reality intermittent; the object of attention is merely a center, the point to which attention returns again and again, to wander from it as often on ever-widening circles. All parts of the object, and then the reflections inspired by these various parts, hold our interest by turns. Even when the attention is fixed on the most trifling material object, it works in just the same fashion." This is entirely in accord with Dr. Bates' statement; it is central fixation.

[1. Ribot, T. *The Psychology of Attention.* See Bibliography.—TRQ]

There are, however, two aspects of concentration to be considered—voluntary and involuntary. Voluntary concentration is an effort and, as Dr. Bates has so clearly shown, cannot be maintained without fatigue.

The highest grades of attention, to which this brief consideration is confined, are involuntary, and involuntary concentration can be defined as "a psychological equivalent of attention minus effort." In ordinary attention, that is, in voluntary concentration—our thought holds the object in focus, whereas in involuntary attention (which we shall consider synonymous with involuntary concentration) the object holds our thought without our volition, perhaps even against our will. "Spontaneous attention is rooted at the very center of our being," and things that hold the attention captive, as in fascination, fixed contemplation, the Hindu's meditation and revery are instances of involuntary concentration, and involuntary concentration is as effortless as the rising sun—it just happens. Then, there are those cases of miraculous quick cures of imperfect sight by one or another of Dr. Bates' methods, where it was enough for the patient to see the better course in order to be able to follow it, the idea and its realization occurring simultaneously, without effort, without volition even. Contrast this with the attitude "No, I see the better course and approve it, but I follow the worse." Involuntary concentration is displayed in the case of the insect, related by Fabre and quoted by Dr. Bates, which in captivity hung downward for ten months, its whole life's span, and in this position performed all its functions, even to mating and laying of eggs, apparently without the least fatigue. Still another instance is that of Napoleon, who could work for eighteen hours at a stretch on one piece of work without the least fatigue. Napoleon speaks of his various affairs arranged in his head "as in a wardrobe." He says, "When I wish to put any matter out of my mind, I close its drawer and open the drawer belonging to another. The contents of the drawers never get mixed and they never worry me or weary me. Do I want to sleep? I close all the drawers, and then I am asleep."

The question, then, may be asked wherein does involuntary concentration differ from relaxation. If involuntary concentration and relaxation are not always one and the same thing, they often are psychological alternatives and not the opponents we think them.

To regard all phases of relaxation as purely passive is as erroneous as it is to say that concentration of the kind under consideration is associated with effort. Relaxation of the passive kind usually ends in sleep or sleepiness, as experienced by many patients after palming. Relaxation combined with action, on the other hand, may also be absolutely free from effort and strain. [Aldous Huxley used the excellent phrase "dynamic relaxation" in his book *The Art of Seeing.*—TRQ]

In any case it is the matter of effort and strain that concerns us most, rather than a question of concentration or relaxation. Victor Hugo speaks of "the calm and intense fixation of the eyes," and surely nowhere is intensity so impressive as in calmness. To be calm is not to be oblivious, and to be intense need not be to strain.

Another thought about relaxation is this: Obstacles to relaxation may prove sources of relaxation. An instance of which is found in the noise that is keeping us awake when wishing to go to sleep. If we sufficiently relax, if we accept the disturbance and sleep in spite of it, not only is the obstacle overcome, but because overcome, it in turn becomes rather pleasantly associated with going to sleep. When again we desire to sleep, we find the noise soothing rather than annoying, and really a source of relaxation instead of an obstacle to it. The following quotation from Jean Kenyon MacKenzie's *Minor Memories* well illustrates how obstacles may become ministering angels. She writes of the stillness of the African forest, "I remember that stillness. Many a time when I am in the subway I remember the ineffable stillness of the forest. I wonder to find myself where I am—so savagely circumstanced—so pressed upon by alien bodies, so smitten by noise. Traveling like this, in white man's fashion, you are certainly safe from the snakes, and the leopards, and the cannibal tribes of that other world where you traveled in other fashions. Now that you are shut up so safely in the guts of Manhattan, your friends feel at ease about you—surely the sun shall not smite you by day nor the moon by night. And yet, perversely, in this perfection of safety you are intimidated. *Suddenly passive* after your desperate adventures with traffic, you feel the hidden things of memory rise and flood your heart; you dream. You remember other times of day than the manufactured night of the subway and other ways of travel. *And suddenly, in the indestructible silence that is the core of that incessant clamor,* you hear a bugle calling in a forest-clearing that is half way around the world." Certainly a remarkable experience—what relaxation, what imagination!

Involuntary concentration without effort is equivalent to relaxation in action. If you can achieve such equilibrium; if you can perform your mental functions without strain as Fabre's little insect performed its physical; if you can, whatever your particular captivity, hang by your feet, head downward without effort, then "be my friend and teach me to be thine."

Note: Some of the quotations in this article and some of its material are from *The Power Within Us* by Charles Baudouin.

Italics mine. [Stanton's.]

ANNOUNCEMENTS

The Work in England

Captain C. S. Price of London, England has been the guest of Dr. Bates for several weeks. Dr. Bates wishes to announce that he finds Captain Price thoroughly capable of curing imperfect sight by his methods.

League Announcement

The speaker of the next Better Eyesight League meeting will be Percival S. Sprinz, D.D.S., who is the attending oral surgeon of the Hospital for Joint Diseases and Chief of the Dental and Oral Surgical Department in the dispensary connected with the hospital. Dr. Sprinz will discuss "Eye Disturbances Due to Local Infection in Teeth and Gums."

The members of the League will welcome information about this important subject, especially when presented by a League member. Dr. Sprinz discarded his glasses a year and a half ago; he is now able to read the photographic diamond type of the small Bible.

QUESTIONS AND ANSWERS

Q–1a. My eyes are swollen and disfigured in the morning. 1b. Although I have eight and nine hours' sleep, it does not rest me.

A–1a. The swelling of your eyes or eyelids in the morning is due to eyestrain when you are asleep. 1b. You may be restless and sleep very poorly and strain your eyes terribly, although apparently you may be asleep for a long time.

Q–2. I have improved my sight by palming, but when I read for any length of time the pain returns.

A–2. When you read and your eyes pain you, it means that you are straining your eyes. More frequent palming may help you more continuously.

Q–3. Explain which "swing" is beneficial, and whether one moves the whole head or only the eyes.

A–3. All swings when done properly are beneficial. When done improperly they are not beneficial. It is necessary for some people to move their head in order to move their eyes and obtain a perfect swing.

Better Eyesight
May 1925—Vol. IX, No. 11

FUNDAMENTALS

1. Glasses discarded permanently.

2. Favorable conditions. Light may be bright or dim. The distance of the print from the eyes, where seen best, also varies with people.

3. Central Fixation is seeing best where you are looking.

4. Shifting. With normal sight the eyes are moving all the time. This should be practiced continuously and consciously.

5. Swinging. When the eyes move slowly or rapidly from side to side, stationary objects appear to move in the opposite direction.

6. Long Swing. Stand with the feet about one foot apart, turn the body to the right, at the same time lifting the heel of the left foot. Do not pay any attention to the apparent movement of stationary objects. Now place the left heel on the floor, turn the body to the left, raising the heel of the right foot. Alternate. This exercise can be practiced just before retiring at night fifty times or more. When done properly, it is a great rest and relieves pain, fatigue, and other symptoms of imperfect sight.

7. Stationary Objects Moving. By moving the head and eyes a short distance from side to side, one can imagine stationary objects to be moving. Since the normal eye is moving all the time, one should imagine all stationary objects to be moving. Never imagine that you see a stationary object stationary.

8. Palming. The closed eyes may be covered with the palm of one or both hands. The patient should rest the eyes and think of something else that is pleasant.

9. Blinking. The normal eye blinks, or closes and opens very frequently. If one does not blink, the vision always becomes worse.

MENTAL PICTURES

By W. H. Bates, M.D.

The human mind is busy as long as we are awake. We remember many things and are consciously or unconsciously shifting from one thing to another. Those things that we remember, we imagine we see. If we imagine we see a letter perfectly, continuously, it is all done easily without effort or strain. If a letter or other object is remembered or imagined imperfectly, it is not remembered continuously, it soon disappears and something else takes its place. When the memory is perfect, it can be demonstrated that no effort is made, and things remembered are imagined as mental pictures easily and continuously.

Mental pictures are very important. For example, if a patient can remember and imagine he sees a letter or other object perfectly, or as well with the eyes open as with the eyes closed, or can remember when looking at the distance a small letter as well as it can be seen at the near point, the patient has a normal eye with normal sight. All cases of nearsightedness, farsightedness, astigmatism, presbyopia disappear momentarily, more continuously, or permanently, when mental pictures are imagined more or less perfectly. It can be demonstrated that when the normal eye with normal vision imagines a mental picture of a letter perfectly, the eye remains normal with normal vision; but if the same patient remembers a small letter or other object imperfectly or imagines he sees it imperfectly, the vision becomes imperfect, a change takes place in the normal shape of the eyeball and the eye becomes imperfect—too long, too short, or of an irregular shape.

The memory of imperfect sight increases the hardness of the eyeball, which can be felt with most cases with the tips of the fingers touching the outside of the upper eyelids. In cases of glaucoma, in which the eyeball is already too hard, the memory of imperfect sight will increase the tension and lower the vision. In these cases, also, the memory of imperfect sight increases pain and produces other disagreeable symptoms.

Negative afterimages: If a patient regards a white Snellen test card with black letters, closes his eyes and has a mental picture of a black card with white letters, it is called a *negative afterimage*. In such cases the symptoms may be modified or corrected by alternately looking at the Snellen test card for part of a minute, then closing the eyes and flashing one of the large letters for a moment, a second, or part of a second. By alternating in this way it is possible to prevent the appearance of negative afterimages.

To obtain perfect mental pictures requires perfect relaxation. If the patient can see at the near point a small letter "o" with a white center whiter than it really is, or whiter than the rest of the white card, it is usually possible to close the eyes and remember or imagine a perfect mental picture of the letter. A small percentage of my patients can remember or imagine one letter or one object as well with their eyes closed as they can see it. The perfect memory of the small letter "o" can be imagined at five feet, ten feet, twenty feet, or farther, by practice as well as it can be seen at the near point.

In one case a child nine years old was brought to me for treatment. The patient had worn very strong glasses for nearsightedness since she was three years old. When first seen she was wearing concave 14 D. S., which improved her vision from 5/200 to 20/100. At school even with her glasses she could not read the blackboard. She was a child with an unusual memory. She could look at one letter of the 10-line of the Snellen test card, see it perfectly when held very close to her eyelashes, close her eyes and remember it as well as she could see it. With her eyes open she could remember perfectly, at first at two feet, then by practice at five feet, and finally at twenty feet. Then she said that she could imagine or saw, or imagined she saw, not only the letter that she had memorized, but also other letters with which she was not familiar.

In a second case mental pictures produced a cure in a reasonable time, about a week. The patient was a man, age thirty-five, who was wearing concave 16 D. S. combined with a cylinder of 2 diopters in each eye, which improved his vision to one-sixth of the normal. After three months of continuous treatment with the aid of palming, swinging, and other methods, he obtained a permanent benefit. His mental pictures were poor for letters and other objects. By practice he became able to remember a small black period just as black with his eyes open as he could with his eyes closed, or as well as he could see it a few inches from his eyes. He was recommended to remember the period perfectly all day long, or at night when he was awake. In the beginning he was very much discouraged, because when he noticed any improvement in his vision he soon lost his mental picture of the period and his vision failed. To prevent the loss of the memory of the period, he was directed to dodge or look away quickly at some other object whenever he was conscious that the memory of the black period was a benefit. This was difficult at first, but by practice he became able to dodge or look at some other object, when his vision was improved, and in this way retained his mental picture of the period. He was very faithful and devoted practically all of his time to his mental picture of the period. In about a week when he walked into the office he said, "Doctor, I am cured."

I tested him at twenty feet, and he told me that he could look at the 200-line letter at the top of the card for a moment without losing the perfect memory of the black period. He also informed me that he could look at the 10-line letters and dodge them just as well without losing his period. Then I said to him, "Can you see anything of the bottom line?" He answered, "I cannot prevent myself from seeing all the letters of the bottom line." I tested him with different cards that he had never seen before and found that he had normal vision.

STORIES FROM THE CLINIC

No. 63: Mental Pictures

By Emily C. Lierman

So many patients tell me when they first start treatment, that they have no mental pictures. They cannot seem to remember or visualize anything while palming. If the mind is under a strain, no amount of palming will improve the vision temporarily or permanently.

A little girl, not quite three years old, came to the Clinic with her mother. The mother told us that after the child had had an attack of measles, her left eye turned in. When I held the card up close, the little girl was able to tell me which way all the "E's" of the pothooks card were pointing. The squint was not so decided either. But when I held the card five feet away front her eyes, the left eye turned in almost completely. that is to say, one could hardly see the iris. I placed her little hands over her closed eyes and told her to think of her best dollie and tell me how it was dressed. I didn't expect her to tell me very much because of her age, but the little tot surprised me. She lisped in her baby talk that her best doll had a pretty pink dress, and that her shoes were black and had straps on just like her own shoes. Her mother held her as she stood on top of a table, for she was very tiny, and when she looked at the test card five feet away, her left eye remained straight temporarily, while she read 5/30 without a mistake. Her mental picture of the doll was perfect. Describing the shoes and dress helped.

At one time I had four boys under treatment at the same time. They were between the ages of nine and twelve, and all were nearsighted. They stood in a row and while palming I talked about baseball. I described the ball, and they described to me just how the field was arranged. After

I had tested each one in turn and improved their vision, they were encouraged to palm more. Their mental pictures were first and second base, a home run, seventh inning, etc. The four boys obtained normal sight in less than two hours that day. Two of them had 10/50 before treatment and improved to 10/10. The other two had 10/40 and 10/30 before treatment and improved to 15/10.

A young mother came to be treated for headaches. Ever since she could remember she had suffered severe pain in the back of her head and eyes. Glasses were put on her when she was a small child but they did not relieve her pain. One of her neighbors where she lived told her how Dr. Bates had relieved her of eyestrain, so she came with a ray of hope. Palming did not give her any relief at first, and always when she came she had an attack of hysteria. When I was able to quiet her, I asked her about her children. She had two girls and a little baby boy. While we were talking she was palming. I noticed the corners of her mouth were drooped, and as she talked she had no control of her tears. I had a strong desire to place my arms about her. When I discovered that her baby boy was much loved in her family, I questioned her about him. I said, "Tell me the color of baby's eyes. I love little boys. Describe him to me."

A smile was noticeable as she answered, "His eyes are brown and his hair is blond; and you ought to see the two dimples he has when he smiles. I must not forget to tell you that he has two teeth, and when he smiles you just have to smile with him." I watched her as she explained all of this. There were no drooping corners to her mouth, but a smile was there all the time. Before I had time to tell her to remove her hands from her eyes, she did so herself. With a great sigh of relief she looked at me and said, "I have no pain just now. I feel so good I want to laugh and sing." A mental picture of her baby boy, remembering and explaining all about him was a relaxation, a benefit to her. She came more than six months to the Clinic for treatment before she obtained normal vision permanently. She had a high degree of myopia when she first came, and her vision was 10/200 with both eyes.

During the first few weeks of treatment her pain would return, but each time it was less severe. When she became able by herself to obtain mental pictures, her pain would disappear and her vision would improve. At times when her mental pictures were imperfect her vision was lowered, and this always caused an attack of hysteria. Later her vision steadily improved, her pain disappeared and toward the end of six months she obtained normal sight, 10/10.

During the six months of her treatment she had to be encouraged very often by her husband or sister, to palm every day. The swing of her body from side to side, while blinking and remembering something pleasant, always helped her pain. To take care of her children and do her household duties was quite enough for any woman, but she made time to practice and she was well repaid.

MAY FAIRIES

By George M. Guild

The merry month of May is expected to be just as full of joy and happiness to the children and grown-ups this year as it has been in other years. The children start the month with a big May Day celebration.

With so much fun going on we know that the fairies are there to keep everybody smiling. The good children in their hearts know they see the fairies and enjoy them. Someone has said that the fairies can turn into all kinds of flowers and in this way escape observation. But you can detect them because if you watch them closely, you can see them blink their eyes. Fairies always have perfect sight and to keep it they have to blink or close their eyes frequently in order to avoid the stare. You see, there are some people who have perfect eyes and, strange to say, their eyes are not conspicuous, and they do not know that they have eyes. Although their eyes are all the time moving, the movement is so short that it is not noticeable. It is a habit which they have, of which they are not conscious, but people who have poor sight are all the time staring and straining in order to see. It is not true that it requires an effort to see. On the contrary, it does require a great deal of hard work, much effort, much strain, in order to fail to see. One nice thing about the fairies is that you never see them staring at you or straining their eyes. No one ever saw a fairy wearing glasses.

Many people ask the question, "Do fairies really exist?" A great many people believe that there are fairies, although they themselves may not have seen any. An eminent scientific man told me that at one time he took some photographs of a flower bed covered with many flowers. He showed these photographs to some children, and right away some of them exclaimed, "Oh! See the fairies!" Neither he nor any of his friends could see any fairies among the flowers.

A man once told me that when he was a child he could remember seeing fairies, many fairies, all dancing together on the grass in the woods; but as he grew older his ability to see the fairies became less. He said that when his wife was cured of imperfect sight she became able to see the fairies, when before her cure she had never been able to see a fairy. From what is known of fairies, it seems that they can, if they wish it, become visible to anyone whom they desire to see them.

Children who have seen fairies have told me that when they saw a fairy and smiled, their sight became unusually good; but if they were disappointed in any way, the fairies at once disappeared. So when you want to see a fairy, be sure to smile. Think of all sorts of pleasant things and thoroughly believe that fairies exist. Children who doubt the existence of fairies never see them.

For some reason or other, the month of May is the best month in the year to see fairies. Most of them have rested all winter long and when the sun comes out and the flowers begin to bloom, the fairies wake up and start to have a good time. I believe that most children like to have a good time, too, just as the fairies do. When a child learns the games that the fairies play, learns to dance like the fairies dance, learns to laugh and sing like the fairies do, that child is very fortunate, indeed. Those children who have seen fairies have told me how they dance around in a ring until they are tired, and then they go and sit on a toadstool and rest. To dance like the fairies dance is a cure for headaches. It is wonderful how long fairies can dance without getting tired. They must do it very easily and without an effort. Fairies have wonderful voices for singing, and you can hear them a very long distance away. They have wonderful eyes for seeing, and can recognize their friends from afar. They have wonderful hearts for loving which explains why they are so popular with children.

GLASSES RETARD PROGRESS

By Edith T. Fisher, M.S., M.D.

This patient, a man age 53, had worn glasses thirteen years for astigmatism. Four years ago his vision became decidedly worse and had been steadily decreasing. Though his glasses had been changed repeatedly by competent ophthalmologists, his vision for distance was not improved to any appreciable degree.

His vision with glasses was 10/70 and the letters were gray and blurred. The diamond type appeared very indistinct, but he was able to read a few words in a very bright light.

Without glasses his vision was 10/200 with both eyes and with each eye separately. The diamond type seemed to be a solid gray blur. The smallest letters that he could read were those of the 30-line and he could distinguish them only when the card was held one foot from his eyes.

First I explained about blinking. I had not seen him blink once since he entered the office. As a child he was taught never to blink while conversing with anyone because it was very impolite, so he had always prevented, as much as possible, any movement of the eyelids. In this way he had acquired the habit of staring. Blinking seemed to require a great effort, but by closing his eyes for a few minutes at a time and then by gradually shortening this period he was soon able to blink easily.

His imagination and memory were very poor, but he could remember the ocean perfectly. As a child he had spent many summers at the seashore and had often sat for hours watching the waves. So I suggested that while palming he imagine himself sitting on a shore watching the waves as he had done in his childhood.

After palming thirty minutes in this way I asked him to glance at the test card and then close his eyes immediately. He saw the "R" in 10/100, but it disappeared before he could close his eyes.

I then held the card where he was able to see the "O" in the 50-line, but he could not remember it. I suggested that he imagine the "O" floating out into the ocean, becoming gradually smaller and smaller. After looking at the "O" again, he closed his eyes and imagined that it was floating away. Then he looked at the test card which was ten feet away and read both letters in the 100-line and they appeared much blacker. The diamond type now appeared as white and black lines instead of the solid gray.

Four days later I saw him again. His vision had not improved. Before I had an opportunity to question him he said, "I know why I have not improved more. It is because I have worn my glasses about an hour a day. Each time after wearing them my sight is just as bad as it was the first time I took them off four days ago."

I had very carefully explained about not wearing his glasses, but he thought I had attributed undue importance to this phase, therefore he had not mentioned that it was absolutely necessary for him to wear them about an hour a day. As the glasses affected his vision so unfavorably and caused the loss of all that he had previously gained, it seemed doubtful that he would ever improve to any great extent as long as he continued to wear them. On days when he did not use glasses, as Sundays and holidays, his improvement was more marked and then, after wearing them, he did not lose quite all he had previously gained; but in this way his progress was exceedingly slow.

He practiced about three hours a day, with the diamond type, palming and sitting in the sun with his eyelids closed. In practicing with the diamond type he derived the most benefit from sitting in the sun and slowly moving the card from side to side, glancing at it casually from time to time and closing his eyes frequently.

In this way he first became able to see the white spaces between the lines very white, then the spaces between the words and finally, in flashes, he could distinguish words. His progress was, without doubt, greatly retarded by his use of glasses, but now, after ten months, he is able to read the diamond type in the sun, and 10/30 on the test card. He is seeing objects at a distance that he had not seen for four years even with his glasses.

REPORT OF THE LEAGUE MEETING

By Mabel A. Young, Secretary

The April meeting of the Better Eyesight League was held Tuesday evening, April 7. The President, May Secor, presided. She stated that, as the body must be regarded as a whole of which the eye is a part, it is planned to have speakers from the outside tell of conditions in other parts of the body which may link up with trouble in the eyes.

Dr. Percival Sprinz was the speaker of the evening. Dr. Sprinz is attending oral surgeon in the Hospital for Joint Diseases, and head of the oral clinic. He is a believer in the Bates Method and a recent member of the League. Dr. Sprinz's talk was very interesting and threw light on many phases of oral infection.

QUESTIONS AND ANSWERS

Q–1. Dr. Bates says that in reading fine print one should look between the lines. Is this not contrary to the principles of central fixation? To see the print best, should one not look directly at it?

A–1. One can look between the lines and shift to the black letters with central fixation. [It is not necessary to look at the spaces between the lines; simply move your attention through the letters along the sentence. See the chapter on reading in *Relearning to See*.—TRQ]

Q–2. If type can be seen more distinctly with the eyes partly closed (squinting), is it advisable to read that way?

A–2. No, it is not advisable to read that way because it is a strain, and alters the shape of the eyeball.

Q–3. Should children read microscopic print?

A–3. Yes, the more the better. Reading microscopic print is a benefit to the eyes of both children and adults.

Q–4. I have attained normal vision, but after reading for a while, my eyes feel strained. Would you still consider I had normal sight?

A–4. If your eyes feel strained you are not reading with normal vision.

Better Eyesight
June 1925—Vol. IX, No. 12

ALTERNATE

It has always been demonstrated that the continuous memory, imagination, or vision of one thing for any length of time is impossible. To see one letter of the Snellen test card continuously, it is necessary to shift from one part of the letter to another. By alternately moving the eyes from one side of the letter to the other, it is possible to imagine the letter to be moving in the opposite direction to the movement of the eyes. This movement of the letter is called a *swing*. When it is slow, easy, short, about one-quarter of an inch or less, maximum vision is obtained which continues as long as the swing continues.

As long as we are awake, we are thinking, remembering, or imagining mental pictures, and are comfortable. To go around blind requires a distinct effort which is a strain on all the nerves and is always uncomfortable. The normal mind alternates its attention from one mental picture to another, which is a relaxation or rest. The memory, or imagination, is best when one thing is imagined better than all other things, central fixation, but constant shifting is necessary to maintain central fixation.

One of the best methods to improve the vision is to regard a letter of the Snellen test card with the eyes open, then close the eyes and remember or imagine the letter better for about ten seconds, open the eyes and regard the letter while testing the imagination of the letter for a moment. By alternately regarding the letter with the eyes open and closed, the imagination of the letter improves in flashes. By continuing to alternate, the flashes improve and last longer until the vision becomes continuously improved.

OLD-AGE SIGHT

By W. H. Bates, M.D.

When most people with normal eyes arrive at the age of forty and upwards, they usually have difficulty in reading books or newspapers, although their sight for distance may be normal. At the age of fifty or upwards, such persons become less able to read at the near point or find it impossible to read even headlines of a newspaper clearly or distinctly. This condition has been called *old-age sight,* although it could be defined more accurately as the imperfect sight of middle age. The medical term for this form of imperfect sight is presbyopia. While imperfect sight occurs quite commonly in middle age, it does occur in individuals under thirty years old and more rarely in children. There are people, however, who even at the age of eighty or ninety are able to read just as well as when they were younger.

The cause of presbyopia is said to be due to the hardening of the crystalline lens of the eye to such an extent that the focus of the eye cannot be brought to a near point on account of the inability of the hard lens to change its shape. Almost every eye specialist believes this theory. In my book *Perfect Sight Without Glasses* I have described the evidence which proves that this theory is wrong.

At one time I was unable to read without glasses. After I found that the lens was not a factor in accommodation, I realized that presbyopia might be cured in some cases. Then, having cured my own eyes, I felt that the old theory of the cause of presbyopia was wrong. Since that time so many patients who were unable to read without glasses have recovered that I feel most, if not all, can be cured. In my experience I have never met with a case of presbyopia which could not be temporarily benefited.

In the treatment of presbyopia most persons experience a decidedly uncomfortable feeling in their eyes when they look at fine print so close that they fail to read it. The more they try to see, the worse it becomes and the more uncomfortable do their eyes feel. By closing their eyes and resting them, their vision becomes better immediately after the eyes are opened, but only for a short time. It can be demonstrated that by staring at one letter or a part of one letter, while trying to see it perfectly, the vision always becomes worse. If the patient alternately closes the eyes and opens them, blinking, the vision may be improved. One can look at the white spaces between the lines and imagine them whiter than they really are, whiter than the margin of the card. When this is accomplished, the black letters become blacker and may be read without any effort, easily, continuously, without fatigue.

Many people can read the newspaper when they hold it two feet from their eyes, although they are not able to read it at twelve inches or nearer. In such cases reading the large letters at two feet and improving the vision at this distance by alternately resting the eyes, enables the patient to gradually shorten the distance from the eyes until it can be read at twelve inches, later at six inches or nearer.

Some years ago a woman, eighty-seven years old, was treated for presbyopia. The eyestrain was so great that she had been unable to obtain glasses which were satisfactory. There was a history of attacks of hemorrhage in various parts of the retina, including the region of the center of sight, the macula. At this time, however, the hemorrhages had all disappeared and the retina was normal.

She was very much worried about her eyes and had a lot to say. Never in my life have I heard anyone talk so rapidly and say so much in so short a time. She repeated herself over and over again, and the constant idea that she tried to emphasize was that she was blind and that no one could give her any relief. It was difficult for me to persuade her to listen to me at first. I had to wait until she stopped for breath and then I handed her some diamond type, which I asked her to read. She very promptly told me that it was impossible, that the print was too small, and that when she tried to read it she suffered from pain, headache, and discomfort.

When my second chance came to speak, I asked her to imagine the white spaces between the lines to be perfectly white. She at once told me that that would not help her, that she could put all the white between the lines that I desired and that she was confident it would not be of any use, although she claimed to have a wonderful imagination. It seemed as though I heard two voices at the same time. One was constantly repeating that it was impossible to read such fine print, while the other voice was reading it at the same time. The audience which had collected around her, relatives, friends and servants, were thrilled, and it seemed everybody was trying to say something, to offer suggestions, and to give advice. Before we could stop her, this elderly woman read the whole card as rapidly as any one could have read it who had normal vision. When she had finished reading, and while she was wondering how she came to do it, I asked her for an explanation.

She answered, "When you asked me to imagine the white spaces between the lines to be perfectly white, I at once recalled white paint. With the help of my imagination I painted these white spaces with this white paint, and when I did that I was able to read."

While it is sometimes very difficult to cure presbyopia, it is, fortunately, very easy to prevent it. Oliver Wendell Holmes told us how to do it in *The Autocrat of the Breakfast Table.* [See the July 1919 issue.—TRQ]

STORIES FROM THE CLINIC
No. 64: Albert
By Emily C. Lierman

Since we have had our private Clinic here at the office, the charity patients come mostly from physicians. Others are sent by ministers of all churches.

Albert, age sixteen, was sent to us by a dentist's assistant who told me of his pitiable condition. His first visit was on December 6, 1924. Albert's sister, who is devoted to him, was present, being anxious to know if we could help him. When he appeared he was wearing a black patch over his left eye because the light troubled him and he suffered intense pain. With the test card the vision of his right eye was normal, or 10/10, but the left eye had only light perception. This is a copy of his prescription for glasses, which he had worn for some time: Right 0.50 D. C. 90 degrees, Left 2.00 D. C. 90 degrees.

Dr. Bates examined him with the ophthalmoscope and found keratitis or inflammation of the front of the eyeball of the left eye. The right eye was normal. While the examination was going on, Albert's sister was weeping. She tried very hard to conceal her tears but in vain. They had been to other doctors and were told that Albert would always have to wear glasses to save the right eye; nothing more could be done for the left eye. The last oculist they consulted said the left eye had cataract and, as there was no sight, there was no use to operate. What a shock it was to his family!

I placed Albert in the sun and focussed the sun glass on his closed eyelid. Then I raised the upper lid and quickly focussed the strong light of the sun on the white part of the eye as he looked down. Immediately he called out to his sister, "I see the light. I can see a sort of web inside of my eye when the light is focussed on it." This made me very happy indeed. I knew then that Albert could be benefited. His sister was overcome.

While the tears flowed down her cheeks she said, "If you can only save that eye there is nothing in the world I would not do for him. Mother and I will take care of him. He need never work again. I can earn enough money for both of us and he can spend all his time taking care of his eye. He must not go blind." The girl was hysterical, of course, but she meant every word she said. She loved her brother. At her age other girls are usually planning a future for themselves, but she was willing to sacrifice herself, so that her brother would not go blind. That is love, indeed.

When we started treatment, Albert became enthusiastic and palmed his eyes for more than a half-hour. He was told to think of pleasant things while palming. Being a perfectly normal boy, he could easily think of such sports as baseball and other outdoor games. He liked to think of the movies and could imagine scenes from the picture called *The Covered Wagon.*

One could hear a pin drop when Albert first looked at the test card with his left eye, still keeping the right one covered. The test card was placed ten feet from his eyes and, while swinging his body from side to side, he flashed the large "C" on the top of the card. I was careful not to have him strain to see more, so he was told to sit comfortably and palm again.

He was with me over two hours that day and I improved his left eye to 10/100 by alternately palming and swinging, and also blinking. When he first removed the black patch, the sclera or white part of his left eye was bloodshot. It looked very much as though blood was ready to pour from it at any moment. There was also a considerable watering of the eye when it was first exposed to the light. The sun treatment instantly stopped this.

Before Albert left us on the first day, Dr. Bates asked me if I had the time to treat him every day. The Doctor said his trouble was so serious that unless we could see him very often he was not so sure that Albert would be cured. I was glad to give the time and I have been repaid. Our dear boy is almost cured. Don't let anyone tell me that prayer does not help. I prayed earnestly every night for Albert and I know that without God's help I could not have accomplished what I did. Albert believes that, too, for he helped me in that way.

Every day that we had sunshine he improved a little with the test card. On January 17, 1925, all the redness of the sclera had entirely disappeared. Then his visits were less frequent. I told him to come once a week, instead of daily. But Albert practiced at home every day for hours at a time. The condition of his eye steadily improved and by the end of February 1925, the vision of the left eye was almost normal.

I am proud of Albert for another reason. He would not allow his sister to support him. He asked me if shoveling snow would make his eye worse again. I said no, as shoveling snow would be practicing the swing, and the exercise would be a benefit.

Then he said, "Please pray for snow. I want to work." Again our prayers were answered. That very night we had a big snow storm, and when Albert came the next day, this is what he told me:

"I stood in line with my shovel and stretched myself as much as possible to look big. I got a job all right, and I will earn $5.00 per day while the snow lasts." We had one snowstorm after another and Albert had much to do.

I believe Albert's case was most remarkable because he did not at any time suffer a relapse. I believe, also, that the sun was the main factor in the relief of his trouble. I cannot understand why so many eye specialists shield the eyes of a patient from the sun. Bandaging them not only frightens the patient, but makes him most uncomfortable. It is true, that when some patients first learn that they are to be treated with a sun glass, they don't like to try it. But just as soon as the light is first thrown on the closed eyelids, they relax and smile and ask for more. The sun is our greatest blessing, I think.

THE SAND MAN

By George M. Guild

The little boy sat on the lap of his mother in a rocking chair. His name was Freddie. He had had a long day and was very, very tired. His mother rocked him back and forth, petted him with her cool hands and quieted him with her frequent kisses. He kept telling her, "Oh, mother, my eyes hurt, my head hurts, my arms hurt, my feet hurt, I am all hurt, and I am all tired out."

While she rocked him back and forth, a little old man came into the room with a bag of sand over his shoulder, the sand man. Freddie did not see him coming and Freddie's mother did not see him coming, but when he threw a little sand into their eyes they both became very sleepy. Freddie sat up and looked around, stretched his arms, and his big tortoise-shell glasses fell from his eyes on to the floor. Freddie jumped down to get his glasses, and then he saw the sand man pick them up from the floor and hold them behind his back where Freddie could not get them. Freddie was very indignant and scolded the sand man for taking his glasses, but the little old man smiled and said, "Do they help you to see?"

Freddie answered, "No, my eyes feel all right until I put them on in the morning, and then things are blurred, and my eyes begin to pain; but the doctor said that if I did not wear them all the time, I would most surely go blind." The sand man said to him, "Would you like to go with me and talk it over with the fairies? They don't like to see little boys or babies wearing glasses."

So the little boy took the hand of the sand man and they ran, skipping and jumping around, out of the room, into the hall, down the stairs, out the front door, through the front gate, and then into the woods. There the moon was shining very brightly through the trees and lighted up a space where thousands of fairies were dancing, laughing, and joking and having a good time. Freddie was so glad to see the fairies because in his heart he knew there were fairies, but all his uncles and aunts and cousins and grown people generally laughed at him and made fun of him for believing in fairies. When the fairies saw him coming, they all ran to him and climbed up on his shoulders and the top of his head, sat on his ears, tickled him under the chin, and made him laugh and he had a good time from the very start

The fairies had some difficulty in teaching him how to dance their way, but they finally got him to go through movements of various kinds. The one he liked best of all was to turn his head, eyes, and his whole body as far to the right and to the left as he possibly could without trying to see the things in front of him, which move in the opposite direction. He never heard fairies sing, but he heard them now and he liked the sound of their voices. He tried to sing with them, but he did so poorly and his voice was so harsh that he could not keep on singing. But the fairies encouraged him, and told him how to hold his lips and his tongue, and how to breathe, and very soon he was singing just as loud and just as musically as the rest of them. This was very strange, indeed, because he sang songs that he had never heard before, that is, consciously. Of course, when he was asleep, he would dream, perhaps, of the fairies singing, but when he woke up in the morning the dreams of the fairies, like all other dreams, were usually soon forgotten.

What surprised him most of all was the fact that his eyes did not bother him. He was no longer sleepy, no longer tired; every nerve in his body was just as happy as he was. There was no pain, only a feeling of delicious joyousness that no words could describe. Not only were his eyes comfortable, free from pain and fatigue, but he was able to see the fairies, the trees, the flowers, the birds, and the toadstools where the fairies sat to rest. It seemed to him that he could see through the trees, that he could see through the ground down into the other side of the earth where China was. He felt as though he could see the Chinese fairies almost as well as he could see the fairies that surrounded him. His eyes never kept still, they were moving in all directions, and the more they moved the better they felt. When his eyes moved in one direction, it seemed as though his hands and feet moved in the other direction, but one could not catch the other. The movement of his eyes was all the time missing the movement of his toes. They seemed like two railroad trains on parallel tracks, which pass each other going in the opposite direction at full speed. He noticed that the fairies were moving in the same direction that his body was moving; the sand man, the trees, the grass, everything was moving with his body, opposite to the movement of his eyes. It seemed a very peculiar thing to him. The strangest thing about it was that for the first time in his life he felt his eyes were rested, although they were moving, and that for the first time in his life also, his body, his nerves were at rest although they were, as he thought or imagined, constantly moving.

The next morning when his mother came to awaken him, she found him looking over toward the trees and smiling. Every once in a while he would laugh out loud, as loud as he could scream. His mother was worried and she said to him, "What is the trouble; why are you up so early? Why are you laughing, and why do you look over toward the trees?"

Then he told her what had happened to him on the previous night when the sand man took him over to see the fairies. She smiled indulgently, as mothers will, but the next question she asked him was the most important one of all, "Where are your glasses?"

Freddie looked up into the face of his mother, who leaned over and kissed him. He threw his arms around her and pressed his cheek against hers and said, "Mother, please forgive me. The sand man took them. The fairies told me how to see perfectly without glasses, so that I would have no pain and would never get tired. I want to get up early in the morning every morning and go over into the woods and play; play where the fairies played, where the fairies cured me of my poor sight."

AN UNFAIR TEST

Editor's Note—*Recently a high schoolgirl wrote me of her experience with a lady school doctor who tested her sight. This may interest the parents of schoolchildren.*

Dear Doctor:

I thought you might be interested in hearing about my "run in" to use a vulgar phrase, with the school physician. She is abominably prejudiced to put it mildly.

She seemed extremely annoyed because you advertised with the aid of your book, *Perfect Sight Without Glasses,* and your magazine *Better Eyesight,* and said something about the fact that she would be put out of the medical profession if she did so. When I told Daddy, he asked if I had said that she probably deserved to be. I failed to think of that in time, but I did tell her that was your only method of giving away your discoveries when nearly all the doctors united to boycott you. That was right, wasn't it? We would have had a very pleasant squabble then but we were interrupted and I had to have my eyes tested. This will either amuse or disgust you, according to your mood. It irritated me at first, and then I saw the funny side and disturbed the entire library by my unseemly chuckles. She, the doctor, is quite six feet tall, and very masculine in appearance. Firmly grasping me by the wrist, she lifted me bodily from the chair and dragged me to the end of the room. I couldn't rebel, for she is most unconscionably strong. She shoved me up against the wall, held my neck tightly, pointed miles away it seemed, and said "Read that card." Honestly, I couldn't see anything, I was so frightened. She helped matters by smacking a large card against one eye. At length I read three lines, and the doctor didn't wait for any more, but said, "Write it down, minus three" whatever that means. Then I read with the right eye, and I went through five lines without a halt or mistake. As I paused for breath, for I had seen it all in one flash, she said "Minus one." I protested I had not finished, and now re-read the lines with my left eye, up to the seventh line, but she did not change the report—probably a lapse of memory, I suppose. Thus ended our historic encounter. Today, though, I had a pleasant surprise. For the first time I saw a picture perfectly. It is one which hangs on the opposite wall, and quite suddenly it sprang toward me more clearly than anything I had ever seen before. Now I know what perfect sight is, and I'll get it again, I am sure.

SUGGESTIONS TO PATIENTS

By Emily C. Lierman

1. Palm in the morning while in bed.

2. Take sun treatment for twenty minutes or longer every day.

3. Mentally or physically, keep up that pendulum-like motion.

4. After sitting in the sun, hold the small card and flash the white spaces.

5. What you do not see immediately, do not worry about.

6. While practicing with the "Seven Truths of Normal Sight," always move the card slowly from side to side as you hold it six or eight inches from your eyes.

7. To induce sleep when suffering from headache or nervous strain, close your eyes, remember the small "F" or "T" of the 10-line of the test card and imagine it is moving

slightly, about one-quarter of an inch, either up and down or to the left and right.

8. There is a right way and a wrong way to blink the eyes while practicing. Children like to hold up their two hands about ten or twelve inches apart, looking first at one hand and then at the other. In this way one blinks when looking at the right hand and again when looking at the left hand. The head should turn in the same direction with the eyes.

9. Nearsighted patients sometimes get along faster in the cure of their eyes by using two similar test cards at the same time while practicing. One card is held in the hand while the other is five or ten feet away. The patient looks at a letter up close and imagines he sees the same letter on the distant card. Then the patient closes his eyes and imagines that letter perfectly. Having seen it perfectly up close, he becomes able by practice to see it just as well on the distant card.

A CASE REPORT

Editor's Note—*Report of a man, 63 years old, who has worn glasses for a great many years. He improved his own vision merely by following directions. Others can do the same.*

I will be 63 years old in July and have not worn lenses since reading *Perfect Sight Without Glasses;* it will be two years the latter part of next July.

I have had monocular vision all my life, congenital convergent squint of left eye producing what has always been called "partial blindness from disuse." I could always see parts of everything but nothing distinctly; enough to get around if I closed my good eye, but could never see to read any printed matter with it.

At first I could not see the big "C" at any distance with the left eye. Now I can see its whole outline at about six inches and all of the letters on the 10-line at three or four feet. In scanning even fine print I can now discern lines and spaces and almost distinguish the letters by holding it close up.

I should add that I have not been at all diligent nor faithful in using Dr. Bates' methods and am surprised at the results obtained by me in spite of that fact. With more devotion I am sure I will get better results.

One patient, a woman of 25 or 30, had worn glasses seventeen years. She was myopic with astigmatism, seeing about half the distance with the left eye as with the right. She had frequent headaches, could not go to the "movies" without great distress. She spent $300 or more on glasses, had no comfort with them, and could not see well with or without them.

She was induced to buy Dr. Bates' book last March. She laid aside her glasses and began to work according to the method, wholly by herself, with most satisfactory results.

Very gratefully yours, Fred W. Morris, D.O., Ridgewood, New Jersey.

QUESTIONS AND ANSWERS

Q–1. When I look at an object and blink, it appears to jump with each blink. Would this be considered the short swing.

A–1. Yes. You unconsciously look from one side to the other of the object when blinking.

Q–2. What are the benefits of each swing?

A–2. The long swing relieves eye discomforts and helps one to obtain the short swing. The short swing improves the vision.

Q–3. Seeing stationary objects moving appears to me to be merely self-hypnotism. I can't do it.

A–3. When riding in a train the stationary telephone poles appear to move in the opposite direction. Of course this is an illusion, but it is a benefit to the eyes to imagine all stationary objects moving.

Q–4. I heard your lecture at the Psychology Club and immediately discarded my glasses. Now I cannot see at all and am worse off.

A–4. You can be cured by practicing relaxation methods when you discard your glasses.

Q–5. You stress palming in your instructions. If I obtain poor results with this exercise should I continue?

A–5. No. Do that which is most helpful.

Better Eyesight
July 1925—Vol. X, No. 1

ASTIGMATISM

By W. H. Bates, M.D.

The word has frightened a great many people. When a patient has astigmatism, it means that the shape of the eyeball is changed from the normal sphere to one that is lopsided. One may be nearsighted and have in addition a certain amount of astigmatism. The same is true in the farsighted eye, which may have at the same time a certain amount of astigmatism. In most cases the front part of the eyeball, the cornea, is the part affected.

In making the diagnosis of astigmatism, the so-called astigmatic chart has been highly recommended. It has been used for more than fifty years and is still popular. The chart consists of vertical, horizontal, and oblique lines. When a patient has astigmatism, the lines running in one direction appear more distinct than the lines running in other directions. I do not consider the astigmatic chart a very good or reliable test, because many patients with no astigmatism have imagined the lines in one direction to be much plainer than the lines at right angles to them. Also, in many cases of astigmatism, all the lines may be seen with equal clearness. Another objection to the test is that when some patients with normal eyes and with no astigmatism regard the astigmatic chart, a high degree of temporary astigmatism has been produced, which was demonstrated by other tests—retinoscope, ophthalmometer.

The instrument for the diagnosis of corneal astigmatism is called the ophthalmometer. When the normal eye was examined with its aid, the curvature of the cornea has been found to be normal in all directions. When the eye was under a strain, the curvature changed, sometimes being more convex in one meridian than in all the others, or one meridian might be flatter than the other meridians. The axis of the astigmatism produced by a strain has been observed to vary, increase or diminish, while the instrument was being used.

When the patient remembered perfect sight, no astigmatism was manifest and the curvature of the cornea remained normal. When a letter or other object was remembered by the patient, one part best—central fixation, no astigmatism was produced. When astigmatism was present, the amount was lessened or it disappeared altogether when central fixation was remembered or imagined. It can be demonstrated that no astigmatism of the cornea can be observed with the aid of the ophthalmometer when the

SWAYING

It is a great help in the improving of vision to have the patient demonstrate that staring at one part of a letter at ten feet or farther is a difficult thing to do for any length of time without lowering the vision and producing pain, discomfort, or fatigue. With the eyes closed it is impossible to concentrate on the memory or the imagination of a small part of one letter continuously without a temporary or more complete loss of the memory or the imagination.

When an effort is made to think of one part of a letter continuously with the eyes closed, the letter is imagined to be stationary. When the imagination shifts to the right of the letter a short distance and then to the left alternately, every time the attention is directed to the right of the letter, the letter is always to the left, and when the attention is directed to the left of the letter, the letter is always to the right. By alternating, the patient becomes able to imagine the letter is moving from side to side, and as long as the movement is maintained the patient is able to remember or imagine the letter. It can be demonstrated that to remember a letter or other object to be stationary always interferes with the perfect memory of the letter. One cannot remember, imagine, or see an object continuously unless it is moving. The movement must be slow, short, and easy.

When patients stare habitually, the eyes become more or less fixed, and are moved with great difficulty. When the patient stands and sways the whole body from side to side, it becomes easier to move the eyes in the same direction as the body moves. No matter how long the staring has been practiced, the sway at once lessens it.

patient is able to remember or imagine letters or other objects by central fixation.

It is also a truth that when things are remembered or imagined to be moving with a slow, short, regular, continuous, easy swing, no astigmatism is present when the cornea is examined with the ophthalmometer. The demonstration cannot be made by an observer who does not understand what is meant by the optical swing.

Rapid blinking also lessens or corrects corneal astigmatism temporarily or more continuously when done properly. When done under a strain, astigmatism may be produced or increased. The ophthalmometer demonstrates the facts.

Sunning, when practiced in such a way as to improve the vision, also is followed by an immediate benefit to the astigmatism, as observed by the ophthalmometer.

It has been noted that after the eyes are closed for some minutes or longer and rested, when they are first opened, an immediate improvement in the astigmatism is manifest.

Any form of treatment which was a benefit to the vision of the patient was also a benefit to the astigmatism, as demonstrated by the ophthalmometer.

The textbooks on the eye have for many years published that most, if not all, cases of astigmatism occur at birth, or that they are congenital. It was supposed to be a permanent condition, but further study of astigmatism has shown that it may be acquired at any age. Schoolchildren have been observed to acquire astigmatism at the age of eight, ten, fifteen years, or older. When the eyes were examined periodically, the astigmatism in many cases had changed. It is capable of increasing or of decreasing. It is an interesting fact that some cases do recover without treatment. This suggests the possibility of successful treatment.

In the normal eye astigmatism can be produced by a strain to see either at the distance or at the near point. At first it is temporary, but later may become more permanent. Astigmatism can always be corrected by relaxation or rest. When the imperfect sight of astigmatism can be corrected by glasses, it is called regular astigmatism, but when the vision cannot be improved to the normal in this way, it is called irregular astigmatism. Many scientific articles have been written on irregular astigmatism which are offered as evidence that it is incurable. The men who wrote these articles did not cure irregular astigmatism and, therefore, being authorities in the medical profession, they stated that nobody else could cure it; and, furthermore, anyone who claimed to be able to cure this form of astigmatism must be a charlatan, and should be expelled from the medical profession.

Irregular astigmatism is produced by eyestrain, and relieved or cured by relaxation or rest. Most cases of ulceration of the front part of the eyeball, the cornea, produce a scar which is more or less opaque. Irregular astigmatism is also caused by ulceration of the cornea.

Patients who cannot stand the light, photophobia, suffer very much from eyestrain. These cases acquire astigmatism which is usually corrected by encouraging the patients to become accustomed to the strong light of the sun. Ulceration of the front part of the eye occurs quite frequently in young children who live in the tenement houses where the light is poor. Astigmatism is found after the ulcerations have healed. Irregular astigmatism has usually been cured by the sun treatment with the aid of the swing, central fixation, and the memory of perfect sight.

Advanced cases of conical cornea have irregular astigmatism, which heretofore has not been relieved by various kinds of operations, glasses, or any other form of treatment. In this disease the front part of the eyeball becomes much thinner and an opening may form with great harm to the eye. In one of my early cases conical cornea occurred in both eyes with one very much worse than the other. It reminded me that when the eyeball is elongated in nearsightedness or myopia, the bulging appears at the back part of the eyeball, which has been called posterior staphyloma. These cases have recovered after a long period of treatment. A temporary cure has been demonstrated with the aid of the ophthalmoscope by the memory of perfect sight. The same is true of conical cornea, which also disappears temporarily with the aid of the memory of perfect sight. These cases become worse by the memory of imperfect sight. Staring always increases the bulging and makes the vision worse.

Conical cornea with its irregular astigmatism, occurs not only in adults but, like nearsightedness, is found also in young children. For such cases the swing has been a great benefit. The mother or nurse can stand facing the child, take both hands and sway from side to side for several minutes or longer. Teaching the child to dance is also a great help. Playing games requiring movement, like running, prevents the stare or strain in most cases. It is well to remember, however, that when the child is moving more or less rapidly from one place to another, the stare is always possible. Encourage the child to look from one place to another. The old-fashioned game of "Puss in the Corner" is a great benefit to the eyes. In this game the child is constantly shifting his eyes from one place to another.

The child should enjoy the games, especially when adults join in the game. Oftentimes a young patient will become quite boisterous and scream with excitement and pleasure. He may be as noisy as he likes. He may play, laugh, and scream, and become very much excited with great benefit to the astigmatism. It is well to exclude all children who carry around with them a grouch, or who make the patient uncomfortable by teasing him.

In my office there have been times when a child made so much noise that my other patients were interested, and too often perhaps, disturbed. Between the mother, the child, and myself, we have had quite a riot with a great deal of noise and loud laughter on the part of the child, but always the astigmatism improved. Anything that helps the child is justifiable. Don't forget that children, as a rule, enjoy themselves more when they are allowed to make a noise than when they are expected to stay quiet. The kindergarten methods of teaching should be practiced. The Montessori system is also a great help in relieving irregular astigmatism from any cause, as well as conical cornea.

One of my worst cases of irregular astigmatism occurred in a woman, seventy-five years old, who gave a history of ulcerations of the cornea, for a long period of years. After each attack, opacity of the cornea appeared, and with repeated attacks the opacities increased until the patient was unable to count fingers. She was recommended to sit in the sun with her eyes closed, holding her head in such a way that the sun shone directly on her closed eyelids [sunning]. Most of the time while she was awake, she practiced the long and the short swing alternately. After a number of months her vision improved so that she became able to thread a needle and do some sewing. She became able to read fine print without the aid of glasses. Her vision for the Snellen test card was also materially improved.

STORIES FROM THE CLINIC

No. 65: Cataract

By Emily C. Lierman

A friend of mine who knows me very well asked me if I ever get tired of Clinic work, do I ever tire of treating obstinate cases—those who take a long time to cure. No, indeed, I do not.

The harder a case is to benefit, the better I like it. I never tire of my patients, but I get tired myself. We appreciate rest all the more when the precious work like ours makes us tired.

Mothers of the Clinic, that is, most of them, are restful to me. I love to treat them. To see the tenderness, the loving expression come to their faces, always brings a perfect mental picture of the Madonna to my mind. When Mother Jones comes, she gives me that mental picture.

Her first visit was on November 1, 1924. She brought with her a note written by her pastor. Dr. Bates had cured many of his friends, so he was sure we could do something for Mother Jones. Her age was sixty-seven and she was troubled with cataract in both eyes. Her vision became defective about four years ago. Dr. Bates' examination with the ophthalmoscope showed a red reflex in the right eye, but none in the left.

After Dr. Bates had left the room, Mother Jones began to talk. I believe as long as I live I shall always remember the sound of her voice. When I compared her with the Madonna, I was not trying to give the impression that Mother Jones is beautiful of face or form. But the impression one receives while looking at her, listening to her tender voice, suggests something holy. She did not know of anyone who had been benefited by the Bates Method, but her pastor had sent her, and that was enough. She is very poor, but her son and family are taking care of her. When I told her that the only way for her to be cured was to practice faithfully every day, and to do exactly as she was told, she promised to do her part. When I tested her sight with the test card, she read 10/70 with both eyes together. Her vision with the right eye was 10/70, but she could not see the card at all with the left eye at ten feet.

She was instructed to palm and to think of something pleasant, something easy to remember. I left her by herself for about ten minutes, and when I returned she had not stirred, and her eyes were still covered with the palms of her hands. I told her to keep her right eye covered, but to open her left eye and tell me what she could see. I held the test card five inches from her left eye, and at that distance she saw the 200-line letter "C." She sighed with relief when she discovered that her left eye was not really blind, but was made so by strain and tension. In this short time the benefit she received from palming proved to her that her cataract was caused by strain.

I placed her in the sun, and while her eyes were closed, I used the sun glass on her eyelids. I could see her relax, and she smiled as she felt the warmth of the sun's rays. I led her back to her chair and told her to open her eyes and read the test card. Her vision had improved to 10/30, reading with both eyes. She was instructed to practice ten minutes many times every day, alternately palming, blinking, and flashing letters on the test card.

Mother Jones came once a week without missing a treatment, and each time her vision improved with but two exceptions, when it remained the same as on the previous visit. On her second visit she read 10/30 after palming, and the third treatment 10/20.

This dear Mother appreciated the sunshine more than any cataract case I ever had. Once when she failed to appear for treatment, I feared she was ill, and I worried about her. I had noticed that her clothes were none too warm during the cold days, and thought perhaps that was the reason for her absence.

While I was thinking about my bank account, a letter came from a private patient who is also one of my adopted mothers. She comes from the state of Ohio where I have many friends. Her gratitude for the great benefit she has received from Dr. Bates prompted her to send a sum of money to be used in making my Clinic family happy. Mother Jones and another poor mother with a big family, and dear old "Pop", who lives in a Home for the Blind, shared in the loving thoughts of my mother from the West.

Mother Jones soon returned to thank me for the gift and to explain why she had been absent. Her son had become a daddy, and both the mother and baby were doing fine. After my joy had been expressed over this great event, I produced a strange test card which she had not seen before, and placed it ten feet from her eyes. Some of our readers may doubt it, but I do believe that the little stranger from heaven had something to do with the improvement in the vision of her grandmother. She read 10/20 with her left eye.

Soon after, I was called upon to take charge of our private practice because of the illness of our dear Dr. Bates. Captain Price of London, England, who is practicing the Bates system successfully in his country, was in our office at the time and offered to help me and my wonderful assistant of the Clinic, Mildred Shepard. I placed Mother Jones in his care. His record showed on February 7, 1925, right vision of the white "C" card 10/20, left vision 10/20. At her second treatment by Captain Price, her right vision was 10/15, left vision 10/15, reading white letters on black card.

Some ophthalmologists would certainly appreciate this, if they would only study and practice the Bates system. What further proof is necessary to convince those of pessimistic minds, that our method of curing people without glasses is a purely scientific one?

Mother Jones is still under treatment, but it will not be long before she will enjoy normal sight. She tells everyone who will listen to her, about how much better she sees and how much better she feels, since she knows how to relax and relieve her eyestrain.

PALMING TESTIMONIES

Editor's Note—*Elisabet D. Hansen of Chicago, a teacher in the sixth grade, has done wonderful things for her pupils. She has taught them palming, which has relieved their nervousness, improved their memory and imagination, and their sight. The testimony of these children is so interesting, that we feel some of it should be published. The children not only benefited themselves, but they also benefited other children, their parents and their friends.*

Palming is the greatest discovery I have read about. It has made me so happy. At first I could not see a thing. I spent money trying to cure my eyes, but nothing could help me. I heard of a great Doctor teaching imagination and memory. So I wished for that Doctor to teach me how it was to be done. My teacher knew of him and inside of a month, palming four times a day, my imagination was getting better and my memory brought back the day when I was younger and I remembered the time I played with my eyes. But when I am old enough I shall travel to all parts of the world to show people how to use and take care of their eyes.—Joseph De Fiore.

I think palming is the best thing in the world, because it makes your eyesight good. I'm sure that if I keep palming all the time my brains and nerve will get better. The first time I never liked to do it, but then I got used to it and now I do it every day and every second I get.

One day while I was going home I met my girlfriend. We were talking about our eyesight and I told her that my teacher teaches all in the room every day. I told her that I would teach her how to do it, if she wanted to. So she took my offer and she said to me, "Come on Margaret, let's go to my house." I went and she said, "Teach me how." I taught her how to swing and palm.

Her name was Marie. She thanked me very much. The next day she brought other girls I knew and I taught them the same thing.—Margaret Micalett.

Palming has done a great deal for me. I can read the smallest letters on the chart. I do much better imagination than I used to do. I have learned better English and can read better, etc.

I have taught my two sisters how to palm. One of them used to get terrible headaches. And since she started to palm she is getting rid of them. I have also taught them to swing and to read the chart. Now they are doing better.—Adeline Valentine.

One day a boy friend of mine dropped a half-dollar. He was looking for it, but could not find it. Of course he had had trouble with his eyes for over a year. I walked out of my yard and asked him what he was looking for and he told me about the half-dollar. I looked on the sidewalk and found it the minute I laid my eyes on the walk. He asked me how I came to have such strong eyesight, and I told him that our teacher taught a lesson to keep eyes in good condition. He asked me to come to his house. I told him that by palming his eyes would be better. He asked me how many times a day. I told him six times or more. Then I heard my mother calling me. I went home. Inside of a week the boy took off his glasses, threw them in a box and told his mother he would never put them on again.—John Marshall.

Many years ago I had poor memory. I was persuaded by all nurses to wear glasses. One day my father bought me glasses. I tried in vain not to wear them, but I had to. Finally I got poorer memory and became sick. I told my father the glasses made me sick. That very minute my father broke them. My teacher taught me how to palm and swing. Soon my memory got to be good. I could see as good as any child in the room. This proves palming and swinging are good for memory and imagination.—Edward Yonan.

THE DREAM KING

By George M. Guild

Georgie was eight years old. He had never seen the Dream King. His mother had promised to tell him all he wanted to know if for one day he did not lose his temper or cry when told to wear his large, heavy spectacles that hurt his nose and made his eyes pain.

One day he succeeded. While his mother sat in her rocking-chair she had a hard time to keep awake. Georgie spoke to her several times, but she did not hear him. While he sat there fretting, he was surprised to see a nice young man, about his own height, walk into the room, take him by the hand, and lead him away. He told him that he was taking him to see the Dream King.

Georgie jumped up and down with pleasure and laughed all the way. Pretty soon they came to Shadowland, where everything was more or less in the shadow, because the only light that Georgie could see was the light of the moon. Every once in a while the person who was conducting him would disappear and someone else would take his place. Sometimes it was a woman, and finally it was a little, old man. He told Georgie that he was the sandman, who went around throwing sand into little boys' eyes to make them go to sleep. But he did not throw sand into Georgie's eyes. Instead, he kept him awake telling him such peculiar things that Georgie quite enjoyed his companionship.

Georgie was sorry to see him go when a blue fairy took his place. She led him to a large open space in a forest, where the grass was cut thin, and on which hundreds and thousands of fairies were having a good time. They were playing a very curious game. They had placed an elderly man on a throne and they crowned him with flowers. He held in his hand a short stick which they told Georgie was the wand of the Dream King. When he waved the wand, touched you, and you wished for something, your wish was granted, first in a dream and then later in reality. Immediately Georgie wished that his eyes would not hurt him any more, and that he could see perfectly without glasses.

The Dream King touched him with his wand and at once Georgie began to sway his body from side to side. His glasses fell from his face, and he found that he could see better without them than he had ever seen with them. It seemed to him as though everything were moving in the opposite direction. The trees, the fairies, and even the Dream King, were all moving in time with his movement. He remembered the faces of the boys that he had played with; he remembered his mother's face—his mother's face which was so tender, kind, and loving.

He became very much interested in what the Dream King was doing. People from various places were bringing all sorts of strange creatures to the Dream King. One fairy brought him a little duck, a few days old, which was about the ugliest duck that Georgie had ever seen. The Dream King touched it with his wand, and at once it became a beautiful swan. He saw caterpillars, ugly, sticky things. The Dream King touched them in turn with his wand, and they became beautiful moths or butterflies which flew away to where flowers were blooming. He saw children who were cripples and were unable to walk without crutches, but after the Dream King touched them with his wand, they threw away their crutches and left his presence laughing, singing, and dancing. It was astonishing to see all the animals, people and bugs who were relieved of all kinds of imperfections and obtain perfect health.

There was a beautiful fairy standing near Georgie. He spoke to her and asked her why she looked so sad. She told him that she had no soul and could never obtain one unless some mortal fell in love with her. Right away Georgie fell in love with her because she was so beautiful and nice. She threw her arms around his neck and kissed him, and thanked him for what he had done because now she had a soul and could be like real people.

Georgie was so pleased that he quickly took her to his mother. When he entered the room where he had left her, he found her still sleeping. He climbed up into her lap, threw his arms around her neck and kissed her. She woke and said, "Oh, Georgie, I had such a curious dream. For a long time I have been worried about you because you had to wear glasses, but in my dream I imagined that the Dream King had cured you. Now that I am awake, I feel that your eyes are troubling you and that you will still have to wear awful glasses."

Georgie laughed and said, "Oh, no. I never will have to wear my glasses again, because the Dream King has cured me. Although it was only a dream, I believe it will come true when you have the fairies to help you." His mother said to him, "But you have no fairy to help you." "Oh, yes I have," he answered, and introduced his fairy to her.

The mother looked so bewildered that he was quite sure she did not see the fairy. "Never mind, mother, I know that you do not see my fairy. I dreamed that I found her, and she is so sweet and lovable that I shall always dream, imagine, or believe that I have her. She has promised to help me keep up the swing, and to remember or imagine perfect sight all the time. I love her very much, I will always love her, and I know that I will never strain, stare, or hurt my eyes again."

DARK GLASSES

Many people when they go from a dark room out into the bright sunlight are dazzled, and feel uncomfortable. If they put on dark glasses for a time, the eyes are more comfortable, and they are tempted to wear such glasses most of the time.

It is a common practice that when a patient goes to an eye doctor, and complains of the discomfort of the strong light of the sun, the doctor will recommend dark glasses, which are usually comfortable in the beginning. Later on, however, the eyes become accustomed to wearing dark glasses, and will feel uncomfortable when the light is good. They are practically in the same condition as they were when they first put them on.

Miners, who work underground who seldom see the daylight at all, always have diseased eyes. There are some diseases which cannot be cured without exposing the eyes to the light of the sun. No matter how strong it may be, while it may prove temporarily uncomfortable, the sun has never produced a permanent injury.

Many people purchase dark glasses along with their other vacation necessities, because they are afraid that the reflection of the sun on the water will harm their eyes. Others have found that by becoming accustomed to the strong light of the sun, their vision was materially improved, but by wearing glasses to protect their eyes, their vision always failed. The proper thing to do is to become used to the sun at all times and in all places. The eyes need sunlight. If they do not get it they become weak.

One of the best treatments is to focus the strong light of the sun on the white part of the eye with the aid of a sun glass, which is kept moving from side to side to prevent the discomfort of the heat, while the patient is looking far down. In many cases sun treatment has accomplished in a few minutes a complete cure of sensitiveness to light.

QUESTIONS AND ANSWERS

Q–1. I have understood that if glasses are not worn, the sight becomes worse.

A–1. After wearing glasses and then removing them, the vision is always worse than if they had never been worn.

Q–2. When people remove their glasses, I notice their eyes look dull and expressionless.

A–2. It is due to the fact that wearing glasses has increased the stare.

Q–3. It is said that defective vision is due to a change in the shape of the eyeball. Does a cure by the Bates Method affect the shape of the eyeball?

A–3. When a person is cured by the Bates Method the eyes become normal and the expression is one of relaxation or rest without any strain. When the eyes are cured, the eyeball becomes normal in shape and is neither too long nor too short.

Better Eyesight
August 1925—Vol. X, No. 2

SCHOOL NUMBER

FEAR

Nearsighted people have frequently been told that it is necessary for them to wear glasses constantly to prevent their eyes from becoming worse. They are afraid that this statement may be true, and one cannot blame them for hesitating to leave their glasses off permanently.

One of my patients stated that she suffered very much from headaches. They were so severe that they made her ill, and confined her to her bed at least once a week. While wearing her glasses, she still was in pain but was afraid, if she left them off, the headaches would become worse. By discarding her glasses, practicing palming, swinging, and the memory of perfect sight, her eyes and head improved immediately. When she resumed her glasses again, she at once became uncomfortable, and the pain returned. She decided to leave them off permanently, and her headaches disappeared.

Some years ago an optician consulted me about his headaches. When I examined his glasses, I found that they were plane window glass. He said that when he wore them his headaches were better, but his wife confided to me that this was not true. He was troubled more when he wore them. He was suffering from fear.

I saw him again a year later and learned that he had permanently discarded his glasses, at my suggestion, during all that time, and was free of headaches.

It has been a habit with me, when patients who suffer from fear of the consequences that might happen if they did not wear their glasses, to have them demonstrate the facts. When the truth is known, fear is abolished. It is very easy in most cases to teach patients some of the causes of headaches.

SCHOOLCHILDREN

By W. H. Bates, M.D.

The August number of *Better Eyesight* each year is devoted to the problem of the imperfect sight of schoolchildren. Every year we have evidence that when most children enter school, their vision is normal. After a few years, most of them acquire imperfect sight. The average is about eighty percent (80%). Of these nearly all have acquired farsightedness and astigmatism. At the age of ten or twelve nearsightedness appears, and farsighted children become less. It is a truth that should be emphasized, that nearly all of the cases of imperfect sight in schoolchildren are acquired after they enter school.

For more than a hundred years, eye doctors have believed that farsightedness is congenital, or is present at birth. They did not believe that it could be acquired. A plausible explanation suggests that young children are more accustomed to using their eyes for distant vision without effort, and for this reason their distant vision is good. However, when they enter school and begin to study from books, they begin to strain at the near point. I have repeatedly published that a strain to see at the near point always produces farsightedness, or hypermetropia. It is not many years before the distant vision becomes imperfect from the strain. Then, when the child makes an effort to see at the distance in order to correct its imperfect distant vision, nearsightedness, or myopia, is produced.

It is difficult to explain why some children strain to see at the near point or at the distance, when others do not strain at all. [Modern right-brain/left-brain concepts explain this; see "Brains and Vision" in *Relearning to See*.—TRQ] I have had children consciously strain and lower their vision either at the distance or at the near point, or, in other words, demonstrate that the strain does not improve their sight. They were unable to tell me why they did it. However, some children profited by their experience and told me that the reason they did not strain was because it lowered their vision. In most cases where the children became conscious that the strain lowered their vision, they told me that the reason they kept on straining was because they did not know what else to do. There are a number of teachers who have suggested to their pupils that since strain causes imperfect sight, why not try resting the eyes, which many of them did with benefit.

However, there is a cause of eyestrain in schoolchildren

which has not been sufficiently emphasized. Children and adults imitate others, consciously or unconsciously. For example, when one person yawns, many others, consciously or unconsciously, yawn also. If in a company of people a feeling of pleasure prevails, each newcomer consciously or unconsciously assumes the same state of mind; but when an objectionable person, who is disagreeable, enters the room, a general feeling of discomfort among those present is felt.

Mothers, fathers, or other relatives affect the minds and the nerves of their children or of other people's children. If one or both parents are wearing glasses for the relief of eyestrain, the children who associate with them a good deal acquire eyestrain and their vision becomes imperfect. In one case I remember where the mother was suffering from eyestrain, accompanied by a high degree of nearsightedness in one eye. She was exceedingly nervous. Her vision was so much improved by treatment that she was encouraged to bring her daughter, who was wearing glasses for nearsightedness. The child was only ten years old, with a history of imperfect sight, which came on gradually and required strong glasses for its relief. With each eye separately or with both eyes, the vision was 10/200. I had her palm for about fifteen minutes. Immediately her vision improved to 10/10, or normal vision. Then I went out of the room and asked the mother to test the little girl's sight while I was gone. When I returned, the child's vision had relapsed to 10/200. I talked to the mother very strongly about the facts, and told her that nearsightedness was contagious. I impressed upon her mind as strongly as I knew how that the child would recover by reading the Snellen test card, provided the mother was not in the same room. The child was not to wear her glasses again.

Some weeks later the mother reported that her daughter had obtained normal vision. She was tested daily by a relative with normal sight who did not wear glasses. One day the mother visited me at my office and was very much depressed. She said that her daughter had had a relapse. I asked her, "Who tested her eyes?" She answered, "I did."

I recommended her never to speak to her daughter about her eyes, and that all the testing should be done by somebody else. This happened five years ago, and I believe the child still has normal eyes and normal sight without glasses.

I have examined the eyes of a great many schoolchildren during the past thirty years. In all classes where the teachers had imperfect sight, or wore glasses, or suffered from eyestrain, a much larger percentage of nearsightedness was found than in those classes where the vision of the teachers was normal, or no eyestrain was present. This fact suggests that teachers should learn how to have normal sight without glasses.

Some of the teachers who were familiar with my methods of curing imperfect sight without glasses taught the children how to palm and rest their eyes frequently during the day. The children were also taught how to avoid the stare by swaying their bodies, their heads and eyes from side to side, alternately closing their eyes, remembering some letter perfectly, and then flashing the Snellen test card. The teachers also taught the children the value of blinking the eyes frequently.

One teacher helped her pupils very much by having them write compositions on palming, swinging, and other methods for improving the sight. Many children were very much impressed by the value of relaxation, and encouraged other children, their parents, friends or neighbors to benefit their eyes in the same way.

Most teachers found that the treatment of imperfect sight improved not only the vision, but also increased the mental efficiency of their charges. It was very remarkable how the children's scholarship improved. Many of them with imperfect sight suffered from headaches and loss of memory. The relaxation exercises were of the greatest benefit in these cases. Some were found whose nerves were so sensitive that, although their scholarship was good, they failed to pass their examinations. In such cases a perfect memory or imagination of a letter or some other object was a complete relief, and their examinations became satisfactory. It was also interesting to learn that ill-behaved or mischievous pupils improved in their general conduct.

Many children suffer so much from headaches and other troubles when attending school, that they acquire a great dislike for their studies and prefer to leave school at an early age and go to work.

I have always had a great deal of sympathy for teachers. They certainly have a great deal to do. So many children are mischievous and seem to take a cruel pride in making the work of their teachers more difficult. In this connection, I wish to call attention to the wonderful work of Ms. Hansen of Chicago, Illinois who has solved the problem, and has published an article in this number, telling how she did it.

This article was written for the purpose of encouraging teachers to practice relaxation methods, which always improve the vision and prevent children from acquiring imperfect sight. If the teachers should, in the presence of their pupils, practice reading the Snellen test card and other relaxation exercises, no doctor and no member of the Board of Education could object.

STORIES FROM THE CLINIC

No. 66: Schoolchildren

By Emily C. Lierman

During the last year many schoolchildren have been benefited and cured of their imperfect sight at our Clinic. Some had been wearing glasses, but a larger number had not worn them. The latter were cured quickly and in a few cases needed only one treatment. The records show that all who were wearing glasses obtained better vision without them. There were no exceptions. For the benefit of those who are interested in eye Clinic work, I shall tell about a number of high schoolboys, all from the same school, who came for treatment.

A director of a Boys' Physical Training Department in one of our largest high schools in New York city heard of our Clinic. About nine-tenths of the boys under his care were wearing glasses. Others struggled along without them, even though they had imperfect sight. The boys were between the ages of 13 and 17 years. Late in the fall of 1924, one of them by the name of Arthur came with a note from the physical director. He accepted him gladly, and he began treatment under the supervision of Mildred Shepard, my assistant. His vision on the first day was 20/100 with each eye. It was noticed that his eyes were partly closed as he looked at the test card. When he was placed in a bright light he had difficulty in keeping them open, and his forehead was a mass of wrinkles. Anyone observing him for the first time would have thought that Arthur never smiled. I thought so myself as he appeared week after week, during the winter months and on through the spring. Recently I treated him and helped him to read 10/10 on a strange card. I also received a shock. He smiled. By closing his eyes to rest them and flashing each letter, he read 10/15 without a mistake. I wanted to stop his treatment then because there were about twenty others waiting. Arthur begged, however, for one more chance. We gave him the sun treatment, and then he returned to the test card and read 10/10. It was at that time I found that Arthur could really smile. Palming, blinking and swinging, with sun treatment, cured him.

The next case was William, whose vision was 10/200 with each eye. I do believe that William practiced faithfully at home and in other places, but he is just one of many cases of myopia who is slow in obtaining a cure. He is not discouraged, and knows that he will eventually have normal vision if he keeps on. His sight improved to 10/40, or one-fourth of the normal, in six months. The physical director wrote to me again, asking if he might send more of his boys who were anxious to get rid of their glasses. We have not the room nor the time to take care of even a small percentage of those who are crying out for help. I read the letter to Dr. Bates. He did not answer right away, but just looked at me. Then he said, "Now, you know how much I love schoolchildren, and you also know how much I disapprove of glasses." I said, "All right, that settles it." My answer was, "Send them along. There's no limit to the number."

Twenty or more came in response to my letter, and all of them were nice boys. How glad I was that I wrote what I did. After they had received their first treatment and I had spent more than three hours with them, Dr. Bates appeared at my room to ask if I were tired. His voice sounded most sympathetic. But I was perfectly relaxed and not a bit tired. As I instructed the boys to palm and swing, I practiced with them. As their vision improved, so did my nerves become more relaxed. I was happy, but not tired. Treating the boys was not easy, but every one of them did as they were told, which made the task lighter.

Samuel had worn glasses about two years. He had a great amount of pain in his eyes and his sight was getting worse. The optician who had fitted him said he would have to wear them all the rest of his life. His vision without glasses was 10/200 with his right eye and 10/100 with the left. He stared continuously, which, I believe, was the main cause of his pain. The first thing I did was to teach him how to blink. This relieved his pain. Palming and the swing improved his vision in both eyes to 10/50 on his first visit. Every time he was treated his vision improved for the test card. At times he did not do so well and he would apologize. Samuel had to have four months treatment before he could read with normal vision, but he was determined, and won out.

Abraham had symptoms of St. Vitus' Dance, with a great amount of pain in both eyes. His vision was: right 10/15 and left 10/10. He had no organic disease of his eyes, but the ophthalmoscope showed eyestrain. After three treatments the symptoms of St. Vitus' Dance had entirely disappeared and he had no more pain. His vision also became normal, 10/10.

Morris hated glasses and wore them but a short time. He had normal vision in his right eye, but only perception of light in the left. I held the test card up close to his left eye and told him to cover the right one. By alternately blinking and flashing the white of the card, he became able to see the letters as black spots. He was instructed to practice with the test card every day, seeing the letters move opposite to the movement of his body. While doing this he was to keep his right eye covered. After his third treatment he read the bottom line of the test card at three feet, or 3/10, with the left eye. He had been told by many doctors that nothing could be done for the left eye, because it was incurably blind. Dr. Bates examined him with the ophthalmoscope and said the trouble was called *amblyopia ex anopsia*, or blindness from effort. Dr. Bates said such cases are usually pronounced incurable. Morris believes that with constant practice, there is no reason why he should not obtain normal vision in his left eye.

Benjamin had never worn glasses. For a long time the constant pain in his eyes made it difficult for him to study. The ophthalmoscope revealed only eyestrain. Right vision, 10/10; left vision, 10/20. After palming a short while and with the aid of the swing, the vision in his left eye improved to the normal 10/10. He had four treatments altogether. On his last visit I helped him to read 20/10 right eye and 20/20 left. He was instructed to practice with very fine print daily and this, I believe, had most to do with relieving his pain permanently. He was more than grateful for the relief he obtained. He had a little brother, named Joseph, who was wearing glasses. Timidly he asked me would I help him, too. "Surely," I said. "Bring him along next time."

Joseph had been wearing glasses for three years, but his sight was not poor without them. Without glasses his vision was 10/15 with each eye. Blinking while he was swaying improved his vision to the normal in five minutes' time. He promised not to put his glasses on again and came to me for four more treatments. These were really unnecessary because his sight stayed normal, 10/10. If our method had been in general use in the schools, this boy and others would not have been forced to wear glasses.

Hyman wore glasses four years for progressive myopia. His vision with his right eye was 10/100, and 10/70 with the left. After his first treatment he was able to read 10/50 with each eye. Constant daily practice, by palming and improving his memory, brought his vision to the normal, 10/10. This boy required only five treatments.

Charles wore glasses about four years, although he had no organic trouble, just eyestrain. His vision was 10/30 with each eye. He was told to close his eyes, and while palming, to remember a small square printed on the test card. He was directed not to remember all parts at once, but to remember or imagine one part best at a time. His vision then improved to the normal, or 10/10. Sun treatment was also given him. Charles was cured in one visit.

Harry had worn glasses one year. His vision was 10/30 with the right eye and 10/70 with the left. Regular daily practice and the sun treatment improved his vision to 10/10 in three visits. Harry vows he will never wear glasses again.

Tobie was a fine, lovable chap and a trifle younger than the rest. His vision was 10/50 with the right eye and 10/70 with the left. Palming and sun treatment improved his sight to normal after three treatments.

The rest of the boys were cured mostly with one treatment. It was only a matter of teaching them how to use their eyes right.

MUSICAL APPRECIATION

By Elisabet D. Hansen

Another year has passed, and Dr. Bates' system of relaxation for the eyes, mind and nerves has again been most successfully tried out.

Every Monday morning the new Victrola record is used as a lesson for open discussion. The composer and artist is the very best, as we wish to instill in the children's minds an appreciation of the beauty, rhythm and style of the music. It is played all through the week, four times daily for five-minute periods.

Before starting the record we devote two minutes to one of the various relaxation exercises, either the long swing, swaying from side to side, the elliptical or variable swing. Next comes the record, and the children, while palming, are to interpret it. This is done sometimes by story, and sometimes, as in an orchestral or string quartet number, they choose one instrument, and follow that through to the end. It is fine to ask them what feelings are aroused, such as gayety, calm, sorrow, noisy street scenes or bravery. They love to do this. Then again the music is only an accompaniment for imaginative stories.

A conservatory in the park was visited by the whole room one day, and they remembered not only the gorgeous color displays, but the temperatures, and what grew best in those places. After their palming lesson, I asked them to write their memory pictures, and it made an excellent composition. What they wrote after palming, on how their pet dogs met them and played with them made interesting stories.

Imagining the clouds as hills of snow, a sled, two boys or girls, usually in bright-colored sweaters and caps, made much fun. They enjoyed counting the little black "o"—remembering their favorite flower blossoms, but, best of all, to watch the fairies dance and play in the woods. (George Guild's Fairy Stories must be read to them every month. It would not do to miss that.)

What you have just read will give you an idea how we vary the palming period. When the music is finished, the children come back very happy, and once or twice a day they read silently the smallest letters of the Snellen test card seen from their seats, both eyes and each eye separately. The card serves two purposes: To keep them from becoming myopic, and also to teach them to print Roman type letters.

It is interesting to see how well and orderly they express themselves in their written composition work, their oral expression, and in the drawing lesson. It is pleasant to see them first look at the flower study or model, close their eyes, and paint as though it were the finest thing in the world to do.

From an educational standpoint, Dr. Bates' system is far-reaching, and can't be bettered in the training of memory and imagination. In silent reading, geography and history, where imagination plays such an important part, it works wonders.

THE MAGIC FROG

By George M. Guild

Once upon a time, a long, long time ago, there lived a young frog who was very fond of travel and adventure. He became tired of sitting in one mud hole, where the only friends he had were other frogs. All the time he was on the move, trying to dodge the ducks and geese who were after him to serve as part of their dinner. He kept moving from one small pond to another until he came to where there was no pond, where there was no mud, and no ducks or geese to dodge. The trees were high and grew closely together, so that the light of the sun was largely cut off. Much to his surprise, he found an open space all covered with nice, short, soft grass.

When the sun went down, the place filled up with fairies. The fairies were surprised to see the frog and crowded around him to see him better. He was just as anxious to see them, and so he hopped on the top of the highest toadstool he could find, and from this elevation he could see thousands and thousands of fairies, all dancing, laughing, and having a good time. The sight of so many fairies in all their bright colors dazzled him so that he was compelled to continually blink his eyes to avoid the glare.

The Fairy Queen was pleased with him, touched him with her magic wand, and transformed him into a Fairy Prince. He wore magnificent clothes, but looked peculiar with his long legs, short arms, and large, bulging black eyes. She gave him a magic white horse to ride. He soon mounted him with a high jump and gave a loud croak. The horse sprang forward and they were off. The fairies cheered and waved their hands. The Prince waved his hat, and they were soon out of sight of the fairies.

In a short time they came to a small house. The Prince got off his steed, tied him to a tree, walked up to the front door, and knocked. No answer. He knocked again and again, without success. Then he opened the door and walked in. Lying on a couch, fast asleep, was a young girl with her eyes covered with bandages. She was suffering great pain in her eyes. Much of the time she cried and screamed in her agony. The Prince was sorry for her and spoke to her kindly and gently. He told her that he was a Fairy Prince who had come to help her. This made her laugh and clap her hands for joy.

"Oh, I must see you," she said. "I have always wanted to see a Fairy Prince." With her permission he removed the bandages with great care. He noted that the eyelids were enormously swollen, the eyeballs very red, and the pupils covered with thick white scars. She was quite blind. When she found that she could not see her Fairy Prince, she took his hand, pressed it against her sore, blind eyes, and began to weep softly.

She said, "You can cure me. Please do it." Then he lifted her in his arms, mounted his beautiful fleet, white horse, and galloped away from the dark woods out into the open fields where the sun shone at its brightest. She complained that the sun hurt her eyes, and pressed her face against his breast to protect her eyes from the glare of the sun. He advised her to hold her face up so that the strong light of the sun could shine on her closed eyelids. At first this was painful, but very soon the strong light felt more and more comfortable, and then the miracle happened. The swollen lids became smaller, the redness of the eyeballs disappeared, and still more wonderful, the white cloud over her pupils melted away and she could see. Her joy was unbounded.

"Oh, how handsome you are!" she said. "But why do you blink your eyes so much, just like a frog?" "That may be," he answered. "I have been told that a long while ago one of my grandfathers was a frog." "I don't care if you were a frog," she replied. "If you let me love you, when I grow up I will marry you."

They then rode on until they came to the woods where the fairies were. The Prince took the hand of the little girl and walked up to the Queen of the Fairies. He told her what he had done and that the little girl and he would like to get married after she had grown up.

Someone shouted, "The frog, he would a-wooing go." At once the Fairy Prince disappeared, and all that they could see of him was a frog, sitting on a toadstool, croaking as loud as he knew how.

The Fairy Queen was so indignant that I am quite sure the flames which started from her eyes would have burned up the speaker. She rushed over to the frog, touched him with her wand, and he again became a Fairy Prince. The

Queen called out in a loud voice, "You shall always be a Fairy Prince, and no one can ever change you back to a frog. When your little sweetheart has grown, be sure to bring her back to the fairies on your beautiful white horse."

The little girl ran to the Fairy Prince and threw her arms about his neck; she swayed from side to side, and when she swayed to the right the trees, the world, and all the fairies moved to the left. When she swayed to the left, everything moved to the right, but it made her eyes feel better, and she kept swaying from side to side for a long time.

The Prince and the little girl were very happy together, and in due time they were married and lived happily ever afterwards.

SIX YEARS OF THE BATES METHOD

By M. F. Husted

Superintendent of Schools, North Bergen, New Jersey

Editor's Note—*It is very gratifying to learn that Mr. Husted obtained such wonderful results in the prevention of myopia in schoolchildren. He has been very enthusiastic about this method during the past six years, and has tested it with great care in a way that is eminently scientific. I believe the evidence he offers to be absolutely true. My experience during the last twenty years substantiates all that Mr. Husted has written.*

Early in October 1919, the North Bergen school nurse, Marion McNamara, tested the sight of all our pupils. A new education was begun, a campaign for "Better Eyesight." In June 1920, a second test was made in order to measure the extent of progress and shows marvelous, practical, and successful results. This new effort in eye-mind education, to prevent and remove strain, adds to the already high educational efficiency of our schools by lessening retardation. Not only does eye-mind education place no additional burden upon the teachers, but by improving the eyesight, health, disposition and mentality of their pupils, it surely lightens their labors and furnishes an additional means of preventing retardation.

During the year 1923-24, every class in North Bergen schools, Grades II-VIII, became a conservation of vision class. Each classroom was visited by the Superintendent, and the values of good eyesight were dwelt upon. Pupils with normal sight volunteered to aid those with defective vision. They have engaged in this work with a helpful enthusiasm, and teachers have renewed interest. As this work is a physical training for the education of the eye-mind, teachers were instructed to use some time assigned to Physical Training or Hygiene to guide the below-normal vision pupils to sufficient proper eye practice for curative effects, and those with normal sight to sufficient practice for the prevention of eye defects.

Our records for 1924 show a startling condition of below normal vision among public school students. It also shows the miraculous results of eye-mind education in relieving strain. Of 129 pupils having glasses, 18 were found with normal vision and 111 had vision below 20/20. It is also shown that out of 4,026 pupils without glasses, 1,133 had below normal vision. The total below normal vision was 1,244 out of 4,155 pupils.

The final results of our 1924 tests are remarkable for the improvement made, and show the wisdom of this special 1924 procedure and the great value of this wonderful discovery. Of 118 below normal pupils wearing glasses, 89 have improved, and out of 1,072 non-wearing glasses pupils with below normal vision, 693 have improved. Out of a total of 1,190 pupils with below 20/20 vision, 782 have improved. Of those that have improved, 342 have even attained normal vision.

Great care has been taken to make these reports accurate. The tests were all made by two nurses assisted by the classroom teachers, and the reports were all made under nurse supervision.

Our 1925 records prove the wonderful effects of eye-mind education in relieving strain. Seventy percent of those wearing glasses improved; 87% of those not wearing glasses improved, and 56% of the entire number benefited attained normal vision.

Conclusions

Because of the prevalence of pupils with defective vision, because of its great simplicity, and because retardation in schools furnished one of the teachers' greatest problems, eye-education is one of the great wonders of this age, and may become a boon of hope to the pupil, a boon of efficiency to the teacher, and a boon of mercy to humanity.

BATES METHOD POPULAR WITH TEACHERS

Throughout the past year a group of teachers in one of the city high schools has been much interested in studying the Bates Method. One afternoon each week, from three to four, we have a "Bates Class." The number attending has varied, sometimes being as many as fourteen. I feel that the total result has been eminently satisfactory. A great deal of enthusiasm has been aroused and many people helped.

Different individuals have, of course, presented different problems. One woman was beginning to feel that her near vision was blurring. She had never worn glasses. It seemed a very short time—perhaps not more than a month—before her eyes improved so that she could read diamond type. At present she is able to see the microscopic print in the little Bible. A man who had worn glasses many years discarded them last December, and says now he has "forgotten how they feel." Another teacher who took off her glasses two years ago, comes to the class once in a while for a little practice with us when her eyes feel tired.

A certain teacher with three diopters of hyperopia and presbyopia has made great strides. She has a vivid imagination and never-flagging enthusiasm. We both feel that her eyes will be normal some day in the near future.

The teachers who come to the class often look very weary. They always say they feel more rested at the end of the lesson. Our procedure is the usual one of palming, swinging, sunning and working with the Snellen test card and fine print.

Some of the teachers who understand the method come to help teach the others. A student in the school whom I have trained always assists at the classes, and that makes the handling of the large group much easier. I am intending to have a similar class next year, and I am sure we are going to accomplish even more.

Better Eyesight
September 1925—Vol. X, No. 3

OPTIMISM

Optimism is a great help in obtaining a cure of imperfect sight. About ten years ago a patient was treated for cataract, complicated with glaucoma. After two weeks of daily treatment, the vision improved very much and the patient became able to travel about the streets without a companion to guide her. Her vision at this time had improved from perception of light to 10/200. After palming, swinging, and the memory of perfect sight, her vision was still further improved. She was very much encouraged and returned home full of enthusiasm to carry out the treatment to the very best of her ability.

Soon afterwards things did not go well at home. The patient became very much depressed and stopped her daily practice. Her daughter was very enthusiastic, and realized that her mother had been very materially improved and that further treatment would bring about a complete cure. She talked to her mother for half an hour or more and encouraged her to continue with her practice. The patient responded favorably, got busy, and was able to bring back much of the sight which had been lost. She made further improvement every day.

At times the mother was very pessimistic. She was continually complaining that she knew very well that she would never get her sight back. Then the daughter would start in with her optimism.

One bright, sunshiny morning the mother got up, took a card with diamond type printed on one side, and was greatly surprised to read it without any trouble. In three months her distant vision was normal.

IRITIS

By W. H. Bates, M.D.

The colored part of the eye, which is visible by ordinary inspection, is called the iris. When the eyes are blue, the iris is the blue part of the eye. When this is inflamed it causes much suffering and, as a rule, the vision is lowered. Many general diseases cause iritis—rheumatism and syphilis are the most common. There are other causes, injuries and sympathetic ophthalmia.

When a foreign body becomes located inside of the eyeball of a healthy eye, more or less inflammation follows, with complete blindness in many cases. Unfortunately, the trouble does not always stop with the loss of vision in one eye. The irritation of the foreign body in one eye may have an effect upon the other. Iritis may then develop and lead to serious consequences. It is said to be sympathetic, meaning that the healthy eye sympathizes with the diseased or blind eye and also becomes diseased. Sympathetic iritis is very treacherous. Cases have been described which became blind from sympathetic ophthalmia within twenty-four hours. The only treatment that is at all efficacious is the removal of the eye containing the foreign body. Sometimes the operation is delayed too long, and after the healthy eye has become inflamed. In such cases removal of the eye with the foreign body may not be beneficial.

Some years ago a lady wrote to me in regard to her brother. She said that at the age of sixteen a bullet from an air gun had entered the inside of the left eye. He was taken at once to the hospital, where he received proper treatment. The surgeon in charge recommended that the eyeball be removed at once. The family refused to have this done so soon and put off the operation as long as they could. But things kept getting worse and worse, and the good eye became affected. The family at once consented to the removal of the eye, but it seemed to be too late. Although he was kept in the hospital a considerable time afterwards, receiving the best of treatment, the vision of the good eye declined more or less rapidly until there was very little left.

At the age of thirty-two he visited me at my office. The vision of the right eye was the ability to count fingers at about three feet. He was unable to see any of the letters of the Snellen test card at any distance. With the ophthalmoscope the eyes showed evidence of previous inflammation, but the interior of the eye was so cloudy that I was unable to see the optic nerve with the retinoscope, I think most men who have seen these cases would agree with me that things were not very promising. The man's sister told me, however, that they had not given up hope and visited every eye doctor who had been recommended. She said that no one was able to help him. The doctors very positively stated that it was impossible for the eye ever to get any better, and it would most likely become even worse.

As a matter of routine, I tried palming and swinging, but without the slightest benefit. When I asked the patient if he had a good imagination, he replied that he thought he had.

With that I took the Snellen test card and held it at less than a foot from his eyes. I told him that at the top of the card was the letter "C," about three inches in diameter.

"Now," I said, "you don't see that letter 'C,' but if you have any kind of an imagination at all, you can imagine the 'C.' Can you not?" "Oh, yes, Doctor," he replied, "I can imagine a sort of a big 'C,' but it is all blurred."

"Well," I said, "remember a letter 'C' that you have seen years ago, that was perfectly black and had a white center which was perfectly white. You can remember having seen such a letter, can't you?" "Oh, yes, I can," said the patient. "I not only can remember a perfect 'C,' but with my eyes closed I can imagine I see it." "Well now, if you open your eyes, can you imagine you see it perfectly? If not, close your eyes and remember, or imagine it, as well as you can."

He practiced this imagination of a perfect "C" with his eyes closed and with his eyes open, alternately, for quite a while. After an hour had passed he said to me, "Doctor, I don't see a perfect letter 'C,' but I believe that now I can imagine I see it when I look at it with my eyes open."

When the "C" was placed more than a foot away, he became able to imagine it just as well as he had up close. With a little more practice he became able to imagine he saw a perfect "C" on a white card at ten feet. Then I asked him, "Can you see any letters at all below the big 'C'?" He said, "Yes, I see two smaller spots below it." Then I told him that the first spot was a letter "R," and that I didn't believe he saw it. He said, "No, Doctor, I don't see it, but I think I can imagine it." "Can you imagine it perfectly?" In a short time he answered, "Yes." "What is the first letter that comes after the 'R'?"

"I don't see it," he answered, "but I imagine it is a letter 'B'." This was quite correct. In a few days his vision improved to 15/10, or more than normal vision.

He demonstrated that when he imagined perfectly a letter that he knew, his sight was improved until he could see other letters that he did not know. I recalled the ophthalmoscopic examination I had made and that the whole interior of the eye was filled with opacities which obscured the retina, and which must have prevented him from having good sight.

The question came up in my mind: In what way did the imagination help his vision? With the ophthalmoscope I saw the opacities in his eye become less when he imagined a letter perfectly; but, when he imagined a letter imperfectly the opacities reappeared.

A second patient had chronic iritis for several years. At times the pain was so great that a number of operations had been performed, without benefit. The vision of the left eye was normal, while the vision of the right eye was only perception of light. He had opacities on the front part of the eye, the cornea, which lowered his vision. The pupil was filled with inflammatory material which obscured the interior of the eye. On some occasions the eyeball of the right eye would be of stony hardness, while at other times the eyeball would be as soft as mush. The eyeball was very hard when I first saw him. With the aid of palming, swinging and sun treatment the discomfort became less.

After the failure of the orthodox treatment for chronic iritis, it is of interest to report the great benefit which followed the "Imagination Cure." Like the other patient described above, the imagination of the known letters with his blind eye helped him to see letters that he did not know and the iritis was very much improved.

STORIES FROM THE CLINIC
No. 67: Iritis
By Emily C. Lierman

Iritis is usually very painful and causes a patient to feel much depressed. A matron of a working girls' home telephoned me to ask if it were possible to treat a young girl who was under her care. This girl, Florence, was not the usual type one finds at the Clinic. We made an exception in her case and admitted her because she was an orphan. Both her eyes were bloodshot and she continually tried to shield them from the light. Even ordinary light hurt her. The trouble began in her right eye, and shortly afterwards the left eye became inflamed. This was about a month before I saw her. She was treated by a number of competent eye doctors, who said she had iritis. They gave her drops to put into her eyes, but the pain still continued. Later, one of these doctors advised her to have her teeth and tonsils examined, but instead of doing this she came to me.

Dr. Bates examined her eyes with the ophthalmoscope. Then he asked me to examine them also and tell him what I saw. When I looked into the pupil of the right eye, I could see the whole area was covered with small black spots. It looked very much like the top of a pepper box. Her left eye was also affected, but not as much as the right.

Her pain was so intense that I did not test her vision with the test card immediately. She was told to palm and remember something pleasant. While palming, she described to me how her room was arranged. She remembered the figured pattern of the draperies on her windows, chairs and bed. She removed her hands and opened her eyes before I told her to, but the pain had disappeared and she wanted me to know it.

I placed her in the sun, being sure her eyes were closed. The strong light was focussed on her closed eyelids for a moment only. She drew away from the light quickly, which is the usual thing for patients to do when they have never had the sun treatment before. I encouraged her to let me try it again. She closed her eyes as she was told and I led her into the sunlight once more. She liked it.

Florence was advised to blink often and to palm her eyes early every morning, and during the day when possible. Six days later I saw her again. The ophthalmoscope showed a decided improvement in the pupil of her right eye. There were only a few small spots on one side of it. The left pupil was entirely clear. Florence said she had been working unusually hard, and also late at night, and feared that the vision of her right eye would not be so good. She read 10/15 with the right eye on a strange card, but the letters were not clear. After she had rested her eyes by palming and practicing the sway, the letters cleared up and she read 10/10. Her left eye had normal vision. Then I gave her the sun treatment again.

The third time I saw her, which was also her last visit, both eyes had normal sight and her pain had disappeared entirely.

Later we had another case of iritis, a woman much older than Florence. She was almost insane with pain in both her eyes. I could not do anything with her for an hour or more because of her extreme nervousness. I placed the palm of my right hand over her closed eyes as she leaned her head against me. Fortunately, she had her little girl, Betty, with her. While I palmed the poor mother's eyes, I held a conversation with Betty, solely for the benefit of her mother.

Betty was telling me how her mother suffered all day long, and at night she had walked the floor because she could not sleep with the pain. Mother love is one of the greatest things in the world. I could feel the mother relax as I held her close. Then she began to talk of Betty's good qualities, and what a great help she was. I placed the mother in the sun, still keeping her eyes covered with the palm of my hand. I held the sun glass in position, so that the strong light of the sun would focus directly on her closed eyelids when I removed my hand.

Knowing that the strong sunlight had been painful to

her during her illness, I did not tell her what I was about to do. I planned to use the sun glass very quickly and not give her a chance to strain. I did it successfully, although I feared I would not. Some patients strain so in their agony that it is difficult to use the sun glass the first time. After the first treatment this patient enjoyed it.

The vision in both eyes was 10/40, but none of the letters were clear. After the use of the sun glass I encouraged her to palm while Betty and I started another conversation. The subject was all about her baby brother. Betty would exaggerate once in a while about some of the things brother did. Her mother would correct her and explain them differently. This was just what I wanted. Anything but the memory of her discomfort would be a help. She was temporarily relieved of her pain when she left the Clinic.

Betty was invited to come with her mother at her next treatment. An eye specialist was visiting us at this time and, after his examination with the ophthalmoscope, he pronounced her trouble to be a bad case of iritis. He was quite positive that she could not be cured in less than six weeks. My patient came every day for one week, and at the end of the second week she was entirely well. During the time that her pain was relieved, her vision also improved. The only methods I used were sun treatment, palming, and perfect memory.

I did not realize how great a help Betty was during her mother's treatment, but after her mother was cured I found out. When patients suffer intensely I seem to feel it. I unconsciously lower my voice and speak as softly as I can. I believe that we all respond to kindness, and this we need most of all when we are ill. Betty repeated to her mother at home a great deal of what she had heard me say at the Clinic. She tried to use the same tone of voice, and also smoothed her mother's throbbing forehead. She even did this during the long nights when sleep was an impossibility. Truly Betty was my assistant in the cure of her mother's eyes.

THE CONGO TREE

By George M. Guild

("The Congo Tree" was written for the benefit of the children. It will help them to obtain relaxation when someone with perfect sight reads it aloud slowly, while the children listen with their eyes closed or when palming. The tree receives its name from a river in Africa, which is a very important river, indeed. It is a magic tree very much appreciated by fairies. The flowers that grow on it are very beautiful and their fragrance is so sweet and delicate that not only do the fairies enjoy it, but also everybody else. Children with imperfect sight and sore eyes, and those who suffer from headaches, are cured at once of all their troubles when they carry away some of the flowers from the Congo tree. The leaves are of great value, too. If a child holds one of these leaves to his ear, the leaf will talk to him in a language that he can understand. It will tell the child how to be happy and enjoy perfect sight without glasses.)

And now the merry jingle
Of fairies dancing single;
Watch them come and watch them go,
Bowing high and bowing low,
Always smiling, singing, glad,
With their laughing, never sad.
Happy, happy, they will be
When they see the Congo tree.
They will climb up to the top,
Swinging, swaying, never stop,
As they move, the earth goes round
With the sky, and with the ground.
Ev'ry leaf upon this tree
Knows a lot of how to see.
This Wonder Tree has a heart
Full of love in ev'ry part.
A tall, heavy tree, all right,
Its top seems out of sight.
The Congo tree is hailing,
To all whose sight is failing,
"Let me help you to a cure,
Come quickly, while it is sure."
Georgie Fairbanks came to see
All about the Congo tree;
It might cure his eyes so sore
Of their pain forevermore.
Without glasses he might play
Ev'ry night as well as day.
The fairies can, they so kind,
Cure his eyes, a long time blind.
The fairies came, took his hand,
Led him forth, a smiling band.
The Congo tree was weeping,
Awake, and yet 'twas sleeping
While Georgie had a strange dream,
Things were not as they might seem.
Blind he was, and yet could see.
Strange, how could that wonder be?
When his eyes were closed tight
All things were as black as night.
He could count up to seven,
Add four, which makes eleven.

The Congo tree sways much more,
A hundred thousand, add four.
The tears it shed made it dry—
Many quarts from each eye.
Wake up, Georgie, do your best,
Shift and swing after your rest.
No more glasses, no more pain,
The Congo tree once again
Is ready to help your eyes.
Hurry, for fast the time flies.
Now it did not shed a tear,
Neither did it have a fear.
Ev'ry leaf and branch could see
All the fairies in their glee.
The Congo tree was talking,
Each special branch knew something,
Its roots on truth were founded,
And they were deeply grounded.
Georgie woke from his dream
And saw things as they might seem.
The fairies told him to read
Fast or slow with some speed;
Also he should often blink,
And as fast as he could think.
Remember what he saw best,
Always taking a good rest.
The fairies came and sat down
Cross-legged on the warm ground,
And then they began to sing
"We have a Queen, but no King."
The only man who was there
Was a youth with curly hair.
While his eyes were on the Queen
A fairy crept close unseen,
Cut away one of his curls,
Decked it with some fine pearls,
Then threw it all in the air,
"A trophy to the most fair."
What a scramble, what a fight
Before 'twas won and held tight!
By a fairy, meek and mild,
But full of fun as a child.
She looked round for her knight,
But he had gone from their sight.
Only Georgie saw him go
With the Queen, and not so slow.
He saw him with the Queen fly
Very fast, toward the sky.
Georgie's eyes were now all right,
Seeing fine by day or night.

THE EFFECTIVENESS OF RELAXATION

By May Secor
Special Teacher of Speech Improvement,
New York City Public Schools

Stammering, stuttering, lisping, and other speech defects may be considered erroneous speech habits which may be corrected by inculcating new, correct habits of speech. This presents a psychological problem. There is, however, another aspect to the work of speech correction—a physiological aspect. Many cases of speech defect are difficult to correct because of the physical condition of the pupils. It is considered an important duty of the speech improvement teacher, therefore, to check up physical conditions and to advise parents to have corrected such defects as eyestrain, unhygienic dental conditions, malnutrition, and excessive fatigue.*

Many stammerers suffer from eyestrain. For years I urged the parents of such children to consult oculists, any oculists of good standing. They did so, and many cases returned with glasses; however, many of these children who used glasses continued to suffer from eyestrain. Upon returning to the oculist they were usually instructed to continue wearing their glasses until they "became accustomed to them." In many cases eyestrain continued, and the correction of stammering was still impeded. I was deeply concerned about the apparent impossibility of eliminating eyestrain.

Finally a friend placed in my hand Dr. Bates' book entitled *Perfect Sight Without Glasses.* At that time I was wearing bifocals, and had used artificial lenses for many years. I read Dr. Bates' book and decided to apply the method to the correction of my own visual defects.

On March 15, 1923, I removed my bifocals. I followed the Bates Method carefully, hopefully, and persistently and have never used glasses since. My near vision and distant vision are excellent and I enjoy great "eye comfort." I have come into contact with many other men and women who have attained normal vision without glasses by means of

*I believe, however, that it is not the province of any teacher, principal, or nurse to advise, urge, or insist upon parents having children operated on. Those in charge of children may, with propriety, advise parents to consult physicians regarding their children. In many cases, however, physicians differ among themselves as to the advisability of operating. I believe that the decision should be made by the physicians and parents.

the Bates Method, after having suffered along with eyeglasses and eyestrain for years.

Convinced of the efficacy of the Bates Method, I became a pupil of Dr. Bates and learned the secret of relaxation. I learned how to relax more completely, and how to help others relax. I began to realize the value of relaxation in education. I made relaxation the keynote of my work in speech correction, and there resulted a harmony that was most helpful to my pupils. It created a pleasant, healthful atmosphere, which enabled pupils to acquire more readily the desired, correct habits of speech. To the stammerer, especially, palming, swaying, swinging, sun treatment, and reading the Snellen card are Godsends.

In April 1925, I began work with the speech defect cases in two new schools. Among these cases were a number who wore glasses, and several of these children were crossed eye. (The term "squint" is frequently misinterpreted.) To induce relaxation and thereby facilitate the formation of new, correct habits of speech, I included in my program palming, swaying with music, swinging, the use of memory and imagination, and sun treatment. Early in June 1925, it became apparent that several pupils, who formerly were very noticeably crossed eye, showed either no defect or a decidedly less acute condition. To verify my observations I photographed these children. I also requested several teachers and a physician to observe them; they did so, and their findings coincided with mine. The following children were among those who entered my speech improvement groups early in April 1925:

Case A. Boy, age 14; myopia and strabismus (crossed eye, called also "squint"); used glasses several years; speech defects, stammering and lisping; known in school as a discipline case. June 1925—marked improvement in speech and strabismus entirely corrected.

Case B. Boy, age 11; myopia and strabismus; used glasses two years; speech defects, stammering, defective phonation, and aphonia. June 1925—marked improvement in speech; strabismus much less acute, and entirely relieved at times, when glasses are not used.

Case C. Boy, age 7; myopia and strabismus; never used glasses; speech defect, lisping. June 1925—speech improved; strabismus relieved—occasional relapse when under strain.

Case D. Girl, age 8; strabismus (but normal vision); wears glasses, constant use; speech defect, lisping. June 1925—lisping corrected; when glasses are removed, strabismus is very evident and child sees "two ladies instead of one"; after removing glasses and relaxing a few minutes, strabismus and double vision disappear; subsequent use of glasses causes return of these two defects, which again disappear after the child removes the glasses and relaxes.

In these cases the relief of visual defects was merely a by-product of educational work, conducted on a basis of relaxation. Would it not be well for us to conduct all educational work in this way, and thus help to relieve eyestrain throughout our schools?

Let us consider the problem of the child having visual defects. What method has been used to help him? He has been urged to wear glasses, and if his eye distress or headaches persisted, he has been urged to continue wearing the glasses until he "becomes accustomed to them." Has this method been successful? Reports of the various sight conservation associations indicate that it has not been successful. What new method may we use to eliminate visual defects among schoolchildren? I suggest the Bates Method for Relaxation. Let teachers remove their glasses, and palm, sway, and swing. Let physicians and principals urge pupils to remove their glasses and practice these helpful exercises. Let us, as educators, be broad-minded and alert. When one method fails let us try another.

THE STORY OF JOHN

By Mary M. Campbell

Most of the books written by eye doctors state that holding the book close is very bad for the eyes. It is also advised that children should read in a good light without leaning over. It has been a very strong belief that when the child leans over to read, the blood gravitates to the eyes and produces imperfect sight.

When my son, John, was less than four years old we believed that his vision was poor and took him to an oculist for treatment. He at once prescribed very strong glasses, and told us that unless we compelled the child to wear them constantly he would most certainly become blind. With this calamity hanging over us all the time, we went to a great deal of trouble to carry out the doctor's orders.

When John was six years old we placed him in the kindergarten. He was quite contented there and enjoyed all the different exercises. The teacher had a long talk with us about his eyes, and told us that she thought that he had perfect eyes and did not need glasses. We consulted another oculist who found that his vision for distance was unusually good and that all of the glasses tried made his sight worse. We asked him if there was any danger of the boy going blind if he did not wear glasses. The Doctor smiled and said, "There is nothing the matter with the boy's eyes; he doesn't need glasses."

Then the Doctor tested his ability to read fine print—diamond type. He read it at about three or four inches from his eyes without any trouble. Then he was asked how far off he could read it, and to our surprise he read the fine print almost as well at arm's length as he could up close. The Doctor said that it was very evident that he did not need any glasses for reading. We said, "But, when John reads a storybook, he always holds it very close to his eyes, and many people have told us that he did it because he was inclined to be nearsighted, and if we permitted him to do this, he would most certainly lose his ability to see at the distance and would have to wear glasses the rest of his life. When he becomes interested in a storybook, he keeps on reading after the light fails. We have seen him reading after dark, just by the light of the moon."

The Doctor told us that it was all right for him to read by moonlight as long as he enjoyed it. He said it could not do John any harm. Since reading Dr. Bates' book I have found that he recommends that young children be encouraged to hold the book as close to their eyes as they desire and to read as much as possible for as long as the child is interested. Near use of the eyes, even when under a strain, always lessens nearsightedness and never causes it. As long as the child can read without discomfort at the near point, that child should be encouraged to continue reading in this way.

One day John came home from school and complained that he had a headache. At once all our old fears returned and we made an appointment with the Doctor to see him the next day. The next morning John's headache disappeared, but we took him to the doctor just the same.

The Doctor asked him, "Did you have the headache in school?" John answered, "No, sir." "When did you get the headache?" "About an hour after I left school," he answered. "What were you doing at that time?" John replied, "I wasn't doing anything." Then his sister, who was present, spoke up, "I saw you with a lot of other boys eating green apples."

John blushed and admitted the facts. The Doctor told us that what we should do was to consult our family physician if anything went wrong with John before taking him to an eye specialist. It seemed a peculiar thing for an eye specialist to say, but we followed his advice, and whenever anything went wrong with John the old family physician relieved him without glasses.

QUESTIONS AND ANSWERS

Q–1a. Does the improvement of the sight by the Bates Method increase the rapidity of reading? 1b. Is slow reading conducive to strain?

A–1a. The better the letters are seen, the more rapidly they can be read. 1b. Yes.

Q–2. Do weather conditions affect the sight?

A–2. They often do. When the eyes are normal the weather does not disturb the sight as much as when the sight is defective.

Q–3. Is cataract curable after an operation?

A–3. After a cataract operation, the crystalline lens of the eye is removed (aphakia). A large amount of hypermetropia is manifest. Strong glasses are usually required to improve the vision. These cases have obtained normal sight for distance and for reading by my method without glasses.

Q–4. How long is it necessary to follow your method before a cure is effected in a case of astigmatism?

A–4. These cases require a variable length of time. Some are cured in a few weeks, while others may require many months.

Q–5. My sight is good, but my vision blurs and the eyes pain. Will glasses relieve this condition?

A–5. I would not expect glasses to give you any relief.

Better Eyesight
October 1925—Vol. X, No. 4

READ FINE PRINT

Many nearsighted patients can read fine print or diamond type at less than ten inches from their eyes easily, perfectly and quickly, by alternately regarding the Snellen test card at different distances, from three feet up to fifteen feet or farther. The vision may be improved, at first temporarily, and later, by repetition, a permanent gain usually follows.

It is a valuable fact to know that when fine print is read perfectly, the nearsightedness or myopia disappears during this period. It can only be maintained at first for a fraction of a second, and later more continuously.

Nearsighted patients and others, with the help of the fine print can usually demonstrate that staring at a small letter always lowers the vision, and that the same fact is true when regarding distant letters or objects.

With the help of the fine print, the nearsighted patient can also demonstrate that one can remember perfectly only what has been seen perfectly; that one imagines perfectly only what is remembered perfectly, and that perfect sight is only a perfect imagination.

A great many people are very suspicious of the imagination, and feel or believe that things imagined are never true. The more ignorant the patient, the less respect do they have for their imagination or the imagination of other people. It comes to them as a great shock, with a feeling of discomfort, to discover that the perfect imagination of a known letter improves the sight for unknown letters of the Snellen test card, or for other objects.

It is a fact that one can read fine print perfectly, with perfect relaxation, with great relief to eyestrain, pain fatigue and discomfort, not only of the eyes, but of all other nerves of the body.

SOME TRUTHS

By W. H. Bates, M.D.

Normal sight can always be demonstrated in the normal eye, but only under favorable conditions.

It has been generally believed that the normal eye has normal sight continuously. This is an error. The normal eye does not have normal sight all the time. It has always been demonstrated that distance, illumination, size or form of the letters or other objects, and other conditions affect the vision of the normal eye, or that conditions favorable to some normal eyes are not favorable to all.

DISTANCE

Most normal eyes have normal sight when reading the twenty foot line of a test card at twenty feet. Of these, a smaller number do not have normal sight at thirty feet or farther. Some others do not see so well at a nearer distance, fifteen, ten, or five feet. Still others may have normal vision when tested at different distances from twenty feet to five feet, and have imperfect sight at more than twenty feet or nearer than five feet. One patient at times could see the moons of the planet Jupiter with normal sight when the eyes were normal; but at twenty feet the vision was imperfect, and remained imperfect for nearer points until tested at six inches, when the vision and the eyes were again normal.

It is a truth that the distance of the test card, when read with normal vision, varied daily, and in some cases within wide limits. These facts suggest that eyes with imperfect sight are improved more satisfactorily when treatment is employed with the test card placed at a distance where the results are best. In myopia, or nearsightedness, with the vision normal at one foot or nearer, improvement in the vision at a greater distance occurs by alternately reading the card at a near point, and a few inches farther off.

It is a truth that when the eye is normal when regarding a letter or some other object at two feet or farther, it may remain or continue normal for part of a minute, and when regarding a letter or other object at a greater distance, it may remain normal for a fraction of a second. By repetition, the flashes of improved vision occur more frequently and last longer.

Illumination

The illumination is important. As a general rule, vision is normal in the normal eye when the light is good. This rule has many exceptions. It is a truth that some normal eyes may have normal sight only in a dim light. One patient suffered from the annoyance of ordinary daylight to an extreme degree. At twenty feet only some of the larger letters were read without glasses. After the light was lessened by screens, the vision improved to the normal. After sun treatment the patient obtained normal vision in a strong light, as well as in a dim light.

Environment

The environment may be favorable or unfavorable. Teachers in the public schools with normal eyes, normal sight without glasses, had more students with normal eyes than those teachers with imperfect sight, or who were wearing glasses. Teachers have cured their students by treatment without glasses while curing their own eyes at the same time. Many people are great imitators. In schools where the students are ambitious to obtain normal sight without glasses, those with imperfect sight are influenced to do likewise—read the Snellen test card, practice the swing and rest their eyes frequently by closing them or by palming.

Schoolchildren with imperfect sight have been treated and cured. The cured children often helped or cured the imperfect sight of other members of their family, their neighbors, and their friends. The facts have been published from time to time in this magazine and elsewhere.

A child, age five, had a well-marked turning of one eye inward toward the nose (crossed eye). The condition was noticed soon after birth. The mother said that the child was very nervous, and when playing with other children who were also nervous her eyes were worse; but when she enjoyed the play, she was not nervous and her eyes were straight. The mother, the child and I played "Puss in the Corner" and made it a very noisy affair. The child screamed with laughter and even the mother smiled. The eyes became straight and remained straight as long as the patient was comfortable. But when the environment of this patient became annoying in any way, the eyes turned. The mother was advised to teach the patient many games which amused or interested her. The object of the treatment was to encourage relaxation.

The cause of death among many aviators has been believed to be due to attacks of blindness from eyestrain. Flying through dark clouds, in storms of wind, rain or snow, the environment may quite readily cause imperfect sight from eyestrain. But even with the weather conditions favorable, aviators have testified that attacks of blindness may occur without the victim knowing the cause.

This subject has been more fully discussed in the *New York Medical Journal* of September 8, 1917.

Strain During Sleep

It is a natural question to ask, "Does sleep secure relaxation of the eyes? How many hours should one sleep to prevent imperfect sight in normal eyes?"

It was a great shock to me to find that patients with normal eyes were under a much greater strain when asleep than when they were awake. I do not know why. It is a truth that when the eyes are normal, there is no strain and they are at rest. Anything that is done is always wrong and lowers the vision, because normal eyes only remain normal when the vision is normal. During sleep one is not conscious of the strain of imperfect sight. But the first thing in the morning the symptoms of eyestrain are very prominent, with headache, pain, and fatigue of the eyes. Many people complain that they have not had enough sleep, although some of them sleep from eight to twelve hours. With all the evidence at hand, I feel that sleep, instead of being a rest to eyestrain, is too often a cause.

A matter of great importance is the prevention of eyestrain during sleep. Some patients are materially benefited by practicing the long swing for five or ten minutes just before retiring. Others enjoy an increased relief from eyestrain by palming in bed until they fall asleep.

Eye-Shades

When the eyes are hypersensitive to light, one usually obtains immediate relief from the discomfort by the use of an eye-shade. This relief, however, is temporary, and very soon glasses are prescribed which seldom are a permanent benefit. The conditions are not favorable for normal vision when using eye-shades.

The normal eye is not made uncomfortable in a good light. An eye-shade makes the eyes more sensitive to light and causes eyestrain. Sun treatment, when used properly, is often followed by quick relief. The patient sits in the sun facing the strong light with the eyelids closed. The head should be moved slowly from side to side. At first there may be slight discomfort which usually disappears in a few minutes. Continue sunning for half an hour or longer. There should be relief at once. By repetition the benefit becomes greater and more permanent.

The Black Bandage

Many people desire to sleep late in the morning without being wakened by the sun. Before retiring they cover the eyes with a black bandage, which is worn until late in the morning. Patients who have used it for some weeks or months acquire a great sensitiveness to ordinary light, lose their good vision for distant letters or other objects, and become unable to read even large print without severe pain, headaches and fatigue.

Summary

It has been demonstrated that the normal eye has normal sight only under favorable conditions, and the conditions favorable to some are not necessarily favorable to all.

STORIES FROM THE CLINIC
No. 68: How Others Help

By Emily C. Lierman

Many reports are received from those students of Dr. Bates who are conducting clinics. It is encouraging to know that this work is spreading so fast. Clinics are being formed not only in America, but in Europe as well, and our representatives deserve the highest praise for their faithful work. A number of patients have taken a course from Dr. Bates, or myself, so they could teach others how to obtain normal vision. Mothers find it a great help to study the Bates Method. Some of them bring one of their children for treatment, and when they see the child obtain normal sight, they become eager to learn how to cure other members of their family. In this way the work has spread. If we could have a Bates Clinic in every town and city, people would be very much benefited.

There are many patients out West who are treating the poor without any compensation whatever. They may not have regular clinics, but it is Clinic work just the same. We have over fifty patients in Cleveland, Ohio, and some of them are helping the poor there. A teacher in one of the public schools has cured many of her little charges who had defective sight. In her reports to Dr. Bates, she mentioned several cases of defective minds that she benefited by palming, blinking and swinging. After a number of her pupils were relieved of mind strain, they were placed in regular classes.

This teacher had to be careful not to offend the authorities or to mention that she was using any system or method. She had the pupils practice for a few minutes every day in her classroom. She can appreciate eye education and common sense, because she is a cured patient.

A few grateful patients, well-known women of Cleveland, go about from place to place, helping unfortunate people who have imperfect sight. While I was visiting at the home of Ms. H. D. Messick, I discovered that she was conducting regular clinic sessions in her home every week. Although she is a busy woman, she gives part of her time to treating patients who cannot come to Dr. Bates. She has done remarkably well with many difficult cases, some of which I would like to report:

A little girl, nine years old, had convergent squint of her left eye. Very little of the iris was visible when I first met her. I was surprised when I saw her again, about six months later. The left eye was almost as straight as the right, and her vision had improved to 10/10 at times, with Ms. Messick's help.

A woman, with atrophy of the optic nerve of the right eye, and myopia in the left, was first examined by me in December 1924. Her face was lined with pain, and she seemed to have no desire to smile. The right eye was nearly blind, and she could not see letters of the test card at any distance with that eye. Her vision was about 10/50 with the left.

She was directed to palm for about five minutes or longer, and then stand and swing her body from side to side, with a slow, easy sway. The vision of her left eye improved to 10/30, and she flashed the large "C" of the test card with her right eye. She was advised not to wear her glasses again and to practice regularly every day. Ms. Messick's efforts in helping this woman were certainly not in vain.

The last report I received was most encouraging, and ought to be so to any patient afflicted as this woman was. The vision of her right eye is now 8/40, and the left eye is, I believe, normal. However, she reads quite a little with comfort, and does not complain of pain any more. Her facial expression has changed for the better and she is very grateful for what has been accomplished.

Another case that I started about the same time was that of a fifteen-year-old boy who was wearing glasses for myopia. His left eye was almost blind, and the vision of the right was 10/30. I taught him to palm and swing, and in less than half an hour his vision became normal, or 10/10, in the right eye. When he covered his right eye, the vision of his left began to improve for the large letters of the card, although they were not clear or distinct. I told him that if he wished to be cured, he would have to practice faithfully every day as he was directed. He promised to do his part. I just gave him a start, but it was Ms. Messick who cured him. I visited him some months later, and found his vision normal when he read the test card with each eye separately. He sees as well with the left eye as he does with the right. He displayed some marvelous drawings of ships, which were done after he was cured. The letter I recently received from him is printed below:

August 26, 1925.
My dear Ms. Lierman:

I am so grateful to you and Ms. Messick for having helped me to follow Dr. Bates' method that I am writing to tell of my experience with my eyes. About December 1924, we were examined by the school doctor. He told me my left eye was nearly blind.

Mother immediately took me to a well-known oculist in Cleveland, and after several visits to his office he prescribed glasses for me, to be worn always. A week had passed when I met you at Ms. Messick's. You told me to discard my glasses and practice palming and swinging, which I gladly did. Some of the teachers knowing I had worn glasses, and seeing that I didn't after I had met you, tried to persuade me to wear them; but I wouldn't, when I noticed how my eyesight was improving. After seeing Ms. Messick once a week, and practicing regularly at home five minutes in the morning and five in the evening, my left eye gradually improved to normal.

With deep gratitude for being spared the great annoyance of wearing glasses, I am. Yours sincerely, Mac.

THE MOVIE MIND

By Jane June

Editor's Note—*The remarkable results obtained by palming are due to the relaxation produced. If a patient will allow his mind to relax, his eyes will be rested and his vision improved. There are many pleasant ways to palm and each patient has his own favorite method. Jane June's idea is very effective.*

When I want to see a picture,
I never need to go
Into a picture-show of any kind.
I've a button in my brain.
I can press it without pain
And release my movie mind.

Anything I've read or seen
Flashes quickly on the screen;
Be it near or far away.
This is what I've seen today:

Out upon the Naples Bay,
White sails softly dip and sway.
The sun is shining clear,
And those ships seem very near,
Although so far away.

Just outside the window-pane,
Which is bright with drops of rain,
There's a robin hopping fast,
For his dinner-time is past;
His head is cock-a-pie
Because he thinks he hears a worm
Crawling underneath the grass.

The brown dog, Nether, is after the cat,
Running hard, though he is fat.
The cat, as mad as mad can be,
Is making for the nearest tree.
When she gets up into that,
Nether, out of breath and feeling flat,
Will have to sit down there below,
Bark offensively—and go.

Oh! there goes a crocodile,
Swimming down the yellow Nile;
Just above him, on a vine,
Feeling very safe and fine,
Swings a monkey—one of nine.
Crocodile says, "Come lower, please."
Monkey says, "I prefer trees,"
And begins to upward climb.

Just you try and you will find
Great fun with your movie mind.

THE BLIND MAN

Editor's Note—*This letter from a school teacher was just received, and seemed so worthwhile that we decided to make room for it in this issue. It substantiates Ms. Lierman's reports that those who know the method can improve the sight of others.*

Dear Dr. Bates:

I cannot resist telling you what my little Edith Collins, age twelve years, has done for a blind man that she picked up on the street.

His eyes were very much sunken. She taught him to palm and sunning. She and a little girl friend visited him in his hovel once or twice a week. Much of the time he was so ill that he kept to his bed, but had this so placed that the sun shone on his eyes. Little by little his eyes came forward. He palmed faithfully and swung a chart that was given to him. A visiting nurse was telling him it was all "bunk" one day, as Edith entered. She spoke to the nurse and informed her it was not bunk, and that if she (the nurse) would come back in two or three months she would find out for herself.

Well, up to July the reports were that he was gradually looking better, and his eyes seemed fuller. When school opened, Edith came into my room and said, "He sees!"

I had forgotten about the man, and for a minute I wondered what she meant. She told me that she had met this man on the street a week or two ago—he was very happy—sees to get around, can read headlines in the papers, and can pick out the smaller words in spots. He has promised her that he will not stop exercising until he obtains perfect sight. He also told Edith that if he had not met her, he would still be a blind man begging for food. Now he intends to find work in some other city.

Isn't this a wonderful thing for a little girl to do? Of course, if it were not for Edith, the man would still have been blind. Children do not discriminate as to whether a man is a beggar, a worker, or worthy. To them there are no differences. They scatter the good into every nook and cranny, and what is more, if it had not been for the revolutionary discovery of this very, very natural way to see and think, I would not have been able to have carried it on to the children, who so unquestionably take to the truth when presented to them.

I have been so excited about this that I had to write you at once!

THE BAT

By George M. Guild

When the city boarders occupied all the rooms and beds of the farm house, little Jimmie was sent to the barn to sleep in the hay. At first the change from the house to the barn was a benefit, but in a few days swarms of mosquitoes invaded the place, and tortured Jimmie. Then The Bat appeared. He was such a homely bat, and has such dreadful habits that he annoyed Jimmie very much. The second night he came, again, very much increased in size, with the same wicked little eyes, and apparently full of plans to annoy Jimmie further. Jimmie grabbed a pitchfork and rushed at The Bat to kill him, not just dead, but very much dead, more dead than any bat had ever been. Before Jimmie reached him, The Bat said, "Have a mosquito?" Jimmie stopped, amazed, and lowered his pitchfork. While he watched, The Bat leaned forward, and dropped a mess of big fat mosquitoes into Jimmie's hands. When Jimmie threw them down in disgust, The Bat looked surprised, because he could not understand how anyone could throw away such a delicacy. He explained to Jimmie that they had a wonderful flavor of sweet flowers and wild honey, and that he was the special Mosquito Catcher to the Fairy Queen. He supplied all the festivals with the choicest mosquitoes.

Jimmie was tired, lay down on his bed of straw, and was immediately fast asleep. He was so grateful to The Bat for clearing the barn of these little pests. Suddenly, he remembered that he had not seen his little crippled playmate for three days, and he became worried. The more he thought of her, the more restless he became. He cried out "'Where is my little crippled blind girl? I want to see her. I want the fairies to help her, because she has such beautiful eyes. She is good and kind, but she is crippled, and her beautiful eyes cannot see. Take me to her Mr. Bat, quick, right away."

The Bat picked little Jimmie up, and flew with him, far away, over mountains, rivers, and woods, and stopped in front of a tiny little cottage on the shore of a big gloomy lake. How did The Bat do it? Easy enough. The Fairy Queen touched him with her wand, and he became large and strong enough to carry Jimmie.

Jimmie hopped off The Bat's back, and looked through the window of the cottage. He saw nothing but a little bare room. Soon a little old witch woman, with a sharp pointed hat, and a broom under her arm walked towards the front door, which The Bat was holding tight shut. The Fairy Queen softly alighted on Jimmie's shoulder, and told him many things. "First," she said, "do not ask questions. The witch is trying to steal the little blind girl, and as long as you do not speak, we can manage her. She is really afraid of The Bat, who threatened to fatten his new mosquitoes on her flesh. I do not want any of the mosquitoes filled with the witch's poison blood at all."

Jimmie listened to all the Fairy Queen told him. Soon the Witch became suspicious and rushed out, straddled her broom, and went sailing toward the sky. Jimmie could not keep still, and called after the old woman as loud as he could, "Goodbye, you old witch!" She heard this, turned back in a rage, and flew straight for Jimmie's face. But The Bat was not idle. He placed himself between Jimmie and the old witch, grabbed her by the neck, threw her to the ground, and swept her with her own broom right towards the lake. When she realized where she was going, she knew she was doomed. She fought back, but The Bat was too strong for her, and in spite of all her efforts she could not stop him. How she did scream, curse and swear. Then she began to cry and beg for mercy, but The Bat kept right on until he swept her into the lake. She slowly sank and finally disappeared. The Bat threw her broom into the water, where it floated on the surface for a few minutes. Suddenly a long, skinny arm, with sharp claws for hands, shot out of the water, grabbed the broom, pulled it beneath the water, and that was the end of the witch.

A company of fairies on the shore of the lake were singing:

"And there she will stay
Ten years and a day—
Good Riddance!"

They all now returned to the cottage to look after the crippled blind girl. She was so glad to hear Jimmie's voice, and thanked them all for saving her from the witch.

The Bat, who was now larger than Jimmie twice over, and strong as a horse, was not satisfied with himself. After much coaxing, the Fairy Queen finally found out that The Bat believed he was too homely and wished to be beautiful. While Jimmie was busy with the crippled blind girl, treating her as advised by the Fairy Queen to cure her, The Bat and the Fairy Queen disappeared. Jimmie did help the little girl and they were playing in the woods, having a most glorious time, for she was not now a crippled blind girl, but one who was cured by the fairies, by The Bat, and by the love of Jimmie.

Suddenly the little girl cried out, "See the beautiful butterfly! It is the biggest that ever was, and on its back is the Fairy Queen!" She clapped her hands with glee and ran to the butterfly. The only way the Fairy Queen could make The Bat beautiful was to turn him into a large butterfly. How proud he was of his beautiful colorings and his soft, silky wings. The admiration of the little girl rewarded him for all his goodness.

Better Eyesight
November 1925—Vol. X, No. 5

MOVING

The world moves. Let it move. People are moving all day long. It is normal, right, proper that they should move. Just try to keep your head, or one finger, one toe, stationary, or keep your eyes open continuously. If you try to stare at a small letter or a part of it without blinking, note what happens. Most people who have tried it discover that the mind wanders, the vision becomes less, pain and fatigue are produced.

Stand facing a window and note the relative position of a curtain cord to the background. Take a long step to the right. Observe that the background has become different. Now take a long step to the left. The background has changed again. Avoid regarding the curtain cord. While moving from side to side, it is possible to imagine the cord moving in the opposite direction. By practice one becomes able to imagine stationary objects not seen to be moving as continuously, as easily, as objects in the field of vision.

When one becomes able to imagine all objects seen, remembered, or imagined, to be moving with a slow, short, easy swing, this is called the Universal Swing. It is a very desirable thing to have, because when it is imagined with the eyes closed or open, one cannot simultaneously imagine pain, fatigue, or imperfect sight.

The universal swing can be obtained without one being conspicuous. With the hand covered, move the thumb from side to side about one-quarter of an inch, and move the eyes with the thumb. Stationary objects can be imagined to be moving.

When walking rapidly forward, the floor or the sidewalk appears to move backward. It is well to be conscious of this imagined movement.

Never imagine stationary objects to be stationary. To do this, is a strain, a strain which lowers the vision.

CENTRAL FIXATION

By W. H. Bates, M.D.

Central Fixation: The letter or part of the letter regarded is always seen best.

With normal vision, a letter or an object cannot be seen clearly or perfectly unless one sees a part of the letter or object best, or better than all other parts.

Central fixation is passive. We do not see by any effort. Things are seen, one part best. Furthermore, it is a condition of relaxation of the eye or mind obtained without any effort.

The normal eye with normal sight is always at rest. Nothing is done. No effort is made. Many cases of imperfect sight have been cured when no efforts were made to see. One cannot relax by working hard, straining, nor obtain rest of the eyes or mind by the help of a strain. When the eyes are normal, they are at rest. When they are imperfect, they are always under a strain.

Central fixation should not be confused with concentration, which is defined by the dictionary to mean an effort to keep the eyes or mind continuously on one point only, and to ignore all other points.

Try it. Look directly, for example, at the point of the notch on the upper right corner of the large letter "C" on the Snellen test card. Keep the eyes open without blinking. In a few seconds, or part of a minute, the mind begins to tire from the monotony. An effort is made to hold the concentration. The effort increases with discomfort or pain. The vision becomes less, the white of the notch looks gray, the black appears less black, less clear and less distinct. The notch regarded is not seen as well as other parts of the large letter not regarded, and central fixation is lost. Not only does the notch appear less clear, but by continuing the effort the large letter "C," as well as all the letters on the card, are seen less and less perfectly. The white of the whole card is also modified and becomes less white. Other objects in the neighborhood of the Snellen test card soon begin to blur and are seen imperfectly. The stare or strain has very much the same effect as if the sun were covered with a cloud or as if the light in the room, or the general illumination, were lessened. When central fixation is practiced, all the objects in the room, including the Snellen test card, look brighter, clearer, just as though the light had increased.

Concentration is trying to see one thing only. It always fails. Central fixation is seeing one thing best, and all other objects not so well. When the vision, memory, or imagination are imperfect, concentration can always be demonstrated. When the vision, memory, or imagination are perfect, central fixation can always be demonstrated.

Central fixation is an illusion. All parts of small letters as well as large ones are printed with the same amount of blackness. We do not see illusions. They are only imagined. When we see best one part of a letter, or other object regarded, we think we see it best, or more accurately, we imagine it best. One can imagine anything desired, and much more easily than to make an effort to see it. This fact should be demonstrated repeatedly and consciously until it becomes an unconscious habit.

With the eyes closed the imagination of central fixation may be much better than with the eyes open. By alternating the imagination of central fixation with the eyes open and closed, both may improve.

Many persons have no mental pictures with their eyes closed. For example: A patient had suffered for many years with almost constant pain and fatigue. With his eyes open his vision was 20/20. He read diamond type as close as six inches, and as far off as twenty inches. He could imagine the white part of large or small letters whiter than the rest of the Snellen test card, but only with his eyes open when regarding the letters. With his eyes closed he could not remember mental pictures of any objects.

He was asked, "Which is whiter, the white center of a large letter of the Snellen test card or the white snow on the top of a mountain?" He answered, "The white snow on the top of a mountain." "Can you shift from one mountain top to another, remembering each one best and the others not so well, or worse?" This also he was able to do. But when he tried to imagine two or more snowcapped mountains simultaneously, he at once was conscious of an effort and lost his imagination of his mental pictures of the snow. The memory of the snowcapped mountains by central fixation helped him to imagine central fixation with his eyes open as well as closed.

A girl, age eight, had imperfect sight not corrected by glasses. The right eye turned in continuously. The vision of this eye was 3/200 with glasses. The left vision was one-half of the normal. She was taught central fixation and became able, in a few days, to imagine one part best of the larger letters. The vision of both eyes improved very much. She demonstrated the value of central fixation, and that she could not distinguish clearly even the large letters with each eye unless she imagined one part best. By repeated demonstrations this young patient acquired speed in the practice of central fixation. She became able to read a newspaper more than five feet from her eyes by artificial light. Fine print, or diamond type, was read rapidly, easily, at one inch from each eye.

She enjoyed the practice of conscious central fixation. It was to me very wonderful to observe her imagine very small letters by central fixation and read them at ten feet or farther. The squint disappeared permanently.

A girl, age twelve, was treated for progressive myopia. The vision of each eye was 3/200. With concave 16 D. S., the sight of each eye was improved to 20/70. The patient was very nervous. Her memory was poor, and she was behind in her schoolwork. Treatment with the aid of palming and central fixation improved her vision slowly. After about six months there came a sudden change for the better. In one day, her vision improved from 10/200 to 10/10 plus. The next day she read the bottom line of each of three strange cards at twenty feet, 20/10. It was remarkable, also, because she read all the letters as rapidly as she could pronounce them. The mother was worried because her daughter had suddenly acquired a habit of running down stairs three steps at a time. She had never stumbled or fallen once. The mother also reported that the patient had acquired much pleasure in coasting and was the most daring of all the children. Her scholarship had improved. The teacher said the patient would read a page of history in a few seconds, and recite it with a perfect memory after a few days, a month, or longer. Her memory for other subjects was equally as good. Immediately after she read the strange cards with normal vision I asked her, "What helped you?" "Starch," she answered.

Then she explained that she had become able to imagine a small piece of white starch perfectly white by central fixation. When her imagination was perfect, her myopia disappeared and her eyes were normal, which made it possible to obtain normal vision. The retinoscope used at the same time demonstrated that her myopia disappeared when she had a perfect imagination of central fixation.

Patients whose sight is very imperfect usually require a much longer time to acquire central fixation than do some others. One should not be discouraged when, after some weeks or many months, their vision remains imperfect. Too many are disappointed because they fail to obtain central fixation after long periods of time, practicing without the help of a competent teacher. One very determined patient devoted many hours daily for over a year without any apparent benefit whatever. She told me that she knew she was curable and was resolved to keep at it the rest of her life if necessary. I wrote her a few suggestions. She followed my advice and was cured in a week.

STORIES FROM THE CLINIC
No. 69: Aunt Mary

By Emily C. Lierman

For a year I have been treating a woman, age sixty-eight, who has cataract in both eyes. In the beginning I saw her about once a week, then later I treated her less frequently because I had so little time. She lives with her sister and family in the country, and everyone who knows her calls her Aunt Mary. She has all the reason in the world to be depressed or unhappy, because with the exception of just a few years, she has been a cripple all of her life. Yet Aunt Mary greets you with a smile and makes you understand that she is happy.

A few years ago her sight began to trouble her, and she was examined by an eye specialist. He said that cataract was beginning to form in each eye and that nothing could be done until they became ripe, when she was to be taken to the hospital for an operation. Then I was consulted by her family and asked to call at her home and examine her eyes. With the retinoscope I saw a clear, red reflex in the right eye, but none in the left. It was evident that her trouble was caused by strain, and her condition was becoming worse because she worried about the outcome.

We placed her in a comfortable chair in the garden where the sun was shining and fastened a white test card on the trunk of a tree. As she looked at the card she began squinting because the bright light bothered her. Teaching her to blink often helped her to look at the card with less discomfort. She could read 10/200 with the right eye and 1/200 with the left, which means that at ten feet the only letter she could see with the right eye was the large letter "C" on the top of the card, and with the left eye she could not see it farther than one foot. With some difficulty, Aunt Mary was able to raise one of her arms so that she could cover her eyes with her palm. She had a good imagination, so while her eyes were covered, we talked about various kinds of flowers she had seen. We also talked of white clouds and a blue sky. As I mentioned one object after another, her mind did not dwell on one thing very long. I spent about an hour with her the first day, and her vision in that time improved to 10/40 with the right eye and 10/200 with the left, improving her imagination of things she had seen, with eyes closed as well as with them open, was the only method I used that day.

There was quite an improvement in her eyes when I saw her again. The vision of her right eye improved to 10/30 and 10/70 in the left. It was impossible for her to stand and swing, so I placed myself before her in an arm chair and moved my body and head to the right and then to the left with a slow movement, and asked her to do the same. While we were doing this, I could not understand why she did not see or imagine things about her moving opposite to the direction in which her head and eyes were moving. Then I noticed that she was staring while trying to follow my directions, even though she was blinking. It did not take her very long to learn how to shift her eyes, and after that she made steady progress. Dr. Bates became interested in Aunt Mary's case and offered to call with me the next time I treated her. He examined her eyes with his ophthalmoscope and said there was not enough opacity of either lens to lower the vision. She was very much encouraged when Dr. Bates told her that her cataract had improved. He also remarked about her cheery disposition, and how her faithfulness in keeping up her daily treatment would help greatly in the cure of her eyes.

There is an enclosed porch where she practices on rainy days or when it becomes too cold to sit in the garden. Her loving family do all they possibly can to make her comfortable, so there is every chance that she will be cured of her eye trouble.

Aunt Mary did not like to practice with the white "C" card because the white background bothered her and made her strain. She likes to practice with the white letter card on a black background, so we use the black card mostly during treatment. In her sunny room hangs a picture which is beautifully colored, but she could not see it clearly. She explained that it seemed to be in a mist always. I gave her fine print to practice with, and she has become able to read it in a fairly good light at six inches from her eyes.

Her confidence in me makes me all the more anxious to cure her. In the last few months she has realized the fact that no operation for the removal of cataract will ever be necessary if she continues to practice. She surprised me one day by reading 10/20 with both eyes, and after sun treatment she read 10/15. Surely, at this time, if her cataracts were as bad as they were in the beginning when I first saw her, her vision would not have improved, neither would she have responded to the sun treatment. Recently I examined her again with the retinoscope, and I saw a red reflex in the left eye, as well as in the right.

A neighbor, who is twenty years younger than Aunt Mary and has presbyopia or old-age sight, was surprised to find out that Aunt Mary had better sight than she had. The fact that her vision was better than a woman so much younger made her anxious to practice more. The last time I visited Aunt Mary she read the bottom line of the test card at ten feet, or 10/10, with her right eye, and 10/20 with the left. She reads the fine print now at all times, and also the newspaper and her Bible without any trouble. When she strains to see at the distance, things seem to blur before her eyes, but when she palms and sways her body as she sits in her chair, the mist clears away and she sees better.

When I first became acquainted with her, I noticed how difficult it was for her to move about with her crutches. To get up from her chair was an effort. Not so long ago, I offered to help her change her position, but she managed very nicely herself and got up with the aid of her crutches without any effort at all. I believe the constant practice of the body swing has not only improved the condition of her eyes, but also her general condition as well.

SONNY

By George M. Guild

Sonny was a manly boy, large for his age and strong with the strength of youth. He was twelve years old. He loved his mother very much and did all that he could to help her. Sonny enjoyed entertaining other boys and was popular with grown-ups as well. His father was very proud of him and frequently talked about his boy to the people he knew. He rather overdid it, and his friends would usually tire of hearing so much about Sonny at home, Sonny at play, Sonny at school, Sonny all the time and every day. His mother was just as proud of her boy and could talk hour after hour about him, if one were polite enough to listen.

There was another member of the family, a sweet young girl, who was sick in bed and who suffered constant pain. She was unable to sit up, and of course unable to walk. Her name was May, and she was eight years old. Recently her sight had become poor, and she was nearly blind. Sonny spent more time with her than one would expect. He invited other boys and girls to visit his sister. He read storybooks to her, all about knights, ladies, kings, queens and the fairies. She liked the fairy stories best of all and wanted very much to see the fairies and talk to them. Sonny was just as anxious as she was to meet the fairies.

One day he went into the flower garden to cry in a place where no one could see him and be annoyed with his tears. May did not seem so well. No one had ever helped her pain, and today she said that her sight was so poor that when she looked at Sonny his face appeared so far away that she could not see it at all. He tried to say something to make her feel better, but his throat had a big lump in it which prevented him from talking. After he had cried for some minutes he felt a little better. One of the flowers seemed more beautiful than any of the others, and while he was looking at this flower it nodded to him and turned into a beautiful fairy. She had bright blue eyes that were full of fun and play. They were kind eyes, too, but mostly they seemed to be laughing all the time. Sonny had never seen eyes which appeared to know so much, to know all there was to know, and to know many things which others did not know, never could know, or would know. Her eyes were indeed full of wisdom.

The fairy danced a few steps, whirled around on her toes, stood still for a moment, bowed low to Sonny, threw him a kiss, and asked a question, "How do you like me?"

"I love you with all my heart," said Sonny. "Why were you crying?" asked the fairy. "I was crying because my sister is sick and becoming blind. No one has helped her. No one can help her." "Would you like the fairies to help you?" "I certainly would," he answered.

Thereupon the fairy blew a gold whistle. In a few minutes the fairies began to arrive. At first slowly, by twos and threes, and then in larger numbers more rapidly. They soon filled the garden. They found places on the lawn, the trees and the outside of the house. They were not silent fairies by any means. It seemed as though all were talking, laughing and singing. Furthermore, they were not still for a moment. Their heads and eyes were always moving in time with their dancing feet. Those people who have seen fairies dancing have said that it is all very wonderful, beautiful and delightful.

Sonny was in a great hurry to have his sister and the fairies meet. He learned that the first fairy he met was the Fairy Queen and beloved very much by all the other fairies. As soon as the Queen met May, she directed the child's mother to lift her from the bed, holding her very gently. Then the mother was told to sway her sick child from side to side, slowly at first, and then more vigorously, but always easily and gently. When done properly, it cured dizziness and many other things.

The Queen insisted that the patient should make believe or imagine that she saw stationary objects to be moving in the direction opposite to the movement of her head and eyes.

May was a good pupil. When her mother swayed her whole body from side to side, she soon became able to imagine the room, the bed and other stationary objects to be moving. The movement did her good. She smiled up to her mother and said, "Mother, dear, the pain in my back is all gone, and I can now see very much better."

The mother kept on swaying the patient from side to side, while May imagined that all the objects she was not regarding were apparently moving from side to side all the time. When the mother tired after half an hour or longer, Sonny took his sister in his arms and continued the swaying. They alternated and continued the swaying for several hours. All this time the fairies were dancing and singing where May could see them. She enjoyed it all and tried to sing the song of the fairies as well as she could, keeping time with their singing.

The Fairy Queen now directed the child to sit up in bed and at first sway herself with the help of her mother and Sonny and gradually do it all without their help. She soon became able to do it alone. Her strength increased rapidly, while her sight also became much better.

The Fairy Queen then advised that she stand on the floor with the help of her mother and Sonny. Her strength continued to improve until, much to the delight of all, she became able to sway herself without any help. Sonny was so happy with her wonderful improvement that he laughed and shouted for joy, while all his mother could do was to smile as the tears flowed from her eyes.

When Sonny's father came home he watched the proceedings approvingly. He did not believe in fairies, consequently he did not see them dancing nor hear them singing. He stood in a corner of the room blowing his nose frequently, although he had no cold.

His daughter soon saw him and, without stopping her swaying, threw him a kiss and called out to him, "Oh, father, my pain is all gone; I can stand on my feet; I can walk. I can see you perfectly; the fairies have cured me. I am perfectly happy. Aren't you glad?"

But he could not speak. He felt so weak that he had to sit down on the edge of the bed. His wife took his hand. She could not speak either. She just smiled, while her tears continued to flow.

Sonny had lost all control of himself. He shouted; he alternately laughed and cried. He danced around the room. He hugged his father, his mother, and the neighbors who came to see the wonderful cure by the fairies. They had to take him to another room, where he flung himself down on a bed, buried his face in a pillow and sobbed as though his heart would break because he was so happy.

The next morning his sister walked into his room and wakened him with a kiss. She smiled and said, "Good morning, Sonny."

THE LIGHT TREATMENT [SUN TREATMENT]

By M. A. Crane

People who live in the dark and seldom or never see the sun, like miners, for example, always have something wrong with their eyes.

In the tenement houses where the light is poor, many children acquire a dislike for the sunlight. They will bury their faces in a pillow and shut out all light. Too many of them are brought to a Clinic with ulcers on the front part of the eyeball. Treatment with antiseptic eyedrops and other measures generally fail to cure. Sending them out of doors in the bright sunlight has been followed by complete relief.

One patient, a man with serious disease of his eyes, had spent much time in a hospital where his eyes were protected from the light by the use of bandages. After some months, his eyes had not improved, and he left the hospital wearing very dark glasses for protection from the light. His eyes became more and more sensitive, although the dark glasses were changed frequently to those that were darker, until he finally wore the darkest glasses that he could obtain. Still there was no relief from the sun. Later, the dark glasses were discarded permanently. The sensitiveness to the light became less after he exposed his closed eyelids to the sun for half an hour or longer, moving his head at the same time slowly from side to side [sunning].

After the eyes have improved, it may be possible for the patient to look down while someone else gently lifts the upper eyelid toward the brow, exposing some of the white part of the eye above the pupil. At first it may be well to shade the eyes from the sun until the patient acquires sufficient control to look down easily, continuously and without strain. With the eyes looking far down, one focuses the direct rays of the sun on the exposed white part of the eye with a strong convex glass, moving the glass continuously to avoid the heat of the condensed sunlight [sun treatment]. One needs to caution the patient to avoid looking directly at the sun while the light is being focussed on the eye. The results obtained from this method have usually been very gratifying. When the eyes are inflamed from disease of the eyelids, the cornea, the iris, the retina, the optic nerve, from glaucoma and other inflammations, the use of the sun glass has been followed immediately by a lessening of the congestion and a decided improvement in vision.

Many people ask the question, "How long does it take to obtain a sufficient benefit to be noticeable?" When the sun treatment is employed, the improvement in the sight may be demonstrated in a very short time. The sun treatment improves the vision of all patients who are wearing glasses for the relief of pain, fatigue, and imperfect sight, no matter what kind of glasses are worn or how strong they may be.

The direct sunlight focussed on the white part of the eye is a benefit in many cases of blindness with hardening of the eyeball (glaucoma), or softening of the eyeball (cyclitis), also in cases of cataract, and of opacities in other parts of the eye. It was interesting to observe the improvement in a large number of patients blind from scar tissue on the front part of the eye, the cornea. They were benefited so much that their sight became normal.

It is good practice to expose the eyes of babies to the direct sunlight not only when they are awake but also when asleep.

The sunlight treatment has never injured the eye nor lowered the vision permanently in a single patient, even when used improperly.

Patients with cataract seem to improve more decidedly from the light treatment than from some other kinds of treatment. Congenital cataract, or cataract present from birth, is benefited and often cured in the same way. Cataract produced by an injury to the eye has improved and occasionally been cured by the effect of light on the eye. So often has the light treatment benefited many kinds of cataract that the use of the light is strongly recommended in all cases.

The beneficial effect of light is largely, if not entirely, due to its mental effect. One evidence that this is true is the fact that the benefit is so quick that there is not enough time for the eyeball to be improved sufficiently to account for the good result. It has been stated by some authorities on the value of sunlight in the treatment of disease, that it should be used out of doors to obtain the best results, and that after it has passed through glass it has lost much of its healing properties This may be true in the treatment of tuberculosis, or other diseases, but apparently not when used for the benefit of imperfect sight.

Strong sunlight in the tropics is as much, if not a greater, relief, as it is in colder countries. Patients who do not wear a hat, or otherwise shield their eyes from the brightness of strong sunlight, have testified that their eyes became much stronger and their vision decidedly improved by the exposure. However, one should first of all accustom the eyes gradually to the light to prevent discomfort.

The question has often been asked, "Is electric light beneficial?" Electric light is beneficial, but not to the same degree as sunlight. Many people have accustomed their eyes to all kinds of electric light and have improved their vision very materially by using the electric light as intelligently as the sunlight.

The sun is the whitest object there is. Many patients complain that it is not white but red, gray, blue, brown, or some other color. It has been described as black when regarded by patients whose eyes were very sensitive to the light, patients whose vision was very imperfect, or who suffered very much from eyestrain.

QUESTIONS AND ANSWERS

Q–1. Why is it that many people feel the need of glasses for near work when they reach middle age?

A–1. When trying to read they strain, which makes the sight imperfect. This may occur before the age of forty or after sixty.

Q–2. How can I prevent the sun from hurting my eyes?

A–2. By becoming accustomed to it. See "The Light Treatment" in this issue of *Better Eyesight.*

Q–3. When should one blink and under what circumstances should stationary objects be imagined as moving, and for what purpose?

A–3. One should blink to improve the sight. Stationary objects should be imagined as moving to avoid the stare which always impairs the sight and causes pain and fatigue.

Q–4. Will you please tell me if results are obtained at all ages or whether there is a limit? If there is, after what age are results unsatisfactory?

A–4. Results are obtained satisfactorily at all ages without an exception.

Better Eyesight
December 1925—Vol. X, No. 6

DIZZINESS

Dizziness is caused by eyestrain. Some people when standing on the roof of a house looking down, strain their eyes and become dizzy. Usually the dizziness is produced unconsciously. It can be produced consciously, however, by staring or straining to see some distant or near object.

Some persons when riding in an elevator are always dizzy and may suffer from attacks of imperfect sight with headache, nausea, and other nervous discomforts.

One lady, age sixty, told me that riding in an elevator always made her dizzy, and produced headaches with pain in her eyes and head. I tested her vision and found it to be normal both for distance and for reading without glasses. To obtain some facts, I rode in an elevator with her from the top to the bottom of the building and back again. I watched her eyes closely and found that she was staring at the floors which appeared to be moving opposite to the movement of the elevator. I asked her the question, "Why do you stare at the floors which appear to be moving by?" She answered, "I do not like to see them move, and I am trying to correct the illusion by making an effort to keep them stationary. The harder I try, the worse I feel." I suggested to her that she look at one part of the elevator and avoid looking at the floors. Her discomfort was at once relieved, and she was soon cured.

In all cases of dizziness, the stare or strain is always evident. When the stare or strain is relieved or prevented, dizziness does not occur. With advancing years attacks of dizziness and blindness occur more frequently than in younger individuals. All attacks of dizziness with blindness are quite readily cured by practicing the imagination of the swing, the memory of perfect sight, or by palming.

SHIFTING

By W. H. Bates, M.D.

Shifting: The point regarded changes rapidly and continuously.

A man with imperfect sight, who had obtained normal vision by my method of treatment without glasses, called about five years later and announced that the cure had proved permanent. His vision was normal when each eye was tested at twenty feet with Snellen test cards which he had not seen before.

He was asked, "What cured you?" "Shifting," he answered.

All persons with imperfect sight make an effort to stare with their eyes immovable. The eyes have not the ability to keep stationary. To look intently at a point continuously is impossible; the eyes will move, the eyelids will blink, and the effort is accompanied by an imperfect vision of the point regarded. In many cases the effort to concentrate on a point often causes headache, pain in the eyes and fatigue.

All persons with normal eyes and normal sight do not concentrate or try to see by any effort. Their eyes are at rest, and when the eyes are at rest they are constantly moving. When the eyes move, one is able to imagine all stationary objects in turn to be moving in the direction opposite to the movement of the head and eyes. It is impossible to imagine with equal clearness a number of objects to be moving at the same time, and an effort to do so is a strain which impairs the vision, the memory, or the imagination. To try to do the impossible is a strain, which always lowers the mental efficiency. This fact should be emphasized.

Many patients have difficulty in imagining stationary objects to be moving opposite to the movements of the eyes or head. When riding in a fast-moving train, and one regards the telegraph poles or other objects which are seen—the near objects may appear to be moving opposite to the direction in which the train is moving, while more distant objects may appear to move in the same direction as the train. [Double oppositional movement.—TRQ]

The above facts may also be imagined when traveling in an automobile. The driver of the car and others occupying a front seat may imagine the road to be moving toward the moving car. When pain, fatigue or other symptoms are present it always means that the individual is consciously or unconsciously trying to imagine stationary objects are not moving. The effort is a strain.

When walking about a room, the head and eyes move in the same direction as the body moves, and the carpet and the furniture appear to move in the opposite direction. However, it can be demonstrated that when the head and eyes are moving forward they are also moving from side to side. Every time the right foot is placed forward the eyes move to the right, while stationary objects appear to move in the opposite direction—to the left; when the left foot steps forward the whole body, including the eyes moves to the left, while stationary objects appear to move in the opposite direction—to the right.

Patients with normal vision are able to imagine this movement more readily than those with imperfect sight. The head and eyes also move upwards and downwards as the foot is lifted and lowered. When you raise your foot to take a step, the eyes go up, and everything else that is stationary appears to go down. When you lower your foot or head, the eyes go down, and stationary objects appear to go up.

Shifting when practiced with the best results is usually unconscious. Very few people with normal sight, which may be continuous for many years, ever notice that they are constantly shifting correctly. One may shift in a wrong way, strain the eyes, and fail to improve the vision. What is the right way? The right way to shift is to move the eyes from one point to another slowly, regularly, continuously, restfully, or easily without effort or without trying to see. The normal eye with normal sight has the habit of always moving or shifting, usually an unconscious habit. When, by practice, the eye with imperfect sight acquires the conscious habit of shifting, the habit may become unconscious. When the shifting is done properly, the memory, imagination, mental efficiency, and vision are improved until they become normal.

It often happens that when one consciously or intentionally shifts in the wrong way, a better knowledge of the right way to shift may be obtained. When the eyes are moved to the right, stationary objects should appear to move to the left; and, when the vision is good, all objects not regarded are seen less distinctly than those regarded. When the vision is imperfect, objects not observed may be seen better, or an effort is made to see them better than those directly observed. In fact, it is always true that in all cases of imperfect sight the eyes do not see best where they are looking, and central fixation is lost. To shift properly requires relaxation or rest. To shift improperly and lower the vision requires an effort. When one stares at a point without blinking or shifting, fatigue, distress, or pain is felt. To continue to stare without shifting is hard work. To see imperfectly is difficult; and, when one regards letters which are blurred or not distinguishable either at the distance, ten feet or farther, or at a near point—six inches or less, the strain on the eyes can be felt. Imperfect sight or a failure to see requires much trouble and hard work. This fact should be demonstrated repeatedly by the patient until thoroughly convinced that rest of the eyes, mind or body can only be obtained by shifting easily, continuously and without effort.

What is true of sight is also true of the memory and imagination. With the eyes closed, one can imagine that he is looking over the right shoulder for a moment and then shift the imaginary gaze over the left shoulder. By lightly touching the closed eyelids with the tips of the fingers he can feel the eyeballs moving from side to side when the shifting is done right. It can be done wrong when one, by an effort, imagines the eyeballs stationary under all conditions.

With the eyes closed, one can imagine alternately looking from one side of a letter to the other. When the imagination of the shifting is done right, the letter remembered is imagined to be moving from side to side. Two letters close together may be imagined or remembered clearly, provided one is imagined better than the other, or when the attention is shifted to each alternately without effort or strain.

Blinking is necessary to maintain normal vision in the normal eye. When blinking is prevented, the eyes become tired and the vision very soon becomes worse. Some persons, without knowing it, will blink five times in one second as demonstrated by the camera. When regarding a large letter of a Snellen test card at twenty feet or one foot, while blinking consciously, the letter appears to move up while the eyelids close slowly, and to move downwards as the eyelids are slowly opened. This apparent movement is caused by shifting the eyes up and down while blinking. Many patients are unable to shift their eyes a short distance with benefit. When blinking, they may fail to obtain relaxation because they too often blink with an effort. It is possible for most patients to demonstrate that the shifting of the eyes up and down improves the vision, when blinking is done easily, without effort. Blinking is very important. It is not the brief periods of rest obtained from closing the eyes which helps the sight so much as the shifting or movements of the eyes. It should be repeatedly demonstrated that the eyes are only at rest when they are shifting.

STORIES FROM THE CLINIC
No. 70: Christmas at the Clinic

By Emily C. Lierman

We had a lively time at the Clinic last Christmas. Many poor souls were made happy at that time, because of the generous contributions received throughout the year for the Clinic fund.

I still keep up the old custom of telling a Christmas story to my younger patients. Every time they come for treatment, I tell them to palm their eyes, and then I try to improve their memory and imagination, which always improves their sight. It is necessary to remind a child of pleasant things, and what is more wonderful to the child mind than a Christmas tree laden with toys and candies? While I am treating boys and girls at the age of twelve or older, I talk about ice skating or sleigh rides, hills of snow, the pure whiteness of the drifts, or I tell them to imagine they are making snowballs. This helps to improve their vision for the test card and relieves tension or pain. Young men and women who work in shops usually find it a benefit to imagine that objects about them are moving all day. I tell them to blink constantly, and shift their eyes while blinking. This stops the stare which causes so much body fatigue. If I have had a hard day treating the most difficult cases, I find it a great help to palm and remember some of my childhood days. I think back to the night before Christmas. Mothers will find it a great help in improving their own sight if they make a daily habit of spending ten or fifteen minutes with their children, palming and resting. Children can easily form mental pictures while palming, especially remembering the Christmas decorations in store windows, the funny mechanical toys, and animals that move about when they are wound up. Recalling or imagining such things while their eyes are closed helps to relieve the mind of school studies, which sometimes cause strain. Adults, especially mothers, listen to me while I am describing such things to the children in the Clinic. When it comes time to treat the older patients, I find it quite easy to have them remember how surprised their children were on Christmas morning, when the tree and toys were discovered.

Many thanks to my friends who make our Clinic family happy at Christmas time.

THE CHRISTMAS FAIRIES

By George M. Guild

The night before Christmas is the time when most little children are happy, wondering how many of the toys they have hoped for will be found under the Christmas tree on Christmas morning. If it were not for the good fairies, Santa Claus would not know what each little child most desires.

The fairies are always with the children, although they are not always seen. They know what the children are thinking, and what they are wishing for. The fairies are eager to help Santa Claus whenever he needs them, particularly on Christmas Eve when he is so busy.

In the country, where the snow does not melt quickly, Santa still travels in his sleigh driven by the reindeers. The jingle bells seem to say, "Good Cheer! Good Cheer !" and arouse merry thoughts in the hearts of all. It is different in the cities, where the snow is taken away as soon as it falls. Santa Claus has to use either his automobile or his airplane.

In a crowded part of the city, where many poor people lived, the boys and girls were sad and lonely at Christmas time. One little girl, whose name was Mary, had no mother nor father, no sisters nor brothers. She had a great deal of trouble with her eyes and could scarcely see. While the other children in the neighborhood were looking in at the shop windows wishing for the wonderful toys, little Mary went to sleep on her cot hopeful that Santa Claus would not forget her. While she slept, the fairies and Santa Claus were very busy. The Fairy Queen gathered all the other fairies together. Some were sent to the woods for the largest Christmas tree that they could find. Others were sent to Toyland to bring back stacks and stacks of toys so that all the children could receive what they desired. All night long the Christmas fairies went back and forth from Toyland to the playground, where the large tree was placed for all to see it. They decorated the tree with strings of popcorn, long golden and silver ropes, and beautiful ornaments. The toys were arranged on all the branches and beneath the tree, too. The Fairy Queen touched the Christmas tree with her wand and many colored lights blazed forth. Just then Santa Claus arrived in his airplane and was very pleased with the work of the fairies. Soon after that the fairies climbed in the airplane with Santa Claus and sailed off to take care of other children.

When daylight came, the children looked out of their windows to see if the snow had fallen in the night. There in the center of the playground stood the beautiful tree. They ran outdoors, calling to their playmates as they went along. Soon an enormous crowd was gathered about the Christmas tree. They were all very excited and made a mad scramble for the toys, and they soon carried off all the presents they wanted. It took Mary longer than the others to reach the tree, because she could not see so well and had to walk slowly and carefully. Then, too, the crowd of children was so large and their eagerness so great that they did not think of little Mary, and she was pushed here and there. Finally, when the children had gone, Mary approached the tree, but she could not see any toys. She sat down and was about to cry when she heard the tinkling of bells and suddenly caught a glimpse of shining lights. She came very close to the tree, and there was one lone toy left among the branches. Mary reached for it and grasped it in her hands. She tried hard to see what it was, but all that she could see were two blinking lights, and each time they blinked they became a more beautiful color. As she continued to look at them, unknowingly she began to blink, too, and all at once she saw a little red and gold jester with cap and bells, and the ugliest face that she had ever seen. That was why all the other children had left it there. But she soon forgot his ugly face when she looked at his eyes again. As they blinked they changed from gold to blue, from blue to yellow, and from yellow to green, and again to a bright scarlet. They danced and twinkled all the while. Then the jester himself began to sway from side to side. This made Mary feel like swaying, and she began to move in time with the movements of the jester. All the while the bells on his cap jingled sprightly tunes for them, making Mary very jolly and gay. Then the jester began to hop up and down, and dance all about, turning 'round and 'round. Mary began to dance, too. They danced here and they danced there, and they danced everywhere. They were circling around the tree when suddenly Mary stood still, surprised. She could see! Everything had become very bright. The jester nodded wisely. He knew it had not happened just then; it had been going on ever since she blinked and swayed and danced with him, but Mary had been too happy to realize the wonderful thing that had happened to her. She looked all about it—the whole playground seemed to sparkle. The Christmas tree had become very green, and she could see even the little needles on the boughs. Mary could not understand all this. The jester chuckled to himself. He knew it was the most natural thing in the world. Fairies just live to help people, and they think nothing of the things that everyone calls miracles.

"Why, I believe it is you who have helped me," Mary suddenly said to the jester. "I do believe you are a fairy!" The jester nodded, bowed, twirled around gaily and then blinked at Mary. "I know," exclaimed Mary, "it is the wonderful things you do with your eyes that have helped me."

The jester nodded twice this time and bowed low. Mary hugged him tightly and ran to tell the other children about the fairy jester. What she did not know was that he was the Prince of the jesters in disguise and went about curing people just as he had cured Mary.

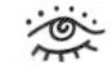

AN OPTOMETRIST'S EXPERIENCE

By Dr. Paul Hotson

Editor's Note—*Dr. Hotson is among the first optometrists to practice the cure of imperfect sight without glasses. This does not mean that he has given up prescribing glasses, but it means that he can now offer his customers a choice of treatment with or without glasses.*

For many years people have been taught to believe that there is no relief from eye troubles except through glasses, and it is hard to make them believe anything else.

Sixteen years ago, I started practicing optometry, and still hold a license. Fourteen years of that time I swallowed and digested the old theory of refraction, although it is full of contradictions which could be demonstrated to the average optometrist in a few minutes.

According to the old theory, nearsighted is incurable, but when you improve the vision of a nearsighted child until it can read two or three lines down on the test card, or even obtain normal vision in one treatment, the old theory falls to pieces. These facts have never been brought to the attention of optometrists in general.

Eyestrain can be cured so easily in the average child by Dr. Bates' method that it should be against the law to fit children with glasses. I predict that within twenty-five years there will not be a child wearing glasses in either the United States or Canada.

A Case Of Chronic Headache

Girl, 16 years old; Right eye 10/10, Left eye 10/10 (with one mistake). Had headache constantly for over a year, medicine did not relieve, and at times she was not able to sleep at night on account of the pain. Right eye had turned slightly in and patient saw double. Headache was completely relieved during first treatment by palming and the memory of a dahlia, which was her favorite flower. She came to my office twice a week and was cured in ten days. The treatment consisted of palming, swinging, blinking and the memory of a small letter "o." Her vision improved to 22/10 and both eyes became straight.

Cured In One Treatment

Child, 10 years old. Vision 10/30. After palming ten minutes, swinging improved the vision to 10/10 in each eye during the first treatment.

AN OCULIST'S EXPERIENCE

By E. F. Darling, M.D.

Editor's Note—*This contribution from an oculist of twenty years' experience in one of the largest Eye Hospitals in the United States is of unusual interest. He is to be congratulated on his perseverance in going without glasses so long before his sight for reading had sufficiently improved to do his work properly. He has not told of the opposition and loss of many of his old friends because he did not prescribe glasses for his patients.*

I have been practicing medicine as an ophthalmologist for the last twenty years. During a period of eighteen years prior to 1923, I spent a large part of my time putting glasses on my helpless patients. However, for the last two years I have been trying to make amends by removing their glasses as rapidly as possible.

The first time I heard of Dr. Bates' work was from an article in one of the medical journals about fifteen years ago. The article made some impression on me, because it was entirely at variance with our accepted views as to the cause and cure of defective vision. In the clinic I attended, at one of the largest eye hospitals, most of the men seemed to know nothing about Dr. Bates. Some thought he was a quack, while others said he was insane.

About three years ago I received notice of the publication of his book, *Perfect Sight Without Glasses,* and at that time I decided to purchase the book and see what it was all about. The thing slipped my mind for another year or so, when one of my old patients came into my office without her glasses on and said she had been working with Dr. Bates. Her vision was much improved, and she wanted to know if I could continue the same kind of treatment with her. I was obliged to confess that I knew nothing about his methods, but I believe I at least volunteered the information that he ought to be in jail.

The next day I went over to the Central Fixation Publishing Company and bought the book. When I reached home, I started reading it and didn't stop until I had finished the whole thing. Here was a plain statement of facts accomplished, and I at once decided to test the matter with my own eyes.

I was wearing convex 2.25 D. S. for distance and convex 4.25 for reading. My distance vision had deteriorated in the eighteen years I had worn glasses, from better than normal to about one-third normal. My near vision had gone back so much that I was wearing the glass which theoretically should suit a person sixty or seventy years old. With the glasses off I could see only the largest headlines on the newspapers. While wearing the glasses, I had occasional headaches and eyeaches, and my near vision was at times very defective, so that I had difficulty in doing fine work of any kind.

The first day I went around without glasses everything seemed blurred, but I felt somehow that I had gotten rid of some particularly galling chains. It was pleasant to feel the air blowing against my eyes, and I walked around the whole afternoon trying to get used to the new condition.

In carrying out the suggestions in Dr. Bates' book, I had a great deal of trouble for the first week or so, especially with the mental images. This was simply due to my extreme eyestrain. In spite of this my vision steadily improved by palming, so that at the end of three weeks I could read the 10/15 line instead of the 20/70 line. I had only an occasional eyeache when I had forgotten to use my eyes properly.

In improving my near vision I had to make several visits to Dr. Bates, and he overcame most of my difficulties at once. I used many of the methods he advocates in this near work, but it was about three months before I could read fine print. It seemed an extremely long, long time to give up reading, but knowing now the advantages after an experience of two years without glasses, I would be willing to go without reading for a much longer period. Many people of the same age get results in a much shorter time than I did. I feel more and more strongly that a person will not have full control of his mental faculties until he gets rid of his glasses. Whether it takes two weeks or two years, the result will pay for the deprivation.

At present I usually read an hour or so in the daytime and three or four hours at night with no eyestrain whatever. Previously I used to walk along with my eyes fixed on the pavement because of the discomfort in taking note of passing people or objects; now it is a great pleasure to examine things minutely. In my work I can go nine hours with about the same fatigue as I felt before in three or four hours. In other words, Dr. Bates' work his changed me from an old man of forty-eight to a young man of fifty. I now enjoy the practice of medicine for the first time since finishing my hospital internship, as I am absolutely certain that if patients will carry out my directions their whole condition will be improved.

In no case can the time required to obtain normal vision be definitely stated. People of the same age and wearing the same strength glasses vary in time required as much as they differ in color of their hair or size of their appetites. Some get quick results, others drag along indefinitely before they get where they should be.

These slow cases require lots of encouragement, and it sometimes takes all their own and the doctor's perseverance to keep them going.

SOME INTERESTING CASES

By Mildred Shepard

Editor's Note—*Ms. Shepard has done much good work in the cure of imperfect sight by treatment without glasses. She came to me as a patient about five years ago and was treated for hypermetropia or farsightedness accompanied by astigmatism. She had suffered with pain and fatigue whenever she used her eyes. After her sight became normal, Ms. Shepard began to treat her friends. She became so interested in curing them of imperfect sight that she decided to take my course.*

Ten days ago a lady came to me after having worn glasses for twenty years. She is now forty-five. Her vision with both eyes was 14/70, and with the left eye she read two letters of 14/50.

Her mental pictures were good, and after palming a while she became able by the use of her memory to read 14/20.

When she came for her second lesson, she could read 14/50 easily, and improved to 10/15. She understands the general principles and wants to work by herself for a couple of weeks. I hope that she will have 14/10 when she comes again.

Another nearsighted young lady of twenty-four, a school teacher, read 14/40 and some letters of 14/30 the first day of her treatment. The same day she improved to 14/20. One week later she read 14/15.

Two of my pupils have gone back to their oculists for examinations, the results of which were rather interesting. In one case the man wanted to get a pair of glasses, which he could use when he sat in the top balcony of the Opera House. When the oculist examined his eyes and compared it with the previous examination, he found so much improvement that he refused to prescribe glasses for him. His vision had improved from 10/30 minus with the right eye and 10/40 with the left to 12.5/10 with both.

In the other case the examination showed 1.50 D of myopia instead of 3.75 D which had been present before.

This man had a pair of still weaker glasses made up, to wear while working under trying and unusual conditions. He hopes soon to discard the glasses altogether. His vision improved from 20/70 to 10/10.

Last spring a young girl of twenty-two came to me. She had worn glasses for nine years. Her vision was 20/200 with both eyes. With the right eye it was not so good. She had six lessons in ten days and became able to read 10/10 on the black card. Six months later she returned. Her vision was still 10/10. She was so enthusiastic that she brought her mother and a friend, both of whom had lessons. She wants to go into the work after she improves her sight still more.

Another girl of fourteen whose vision was 7.5/100 last February can now read 8/10 on the black card, and when she once masters central fixation I know she will get back to normal vision.

Another has improved from 6/200 to 5/30. She still has a long way to go, but she is faithful, and we both are hopeful.

I might go on indefinitely giving other cases, some similar and some quite different.

Better Eyesight
January 1926—Vol. X, No. 7

THE PERIOD

The perfect memory or imagination of a period is a cure for imperfect sight. Only the color needs to be remembered. The size is immaterial, but a small period is remembered with more relaxation than a large one. It is true, however, that with perfect sight one has the ability to remember all things perfectly.

One cannot remember a period perfectly by any kind of an effort. It usually happens that one may remember a period for a time, and then lose it by an effort. To remember a period stationary is impossible. One has to shift more or less frequently in order to remember a period perfectly all the time, or one has to imagine the period to be moving, or one has to remember the period by central fixation—one part best. By shifting is meant to look away from the period and then back, but to do it so quickly that it is possible to remember the period continuously, although you are not looking at it all the time—this with the eyes closed. Every time you blink, you shift your eyes. You can blink so rapidly that it is not noticeable. When you close your eyes and remember a period, you cannot remember it unless you are, with your eyes closed, going through the process as though you were blinking, looking away from it and back again, but so quickly that it seems as though you were looking at the period continuously. You cannot remember the whole of the period at once. No matter how small the period is, you cannot see or remember it perfectly, all parts equally well at the same time. You cannot remember the period perfectly by any kind of an effort. When the memory of the period is perfect, the mental and physical efficiency is increased. A perfect memory of the period does not necessarily mean that one should think only of the period.

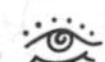

SWINGING

By W. H. Bates, M.D.

When the eyes move slowly or rapidly from side to side, stationary objects appear to move in the direction opposite to the movement of the head and eyes.

People with normal vision are not always conscious of the swing. When called to their attention, however, they can always demonstrate it, and are always able to imagine all stationary objects to be moving. In imperfect sight, the swing is modified or absent. This is a truth which has been demonstrated over a long period of years by a great many people, and no exceptions have been found.

The normal or perfect swing is slow, short, easy and continuous. When the swing is normal, it is always true that not only is the vision normal or perfect, but also the memory, the imagination, or the mental efficiency correspond. When the memory is imperfect, the imagination, the mental efficiency, and the sight are also imperfect.

All cases of imperfect sight from myopia, or nearsightedness, become normal when the swing becomes normal. The same is true in cataract, glaucoma, diseases of the optic nerve and retina. For example, a woman, aged sixty-three, was treated for imperfect sight from cataract. Her vision was 10/200, and was not improved by glasses. For twenty years she had not been able to read a newspaper with or without glasses. In three visits, with the help of the normal swing, her vision improved to 10/10 minus, with flashes of normal vision, and she read diamond type at twelve inches rapidly without glasses. Other similar cases have been relieved as promptly.

It is important to understand how the swing can be imagined. Some people with mild cases of imperfect sight can imagine a letter or other object to be moving when they see or remember it perfectly. There are many others who fail. Severe pain, fatigue, or worry often prevent the demonstration of the swing. Blinking and palming are helpful in demonstrating the swing. The distance of the object regarded is important. The patient should be placed at a distance at which he can best demonstrate the swing. The distance varies with the patient.

It is unfortunate that many patients consider the swing complicated or impossible. However, they can usually demonstrate that a stare or strain lowers the vision. When holding a test card at a convenient distance from the eyes, patients may be convinced that the test card is seen better when moving. They may not profit by their experience, but continue to stare or strain, which always lowers the vision.

One patient was unable to imagine any kind of a swing. He was suffering from pain, mental depression, and imperfect sight for the distance. Reading the newspaper, even with glasses, was impossible. Since nothing he tried gave him any relief, I suggested that he stop trying to see and make no effort to imagine stationary objects to be moving. He practiced this while sitting in my waiting room. He paid no attention to the apparent movement of stationary objects, nor did he look at any object more than a fraction of a second. His vision after that improved from 20/50 to 20/10. He became able to imagine the movement of objects and demonstrated that all his pain and mental depression were caused by a stare or an effort to see all things stationary when he regarded, remembered, or imagined them. He was comfortable when he imagined objects moving or swinging, but very uncomfortable when he made an effort or imagined them to be stationary.

Recently, I tested the sight of a girl about ten years old. She read the Snellen test card at ten feet with normal vision. She was asked, "Do you see any of the small letters moving from side to side?" "Yes," she answered, "they are all moving." "Now can you imagine one of the small letters stationary?" At once she quickly looked away and frowned. "Why did you look away?" her father asked her. She replied, "Because it gave me a pain in my eyes and head, and the letters became blurred. Don't ask me to do it again."

The experience of this child is the same as that of everyone, young or old, with perfect or imperfect sight. When the sight is normal and continuously good, to try to stop the swing of a letter or other object necessitates a strain—an effort which always lowers the vision and produces discomfort or pain in one or both eyes.

It has been repeatedly demonstrated that a letter or other object cannot be remembered or even imagined perfectly and continuously, unless one can imagine it to be moving or swinging. Not only does the sight become imperfect, but also the memory, imagination, judgment, and other mental processes are temporarily lost. These facts should be known to teachers because they greatly affect the sight, the mental efficiency, and the scholarship of their pupils.

When the memory, imagination and vision are normal, the eyes, the brain and the entire nervous system are at rest. The reverse is also true, for when the muscles and nerves of the body are not at rest, the sight, memory and imagination are imperfect, and the mental efficiency is lessened or lost.

It is impossible to imagine pain, or any symptom of disease and the normal swing at the same time. Children with whooping-cough have been immediately relieved by the relaxation obtained from the swing. Many patients suffering from severe attacks of bronchitis have been promptly relieved in the same way. Angina pectoris, pneumonia, trifacial neuralgia, and other serious diseases have also been relieved after relaxation or rest was obtained with the aid of the swing.

The swing is generally beneficial. Some patients obtain more relaxation from one type of swing than from another. The long swing, however, is most helpful in a great many cases.

Long Swing

Stand with the feet about one foot apart. Turn the body to the right, at the same time lifting the heel of the left foot. The head and eyes move with the movement of the body. Do not pay any attention to the apparent movement of stationary objects. Now place the left heel on the floor, turn the body to the left, raising the heel of the right foot. Alternate. Pain and fatigue are relieved promptly while practicing this swing. When done correctly, relief is felt in a short time. The long swing, when done before retiring, lessens eyestrain during sleep.

Variable Swing

Hold the forefinger of one hand six inches from the right eye and about the same distance to the right. Look straight ahead and move the head a short distance from side to side. The finger appears to move in the direction opposite to the movement of the head and eyes.

Drifting Swing

The patient does not think of nor regard anything longer than a fraction of a second. It is helpful in doing this for the patient to imagine himself floating down a river. He may be able to imagine the drifting movement of the boat in which he is floating, better with the eyes closed than with them open. In this case, alternate the imagination with the eyes open and with them closed. The imagination may be improved in this way.

Short Swing

When the sight is normal, one can demonstrate the short swing. When it is imperfect, one can demonstrate only the longer swing. When a patient with imperfect sight regards the Snellen test card at ten or fifteen feet, he may be able to imagine one of the letters on the card to be swinging a quarter of an inch or less. The imagination of a shorter swing always improves the sight. Some patients can imagine the short swing better with their eyes closed than with them open. Alternate the imagination of the swing of the letter with the eyes closed and with them open. By repetition, the vision of the letter with the eyes open will improve (at first in flashes, later more continuously), if the memory of the short swing is perfect with the eyes closed.

Universal Swing

When the eyes are at rest, they are always moving. When the body is at rest, it can always be imagined, one part in turn, to be moving or swinging. The chair on which the patient is sitting is swinging. The floor on which the chair rests is also swinging. The walls of the room also swing when the floor swings. When one part of the building swings, one can imagine the whole building to be swinging. The ground on which the building stands is also swinging. When the ground swings, other buildings connected with it swing. One can imagine the whole city to be swinging, this continent and all other continents on the earth can be imagined swinging. In short, one can imagine not only that the whole world is moving, but also the universe, including the sun, the moon and stars. The practice of the universal swing is of the greatest benefit, for in this way one can obtain the maximum amount of relaxation.

STORIES FROM THE CLINIC
No. 71: Partial Paralysis of the Third Nerve

By Emily C. Lierman

George, age five years, was sent to me by a physician who diagnosed his case as paralysis of the third nerve of the right eye. A number of eye specialists said that he could not be cured. One gave him internal treatment for about six months and used electricity on the eye without much permanent benefit. When a nerve is paralyzed, its function is lost. In other words, the nerve is not able to bring about a contraction of the parts supplied by the nerve. To explain further, that branch of the third nerve distributed to the muscle which raises the lid had lost its function. In general, it has been believed for many years that a paralyzed nerve is relaxed. After many years of observation and experimental work, it was demonstrated that a paralyzed nerve was under a great tension. Treatment which relieved the tension and brought about a sufficient relaxation was a cure for the paralysis.

In Dr. Bates' book is an illustration of a patient with paralysis of the seventh nerve. One of the functions of the seventh nerve is to close the eyelid. When it is paralyzed, the eye remains open. Not only does the eye remain in this way, but the lips are separated. The patient is not able to close the lips sufficiently to whistle. By palming and swinging, relaxation is obtained—the patient becomes able at once to close the eyelid and to close the lips sufficiently to whistle. These cases of paralysis do not need electrical nor other stimulation. They are cured by rest. I believe that electricity is a valuable remedy, but it has lost much of its prestige by being employed in cases where it was not needed.

Georgie's mother has unusual intelligence, and she came to us confident we could relieve or cure Georgie's eyes. This is the history of his case as she described it: When he was born his right eye was wide open, and the child was unable to close the eye. About three months later the eyelid closed, and the child was unable to open his eye. Several eye specialists in Brooklyn told the mother that the eye could not be cured.

From the very beginning, Georgie was a source of pleasure to me. He seldom spoke above a whisper and preferred to go through each treatment without speaking at all, if possible. At such times he was given the card with the letter "E" pointing in different directions. When I asked him which way the "E's" were pointing, as I pointed to each one with my pencil, he would say left, right, up, down. But if he were not in the mood, he would raise his hand and indicate the direction in which the "E" was pointing. In the beginning, this card was the only one used in his treatment because he did not know all the letters of the alphabet. After he was admitted to the kindergarten school, he asked for the alphabet card, and also a figure card, which children favor a great deal for testing their sight. When Georgie's first test was made, he was unable to open his right eye. The left eye was normal, or 10/10.

I taught him to palm, and while he sat quietly, I began to talk to his mother. The conversation was solely for his benefit, so I talked about him. Like all mothers of her type, she praised her little boy and informed me of all the wonderful qualities of his mind, and that he was most obedient. I saw him smile, and for a moment he peeped a little through his fingers. After he had rested his eyes for ten minutes, I told him to keep his left eye covered, and look at the card with his right eye. His mother sat facing him with her eyes wide open with astonishment, as she saw the eyelid open just a trifle. He was able to keep his right eye open long enough to read 10/70, then the eyelid dropped again. His mother obtained a number of different Snellen test cards and used them at home for the daily treatment of the paralyzed eye.

I treated Georgie again, one week later, and I immediately had him practice the palming. So many patients have failed to palm successfully because they stare even with their eyes closed. Georgie palmed successfully because, at my suggestion, he remembered the things that were pleasant and easy to recall. If I could not think quickly enough of a story to tell him, I would show him something in my room which pleased him. Then he would palm and describe it to me. At one time I showed him a box of bonbons, which were attractively arranged, and promised him some if he would sit and palm for a long time. His mother and I were amused because he was unusually quiet when he remembered the candy. After he had palmed awhile, I suddenly asked him what he was thinking about. He opened his eyes long enough to say the word "candy" and then closed them again. The vision of his right eye improved from 10/70 to 10/50 that day, and the eyelid was more open than before. The left eye improved to 12/10.

At every visit his vision was improved, while the paralysis diminished with the increased relaxation of his eye. I noticed that occasionally he would forget to blink, and then he would stare and strain, which lowered his vision and increased the paralysis. His eyelid has opened more, and his vision has improved since he became the owner of a little puppy. Whenever he played with the little dog, his mother noticed that both eyes would blink. This is evidence that things seen in motion are seen best. The vision of his right eye was improved to more than 10/10, while that of his left eye to 18/10, which is very unusual in a child six years old. He had been under my treatment for about a year.

THE BLINKING KNIGHT

By George M. Guild

Inside a dark, dingy, little shop, a group of children bent over their work. Outside, New Year's revelry echoed along the streets, but the day held no joy nor merriment for these little workers. It was just like every other day. It meant sitting from early morning until late at night stringing countless numbers of little beads together to make ornaments. They stooped over their tasks until their sight grew dim and colored spots danced before their eyes. They could not stop their work nor rest for even a moment, but the angry proprietor prodded them on.

Today, fear and dread settled in the hearts of the poor children. Had they not been told that their work was very bad and that they would be dismissed? They knew it was, because they could not see to match the beads in the dull light of the shop. Perhaps glasses would help them, but where was the money to come from?

As evening approached, the light grew dimmer and dimmer. It seemed to the children that they could no longer go on, when from a dusty corner they heard a voice say, "Good evening, children." As they looked, they saw a light shining. The light grew stronger and stronger and seemed to fill the room. The little workers almost shouted aloud with joy. Suddenly a little man with a flaming sword jumped out to the center of the room. On his head he wore a soft velvet hat with a very large brim; a cluster of huge diamonds shone on the front, while smaller ones covered the hat band. His coat had a long tail, which swayed with every movement he made. The many glittering buttons were immense diamonds. His yellow vest, which contained a great many more pockets than any vest the children had ever seen, was decorated with diamonds, rubies, emeralds, and sapphires. His violet trousers reached only to his knees, and they too were covered with jewels. He wore long stockings of fiery red, and his low patent leather shoes were trimmed with large silver buckles. The belt of the scabbard for his sword sparkled with jewels.

When the children gazed on this knight, they became very quiet and curious to know who he was. His eyes were sympathetic as he smiled good-naturedly on them. When he spoke, his voice was like music to their ears and made them all feel comfortable and at peace with the world.

"Children," he said, "the fairies have sent me to help you to be happy. I love each and every one of you and want to cure your eyes so that you will be able to have perfect sight all the time. You will be able to see even in the dimmest light without glasses. All of you are working too hard. Make believe that you can see fairies, that you can talk with them, dance with them, and be like them. When I was a boy, I wanted to be a fairy, but when I grew up, the king made me a knight. One day, while riding through a wood, I saw some blue flowers. They were so beautiful and fragrant that I said aloud, 'Oh, you lovely blue flowers, how I wish you were all fairies,' and then, much to my surprise, every flower turned into a blue fairy. They climbed upon my steed and urged him to canter as fast as he could. Very soon we came to a field of beautiful yellow flowers. While I looked at them, entranced, myriads of little yellow fairies danced gaily from the petals and mingled and danced together, leading us on until we reached a meadow of violets nodding in the breeze. They were even more beautiful than the others. I wished that they too were fairies. All at once the violets turned to violet fairies and they frolicked with the other fairies."

The knight ceased to speak for a moment and then suddenly held up a bouquet of blue, yellow and violet flowers. The children saw him leap to the middle of a large table in center of the room. There he began to dance, and as he danced he blinked his eyes and waved the flowers around his head, crying out to the children, "Make believe that these flowers are fairies. Remember the colors perfectly. Blink your eyes as you see me blinking, and never forget what you will see now." Immediately the flowers all turned to fairies of the same color.

At once they all began to dance around the blinking knight, laughing, shouting, and enjoying themselves. The knight touched each child in the shop with his wonderful sword, and each child, as soon as she was touched, turned into a fairy. Some blue, some yellow, and some violet, and all blinking as frequently as the blinking knight.

"Now that you are all fairies," he said, "you must think, remember, imagine, and believe all things which are good. Tomorrow morning, you will all waken and believe that all this was a dream. I want to tell you that I was born a thousand years ago. I speak with the wisdom of the ages when I say to you, that if you will only remember me and make believe that you are fairies, you will always be happy and good the rest of your lives."

HOW ESTELLE HELPED

By Beatrice Smith

There are many cases of imperfect sight, many cases of pain and fatigue, which can be cured by other patients who have obtained normal sight without glasses by practicing relaxation methods.

About three years ago, a young man, age seventeen, suffered very much from pain in his right eye. The pain increased quite rapidly and finally became so severe that in order to get any relief, he was compelled to take morphine. As time passed, the dose of morphine was increased and increased with unusual rapidity. The outlook seemed dismal. The eye specialists in some of the large cities prescribed glasses for him, but without benefit. One day while walking along the street, he met a lady whose daughter had been cured by the treatment of imperfect sight without glasses, discovered and practiced by a physician living in New York City. The lady recommended him to practice palming, swinging and some other methods described in a book called *Perfect Sight Without Glasses*. The palming gave instant relief. By palming for fifteen minutes every night and morning, the pain was relieved or prevented. This treatment was continued for some months, usually about three times daily for fifteen minutes each time. As the days went by without a return of the agonizing pain, he practiced palming less frequently until, after three months of not having had an attack of the pain, he stopped the palming and forgot all about his right eye.

The patient lived in one of the large cities of the West. It was interesting to learn of the great number of people who followed the treatment of this case of pain and kept in mind all the particulars. When the boy began to lessen the number of treatments by palming, some of his friends were very much concerned for fear that he was stopping the treatment too soon. When he remained free from pain for some time, they were relieved, but still more or less apprehensive. I believe the boy felt deep down in his heart that if that pain ever came back, he would know how to handle it.

The patient who recommended the boy to palm had a daughter about ten years old, who had been to New York, taken the treatment and been cured of imperfect sight without glasses. This little girl kept after the young man in the early days of his treatment and insisted that he practice all those methods which were beneficial, repeatedly and continuously. I believe it was the efforts of the little girl which did more than anything else to benefit the patient. True, he was willing to palm and did palm, but there were days when he would forget and she kept after him until he was cured. I believe that she had more to do with the cure of the boy's pain than did the supervision of other people.

A STUDENT'S EXPERIENCE

By Margaret Robinson

Author's Note—*Dr. Bates has asked me to send some report in regard to my teaching of his methods in Bloomington, Illinois. Converts to the truth of Dr. Bates' explanation of eye troubles are persuaded that glasses, for the average person, are unnecessary, and also that the vision is lowered as a result of their use. It is appalling to find how many people are actually struggling with glasses which, they have been told, would relieve their strain and save their vision. If, in my very limited experience, I have found so many of this type, there must be a great number of such unfortunates in every community. The three following cases illustrate what I mean:*

Ms. I., age thirty, had worn glasses since she was ten years old. In the past two years, since a goiter operation, she said she had visited the oculist at least once a week. He had changed her glasses four or five times during this period, had stopped all reading, and was putting medication in her eyes to relieve a distress, which she said was almost constant. He seemed uncertain what to do next, as her vision was steadily growing worse. With her glasses she read 10/30 with both eyes and 10/200 with the right eye alone. After taking off her glasses and palming for a short time she read better than 10/20 with both eyes, and almost 10/70 with the right eye. The near vision of the right eye was also impaired. On the first day she could not read ordinary type with this eye alone. In two weeks she lost all sense of strain and read 10/10 with both eyes and began to read 10/50 with the right eye. She read diamond type readily with both eyes together, and slowly with the right eye alone, at six inches. She reported that she was able, without fatigue, to read two hours or more at a time, day or evening. She looked and acted ten years younger.

Ms. J., age forty-two, was very much frightened about her eyes, and very loath to give up the large glasses, behind which her eyes looked so tired and drawn. She had been forced to give up her position at an embroidery counter because of the failure of her vision. In eight months she had had three different pairs of glasses, and said that the oculist told her frankly that he was much puzzled as to how to relieve her very serious strain. Four lessons, with her intelligent cooperation, and less than a month's time, relieved the situation. Her eyes were comfortable and she was able to see satisfactorily for reading and sewing, as well as at a distance. The look of relief on her face was very gratifying.

Ms. W., age forty-nine, had suffered with very severe eye difficulties for twenty years. She had been forced to give up her piano work, could do practically no reading, and said, in fact, that many of the interests of her life had been dropped because of her eyes. Bright lights and use of her eyes for close work produced a sharp pain in her head which she had learned to greatly dread. For about a year she was allowed to use "very strong" glasses ten minutes at a time. Of late she had used them longer than that, but it made her eyes very tired to do so. There were dark rings under her eyes and she was very nervous. Without her glasses she was able to read 10/15, and also large clear type at reading distance, but better at an arm's length. She did this, however, with fear and trembling, often stopping to close her eyes. In two weeks she was reading 10/10 readily without fear, and also getting flashes of clear vision when practicing with the diamond type card held at six or eight inches from eyes. She was comfortable, had lost all dread of bright lights, did not get the pain in her head anymore, and was losing the dark rings under her eyes. She stopped taking lessons at this point, but continued to improve, according to reports which reached me several months later.

In each of these cases, glasses were not only useless, but actual torture. In each case the individual had given up what she wanted to do because of her eyes. In each case a couple of weeks without glasses, combined with learning how to relieve the eyestrain, made life, as each wanted to live it, possible. It seems incredible that the value of such facts is not more quickly and more generally accepted.

QUESTIONS AND ANSWERS

Q–1. I can read with no trouble but cannot distinguish things at a distance, especially the features of people. What would you suggest?

A–1. You are nearsighted. The imagination cure is the quickest and most satisfactory cure of myopia. Use two Snellen test cards, one held at one foot or nearer, or at a distance where you can see it best; the other placed at five feet or farther. Look at the first letter of one of the lines of the near card and with the eyes closed remember it for half a minute or longer. Then look at the same letter on the distant card at five feet or farther and imagine that letter for not longer than a second. Then look at the near letter again for part of a minute, close your eyes and remember it, and then glance at the same letter on the distant card for not longer than a second, and imagine it as well as you can. Alternate. When you become able to see the bottom line on the distant card, place it a few inches farther off and repeat.

Q–2. What method is most helpful in myopia?

A–2. Palming, swinging, and the use of the memory or imagination (described above), are most helpful.

Q–3. Can you tell me what to do for inflammation of the white of the eye (sclera)?

A–3. The light treatment is beneficial. Sit in the sun with the eyes closed and let the sun shine directly upon the closed eyelids. Move the head a short distance from side to side. Practice sunning for half an hour or longer three times daily when possible.

Q–4. Will you kindly tell me what I can do in order to read as well with the eyelids fully open as I can when they are slightly parted (squinting)?

A–4. Improve your vision with the aid of the imagination cure as described above in answer to Q—1. When your vision improves, your eyelids will be more open.

Q–5. Is there any exercise or any particular method of relaxation that will help double vision?

A–5. Closing the eyes and resting them is a cure for double vision. Blinking frequently, just as the normal eye does, is also beneficial.

Q–6. Please explain the elliptical swing.

A–6. In the elliptical swing, the head and eyes are moved continuously in the orbit of an ellipse or a circle. The continuous movement of the head and eyes prevents the stare or strain, since staring requires that one try to keep the eyes from moving.

Q–7. How many times a day should the sun treatment be given?

A–7. The sun treatment should be given for half an hour or longer three times a day, or more often, when possible. The more sun treatment, the better, as it rests and strengthens the eyes.

Q–8. What treatment helps most people?

A–8. Palming is generally most helpful.

Q–9. Is it possible for some people to be cured by the help they may obtain from your book *Perfect Sight Without Glasses*?

A–9. Yes. By practicing the methods recommended in my book, many readers have improved their vision without my supervision. It helps to have someone with perfect sight supervise your treatment.

Q–10. Is myopia hereditary?

A–10. No. It is, however, contagious in many cases. When parents are cured of myopia, their children may recover without treatment.

Q–11. How long does it take to cure an average case of myopia?

A–11. Some patients are cured more quickly than others. The length of time is uncertain, as patients differ in their response to treatment.

Better Eyesight
February 1926—Vol. X, No. 8

DEMONSTRATE: EFFORT, BLINKING AND PALMING

EFFORT

That an effort to see always lowers the vision. Look at the Snellen test card at a distance of twenty feet. It may be possible for you to see the large letters and read them without any apparent effort, while the smaller letters produce a strain which you can feel. If you consciously increase the effort to see the smaller letters, your vision becomes more imperfect. It is not easy for you to realize that effort is always present when the vision is lowered. Knowing the cause of your imperfect sight is a great help in selecting the remedy.

BLINKING

That the normal eye blinks very frequently. In order to have normal sight, the eyes must blink. One can demonstrate that when the patient looks at one letter at the distance with normal sight, or looks at one letter at a near point where it is seen clearly, keeping the eyes continuously open without blinking for a minute or longer always lowers the vision for the distance or for the near point. This should convince the patient that blinking is absolutely necessary in order to obtain good vision.

PALMING

That palming, when done correctly, improves the vision. When the closed eyes are covered with one or both hands, and all light is excluded, the patient should see nothing at all, or a perfect black. This is a rest to the eyes and always improves the sight at least temporarily. Palming can be done wrong. When it is practiced incorrectly, the field imagined by the patient contains streaks of red, white, blue, or other colors. The eyes are under a strain, and the vision is not materially improved by the wrong method of palming. It can be demonstrated that palming for half an hour or longer is a greater benefit than palming for only a few minutes.

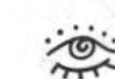

MEMORY

By W. H. Bates, M.D.

When the sight is normal, the memory is perfect. The color and background of the letters or other objects seen are remembered perfectly, instantaneously, and continuously.

One of the quickest cures of imperfect sight has been gained through the use of the memory. When the memory is perfect, the eyes at once become normal with normal vision. A perfect memory changes the elongated eyeball of myopia into the shorter length of the normal eye. No matter how high a degree of myopia one may have, when he has a perfect memory of some one thing, he is no longer myopic, but has normal eyes with normal vision.

An imperfect memory or an imperfect imagination may produce organic changes in the eyeball. The organic changes, which are present in many diseases of the eye, have been relieved with the aid of a perfect memory. In some cases the vision has been reduced to perception of light from scars on the front part of the eyeball. Perfect memory brings about the absorption of such opacities. A perfect memory has cured these obstinate cases.

Conical cornea is a very serious disease. Neither operation nor the use of drugs relieves or cures it. A perfect memory gives instant relief, the curvature of the cornea becomes normal, and the patient obtains normal vision.

Glaucoma has been referred to as a very treacherous disease of the eye because symptoms of blindness may become apparent at unexpected moments. The pain of glaucoma may be very severe. In most cases, the eyeball becomes very hard. The vision fails in a few hours, and all perception of light may be lost. These very severe cases are usually not benefited by operation nor drugs. The practice of a perfect memory has relieved all the disagreeable symptoms, and the vision has returned to normal.

There are patients who suffer from paralysis of one or more of the nerves connected with the eye. By resting the nerves or the muscles to bring about a condition of relaxation, which is best obtained by a perfect memory, the symptoms of paralysis are relieved. Paralysis of the nerves of the eye is caused by too great activity and is relieved by relaxation.

When one of the eyes has been injured or has a foreign body in the inside of the eyeball, the good eye may become affected and, in rare cases, may even be lost before the eye that has been injured is lost. This is called sympathetic ophthalmia. Through the use of the perfect memory, these cases, although of many years' duration, have been benefited and normal vision obtained. To be able to demonstrate a perfect memory habitually or unconsciously, it is necessary first to consciously remember with the eyes closed or open one thing perfectly until an unconscious habit is formed.

A person can remember what his own name is without having a mental picture of each letter of the name. This is an example of what is known as an abstract memory. A concrete memory is a more perfect memory because one remembers a mental picture of the object with the eyes closed, as well or better than he can see it with the eyes open. One can remember perfectly only that which is seen perfectly. When a letter is seen perfectly, the whiteness of the card or page in the neighborhood of the black letter is imagined whiter than the rest of the card or page, or that part in which there are no black letters. The whiter that one can imagine the white in the neighborhood of a letter, or inside of the letter, enables one to see the blackness of the letter blacker than before. In other cases, where the whiteness in the neighborhood of the letter is apparently of the same whiteness as the rest of the card, the memory or the imagination of the black letter is imperfect.

Mental pictures are imagined perfectly when the memory is perfect. A great many patients complain that they are unable to remember mental pictures of the letters of the Snellen test card. They can remember what the letters are but have no mental pictures of them. To obtain perfect mental pictures, it is necessary that the sight should be continuously good. Most people, when they fail to imagine mental pictures, try to remember too much at once. When remembering a letter, it is not necessary to recall all parts of the letter. The memory of the color or one small portion of the letter is sufficient. The smaller the part of a black letter that you remember, the blacker it is, and the easier it is to recall. It should be emphasized that when one has a perfect memory, central fixation can always be demonstrated. When central fixation is absent, the memory of the letter, as well as the imagination or the sight, is always imperfect. One can regard a point or a small part of a letter by central fixation for only a short time, not longer than a few seconds, without the memory becoming imperfect. Shifting is necessary to maintain a perfect memory, which is continuous. In other words, when practicing central fixation, the point regarded changes frequently.

After a demonstration that central fixation is necessary for a perfect memory, one patient became able to imagine, with his eyes closed, a small letter "o" with a white center as white as snow, starch, or any other white object that he had ever seen. He had no trouble in doing this. He said that he could remember it easily and quite continuously. Then I requested him to remember an imperfect "o," which was a shade of light gray instead of black. It had no white center, but was covered with a blur or a fog. He was able to remember it quickly, easily, for a few seconds, but when he was requested to remember the imperfect "o" for a minute or longer, the gray shade became darker and, at times, lighter, and the memory of the imperfect "o" became very difficult. In spite of all the efforts he made, he was unable to remember the "o" continuously. In strong contrast to the memory of the perfect "o," the memory or the imagination of the imperfect "o" was difficult. He agreed with me when I told him that in order to fail to see perfectly, he had to stare, strain, and make a tremendous effort. On the other hand, the memory or the imagination of the perfect "o" was spontaneous, easy, and continuous, and he experienced a feeling of general comfort in all his nerves. He was able to demonstrate that he could remember the perfect "o," provided he imagined it was moving, and that he could not remember it when he tried to imagine it stationary.

Flashing is a great help in improving mental pictures. With the eyes open, one may see a letter quite perfectly and have a mental picture of that letter with the eyes closed for a fraction of a second. By repeatedly flashing the letter in this way, the mental picture becomes more frequent and lasts longer. When the sight becomes more continuously good, the memory is also benefited, and with this improvement in the memory, the mental pictures become more perfect. The converse is also true. When the memory is improved, the sight is improved.

You cannot have a perfect memory by any effort or strain. The more perfect your memory, the greater is your relaxation, and the more perfect is your sight.

STORIES FROM THE CLINIC

No. 72: Jane

By Emily C. Lierman

A year ago, a little girl named Jane, age twelve years, came to me for treatment. She had worn glasses approximately four years for progressive myopia. Progressive nearsightedness is a very serious disease in which the sight becomes worse more or less rapidly. With the increase in degree of nearsightedness, the retina becomes inflamed, and the vision is ultimately lost. [There is a high correlation between high degrees of myopia and detached retina. See "Detachment of the Retina" in the November 1926 issue.—TRQ] This disease cannot be relieved by glasses nor by any known method of treatment, other than that recommended by Dr. Bates. Jane was also troubled with astigmatism.

When I first saw her, I was deeply impressed by her personality. She had unusual intelligence. Her parents were willing to make any sacrifice in order that Jane might be cured without glasses. She loved music but was ready to give it up temporarily so that she could faithfully practice the daily treatment outlined for her.

When her vision was tested, she read 15/70 with the right eye, and 15/50 with the left. After the first treatment, her vision with each eye improved to 15/40. The circular swing, which has proved so helpful in the cure of many patients, was her main treatment at the first visit. In this swing the head and eyes move in the orbit of a circle. They move continuously, and there is no opportunity to stare or strain, as there may be when the head and eyes are just moved from side to side. The diameter of the circular swing should be as short as possible because the greatest degree of relaxation can be obtained if a short circular swing can be practiced. There is this objection, however, that when the orbit of the swing is short, the patient may unconsciously stop the swing, and a stare or strain results. In a circular swing, in which the diameter of the circle is longer, relaxation is always obtained. The circular swing can be practiced with the patient standing or sitting. The results vary from time to time. At one time, the greatest benefit may be obtained while the patient is sitting, at another time while he is standing.

Having worn glasses steadily for four years, it was not so easy for Jane to go without them in the beginning. The second time she was treated she complained of a headache. This was immediately relieved by the circular swing, and her vision improved to 15/20. After this visit, she practiced the treatment at home for six months or longer, but she never failed to report the condition of her eyes.

About a month after her first treatment, her vision for the test card had improved to 15/10. In the treatment, we used a card with numbers, another with "E's" pointing in different directions, which is called pothooks, and still another with different letters. She found no difficulty in reading all the letters and figures on these cards at fifteen feet. It was noticed, too, that her little nervous habits disappeared. I gave Jane several treatments, and in all her eye tests she did not make a single mistake.

Other test cards, unfamiliar to Jane, were then used. I placed Jane thirty feet away from the card and, without any hesitation or one mistake, she read every letter. She did not have to be reminded to blink her eyes regularly, because it had become a habit. Blinking helped so much in keeping her relaxed. Our small fundamental test card, pocket size, was then used. We placed it in a good light, and Jane surprised me by reading the "R Z 3" line at six feet. This is read by the normal eye at three feet.

This article ought to convince any patient that progressive myopia is curable. It should encourage those who have given the method a trial, to keep on practicing as Jane did and win out as she has. At no time have I met a more wonderful child. She loved to practice the method every day. I shall always remember the last precious hour I spent with her. Her last words to me were, "There is one thing I am certain about and that is none of my children, nor grandchildren, nor great grandchildren need ever wear glasses."

THE MAGIC KITTEN

By George M. Guild

Once upon a time, a small black kitten strayed about the streets. The city seemed a huge world, peopled with giants who pushed and shoved him here and there. He tried to escape them, but their enormous feet seemed everywhere. Finally, he came to a crooked alley which was quiet and peaceful. He crept behind an ash barrel, glad to be away from the terrifying crowds. He grew drowsy and was falling asleep when suddenly a loud crash sounded in his ears. His heart began to pound faster and faster, and he wondered what would happen next. He was so frightened that he could not move. When nothing happened his fear left him and, like all little kittens, he became curious. He poked his nose from behind the barrel, but could see no one. Then he grew very bold and jumped to the top of the barrel, where he saw only a broken flower-pot with some faded roses scattered among the fragments. With his paw, he gently touched one and then another of the faded blossoms. They all seemed to move. He jumped down, and in his excitement pushed one to the ground. He ran a little way off and then cautiously approached to look at it.

Slowly the petals unfolded. In the center appeared a tiny golden fairy waving a beautiful wand. She danced gaily upon one of the petals and beckoned to the little kitten to come closer. He was frightened, but he felt a magic power drawing him nearer and nearer. As he came toward her, she bent over and gently touched him with her wand. How strange he felt! Happy and contented, not like the little stray kitten that stole about the streets looking for shelter.

"Now you are a beautiful kitten, golden as the sun. Gone is the ugly, black creature that you were. Favored of the fairies, scamper away and make others happy as I have made you!" Saying this, the fairy hopped into the center of the flower, and the petals folded about her.

The kitten ran off as fast as he could go to carry out the bidding of the fairy. Soon he came to a group of boys and girls at play. The children stopped their games to look at the little golden kitten. As they crowded about him he danced merrily, swinging his tail in time with his steps. The children clapped their hands with glee. The more joyous they became, the more sprightly did he dance.

Suddenly he stopped before little Eppie who had been trying to see him dance. Poor little Eppie's eyes were crossed, and it was difficult for her to see anything, even with her spectacles on. The kitten began to sway rhythmically from side to side. Eppie watched him without moving her eyes. She tried so hard to see him and stared so much that he seemed only a blur of gold. She wanted to see him so badly, but the more she tried, the less she saw. Finally, Eppie could no longer keep back her tears. Seeing her tears, he danced over to her and gently touched her with his paw. As she bent over to pet him the magic kitten reached up and pulled off her glasses and let them fall to the ground. He stood up on his hind paws, grasped both of Eppie's hands and began to sway slowly from side to side.

He then dropped her hands and scampered off a short distance. Eppie followed him and looked down into his shining eyes. He kept blinking up at her, looking very wise. Eppie blinked back at him, and all at once she realized that she could see him perfectly. He turned three somersaults in the air, landing gracefully on his feet, and stood before her swinging his beautiful tail. Eppie watched the movement of his tail, swaying her body in rhythm with it.

The children all cried, "Oh, look at Eppie's eyes! How straight they are, and she hasn't her glasses on, either!" Then, they too started to sway from side to side as they watched the swinging tail of the golden kitten.

By this time it had grown dusk and the children had to go home. They all wanted to take the kitten home, but he clung close to Eppie. When the other children tried to touch him, a tongue of golden flame shot from his mouth and they quickly withdrew. Eppie held him tightly in her arms and ran home to tell her mother and father the glad news.

Before she had a chance to tell them all about her wonderful experience, they cried out in amazement at her changed appearance. Eppie told them breathlessly about the magic kitten, and what he had done for her. At the mention of him the kitten jumped out of her arms and began to swing his golden tail. With one accord, they all swayed in time with its motion. And so they became very jolly and happy.

The next morning, when Eppie awoke, the kitten had disappeared. Disappointed, she set out for school. Much to her surprise, there at the door of the schoolhouse stood the golden kitten, waiting for Eppie. He ran ahead of her and jumped up on the teacher's desk. He stood there swinging his tail to and fro. The children who were waiting in their seats for the arrival of the teacher took great delight in the kitten's performance. They felt impelled by his mystic power to sway in time with the swing of his tail.

In the midst of their merriment, the teacher entered the room. The children stopped in fear, but the magic kitten became even more animated. The teacher approached her desk, and as she leaned over to see the kitten, her glasses dropped off her nose and broke in a thousand pieces upon the floor. She became angry and was about to throw the kitten from the desk, when she too felt the magic power of his swinging tail. In spite of herself, she swayed from side to side. Her anger left her, and she forgot her broken glasses.

The children looked at her in amazement, for they or anyone else had never seen her without glasses. The teacher was just as amazed as the children, for she suddenly became aware that she could see her class clearly. She was as joyous as the children had been.

"Surely this must be the magic kitten we read about yesterday!" she exclaimed. While she was speaking the kitten jumped down from the desk, flourished his tail and disappeared. The children were dismayed, but the teacher said, "Even though the magic kitten has gone, we shall always remember what he has taught us. We will set aside a time each day to practice the swinging movements of the magic kitten."

CASES BENEFITED

By Dr. Clara C. Ingham, Portland, Oregon

Cataract. A lady sixty-five. Vision of right eye 20/200; left eye 20/100. Unable to do any reading. Six months treatment gives vision 20/20. Can read diamond type print.

Strabismus. Child of ten years. Vision 20/40. After eight months' treatment, vision is normal and eye straight.

Extreme strabismus and oscillation (nystagmus). College student afflicted from childhood. One of the most difficult cases for correction that ever entered my office. Sight in strabismic eye 2/200; in the straight eye 20/50. At the present time the oscillation has practically ceased while the strabismic eye is straight much of the time. Patient still comes about twice a week and while not yet normal, the vision of both eyes is greatly improved. This young man's mother is a teacher in the schools, and her son's restoration has done much to place Dr. Bates' method before the schools.

Pain. A man of thirty-two. Vision 10/200. Severe pain

in eyeballs and temples. Eye troubles from childhood. Says he was never conscious of absolute freedom from pain. After a year's treatment, is one of our greatest enthusiasts for good eyesight. He is an instructor in a college and will gladly spread the gospel.

Nearsightedness. Grammar schoolgirl about fourteen, nearsighted from straining to see the blackboard. Vision in right eye 10/100; in left eye 10/70. After two months normal sight, and has learned how to protect herself against eyestrain in school, so has no fear of a recurrence of the trouble.

Acute Glaucoma in right eye, the left eye having been completely lost by the same disease more than a year previous. The right eye responded very readily to treatment, as has the left also, though seemingly past help when the patient first came.

EYESTRAIN

By W. H. Bates, M.D.

Eyestrain is the cause of many serious diseases of the eye. It is always manifest when imperfect sight is present. The normal eye does not ordinarily have eyestrain. When it is acquired, the sight always becomes imperfect. When the sight is imperfect, the eyes are under a strain. They are staring—making an effort to see. This condition is not cured by glasses. The fact that wearing glasses always increases eyestrain can be demonstrated.

After treatment has been instituted, it is soon found that the use of eyedrops or drugs is of no avail. Bathing the eyes with a solution of boric acid or other similar remedies does not give the desired results. Attention to general health, physical exercise, and diet does not relieve symptoms of eyestrain. It is commonly a chronic condition. Patients who are suffering from this malady have usually acquired a habit of continually making an effort to see. One cannot correct this bad habit of strain without substituting in its place the beneficial habit of practicing relaxation continuously.

The normal eye is always moving. To demonstrate eyestrain, one must first imagine the eyes stationary or actually force them to be stationary. This should prove to the patient that the eyes are under a strain when stationary, or when stationary objects are imagined to be stationary. The normal eye maintains the habit of relaxation—of always moving. When the eyes move, stationary objects are imagined to be moving in the direction opposite to the movement of the head and eyes. When the normal eye has normal vision, the head and eyes are continuously moving. This is a rest to the eyes, and a habit which can be more easily practiced than the habit of straining the eyes in an effort to keep them stationary.

Many people state that they have no time to practice the method which will bring about relaxation. This objection is answered by the fact that everyone has as much time to use his eyes correctly as he has to use them incorrectly. When the eyes are used correctly, the patient feels more comfortable, which should encourage him to use his eyes properly. When the eyes are not used correctly, discomfort is felt. Pain, fatigue and other nervous symptoms are produced.

Subjective conjunctivitis is a very painful symptom of eyestrain. The eyes burn and smart and the patient suffers from pain, fatigue, and many other disagreeable sensations. Later the eyelids become inflamed.

In the year 1884 I roomed with a young medical student who was suffering from this form of eyestrain. During the examination period he could not read more than five or ten minutes before his eyes became so sore and painful that he was unable to read at all. His physician prescribed a spray which had no apparent benefit. Another doctor prescribed flesh gloves to be used in rubbing the skin all over the body. He derived temporary benefit from this treatment, but it had to be repeated at frequent intervals. It seemed to me at the time that the eyestrain was relieved by the massage, but a more thorough observation later proved that this was untrue. The relief was manifest when the massage was delayed or postponed, or when he had rested his eyes.

One evening while I was reading he said to me, "Why do you blink so often?" "Because it is an easy way to rest my eyes," I answered. He practiced blinking and obtained complete relief. "My eyes are cool and comfortable, my sight is perfect, and best of all, I can remember what I read more easily," he stated.

We investigated the facts. He demonstrated many times that when he read without blinking the symptoms of eyestrain soon appeared, and his vision became worse. Other students tried it as well, and we all were positive that staring or trying to see without blinking always caused eyestrain. When the blinking was practiced relief was always obtained. There were no exceptions.

QUESTIONS AND ANSWERS

Q–1. It is difficult for me to find time enough to gain perfect relaxation. What would you suggest?

A–1. You have just as much time to relax as you have to strain. Practice relaxation all day long. Whenever you move your head or eyes, notice that stationary objects move in the direction opposite to the movement of your head or eyes. When walking about the room or on the street, the floor or pavement appears to come toward you, while objects on either side of you move in the direction opposite to the movement of your body. Remember to blink frequently just as the normal eye does. Constantly shift your eyes from one point to another, seeing the point regarded more clearly than all other parts. When talking with anyone, do not stare. Look first at one eye and then the other, remembering to blink. Shift from the eyes to the nose, to one cheek and then to the other, then to the mouth, the chin, and back to the forehead.

Q–2a. Why is it that I have perfect vision only in flashes? 2b. Can these flashes become permanent?

A–2a. You have not yet lost your unconscious habit of straining. 2b. When relaxation methods are practiced faithfully at all times, the flashes of improved vision become more frequent and last longer until the vision becomes continuously good.

Q–3. What causes twitching eyelids?

A–3. Strain causes twitching eyelids and is relieved by rest and relaxation. Palming, sun treatment, swinging, and blinking are very beneficial.

Q–4a. Is working or reading under electric light harmful? 4b. Should a shade be worn?

A–4a. It is not harmful to read by electric light if the eyes are used properly. 4b. Do not wear a shade or any other protection for the eyes. Practice sun treatment.

Q–5. When remembering a black period, I see a bright disk with a small black center. Is this seeing a period?

A–5. No, you are straining. The period that you imagine is very imperfect because to remember the period, and at the same time a very bright disk, is an unconscious strain. You cannot strain and remember the bright disk, and simultaneously relax and remember a black period. When your bright disk is prominent, everything else is remembered under a strain. You cannot strain and relax at the same time.

Better Eyesight
March 1926—Vol. X, No. 9

DEMONSTRATE: CENTRAL FIXATION

That central fixation improves the vision. The normal eye is always at rest and always has central fixation. Central fixation cannot be obtained through any effort. When an effort is made by the normal eye, central fixation is always lost. In central fixation, one sees best the point regarded, while all other points are seen less clearly.

Look at the upper left-hand corner of the back of a chair. Note that all other parts of the chair are not seen so well. Look at the top of a letter at a distance at which it can be seen clearly. Then quickly look at the bottom of the letter. Alternate. When the eyes go up, the letter appears to move down. Then the eyes move down, the letter appears to move up. Coincident with this movement, you can observe that you see best the point regarded and all other points less clearly or less distinctly. When you can imagine the letter to be moving, it is possible for you to see best where you are looking.

The size of the letter or object seen does not matter. Central fixation can be demonstrated with the smallest letters which are printed, or the smallest objects. Close the eyes and remember or imagine how the small letter would look if you imagined one part best. By shifting from one part of the letter to another, central fixation with the eyes closed may be made continuous for one-half minute or longer. Then with the eyes open, it is possible for one second or less to see, remember, or imagine the same small letter or other objects in the same way—one part best. Note that when the letters are read easily and clearly, they are always seen by central fixation, and relaxation is felt. Central fixation is a rest to the nerves and when practiced continuously, it relieves strain and improves the vision to normal.

[While I was teaching centralization in one of my classes, using two pencils separated approximately 14 inches from each other, one of my students said, "Well, *of course,* the peripheral pencil is less clear—*because I am not interested in it."* The implication was that if he had just as much interest in the peripheral pencil, he should be able to see it just as clearly as the pencil he was centralizing on, simultaneously.

I had to think about this one for a while.

The next class I explained to him that the reason the peripheral pencil was less clear was *not* due to the fact that he was less interested in it. To prove this, I had him centralize on one of the pencils, and then I asked him to have just as much interest in the peripheral pencil as the pencil he was centralizing on (without looking directly at the peripheral pencil). When he did this, he agreed that the peripheral pencil was not as clear as the pencil he was centralizing on.

The reason peripheral objects are less clear is due to the rods that are located in the peripheral parts of the retina; rods are incapable of perceiving sharp details. Only the cones, located in the center of the retina, can pick up sharp details. People with imperfect sight have eccentric, diffused, or "spread out" vision. They try, usually subconsciously, to see all objects—even the objects picked up with the rods—clearly at the same time. This, of course, is impossible to do and is a tremendous strain on the visual system.—TRQ]

IMAGINATION

By W. H. Bates, M.D.

Imagination is good. One may even see the white part of letters whiter than it really is, while the black is not altered by distance, illumination, size, nor form of the letters.

Imagination is good in normal sight. When the sight is normal, the imagination is normal. The converse is also true—when the imagination is normal, the sight is normal. A cure is obtained when the imagination is improved to the normal. One may imagine a letter of the Snellen test card very well while regarding it with the eyes open. When the sight is normal, the imagination may be as good and usually much better with the eyes closed than with the eyes open. When the sight is perfect, one can imagine with the eyes open, objects of all sizes and forms, familiar or strange, just as well as he can with the eyes closed. Under favorable conditions of environment, namely light, distance, and restful surroundings, the imagination is usually good. A perfect imagination can only be obtained when the memory is perfect. When the memory is perfect, the consciousness of the movement of all things remembered or imagined can always be demonstrated. The eyes are constantly shifting when the imagination is good. After the shifting stops, the perfect imagination is modified or lost.

It is not possible to have a perfect imagination and an imperfect one at the same time. For example, one cannot remember a black color perfectly black and a white color imperfectly white simultaneously. When a black letter with a white center is imagined perfectly, both the white and the black are perfect. It is impossible to imagine the letter with a perfect white center and an imperfect or gray-black outline. When the imagination is perfect for one thing, it is also perfect for all things. When a patient makes his first visit, the vision of each eye is tested for the Snellen test card at about fifteen feet. If the large letter of the Snellen test card cannot be distinguished at this distance, the card is brought closer until the letter is clear enough to be recognized. Experience has demonstrated that trying to improve the vision of such patients at fifteen feet or farther is disappointing, but when they practice with the card at ten feet or nearer, the vision usually improves immediately. Some nearsighted patients have good sight at six inches, but not at twelve inches. By having them read as well as they can at six inches and then look at the card at twelve inches for a moment, the vision usually improves. Some patients can see very well at five feet for a short time. They are instructed to always close their eyes when their sight becomes imperfect, and when they open them, to keep them open for just a moment or a flash. This alternate resting the eyes by closing them and looking at the letters just for a second is a benefit to a great many. There are, however, a large number of patients who are not benefited at all by this method, because as soon as they open their eyes or even before that, they stare or strain and make an effort to see.

It helps very much to suggest to the patient that he use the word "imagination" and not the word "sight." To most people, to improve the imagination seems easier than to improve the sight, and quite a number believe that when they know what the letter is, although they may not see it, they can always imagine it. It is interesting to observe that when the imagination of a letter is improved by resting the eyes, other letters on the card not regarded become blacker and the whiteness of the card whiter. It is frequently demonstrated that one of the best ways of improving the sight is to improve the imagination of letters that are known. Often a patient says that he can imagine a known letter and sometimes thinks that he sees it, but he and his friends are usually very suspicious of the vision obtained when regarding a familiar card whose letters are known. It is necessary to demonstrate in various ways that when the imagination is improved, the vision is improved. This statement, however, does not convince the patient. The only test that is convincing is to test the patient with an unfamiliar card. It is oftentimes quite a shock to him to find that he can quite frequently read an unfamiliar card with much better vision than he is able to imagine or see the card that was familiar.

If a patient is unable to read fine print at twelve inches from the eyes or nearer, great benefit is derived from imagining the white spaces between the lines to be whiter than the rest of the card. When the white spaces are imagined perfectly white, the black letters are imagined perfectly black. When the imagination of the white is perfect enough, the imagination of the black letters is also sufficiently perfect, so that the letters are read easily without effort or strain, and without consciously looking at the letters. It is good practice to have a patient decide to imagine the white spaces perfectly white. If the letters improve, one should not try to read them. It is exceedingly difficult for most people to do this. With the slightest improvement in the white spaces coincident with a corresponding improvement in the blackness of the letters, the temptation to forget the white spaces and try to read the letters is very great. To play the game, one must play it fairly and not be in a hurry to read the fine print when the imagination of the white spaces improves. In some cases it is well for the patient to close the eyes and remember the whitest white he has ever seen. This may be white snow, a white pillow, or whitewash. Then open the eyes and flash the white spaces, imagining them to be as white or whiter than the object remembered.

The imagination is not modified by the illumination. It is very interesting to find patients with good sight who can imagine things perfectly in a dim light. When this is accomplished, the clearness of all things seen gives one the impression that the light has increased. For example, there are many people who, after the lights have been dimmed in the theatre, can read the program apparently as well as they can when the light is good. Patients with imperfect sight are troubled by the dim light more than are patients with normal vision.

Other environmental conditions affect the vision—excitement of various kinds, unexpected noises and unusual occurrences. When some people go to a circus, they may become very nearsighted in a few minutes, although when attending a performance at the theatre their eyes do not trouble them. Others cannot see well at the opera, because they are not accustomed to observing people's faces so far away, and yet on the street in all kinds of light they may have normal vision. When people with imperfect sight try to find their way about in dark places, they strain their eyes to such an extent that they suffer pain, headache, and become exceedingly nervous. People with normal eyes and normal sight maintain a perfect imagination in strange as well as familiar places.

The normal eye is able to imagine the white centers of black letters whiter than they really are. Other people with imperfect sight imagine the white center of a letter "O," for example, of the same shade of white or less white than the rest of the card. The use of a screen helps such patients to improve their imagination. Use a card or piece of paper with an opening slightly smaller than the white center of the letter "O." Cover the black part of the letter with the card, exposing the white center. By alternately closing the eyes and resting them, the patient becomes able to see or imagine he sees the center of the "O" less white than it appears to be when the black part of the letter is exposed.

No patient is cured until he becomes able to imagine a letter at ten feet or farther as well as he can see it at one foot or less. In this connection, it is well to emphasize the fact that the cure of imperfect sight can only be accomplished without effort. Too many patients believe that the cure of imperfect sight is very complicated, and that they have to make a great effort. It is only when they become convinced that the one way they can obtain perfect sight is by rest, or that when their sight is imperfect a strain is necessary to keep it imperfect, that a permanent improvement is obtained. A sufficient improvement of the imagination is a cure of imperfect sight. Patients with perfect sight have a perfect imagination of the things that they can remember. Patients with imperfect sight always have an imperfect imagination.

So many people look with contempt on the imagination, especially when it comes to treatment of the eyes. Most people do not associate imagination with perfect vision. They are of the opinion that they can imagine they see something without actually seeing it. This is not so. Perfect imagination and perfect vision are identical.

Of all the discoveries that I have made, there is none of so much practical value as the discovery of the importance of the imagination.

STORIES FROM THE CLINIC
No. 73: Margaret Mary
By Emily C. Lierman

Margaret Mary is not yet five years old. Her mother told me that an eye specialist prescribed glasses for her when she was two years old to be worn constantly for the cure of squint, which she had contracted after an attack of whooping-cough. The squint was alternate, sometimes the right eye turned in, at other times the left.

When I tested her sight at the first visit, October 24, 1925, the vision of each eye was one-fifth of the normal. She is an obedient child and did what I told her. At my request, she covered both eyes with her hands. I asked her to remember her dollie. She smiled and asked, "Which one?" I answered, "Your best dollie."

I found that Mary had a good memory for colors. When I asked her what the color of her best dollie's dress was, she answered, "Pink." As she, herself, was wearing a blue dress, I tested her memory for colors by asking her if the dollie's dress were the same color as the dress she was wearing. She peeped between her fingers, looked at me and said, "No, my dress is blue." I asked her if the dollie had black shoes like hers. She answered, "No, she hasn't any shoes."

All these questions were necessary in order to encourage the child to imagine perfect mental pictures and obtain relaxation. After she had palmed five minutes, I told her to remove her hands from her eyes and look at the card. Her vision, when tested, had improved to one-half of the normal.

I taught the child how to sway her body from side to side, as I held her hands and moved with her. While we were doing this, Mary's mother looked on. She was amazed when the eyes became straight from the swaying. Then I told the mother how important it was to have the child practice the swaying several times every day. She has a Victrola in her home, and I advised the mother to play a waltz, if possible, when the child was swaying.

When Mary returned a week later, I noticed that the squint was much better. She placed her arms about me and said she loved me because I removed her glasses. I tested her sight and found that it had improved considerably. When she was reading the card for me, there were times when she sighed. This was a signal that she was tired. I would then lead her to the drawer in which some candy is kept. If parents do not object, I give my little patients some good candy while they are practicing. In my experience, nothing has relieved eye fatigue in children so much as a little candy.

During a treatment, in which her eyes were perfectly straight, two boys came into the room. I watched Mary and noticed that her left eye turned in considerably. I immediately placed the boys in another room. When I returned and spoke kindly to Mary, her left eye became perfectly straight again. Her aunt who had brought her was amazed at the quick relief of the squint. It was evident that the unexpected presence of the two boys had caused a strain which produced the squint.

Before she left me that day, her vision had improved to four-fifths of the normal. On January 16, 1926, her vision had improved to the normal with the eyes straight. Up to this time, we had been using the card with the letter "E" of different sizes pointing in various directions. As she did not know numbers, I taught them to her with the aid of a Snellen test card consisting of figures up to ten, while holding the card about one foot from her eyes. She was delighted with the change and her eyes remained straight all the time. Her joy was unbounded when I told her that she could take the card home with her. One week later, she was able to tell every figure on the numeral card.

This case was interesting. The child had been wearing glasses prescribed by a competent doctor for two years without relief. The squint was not cured nor benefited by them because it returned just as soon as the glasses were removed. Even while wearing them the squint was usually evident, and the vision was not improved. A study of her treatment and the results showed that the cause of the squint and the imperfect sight was a nervous strain. Many children as well as adults can produce a temporary squint by a stare or strain.

Investigation has proved that this fact should be emphasized. For more than one hundred years ophthalmologists have declared repeatedly that the imperfect sight of a squinting eye is usually incurable. Many writers make the statement that children are born with squint. In these cases, the blindness is usually more marked at the center of sight, and yet with the ophthalmoscope the center of sight may look perfectly normal. One celebrated writer tried to explain the facts in a few words by stating that the blindness of squint was a condition in which neither the patient nor the doctor could see anything, meaning, as was stated above, that although the sight of the squinting eye may be very poor or entirely absent, the ophthalmoscope shows no evidence of disease of the retina. All cases of squint are cured by treatment which eliminates strain.

FUNDAMENTALS

By W. H. Bates, M.D.

Glasses Discarded

Glasses must be discarded permanently because it is a truth that one cannot be cured while wearing them, even occasionally. [Students *have* succeeded by using reduced prescription glasses; they must be used *only* when essential.—TRQ] Dark glasses and other measures to protect the eyes from the strong light are also objectionable. The eyes become more sensitive to light with a loss of vision. Magnifying glasses lessen the clearness of all colors, including black and white. The size and form of objects are modified by all kinds of glasses. Glasses for the correction of farsightedness may, and usually do, give the wearer the impression that objects are larger than they really are; while nearsighted patients when wearing glasses are impressed with the fact that objects look smaller than they actually are. Glasses for the correction of astigmatism may cause dizziness.

In wearing any glasses, it is necessary to look directly through the center of the glass in order to obtain maximum vision. If one regards an object by looking in a slanting direction through the glasses, its form and location are changed. Many people, when they first put on glasses, feel as though they were a long distance from the ground. With other glasses, they have the sensation of being shorter, or that the distance from their eyes to the ground has become lessened.

The discomfort of glasses is very great with a large percentage of people who wear them. Frequently, when they complain to their ophthalmologists or to the opticians who supplied the glasses, they are advised that by perseverance their eyes will become fitted to the glasses. This does not seem quite satisfactory because people feel that the glasses should fit their eyes, and not that they should struggle along with all kinds of discomforts in order to make their eyes fit the glasses.

Tinted glasses, red, yellow, blue, green, or black, when worn constantly, usually feel comfortable to the patient because the amount of light is lessened. At the seashore, when the reflection of light from the water affects the eyes badly, causing pain and discomfort of all kinds, the wearing of colored glasses is, for the time at least, often a great relief. However, constant wearing of such glasses is later followed by sensitiveness to the light and the necessity for stronger glasses to obtain a sufficient amount of relief. The protection of the eyes by dark glasses, shades, and other measures has caused inflammations of the eyeball and of the eyelids. Pure sunlight is necessary for the health of the normal eye, and when people live in dark rooms, they usually find their eyes are weakened.

The shape of the eyeball is changing frequently. Sometimes the eyes are focused for distant vision and other times for near vision. Glasses which correct the sight for reading very seldom enable the patient to see at the distance as well as without them. On the other hand, nearsighted persons whose vision is poor for distance, when wearing glasses to enable them to see distant objects, find that their ability to read with maximum vision is impossible with such glasses. When the glasses do not correct the vision for all distances, the eyes strain and try to overcome the bad effect of the glasses. Without glasses, the eyes may strain, but the wearing of glasses increases the strain. Glasses correct the eye trouble to a certain degree, but when the eye trouble varies, or the strain varies, the glasses do not relieve the wrong focus of the eye at all times. For example, the glasses that correct the imperfect sight, or the strain of imperfect sight at ten feet, may not do it when the eye strains and is focused for a nearer point, or for a more distant point. Many people complain that they do not get relief from wearing glasses at all hours of the day, because strain and inflammation of the eyeball produced by the strain is so variable. When the eye becomes normal, or when it becomes able, as the result of treatment, to change its focus without difficulty, the patient is comfortable and can only be comfortable without glasses.

Central Fixation

Central fixation is seeing best where you are looking, and at the same time seeing worse where you are not looking. The letters of the Snellen test card, when seen clearly, are always seen by central fixation. Diamond type, when read slowly, or when one letter is seen clearly, continuously, for part of a minute, requires central fixation.

Concentration is an effort to see where you are looking and not to see at all where you are not looking. This is impossible without a strain. An effort to concentrate always fails to improve the vision. All persons with imperfect sight try to concentrate. When the vision improves, the effort to concentrate becomes less. Persons with normal sight never try to concentrate. [Centralization is *effortless* concentration.—TRQ]

Favorable Conditions

Light may be bright or dim. Some persons are unable to see in a bright light. Their vision is usually improved by the sunning. They sit in the sun with the sun shining directly on their closed eyelids as they slowly move their heads a short distance from side to side. This is practiced for half an hour or longer whenever possible. The eyes are rested and strengthened, and gradually grow accustomed to the strong light of the sun.

Individuals who cannot see so well in a dim light as in a bright light are benefited by the imagination of the halos, that is, the imagination of the centers of round letters to be whiter than the rest of the card. The memory of perfect sight also helps one to see in a dim light. By the memory of perfect sight is meant the ability to remember or imagine perfectly a letter or an object which has been seen perfectly.

The distance of the print from the eyes, where seen best, also varies with individuals. In some cases, the letter or object regarded and seen clearly may be, as in nearsighted eyes, one foot or less from the face. To be able to see farther off, requires practice. When things are not seen at a greater distance, two feet or farther, the vision usually is improved by remembering one letter of the Snellen test card perfectly with the eyes closed. Then when the eyes are opened for a fraction of a second, it is possible to imagine the known letter at two feet or farther.

Many middle-aged people can see well at twenty feet or farther, but are unable to read the newspaper at two feet or nearer. The same principle holds true in these cases, as in those of nearsightedness, except that the distance of the print from the eyes is gradually decreased until it is read without effort or strain at twelve inches.

Shifting

In normal sight the eyes are moving all the time. It is necessary when the eyes are at rest, that they keep moving to avoid the stare. To stare, the eyes must be stationary. Shifting prevents the stare. When the sight is imperfect, the eyes strain or stare by regarding one point all the time. All patients with imperfect sight, when they look at a letter, see it stationary. They look at a part of the letter or the whole of the letter, and see it all alike. The vision always becomes imperfect when this is done.

There are various ways of obtaining the habit of shifting. One has to first obtain the conscious habit. Shifting a long distance is readily accomplished, but when one shifts a very short distance, it is not always easy to be conscious that the eye really moves. One can be sure that the eye is moving when objects, not directly regarded, appear to move at the same time. No matter how great the strain of the eyes may be, it is always possible to shift a long distance, usually by turning the head in the same direction as the eyes move. The long shift is always some relief. When the shifting is shortened to one-quarter of an inch or less, when regarding small letters, the eye with imperfect sight may have difficulty in imagining the letter to be moving so short a distance. Nearsighted people who have good vision close to the eyes, at one foot or less, and can read the finest print, are able quite readily to imagine the eyes shifting as short a distance as the width of one of the small letters. The short shift is more difficult, but when it is successfully practiced, one obtains a greater amount of relaxation than can be obtained from the long shift. I wish I could emphasize the value of shifting. About five years ago, a patient whom I had cured of nearsightedness some years before called to see me. His vision was normal not only for a familiar card, but he could read with normal vision letters of an unfamiliar card.

"Did you have a relapse?" I asked him. He replied, "I have never had any relapse." "What do you think has cured you?" His answer was, "Shifting."

Swinging

When the eyes move slowly or rapidly from side to side, stationary objects appear to move in the direction opposite to the movement of the head and eyes. Some people have a very painful and disagreeable time in becoming able to imagine that stationary objects appear to move when the eyes move. If one stares directly at a stationary object, it does not move. This suggests very strongly that one should not expect stationary objects to move when he looks directly at them. When one shifts a long distance from one point to another without effort or without strain, or without trying to see, it is possible to imagine stationary objects not regarded to be moving. Some people tell me that when they look out of a car window of a railroad train, they do not imagine the telegraph poles to be moving opposite to the movement of the train. On the contrary, they feel that they are moving and do not like to imagine the illusion of the telegraph poles to be moving. One has to treat such patients with much ingenuity. One patient could imagine things moving while she was running, but not while she was walking. I had her run around the office one morning until she obtained considerable improvement in the swing. Later, she became able to obtain the swing of stationary objects when she did not run so fast or so long. At first she practiced a fast walk, and then a slower walk until she became able to imagine stationary objects to be moving by just moving her head and eyes.

QUESTIONS AND ANSWERS

Q–1a. When one uses an electric light in place of sunlight, how strong a light is it proper to use? 1b. Because of the heat, how close to the light is it advisable to sit? 1c. How long is it advisable to sit at one time? 1d. How much time should be given to it in a day?

A–1a. One can use an electric light of 1000 watts with benefit. 1b. Sit five feet or farther away from the light to avoid any discomfort from the heat. 1c. Practice for a half-hour or longer. The more light treatment taken, the better. 1d. Devote at least a half-hour a day to the sun or light treatment.

Q–2. Is the effect of the sun glass and that of sunshine falling on closed eyelids different, so that one needs both kinds each day?

A–2. The sun treatment with the sun glass is more intensive than without it. At first, patients become accustomed to strong light by sitting in the sun and allowing the sun's rays to shine directly on the closed eyelids, as they slowly move their heads a short distance from side to side. Then, with the sun glass, the strong light of the sun is focused on the closed eyelids, and when the eyes are accustomed to that, one can consider the advisability of focusing the direct rays of the sun upon sclera of the eyeball itself. This is done by lifting the upper lid while the patient looks down. When the sun is focused upon the white part of the eye, one should keep moving the glass from side to side, and for a short time only, so as not to produce discomfort from the heat.

Q–3. If one practices reading fine print for a time each day, is it harmful to read print like that of the *Forum* (usual magazine type)?

A–3. No, the more you read, the better, even though you read with imperfect sight. Large print can be read with a strain, but fine print can only be read when the eyes are relaxed. It is all right to read print of any size if one reads it with perfect sight. When read with imperfect sight, the eyes are under a strain. Imperfect sight is always caused by a stare or strain, and one can stare or strain when regarding a large letter, blurring it to a considerable degree, and yet be able to tell what the letter is. The same amount of strain, which produces as much of a blur, when looking at a small letter, may make it impossible for one to read the small letter perfectly, although he can still distinguish the large letters. Any size type can be read without strain if blinking, shifting, and central fixation are practiced.

Q–4. In viewing movies, is it not more beneficial to sit as far back as one may and not strain, than to sit farther forward?

A–4. Sit at a distance from the screen at which you are most comfortable, i.e., where you can see the picture with the least discomfort. One can strain the eyes when sitting at almost any distance from the screen. To avoid the stare and strain as much as possible, it is necessary to keep shifting the eyes from one part of the screen to another, or to look off into the darkened room from time to time to give the eyes a rest. Some people are benefited by palming for a few seconds or longer, and in this way prevent the strain.

Q–5. When palming and seeing mental pictures, I almost never think whether it is black before my eyes or not. If I turn my attention to it, it is usually dark, more or less, but not a black black. Am I right not to think at all about it?

A–5. When palming, do not try to think of anything. Just think of something pleasant, something that you remember perfectly, and let your mind drift from one pleasant thought to another.

Better Eyesight
April 1926—Vol. X, No. 10

RETARDATION NUMBER

DEMONSTRATE: THE OPTICAL SWING

Demonstrate that the optical swing always improves the vision.

Stand before an open window with the feet about one foot apart. Sway the whole body, including the head and eyes, from side to side. When the body moves to the right, the head and eyes also move to the right, while at the same time the window and other stationary objects are to the left of where you are looking. When the body sways to the left, the window and other stationary objects are to the right. Be sure that the head and eyes are moving from side to side with the whole body, slowly, without an effort to see. When the swaying is done rapidly, it is possible to imagine stationary objects are moving rapidly in the opposite direction. While the swinging is being practiced, notice that the window and other stationary objects which are nearer appear to move in the opposite direction to the movement of the body, head and eyes. Objects beyond the window may appear to move in the same direction as the body, head and eyes move. [Double oppositional movement!—TRQ]

Note that when the body is swaying rapidly, the window and other objects are not seen very clearly; but when the swaying is slowed down and shortened, so that parts of the window move one-quarter of an inch or less, the vision is improved for those parts of the window regarded. More distant objects, which move in the same direction as the movement of the body, head, and eyes, are also improved with the slow, short, easy swing.

After you have become able to imagine the window to be moving, practice on other objects. All day long, the head and eyes are moving. Notice that stationary objects are moving in the opposite direction to the movement of the head an eyes. To see stationary objects apparently stationary is a strain which lowers the vision and may cause pain, fatigue, and other discomforts.

RETARDATION

By W. H. Bates, M.D.

When pupils in school fail to maintain the scholarship of other and normal children of the same age, their mental efficiency or their standing is said to be retarded. Such children may remain in the same low grade for several years with no apparent improvement in their scholarship, and are seldom promoted. The cause is rarely due to an impaired mentality. The fact that all of those observed have been benefited or cured by eye-mind education is convincing evidence that retardation is functional.

Imperfect Sight

Imperfect sight is usually associated with retardation, which is very prevalent. When these cases improve, their vision always improves. One principal reported that all the schoolchildren in the rapid advancement classes under her jurisdiction had normal sight without glasses. In all the other classes the percentage of retardation was very high, and in some classes all the pupils were suffering with retardation. It was customary to separate the children whose retardation was extreme and put them all in one class under the control of one teacher. The teacher told me that after she had improved their vision, their scholarship advanced and they were transferred to the usual grades.

Retardation Cure

For many years, retardation has been studied by competent people; all sorts of causes have been ascribed to this condition, and remedial measures have been practiced which have heretofore not been of the slightest benefit. The method which I suggested was very simple. A Snellen test card was placed in the classroom in a place where it could be seen by all the children from their seats. Sometimes two or more cards were placed upon the wall. Every day for a short time under the supervision of the teacher, all the children read the card, first with one eye and then with the other, while one eye was covered with the palm of the hand in such a way as not to press upon the eyelids.

Benefits

The teacher told me that the use of the cards in this way after a few weeks or months was followed by an improvement in the sight, when the retardation became less. One benefit of this practice was that it relieved or prevented headaches and other discomforts. The ability of the children to study was stimulated. The memory, imagination, judgment and other phenomena of the mind were very much benefited. It was also encouraging to note that, with the improvement in their retardation, a larger number of children continued in school than ever before. In the beginning, many of these children were so unhappy and so uncomfortable in school that they were usually anxious to stop school and go to work. After their retardation was improved and their vision benefited, they said that they could look at the writing on the blackboard and read it without discomfort. They also said that they could study without getting headaches. Furthermore, they seemed to become able to remember and understand what they read or what they studied.

Truancy

Truancy was very common among the children who were suffering from retardation. After the retardation was relieved or cured, truancy became very much less and the children volunteered the information that after they became able to read or study without discomfort, they could understand better the lessons that were assigned to them. Children who were very restless and mischievous, so-called bad boys or bad girls, became model pupils and very easy to handle.

Stare

The evils of retardation were numerous. The cause was always a stare, a strain, or an effort to see. The cure was accomplished by teaching the children how to use their eyes without staring or straining. While reading the Snellen test card in the way just described was a great benefit, there were other methods practiced by some children which were an added benefit. One teacher from the northern part of the State of New York was exceptionally good and was able to keep order in her classroom when other teachers failed. She wrote me that she always began the day by having the children palm, or cover both closed eyes with the palms of the hands in such a way as to exclude all light. This the children did for fifteen minutes and then they started in with their work feeling rested and comfortable. When she noticed them becoming fatigued she had them practice swinging, and the result was that they continued their work without becoming restless.

Memory

Another teacher, living in Chicago, found it an advantage to teach the children how to remember. This was accomplished in some cases by having the children remember their own signatures at first, as well as they could. They improved their memory by alternately looking at their signature and then closing their eyes while remembering it. The children were able to demonstrate that it was easier for them to remember one word of their signature than three or more words. They also found that they could remember one letter of their signature better than the whole word. By practice, they became able to remember a part of a letter better than the whole letter, and the smaller the part remembered, the more perfectly was it accomplished. Many of them became able to remember a small period perfectly black, as well with their eyes open as they could with their eyes closed.

Imagination

This teacher also improved the imagination of her pupils. Someone would read a story. Then all the children would palm and remember the story as well as they could. After opening their eyes, they would illustrate the story in various ways. The teacher sent me about forty illustrations, and I found them very interesting. They were unusual, but the teacher claimed that doing these unusual things was a great benefit to a large number of children who were suffering from retardation. Coincident with the improvement in the memory and the imagination was a corresponding improvement in the sight. There were other benefits just as important in value.

Adults

Adults also suffer from attacks of retardation. For example, a portrait painter may do good work for a longer or shorter period, but at intervals his work becomes decidedly poor, unsatisfactory, and a failure. Writers, financiers, inventors, teachers and professional people of all kinds have attacks of retardation when their mental efficiency is lost or impaired, usually suddenly, for longer or shorter periods of time.

Automobile Drivers

It is an interesting fact that people who drive automobiles suffer greatly from eyestrain. Taxi drivers are under more or less of a nervous strain. I am very fond of talking to these people about their work because, being very observant, they teach me a lot. Many of them have told me that when they had an accident, it was difficult for them to believe that it was their fault.

At one time a taxi driver ran into another, broadside on. There was quite a smash-up and a number of people were injured. The taxi driver was not detained very long, and later he came to see me about his eyes. Among other things he said, "Doctor, I never saw the automobile that I ran into. I never knew it was there until after the smash. Do you think there is anything wrong with my sight?"

I tested him very carefully and found that his vision was 20/20 with each eye. I examined his eyes very carefully with the ophthalmoscope and finally I said to him, "You have perfect eyes, but you don't always see with them." "What do you mean?" he asked. "I mean this—that while your sight is perfectly good usually, there are times when you become totally blind. Everybody with perfect sight does not have perfect sight all the time." "Well," he asked, "what am I to do?"

After talking to him for a while and explaining what I meant by the stare, the strain, or trying to see, and how one always stared when one had imperfect sight, I told him that the remedy was to use his eyes in such a way that he did not stare. Riding all day long in a car, he should notice that the road in front of him comes toward him, while objects on either side of him move in the opposite direction. In this way he would not stare so much and the attacks of imperfect sight would be eliminated.

Sailors

A sea captain called on me one day with a history of imperfect sight at irregular intervals. When his sight was tested with the Snellen test card at twenty feet, his vision was normal. I told him that he had perfect sight.

I examined him with the ophthalmoscope and told him that he had perfect eyes. "Well," he asked, "why do I have those attacks of blindness when I cannot even see a big lighthouse, and when I cannot see a large vessel coming towards me sufficiently clearly to avoid a collision?" I talked to him the same way I had to the taxi driver and he, very grateful, left the office.

Stories from the Clinic
No. 74: Retardation
By Emily C. Lierman

About seven years ago, a girl age sixteen, was treated for a severe inflammatory trouble with her eyes. She was brought to me by her father. Her eyes were paining her continuously and her vision was very poor. To protect her eyes from the light, she was wearing glasses which were so thick that her vision was lowered to a great extent by them. The suffering of the girl was pitiable. It was impossible for her to do any reading whatever, and she had been compelled to stop school two years previously.

The first thing we did for her was to give her the sun treatment with the aid of the sun glass. Before she was placed in the sun, she was instructed to close her eyes and keep them closed until she was told to open them. She was then placed in a chair where the sun shone directly on her closed lids while she moved her head continuously, a short distance from side to side. After ten minutes, her eyes had become somewhat accustomed to the sunlight. With a little encouragement, she succeeded in opening her eyes while looking far down. The upper lid of each eye was gently raised sufficiently to expose the white of the eye to the direct rays of the sun. Her eyes rapidly became more and more accustomed to the strong light, until she was able to stand the light focused in flashes on the white part of the eye with the sun glass. Her vision at times was 10/200. Best of all, she was able to open her eyes without discomfort. It seemed like a miracle. For the first time in two years she was free from pain. Both she and her father were very happy. Whereas at the beginning her father had led her in the room, she led him laughingly out without the thick dark glasses on. Being of a nervous temperament she would, at times, become hysterical as her vision improved; but after she was entirely cured she seemed like a different person. Her nervousness disappeared and her manner was calm. As she became more accustomed to the strong light, her vision gradually improved to the normal.

Palming helped her very much. Imagining stationary objects to be moving, whenever she moved her head and eyes, relieved or prevented the stare or trying to see. The memory or imagination of perfect sight enabled her, at the same time, to read the Snellen test card with normal vision, at first in flashes, and later more continuously. The greatest benefit she obtained from the eye treatment was that her mind became able to do things with much greater efficiency and her memory was decidedly improved. She became able to remember a small black object, or a small black period, as well with her eyes open as she could with her eyes closed. Formerly, when she read a page of history, she had to reread it half a dozen times before she could understand any page that she read. In three months time, her trouble had entirely disappeared; she returned to school and her friends and teachers were amazed at the great change in her. After her eyes were cured, she read the pages in her history book only once, and not only grasped the meaning but also was able to remember it for six months or longer without having to read it again just before examination time. At one examination, the questions were written on the blackboard and, after she read them, she was shocked to find that she could not answer a single question. Fortunately, she remembered her eye treatment and the little black period. With the help of palming, swinging, and the memory of perfect sight, she remembered the answers to all the questions.

This experience that she had is very valuable because she was cured of an attack of retardation by simple methods which could be employed in all schools, colleges or elsewhere in the business world.

The principal of this school visited Dr. Bates to learn more about our method of treatment and also placed herself under his care until she was cured without glasses. She had been wearing them for presbyopia.

Some years ago I wrote about a group of children who were suffering from retardation. Their teachers could not understand so many failures. After it was discovered that they had imperfect sight, the school nurse sent them to the optician to be fitted for glasses. Later, it was noticed that even though they were wearing glasses, the retardation still continued. A little girl from the same school, who wore glasses, came to our Clinic and was cured without them. She encouraged other children to come to us. The little girl who encouraged them to come, was a very good assistant for she knew exactly how to start each one with the treatment. With her help, all of them were cured without their glasses.

This happened in the spring when the thought of being promoted was uppermost in their minds. Through one of their teachers, who was cured of her myopia by Dr. Bates, I learned that all were promoted with the exception of one little boy. Not one mother of any of those dear children was any happier than I when they brought the joyful news to me. I was proud of my work and proud to tell it, too.

During that vacation, two public school graduates, who were under treatment for their sight during the previous spring and had obtained normal vision, told me how they had successfully passed all their tests.

One of them said, "If it had not been for the memory of a little swinging black period which I never forgot, I am sure that I would have failed." The other graduate said, "I did not need to remember anything in particular when the tests were easy, but you bet I never forgot the movement of a small black period when the test was difficult." I believe retardation will no longer exist when imperfect sight is avoided and eyeglasses are a thing of the past.

RETARDATION

By M. F. Husted
Superintendent of Schools, North Bergen, New Jersey

It has been found by educational experts that certain norms for the Age-Grade location of pupils should exist. Pupils above this age for the grade are classed as Over-Age for their grade and pupils of this age are classed as Normal Age and pupils below this age are classed as Under-Age. Classes, schools and school systems are considered in good condition when the number of over-age pupils does not exceed the number of under-age pupils. It is considered by administration experts that this standard test of a school system affords the best single test of the value of the schoolwork done. The normal ages are determined by expert educational authority to be used as follows:

Grades	I	II	III	IV	V	VI	VII	VI
Normal Ages	6–7	7–8	8–9	9–10	10–11	11–12	12–13	13–14

Pupils who are over this age are known as "Retarded" or as "Repeaters."

REASON FOR RETARDATION

1. All experience shows that "All men are *not* created equal."

2. Parents change places of residence and pupils change schools. These pupils are not promoted at the end of the term, as are pupils who have spent the entire year in one school.

3. Ill health of a pupil or in a family, irregular attendance, prevents the receiving of the usual amount of instruction.

4. Entering school so late as to produce over-age.

5. Misfits for a grade for a time—those who do not speak English.

6. Changes of teachers are too frequent.

7. The quality of teaching is too low because teacher training is too little.

The Boston National Educational Association Meeting in July 1910, which the writer attended, contributed the following, "Children who make rapid progress (under-age) through the grades shall at least equal in number those who make slow progress (over-age). At the present time this condition does not exist commonly, if indeed it does anywhere. It is probably a most conservative statement to say that in the average city there are at least ten times as many children making slow progress as there are making rapid progress. *To change this condition is the great school problem:*

"Develop and perfect measures:

1. For conserving and increasing the physical soundness of pupils.

2. For discovering and excluding cases of contagious disease.

3. For finding and having remedied physical defects.

4. For making the entire school and its surroundings happier, healthier and more wholesome.

5. For that sort of record-keeping that shall enable the school to keep track of each individual child from the time he enters school until he leaves and to tell when he fails and why he fails and guide in preventing him from failure.

6. For changing our courses of study or our methods of grading and promotions so that the children who make rapid progress through the grade shall be at least equal in number to those who make slow progress."

One of the important remedial measures in solving this great problem is not emphasized, namely: better and more efficient methods of teaching, this is what North Bergen has relied on to produce its progressive betterments in age-grade conditions.

Because "Retardation" means a below normal standard of attainment for pupils, and a higher standard of cost for communities, North Bergen, New Jersey has, since 1907, given this problem special attention.

The factors used in reducing this educational waste of time and money, and waste in community progress, are:

1. Better methods of teaching.
2. Closer supervision of schoolwork.
3. Better cooperation of parents.
4. Better school attendance.
5. More of the play spirit in class work.

TABLE A
PERCENTAGE OF RETARDATION DIMINISHES

	1913	1916	1917	1918	1919
Under-Age	19	23	28	29	29
Retarded	27	19	16	13	13
	1920	1921	1922	1923	1924
Under-Age	29	30	30	30	29
Retarded	14	13	14	13	14

According to Dr. Ayres, the founder of the age-grade method of measuring school progress, Table A, above, indicates a high standard of school attainment. Under-ageness of 19% in 1913 was gradually increased until in 1921 the table shows a 30% distribution. Retardation of 27% shown in 1913 is gradually further reduced and shows only 13% in 1918.

The excellence of these conditions is also seen from a comparison of North Bergen with other systems.

TABLE B
COMPARATIVE DATA FOR NINE CITY SCHOOL SYSTEMS
(American Ed. Digest, May 1924)

City	Percent Under-age	Percent Normal	Total Under-age Plus Normal	Percent Retarded
New York, NY	14.0	46.0	(60.0)	40.0
Seattle, WA	10.5	47.6	(58.1)	41.9
Newark, NJ	14.3	40.7	(55.0)	45.0
St. Paul, MN	6.7	45.9	(52.6)	47.4
Reading, PA	7.2	44.9	(52.1)	47.9
Grand Rapids, MI	9.0	43.0	(52.0)	48.0
Omaha, NE	5.0	37.0	(42.0)	58.0
Portland, OR	4.0	31.0	(35.0)	65.0
Birmingham, AL	1.3	19.0	(20.3)	79.7
North Bergen, NJ	29.0	57.0	(86.0)	14.0

Nine cities are ranked in the order of highest efficiency as shown by the combined number of under-age and normal pupils (column 3).

The excellence of these conditions is also found in the fact that Americans exploited the efficiency of German schools—exploited by Germans to American pedagogues visiting the German Empire and they in turn to American Educators. Their schools contained 50% of retardation but this was not revealed until statistics leaked out after the war.

Eye-Mind Education

After working ten years upon the solution of the problem of Retardation, I found that we had about reached its maximum reduction for several reasons:

Teacher and pupil morale waned and effort accordingly, because:

1. Retardation problem was no longer a stimulation.
2. Because of the disorganization due to influenza epidemic.
3. Because of emphasis given to well-known differences in pupils.
4. Because of emphasis given to intelligence testing.
5. Because of unsatisfactory salary conditions.

In the midst of these perplexities, salaries were raised and Eye-Mind Education was practiced for the purpose of maintaining the high standards we had attained. After careful analysis, observation, and personal tests, I became convinced of its great educational values. After seven years' experience with Eye-Mind Education, I class it as one of the marvelous discoveries of the present age, second only to that of radio waves and their control. The Bates Method of Educating the Eye-Mind, to prevent and remove eye and mental strains, to prevent and lessen Retardation in schools, is soundly established. Its contributions to the happiness of mankind is unspeakable.

Since 1920 our records of progress in Eye-Mind Education have been carefully made.

Not only does Eye-Mind Education place no additional burden upon the teachers, but by improving the eyesight, health, disposition and mentality of their pupils, it surely lightens their labors and furnishes an additional means of preventing retardation.

In 1924, out of 129 pupils wearing glasses, 18 were found with normal vision and 111 with vision below 20/20. Out of 4,026 pupils without glasses 1,133, or 28.1% had below-normal vision. The total below-normal vision was 1,244 out of 4,155 pupils or 29.9%.

In this year, out of 118 below-normal pupils wearing glasses, 89 or 75.4% improved and of 1,072 pupils not wearing glasses but having below-normal vision, 693 have improved, or 64.5%. Out of a total of 1,190 pupils with below 20/20 vision, 782 improved, or 65.8%. Of those who improved 342 even attained normal vision, or 43.7%. This is indicative of what may be attained by this educative process under more systematic and persistent procedure.

Dr. William M. Carhart says in the *Medical Times*, *"Not all retarded children are so retarded from eyestrain, but the effects of eyestrain are one of the main causes of such retardation."*

The vision tests of 1925 showed that 17% of pupils with glasses had normal vision and 64% without glasses had normal vision. The year's work produced wonderful effects in Eye-Mind Education. The records show 70% of those wearing glasses were improved, that 87% of those not wearing glasses improved, and that of those improving, 56% attained normal vision.

The writer had 24 years' personal experience in wearing glasses, most of the time with bifocals. After this 24 years' knowledge of the advantages and disadvantages of glasses, they were laid aside on August 15, 1924, and have not been worn since.

Owing to attained age and 24 years of Eye-Mind strains being physically recorded, Eye-Mind improvement was slow but marvelous and my visual difficulties are now confined to poor print, poor type and poor light. I have attained wonderful improvement in this one and a half years of Eye-Mind practice. On many occasions truly miraculous conditions prevailed. They were periods of reflective, very free thinking, when thought flowed and was created as fast as pen could write. There was ease, relaxation of eye and mind. A noted experience of this occurred on the morning of November 3, 1925, after I had read some article upon schoolwork. I was seeing thoughts with my mind's eye. Near and distant vision was wonderfully free and clear. These experiences and phenomena have occurred many times during the past six months. The thrill of ecstasy, and feeling of freedom during these periods, arising from a complete emancipation from the thraldom of wearing glasses and their effects, are indescribable. They indicate an intimacy of relationship between the mind and matter never fathomed, and they also indicate that man is still a free agent to search out truth and happiness, and if he wills to use and uses his intelligence and available scientific data, he may carve out a new birth of freedom and progress for the human race. Man creates his own destiny.

Eye Education as an ally of mind development, of eye and physical health conditions and of human efficiency and happiness, should be practiced in every American school. Excepting radio, it is the miraculous wonder of the great age in which we live.

QUESTIONS AND ANSWERS

Q–1. At intervals, sometimes months apart, I find my eyes twitching but it is hardly noticeable to an observer. What is the cause and how can I overcome it?

A–1. This is caused by mental tension which has a direct effect on the eye. Practice relaxation methods, palming and swinging.

Q–2. Why does eating ice cream hurt my eyes?

A–2. Because the nerves of the eye are in direct relationship with the roof of the mouth, and the sudden chill makes the nerves sensitive.

Q–3. If I am worried at night and lie awake, my eyes burn and pain, and I have a feeling that a magnet is drawing my eyes through my head. What causes this and what is the cure?

A–3. This is caused by the tension of the mind. Just before retiring and the first thing in the morning, practice the long swing.

Q–4. If I am sitting in the sun reading, I can see the print perfectly and my eyes do not trouble me, but if I raise my eyes and look at any other object, everything seems blurred and there are colored spots before my eyes. Is this caused by the sun or the manner in which I read?

A–4. The sun is beneficial to the eyes but the glare of light on the white page produces a tension of the nerves. Sunning should help you to become accustomed to the strong light. Sit in the sun with the eyes closed, allowing the sun's rays to shine directly upon the closed eyelids as you slowly move your head a short distance from side to side. Practice this daily for half an hour or longer.

Better Eyesight
May 1926—Vol. X, No. 11

PRESBYOPIA NUMBER

DEMONSTRATE: THE LONG SWING

The long swing not only improves the vision, but also relieves or cures pain, discomfort and fatigue.

Stand with the feet about one foot apart, facing squarely one side of the room. Lift the left heel a short distance from the floor while turning the shoulders, head, and eyes to the right, until the line of the shoulders is parallel with the wall. Now turn the body to the left after placing the left heel upon the floor and raising the right heel. Alternate looking from the right wall to the left wall, being careful to move the head and eyes with the movement of the shoulders. When practiced easily, continuously, without effort and without paying any attention to moving objects, one soon becomes conscious that the long swing relaxes the tension of the muscles and nerves.

Stationary objects move with varying degrees of rapidity. Objects located almost directly in front of you appear to move with express train speed. It is very important to make no attempt to see clearly objects which seem to be moving very rapidly.

The long swing seems to help patients who suffer from eyestrain during sleep. By practicing the long swing fifty times or more just before retiring and just after rising in the morning, eyestrain during sleep has been prevented or relieved. It is remarkable how quickly the long swing relieves or prevents pain. I know of no other procedure which can compare with it. The long swing has relieved the pain of facial neuralgia after operative measures had failed. Some patients who have suffered from continuous pain in various parts of the body have been relieved by the long swing, at first temporarily, but by repetition the relief has become more permanent. Hay fever, asthma, seasickness, palpitation of the heart, coughs, acute and chronic colds are all promptly cured by the long swing.

PRESBYOPIA

By W. H. Bates, M.D.

Presbyopia, or old-age sight, occurs in people after the age of forty. Although the sight may be good for distant vision, it is always poor at a near point. While, in most cases, it occurs after middle age, there are exceptions in which it appears before the age of forty and even in young children.

Generally Accepted Cause

The cause is said to be due to a hardening of the lens, and the belief is that with advancing years the ability to read at the near point becomes much less, because with increased hardening of the lens accommodation is difficult or impossible. The lens, I believe, is not a factor in accommodation. In my book, *Perfect Sight Without Glasses,* I have described the evidence which proves that the change in the focus of the eye is not brought about by a change in the form of the lens.

True Cause

The true cause of presbyopia is a strain or an effort to see. When a person with presbyopia tries to read without glasses and fails, the patient feels that an effort or strain has been made. When this effort to see is increased, the vision, instead of being improved, becomes much worse. One can demonstrate that it is not possible to improve the ability to read fine print by any kind of an effort. When a patient with presbyopia rests the eyes by closing them or by looking away from the page and then looking back at the reading matter, the vision is temporarily improved. Some people have been cured by resting their eyes at frequent intervals during the day without trying to see. After resting the eyes, the vision is usually momentarily improved. In other cases it can be demonstrated that the patient is trying to concentrate. Let me suggest that the reader look at the upper left-hand corner of a letter "F," which is of sufficient size to be distinguished. Try to imagine a small area of this corner to be the blackest part of the "F." Without shifting your eyes or closing them, keep on concentrating, or trying to concentrate on this one point. Note that for a few seconds it is readily done, but very soon one feels a strain, and that to keep the eyes fixed on this one point becomes more and more difficult. The eyes feel uncomfortable and every once in a while the eyes shift and the upper left-hand corner of the letter becomes blurred and is frequently lost altogether. The whole letter, in fact, becomes imperfect and blurred while trying to concentrate on the upper left-hand corner. It is usually a relief to look away from the "F" and think of something else. It can be demonstrated that trying to concentrate on one point can only be accomplished for a short time. In other words, concentration for any length of time is impossible. This experiment is of great importance because persons suffering with presbyopia fail to read because they try to concentrate. Concentration may be all right on numerous occasions, but it is of no value in improving the sight. There are people who are able to help themselves when they find out what is wrong. Knowledge of the true cause suggests the cure. For this reason some people have cured themselves of presbyopia by just resting their eyes without trying to concentrate.

Treatment

When a patient with normal sight reads fine print, it can be demonstrated that while the letters are blacker and clearer, the white spaces between the lines appear whiter than they really are. If one looks at the letters, eyes seem to become tired and the vision fails. If, on the other hand, one looks at the white spaces between the lines from one side of the page to the other, it is possible to imagine the white spaces much whiter than they really are without discomfort, fatigue, or loss of vision. Whenever one fails to read at the near point, the attention is not attracted to the white spaces between the lines, but an effort is being made to look directly at the letters. When one regards the white spaces, the whiteness may be improved by closing the eyes and remembering something else that is much whiter, such as white snow, white starch, whitewash. Now, when the eyes are open, the first glance at the white spaces enables one to imagine them whiter than before, but only for a short time, a second or a fraction of a second. Then close the eyes and remember the white as before. When the memory has become perfect with the eyes closed, again regard the white spaces with the eyes open, and note that there are times when the white spaces become intensely white. When the imagination of the white spaces improves, the imagination of the black letters also improves. By continuing to look at a white space, shifting from one side of the page to the other, after the imagination of the white space becomes more nearly perfect, the black letters are read correctly, easily, without any effort or fatigue.

The Thin White Line

When the imagination of the white spaces has improved, it often happens that one can see or imagine he sees a thin white line much whiter than the white spaces, a line which extends from one side of the page to the other, which is located between the bottom of the letters and the upper part of the white space between the lines. The consciousness of this thin white line is a wonderful help. Most people are cured of presbyopia when they become able to imagine they see this white line. It is bright, clear and distinct. It gives a restful, pleasant feeling in all the nerves of the body when the thin white line is seen, remembered or imagined. In cases of inflammation, when one is able to imagine the thin white line, pain in the eyes, head or other parts of the body disappears as though by magic.

[The thin white line below each sentence is due to the combination, or merging, of the white halos around each letter. In other words, the bottoms of the halos around each letter appear to form a thin, white stripe just underneath the baseline of a sentence. This thin white line can often be seen along the very edges of the paper as well.—TRQ]

Failures

There are a number of causes of failures, and this number is oftentimes multiplied when different individuals become able by some ingenious method to bring about a failure.

Some patients keep their eyes open continuously without blinking. When resting the eyes by closing them, it is not always easy to help the patient to keep the eyes closed a sufficient length of time, or until one becomes able to remember a perfect white. When the memory is perfect, the eyes, mind, and all the nerves of the body are at rest. Rest of the eyes and mind increases their efficiency.

When the eyes are open, and the white spaces between the lines are imagined, it is necessary that they be closed in about a second. Too many patients close their eyes for too short a time, and when they open them they are very apt to keep them open too long a time. It is really remarkable how difficult it is for some people to close their eyes for part of a minute and then to open them for just a second. They seem to forget everything they know as soon as they test their sight.

Over and over again, I have had them prove that testing the sight causes a strain which always lowers the vision. Testing the imagination is different and is less apt to cause a strain. A patient with presbyopia can look up at the ceiling or a white cloud in the sky, and remember or imagine a mental picture of a perfect white color, and do it without any conscious strain or effort. Just as soon as they look at the fine print they forget their imagination and fail by making an effort to see. One might suggest that in the cure of presbyopia one should first find the principal cause of failure. It is necessary to be on the lookout for more than one cause. Some patients can produce many causes of failure in a short time. The ingenuity they exhibit is oftentimes very remarkable.

After some of my tests, the patients ask questions or make statements which convince me that they pay no attention whatever to my directions for avoiding the strain. Many patients' minds seem to be bewildered by the numerous thoughts that they have about presbyopia, which have been told to them by other people. They have a bad habit of outlining their own plan of treatment, which they may practice unsuccessfully.

A Presbyopia Cure

A patient over sixty years old came to me recently wearing convex 3.50 D. S. in each eye for distant vision and convex 6.50 D. S. in each eye for reading. Although these glasses enabled him to read fine print, they caused him continuous pain, discomfort and fatigue. His eyes were so bad that looking at the Snellen test card even at a distance gave him pain. Without his glasses, his vision was about 10/40 in each eye.

By looking at the spaces between the lines of black type of the Snellen test card at ten feet or farther, he felt no pain; but when he looked at the letters, he very soon was able to demonstrate a strain which blurred the letters, produced double vision and caused him much discomfort. By practicing for several hours, his vision improved until he became able to read the bottom line in flashes at one foot and the 20-line of the Snellen test card at ten feet.

He was given a Snellen test card to hold in his hand at about one foot and was advised to regard the figure "2" in flashes, alternately closing his eyes and resting them. In about half an hour, he became able to flash the "2" at every trial. At first he could see it only for a fraction of a second, but finally became able to see it almost continuously for part of a minute. A card with fine print was fastened to the Snellen test card just below the figure "2" at about one foot from his eyes. By alternately seeing the figure "2" quite perfectly and flashing the fine print for about a second, he became able to see some of the words of the fine print without losing the figure "2."

There have been other patients who have been cured of presbyopia by similar methods.

STORIES FROM THE CLINIC
No. 75: Presbyopia
By Emily C. Lierman

For some time I have been treating a woman, age eighty, for presbyopia. She also has imperfect sight for distance which cannot be improved by glasses. This condition has been described by eye doctors as very difficult or impossible to cure. The retina, optic nerve, and all other parts of the eye, are seen to be normal when the ophthalmoscope is used. Recent observations have demonstrated that the cause is due to eyestrain. When the strain is relieved, the vision always improves and the sight may become normal.

Two years ago, when this patient's vision was first tested with the Snellen test card, she read 10/100 with the right eye and 10/70 with the left. She was unable to read fine print with either eye, at any distance. After resting her eyes during treatment, by just keeping them closed, she read 15/30, but some of the letters on the 30-line appeared double. Palming relieved the double vision.

Double vision is, of course, only an illusion and is caused by strain. The quickest cure for this is to cover the closed eyes with the palm of one hand, and only uncover the eyes to open them long enough to see one letter of the test card at a time. After doing this, quickly close the eyes and cover them again with the palm of one hand. In this way, the patient does not keep the eyes open long enough to strain or produce double vision.

Later, this patient had a relapse and was discouraged to find that she could not read the test card so well. I soon learned that, although the patient had practiced many times a day, she had been making an effort to see better, and had made her sight worse. At a subsequent visit, she became able to read small print by rereading large familiar letters. Her vision for the test card also improved to 12/30 after closing her eyes for ten minutes or longer. This time she read the letters without seeing them double. From the beginning of her treatment up to the present time her visits have been irregular and, because of this, it has taken her much longer to be cured.

When most patients grow older, they are very apt to strain more than when younger, and they are not conscious of the strain produced while reading, sewing or seeing at a distance.

[More accurately: many left-brain-dominant children tend to strain to see the distant blackboard and become myopic; many right-brain-dominant adults, after age 40, tend to strain while reading up close and become presbyopic. See Chapter 19, "Brains and Vision," in *Relearning to See.*—TRQ]

The sunlight helped this patient tremendously. Whenever possible she was placed in the sun, and the sunlight was focused on her closed eyelids with the sun glass. This always improved her vision. When there was no sun, I placed her close to a strong electric light for a half-hour or longer. She liked this treatment because the sunlight was so restful to her, and she could read the test card at ten feet.

I have been treating another patient, a man age sixty-four, with presbyopia. The vision of both his eyes was the same, namely 15/30. He could not read newspaper nor magazine type at all without glasses. When he looked down, he had double vision in the left eye.

Very little could be done for him in the beginning of the treatment because he had a bad habit of unconsciously staring. He also made a great effort to concentrate while reading or while otherwise occupied. What a surprise it was to him when he learned that when he tried to concentrate, his vision was lowered. This also produced a great deal of pain and discomfort in his eyes and head, causing a general depression for hours afterward.

I advised him to close his eyes in order to rest them, and to remember something he had seen perfectly. At first he could only remember his pain and discomfort, but by showing him the Snellen test card, illuminated by a strong light and held about one foot from his eyes, he became able to see or imagine the whiteness of some of the halos. Then, when he closed his eyes, he remembered the halo for a moment. By alternately looking at the halo, closing his eyes and remembering it, he became able to flash the halo or to see it for a few moments. By practice, the white halo was imagined more frequently until his memory became almost continuously perfect.

The pain was soon relieved. It was an easy matter to treat him after that. Blinking became a habit, and he learned to shift quickly and easily. I find that some patients stare even though they do blink often. They keep their eyes fixed in one direction or on one thing. In this way they do not get any relief and the vision does not improve. The normal eye shifts about a quarter of an inch or less while blinking, but it is not noticeable. People who wear glasses, seldom shift their eyes. That is the reason why eyeglasses become tiresome to so many people.

At a recent visit, my patient became able to read 10/20 with the test card, and he was no longer troubled with double vision. Closing his eyes often to rest them helped. Now that his distant vision had improved so much, I was anxious to help him to read fine print or diamond type. During one of his previous treatments, I helped him to read newspaper and magazine type, which was an encouragement to him. When the fine print was placed about eight inches from his eyes, he asked, "You don't think I will ever be able to read such fine type as that, do you?" This question amused me because most patients with presbyopia ask the same question. I answered, "Yes, I know you will."

With a great deal of doubt in his mind, he followed my advice. He was given a booklet which contains microscopic print, and told to hold it about eight inches from his eyes. Then directly above this print was placed the small diamond type card, which describes the "Seven Truths of Normal Sight." Then above this was placed another, a little larger in size, describing the Fundamentals of treatment by W. H. Bates, M.D. This card is made up of different sized type which starts rather large at the top and graduates down to fine reading type at the very bottom of the card. The patient was directed to look at the white spaces between the microscopic type; then blink and shift his eyes to the white spaces of the diamond type; then blink and shift again to the larger white spaces of the Fundamentals card. In this way, my patient read sentence after sentence of the Fundamentals until he had read the very small print at the bottom of the card. The patient is grateful for learning how to use his eyes normally.

[See Appendix F, "Snellen Eyechart and Test Cards," for the Fundamentals card.—TRQ]

"THE FOUNTAIN"

By James Russell Lowell

Editor's Note—*The little poem below called "The Fountain" applies to the normal eye. The eye at rest is constantly moving just as the water in the fountain.*

"The Fountain"

Into the Sunshine,
Full of the light,
Leaping and flashing
From morn till night;

Into the moonlight,
Whiter than snow,
Waving so flower-like
When the winds blow;

Into the starlight
Rushing in spray,
Happy at midnight,
Happy by day;

Ever in motion,
Blithesome and cheery,
Still climbing heavenward,
Never aweary;

Glad of all weathers,
Still seeming best,
Upward or downward,
Motion thy rest;

Full of a nature
Nothing can tame,
Changed every moment,
Ever the same;

Ceaseless aspiring,
Ceaseless content,
Darkness or sunshine
Thy element;

Glorious fountain,
Let my heart be
Fresh, changeful, constant,
Upward, like thee!

—James Russell Lowell

AHIJAH'S STARING

1 Kings XIV-4.
"But Ahijah could not see; for his eyes were set."

EFFECTS OF PRESBYOPIA

By W. H. Bates, M.D.

Patients who have been cured of presbyopia, which is caused by eyestrain, are able to do more satisfactory work than those who have imperfect sight and wear glasses. We receive many reports from patients who have had difficulties in their special line of work and have found that they accomplished more and were more accurate after their presbyopia was cured. Frequently, people of fifty years or more, lose their positions because of mistakes made in figures or whatever their work may be. They are not always told the reason for their dismissal. They are simply discharged and a younger man put in their place.

One of my patients, sixty-four years old, told me that after having worked faithfully and steadily for forty years in one place, he had been informed that he could no longer figure accurately. It was a shock to him when he was placed on half pay and sent to another department. He was presbyopic, but was cured by treatment without glasses. During the absence of the younger man, he was temporarily placed in his former position. His work was so accurate and efficient that he was reinstated permanently.

Artists have the same experience with colors. It can be demonstrated that colors, when seen under a magnifying glass, become less distinct. White becomes a shade of gray; black becomes a lighter shade of black. It can also be shown that objects seen through glasses do not appear to be of the same size as the same objects viewed with the naked eye. Many artists are disappointed with their work because, for some good reason, they feel that it is not appreciated. The great mistake they make is that, like other people suffering from presbyopia, they believe that because their ability to read is improved with glasses, their perception of colors and form is also benefited. It is not always easy to convince artists that glasses actually lower their vision not only for colors, but also for form.

QUESTIONS AND ANSWERS

Q–1. Why do albinos always have poor eyesight?

A–1. They do not all have imperfect sight. It is because their mental equipment is imperfect that some have imperfect vision. When the memory or imagination is improved, the vision also improves.

Q–2. What color eyes are the strongest? I have been told that color matters, why?

A–2. The color of the eyes has no effect upon the strength.

Q–3. Doesn't it hurt to wear eyeglasses for near work during the interval of eye practice?

A–3. You should use your eyes correctly all day long, no matter what you may be doing. Practice blinking shifting, central fixation, and imagining stationary objects to be moving opposite to the movement of your head and eyes. Wearing glasses for any purpose whatever retards your progress and lowers your vision.

Q–4. What is the movement of the thumb and forefinger, and how does it help?

A–4. Let the ball of the thumb rest on the ball of the forefinger. Move the thumb in a circle, about one-quarter of an inch in diameter. When the thumb is moving continuously, one can imagine that all the nerves of the body are moving with the thumb. This prevents the stare and strain. This movement of the thumb can be practiced when in a room or on the street. When the right foot moves forward let the thumb move in the same direction. Then, when the left foot moves forward, let the thumb move backward. Alternate. When practicing the long swing, the movement of the thumb is a help. When you turn your body to the right, move your thumb in the same direction. When you turn your body to the left, move your thumb to the left. Let the movement of the thumb be a continuous movement.

When you practice the short swing and the slow, short, easy, circular, continuous movement of your thumb in the same direction as the movement of your head and eyes, it helps you to see better, to remember better, and to imagine better.

Q–5. I am forty-five years old and have worn glasses for eighteen years. As my eyes have pained me for so long, is it too late to expect help or to discard my glasses?

A–5. It is certainly not too late to discard your glasses and improve your vision. When relaxation methods are employed, the pain disappears and the vision improves. I suggest that you palm for five minutes ten times daily, or more often if possible. Practice the sun treatment for a half-hour, one hour, or longer, every day that you have sunshine. The circular movement of the thumb, as described above, relieves pain almost immediately.

Better Eyesight
June 1926—Vol. X, No. 12

CATARACT NUMBER

DEMONSTRATE: STARING

1. Demonstrate that when the eyes are stationary, they are under a tremendous strain. Stand before the Snellen test card at a distance of fifteen or twenty feet. Look directly at one small area of a large letter which can be seen clearly. Stare at that part of the letter without closing the eyes and without shifting the eyes to some other point. The vision becomes worse and the letter blurs. Stare continuously, and note that the longer you stare, the more difficult it is to keep the eyes focused on that one point or part of the letter. Not only does the stare become more difficult, but the eyes become tired; and by making a greater effort, the eyes pain or a headache is produced. The stare can cause fatigue of the whole body when the effort is sufficiently strong and prolonged.

2. Demonstrate that when the eyes are moving from one point to another, frequently, easily and continuously—the stare, the strain, or the effort to see is prevented and the eyes feel rested. In fact, the eyes are not at rest except when they are moving. Note that when you look at a letter on the Snellen test card and alternately shift from the top to the bottom of it, the vision remains good or is improved. When the letter is seen perfectly, the eyes are shifting; and when seen imperfectly, the shifting stops.

3. Close your eyes and remember your signature. This can usually be done quite perfectly. Try to remember the first and the last letter of your name simultaneously. This is an impossible thing to do and requires a strain. If you shift from one letter to another, you can remember your signature, one letter at a time; but if you make an effort to remember it, the memory and the imagination of your signature disappears.

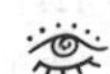

CATARACT

By W. H. Bates, M.D.

Defined

Cataract is an opacity of the lens of the eye. The lens of the eye is located in the pupil just behind the colored part of the eye, the iris. The lens is about the size of an ordinary pea. It is curved more on the front part than on the back. It is suspended in the eye by a bag-shaped structure, called the capsule. The capsule is a thin membrane. Covering the inside of the front part of the capsule is a layer of cells resembling in form and structure some of the layers of the skin of the body. The cells of the front part of the capsule are believed by some authorities to cause a secondary cataract after the lens has been extracted. Some years ago, I demonstrated by a long series of experiments that secondary cataract is not caused by these epithelial cells, but by scar tissue. The lens is composed of a number of layers of transparent tissue, which lie parallel to each other. When one places a number of sheets of plane window glass in a pile, with each pane of glass parallel to all the others, the pile of glass is transparent; but if one sheet or more is at an angle, that is, not parallel, the pile of sheet glass is clouded. This is a simple description of what takes place in the lens of the eye when it becomes opaque. When the lens is clear, its layers are parallel to each other. When the lens is opaque, one or more of the layers is at an angle to the rest. Some patients with normal eyes are able by means of an effort to consciously produce a cataract. When the cataract is beginning to show, it can be increased consciously by the memory of imperfect sight, which requires an effort with a resultant contraction of the muscles on the outside of the eyeball. When one group of eye muscles contract, the eyeball is lengthened and myopia is produced. When another group of muscles contract, the eyeball is shortened with a production of hypermetropia. When all the muscles of the eye contract sufficiently, the eyeball is squeezed in such a way as to change the parallelism of the layers of the lens with a consequent loss of its transparency.

Occurrence

Senile Cataract. There are various kinds of cataracts. The most common form is called senile cataract, because is usually occurs in elderly people after the age of fifty. Exceptions, however, are found in which the cataract may occur at a much earlier period. In the senile cataract at the beginning of the cloudiness of the lens, one sees opacities extending in nearly straight lines from the periphery, or the outside margin of the lens, to the center. Later on, the parts of the lens between these lines of opacities become clouded until the whole lens becomes totally opaque. A lens is said to be ripe when its whole structure becomes opaque, when the patient's vision becomes so poor that he is unable to count his fingers held about a foot from the eyes.

Congenital Cataract. When a child is born with an opacity of the lens, such a cataract is called congenital.

Traumatic Cataract. A traumatic cataract is caused by some mechanical injury like a blow or the puncturing of the lens by a sharp object. Being struck by a baseball or having a sharp object, such as a stick or a toy thrust in the eye is a common cause of traumatic cataract.

Complicated Cataract. When in addition to cataract, the patient has some disease of the eye, glaucoma, atrophy of the optic nerve, or serious inflammation of the interior of the eyeball, he has what is called complicated cataract. In these cases, the patient is usually unable to distinguish light in some parts of the field.

There are other kinds of cataract which occur less frequently.

Symptoms

Occasionally, a cataract may be sufficiently prominent to be recognized with the naked eye. In most cases, however, one cannot discover the cataract without the aid of the ophthalmoscope. When cataract is far advanced or the lens becomes totally opaque, the red reflex of the normal eye is not seen in the area of the pupil. If the cataract is only partially developed, one sees a red reflex shining through a clear part of the lens, while other parts of the lens are more or less opaque.

Demonstrations

Some years ago, when I was attending lectures at a medical college, an experiment was performed which was so convincing that I have always remembered the details. A professor was talking about the eye. He showed us an enucleated eyeball of a cow and called our attention to the fact that when he held the eyeball loosely in his fingers, the pupil was perfectly black. Then, when he squeezed the eyeball, almost immediately the pupil of the cow's eye became distinctly white from the pressure exerted upon the lens. Then, when the lecturer relaxed the pressure of his fingers, the pupil at once became perfectly black as it was before, and the cataract disappeared. The experiment was repeated a number of times. The pressure on the eyeball always produced cataract; relaxation of the pressure was always followed by the disappearance of the cataract.

Some years ago, I performed an experiment on a rabbit which had just been killed by chloroform. By dragging upon the muscles on the outside of the eyeball, it was possible to obtain pressure on the lens and produce a temporary cataract. When pressure on the eyeball was released, the cataract disappeared. By advancing the muscles and fastening them permanently to the back part of the eyeball with the aid of sutures, the cataract which appeared in the pupil was permanent so long as the pressure was maintained by the advancement of the muscles. The facts demonstrated very conclusively that cataract in the rabbit's eye can be produced by pressure on the eyeball with the aid of the muscles on the outside of the globe.

Treatment

If cataract can be produced in a rabbit's eye experimentally, one would expect the same thing to occur in the human eye. Treatment which relieves pressure on the eyeball is always beneficial. It is very interesting to discover that all cases of uncomplicated senile cataract have been benefited by relaxation or rest, at first temporarily, later more continuously or permanently.

There are a great many methods of treatment which bring about relaxation in the cure of cataract. The measures employed are not injurious. In fact, there is no possibility of making the condition of the eye worse. It is well to emphasize the fact that the same method of treatment to obtain relaxation is not a benefit in all cases.

1. Rest. Closing the eyes and resting them, or covering the closed eyelids with the palm of one or both hands, without exerting any pressure on the eyelids, has improved the majority of my patients. In my book, I report a case of cataract which was cured permanently by palming for a long period of time, twenty hours continuously. Palming for five minutes hourly is usually beneficial. With the eyes closed and covered, it is well that the patient allow his thoughts to drift from one thing to another without trying to remember one thing in particular all the time. By thinking of pleasant things, it is often possible for the patient to forget that he has eyes and in this way a larger amount of relaxation is attained.

2. Swinging. Swinging is very helpful in the cure of cataract. This swinging of the body can be done with the patient standing or sitting. Some patients have practiced the swing while sitting in a chair for many hours during the day. When tired, they would alternate with palming. When the swinging is done correctly, it is restful and a benefit not only to cataract, but to other conditions of the eye. In swinging, one moves the body, head and eyes from side to side. When the body sways to the right, the head and eyes move

in the same direction. When the body moves to the left, the head and eyes also move to the left. When the eyes move to the right, all objects not regarded are to the left of where the eyes are looking. When the eye moves to the left, all objects not regarded are to the right. By practicing the swinging exercise, many patients soon become able to imagine stationary objects to be moving in the opposite direction to the movement of the head and eyes. The great benefit derived from the sway is that the stare, the strain, and concentration are prevented. One cannot sway, move the eyes, and at the same time hold the eyes stationary in order to stare or concentrate.

The normal eye with normal sight never sees anything with perfect sight continuously unless it can become able to imagine it to be moving. This movement is usually about one-quarter of an inch from side to side. Things imagined to be stationary soon become imperfect.

3. Memory and Imagination. It is not possible to remember a letter of the Snellen test card perfectly unless it is seen perfectly. It is not possible to imagine a mental picture of the letter perfectly unless it is remembered perfectly. Furthermore, it is not possible to see the letter perfectly unless one has a perfect imagination of a known letter or other object as well with the eyes open as with the eyes closed.

One of my patients had normal sight with the right eye, but only perception of light with the left eye which had a ripe cataract, or a cataract in which the whole lens was opaque. With the right eye, she could remember or imagine perfectly the letters that she was able to see perfectly. When she covered the good eye with a screen, she told me that she could imagine the small letter on the Snellen test card as perfectly with her left eye as she could with her right. She was told that because of her poor sight in the left eye, she was unable to imagine perfectly at the same time with her left eye open. She remonstrated with me and was very positive that she could imagine as well with her left eye open as with her right. Finally, I asked her how much she could see on the strange card, and much to my surprise she read it with normal vision. When the eye was examined with the ophthalmoscope at the same time that she said her vision was normal, the cataract had disappeared. She was right and had demonstrated the truth that when her imagination was perfect, her sight was also perfect and in order to have perfect sight, it was necessary for the cataract to disappear, which it did. This case was one of the strongest evidences that imagination treatment is one of the best methods that can be employed to cure cataract. It interested me so much and emphasized the value of the imagination so greatly that it has become a routine treatment for my other cases. While it is beneficial in most cases, it is seldom curative because very few patients have so perfect an imagination.

I treated a woman, age fifty-six for the first time on November 7, 1923. The right eye had incipient cataract with a vision of 15/70. The left eye had a ripe cataract with a vision of only perception of light. The numerous eye doctors whom she consulted all advised an operation for the removal of the cataract of the left eye, and told her that no other treatment would be of any help. The patient was benefited by palming, by swinging, and most of all by the use of her imagination. When her imagination, with the right eye open, improved, her vision improved to the normal. With her left eye open, her imagination was not so good, but even with an imperfect imagination her vision at once improved to 15/200. After two weeks of treatment, there were days in which her imagination became, with the left eye open, as good as with her right eye open, with normal vision in each eye. After some months of treatment without my supervision, the vision of the right eye became permanently normal and the cataract disappeared. By continuing the treatment at home, the left eye obtained normal vision for short periods of time only. Since she obtained normal vision with the left eye, although temporarily, it is possible for the temporary improvement to become permanent.

The memory of perfect sight is a rest to the eye, with a coincident relaxation of all tension or strain of the muscles of the eye.

4. Fine Print. Cataract patients become able to read fine print at six inches or nearer to their eyes more quickly than do patients with imperfect sight from other causes. By reading fine print frequently, or for long periods of time, the cataract becomes less.

5. Sun Treatment. The eyes need sunlight. People who work in mines, where there is no sun, sooner or later develop inflammations of the interior of the eyes. The cloudiness of the lens from cataract is lessened by exposing the eye to the direct rays of the sun. When using the sun treatment, it is best to let the eyes become accustomed to the sun by mild treatment at first. Have the patient sit in a chair with his eyes closed and his face turned toward the sun. He should slowly move his head a short distance from side to side. The movement of the head prevents concentration of the sun's rays on one part of the eye. After some days of treatment, or when the patient becomes more accustomed to the light, one may use the sun glass with added benefit. Direct the patient to look far down and while he does this, lift the upper lid—gently, exposing to view the sclera, or white part of the eye. Now, with the aid of the sun glass focus the sunlight on the forehead or on the cheek, and then rapidly pass the concentrated light over various parts

of the sclera. This requires less than a minute of time. It is not well to be in a hurry. One should wait until the patient becomes sufficiently accustomed to the sun to permit the upper eyelid to be raised while he looks far down, exposing the sclera only. It is important that the patient be cautioned not to look directly at the sun.

PROGNOSIS

The cure of cataract is usually accomplished more quickly than the cure of some other diseases of the eye. My assistant, Emily C. Lierman, has had unusual success in treating cataract cases, as she adapts my methods to each individual case.

STORIES FROM THE CLINIC
No. 76: Cataract
By Emily C. Lierman

Many patients, after being cured of imperfect sight, go their way and we never see them again. However, many come back, even after a period of five years or more, to report, or to show their gratitude.

If a patient is cured quickly, he is very apt to forget that he ever had eyestrain. Normal vision helps him to forget, and he is able to go on with things that interest him without tension or strain. There is nothing that affects the whole nervous system more than eyestrain.

I have deep sympathy for patients suffering from cataract. Some of these have told me that, when they first discovered or were told that they had acquired cataract, the shock was so great it sometimes made them very ill. I have often wished that I could broadcast to every human being troubled with cataract that they need not worry about an operation, nor fear blindness.

While treating patients at the Harlem Hospital Clinic, Dr. Bates placed under my care many patients with cataract. Some of them were children who were born with it, while others acquired it from an injury of some sort. If they faithfully practiced the daily treatment for their particular case, they always improved. There were no exceptions, although in all cases where the patient did not practice enough, it took much longer for a cure. Adults were also cured quickly when the directions for home treatment were faithfully carried out. Age made no difference.

A mammy, who was a faithful servant of one of our private patients, came regularly, three days a week for many months, and was treated for cataract. In the beginning of her treatment, she could not see the letters of the test card at five feet. As she explained it in her dialect, "Do you know, ma'am, I can see nothin', no ma'am, nothin' at all at the distance!"

Long periods of palming, early in the morning and late in the afternoon when her work was done, helped her sight. In the Clinic she was taught to sway her body slightly from side to side and to blink all the time. The swaying helped her to see things about the room moving opposite to the movement of her body. The blinking prevented the stare, which is usually the cause of cataract. The quickest way to obtain a cure is by palming, and I advise my private patients to practice it for several hours or many times each day. It would be impractical, however, to advise a Clinic patient to use the same method, because they cannot spare the time from their work, nor can the employer spare them. If such advice were given them, their answer would surely be, "This treatment is only for those who can afford the time." Dr. Bates often tells them that it takes less time to use their eyes correctly than it does to use them incorrectly.

Clinic patients, as well as private ones, are advised to relax all day long. Mammy was to see things moving all day by watching her broom as she swept the floors; the washboard as she washed the clothes; the clothes-wringer as she turned the handle; and the dishes as she dried them and put them in the cupboard. We treated her many times, but occasionally she had a relapse.

As time went on, she obtained normal vision with the use of the test card, and became able to read very fine print and to thread a needle. We left the Harlem Hospital Clinic, never thinking that we would hear from her again. Six years had passed, and new patients were coming and going from our own Clinic, when one day about three months ago, we received a letter from mammy. All through the letter were words of gratitude and praise for what we had done for her. She is now seventy-eight years old, and can still read her newspaper and thread a needle. She asked for permission to come to see us. She wanted the Doctor to look at her eyes to prove that her cataract had entirely disappeared. We, of course, were anxious to see her. When she came both of her eyes were examined and no sign of cataract was found in either eye. Her vision with various test cards was 10/10, and she read fine print without any difficulty because she did as she was told. She was cured. It was not always easy for her, as her work at times required good eyes. Her madam had patience with her for she also was under treatment. During mammy's last visit, she said, "Ah jest know that ah was cured 'cause ah could see de crumbs on de carpet to brush up, and ah could see de dust all ober de furniture and ah cleans better. De sun is clear now an' not in de mist no more."

About a month ago, another patient came with a report

of good vision. She is over eighty years old and has a disposition just as cheery as she had when I first knew her, about eight or nine years ago. Perhaps our readers will remember an article I wrote about her. She was the patient who was employed in an orphanage. [See the March 1920 issue.—TRQ]

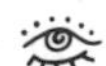

A RADIO TALK

The following lecture was delivered at Station WMSG, Madison Square Garden, on Tuesday, May 18, by W. H. Bates, M.D.

For a few minutes this evening, I wish to talk to you about your eyesight. So many people are troubled with their eyes that I feel that anything that is a benefit to them should be broadcasted. In the first place, it is an error to believe that perfect sight requires hard work or an effort. Perfect sight comes without an effort. This is very easily tested. All you have to do is to look at a small letter in a book or a newspaper and note that when seen perfectly, it is seen easily. If you do something that is wrong, by trying to see this letter better or making an effort to improve it, your vision fails. If the efforts are continued and you concentrate on just one point of the letter, the vision not only fails, but your eyes begin to feel uncomfortable. Pain and headaches often occur when the eyesight is imperfect. People who have perfect sight are usually more comfortable than people who have imperfect sight.

It is generally believed that the normal eye has perfect sight all the time. A scientific study of the facts has convinced me that this impression so generally believed and taken for granted is far from the truth. After forty years' special study of the eye under different conditions, I am convinced that the normal eye has imperfect sight most of the time. Age is no exception, young and old are equally affected.

There is but one cause of functional imperfect sight, and that is a strain or effort to see. The strain may be an unconscious one or it may be conscious and manifest itself by pain, fatigue, or other discomforts.

Light has a very important effect on the vision of the normal eye. The vision of all persons is imperfect when the eyes are first exposed to the strong light of the sun or to strong artificial light, but people who are supersensitive to the light of the sun should not dodge it, but should gradually accustom the eyes to the sunlight.

Movies usually produce temporary defective vision. Some people have complained that they always suffered with pain and had poor sight whenever they regarded the screen with its flickering light. I believe that some years ago, when photography was less perfect than it is now, the pictures produced a great deal of eyestrain, much greater than at the present time. I always advise my patients under treatment for the cure of defective vision, to go to the movies frequently and gradually become accustomed to the flickering light. After this is accomplished, no other lights seem to bother them.

Noise is a frequent cause of defective vision of the normal eye. All persons see imperfectly when they hear an unexpected loud sound. Familiar noises do not lower the vision usually, but unfamiliar, new, or strange noises always do, at least temporarily.

Artists, bookkeepers, lawyers, physicians, writers, mechanics, and others found their mental ability or efficiency increased many times with the aid of eye training. Many recruits for the Army and Navy were found to have imperfect sight and were rejected, although their eyes were normal. Eye training improved their sight.

The cadets at West Point and the midshipmen at Annapolis have been well trained to obey orders, and any method that was employed to improve the sight of the soldiers and sailors was grasped and practiced with unusual intelligence. One great difficulty, if not the greatest difficulty in helping the sight of the soldiers and sailors, was that those who had inquiring minds wanted to know the whys and wherefores of everything. They were slow in obeying orders and were, on the whole, difficult to cure; but those who were benefited usually had no questions to ask, no arguments to offer. They were sure to be benefited; they were sure to do as they were told, and because they did as they were told without any discussion, they obtained normal vision as a general rule at the first visit. The soldiers and sailors who were treated successfully improved at the very beginning and improved so rapidly that most of them were cured in about an hour of eye education. Those who were cured became able to cure others.

The most important method employed was to have the patient sit with his eyes closed and rest them for half an hour or longer. Then, when he first opened his eyes, the vision was usually improved temporarily. It had a good effect when the patient was taught that a stare, a strain, or trying to see always lowered the vision, and often produced pain, headache, fatigue; or other nervous troubles. The demonstration that staring lowered the vision helped the patient to avoid the stare. When he knew what was wrong with him, it made it possible for him to practice in such a way as to avoid the stare.

Blinking was a great help. The normal eye blinks, or opens and closes, unconsciously very often. It has been demonstrated that blinking consciously gives one temporary improvement in the sight.

A young man came to me soon after war was declared, begging me to help him, if possible, so that he could enlist in the Marines. He told me that he had tried to enlist a number of times, but he was always rejected because of his poor eyesight. In order to be accepted, it was necessary for him to have perfect sight in each eye without the use of glasses. He proved to be an apt pupil, and by using his eyes without effort or trying to see, his vision soon became normal. The next time he applied for enlistment, he was at once accepted because he had perfect sight. He wrote me a letter while he was in France, in which he reported that he went on the rifle range and made a score of 251 out of a possible 300 points. He was the second highest qualified man in his company, and was awarded a sharpshooter's medal. His best ranges on record day were the 600 yard slow fire and the 200 and 300 yard rapid fire. On the 600 yard range, he made six bull's-eyes and four four's. The bull's-eye for the 600 yard range was twenty inches in diameter. He had not been in Brest, France very long before a call came for fifty men from each company who had high rifle range records to go at once for quick preparation to enter the lines as machine gunners. He was among those selected.

The aviation branch of the Army requires very good sight. It is interesting to note that while aviators may have normal sight when they first enlist, in the course of a few weeks their vision may begin to fail. They complain that at irregular intervals they suffer from attacks of blindness. At first these attacks are not severe, but later on they become worse. During one of these attacks of blindness, the pilot will lose control and the machine will fall to the ground unless the aviator can recover his vision before it is too late. A number of aviators have told me that they did not know of one man whose sight was continuously normal. It is for this reason the death rate among aviators has been so high.

These facts have led me to the following conclusions:

First: All persons with normal eyes and perfect sight do not have normal eyes and perfect sight continuously.

Second: The cause is always an effort or strain to see.

Third: That treatment by eye training is successful when distant, small, familiar letters are read a few moments at least every day.

Fourth: The good results obtained justify the use of this method in all schools, the Army, Navy, Merchant Marine, and on all railroads—in short, by everybody who desires or needs continuous perfect sight.

If any of you are interested in the preservation of your eyesight for yourself, your family, or your children, I shall consider it a privilege to answer any question sent to me at this station.

Better Eyesight
July 1926—Vol. XI, No. 1

MYOPIA NUMBER

DEMONSTRATE: CENTRAL FIXATION

1. The smaller the object regarded, the easier it is to remember. One can, with time and trouble, become able to remember all the words of one page of a book. It is easier to remember one word than all the words of a page. It is still easier to remember one letter of a word better than all the letters. Regard a capital letter. Demonstrate that it is easier to see or remember the top of the letter best, and the bottom of it less clearly than to remember the top and bottom perfectly and simultaneously. Now look directly at the upper right-hand corner and imagine one-fourth of the letter best. Then cover the remaining three-quarters of the letter with a piece of paper. It is possible to look directly at the exposed part of the letter and imagine half of it best. Cover the part that is not seen distinctly and demonstrate that half of the exposed part of the letter can be seen or imagined best, while the rest of it is not seen so clearly. With the aid of the screen, an area as small as an ordinary period may finally be imagined. Demonstrate that the imagination of a perfectly black small period, forming part of a small letter at fifteen feet, enables one to distinguish that letter.

2. With the eyes closed, a small black period can be imagined blacker than one that is three inches in diameter. If this fact cannot be readily demonstrated with the eyes closed:

Stand close to a wall of a room, three feet or less, and regard a small black spot on the wall six feet from the floor. Note that you cannot see a small black spot near the bottom of the wall at the same time.

Place your hand on the wall six feet from the floor, and note that you cannot see your hand clearly when you look at the bottom of the wall.

MYOPIA

By W. H. Bates, M.D.

Definition

Myopia has been called nearsightedness because the vision is usually very good for objects which are seen at a near point, while very dim or blurred for objects at ten feet or farther. In myopia, the eyeball is elongated. The normal eye, when reading fine print, becomes elongated, or myopic, during the time that the eye is focused for reading.

Acute Myopia. When myopia is acquired, it is called acute myopia in the early stages. When treated at this time, it is readily curable without glasses. The practice of prescribing glasses in these cases leads to a permanent use of them.

Progressive Myopia. In these cases, the myopia increases quite rapidly, and may be accompanied by much discomfort, pain, fatigue, and loss of vision. In advanced cases, many become unable to see as well with very strong glasses as they can without them.

Complicated Myopia. Many authorities have stated that the myopic eye is usually a diseased eye. It may be complicated with cataract or other eye diseases, or it may not. The exceptions are so numerous, that it can usually be demonstrated that diseases of the eye have nothing whatever to do with the cause of uncomplicated myopia.

Occurrence

Myopia usually occurs at about twelve years old. It is rarely congenital. Some become myopic at the age of four, fifteen, seventy, or any age, earlier or later. Some children with normal vision may go through life without becoming myopic. Risley, after a careful study of the eyes of schoolchildren, believed that myopia was only acquired by children with astigmatism or with hypermetropia (farsightedness). At one time, statistics were quoted that children living in large cities had myopia to a greater extent than those who lived in the country. I believe statistics are uncertain, because one can generally obtain statistics which prove the contrary.

It is a popular belief that habitual use of the eyes for reading, sewing, or for any other use at a near point, promotes the increase of myopia. Simultaneous retinoscopy always demonstrates that near use of the eyes—even under a strain in a poor light—instead of producing myopia, always lessens it or corrects it altogether.

Another theory, that individuals who use their eyes repeatedly for distant vision suffer less from myopia, has also been disproved by simultaneous retinoscopy. A strain to see at the distance always produces myopia. During the late war, it was unusual to find sailors or aviators with normal vision, or normal eyes without eyestrain. In order to obtain recruits for these branches of the service, because of the general prevalence of myopia, the standard of the requirements for admission had to be repeatedly lowered.

Symptoms

Myopia is always accompanied by a strained look of the eyes, when regarding objects. Partly closing the eyelids, a form of squinting, is often observed in myopia. When the sight is imperfect, this practice may improve distant vision for a few seconds; but at a near point where the sight is good, about five inches from the face, squinting always lowers the vision, especially when one eye is covered.

Cause

Staring can always be demonstrated to be the principal cause, if not the only cause of myopia. There are no exceptions. We may say, "It is a truth that the cause of myopia is the stare." Contributing causes are numerous. Any child with normal eyes and normal sight will at once become temporarily myopic if you scold him severely. Teachers with normal sight and normal eyes are usually relaxed, and do not stare or strain. On the other hand, teachers who wear glasses for myopia are under a strain. This strain is contagious, and children under their care are more apt to acquire myopia than those who are under the care of teachers with normal eyes and normal sight.

Treatment

The cause suggests the cure. Since the stare or strain produces myopia, the cure would naturally be rest or relaxation. This is obtained by palming, swaying and improving the memory and imagination. [These topics have been covered repeatedly and at length in previous issues. They have been omitted here.—TRQ]

Prevention

In order to prevent, as well as to cure myopia, it is necessary that you use your eyes correctly all day long.

1. Blink frequently, just as the normal eye does. Staring is a strain, and always lowers the vision.

2. Shift constantly from one point to another, seeing best the part you are looking at, and other parts not so clearly.

3. All day long, your head and eyes are moving. It is important that you notice stationary objects to be moving

in the opposite direction to the movement of your head and eyes. When you walk around the room or on the street, notice that the floor or pavement appears to come toward you, while objects on either side of you appear to move in the opposite direction to the movement of your body.

4. Practice daily with the Snellen test card for five minutes or longer.

Shifting, blinking, and imagining stationary objects to be moving, can be practiced at all times and in all places, no matter what you may be doing.

STORIES FROM THE CLINIC

No. 77: Myopia

By Emily C. Lierman

Many times I have been called upon to answer the question, "How do you treat or cure myopic cases?" This has been asked not only by laymen, but also by physicians. It is not an easy question to answer because myopic cases vary in their response to treatment, and each requires an individual application of the method. Some patients with a high degree of myopia improve or recover in a reasonable length of time, while others with only a slight degree become despondent because it takes so long to be cured. These patients fail because they are unable to refrain from making an effort to see. Myopic cases are cured quickly when they do exactly as they are told instead of straining their eyes by trying to see.

Progressive myopia is generally believed to be incurable, and to my knowledge there is no method of benefiting or curing it other than the Bates Method.

A man, seventy years old, called on me recently to learn what he could about the method. He said that he had been myopic since birth. Several eye specialists had told him that he could never be cured. Opticians had also told him the same thing. His eyeglasses were changed every two or three years, and each time he was given stronger ones. When he was examined with the ophthalmoscope it was found that he had incipient cataract in both eyes, in addition to myopia. When I told him about the cataracts, he said that other doctors had also informed him of them. He asked if I could help him when so many others had attempted to do so by fitting him with glasses and had failed. I told him glasses were not necessary and suggested that he try the Bates Method. With much hesitation, he finally consented. He said that he would believe in the treatment if I could improve the vision of either eye for the distance in one visit. At ten feet from the test card, he could see only the 200-line, or the letter "T," but he said even that looked very much blurred.

I taught him to palm, and while he was resting his eyes in this way, asked him if he could remember a favorite chair in his home, or the title of a book he had read. I reminded him of a sunset, and a white cloud in a blue sky. He visualized the mental pictures described, and nodded his head as I mentioned one thing and then another. I continued this method for half an hour and then asked him to remove his hands from his eyes, but not to open them. I told him to stand with eyes closed, and sway his body a short distance from side to side, just as an elephant does. This made him smile, but he did as I told him. He was then directed to open his eyes and to blink frequently as he swayed. While moving his body from left to right, he was able to flash the letters of the test card and, without stopping, he read 10/50 with both eyes.

His face expressed his pleasure, and his eyes twinkled as he remarked, "I'm coming back for more treatment and will prove to those who gave me no hope that I am cured!"

Another patient, a woman, thirty-five years old, was cured of myopia in two months' time. Her vision of the test card was 5/40 in each eye. During her first treatment, she made very little progress because she strained so hard to see beyond two feet from her eyes. Palming seemed to tire her instead of help her. She frequently removed her hands from her eyes, although she still kept them closed. I decided to have her sway her body from side to side, first while sitting in a chair, and later while standing. To help her to sway rhythmically, I practiced with her and reminded her to blink all the time. When she became able to imagine things about the room to be moving in a direction opposite to the movement of her body, I told her to flash one letter of the test card at a time. When she saw things moving in an opposite direction about the room, her eyes remained open in a natural way. Just as soon as she glanced at the letters of the test card, she squeezed her eyes, practically closing them, and the muscles of her face became tense. When she was again seated in her chair and had closed her eyes, I placed three large test cards, all similar, at different distances from where she was seated. I placed the nearest about one foot away, the second three feet, and the third five feet from her eyes. We again started the standing sway and, while blinking, she was directed to look at a letter on the card nearest her, then to flash the same letter on the next card, and to repeat this with the distant card. This method was successful, and she was overcome with joy as she flashed each letter in turn on the cards.

Eight weeks later, she read 10/10 on different test cards. The retinoscope showed no more eyestrain, and the patient has not had a relapse since.

THE GREAT DELUSION

"Wearing Glasses to Strengthen the Eyes—A Billion Dollar Industry Based on an Error!"

By Dr. Wendell A. Diebold

Tens of thousands make their living in a profession whose basis is founded on a misconception! Strong statements I grant you, yet the saddest part is that they are only too true.

Fitting of glasses to aid our vision on the theory that the lens of the eye is a factor in accommodation is the present practice. It is true that glasses do enable some people to see better—for a time—just as any crutch may help a lame man to get about, but when his lameness is gone or his broken leg has mended, he can throw away his crutch. Not so with the crutches of the eye. The longer, in most cases at least, glasses are worn, the poorer becomes the vision and the stronger must the lens be. In other words, the eyesight gradually becomes less acute—its keenness diminishes.

If glasses really strengthened the eyes, why should stronger and stronger lenses, ever so often, be required? If the theory that we are born with defective organs of sight (a rare condition) were correct, there might be some justification for the enormous number of folks with glasses, but all errors of refraction are functional, and therefore curable by the proper methods.

The general teaching regarding the eye has been that it is more or less of a fixed organ. It is supposed that some are born with short eyes and therefore they are apt to have various degrees of farsightedness, and astigmatism—while others are supposedly born with long eyeballs, and therefore they are doomed to shortsightedness or nearsightedness, technically known as myopia.

Now, while the rank and file of the eyeglass fraternity have blindly accepted the teaching handed down to them in their colleges and schools, there have been many experiences in their actual application that have not coincided with their theory. A classical example is the cases of people who have had their lenses removed through a cataract operation and still have been able to acquire the ability to accommodate without a lens. This could never have occurred if the lens were the factor of accommodation. [The observation that a lensless eye can still accommodate (most likely by the action of the oblique muscles) does *not* prove that the lens cannot accommodate. Can *both* the oblique muscles *and* the lens accommodate?—TRQ] Again, tens of thousands of cases of nearsightedness, farsightedness and astigmatism have been corrected and normal vision secured. It is evident that these results could not have been secured if the error of refraction were a fixed thing—something people were supposed to have been born with, and not a functional condition as first maintained by Dr. W. H. Bates of New York City.

Dr. Bates, as long ago as 1886, cured cases of myopia by a simple method based on a principle that he later demonstrated scientifically. He was one of the few who was not satisfied with the usual explanations, and when he found that he could by some simple methods secure correction of "errors of refraction," he realized that the old theory must be wrong. What did he do? He tried to prove, by reenacting the same experiment that Helmholtz performed, that the lens accommodation theory was correct. He worked almost continuously for two years, and every experiment made proved that the theory was wrong, due to a mistaken interpretation of certain facts. Then he had to prove his own theory, which is, that the extrinsic muscles that move the eyeball also control its shape. The oblique muscles in contracting elongate the eyeball, producing myopia; and the recti muscles in contracting shorten the eyeball and produce hypermetropia. He made many thousands of experiments on animals of all kinds. He found that by cutting the superior oblique muscle that the retinoscope would not show any focusing of the eye. [The fact that Dr. Bates was unable to produce accommodation when the superior oblique muscle was cut does not prove that the lens cannot accommodate.—TRQ] When it was sewed together again, the eye focused normally as before. This proves that the tension of the extrinsic muscles determines the shape of the eye, therefore, its focusing. [Dr. Bates proved that the extrinsic muscles are capable of accommodation.—TRQ] So, on this basis, Dr. Bates says that the bad habit of staring and straining to see (and other conditions of mental and bodily strain) causes an undue tension on the extrinsic muscles, which does not allow the eyeball to accommodate through shortening or lengthening at will, as it should, and therefore give us perfect vision. Now the proof of the pudding is in the eating; not only has Dr. Bates, for many years, corrected all kinds of defective vision in tens of thousands of cases, but many other physicians all over this country and England, by using his methods, are securing the correction of farsightedness, nearsightedness, "old-age sight," astigmatism, crossed eyes, and even cases of cataract and glaucoma.

[Regardless of mechanism(s) of accommodation, Dr. Bates' research proved that when the external eye muscles release their tension, the eyeball returns to its normal shape, with the resultant elimination of myopia, hyperopia, astigmatism, strabismus, and many other vision problems.

Since the lens supposedly accommodates perfectly up to age forty, according to the orthodox, obviously imperfect eyesight before the age of forty, and imperfect sight other than presbyopia after age 40, must be due to other causes than the lens becoming inflexible.—TRQ]

Dr. Bates' work and research are undoubtedly one of the greatest boons of this century that has come to suffering mankind. Generations unborn will do homage to him. He at last has made it possible for nearly everyone to regain normal sight. The practice of a few of his simple rules will positively prevent children from ever developing defective vision. From a lifetime of study and practice, he asserts with the conviction of one who knows whereof he speaks, that to put glasses on children is a crime. My own experience convinces me that children and young people can regain perfect vision if they have lost it, or maintain it if they are now blest with it. The results in at least seventy-five percent of adult cases have been more than gratifying in that their vision has been restored to normal. Even the cases where restoration could be only partially accomplished, because of the great degree of degeneration that had taken place, have been much improved. All cases can secure improvement by these methods.

A RADIO TALK ON BETTER EYESIGHT

By Emily C. Lierman

I believe that most people are interested in knowing how to prevent eyestrain. Strain is the cause of much discomfort, pain, and fatigue. I want to reach those who must use their eyes all day long, those who are employed in offices, factories, stores, shops and, in fact, wherever good eyesight is required.

I would like to say a few words to the business man who really needs good sight for the work he does. If he can accomplish his work without the aid of eyeglasses, it is done with less fatigue and in less time than when glasses are worn. Reports which have been received from those who have been treated verify this fact.

When glasses are worn, the eyes and the mind are not at rest. When the eyes and mind are under a strain, it is difficult to work efficiently. When the business man or woman is arranging a business deal, unless the mind and body are relaxed, mistakes are made which may mean a great loss.

Eyestrain is contagious. This is particularly obvious in the department stores. While waiting at a sales counter to be served, I have watched the person ahead of me straining her eyes as she explained to the saleslady just what she wanted. Unconsciously, the saleslady feels the strain of the customer and, not realizing the cause, suffers throughout the rest of the day unless she knows how to relax. The saleslady, in attempting to please, tries so hard that she often fails to make a sale because of the tension of all the nerves in her body. She does not know that this is caused by eyestrain. In five minutes' time she can be relaxed if she knows what to do. If she will remember to blink her eyes frequently, just as the normal eye does all day long, she will feel relaxed and rested. When she talks to a customer she should shift her eyes from one part of the customer's face to the other, remembering to blink as she shifts from one eye to the other—to the nose, from one cheek to the other, the chin, the mouth, and back to the forehead. In this way she feels no fatigue whatever. I am not thinking so much of her sales ability, as I am of the restful feeling she desires to have when her working hours are over.

This applies not only to those who work in department stores and shops, but also to office workers. The stenographer who has to listen sometimes for hours at a time, taking dictation from the nervous employer who perhaps finds it hard to be pleasant, also needs all the pleasure and recreation that she can get. While she is taking the dictation, she must be careful not to be affected by the strain in the sound of the voice dictating to her. If she is not careful, she will make mistakes or be in a much strained condition of mind and body when she leaves the office. Her strain can be relieved by watching her pencil move as she writes, being sure to blink frequently. Her employer appreciates her efficiency much more when she is able to take dictation without tension or strain.

Most people strain their eyes while they are asleep. Indications of strain are swollen eyelids upon rising in the morning, a feeling of heaviness and of not having had enough sleep. Early morning headaches are usually caused by eyestrain during sleep. This strain can ordinarily be relieved or prevented by palming. By this, I mean to close the eyes and cover them with the palms of both hands in such a way as to exclude all light, without exerting any pressure on the closed eyelids. If this is practiced before retiring and immediately upon rising in the morning, the eyes become relaxed sometimes within a period of five minutes.

Have you ever noticed an elephant as he sways his body from side to side? Sometimes he is looking straight ahead of him, or he is watching his trunk as he sways his body. It means everything to the comfort of the elephant to keep swaying from side to side. This gives him a feeling of rest and relaxation and prevents him from becoming discontented.

The lion and tiger in captivity are always pacing up and down their cages. They are contented knowing that sometime or other the keeper will satisfy their appetites. They keep moving all the time they are awake, because in this way they obtain rest and relaxation. As the animal receives rest and relaxation, so may the human being, by swaying from side to side without effort or strain.

The long swing is particularly beneficial in improving the vision, and invariably helps those who do not sleep well.

I would like to encourage the tired mother who stands on her feet most of the day, performing duties of the household which are seemingly endless. It is not always the small baby that tires her most; but the strain and tension caused by her concern for the comfort of her husband and other members of the family. Her desire to attend to all of her duties sometimes causes a great deal of eyestrain. This is more noticeable to her when she is called upon to thread a needle or to sew. Before she tries to thread a needle, she should close her eyes and rest them for just a second or two, holding the needle in place so that when she opens her eyes, she may see the eye of the needle. By blinking she will soon become able to thread the needle without her glasses. She should remember, while attending to other duties in the household, to blink her eyes and sway her body slightly from side to side. She can do this all day long, no matter what she may be doing, whether cooking or sweeping the floor, washing dishes, or anything else, and she will feel relaxed and happy.

It is a wise mother who keeps a rocking chair handy to rock her baby to sleep. The swaying back and forth gives rest to the baby and peace of mind to the mother. If she has children who attend school, she can easily teach them to relax by palming XE "palming" and swaying for a very short time before school. The mother can remind her child to blink the eyes often and not to stare at the blackboard or at the teacher. The child will soon notice that his vision becomes better.

For the benefit of those who desire to improve their eyesight and to work without the aid of eyeglasses, I shall be glad to answer any question addressed to me at this station, WMSG.

Better Eyesight
August 1926—Vol. XI, No. 2

SCHOOL NUMBER

DEMONSTRATE: IMAGINATION

Vision is always imagination, either perfect or imperfect. What we see is only what we think or imagine we see. The white center of the letter "O," when seen perfectly, appears to be whiter than it really is, or whiter than the rest of the card. That part of the center of the "O" which is in contact with the black appears to be the whitest part of the white center. By covering the black part of the "O" with a screen which has an opening in the center, the whiteness of the center of the "O" appears to be the same shade of white as the rest of the card. Now remove the screen, and at the first glance the center of the "O" appears for a short time to be much whiter than it really is. In other words, one sees something which is not really seen, but only imagined.

When one looks at the upper right-hand corner of a large letter of the Snellen test card, it is possible to see that point best and all the rest of the letter not so black. The part seen best appears blacker than it really is. The part seen worse appears less black than it really is. Things seen more perfectly than they really are, are not seen, but imagined. Things seen less perfectly than they really are, are not seen imperfectly, but are imagined imperfectly.

SCHOOLCHILDREN

By W. H. Bates, M.D.

Most children have normal eyes when they enter school. In a few years, their sight may become imperfect. Acute cases are usually benefited or cured by prompt treatment without glasses.

Causes of Imperfect Sight

I have frequently called attention to the fact that in all cases of imperfect sight, *staring* is present, and can usually be demonstrated. It is the cause of imperfect sight. When treatment corrects the habit of staring or trying to see with an effort, the vision becomes normal.

The surroundings have an important effect upon the vision. It is possible to lower the vision of any child by an unexpected noise or by punishment, either physical or mental. The vision is usually affected by the temperament of the people with whom the child comes in contact. When a child is comfortable, the sight is good. When a child is nervous, the vision is lowered.

The following case illustrates these facts. A half-hour after birth, a child was observed to squeeze its eyelids, wrinkle up its forehead and, in fact, contract the muscles of its whole body. The child's eyes were examined with the retinoscope, and when it was straining so terribly, it had a high degree of nearsightedness. A drop of strong atropine solution was put into both eyes. Atropine is supposed to lessen the eyestrain which causes myopia. This child, however, was not benefited in the slightest—the pupil dilated, but the nearsightedness continued. The remarkable fact was repeatedly observed that, in spite of the atropine, the child produced at about fifteen minute intervals or more often, all the errors of refraction known for which glasses are prescribed. Sometimes it was farsighted in both eyes; sometimes farsighted in one eye and nearsighted in the other. Astigmatism would come and go—and the degree, as well as the axis, was variable within short periods of time. Sometimes the retinoscope demonstrated that the eye had mixed astigmatism, that is, it was flatter than normal in one meridian, while the one at right angles to it was more convex than in the normal eye.

The nurse, who was not a graduate of any hospital, took the child in her arms and began to rock it from side to side. Watching the child's face, one could see the muscles begin to relax, the wrinkles become less, the contraction of the muscles of the arms, limbs, and of the whole body, become relaxed. The little one opened its eyes and smiled; at this moment both eyes were normal. Then it turned its face to the nurse's breast and promptly went to sleep.

The child was examined daily for about a week, then less frequently, about twice a week for several months, and then only occasionally. When she was four years old, her eyes were normal. She was sent to kindergarten, and after being there for about a month, the retinoscope showed that she had myopia in both eyes, which strong atropine drops did not correct. I asked the teacher to encourage this child to dance and run as much as possible while at school. After two weeks, the child was examined again with the retinoscope and the eyes were found to be normal, with no myopia nor astigmatism whatever. At this time, the eyes were straight. A month later, the child was again examined. The right eye was normal, but the left eye was very farsighted and turned in toward the nose. With the right eye open, the child could distinguish her parents, relatives, and some of her playmates across the street, at a distance of more than fifty feet. With the right eye covered and looking with the left eye, she could not recognize her acquaintances farther off than fifteen feet. It was very evident that the sight of the left eye was imperfect.

Not long afterwards, I visited the kindergarten and was much shocked to find that the child was wearing glasses for the correction of the squint. It annoyed me so much that I at once called on the parents and had a heart to heart talk with them. The father was a friend of mine and teased me a little for taking the matter so seriously. The mother remembered how much time I had spent on the child previously, and was willing to have me treat the child. The child's glasses were removed permanently and she practiced shifting, swinging, and palming. Reading a Snellen test card (the pothooks card with "E's" pointing in different directions) for about five minutes each day was a benefit. In a short time, the eyes became straight and the vision of both eyes became normal at the same time.

Later, the child had a relapse which was evidently caused by being annoyed by a girl who had joined the kindergarten class during the previous month. It so happened that the child who annoyed the patient went away for a visit, and while she was gone, the patient's eyes became straight and remained straight. When the irritating child returned to the school, the patient again had a relapse. I recommended that the patient be taken out of the kindergarten and kept in agreeable surroundings with children and others who did not make her nervous. The child outgrew this nervousness and ten years later there had been no return of the squint.

Treatment

1. Age. One of the first questions that people ask is "How old should a child be before it can be treated?" The answer is that the younger the child, the more successful is the treatment.

2. Frequency. Another question frequently asked is "How long does the child have to be treated before good results are obtained?" My habit is to ask the parents to wait and see the results of the first treatment. I am then usually able to tell them that the child has a temporary cure and does not necessarily need to come to see me again. If the child is only partially cured, however, it may be advisable to have him come for a few days, a week or longer, until he

becomes able to improve his sight without my supervision. Then he may continue to practice at home until cured. If the cure is delayed, it may be necessary to take more treatments under my personal supervision.

3. Palming. When palming, the patient closes the eyes and covers them with the palm of one or both hands, in such a way as to avoid pressure on the eyelids. Babies, three years old or younger, have been taught to palm. When they find that the discomfort in their eyes or head is relieved by the mother covering their closed eyelids with the palms of her hands, the children may acquire the habit of doing it themselves. I have had cases of whooping-cough, in which children three years old have stopped the cough by palming, after they had obtained benefit from palming done for them by an older person.

While nursing her baby, whose sight was imperfect and eyes inflamed, one mother was observed to cover its eyes with her hand. She said that the palming relieved the pain in the eyes, improved the sight, quieted the child, and promoted sleep.

4. Swinging. One of the best methods for preventing staring is to practice the swing. We often see babies laugh or scream with delight when someone swings them sideways or up and down. They open their eyes wider, breathe more deeply, and the muscles of their arms, limbs, and whole bodies relax with pleasure and happiness. It is not conceivable that a baby so happy could have pain, poor sight, or be crossed eye. Children and babies are forced to wear large tortoise-shell rimmed glasses which invariably kills the joy in their hearts. They seldom smile, the eyelids contract, wrinkles appear on their faces, and the world becomes a place in which to be sad. Let us bring back the rocking chair, the swing, the cradle, and encourage mothers to swing their babies in their arms as they love and pet them.

5. Rest. Children of all ages are benefited by resting their eyes and minds for a few minutes, several times a day. Teachers realize the benefit of rest in the schoolroom, and books are laid aside, windows opened, and a few exercises with deep breathing, are practiced. I am not aware that the school authorities have ever been criticized for devoting this daily amount of time to rest.

A more effective method for obtaining relaxation of the mind is as follows: A Snellen test card is permanently placed on the wall in front of the children, where it can be read by all of them from their seats. Twice each day or more often, the children read the card with each eye separately as well as they can. When practiced properly, reading the Snellen test card with both eyes open, or alternately with each eye, the other being covered, has improved the vision in all cases. In some cases, the vision became normal in two weeks or less, while others required a longer time to obtain this result. Practically all of the children were temporarily cured in three months.

It rests the eyes to read the Snellen test card with good vision. To fail to read it perfectly requires a strain or an effort. When these facts are demonstrated and the child realizes the cause of its imperfect sight, much good may follow. When children do not know the cause, they have more trouble in obtaining relief.

STORIES FROM THE CLINIC

No. 78: Schoolchildren

By Emily C. Lierman

During the last year, I have had more squint cases under treatment than any previous year. My records show that all of these cases also had imperfect sight. All, with the exception of two little boys who were in the second and third grade, were too young to attend school. At the close of the Clinic in June, it was not necessary to send them to kindergarten, as every one of them was ready for the first grade.

I am very sure that parents who have children with squint, or crossed eyes, want to know what to do to correct the trouble.

Many of them who visited us were unwilling to have their girls or boys operated upon for the cure of squint. If the patients are faithful in the daily practice, we can assure them of a cure. In some cases where the sight of one eye is imperfect, while that of the other eye is normal, we advise a black patch to be worn over the good eye, especially during practice. This is done only when the eye with imperfect sight turns in or out.

It is always encouraging to the patient if he can see the eyes improve, or become straight while under treatment. If I notice a decided improvement while treating such a case, I place my patient before a large mirror and direct him to closely follow my instructions. I then quickly draw his attention to his eyes, and before he has a chance to strain, he notices the improvement. This usually encourages them to continue their practice until they have a permanent cure. Other patients who are not troubled with squint, but have imperfect sight, are treated in a different way.

When children are too young to read the alphabet or figures, we use a pothooks test card with the letter "E" pointing in various directions. This card is placed at five or ten feet from the patient, and he is requested to tell in which way the letters are pointing. When the letters become smaller, they begin to look blurred. Then it is best to advise palming for five minutes or even less. When the patient again reads the test card, the vision is usually improved for one or more lines of letters. The child is then shown how to sway by standing and gently moving the whole body with the head from side to side. Most patients must be reminded to blink, so the child is frequently encouraged to blink while swaying, just flashing the card and seeing one letter at a time. When children understand the great benefit derived from the sway of the body, there is no difficulty in curing their imperfect sight or squint. Most of the patients have some kind of music at home, and children as well as adults enjoy keeping time with it as they practice the sway, which helps the patient to relax. Relaxation being the only way to improve the sight, the patient is thus benefited by the sway.

I am always able to teach my tiny tots their letters and figures by playing a game with each one. If he has squint, I place the card close to the eyes and point to the largest letter and ask what it is. He may say, "I don't know," and then I mention whatever the letter is. After this, he is directed to play peek-a-boo, which means to look quickly, repeat the letter after me, and then close the eyes. This is exactly the same method used for adults, only it is not a game of peek-a-boo. When a child is instructed in this way, the second treatment becomes more interesting, and each time he is taught a few more letters.

I never forget to praise my little patients after each treatment, as it makes them more anxious to help me when treating them. The little Fundamentals cards play an important part in the treatment and cure. They help grown-ups, as well as children.

Mothers may at first find it a task to devote the necessary time and care to their children with imperfect sight, but the result is worth the effort. Children can practice the sway at home for five minutes before they go to school. When they read letters or words written on the blackboard, their vision always improves, providing they do not stare at the letters. Blinking frequently relieves all tension and strain. When no effort is made, children can read from their books, feeling relaxed and rested, both in mind and body. Boys and girls from the high schools who have been treated and cured appreciate this fact. Many schoolchildren whose defective vision has been cured have interested their teachers in the matter. As a result, they came to Dr. Bates for treatment and were also cured. Dr. Bates and I realize the strain under which teachers of the public schools work. Many of them do not know how to relax, and their anxiety to instill knowledge in the minds of the children keeps them constantly tense.

A young man who was just about to enter Columbia College recently told me that every morning for one whole year after he was cured, he never missed an hour's practice with his eyes. He said it helped him to keep relaxed during school hours, and he noticed that his mind was benefited. He could think easier and his memory, which was very poor while he was wearing eyeglasses, was so much improved that he found no difficulty in studying his mathematics and history. More boys than girls seem anxious to cure their imperfect sight. I believe this is because boys and young men are interested in more strenuous sports. Eyeglasses are useless to the oarsmen, football and baseball players and, for the sake of these sports, they are willing to practice faithfully to bring about a cure.

WHAT THE BATES METHOD DID FOR ONE SCHOOLBOY

By May Secor

Special Teacher of Speech Improvement, New York City Public Schools and Pupil of Dr. Bates

John was crossed eye; the taunts of his schoolmates kept him well aware of this. When he looked at an object directly in front of him, the pupil of his "lazy eye" was only partly visible; with this eye he could see the large "C" of the Snellen chart only when he was within sixteen inches of the chart. John was nearly seven years old; he was retarded at school, having been obliged to repeat Grade 1A. He was a neurotic child—extremely erratic in his behavior at school and at home.

During the latter part of his second term in 1A we began to instruct him in Dr. Bates' method of Eye Education. We aimed to keep John relaxed and happy; to present each exercise as a game; to suggest each game in such a way that he would be anxious "to try it"; to foresee an outburst of passion when it was brewing, and ward it off; in general, we aimed to instruct John in methods of relaxation, keeping him busy with happy, healthful thoughts and activities, thus avoiding correction and possible outbursts of passion. We admit that the case was difficult and required much time and study. We used the following methods:

1. Instruction to Parents and Teachers. Teach the child's parents and teachers the principles underlying the Bates Method, and gain their sympathy and cooperation.

2. Rest Periods. Enjoy two rest periods each day—after lunch and after school or work. Go to your bedroom, open the window, remove your shoes and other tight clothing, and lie down and sleep.

3. Blinking. Notice how gently and often a tiny baby blinks. Close your eyes and remember a baby blinking, and

gently blink as a baby does. Blink as you read an eye chart or a book, play cards and other games, watch automobiles pass, or enjoy physical exercises.

4. Swaying. Watch the moving pendulum of a large clock. Close your eyes and remember the pendulum moving. Gently sway as the pendulum does, and see things moving in the opposite direction as you blink. Vary your position. Stand with your feet slightly apart as you sway your body. Sit in a comfortable chair and gently sway the head and body from side to side.

5. Swinging. Enjoy the long swing, the memory swing, and the variable swing fully described on the Fundamentals cards. As you shift, see letters and objects swing.

6. Palming. Lie down or sit in a comfortable chair, and rest your feet and legs on a stool, which is as high as the seat of your chair, and tuck a pillow under each elbow. Gently close your eyes; cup your hands, and place them gently over your eyes, and enjoy the following: See something which is very black (a black cat, a black overcoat, or black velvet). Practice the memory swing as you make believe that you are swaying, reading the chart, looking at a certain picture, watching automobiles pass or playing a game.

7. Reading Test Cards. Stand and sway, or sit in a comfortable chair, and rest your legs and feet on a stool which is as high as the seat of your chair. Read the Snellen test card lazily, comfortably, and gently blink as you read. Read the test card with your better eye and then palm. Read the test card with your worse eye and then palm. Read the test card with both eyes together and then palm. Practice with the pothooks chart as follows: Name or indicate with the hand the direction in which the letter points. Copy the chart, using white paper and black crayon. Read it with the "lazy eye" (eye patch on other eye). Copy a line at a time with black kindergarten splints which have been cut in corresponding lengths.

8. Memory. While you palm, practice the memory swing. Recall the face of a friend, a certain picture, the odor of a rose, or the tune of some song you like.

9. Imagination. While you palm, imagine you are taking a trip to the country or that you are drawing a small picture of a house or a dog.

10. Sun Treatment. Learn how to sway and blink with relaxation before using the sun treatment. Enjoy the sunshine; walk, play, or lie in it. Stand or sit in the sunshine, and gently blink, sway, and see things moving. Enjoy the long swing.

11. Reading Books. Read any book which is "easy for you to read" with fairly small print. Sit in a comfortable chair with legs and feet on a stool, and gently blink and read. Occasionally palm for a few minutes. Let the mind drift and visualize some episode in the story.

12. Learning New Exercises. Begin by learning how to relax, blink, and sway, and then very gradually add other exercises.

13. Use of Eye Patch. Wear an eye patch over the better eye at first for a half-hour, and then gradually increase the length of time.

14. Environment. Enjoy your lesson at patient's home, indoors or on porch, at instructor's studio, on a pier (if fond of boats), or in a park. Select cheerful, pleasant people as companions.

15. Sleep. Before retiring, sway, blink, palm, and read the chart. Open bedroom windows, and if possible, retire at eight-thirty and remain in bed until six-thirty or seven a. m. If wakeful during the night, palm and practice the memory swing.

In this way, we applied Dr. Bates' method of Eye Education to John's case. We treated John for seven weeks. He then spent two months in the country without treatment. Upon his return, we again took up the work.

The muscular control in the crossed eye improved from the second lesson on. The vision improved greatly, and the crossed eye gained the ability to fixate. But this was not all. In the fall, John's mother reported that he was "made over." At home John was pleasant and obedient; and whereas he had formerly been retarded at school, his record is as follows since he has been under our care:

June 1925—Promoted to 1B; October 1925—Advanced to 2A; February 1926—Promoted to 2B.

John has been re-educated—from the standpoint of vision, of nervous make-up, of behavior, and of intelligence. Since Dr. Bates' method has accomplished this for John, may we not apply it with equal success to other cases?

QUESTIONS AND ANSWERS

Q–1. My sight is good, but I am suffering from eyestrain caused by muscle imbalance. No oculist has been able to help me. I have had to become a cook from being a typist and dressmaker. If I focus my eyes on my fingers for more than a moment, terrific pain shoots through my eyes. I cannot stand light and have to cover the kitchen tables with a dark cloth. Please tell me what to do. Is it possible for me to discard the dark glasses I wear?

A–1. It is evident that when you look at your fingers for more than a minute, you stare, strain, and make an effort to see. Practice the variable swing. Hold the forefinger of one hand six inches from the right eye and about the same distance to the right. Look straight ahead and move the head a short distance from side to side. The finger appears to move, and the stare is prevented. In order to overcome your sensitiveness to light, I suggest that you obtain as much sun treatment as possible.

Q–2. Often, when I am trying to see a thing, it will come to me, but my eyes will commence to smart, and then I blink and lose it. What shall I do to overcome that?

A–2. Blinking can be done correctly, and it can be done incorrectly. You strain while you blink. The normal eye blinks easily and frequently. Strain is always accompanied by the stare. By standing and swaying from side to side so that your whole body, head and eyes move together, the stare is lessened. The swing and the movement of the eyes lessens the tendency to stare.

Q–3. What does "seeing things moving all day long" mean?

A–3. Your head and eyes are moving all day long. Notice that stationary objects appear to move in the opposite direction to the movement of your head and eyes. When you walk around the room or on the street, observe that the floor or pavement appears to come toward you, while objects on either side of you, appear to move in the opposite direction to the movement of your body.

Q–4. Could cataract be caused by diseased teeth?

A–4. While it is possible for abscesses of the teeth to cause cataract, most cases are caused by eyestrain, and are curable.

Better Eyesight
September 1926—Vol. XI, No. 3

REST NUMBER

REST

By W. H. Bates, M.D.

Rest and relaxation of the eye and mind is perfect when the vision is perfect, and can always be demonstrated.

When the eye is at rest, it is always moving. To demonstrate this, instruct the patient to close his eyes and imagine that he is looking first over his right shoulder, then over his left shoulder. By alternating quite vigorously, the eyeballs can be seen to move from side to side. While the eyes are still closed, one can place the fingers on the closed eyelids and feel this movement. Now instruct the patient to imagine a shorter movement of the eyes from side to side, that is, look a shorter distance from right to left while the eyes are closed. The movement can usually be felt, but it is not so manifest to the observer as it is when the wide movement of the eyes is made. However, after a little practice, five minutes or more, when the patient is imagining the eyes are moving, one can feel the movement even though it may be very short, one-quarter of an inch or less. If the patient stares at a part of an imaginary letter with the eyes closed, the memory or the imagination of the letter becomes blurred and the movement of the eyeball is not continuous. On the other hand, if the patient remembers a letter perfectly, the eyeball appears to move continuously a short distance in various directions.

When central fixation is practiced, that is, when one remembers or imagines one part of a letter best, the eyeballs move. If one tries to remember or imagine a letter, all parts equally well, the movement of the eyeballs cannot be seen or felt, and the eyeballs appear stationary. One can demonstrate the movement of the eyeballs very well with the aid of the ophthalmoscope. When the optic nerve is regarded with this instrument, one can always see the movement of the pigment of the eye or of the blood vessels of the retina when the sight, memory, or imagination is normal. This movement is slow, short, easy and continuous. When the sight, memory, or imagination is imperfect, the eyeball may move very irregularly, with frequent periods when it is stationary.

In nystagmus, the eyeballs move from side to side, usually continuously, a distance so great that it is conspicuous. The rapidity of this movement may vary. It is always stopped after closing the eyes and resting them a sufficient length of time, several minutes or longer, or by practicing the slow, short, easy swing.

Nystagmus is generally believed to be difficult to cure. In fact, it is so difficult that very few cases have ever been reported as benefited by orthodox methods of treatment. It has usually been considered an incurable symptom of disease of the eye. Nystagmus is, however, to a greater or lesser degree, under the control of the mind of the patient. Some people are able to stop the movement at will. These cases, however, are rare. Some children acquire the ability to practice nystagmus just as they learn to look crossed eye. Nystagmus requires a strain. When practiced either consciously or unconsciously, the vision is always lowered. When the nystagmic movements are lessened or stopped altogether, the vision improves and has frequently become normal, either temporarily or permanently.

Some years ago I treated a boy, age ten, for the cure of nystagmus. His mother told me that she had visited many physicians and had sacrificed a great deal financially in order to obtain a cure for her son. I tested his vision and found it normal at times, when the nystagmus would stop. Repeated tests demonstrated the fact that his vision was always worse when he had the nystagmus. While he was reading with almost normal vision, I said to him, "Stop the movement of your eyes!" Much to my surprise, he did what I told him and then read the card with normal vision. Then I said to him, "Start it up again and read the card." This he did very promptly, but he was unable to obtain normal sight. Again I asked him to stop the nystagmus and his vision became normal and remained normal as long as he had no nystagmus.

The mother paid close attention to the conversation. She realized that the boy was able to produce or stop the nystagmus at will. He seemed to be pleased by the attention he received when he showed off his control of it. The mother asked me no questions. There was no need of questions after the convincing demonstration that the boy gave of his ability to control the movement.

It can be demonstrated that when the eyes are not at rest, the vision is always imperfect. When the memory or imagination is perfect with the eyes closed, the vision is improved when the eyes are opened. Usually the improvement of the vision is only temporary, and may last for only a second, or in flashes. In these cases, the memory soon becomes imperfect with the eyes open. By alternating perfect memory with the eyes closed, the memory with the eyes open usually improves. By practice, many patients become able to remember or imagine with their eyes open a small area of black or white, as well as they can imagine it with their eyes closed. When such patients look at a blank wall, where there is nothing in particular to see, no effort may be made to see and the vision improves. One can practice with the Snellen test card and remember for a moment one known letter of the card, with the eyes open, as well as one can for a longer time with the eyes closed. When one letter of the Snellen test card is improved, all the letters and other objects are also improved. The perfect memory of a known letter with the eyes closed is perfect rest, while an imperfect memory or imagination with the eyes closed or open is always a strain. It is a great help to many people with imperfect sight to demonstrate that rest improves the vision, while the stare or strain always lowers it.

To fail to see requires an effort. When the patient regards the letters which are so blurred and indistinct that he cannot tell what they are, he is always straining, trying to see, either consciously or unconsciously. People are cured of their imperfect sight when they cease to strain, stare, or make an effort to see. When I explained this to one of my patients, she said that I was wrong, that the only way she could see was by means of an effort. I had her test the facts. When she looked at the Snellen test card at ten feet, she could not read it with normal vision. At five feet her vision was better, but when she made an effort, her vision became much worse. The same was true when she regarded letters at a nearer point, three feet, two feet, or even one foot. An effort to see always made her sight worse. She had to demonstrate the facts repeatedly before she was finally convinced that her vision was good only when her eyes were at rest and no effort was made.

Blinking, when practiced properly, promotes relaxation or rest. The normal eye blinks continuously all day long when the patient is awake. At night, when the patient is asleep, a movement of the eyeballs can be seen which resembles the movement of the eyeballs when the eye blinks. When the eye blinks slowly and the upper eye lid is slowly closed, distant objects appear to move up.

When the eyelids slowly open, objects appear to move down. This movement is usually accompanied by an improvement in the vision. Blinking is absolutely necessary in order to obtain continuous normal vision. The normal eye blinks unconsciously, easily, sometimes with great rapidity and at other times rather slowly. It is impossible to stop the blinking of the normal eye. Any effort to do so is a strain, which lowers the vision and, if kept up for some minutes or longer, produces pain, fatigue, dizziness, and other nervous symptoms.

The normal eye is shifting or looking from one point to another continuously, not only when one is awake, but also when one is asleep. This continuous movement of the eyes brings about a condition of perfect rest. To stare at one point for a few seconds or part of a minute is a difficult or painful thing to do. It requires a great effort which lowers the vision. It is not possible to see two black periods perfectly black at the same time. The only way that they can be seen perfectly black is to shift from one to the other alternately. It is not possible to see a large letter or a small letter perfectly without shifting or looking from one part of the letter to another part. It is well to realize that the human mind is not made to see more than one thing perfectly at a time. To see two or more things perfectly at the same time is impossible, but one can shift from one thing to another and alternately see each perfectly for a short time.

When regarding a person's face, it is impossible to see the whole face perfectly at once. It is necessary to shift from one part of the face to another to see those parts perfectly. If the shifting is more or less rapid, one gets the impression of seeing the whole of the face at once, when, as a matter of fact, only a small area is seen at a time.

One of my patients had normal sight in one eye and one-half normal vision in the other. He was very positive that he could see every letter of the Snellen test card perfectly at the same time. He was not aware that he shifted from one letter to the other, or that he shifted from one part to another of large and even small letters in order to see them clearly, or to be able to distinguish them at all. When he covered his good eye and looked with the poor one, he could read only one letter at a time. He was quite conscious that he did not see even the large letters perfectly; but when he practiced shifting with his poor eye, his vision improved not only for the large letters, but also for the small letters. It required considerable time and much patience to convince him that it was impossible for him to see all parts of any letter perfectly at the same time. When he demonstrated that staring lowered his vision, and that shifting improved it, he obtained normal vision in each eye.

When palming is done correctly, the vision, memory, and imagination always improve. By palming is meant to close the eyes and cover them with the palm of one or both hands without exerting any pressure on the closed eyelids. Think of something pleasant, something that you can remember perfectly. Then let your mind drift from one pleasant thought to another. This should be practiced for five minutes ten times daily, or more often when convenient. Some people obtain more benefit by palming for a half-hour, an hour or longer.

There are patients who have difficulty in palming, that is, they strain and make hard work of it. For them it is easier to simply close their eyes and in this way rest them. Other patients obtain relaxation by closing their eyes for part of a minute, then opening them for part of a second, and quickly closing them again. This is called flashing, and usually improves the vision immediately.

It is true that when the eye is perfectly at rest, the sight, memory, and imagination are always normal. Conversely, it is impossible for the sight to be imperfect when the eyes are perfectly at rest. Not only are all errors of refraction benefited and cured by rest, but also organic diseases of the eye—glaucoma, cataract, opacity of the cornea, disease of the retina, choroid, or optic nerve are cured by rest and relaxation.

STORIES FROM THE CLINIC

No. 79: Relaxation Effective

By Emily C. Lierman

When some of my patients are told upon their first visit that glasses will not be prescribed, they wonder what kind of treatment they will receive and they become very much frightened. During my first year of study in Clinic work, I noticed that adults, especially, were so frightened that it was difficult to test their sight. Under these trying conditions, a fair test could not be made. Each time the patient was told to read the test card, the retinoscope showed a change in the shape of the eyeball. As I studied each case under treatment, I became convinced that mind strain had a great deal to do with eyestrain. I planned a way to approach such patients and put them at ease, and found it effective with adults and children.

I have had many schoolchildren under my care who, for no apparent reason, became nervous as soon as they entered school. When I questioned them about their teachers, the answer was usually a favorable one. Sometimes they would complain about some boy or girl whom they feared, and I was able to help them solve the problem. I would find out sooner or later that my patient was suffering from mind strain and fear. It was necessary to convince the patient, after an eye test with the Snellen test card, that it was eyestrain and undue effort to improve in school studies that caused the trouble. After the vision was improved, there were no more complaints from either the patient or the school officials.

An interesting case was that of a housepainter who spent most of his working hours on a scaffold, painting the outside of high buildings. He would become so dizzy that he was finally compelled to give up his work. Other jobs were not so easily obtained, and he began to worry because there was no income for his wife and family. He called on a doctor about the dizzy spells and was advised to go to our Clinic to have his eyes examined. With the ophthalmoscope, Dr. Bates could find nothing organically wrong with either eye. Dr. Bates said that apparently the man was in general good health. I questioned the patient about his former position as a painter. He told me that his fellow workman on the scaffold had lost control of himself, had fallen to the ground and been killed. Since that time, the patient had had attacks of dizziness.

Palming seemed to give him relief almost instantly, even though he had his eyes covered for a very short time, a period of five minutes or less. At fifteen feet from the test card, he easily read down to the 40-line, but beyond that line the letters were blurred and the dizziness returned. He was instructed to palm again, and while doing this, I told him to remember moving objects. He said it was easy for him to remember an automobile moving slowly, or a streetcar stopping at a corner, letting off passengers and taking on others. He could imagine boats moving up and down the Hudson River. In this way, we passed on from one thing to another, and after a few minutes of palming, he read the whole card without stopping and without a mistake. I placed my forefinger on the card to guide him in seeing the white spaces between each letter and reminded him to blink as he flashed each letter. The dizziness disappeared and he said that he felt as though a great load had been removed from the top of his head.

During each treatment, I was careful not to mention the scaffold or the accident, but we did talk about paints and colors as he sat with his eyes closed. He seemed eager to explain and I encouraged him to do so. It was interesting to hear him tell how colors were mixed to produce the correct shades desired. His mind became free from strain and his dizziness disappeared entirely. Test card practice was continued both in the Clinic and at his home. Later, I added the swing to be practiced with eyes open and with them closed.

One day he came with an interesting story of how he had treated and cured his little son, nine years old, who was nervous and destructive. Punishing him seemed to make him worse. When his father first practiced the swing, the boy imitated him in fun. Later, it became a natural thing to see both of them swaying and keeping time with the Victrola music. Other practices of the Bates Method also became a daily habit to the boy. He especially enjoyed keeping his eyes closed while his father told him of a farm out west where he had lived as a boy.

Faithful practice has given the father normal vision and a relaxed mind, and he has returned to the scaffold and painting with no more attacks of dizziness.

Recently, while crossing the river on a ferryboat, I stood where I could see the pilot at the wheel and watched him carefully. He was a man about the age of fifty, and did not wear glasses. As we started out of the ferry-slip, we moved slowly. The pilot looked straight ahead and I observed that he blinked his eyes frequently. At first I counted five blinks to the second; then he blinked so often and so irregularly that I could not keep count. I continued to watch him, however, as we crossed the river, and noticed that his head moved about half an inch from side to side and that he blinked his eyes all the time. It particularly interested me to note that when he changed his position a little, perhaps to stand more comfortably, he kept on swaying his body and blinking. The ferryboat went into the slip as though it were sliding on ice, and there was not the slightest jar as the boat touched the sides of the ferry-slip. The pilot had good vision.

Near our office building there is a traffic policeman who manages a steady flow of traffic. He sees things moving all day long. Sometimes his right hand is raised and other times the left, as he halts traffic. He turns his body to the right or to the left, whichever way the traffic is going. His eyes serve him well because he keeps them moving. His whole body appears to be perfectly relaxed, and he demonstrates the efficiency of a relaxed mind.

RADIO TALK

Eye Education: Blinking

By May Secor

The following radio talk was broadcasted from Station WMCA, Hotel McAlpin, on Thursday, July 8, at 4:15 p.m.

Have you a tiny baby in your home? If so, he will teach you how to use your eyes with relaxation. Notice how gently he blinks his eyes—and how often! If you have no baby in your home go to the park tomorrow, and learn your lesson from a baby there. You will notice that when baby blinks, his eyelids simply drop. He blinks very, very gently.

Now, will you please sit in a very comfortable chair. Rest your feet and the calves of your legs on a stool which is as high as the seat of your chair.

Let us all palm. Gently close the eyes. Cup the hands and place them gently over the eyes. Think of something that is very, very black. Now imagine that you are watching a tiny baby as he lies in his carriage. See how gently he blinks! And how often! Now place your hands lazily in your lap. Gently blink, slowly turn your head to the right, as you—

Blink, blink, gently blink, slowly turn your head to the left, as you blink, blink, gently blink; very, very gently blink. Slowly turn your head to the right, and blink, blink, gently blink; very, very gently blink. Slowly turn your head to the front, and blink, blink, gently blink; very, very gently blink.

QUESTIONS AND ANSWERS

Q–1. Are all cases of squint curable without glasses or an operation?

A–1. All cases of squint, or crossed eyes, are curable by the Bates Method.

Q–2. Is it possible to cure squint in a child under two years old by the Bates Method, and what is the treatment employed?

A–2. A child, two years old or younger, can be treated and cured of squint, with or without imperfect sight, by the Bates Method. The treatment is varied. The swing can be practiced by the mother holding the child in her arms. If the child is able to stand or walk, it is held by the hands and the sway is practiced with the child moving from side to side. Keeping time with music encourages the child to continue the swaying for a longer time.

Improving the memory and imagination of the child is also recommended. The child is encouraged to play with toy animals and is taught the names of the different animals. Usually the animals are placed on the floor in groups and the child is asked to pick up the animals as they are named. As the child reaches for one and then another, the parent may observe whether the child goes directly toward the toy or reaches to either side of it. This method is used in extreme cases of squint where the child does not see perfectly where it is looking.

Colored yarns are also used in these cases. The child is taught names of the different colors. An improvement is always noted after such treatment because the child is constantly shifting his glance from one colored skein of yarn to the other as he selects the one called for. The problem is to educate the eyesight. The more the eyes are used, the better.

Palming is beneficial in the cure of squint. If the child is told that it is just a game of peek-a-boo, he immediately becomes interested and enjoys it. Reading a story to the child as he palms is usually beneficial, and improves the squint.

With children three years or older, the pothooks card is used. This is a test card with the letter "E" pointing in various directions. The child tells whether it is pointing up or down, left or right. If a mistake is made, palming is introduced in order to rest the eyes.

Children with squint are usually unruly, disobedient, or destructive. When the squint is improved, a change in their conduct is also noted. They become quiet, obedient, and their mental efficiency is improved.

Q–3. Is diabetic cataract curable?

A–3. Diabetic cataract is curable when the general disease of diabetes can be relieved by treatment.

Q–4. After a serious illness eight years ago, my pupils became very large. Is there anything you can suggest that will help them to contract?

A–4. Dilated pupils are not usually symptoms of disease of the eye. The sun treatment is beneficial.

Better Eyesight
October 1926—Vol. XI, No. 4

DEMONSTRATE: STRAIN AND MEMORY

1. A strain to see at the distance produces near-sightedness.

Look at a Snellen test card at twenty feet and read it as well as you can. Now strain or make an effort to see it better, and note that instead of becoming better, it becomes worse.

2. When a mental picture is perfect with the eyes closed for part of a minute or longer, a perfect mental picture can be remembered, imagined, or seen for a second or less with the eyes open.

Remember a black kitten. If your mental picture is gray or an imperfect black with the eyes closed, imagine that you are pouring black ink or black dye over it. Note that the clearness of the mental picture improves.

Look at a page of fine print. Then close your eyes and imagine the white spaces between the lines to be perfectly white. If they appear to be a grayish white, imagine that you are painting the white spaces between the letters, inside the letters, and between the lines, with white paint or whitewash. Then open your eyes for a fraction of a second and note that the white spaces between the lines will appear whiter, if you do not make an effort to see either the black letters or the white spaces.

LORD MACAULAY

By W. H. Bates, M.D.

Lord Macaulay, who will always hold an eminent place among English men of letters, was born October 25, 1800 and died December 28, 1859. Before he was 30 years old, he became a member of the House of Commons, and later held positions of trust and importance which required him to visit different parts of the world. At one time he wrote a code of laws for the benefit of the people of India and devoted considerable time to the work.

Lord Macaulay was said to be the most rapid reader on record, and had the ability to remember perfectly what he had read ten or more years previously, without refreshing his memory by re-reading it. He was able to read a page of five hundred words in one second. Not only could he remember the words that were spelled correctly, but also those words which were spelled incorrectly. He was able to remember the page on which they could be found, the line of the page, the location of the words on the line, and how each word was misspelled. For example, if the word "which" were misspelled, he could remember that it was the fourth word on the fifth line on page 120, and that it was spelled "whiche." This seems a remarkable statement to make, but I have had patients who became able to read almost as rapidly as Lord Macaulay after a course of eye education. This training consisted of central fixation and the imagination of the halos, i.e., the white spaces inside the letters, between the letters and between the lines of letters.

Central fixation is the ability to see best where you are looking and not so clearly where you are not looking. This requires shifting from one part of an object to another part. To have perfect sight, Lord Macaulay unconsciously practiced central fixation. If he had consciously tried to see a letter or to keep his attention fixed on one part of a letter, or if he had tried to see all parts of a letter at once, his vision would have been imperfect. To see the top of a letter perfectly, it was necessary for him to look at and see the top of the letter best, and the rest of the letter not so well. To see each of the other sides perfectly, it was necessary for him to look at and see each side best, and the rest of the letter not so well. Since the average number of letters in each word is five, he shifted four times five, or twenty times, to see each word with maximum vision. To recognize five hundred words, it was therefore necessary for him to shift five hundred times twenty, or ten thousand times in one second.

In order to see perfectly, it is necessary that one imagine perfectly. Macaulay remembered or imagined the white spaces between the lines to be whiter than they really were. When the white spaces were imagined perfectly white, the black letters were imagined perfectly black, because the white spaces could not be imagined perfectly, without the black being imagined perfectly at the same time. For the same reason, when the blackness of the letters was imagined perfectly, the form of the letters was also imagined perfectly. It has been demonstrated that trying to see the black letters is a conscious strain, or is attended by a conscious strain, and always lowers the vision.

It is a truth that one cannot remember a letter perfectly unless it has been seen perfectly. When the memory for one letter is perfect, the memory for all letters is also perfect. A letter cannot be imagined perfectly unless it has been remembered perfectly. It cannot be seen perfectly unless it has been imagined perfectly. We see only what we imagine we see. The speed of reading is greatest when the vision is perfect.

After a course of eye training, some of my patients were able subconsciously to remember large letters of the Snellen test card, which they had previously regarded, without being conscious of distinguishing any of the letters. Many of these patients have become able to remember or imagine small letters of the test card at thirty, forty, or fifty feet. I have had some patients glance for a few seconds at a page of diamond type at ten feet or farther, without consciously reading any of the letters. With their eyes closed and covered with the palms of their hands, some of them became able to remember or imagine one or more letters of the fine print. They must have unconsciously seen the fine print to have been able to imagine the letters, because one cannot imagine something not remembered, and one cannot remember perfectly unless one has seen perfectly. Therefore, in order to imagine a letter perfectly, it is necessary that the letter be seen previously, either consciously or unconsciously.

The method of rapid reading practiced by Macaulay is invaluable and should be more widely employed.

In my writings I have remonstrated against the methods employed to teach rapid reading. The usual procedure was to encourage the student to see all of the letters of a word at once, or to see all the letters of a paragraph of words at the same time. This was accepted as the correct method and very intelligent scholars have recommended it. My research has proved that there is nothing more injurious to the eyes than to make an effort to see a whole letter or a whole word, all parts equally well. If one looks at the first letter of a word, the last letter is not seen perfectly at the same time. If an effort is made, the whole word becomes blurred and may not be distinguished. The stronger the effort that is made, the more injurious it is to the mind and eyes.

In the public schools of the City of New York, teachers are advised to practice this method of rapid reading with young children. Although the result is unsatisfactory, many teachers still persist in their efforts to teach the impossible. It is interesting to know that children who have perfect mental pictures of letters, or other objects, have a normal memory or a memory that is just as perfect for letters or objects. The scholarship of such children is much better than that of others whose memory or mental pictures are imperfect. A number of schoolchildren have told me that at the time of their examinations, they could read a question on the blackboard and have no conception of what the answer might be, but if they closed their eyes and remembered the first letter of the question perfectly, it helped them to remember the answer to the question.

One teacher with a class of children who were mentally deficient found that the practice of central fixation, palming, and the use of the imagination was of great benefit to the minds of those children. A school teacher in Chicago has made a practice of teaching her pupils how to imagine things perfectly, with the result that no matter how ignorant they may be at the beginning of the school term, it is not long before they become able to make the same progress as other children in the rapid advancement classes.

The dean of the department of metaphysics of one of our prominent universities came to me and complained that he was suffering with all kinds of mental and eye troubles because he had lost the power of concentration. The strain was so great that he was compelled to give up his work. Glasses were of no benefit. He demonstrated that to concentrate on one letter or one part of a letter it was necessary for him to make an effort, and in a few seconds his vision became very imperfect.

With perfect sight, no effort is made and the eyes and mind are at rest. There is no fatigue, and one can read with great rapidity for many hours continuously, without being conscious of having eyes.

STORIES FROM THE CLINIC

No. 80: Fear

By Emily C. Lierman

Fear is one of the many symptoms which accompanies imperfect sight. This is more noticeable in adults than in children. If pain results from imperfect vision, the fear is much greater. Many of our patients have been to other clinics, or other doctors, and were told that if glasses were not worn, they would go blind. Sometimes they were told that they had an organic disease of the eyes, such as glaucoma, iritis, keratitis, atrophy of the optic nerve, or cataract. The patient has cause to fear. It is my belief that the doctor should tell his patient what the trouble is; but when he is not absolutely sure of his diagnosis, he commits an error in telling the patient something which he himself would be afraid to hear. Such cases are numerous, and Dr. Bates and I both know that they come to us feeling that it is their last hope. Their fear is always noticeable.

A case which is worth mentioning is that of a woman over fifty years old, who came with little hope of being cured. She had been treated and fitted with glasses by several eye specialists without any relief of pain or improvement in her sight. Two doctors who had examined her said that all her pain was caused by glaucoma, which she had in both eyes. She said that she had a constant fear of going blind, and many times had a strong desire to end her life. The effort to conceal this desire from her family, who loved her dearly, produced more tension and strain.

Dr. Bates examined her eyes thoroughly and said that there was no opacity of the lens or other parts of either eye. Both optic nerve and retina were normal. Her vision of the test card, with each eye separately, was 10/40. Although the letters were blurred, she could tell what they were. I noticed that she stared a great deal as she explained her trouble to me. Since palming usually stops the stare with most patients, I taught her to palm, being sure to keep up a steady flow of conversation in order to distract her attention from her eyes.

I knew that she had been studying Dr. Bates' book, *Perfect Sight Without Glasses,* and I asked her what she thought the Doctor meant in his book by mental pictures. She said that she had no mental pictures while her eyes were closed and covered. I knew then that she made an effort to imagine things with her eyes closed, so I did not mention mental pictures again. However, I did not get away from the subject, but while talking I mentioned the color of the dress which she wore and asked her if she could remember the design in the trimming of her dress. She explained the design accurately. Then I asked her which she thought was the whitest white, a white cloud in a blue sky or a drift of snow. She answered that she could think of nothing whiter than the white of snow. All this time, I believe that she had had mental pictures of the white cloud and the snow, as well as the design in the trimming of her dress. While her eyes were still covered, I asked her if she had any pain. She said no, that she had forgotten all about it.

She was then taught to sway her body while standing with her feet about one foot apart. She did this very gracefully. I told her to keep up a constant blinking of her eyes as she swayed from side to side, getting a glimpse of the letters of the test card ten feet away. She was instructed to look at only one letter at a time and to quickly look away from the card to avoid the tendency to stare or strain. We continued to practice this for ten minutes and, in order to keep up her interest, I swayed with her all the time. Her vision improved to 10/20 and she said every letter was clear and distinct.

In treating her again the next day, I used a different test card, the pothooks card with the letter "E" pointing in various directions. She had faithfully carried out instructions which had been given her for home treatment, otherwise she could not have gained as much as she had in so short a time. Her vision with each eye separately was 10/15. Other cards were used, but she did not read them so well. Sometimes this happens, especially with patients as nervous as she.

It is strange that some of us have likes and dislikes, even with an ordinary test card. This fact ought to convince school nurses and doctors that when children's eyes are being examined with the various test cards, they cannot do so well with some cards as they can with others. A person with an unsympathetic mind would scoff at the idea that a test card could make a difference in the vision, but it is a fact which can be demonstrated.

To vary her treatment, I used a small test card with the Fundamental principles of the method, written by Dr. Bates, on the opposite side. The letters on this card are printed in unusually large reading type at the top of the card, and they gradually decrease in size to very fine print, or diamond type, at the bottom of the card. When she first took the small card, she held it at arm's length in order to read the largest type on the card. Rather than worry her by telling her to hold the card closer, I took her out in the sunshine, told her to close her eyes, and gave her the sun treatment with the sun glass. At first she drew her head away, indicating that she did not like it. In a soft tone of voice, which I had used from the beginning and which I realized helped to alleviate her nervousness and fear, I suggested that she let me try it again. I told her that babies enjoyed the sun treatment when the sun glass was used on their closed eyes. I explained how many of our boys who returned from France after the war enjoyed this wonderful sun treatment which Dr. Bates had discovered was so beneficial for all sorts of eye troubles. During all the time that I talked with her, I used the sun glass on her eyes. I noticed that she responded, because her body relaxed and she settled in a more comfortable position in her chair. When I stopped the movement of the sun glass for a moment, she immediately asked for more, so I continued using it on her closed eyes for more than twenty minutes. After this treatment she read three sentences of the Fundamentals card, at eight inches from her eyes. The type of the third sentence is about the size of book type.

During her third treatment, she smiled most of the time, whereas she had been very sad before. She suggested that I test her sight with a strange test card. By swaying her body from side to side as she stood twelve feet from the card, she read the 10-line letters, one at a time, looking away from the card after seeing each letter.

Having watched her carefully, I noticed that at times she forgot to blink. When she finished reading the card and complained of a burning in her eyes, I reminded her that she had not been blinking often enough while reading the test card. She then practiced blinking often, just as the normal eye does.

I believe she will always remember the next treatment she had. The balcony which surrounds our office is a delightful place on sunny days, and I gave her sun treatment there for almost half an hour. Then we turned our backs to the sun, and I placed my book, *Stories from the Clinic,* in her lap. Before she started to read, I took one of the small black test cards, with white letters, and put it on the opposite side of the page which she was reading. By looking at a white letter of the test card, she began immediately to read sentence after sentence of the book. For the first time in twenty years, she was able to read book type without glasses. During her last treatment, she read words and numbers in the telephone book. Her pain was gone; she no longer wished to die, and she is now a happy woman, because she can read her books without the aid of glasses.

LETTERS AND REPORT

BLIND AUNT KATE

Editor's Note—*We take pleasure in publishing the following letters from a patient of Dr. Bates.*

My dear Dr. Bates:

May I take a few minutes of your time to read something very interesting which I am eager to tell you?

It is the case of a smart old lady of 86. She is called "Blind Aunt Kate" and I thought when I met her, that she must be totally blind, as I saw her grope her way along. She was unable to distinguish me from someone else, although my face was within six inches from her face. A week ago today, August 29, I tested her eyes outdoors in the sunlight. At first she was unable to see the large "E" on the black card; then she read it at eight inches, and later at eighteen inches. After palming for five minutes, she distinguished it at twenty-eight inches and at thirty-six inches; after palming again, the "F" and "P" came out at eight inches, and after palming again, at twenty-six inches. The following day she saw "L P E D" at thirty-five inches and the large "E" at sixty-six inches. Also she was able to see all the rest of the lines at various distances and two letters of the very last line at six inches. Today is dark and rainy, but she showed great progress after one week's work. Indoors, she could distinguish the large "E" at seventy-six inches; "F P" at sixty inches; and "T O Z" came out still more clearly at sixty-nine inches. Also, through the rain she could see the barn, a wagon in the yard, the path and road and a stone fence following the road, things which she hasn't been able to see on a bright day for over a year. She also distinguished different faces, including mine, half way across a large room.

She is so happy over her week's improvement, she says if she can see this well for the rest of her life, she won't complain. She is very faithful in her work and would gladly do anything more that I would suggest. I have done nothing but have her palm, blink frequently (she has been staring so persistently), swing her eyes horizontally, and see things moving by as she walks.

Her eye doctor here used to call her trouble an enlargement of the eyeball and said glasses would do her no good. She wore glasses for forty-five years and took them off a year ago. She has not read even coarse print in four years. She says for the past two months her eyes had failed so rapidly that she was trying to resign herself to utter blindness. She is a very sweet, patient old lady and is quite unhappy from outside influences, so I am very eager to give her all the help for her eyes I can. It almost seems as if my mother's spirit has led me right to her. If you could give me some special exercises for her to follow, I could help her even more, I'm sure, in the two weeks remaining of my vacation. On a bright day she can see every letter of the black "E" card. I am just beginning to work with her on the white card, but today indoors she could read the first three lines as far off as on the black card. I did not test her on the rest of the lines.

Hoping I am not asking too much of an already busy man, and thanking you, I remain, Alice Avery Price.

The following letter came a few days later:

Dear Dr. Bates:

Your very encouraging letter was received and made both Aunt Kate and myself very happy. I should be very glad indeed to have you publish her story, and she says too, that it would make her so happy if she thought someone else might be helped through her experience.

She has been ill for two days so that I had to discontinue the work on the card. She has, however, kept resting her eyes and at 6 o'clock this evening, when it was very gloomy, we sat at an upper window together and she suddenly remarked, "Now, I can see that old stone wall across the road so plainly!" I hope tomorrow we can resume the work with the card.

I wrote you on September 5, which was, I believe, a dark day and just one week from the day I first tested her eyes. The next day was sunny again and I tested her eyes with this result, which you will agree was splendid. The large "E" she saw at 174 inches; "F P" at 136 inches; "T O Z" at 142 inches; "L P E D" at 78 inches; "P E C F D" at 53 inches; "E D F" etc. at 41 inches (all but "Z," which she saw at 35 inches); "D E F P" etc. at 13 inches. The last two lines she made out entirely by holding the card closer to her eyes.

So, according to my most careful measurements she saw the various lines at from five to ten and seventeen times the distance she saw them eight days previous.

I am telling you this in such detail so that you will realize there is no mistake in my previous story. I measured the distance so carefully on each occasion. You may also make use of these latest figures in your magazine account of Aunt Kate if you wish.

Sincerely yours,

Alice Avery Price, White Plains, New York.

Cured in One Visit

A report from Anna Woessner, Teacher of Dr. Bates Method.

Madeline, age 12, had very poor vision for things up close, and in school was unable to distinguish figures on the blackboard. Outdoors, all objects at 20 feet or farther were blurred to her. She had worn glasses for a year and they constantly annoyed her. When she heard about the Bates Method of treatment and that I was treating patients, she was eager to obtain help from me so as to discard her glasses, if possible. When I met her, the only test card available was a small letter card with the "Fundamentals" by W. H. Bates, M.D. printed on the opposite side. The test card begins with the letter "C" which can be seen clearly with the normal eye at fifty feet. Madeline could not see even this letter clearly at five feet. While palming I asked her to describe her doll to me. Then she told me about her bicycle and imagined it was moving with her as she was riding. Before she opened her eyes to look at the card, I put it off at a distance of eight feet and told her to stand, open her eyes, sway her body, and while blinking to look at the card, then at a birdcage nearby. Without a stop she read up to line 5, "C G O," or the letters which are seen by the normal eye at fifteen feet. With more practice of this kind, her vision improved from the third to the bottom line at nine feet away. These letters are read by the normal eye at four feet.

Sun treatment was given her which she enjoyed, and this helped to improve her near vision, so that she could read the finest print of the Fundamentals on the opposite side of the small test card. Madeline had just one treatment. Greatly encouraged, she promised to practice often every day and not put on her glasses again. One month later I saw her again, but she did not need another treatment. Her vision was normal at the near point as well as for the distance.

Madeline's sister Regina is 15 years old. She has congenital astigmatism and, although she has worn glasses for ten years, she still "hates them." Without glasses, her eyes were mere slits. Her vision was 10/40 with the left eye and 10/30 with the right.

After impressing her with the importance of shifting and blinking, which she had been very careful not to do, I gave her a short period of sun treatment. At first this was distressing, as she was unable to open her eyelids for even a moment. After swaying, with closed eyes, this was overcome, and at the end of the treatment she read the greater part of the 10-line.

After several more treatments, her vision became practically normal. She is continuing her treatment under my supervision, and after a few more I feel confident that her vision will be normal.

"THE SWING"

By Ms. A. J. Campbell

All things are in Motion;
Let's fall into time,
And Swing along with them,
While chanting this rhyme.

We'll keep our swing steady,
By Grandmother's Clock,
Its pendulum swinging,
Its measured tick-tock.

In Memory I'm seeing
A fine old elm tree;
Its low-hanging branches
Seem beck'ning to me.

A brown bird sits rocking
On that topmost limb.
I wonder who taught
The Bates System to him.

With eyes all a-sparkle,
Face turned to the Sun,
His head ever turning,
His day is begun.

White clouds float above him
In limitless blue;
His wee throat is swollen
With song, the day thru.

Teach us, then, oh brown bird,
To start our day right;

That our Eyes like yours,
May be sparkling and bright.

—Ms. A. J. Campbell, patient of Dr. Jean B. Claverie, Chicago, Illinois.

QUESTIONS AND ANSWERS

Q–1. What causes redness and smarting sensation of the eye even when plenty of sun treatment has been given? Should one continue with sun treatment under the circumstances?

A–1. Take the sun treatment frequently for five or ten minutes at a time daily, increasing the length of time until the eyes become accustomed to the sun. The eyes should always be benefited after the sun treatment, and one should always feel relaxed. When done properly, the redness and smarting should soon disappear. If the eyes are not benefited, it is an indication that you strain while taking the treatment. Alternate the sun treatment with palming or closing the eyes to rest them.

Q–2. What makes the eyes seem extremely heavy upon rising in the morning?

A–2. Eyestrain while sleeping. See the May number of *Better Eyesight* on Presbyopia.

Q–3. Is it harmful to sit facing the sun, while reading a book in the shade, thus getting sun treatment?

A–3. To sit facing the sun, while reading a book, is not injurious to the eyes, provided the patient is comfortable. Some people become uncomfortable, which produces a strain, and the sun is of little benefit under such conditions.

Q–4. Does sun treatment have to be continuous to be effective, or can short spells be substituted?

A–4. Sun treatment does not have to be continuous. Short periods are equally beneficial.

Q–5. Is resting the eyes by palming a more effective cure for smarting of the eyes than the sun treatment XE "sun treatment"?

A–5. This depends upon the individual. Some are benefited more by palming, while others receive more benefit from the sun treatment.

Q–6. Should sun treatment be moderated due to the heat of the sun—as in the tropics.

A–6. Take as much sun treatment as you can with the eyes closed while slowly moving the head a short distance from side to side to avoid discomfort from the heat. Should it make you uncomfortable and nervous, lessen the length of time that the sun treatment is employed.

Better Eyesight
November 1926—Vol. XI, No. 5

DEMONSTRATE: IMAGINATION

By practicing you can imagine a letter at ten feet as well as you can see it at one foot.

Regard a letter of the Snellen test card at a distance where it cannot be readily distinguished and appears blurred. Now look at the same letter on a card at the near point, one foot or less, where it can be seen perfectly. Then close your eyes and with your finger draw the same letter in the air as well as you can remember it. Open your eyes and continue to draw the imaginary letter with your finger while looking for only a few seconds at the blurred letter on the card at ten feet. Then close your eyes again and remember the letter well enough to draw the letter perfectly in your imagination with your finger. Alternate drawing the letter at ten feet in your imagination with your eyes open and drawing it with your eyes closed as well as you see it at one foot or nearer. When you can draw the letter as perfectly as you remember it, you see the letter on the distant card in flashes.

By repetition you will become able not only to always imagine the known letter correctly, but to actually see it for a few seconds at a time. You cannot see a letter perfectly unless you see one part best, central fixation. Note that you obtain central fixation while practicing this method, i.e., you see one part best. Drawing the letter with your finger in your imagination enables you to follow the finger in forming the letter, and with the help of your memory you can imagine each side of the letter best, in turn, as it is formed. By this method the memory and the imagination are improved, and when the imagination becomes perfect, the sight is perfect. You can cure the highest degrees of myopia, hypermetropia, astigmatism, atrophy of the optic nerve, cataract, glaucoma, detachment of the retina and other diseases by this method.

DETACHMENT OF THE RETINA

By W. H. Bates, M.D.

Occurrence

In detachment of the retina, the inner coat of the three coats of the eyeball become separated from the other coats. At first only a small part of the retina may become separated, but later the detachment may increase in extent until the whole retina is separated from the other parts of the eye. In the early stages, the sight may be good and remain good for some months and even for some years. Usually the patient complains of a loss of vision almost from the beginning.

Detachment of the retina occurs frequently in high degrees of myopia. Some statistics report that one-third of all cases of extreme myopia sooner or later develop detachment of the retina, at first in one eye and afterwards in the other eye. However, it may occur in normal eyes without any inflammation of the other coats. The detachment, which is observed covering tumors of the eyeball, usually presents a different appearance from other forms of detachment. Detachment of the retina is a rare disease. "Galezowski found it in 5/10 of 1% of ophthalmic cases. It is supposed to be caused by muscular exertion, coughing, sneezing, vomiting, anger, or fear. Injuries of the eyeball cause a small proportion of cases." (Ball.)

I believe that mental or ocular strain is the principal cause.

Symptoms

"In the beginning, the symptoms of detachment are periodical dimness of vision, flashes of light and the appearance of sparks, dust or soot before the eyes. The field of vision becomes less and there may be the appearance of a cloud or floating specks before the eye. Patients have complained that they can see only a part of an object at a time. So long as the center of sight is not involved, the vision of objects straight ahead is good. Sometimes the detached retina may be functional for a time, producing vertigo. In uncomplicated cases, there is no pain." (Ball.)

Orthodox Methods Of Treatment

Ball in his *Modern Ophthalmology* states, "The treatment of retinal detachment is an unsatisfactory—in fact, almost hopeless—task. While in a few rare instances the retina has become reattached spontaneously, and a few recoveries have followed the administration of saline purgatives, and some cures have followed the internal use of mercury, iodide of potassium, and salicylic acid, the majority of successful results thus far reported have been attributed to surgical intervention. Surgical intervention, proposed by Sichel in 1859, has assumed numerous forms: simple puncture of the sclera and choroid (Sichel), discission of the retina (Von Graefe), drainage by a fine gold wire passed to the choroid by means of catgut (Galezowski), dislaceration with two needles (Bowman), iridectomy (Galezowski and others), injection of iodine into the subretinal space (Galezowski, Gelpke, Scholer), electrolysis (Gillet de Grandmont), cutting of vitreous bands and transfixion of the eyeball (Deutscbmann, Jaencke), injection of a 3.5 percent strength solution of gelatin in a physiologic salt solution between the sclera and capsule of Tenon (de Wecker), puncture of the eyeball with the galvano-cautery (Galezowski, Abadie), injection of normal salt solution into the vitreous after evacuation of subretinal fluid (Walker), and injection of air into the vitreous (Jensen). Most of these procedures should be ruled out of the domain of modern ophthalmology. All are dangerous to the integrity of the globe, and one of them, intra-ocular injection of iodine—has been followed by meningitis and death."

Holth (*Wien. Med. Woch.,* February 3, 1912) claimed that in cases of detachment of the retina, a piece of the sclera was excised from the eye without injuring any of the coats of the eye (choroid). The hardness of the eyeball was then diminished for some weeks or months, and in two cases the detachment of the retina disappeared and the field of vision became enlarged, but vision itself did not improve. The most important point was that in one case the myopia decreased from 18 diopters to 5 diopters, in another from 16 diopters to 10 diopters and in a third case from 12 diopters to 5.5 diopters.

The author explains the effect of the operation as follows, "In the first months after the operation, subchoroideal lymph oozes through the opening in Tenon's capsule and on account of this the absorptive capacity of the choroid is increased. By the traction of the outer eye muscles, the walls of the myopic eye become compressed, and the myopic refraction becomes diminished."

The Writer's Method Of Treatment

The results of the preceding methods of treating detachment of the retina, as well as of many other methods which are not reported, have been practically of no benefit. It is my desire to call attention to the fact that detachment of the retina is curable because it has been cured. In the course of a lifetime, most ophthalmologists have seen one or more cases of detachment which recovered spontaneously, or without any treatment. This fact suggests that if some patients recover without treatment, detachment is curable under certain conditions. It can be demonstrated that the cause of detachment of the retina is a mental strain and is not necessarily due to an injury to the eye by a blow. If it is due to mental strain, relaxation of the mental strain should be followed by a benefit. In all cases of retinal detachment which I have observed, relaxation methods of treatment have always been followed by an improvement or a cure of the detachment. These methods of obtaining relaxation are those which are unconsciously practiced by the normal eye when the normal eye has normal vision. For example, the stare or the effort to see distant or near objects, always causes imperfect sight. Rest or relaxation of the eyes is always a benefit to those with imperfect sight. The normal eye is moving all the time, and an effort to keep the normal eye stationary is always followed by imperfect sight. People with normal eyes and normal sight are always moving their heads and eyes from one point to another, and do not look fixedly at any one point continuously.

One can rest the eyes by blinking without necessarily staring or straining. To keep the eyes wide open continuously always makes the sight worse. Patients with detachment of the retina use their eyes in the wrong way, just as nearsighted people use their eyes incorrectly. In many cases of detachment, the patients suffer from the annoyance of bright sunlight. By gradually accustoming the eye to the sun, the symptoms of retinal detachment usually improve.

Cases

A sharpshooter came to me for treatment of detachment of the retina. He said that when he saw the bull's-eye at 1000 yards, it appeared to be moving. When he tried to stop the movement, the effort made him very nervous and his sight became so imperfect that he could not see the bull's-eye at all. When he allowed the bull's-eye to move, the score was better. At that time, he spent so many hours at target practice that he became very nervous and tired. The interesting fact was that the left eye which was not used in aiming, developed detachment of the retina while the right eye, which was used almost constantly, remained normal. If the detachment were caused by eyestrain, we would expect the eye which was used to be affected. On the contrary, the eye that was not used developed detachment of the retina. It was the strain of his mind, and not the strain of his eyes which caused the retinal detachment.

The dark glasses which he was wearing to protect his eyes from the sun were so strong that they seriously interfered with the vision of his good eye. The left eye had very disagreeable symptoms. He imagined he saw red, blue and other colored lights. All the treatment that he had received in the hospital had not relieved these sensations. These lights disappeared after he had practiced the various swings for many hours daily. Subjective symptoms disappeared first, and when he became able to obtain a considerable amount of relaxation, the objective symptoms of detachment then disappeared. The treatment which brought about this result was much the same treatment that is employed in the cure of myopia, astigmatism, farsightedness, or squint. Relaxation or rest was very beneficial. Palming was particularly helpful. Any treatment which promoted relaxation was always followed by an improvement in the detachment of the retina.

A patient suffering from a high degree of myopia which was progressive was suddenly afflicted with detachment of the retina in one eye. He received the usual orthodox treatment from a number of ophthalmologists living in Pittsburgh, New York, Chicago, and other places, but without any benefit. When he finally came to me and was treated by relaxation methods for the relief of the high degree of myopia, the detachment became less and the myopia decreased. Considerable relaxation was obtained by the practice of the optical swing, which has been described many times in this magazine. He was first treated on July 30, 1925. The vision of the right eye was 8/200, while that of the left eye, which had the retinal detachment, was only 1/200. Looking straight ahead with his left eye, his vision was imperfect. At times he had some vision, for a few seconds only, while looking straight ahead.

His visits to the office were irregular. On October 17, 1925, after three month's treatment, the vision of the right eye had improved to 15/200, while that of the left eye was 15/200 plus. After the long swing, the vision of the right eye immediately improved to 15/100, while that of the left eye improved to 15/100 plus. With the ophthalmoscope, the retina appeared reattached and was otherwise normal. The field of vision was normal.

The patient returned home very much pleased. However, he made a mistake, I believe, in calling on some of the eye specialists whom be had previously consulted and who had all pronounced his imperfect vision from the detachment to be incurable. Some told him that they must have made a mistake in diagnosing his case, because if he had had detachment of the retina, the eye would not have recovered. They believed that all the other men who had made the diagnosis of the detachment of the retina had also made a monumental blunder. This would have been perfectly satisfactory, but unfortunately the patient neglected the treatment I had prescribed and had a relapse. He again visited the same eye specialists without being encouraged, and when he came back to me, he was very much discouraged.

I believe that he would have returned sooner had not the other ophthalmologists influenced him against the relaxation treatment.

After studying these and other cases, I believe that the cause of detachment of the retina is usually some form of mental strain. It is gratifying to have proved that when this strain is relieved, the detachment of the retina disappears and the eye becomes normal.

STORIES FROM THE CLINIC

No. 81: Mind Strain

By Emily C. Lierman

There are many causes of mind strain and hundreds of people suffer from its effects without realizing it. People who have difficult problems to solve are subject to mind strain. Business and financial worries also cause mind strain, which is usually accompanied by eyestrain. If these people are taught the proper way to relax, mind and eyestrain can soon be relieved. It is not easy to relax. Osteopathy helps some people, but the difficulty lies in being able to continue the relaxation methods after the doctor has completed his treatment. This is true of the Bates Method of relaxation. Most patients who have been treated for eyestrain leave the office after their first treatment feeling entirely relieved of pain, fatigue, and mind strain, and with decided improvement in their vision, either for the distance, the near point or both. Such patients obtain normal vision permanently by carrying out at home the advice given by the Doctor.

Many patients ask why their pain or other discomforts return after treatment. The answer is obvious. It is caused by a patient not continuing the practice, or by trying too hard while practicing. We are very apt to forget that which is most essential for obtaining better eyesight—relaxation and rest of mind and body. Always remember that the eye is at rest only when it is moving. Dr. Bates emphasizes this fact because patients so often forget. When the mind is under a strain, it is difficult to solve a problem or to think clearly.

A well-known business man from the West called to see Dr. Bates not long ago. He had been warned that Dr. Bates was not sincere nor scientific. The man was too busy to experiment with new ideas in eye treatment, so he went to Europe hoping to find a doctor there who could cure his eyestrain and the intense pains in his head. Opticians in Europe did their utmost to relieve him. When specialists in England failed to help him, he tried Germany, France, Switzerland and Italy. Had his search only carried him to Spain, he might have found Dr. Ruiz Arnau of Madrid, who is now there introducing Dr. Bates' method into schools, and to those medical doctors who desire to learn a better way of obtaining perfect vision than the use of eyeglasses. Dr. Arnau became interested in the Bates Method some years ago when he himself was suffering with continual headaches and other discomforts caused by mind and eyestrain. He came from San Juan, Puerto Rico, leaving a good practice to seek the only Doctor who could help him. Dr. Arnau has shown his appreciation for what Dr. Bates has done for him by writing a book entitled, *El Uso Natural de la Vision,* which he dedicated to Dr. Bates.

Many other doctors, who were seemingly incurable, have come to us and were cured. They in turn help their patients so that eyeglasses can be discarded, or not become necessary.

The Westerner came back to America feeling very much discouraged, and with no hope of being cured. In a skeptical frame of mind, he came to Dr. Bates, as a last resort. After one treatment, in which he was entirely relieved of pain, he placed himself in Dr. Bates' care and in less than two weeks of daily treatment, was able to read letters, newspapers, and book type without the aid of eyeglasses. Many patients have visited Dr. Bates, through his recommendation, and his letters to Dr. Bates are full of gratitude for the cure of his mind and eyestrain.

When patients learn how to do their work without effort or strain, regardless of the nature of the work, their mind, memory, and most of all their imagination is improved.

During the summer months of this year, I cured a woman with a terrific amount of mind strain. She obtained no relief until she realized that making an effort to see, in reading, sewing, or doing other things, prevented a cure. "Take things easily," is only a short sentence of three words, but I repeated that sentence to her seventy times seven before she realized its great significance. I gave her a treatment daily for some weeks and when she left for her home, many miles from New York, she said she felt like a new woman, and would always be grateful for the results I had helped her to obtain. She now reads her books without the aid of eyeglasses, which she had worn constantly for more than twenty years. Palming, the long swing of her body, and reading the test card one letter at a time, helped. Constantly reminding her to blink was most necessary.

Mind strain causes many things. It destroys the finest nature and many an innocent human being, and often drives people far away from pleasant surroundings, killing quicker than any electric storm.

It is not always easy to treat severe cases. When a patient has been under a strain for a length of time, it is sometimes difficult to relieve the strain permanently in a short time.

Patients vary in their response to treatment. While some obtain permanent relief in a few visits, others find it necessary to place themselves under treatment for a longer period.

QUESTIONS AND ANSWERS

Q–1. Is age a factor in the cure of imperfect sight without glasses?

A–1. Age is not a factor. I have cured hundreds of patients past sixty.

Q–2. What method is best to relieve the tension in the back of the neck?

A–2. The variable swing.

Q–3. Is the swing apt to cause nystagmus?

A–3. No; the swing relieves strain, whereas nystagmus is caused by eyestrain.

Q–4. What causes the lids of the eyes to itch and sometimes become scaly?

A–4. This is due to strain. Practice relaxation methods all day long—shifting, blinking and central fixation. Get as much sun treatment as possible.

Q–5. What causes my vision to improve for a day or two, and then relapse?

A–5. This is caused by lack of practice and by straining your eyes. When the vision is good, you are relaxed.

Q–6. In palming, should one close the eyes tightly?

A–6. No; easily, lazily and naturally at all times.

Better Eyesight
December 1926—Vol. XI, No. 6

DEMONSTRATE: EFFORT

It requires an effort or a strain to produce imperfect sight.

Look at the notch at the top of the big "C" of the Snellen test card at fifteen feet. Keep your eyes fixed on the notch. Make an effort to see it and increase that effort as much as you possibly can. Notice that it is difficult to keep your eyes and mind fixed on that one point. Notice also that it is tiresome and makes your eyes pain. If you keep it up long enough, your head begins to ache and all the nerves of your body are strained.

If you look at some of the letters on the lower lines which are much smaller than the big "C," they may appear so blurred that you are not able to distinguish them. Trying to see these small letters blurs them still more.

Now hold the test card in your hand about one foot from your eyes. The big "C" is seen plainly and without any effort. Try to see the top and the bottom of the big "C" perfectly black at the same time. Notice that the "C" becomes blurred and the strain which blurs it also gives much discomfort.

From this evidence, we can conclude that perfect sight comes easily, without any effort or strain, while imperfect sight is always produced by a strain or an effort to see.

ASTIGMATISM

By W. H. Bates, M.D.

Many people who have astigmatism often talk about it in a boastful way as though it were a mark of distinction. This is not so strange, considering the fact that so many eye doctors claim that astigmatism does more harm to the eyes and nerves than any other condition. They tell their patients that in order to prevent serious eye diseases, glasses should be worn constantly. Such patients, accordingly, become much worried and are in constant fear of serious eye trouble developing and probable blindness resulting. It is true that the glasses prescribed may give temporary relief, but no patient under my observation was ever cured or benefited very much by glasses.

Definitions

The normal eye is spherical in shape and all the meridians are of the same curvature. The curvature of the cornea is like that of a segment of a sphere; but when astigmatism is present, it is said to be lopsided; that is, one principal meridian of the curvature is more convex than the meridian at right angles to it. With an instrument called the ophthalmometer, it is possible to measure all the meridians of the curvature of the comes.

Astigmatism may be simple hypermetropic, simple myopic, compound hypermetropic, compound myopic, mixed or irregular.

In Simple Hypermetropic Astigmatism, one principal meridian of the cornea has a normal curvature, while the meridian at right angles to it is flatter than all the other meridians.

In Simple Myopic Astigmatism, one principal meridian of the cornea has a normal curvature, while the meridian at right angles to it is more convex than all the other meridians.

In Compound Hypermetropic Astigmatism, the two principal meridians are flatter than the meridians of the normal eye, one being flatter than the other.

In Compound Myopic Astigmatism, the two principal meridians are more convex than a normal meridian, one being more convex than the other.

In Mixed Astigmatism, one of the principal meridians is flatter than a meridian of the normal eye, while the other principal meridian is more convex than a meridian of the normal eye.

In Irregular Astigmatism, the meridians of the curvature of the cornea are so malformed that no glasses can correct the astigmatism.

Occurrence

Astigmatism is the most common defect of the human eye. Most people with astigmatism have had it since birth. In some cases it may increase, while in other cases it may become less or entirely disappear.

Nine-tenths of the cases of astigmatism are due to imperfect curvature of two or more meridians of the cornea. The other cases of astigmatism are due to imperfect curvature of the lens, or less frequently to a malformation of the eyeball.

Symptoms

When a high degree of astigmatism is present, the vision is appreciably lowered. Usually when vertical lines are regarded, they may appear more distinct than horizontal lines, or the reverse may be true. It was found that so many patients with astigmatism failed to see vertical lines as well as horizontal lines, or had trouble in seeing oblique lines, that a card, called the clock-faced card, was designed with lines at various angles. At one time it was believed that astigmatism could be diagnosed when the patient was able to see horizontal lines on this card better than the vertical lines or vice versa. Some patients with astigmatism could see distinctly the line pointing to five o'clock, while the line at right angles to it could not be seen so well. With increased experience, however, it was found that some patients with astigmatism could see horizontal and vertical lines equally well. On the other hand, patients with normal vision have complained that they did not always see vertical or horizontal lines equally well.

A man, sixty years old, was found to have unusually good vision without any symptoms of astigmatism; but when he regarded a number of vertical, horizontal, and oblique lines, his vision immediately became very imperfect with a production of six diopters of astigmatism. When he closed his eyes and rested them, his vision soon became normal and the astigmatism disappeared.

Cause

The cause of astigmatism is always associated with an effort or a strain. In all cases the stare can be demonstrated. An imperfect memory requires an effort or a strain and always produces astigmatism. An imperfect imagination also requires an effort or strain and always produces astigmatism. A mental strain of any kind always causes astigmatism. In the normal eye, astigmatism can be produced with a very slight amount of strain or effort to see. In those cases, however, where a great effort is made for a length of time, the astigmatism becomes very much increased, and may be more or less permanent. Irregular astigmatism is caused by the contraction of scar tissue, either from ulcerations of the cornea or from an incised wound.

Treatment

Some years ago, I published an article in the *Archives of Ophthalmology* with the title, "A New Operation for the Cure of Astigmatism—A Preliminary Report." In this article, I described an operation in which the more convex meridian of the cornea was incised at right angles to its curvature, but not penetrating into the anterior chamber. The scar produced by the cut of the knife usually healed very promptly, and the traction of the scar tissue flattened the curvature of this principal meridian. A number of cases were reported with good results. It was not very long, however, before I had some unsuccessful experiences in which, for some reason or other, the operation failed. The theory was so good that I expected the facts to verify it. I became disappointed with my operation and did not investigate the facts any further after the first six months. A year or two later, my operation was performed by someone in England, and a report of some interesting cases that were apparently cured was published in an English medical journal. Other articles were published in medical journals, confirming my earlier claims and giving me due credit.

I no longer believe that an operation of any kind should be performed because all forms of astigmatism can be demonstrated to be always temporary. Astigmatism is not organic; it is always functional, even when scar tissue is associated with it.

Scar Tissue

It is very interesting to observe cases of astigmatism in which scar tissue of the cornea is a complication. Scar tissue, as is well known, is composed largely of new connective tissue. With the aid of the memory and the imagination, this connective tissue sometimes disappears in a very short time. When the memory is perfect for some letter, color, or object, the scar tissue disappears. When the imagination is perfect for a letter or other object, the scar tissue disappears. Imagination or memory of perfect sight is a cure for astigmatism.

Conical Cornea

The most serious effect of astigmatism is to produce conical cornea. In this disease, the front part of the eyeball becomes more conical in shape, and after some years the apex of the cone becomes ulcerated. This ulcer becomes steadily worse with an increase of the astigmatism. Not only is the vision progressively lowered, but the patient may also suffer from severe pain. There is no operation which has been generally accepted which is satisfactory in correcting conical cornea, nor has any treatment heretofore practiced been curative or even beneficial.

The treatment in my experience which has yielded the best results is the practice of the variable swing. The patient holds the forefinger of one hand about six inches in front and to one side of the eyes. When he moves his head a short distance from side to side, the finger appears to move in the direction opposite to the movement of the head and eyes.

While practicing the variable swing, the patient is directed to regard one known letter of the Snellen test card at ten or fifteen feet, and imagine it as well as he can with his eyes open for a few seconds. The eyes are quickly closed while the patient remembers the same letter more perfectly than it was seen. He then opens his eyes and imagines the known letter on the card as well as he can for a few seconds. The patient alternately remembers the known letter perfectly with the eyes closed and imagines it with the eyes open for a few seconds, until he becomes able to imagine he sees the known letter nearly as well with his eyes open as he can remember it with his eyes closed. By this method, the patient can improve his vision for each known or unknown letter of the Snellen test card. It is remarkable how promptly the conical cornea subsides when the variable swing is practiced in this way. Some patients have obtained normal vision in a much shorter time than one would expect.

Case Reports

Recently a man, age sixty, was treated by me for the relief of eye troubles, caused by one-quarter of a diopter of astigmatism. He suffered intensely from strong light and complained of floating specks. He was not able to read fine print with or without glasses for any length of time without pain and fatigue. It seemed very strange that he should suffer so much from so low a degree of astigmatism. His distant vision was almost normal, while his ability to read was only slightly impaired by the pain. When his astigmatism was corrected by treatment, his vision with each eye for distance improved until it became normal and the floating specks disappeared. After practicing the swing and improving his vision for the Snellen test card, the fatigue which he had felt when working and reading was also lessened. He no longer suffered from discomfort in the strong light of the sun after he had received the sun treatment with the sun glass.

Hypermetropic Astigmatism

About a month ago, a fourteen year old girl came to me for treatment. She had about three diopters of hypermetropic astigmatism in each eye. The vision of each eye was one-half of the normal. After practicing rest and the short sway of her body for an hour or longer, her vision became almost normal without glasses.

Without any treatment, she read the fine print imperfectly at twelve inches. She was directed to close her eyes and to imagine the spaces between the lines to be as white as snow, white starch, whitewash or a white handkerchief. With her eyes open and moving her head a short distance from side to side, she became able to imagine the white spaces between the lines to be more perfectly white. By alternating, her imagination of the white spaces increased, until she became able to read diamond type at six inches or less, without any fatigue or discomfort. Her ability to read had been improved by her imagination. When her symptoms were relieved by this treatment, it was found with the aid of the retinoscope that the astigmatism had disappeared.

Compound Myopic Astigmatism

Another patient was a girl, age fifteen. The vision of the right eye was one-third of the normal, while that of the left eye was one-fifth of the normal. She was wearing glasses for the correction of compound myopic astigmatism, in which the astigmatism in each eye was less than one diopter. With the aid of palming, swinging, and the use of her imagination, her vision became normal in each eye and the astigmatism disappeared.

This patient had but one treatment and obtained a quick cure, which is very unusual.

Simple Hypermetropic Astigmatism

On June 1, 1924, a man, thirty years old, became a patient. The vision of his right eye was 10/70, while that of the left eye was 3/200. For the correction of astigmatism he was wearing a convex 5.00 D. C. in the right eye and convex 5.50 D. C. in the left eye. His glasses were not satisfactory, and he suffered from double vision.

He could not remember mental pictures or read fine print. After palming, swaying, flashing and blinking, his vision was temporarily improved and the double vision disappeared. He obtained a considerable amount of rest from the drifting swing. The universal swing was also a great benefit. His ability to read was improved by having him imagine the white spaces between the lines of black letters to be whiter than they really were. It helped when he imagined that he was painting the white spaces with white paint, alternately with his eyes closed and with his eyes open. [My students pretend they use a nose-paintbrush.—TRQ] His vision was very much improved by the imagination of the white centers of most letters to be whiter than they really are.

His visits were irregular. Nevertheless, on October 22, the vision of the right eye had improved to the normal, while the vision of the left eye had improved to 15/70. With the aid of the retinoscope, it was demonstrated that the astigmatism of the right eye had entirely disappeared, while that of the left eye was very much reduced.

The histories of these cases indicate the possibilities of relieving all degrees of astigmatism without the use of glasses.

STORIES FROM THE CLINIC
No. 82: The Christmas Party
By Emily C. Lierman

The same Christmas spirit prevailed at our Clinic last year as it had in other years. This time our tree was more beautiful than ever. . . .

Among the children was a boy, age ten, whose father was a foreigner and could not speak very good English. This little chap had been coming to the Clinic for some time before Christmas and was being treated for hysterical blindness. A note from his teacher explained why she had sent him to me. The school nurse said that he was mentally deficient. He knew the alphabet and could read numbers, but could not spell a word. The nurse and teacher were under the impression that glasses might help the condition of his mind, as well as his sight. His name was difficult for me to remember, so I called him Bobby. Bobby always kept his head lowered and his eyes almost closed while I talked to him. Until his third visit, his answers to my questions were unintelligible. His father was always ready to reply to the questions I asked Bobby, but I could not understand him either.

After many failures in trying to interest Bobby in the test cards with various letters and numbers, I turned to a large geographical globe in my room and began to turn it, at first slowly, and then more quickly. He watched me, raised his head and opened his eyes wide. I observed him closely as his staring eyes, scarcely blinking, followed the turning of this strange thing that fascinated him. His facial expression changed and I knew that he was interested. Slowly he came toward the globe and gave it a turn or two himself. I was hoping he would do that, but his father apparently did not want him to touch it. He rose quickly from his chair and in a rough voice ordered Bobby to be seated. Bobby's eyes again lowered and his head dropped. I had discovered one cause of Bobby's trouble. His father's harsh manner reacted upon the child's eyes. During my many years of clinical work, I have seen other fathers like him and, I am sorry to say, some mothers, too. Poor Bobby! I could not say much, but I would like to have requested the father to wait outside during the treatment, but he would not have understood.

Later Bobby made progress with the use of the pothooks card. After the third visit, Bobby's sight continued to improve and he learned to pronounce words and read them correctly.

Among others at our Christmas party, was a man who had been a brakeman on a train for some years. When his vision became so poor that glasses no longer helped him and the loss of his eyesight endangered the lives of others, he was discharged by the company for which he worked. His family of five were in want and he could not find steady work.

He had come for his first treatment, two months before Christmas. He had progressive myopia, and even with glasses he could not see clearly beyond six feet. His vision was 10/100 with each eye. Toward the end of March, less than six months later, he was again working on the freight trains without glasses, and with almost normal vision. On his last visit, his sight had improved to 10/10 and his nervous condition was benefited at the same time.

THE CROSSED EYE FAIRY

By George M. Guild

Fairies are magnetic, attractive and pretty. They are usually free from care and trouble, and spend most of their time in dancing, singing and playing with nice little boys and sweet lovable girls. Their eyes are usually bright, sparkling, loving and kind. It is very unusual for a fairy to have any eye trouble. One warm summer night while I was asleep, someone whispered in my ear, "Have you seen the crossed eye fairy?" Of all the fairies I had seen, and I had seen many thousands, not one could I remember who was crossed eye.

The whisper was so faint that it did not wake me, but it was sufficient to startle me and make me very restless. I imagined that I saw a fairy with crossed eyes and not only was one eye crooked, but her nose was also turned out of line. I tried many times, but it was not possible for me to get hold of the nose in order to twist it back to where it belonged. The fairy ran away, dodging behind bushes, trees, and flowers, just like a will-o-the-wisp. I searched everywhere in my dreams for the little sprite, but in vain.

When I woke up, I decided to visit the fairies and, if possible, have a talk with the crossed eye fairy that evening. There was a full moon so bright that I knew that the dell where the fairies assembled would be almost as bright as though it were daylight. Soon after I arrived where the fairies were gathered, I sought the Fairy Queen and found her. When she saw me, she asked me if I had seen the crossed eye fairy. I told her that nothing could interest me more than to meet her. "Would it make you love the little fairy less," she asked, "if you saw her with crossed eyes?"

I answered, "No, please let me see her." "Perhaps you would try to cure her by an operation?" she asked. "Oh, no," I replied, "I would never do that" "Do you think glasses would help her?" she asked.

The thought of a pretty fairy wearing large heavy glasses was repugnant to me. I told the Queen that I had never known of anybody with crossed eyes who was cured by wearing glasses. I had seen many cured, but they had all recovered without the use of glasses and needed no operation.

The Queen then led me to a part of the forest where the crossed eye fairy had sought refuge from the pitying eyes of her friends. I had noticed that most crossed eye people were extremely unhappy, and I had always tried to cure them and make them happy. The Queen of the fairies remembered that I had always done something to relieve fairies who were unhappy. I had found that fairies suffered just as much as anybody else and needed some help as well as mortals. The Queen then took me to the crossed eye fairy who lay on a soft bed of moss with her head and face turned away from the fairies who were curious. When I arrived, she was crying and sobbing continuously, suffering as only a sensitive fairy can suffer. Many of the other fairies tried in vain to comfort her. We were all overwhelmed with a great pity, but it was difficult to know what to do.

"How did she become crossed eye?" I asked. One fairy answered that she caught it from Mary, a four year old child who had visited her. I asked where Mary lived and went to see her. I found her living in a cottage on the shore of a lake. Her father and mother and brothers and sisters were all very nervous, so I persuaded them all to dance and play. Mary enjoyed being thrown around in a circle fast and then faster until her feet could not touch the floor. One of the older boys held her hands in his while he played this new game of swinging her feet clear of the floor. When she practiced this swing, it made her laugh. She enjoyed it so much that she begged everybody to swing her.

While swinging I told her to look upwards and her eyes

became perfectly straight, temporarily. By practicing the swing more continuously her eyes remained straight for a longer time. She said that her eyes were not tired any more and she felt rested. I swung with her for hours, and then her father, mother and others relieved me and swung her feet from the floor until late in the afternoon.

Before the moonlight appeared, I took Mary to visit the crossed eye fairy. There she was, still lying on her face and crying bitterly. Mary told her how she had been cured by the swing. The crossed eye fairy stopped crying and listened attentively. All the other fairies listened, too, and then began to swing her until her feet were flying around without touching the ground. They all enjoyed this new game and were very gay. The fairy with the crossed eyes enjoyed it most of all and kept begging for more. She said that her eyes became straighter and straighter until they were almost cured. She said that it made her eyes feel better and she felt relaxed all over.

All the fairies became so happy over this that they led me to a nearby hamlet where dozens of boys and girls had crossed eyes. At once the Queen caught hold of a crossed eye boy and swung him in a circle until his eyes became straight. I did the same to others until all were temporarily cured. Then a wonderful thing happened. The crossed eye fairy swung another child, the last one of all, until the eyes became straight, and then they were all completely cured, including the crossed eye fairy. I visited them the next and many days later and found all of them completely and permanently cured.

Years later I returned to the little hamlet and found no more children with crossed eyes and everybody there was very happy.

QUESTIONS AND ANSWERS

Q–1. What causes my vision to become blurred upon sudden confusion or when I have a number of activities coming at once?

A–1. The fact that your vision becomes blurred at such times is proof of your eccentric fixation. Do not try to see or do several things at once. Practice central fixation, seeing the part regarded best and other parts not do clearly, all day long.

Q–2. If poor eyesight is caused by some physical ailment, will your methods help?

A–2. Yes, relaxation is always a benefit, not only to the eyes, but to all the nerves of the body.

Q–3. My daughter, age 10, is practicing your method for the cure of crossed eyes. Would it help to cover her good eye with a patch, which is easy for her and keeps the left eye straight for a certain period of time, besides making it work? It helped her so much when she wore glasses, that I thought it might help her without them in the same way.

A–3. It is first necessary to improve to normal the vision of both eyes, when used together. Then cover the good eye and practice improving the vision of the crossed eye.

Q–4. I am sixty-five years old and, in addition to bifocals, I am wearing strong prism glasses for reading. These tire me and strain my eyes. Am I too old to be helped by your methods, and would the adjustment of my eyesight increase the dizzy attacks which I have had and which I dread most of all?

A–4. Age is not a factor in the cure of imperfect sight by my methods. Patients, eighty years and older, have become able to read fine print at six inches and have obtained normal sight for distance. Relaxation prevents dizziness and is beneficial to the entire system. See the December 1925 number of *Better Eyesight* on "Dizziness."

Better Eyesight
January 1927—Vol. XI, No. 7

DEMONSTRATE: MOVEMENT AND THE CIRCULAR SWING

MOVEMENT

Perfect sight is not possible unless one imagines a letter to be moving, and that an effort to imagine a letter stationary always fails.

Close your eyes and remember a small letter of the Snellen test card. Imagine that someone is moving the test card a short distance from side to side so that all the letters on the card appear to be moving with the movement of the card. Remember the small letter moving. You can remember it, provided you imagine it is moving. Now try to stop this movement by staring at one part of the small letter and imagining that it is stationary. The letter soon becomes blurred.

THE CIRCULAR SWING

The circular swing prevents the stare and relieves pain and fatigue.

Hold the forefinger of one hand about six inches in front of one eye and a few inches to the outer side of the face. By moving the head and eyes in a circular or an elliptical orbit, notice that the finger appears to move in the direction opposite to the movement of the head and eyes.

HYPERMETROPIA

By W. H. Bates, M.D.

DEFINITION

By hypermetropia is meant a shortening of the diameter of the eyeball so that images are focussed behind the retina instead of in front of it as in myopia. The vision for distant objects may be imperfect. Some writers have defined the hypermetropic eye as a farsighted eye, because near vision is usually imperfect, while distant vision is usually good.

OCCURRENCE

Hypermetropia is acquired by persons who strain their eyes to see at the near point. After the removal of the lens, as in cataract extraction, a high degree of hypermetropia is produced. It is not unusual for people to acquire hypermetropia at the age of forty or fifty, when presbyopia is prevalent. With few exceptions, all persons fifty years old have acquired hypermetropia to such an extent that they are unable to read without glasses.

[Since Dr. Bates did not believe the lens accommodated, presbyopia was, in his opinion, actually hypermetropia.—TRQ]

SYMPTOMS

Hypermetropia may cause much pain, headache, fatigue and other nervous troubles. The vision at the near point is not so good in hypermetropia as in the normal eye, while the vision for distance is not impaired to the same extent. There are, however, a great many cases of farsightedness in which the vision for distance is much less than some cases of myopia. To classify cases of hypermetropia as being farsighted is not always correct. The hypermetropic eye is not always a farsighted eye.

[In other words, if the eyeball is short a small amount from front to back, only the close vision is blurred; but if the eyeball becomes very short, the blur extends into the distance.—TRQ]

CAUSE

Hypermetropia is usually a functional condition of the eye, i.e., it is caused by a mental strain. There are, however, cases of hypermetropia which occur after the removal of the lens, as in cataract extraction; but even in these cases, mental strain to see at the near point always increases the hypermetropia. In all forms of hypermetropia, relaxation at the near point lessens the hypermetropia, whatever the cause may be. Knowing that the cause is due to a mental strain at the near point, the successful treatment of all forms of hypermetropia is suggested.

TREATMENT

All measures which prevent strain and promote relaxation are always beneficial. Hypermetropia responds to "strain" almost immediately. A strain at a near point always increases the amount of hypermetropia or produces it in the normal eye. When the lens is removed in the normal eye, the hypermetropia produced is still functional and curable. [The lens accounts for approximately 20% of the refraction needed to see clearly; the cornea accounts for the remaining 80%.—TRQ]

The cure of hypermetropia is accomplished by lessening or correcting the strain to see at the near point. The correction of the distance strain is usually more readily accomplished. With perfect sight, there is no strain. The eyes are at rest. Any effort that is made to improve the vision is always wrong and never succeeds. When the vision is normal, the eyes are at rest.

Imagination

Demonstrate that perfect sight is accomplished when the imagination is good, and that you see only what you imagine you see. Take a Snellen test card and hold it at a distance from your eyes at which your sight is fairly good. Look at the white center of the large "O," and compare the whiteness of the center of the "O" with the whiteness of the rest of the card. You may do it readily; but if not, use a screen, that is, a card with a small hole in it. With that card, cover over the black part of the letter "O," and note the white center of the letter which is exposed by the opening in the screen. Remove the screen and observe that there is a change in the appearance of the white, which appears to be a whiter white when the black part of the letter is exposed. When the black part of the letter is covered with a screen, the center of the "O" is of the same whiteness as the rest of the card. It is, therefore, possible to demonstrate that you do not see the white center of the "O" whiter than the rest of the card, because you are seeing something that is not there. When you see something that is not there, you do not really see it, you only imagine it. The whiter you can imagine the center of the "O," the better becomes the vision for the letter "O," and when the vision of the letter "O" improves, the vision of all the letters on the card improves. The perfect imagination of the white center of the "O" means perfect imagination of the black, because you cannot imagine the white perfectly without imagining the black perfectly. By practice you may become able to imagine the letter "O" much better than it really is, and when this is accomplished, you become able to actually see unknown letters.

Test Card Practice

Practice with the Snellen test card at ten feet. Regard the known letter and imagine that you see it. Your imagination of the letter may be imperfect with your eyes open. Then close your eyes and the letter may be remembered more perfectly. Open your eyes for a second and imagine the known letter on the card at ten feet, close the eyes quickly and remember the known letter better for part of a minute. Then when the known letter, with the eyes closed, is remembered perfectly, open your eyes and imagine it on the card. By doing this alternately, the imagination of the known letter, with the eyes open, improves until you become able to imagine you see the known letter clearly enough to tell what it is. If you become able to imagine you see the known letter quite clearly, you actually can see the unknown letters and read the whole line.

Swinging

It is also beneficial while practicing this method to sway the body, head and eyes a short distance from side to side, and imagine the card and the letters to be moving in the opposite direction. It may help you to imagine the card moving by regarding the background close to one vertical edge of the card. By swaying from side to side, the edge of the card appears to move over the background. The shorter the movement of the body, head and eyes, the shorter is the movement of the card and the better is it remembered, imagined or seen. The short swing is more beneficial than the long swing. It is necessary to realize, however, that it doesn't require much of a strain to stop the short swing and blur the whole card. When the short swing stops, you should increase the swing or the swaying of the body from side to side until the card can be again imagined to be moving. This combination of swaying, memory with the eyes closed, and imagination with the eyes open, is a cure for hypermetropia.

Fine Print

When the vision for distance becomes nearly normal, the vision at the near point can then be improved to normal. Hold a card of fine print about ten inches from the eyes. Do not look directly at the letters. Imagine that where the bottom of the letters comes in contact with the white space between the lines, that the whiteness is increased, and with practice you can become able to imagine a thin white line, which is below the letters and whiter than the rest of the white space. When this thin white line is imagined white enough, the letters are imagined black enough to be read.

If you fail to imagine this thin white line with your eyes open you may be able to imagine it with your eyes closed. Then open your eyes and imagine it as well as you can. Close your eyes and remember or imagine the thin white line whiter. Then bring the card up an inch or two closer and imagine the thin white line as well with the eyes open as you can remember it with the eyes closed. By alternately remembering, with the eyes closed, the thin white line quite perfectly at ten inches, it becomes possible to imagine it with the eyes open at nine inches or six inches, or even nearer, and to imagine it as well with the eyes open as with the eyes closed. When you become able to imagine the thin white line as well at six inches with the eyes open as you can remember it with the eyes closed, the hypermetropia is usually corrected. This treatment has cured hypermetropia of 16 D. S.

Central Fixation

The following case illustrates the possibilities of the cure of hypermetropia by treatment without glasses.

Mr. George, age thirty-five, was employed as an assistant in a library. His vision without glasses was only 5/200, with convex 16 diopters his sight was improved to 20/50. A second pair of glasses, convex 20 diopters was required to enable him to see to read and do his work.

An operation had been performed some years previously for the removal of congenital cataract. This case was apparently one which was not curable. However, he was given relaxation treatment to find out how much benefit could be obtained.

After closing his eyes and resting them for half an hour, his vision without glasses improved to 20/200 which continued only for a very short time, a few seconds. He demonstrated that concentration, trying to see by an effort, always lowered his vision very quickly. Blinking frequently, or palming, i.e., covering his closed eyes with the palms of both hands, was restful and his sight improved temporarily. He became able to imagine one part best of a large letter, while the other parts of the letter were seen worse, i.e., central fixation. He demonstrated that the practice of central fixation was restful, easy, required no effort, and always helped his sight.

After he regarded a Snellen test card which was moved an inch or less from side to side, he became able by practice to imagine the small letters of a stationary Snellen test card to be moving or swinging. With the help of this movement, central fixation was demonstrated until his vision improved continuously to 20/40, a vision which was better than that with his strong glasses.

This unusually good result was an encouragement to attempt to improve his vision for reading. When tested with the fine print, diamond type, he demonstrated that with the card held at two feet he read no letters, but the white spaces between the lines of black letters could be imagined whiter than the rest of the card and without effort or strain. By practice, with his eyes closed, his memory or imagination became better than with his eyes open. It was suggested that he keep his eyes closed for part of a minute while remembering the whiteness of snow and to imagine it with his eyes open for only a short time. By alternating, his imagination with his eyes open improved for the whiteness of the white spaces and for the blackness of the letters. His vision became better for the diamond type at six inches than at twelve inches.

[The debate over the mechanism(s) of accommodation is not of much interest to hypermetropic and presbyopic students who have eliminated their reading glasses.—TRQ]

STORIES FROM THE CLINIC

No. 83: The Swing

By Emily C. Lierman

Recently I had the pleasure of talking to a large gathering of people in Chicago who were interested in the Bates Method. I was very much impressed by the fact that there was not a corner or part of the large room that was not lighted. As I watched the people coming in, I noticed an air of cheerfulness about them which attracted me. The meeting was held in the office of Dr. Jean Claverie who is very successful in treating and curing patients by the Bates Method. A number of doctors mingled with patients and their friends in the audience. After the lecture, several important questions were asked which helped all of those present to better understand the Bates Method. It was not difficult to determine those in the audience who knew nothing about the Bates Method, and the benefits that could be derived from it, as they were wearing glasses and the more I talked, the more they stared at me. This staring was an unconscious act on the part of these people. I told them about the various ways in which patients could be relieved of their eyestrain, and spoke of those who stare and the suffering it caused. I added that there were quite a number who were listening to me who forgot to blink their eyes. It was interesting to watch the blinking habit begin. I mentioned the fact that those who did not have trouble with their eyes, blinked unconsciously and irregularly all the time, except when they were asleep. It was surprising to me and to Dr. Edith T. Fisher and Ms. Elisabet to note how few there were who continued to stare after I brought this fact to their notice.

There were several school teachers there who asked me questions which I enjoyed answering, not only for their benefit but also for the benefit of others whom I knew were skeptical by the expression on their faces.

One teacher asked, "Should I apply the swing to the class in general or instruct each pupil separately?" I answered, "Have them all stand up and sway together with you. Be sure to have them blink their eyes as they sway."

Benefits

The body swing, which is so relaxing and helpful in relieving all strain of the body as well as of the eyes, is similar to the movement of the eyes themselves. When the eye blinks, it also moves slightly from side to side without effort or strain. Dr. Bates has proved that when the eye is at rest, it is moving. I have observed many people in great pain and have recognized the fact that they do not blink often enough. Not knowing that blinking is a good habit, they stare and make their condition worse. Staring brings on more tension, therefore the pain becomes more intense. When the patient is reminded not to stare and is told to move the head slightly from side to side, even though he cannot move the rest of his body, he becomes relaxed and soon falls asleep. Moving the head from side to side on the pillow is in the nature of the swing. Many patients erroneously believe that they have to sway the whole body in order to produce the relaxation necessary for the relief of eyestrain. I believe that the swing is just as essential to the human body as it is to animals. It is a good plan to watch the animals and learn a lesson from them. The tiger and lion as well as other animals move most of the time while they are awake and are, therefore, relaxed. The elephant sways his bulky body from side to side, because it rests him.

People who work in offices, department stores and other places of business can practice a short, easy swing of their bodies. The movement can be so slight as not to be conspicuous to others. It is always interesting to watch soldiers march and observe the sway of their bodies in unison with the rhythm of the music. A mother who is busy with her household duties is always grateful for the few minutes of rest and relaxation she obtains when rocking the baby. A baby in its cradle enjoys the movement of the rocking. If the heart stops beating, which is really a sway inside the body, the blood no longer has a chance to flow nor the pulse to beat. If the pendulum of the clock stops, the clock does not tell the time. In my opinion the swing is as great a blessing as the sunshine. Just as the benefit of the sun is lost when wearing dark glasses, so is the swing lost by staring and straining.

TEMPERAMENTAL STRAIN

By Lawrence M. Stanton, M.D.

It is more natural to do things, both good and bad, unconsciously than consciously. Yet the road of progress is the reverse of this, and perhaps there is no felicity greater than that of translating unconsciousness into consciousness.

Dr. Bates has well said—and what does he not say well?—that it is easier to strain unconsciously than consciously, and in order that we may deplore and so correct it, he advises us to prove it for ourselves. Ninety-nine percent of those who suffer from poor vision are unaware that they strain in seeing and to convince them of it is not an easy task.

In spite of what has been written of strain and relaxation, we are still far from able to accomplish the one and avoid the other. In the matter of relaxation relating to vision, we practice the exercises given us in the Bates Method. That is, after learning what the eye does and does not do in order to see, we consciously imitate the unconscious behavior of the normal eye. As perfect sight is due to the absence of straining to see, we speak of these exercises as relaxing exercises. But on observing the vast difference in the results of these exercises upon our patients, we ask why this difference? Why is it that we get quick cures, rapid progress in one case and not in another, when apparently the exercises are practiced by both equally well? Dr. Bates repeatedly states, whether speaking of palming, shifting or swinging, that the practice can be done in the right or in the wrong way. In the successful case, the patient overcomes his strain and does the exercises easily, while in the unsuccessful case, the element of strain remains—he does not do the exercises easily, his straining is yet to be realized, to be brought from unconsciousness to consciousness and dealt with. One who has only the strain in his eyes to contend with progresses rapidly, while one who has to detect the strain in himself has a harder task.

There are, then, two avenues of approach to normal sight, one through one's eyes and the other through one's self. The subject of strain in one's self, the temperamental strain, is vast, and to do more than call attention to it in this article for *Better Eyesight* is impossible. I will, however, relate a few cases and some of my own experiences that may be suggestive. The experiences point to temperamental and the patients to simple visual strain.

On returning city-wards one evening, I had been reading comfortably on the train. When nearing the station, the train was delayed for some time by the home-going commuters. My eyes soon began to trouble me in an unaccountable way. I asked myself what was the matter, since they should have hurt me less in a quiet than in a jolting car. I found that while giving attention to what I was reading, I was at the same time anxious over the thought that I would be late for dinner, and that I had promised the cook an early dinner with an evening out; also that I had to visit a patient before returning home to my belated meal. In other words, I was mentally trying to give equal attention to several things at the same time. I was straining. It was as disrupting as trying to watch a Three-Ring Circus. I could in a moment produce discomfort in my eyes not only by anxious thought, but by ungoverned, disorderly thinking.

[Bates teacher Clara Hackett, author of *Relax and See,* once stated, "Diffusion is confusion."—TRQ]

On another occasion when reading a sign across the car there was one word I could not see in spite of blinking, swinging, etc. Suddenly the lights went out for an instant and when they came on again, I instantly saw the unseen word. The momentary rest to my vision gave me the relaxation I had not otherwise obtained. I had been straining, but when the matter was taken out of my hands, the strain vanished and I saw.

A boy, ten years old, with slight convergent squint and a history of very marked squint when younger, could read 10/10 with the left eye, but only 10/70 with the right. The diamond type card he could not read at any distance with the right eye. With the left eye covered, the letters below 10/70 were seen gray with the right, the amblyopic eye; but when he imagined the letter swinging, which he very *easily* could do, he saw them black and soon could read the 30-line. It was the "easily" in his case that worked the miracle.

Another boy could not form a mental picture of his dog, but when he remembered one of the dog's legs, then another, when he thought of his back, then of his tail, and told me whether the latter was straight or curled, whether the color of the tail was the same as that of the back, his mental picture was much improved and so was his vision. The delight that this boy *felt* in his reconstructed dog was an important factor in his mental picture.

Now let us suppose two other cases with refractive errors paralleling the two just mentioned but in respect to temperament quite different. The first boy, we will say, cannot easily swing the letters, seeing them black, nor can he do anything with ease; the second boy's dog is not his comrade and he has no delight in a mental picture of him. Here we have psychological problems, temperamental insufficiencies, to meet before the relaxation is established that cures the imperfect vision of these patients, and yet physical sight is no whit worse in the latter than in the former group.

If only we could give up, let go, let the thing be done for us, of how much strain would we rid ourselves! What a difference between trying to do a thing and doing it; between trying to see and seeing!

USE OF THE SUN GLASS

In using the sun glass, it is well to accustom the eyes of the patient to the strong light by having him sit in the sun with his eyes closed, and at the same time he should slowly move his head from side to side in order to avoid discomfort from the heat. Enough light shines through the eyelid to cause some people a great deal of discomfort at first, but after a few hours' exposure in this way, they become able to gradually open their eyes to some extent without squeezing the lids. When this stage is reached, one can focus, with the aid of the sun glass, the light on the closed eyelids, which at first is very disagreeable. When the patient becomes able to open the eyes, he is directed to look as far down as possible, and in this way the pupil is protected by the lower lid. Then by gently lifting the upper lid, only the white part of the eye is exposed, while the sun's rays strike directly upon this part of the eyeball. The sun glass may then be used on the white part of the eye. Care should be taken to move the glass from side to side quickly. The length of time devoted to focusing the light on the white part of the eye is never longer than a few seconds. After such a treatment the patient almost immediately becomes able to open his eyes widely in the light.

Better Eyesight
February 1927—Vol. XI, No. 8

SQUINT

By W. H. Bates, M.D.

Squint, also known as strabismus, is a condition of the eyes in which both eyes do not regard one point at the same time. It is very common, and more prevalent among children than adults. Many cases improve with advancing years, while others may become worse. Squint may occur at the same time with myopia, astigmatism, or hypermetropia, or with any disease inside the eye.

Symptoms

In squint, one eye does not look in the same direction as the other. For example, the left eye may look straight at the Snellen test card with normal vision, while the right eye may turn in toward the nose, and have imperfect sight. The squint is variable in some cases. At times it may be less or disappear altogether, while at other times it may be more pronounced. In some cases of squint, the patient is conscious of the strain. When the eyes turn in, he may be conscious that his eyes are not straight. When the eyes are nearly straight, he is usually able to realize that the eyes are not so strained.

Cause

The cause of squint in all cases is due to strain. When the eyes are under one kind of strain, they may turn in, and with a different strain they may turn out, or one eye may be higher than the other—all caused by strain. The relief or cure of one kind of strain relieves or cures all forms of strain. Squint in any form is always benefited by rest.

Rest

The best treatment for squint is mental rest. Many patients with squint suffer very much from eyestrain. By closing the eyes and resting them, or by palming for a few minutes or longer, about ten times a day, most of these cases are cured without other treatment.

Patch

In many cases, the squinting eye has imperfect sight. When the eyes are examined with the ophthalmoscope, no change can usually be discovered in the retina. Such cases have what is called *amblyopia ex anopsia.* Some cases are benefited by wearing a patch over the good eye, so that the patient is compelled to use the squinting eye for vision. After several weeks or months, the vision of the squinting eye may become normal by constantly wearing a patch over the good eye. Many cases of squint are cured in this way.

Swinging

The strain, from which so many of these patients suffer, is benefited by the swing. Almost all squint cases can be taught to imagine, while the good eye is covered, that stationary objects are moving. In cases where the swing of stationary objects is not readily accomplished, any of the following methods may be effective:

1. The forefinger is held about six inches in front of the face, and a short distance to one side. By looking straight ahead and moving the head from side to side, the finger appears to move. This movement of the finger is greater than the movement of objects at the distance, but, by practice, patients become able to imagine not only the finger to be moving, but also distant objects as well.

2. The patient may stand about two feet to one side of a table on which an open book is placed. When he steps one or two paces forward, the book and the table appear to move backward. When he takes two or more steps backward, the table and the book appear to move forward.

3. The patient stands in front of a window and looks at the distant houses. By swaying his body from side to side, the window, the curtains, or the curtain cord may be imagined to be moving from side to side, in the opposite direction to the movement of his body, and the more distant objects appear to move in the same direction [double oppositional movement] that he moves his head and eyes.

4. The patient stands ten feet or less from the Snellen test card and looks to the right side of the room, five feet or more from the card. When he looks to the right, the card is always to the left of where he is looking. When he looks to the left side of the room, the card is to the right of where he is looking. By alternately looking from one side of the card to the other, the patient becomes able to imagine that when he looks to the right, everything in the room moves to the left. When he looks to the left, everything in the room appears to move to the right. After some practice, he becomes able to imagine that the card is moving in the opposite direction to the movement of his eyes. This movement can be shortened by shortening the movement of the eyes from side to side.

5. When the patient regards the Snellen test card at fifteen feet or nearer, and looks a few inches to the right of the big "C," the letter is always to the left of where he is

looking. When he looks a few inches or farther to the left of the "C," it is always to the right of where he is looking. By alternately looking from right to left of the "C," he becomes able to imagine it to be moving in the opposite direction. By shortening the distance between the points regarded, the swing is also shortened. The patient is encouraged to practice this swing with the good eye covered. When the swing is practiced correctly, there is always a benefit to the vision and squint.

Memory

Some patients are very much benefited by being encouraged to remember the letters on the Snellen test card perfectly, i.e., to remember the black part of the letter perfectly black and the white part perfectly white. When the memory is perfect, it is possible for the imagination to be perfect. This being true, the patient becomes able, by practice, to imagine he sees each and every letter of the Snellen test card, and to imagine them to be moving. The movement of the swing can be stopped by staring at one point of a large or small letter, with the result that the vision is always lowered and the squint becomes worse. When the patient becomes able to imagine known letters perfectly, he is soon able to imagine the letters of a strange card perfectly. When the letters are imagined perfectly, they are seen perfectly. Practice with a familiar card, or with a card whose letters are remembered, is one of the best methods known for curing the imperfect sight of squint and the squint itself.

Central Fixation

Another satisfactory method is to have the patient practice central fixation, or seeing best where he is looking, and seeing worse where he is not looking. In practicing central fixation, it is necessary for the patient to shift constantly and to blink frequently. To teach a patient central fixation, his attention is called to the fact that when he looks at the top of the card, he can distinguish the large letters, but the letters on the bottom of the card cannot be distinguished. When he looks at the bottom of the card, he sees the small letters where he is looking better than the large letters on the upper part of the card where he is not looking.

Eccentric Fixation

Some patients have what is called eccentric fixation, which is the opposite of "central fixation." Such patients see best where they are not looking. Eccentric fixation can always be demonstrated to be present when the vision is imperfect, or when the squint is manifest. To cure eccentric fixation it is necessary to demonstrate these facts, and by practicing with the small letters, the results are usually good. The patient is told to look at the first letter on the bottom line of the Snellen test card, which may be read at ten feet or nearer, and have him note that the letters toward the right end of the line are blurred or not seen at all. By alternately shifting from the beginning of the line to the end of the line and back again, the vision is usually improved, because eccentric fixation is lessened by this practice. Sometimes it is necessary for the instructor to stand behind the card and watch the eyes of the patient, who may look a foot or more away from the letter that he is requested to regard with the squinting eye, while the good eye is covered. He may look a foot above or a foot below, or at some point a foot or more away from the letter which he is asked to regard. The instructor is usually able to tell when the patient is not looking at the letter desired. The instructor directs the patient to look down when he sees that the patient is looking too far up. The patient is directed to look to the right, when it is observed that he is looking too far to the left, and by watching him closely, the eccentric fixation can be corrected to such an extent that the vision becomes normal and the squint disappears.

Fixing Eye

A great deal has been said about the "fixing eye" [more commonly called the "fixating eye" today—TRQ] in squint, i.e., the eye that looks straight. Sometimes the vision of the squinting eye may be very poor, and one would expect the patient to focus with the eye that has better vision. This is not always the case because some patients with a high degree of myopia in the left eye will turn the right eye in and look straight with the left eye. These cases are very interesting; no two are exactly alike and one needs to study the individual case in order to obtain the best results.

Imagination

There are some rare cases where the vision is perfect in each eye, and yet the patient will suffer from squint. One may have considerable difficulty in finding the method of treatment which will cure or relieve these cases. One of the best methods is to have the patient practice the imagination cure. The patient can look at a page of a book twenty feet away and not read any of the letters. If the letter "O" is the second letter of the fourth word and on the 10th line, the vision may not be good enough for the patient to recognize the letter, but he may become able to imagine it. If he imagines that the left side is straight, it makes him uncomfortable and the left side is not imagined perfectly black. If he imagines that the left side is curved, he feels comfortable and the left side appears clearer and blacker. By imagining each of the four sides of the letter "O" perfectly, the imagination of the letter is improved, but if one or more sides are imagined imperfectly, the patient is uncomfortable and the vision or the imagination of the "O" becomes imperfect. Some patients are able to imagine perfectly and are conscious when they imagine imperfectly.

In one case, a girl eleven years old was able to look for half a minute at diamond type which was placed ten feet away, at a distance where the patient could not distinguish the letters. She then closed her eyes, palmed, and imagined correctly each letter that her mother designated. For example, her mother picked out the capital letter "M," the first letter of the fourth word on the 10th line. While palming with her eyes closed, the patient imagined the left side straight, the right side straight, the top open and the bottom open. I asked her if it could be an "H." She answered that it could, but that she could imagine an "M" better, which was correct. Some patients are able to use their imagination correctly and imagine small letters just as well as capital letters. In order to obtain perfect results, it is necessary that the eyes be perfectly relaxed, and when the eyes are relaxed, all the nerves of the body are also relaxed. Those cases of squint which become able to do this are soon cured.

Imagination of crossed images with the eyes closed is characteristic of divergent squint, i.e., squint with the eyes turned out. The patient imagines the crossed images alternately with the eyes open and with the eyes closed. When, by practice, the imagination becomes as good with the eyes open as with the eyes closed, the squint is usually corrected.

Double Vision

If the usual treatment of squint has failed, it is well to teach such cases to see double. When the right eye turns in toward the nose and the left eye is straight, the letter or other object seen by the left or normal eye, is seen straight ahead, while the image seen by the right or squinting eye, is suppressed by an effort and is not seen at all (amblyopia). To teach the patient to see with both eyes at the same time requires much time and patience. When double vision is obtained, the image seen by the right eye is to the right, while the image seen by the left eye is to the left. We say that the images are seen on the same side as the eye which sees them. With the eyes closed, the patient is taught to imagine a letter, object or a light to be double, each image imagined to be on the same side as the eye with which the patient imagines he sees it. With an effort, the two images may be made to separate to any desired extent. By repeatedly imagining the double images with the eyes closed, the patient becomes able, with the eyes open, to imagine the double images to be separated a few inches or less, a foot apart or farther.

Patients become able not only to imagine images with the eyes closed, apparently seen on the same side as the eye which imagines them, but also—and this suggests curative treatment—to imagine crossed images, that is, the right eye image is imagined to the left, while the left eye image is imagined to the right. With one or both eyes turned in, each of the double images is imagined on the same side as the eye which imagines it. When the images are crossed, the convergent squint is over corrected and the eyes turn out.

All this can at first be accomplished more readily with the eyes closed than with them open. When the patient controls the separation of the images with the eyes open as well as with the eyes closed, the squint is benefited.

Case Reports

1. A boy, two years old, had developed squint in his right eye several months before I saw him. He was just beginning to walk. At his first visit, I took hold of his hands and swung him round and round until his feet were off the floor, and had him look up toward the ceiling. While doing this, his eyes became straight. The father and mother also took turns in swinging the child, and when he looked up into their faces, his eyes were straight. Every day, one or more members of the family would swing the boy around for at least five minutes. A year afterwards, the squint had not returned.

2. A girl, age fourteen, had an internal squint of the right eye. The vision of this eye was very poor, and she was unable to count fingers at one foot from that eye. The vision of the left eye was normal. She was encouraged to use her right eye by covering the left with a patch. She did not like the patch, so the lenses were removed from their frame, and an opaque glass was placed in the frame for the left eye. The girl was very nervous and wearing the glass gave her continual trouble. Her playmates teased her so much that she deliberately dropped them in the snow. Her father talked to her and insisted that she wear the frame with the opaque glass all the time. When she realized that she must keep the good eye covered until she was cured, her vision immediately began to improve. In less than a week, she became able to read the 10-line on the Snellen test card at twenty feet with each eye. She also became able to read fine print with the right eye just as well as she could with the left. The realization that she would have to wear the glass until she was cured was an incentive for her to practice those methods which improved her sight. When she looked at the Snellen test card at one foot, and remembered that the large letter at the top was a "C," with the aid of her imagination she became able to see the "C." When she closed her eyes and remembered a better "C," she was able, with her eyes open, to imagine it at a greater distance, three feet. In a short time, her vision improved to 20/200

by alternately remembering a better "C" with her eyes closed, and imagining it as well as she could with her eyes open in flashes. Palming was a help and improved her vision to 20/40. A few days later, her vision had improved to 20/20 with the aid of the swing.

3. A young woman, twenty-four years old, called to see me about her left eye which was causing her more or less pain. The left eye became very much fatigued when she tried to read. Her vision in that eye was 20/40. Her right eye had no perception of light and was turned in. A great many doctors had told the patient that the blindness was hopeless, and that nothing could be done to improve the vision of the right eye.

I had the patient practice the usual relaxation exercises, swinging, palming, etc. The vision of the left eye improved very rapidly and, much to my surprise, the vision of the right eye also improved, After two weeks, during which the patient had received about six treatments, the vision of both eyes became normal. The right eye which had had no perception of light was sensitive now to a light reflected from the ophthalmoscope into her pupil. The pupil of the right eye always contracted when the light was turned into either eye.

The squint disappeared and she was able to see the same object, with both eyes, at the same time.

STORIES FROM THE CLINIC

No. 84: Case Reports

By Emily C. Lierman

Before knowing about the Bates Method, I did not think it possible that a person of seventy or more years could see without the aid of eyeglasses. After practicing the Bates Method, I discarded the glasses, which I had worn for thirteen years, and I have had good sight ever since.

Dr. Lilian Wentworth, of San Diego, California, who is now taking a course in the Bates Method, has brought several interesting facts to my attention. Her grandfather discarded glasses at the age of seventy-five because he could not see with them. Living in the country, it was difficult for him to be fitted with suitable glasses for reading or distant vision. After being without glasses for a few weeks, he would read large print to while away the time. He had in his possession a book of Psalms which was printed in rather large type, and he read this print daily to amuse himself. He then started reading the headlines of newspapers. This was very thrilling to him and the knowledge that he could do without his glasses caused him to boast to his friends about it.

Dr. Wentworth believes that we would be much happier if all of us would find something to occupy our minds. She urged her mother to take up glove mending at the age of seventy-five and her mother soon became successful with the work. At the same time, Dr. Wentworth's mother conceived the idea of leaving off her glasses. She thought that she might become able to see and read without them just as her father had done at that age. An oculist had told her ten years previously that she had incipient cataract of both eyes and that, in time, she would undoubtedly be forced to have the cataract removed by an operation. From the time she began mending gloves until she died, at the age of eighty-two, she did not use glasses again.

An operation had not been necessary because the cataract had either disappeared or become absorbed. That which interests me most in her case is the fact that in glove mending it is necessary to use the finest silk or cotton thread obtainable. It was necessary for Ms. Wentworth to make very fine stitches in mending the gloves or she would have failed. At all times her work was satisfactorily done and she was highly praised by those who gave her their work to do. Although she did not use glasses while working or reading, she put them on from time to time to test her ability to see with them. She complained that they did not fit her. In order to test her vision, she tried several times to find someone who could fit her with glasses, but was unsuccessful. She was always informed that there was nothing wrong with her sight.

I told Dr. Wentworth that I believed her mother had actually cured herself of cataract by doing this fine sewing. It is generally believed that fine work causes eyestrain, but it proved a benefit to her sight. Dr. Wentworth's mother enjoyed doing this work in her old age, and enjoying it, did not strain her eyes. I believe she forgot all about her eyes while using a fine needle and in making fine stitches.

Fine sewing is like fine print. If one strains to read fine print, one always fails; so it is with fine sewing. The more effort one makes while reading or sewing without the aid of glasses, or even with glasses, the more trouble one has in seeing. People with whom I have come in contact, who have had trouble with their eyes when reading, sewing or doing any kind of work with their glasses, were always better off without them, even though their vision was not good.

One of my patients, a woman age sixty-five, had myopia and cataract. Her vision was 6/50 in both eyes; in other words, she read the letters on the fifty-foot line of a test card at six feet. Palming seemed most difficult for her to do. Closing her eyes to rest them helped temporarily, but when asked to read the same line of letters that she had just read after having her eyes closed for a few minutes, she was unable to see the letters clearly enough to read them. I then realized that I must use another method, so I tried shifting. I had her stand with her feet about a foot apart and swing her body to the left as she looked out of the window off in the distance, then back to the test card, looking only at one letter that I was pointing to and then swinging her body as she looked out of the window again. Her vision in both eyes improved to the 40-line. Shifting quickly from the test card, thus avoiding the stare, helped her to see all the letters clearly on that line. As she was a nervous person, I did not have her keep up this exercise very long. I decided to teach her to swing back and forth, first placing the right foot forward, and swinging her body toward the test card; then after a few moments of this, she was told to reverse the movement and put the left foot forward. In this way, while seeing things move in the opposite direction, she read the 30-line letters, but she did not see them continuously.

She complained of being tired, so I placed her in a chair and gave her a footstool to rest her feet, as I wanted to be sure that she was comfortable. Then I taught her the thumb movement exercise, i.e., making a small round circle with the thumb on the tip of the forefinger of her right hand. After she had practiced the thumb movement for a few minutes, I gave her some white thread and a needle with a large eye and asked her to thread it. I told her to imagine one of the letters of the test card perfectly black as she held the needle and thread in place. She failed to accomplish what I asked her to do. I found I could do nothing more for her at that time, so I instructed her to keep up the thumb movement whenever she read her test card or practiced any other part of the method.

At her next lesson her vision was 10/30 with both eyes and she saw all the letters clearly. Shifting and swinging helped. She read some of the letters of the 20-line as she looked from the test card to a design on the floor, which she had previously remembered and described to me when her eyes were closed.

She was told to resume the thumb movement and blink as she looked at the 20-line letters. By looking down in her lap at her black dress, then glancing at the test card while blinking, she read the whole of the 20-line letters, one letter after another without stopping.

At her third lesson, she became able in a few minutes time to thread a needle without any trouble. I placed her in the sun and had her move her head from side to side, allowing the warm sun to shine on her closed eyelids. In less than an hour's time, her vision had improved to 10/10 in flashes.

QUESTIONS AND ANSWERS

Q–1. In practicing the universal swing, beginning with the finger, then the hand, the chair, and so on until one gets to the sky, ought one to hold continuously in mind each object added together with the sky, or just the sky moving with the finger?

A–1. Imagine only one thing at a time moving with your finger.

Q–2. Will relaxation methods alone remove a blood clot from the vitreous humor?

A–2. Yes, provided the patient practices my methods correctly and faithfully.

Q–3. How is it possible to get sun treatment when there has been no sun for days?

A–3. I should advise you to purchase a 250- or 500-watt electric light and sit in front of it with your eyes closed. It would be well to use the sun swing at this time which is moving the head a short distance from side to side. See the Questions and Answers column in the October 1926 issue of *Better Eyesight.*

Q–4. When you suggest new methods do you mean to discontinue with the old?

A–4. Not necessarily; all the methods I recommend have relaxation for their object. It is for the patient to determine which treatment is most beneficial and to continue its practice faithfully. Some patients tire easily when one thing is done continuously. For this reason several are suggested in order to vary the practice.

Q–5. I have been able to improve my vision in one eye but not in the other. Can you give me a reason for this?

A–5. This is caused by imperfect imagination. If you will practice my methods of memory, imagination, blinking and shifting, your other eye will also improve. I suggest that, when both eyes together are improved to normal, you wear a patch over the good eye as often as possible and practice until your other eye is also improved to normal.

Q–6. I am told that I am losing my "central vision" [macular degeneration—TRQ]. Is it possible to regain what I have already lost or to forestall the loss of the remainder?

A–6. Yes, it is possible by faithful practice of my methods.

Better Eyesight
March 1927—Vol. XI, No. 9

DEMONSTRATE: MEMORY AND IMAGINATION

Memory and imagination improve the vision.

Look at the large letter at the top of the card and note that it may be more or less blurred. Close the eyes and remember or imagine the same letter perfectly. Then open both eyes and imagine it as well as you can. In a second or less, close your eyes and remember the letter perfectly. When this is accomplished open the eyes and imagine it as well as you can. Close them quickly after a second or less. Practice the slow, short, easy swing and alternately remember the large letter with the eyes closed for part of a minute or longer, and then open the eyes and imagine it as well as you can.

When done properly, you will be able to improve your vision of the large letter until it becomes quite perfect. Then practice in the same way with the first letter of the second line. Improve your imagination of the first letter of the second line in flashes until it improves sufficiently for you to recognize the next letter without looking at it.

Improve the sight of the first letter of each line by alternately remembering it with the eyes closed for part of a minute and then flashing it for just a moment, a second or less. You should be told what the first letter of each line is. With your eyes closed remember it as perfectly as you can. Then open your eyes and test your imagination for the letter for a very short time, one second or even less. Keep your eyes closed for at least a part of a minute, while remembering the known letter. The flashes of the known letter with the eyes open become more frequent and last longer, until you become able to see, not only the known letter, but other unknown letters on the same line.

BLINKING AND SHIFTING

By W. H. Bates, M.D.

Blinking

By blinking is meant the opening and closing of the eyes more or less rapidly. The normal eye with normal vision blinks almost continuously. Sometimes the upper lid just covers the pupil while in other cases both lids may be completely closed. With the aid of the movie camera it has been demonstrated that one may blink five times in one second without being conscious of it.

When an effort is made to stop blinking, whether successful or not, the vision is always lowered. When the eyes are permitted to blink regularly, easily, continuously, the vision is usually benefited. The camera also shows that the lower lids move up with a strong contraction of the muscles.

In many cases of normal vision, especially in those cases which are even better than the average normal vision, blinking is sometimes practiced with incredible rapidity, and on other occasions the eyes may blink infrequently. The blinking of the normal eye varies or is different from the blinking of the eye with imperfect sight. The blinking of the eye with imperfect sight is usually very irregular and jerky and is accompanied by a manifest strain of the muscles of the eyelids. With imperfect sight an effort is always being made to hold the eye stationary and to stop the blinking. If the eyes are allowed to shift and to blink, the vision improves.

Blinking is fundamental and very important, because one cannot shift frequently or continuously with improvement in the vision unless the eyes blink often. [Every 2-3 seconds on the average.—TRQ] To keep the eyes open without blinking requires an effort, a stare or strain. The patient becomes unable to shift easily or rapidly, and the vision always becomes imperfect.

The best way to rest the eyes is to close them while many things in turn are remembered or imagined. Blinking is a rapid method of resting the eyes and can be practiced unconsciously all day long, regardless of what one may be doing.

It is interesting to observe some people's eyes when they are asleep. One may note that the eyelids are blinking, which prevents the eyes from staring or straining, although the patient is unconscious of his eyes.

It is a well-known fact that when people are asleep the eyes are often under a terrific strain. The first thing in the morning, after such a patient opens the eyes, he may find that his sight is very imperfect. He may suffer from pain in the eyes, pain in the head or in other parts of the body, or from extreme fatigue, as if he had been awake and hard at work all night long. When first opening the eyes, the patient may experience a feeling of dizziness, after the eyes have been straining during sleep. It is not an easy matter to recommend successful methods of obtaining relaxation to such patients so that instead of working hard during sleep the eyes may be completely relaxed and rested.

In some cases, the patient may have fairly good vision when he first opens his eyes after a good sleep. However, such cases are uncommon.

When the normal eye has normal vision it is always at rest [and moving.—TRQ] During sleep, however, with the aid of simultaneous retinoscopy it has usually been demonstrated that the eyes are straining, staring or making an effort to see. The unconscious blinking is nature's method of resting the eyes during sleep.

Shifting

When the normal eye has normal vision it is always shifting or moving from one point to another. This is true with the eyes open as well as with the eyes closed. The shifting with the eyes open may be from side to side, from above downward, or in any other direction. The horizontal shifting is practiced more than the other forms of shifting. The eye is never stationary. When the vision is imperfect, the shifting is also imperfect and may be jerky. It may result in discomfort of the eyes, the head or in any other part of the body. The shift of the normal eye varies and is more or less irregular.

To know the proper way to shift the normal eye, in order that the vision may be continuously normal, it is well to demonstrate the wrong way. When the shifting is practiced or the eyes move from point to point, the vision is usually benefited, provided one shifts slowly, easily and continuously.

Advise the patient to look directly at one point or one part of the smallest letter which can be distinguished. When he does this for a few seconds, he usually becomes able to feel that an effort is being made, and when the effort is continued or increased, much discomfort is felt and the vision always becomes imperfect. The patient is encouraged to prove that concentration does not last long, and that it is impossible for the eyes, memory or mind to see perfectly, remember perfectly, or imagine perfectly, when an effort is made to concentrate. When the eyes shift from one point to another, a feeling of relaxation soon follows and the vision improves. When the eyes do not shift from point to point, it can always be demonstrated that the vision becomes worse and that the eyes, mind and all the nerves of the body are uncomfortable and may be conscious of an effort or strain.

To constantly stare at one point of a letter or other object is wrong because it lowers the vision and causes discomfort to the eyes. Perfect sight is not possible and cannot be imagined continuously unless the shifting is continuous. The movement of letters or words, which can always be demonstrated in normal vision, depends upon the shifting.

When the eyes stare and do not move, or when an effort is made to imagine letters or other objects to be stationary, the shifting stops, and if things seen are imagined to be stationary without shifting, or an effort is made to stop the shifting, the vision always becomes imperfect.

With the eyes open, it is possible to shift from the first letter of a line of the Snellen test card at fifteen feet to the end of the line and improve the sight. In most cases a known letter of the Snellen test card can be remembered more or less perfectly with the eyes closed, but only when the eyes or the mind shift from one letter to another, or from one part of one letter to another part. The letter remembered can be imagined or a mental picture of the letter obtained only by constant, slow, short, regular, continuous, easy shifting. When the patient can remember or imagine letters or other objects perfectly with the eyes open as well as with the eyes closed, the vision is always benefited. If shifting is not practiced, the vision always becomes worse.

Many people with imperfect sight are not able to shift or move their eyes without an effort. They complain that they lose their mental control because they are unable to shift easily or continuously. Much better vision is obtained with a short movement or shift of the eyes than with a long shift.

It is necessary for those who have imperfect sight caused by a stare, a strain or an effort to see, to become able to shift in such a way as to benefit their vision. Keep the eyes closed for a large part of a minute and open them for a short time, a second or less. It takes time to stare, concentrate or make an effort to see. It is not possible to stare and lower the vision in a fraction of a second. Perfect sight is inconceivably quick. It is easy, regular and continuous. When shifting is practiced rapidly, easily and continuously, the symptoms of imperfect sight and other symptoms caused by strain are relieved at once.

Shifting is very often practiced wrongly and the vision becomes lowered or no benefit is gained. To shift rapidly, look up for a moment and then look down quickly, rest the eyes for part of a minute; then repeat, look up and down quickly without paying much, if any, attention to the sight. While looking down again, rest the eyes for part of a minute. Alternate until the shifting up and down can always be accomplished rapidly or rapidly enough to avoid testing the sight. When the eyes move up, the test card or other stationary objects move down. When the eyes move down, stationary objects move up or in the opposite direction to the movement of the shifting eyes.

Normal sight cannot be demonstrated continuously unless the eyes are continuously shifting. The patient is usually unconscious that he is shifting rapidly when he believes that he can see one letter of the bottom line perfectly and all the time.

Many people have said that they can see a letter with normal vision at fifteen feet or farther without moving their eyes, and without imagining the letter to be moving. In other cases where some people thought they could regard one letter with normal vision without shifting, it was found that while doing this the eyes, when observed at the near point, a few feet or farther, could be seen to move very quickly, up, down, from side to side or in other directions. The movement of the eyes was so rapid that it was not noticeable, unless the patient was observed very closely.

When the top of a large letter is regarded, that part may be seen best for a short time, while the rest of the letter is seen worse, i.e., central fixation. One cannot see with central fixation and have normal vision unless one is continuously shifting. When the bottom of the letter is regarded, it may be seen best, while all the rest of the letter is seen worse. By shifting alternately from the top to the bottom of the large letter, the vision is usually improved. At the same time, the uncomfortable feeling in the eyes or head is relieved and all pain is benefited.

One patient with very unusual vision read the bottom line marked "10" not only at ten feet but at a much greater distance. In a good light she claimed that she could see one letter of the 10-line at fifteen feet, 15/10, continuously without blinking and without shifting. Although she was not conscious of the fact she must have been blinking or shifting because the movie camera has always demonstrated that no one could see one letter of the Snellen test card continuously without rapid blinking or shifting.

It requires time for one's sight to become imperfect. The habit of staring or straining cannot be accomplished in a second. It takes a longer time to fail than it takes to succeed. Perfect sight can only be obtained quickly without effort or strain. The cure of imperfect sight, then, is to stop all effort. It is not accomplished by doing things; it can only come by the things that one stops doing.

STORIES FROM THE CLINIC

No. 85: Case Reports: Four Boys and a Girl

By Emily C. Lierman

During my many years of Clinic work with children, I have found that boys are easier to treat and cure of imperfect sight than girls of the same age.

Robert, age eight, was one of the first of a group of four to be tested with the Snellen test card. His mother had noticed during the last year that his left eye was beginning to turn in. The school nurse had also noticed this and had recommended glasses for him. Robert had refused to be fitted with them. He said if he were compelled to undergo an examination for glasses and they were purchased, he would refuse to wear them.

I knew before I started treating Robert that I would have no trouble in improving his sight, if it were necessary. I was doubtful about his having imperfect sight because I had watched him as he moved about, before I began treating him. I did notice, however, that he had a habit of keeping his head more to one side, which caused an unnecessary strain and prevented him from seeing with both eyes straight. I noticed that, at intervals, he had a slight convergent squint of the left eye.

Robert read 10/10 with the test card with each eye separately. While he was reading the card, I had his mother sit where she could watch his eyes. He read the test card so fast that it was hard for his mother to keep up with him, to notice whether he had made a mistake in reading the letters or not. He read up to the 20-line of the test card with his eyes perfectly relaxed. Then, as he read from the 20- to the 10-line of letters, he began to frown and stare. It was then that the eye turned in. His mother was quick to observe this and commented on it. I asked her if she could describe to me what he did after he had read the 20-line letters. She said she noticed that he frowned and that the eye turned in, but that was all. I asked Robert if he could tell me what he did that was wrong when be arrived at the 20-line letters. He did not know, so I explained to him and his mother that he had not blinked once until he had read the last letter of the card.

When Robert first began reading the card, I noticed that he blinked only twice from the time he started with the large 200-line letter until he arrived at the 20-line. I explained to both of them that this was not enough; that the normal eye blinks often, irregularly and in an easy way, and that it is done unconsciously by persons with normal sight. I explained how necessary it was for Robert to consciously blink often, all day long, no matter what he was doing.

I taught him to palm, asking him to tell me what he was most interested in. I meant his schoolwork, but did not tell him so. Before I had an opportunity to say that I meant schoolwork, Robert cried out, "I like to play best." It was evident from his mother's expression that she thought I would be displeased with his reply, but it is natural for boys to enjoy and to like their play most. I told Robert to imagine he was playing basketball in the gymnasium, which I knew was part of his school routine.

While he palmed, I asked him to remember how he held the basketball, then threw it in the air, and finally made the basket. He smiled as I described this to him. After he had removed his hands from his eyes he was instructed to stand and sway, and by reading one letter at a time, blinking for each letter, he read the whole card without frowning and with both eyes straight. His mother said I had performed a miracle. I told her that the cure was only temporary and that Robert would unconsciously stare again and the eye would, undoubtedly, turn in. This would happen at irregular times, from day to day, until Robert made it a habit to blink and shift, as the normal eye does.

The next time I saw Robert and his mother they informed me that I had made a mistake. Robert's eye did not turn in again, neither did he forget to blink regularly and often. His second test was better than the first one. I had him stand fifteen feet from a strange card which he had not previously read. He read every letter of the card with each eye separately and with both eyes together, not forgetting to blink and shift, and at all times both eyes were straight. Just saying to Robert's mother that he would forget to blink and that the eye would without a doubt turn in again made him determined to remember to use his eyes right.

Two other boys of this same group are brothers. One is nine and the other twelve years old. James, the younger of the two, is keener, but more nervous. He read the whole test card, 10/10, without a mistake. Having watched Robert during his test, he knew exactly what was required of him. It was amusing to see how serious James was during the whole procedure. I had explained previously to Robert that the elephant has intelligence enough to sway his body in order to obtain relaxation and prevent strain. I explained that the elephant must sense that standing still is not good for him because it makes him uncomfortable, therefore, he keeps moving. James was anything but graceful; he swayed like a little elephant in reality. Everyone in the room watching him laughed, but not a smile out of James. At first I thought he was going to cry because he became so excited and nervous. I stood quite close to him and directed him to hold my hands and sway with me. After swinging with me for a short time, he learned to swing by himself. He had to be reminded that blinking alone was not sufficient. James began his lesson by blinking but not looking away. He stared at every letter until I stopped him. After he realized that it was necessary to shift, I had very little else to do for him. Looking out of the window and then back at the card, seeing one letter at a time, swaying, in this way for each letter, his vision improved to 15/10. His second test was even better. He stood twenty feet from a card that he had not seen. He read straight through it without a mistake, with each eye separately, 20/10.

James' grandmother, who was with him, noticed that his nervous twitching ceased. Before, he had not been able to sit still in his chair longer than five minutes at a time, but now he could sit quietly with a book in his hand and read in any kind of light, and not move until it was bedtime.

Jack, James' brother, acted as though he were a grown-up. He very readily stood ten feet from the card and read it through like a racehorse, staring all the while he did so. He had either forgotten that it was wrong to stare, or did not realize that he was staring. After he had finished reading the card, I asked him if that was the way he read his books, or the blackboard at school. "Oh, Yes," said he, "I can read even faster than that." Jack evidently thought that speed was what counted in the test. He was waiting patiently for praise and looked very forlorn when I found fault with him. He soon realized that the way he read the card was not correct, and that he was under a tension and strain when reading so rapidly. For a half-hour I impressed upon his mind that he must not look at more than one letter of the test card at a time without blinking and looking away, which means shifting from the card to a blank wall, or some other place where there are no letters. He asked me why it was necessary to look away from the card after seeing each letter. I told him that when he looked away from the card after seeing each letter, he prevented any strain of his eyes by looking at something that was not hard to see. In other words, shifting is something the normal eye does all the time, only people with good eyes do not notice that the eyes shift because it is done unconsciously.

The next time I saw Jack, I had him stand twenty-five feet from a strange card, and he read it correctly by seeing one letter at a time and looking away. Later he read each line of the card backwards, not looking at the card, but shifting from one side of the card to the other. I asked him to read from one of his books that he had with him, and show me how he read so that I could guide him if he did not read it correctly. After each sentence or two, he would look on the opposite page and see a capital letter at the beginning of a sentence, blink and then proceed with his reading. He told me he could read this way, without any feeling of fatigue, if he blinked his eyes, which he usually remembered to do.

Harold, age eleven, was the tallest and stockiest of the group. His eyelids were swollen and very red, but his vision for each eye was 10/10. He had a habit of keeping his eyes open for a long time without blinking at all. Blinking was one of the first things I encouraged him to do. I had him stand by himself in a corner of the room, and told him not to remove his hands from his eyes until I told him to do so. He nervously wiggled about in his chair after sitting a minute or so. I suppose that five minutes of palming seemed like five hours to him. When a boy of his age has imperfect sight but is perfectly healthy otherwise, it is almost impossible to expect him to be still, even for so short a time. I wanted to see whether palming would relieve the redness of the eyelids and I was glad to see that there was less redness, after he stopped palming. I then had him stand twenty feet from a strange test card and he read the 10-line with each eye separately, 20/10. He whispered in my ear that he was just a little afraid that the other boys would get ahead of him. There was a little sun streaming in one of the windows of the room. He stood there and closed his eyes while I used a sun glass on his eyelids. At first he was a bit frightened for fear that I would harm him, but after I had focused the sun's rays through the glass on his hand, he was reassured. The sun was most beneficial to his eyelids, and the redness disappeared before he left. I feel that the redness of his eyelids was not wholly from eyestrain, but from eating much candy and other sweets, which he confessed he was fond of. If Harold follows my advice, I am sure that the condition of his eyelids will be normal the next time I see him.

Anne, a girl age twelve, who has myopia was my next patient. She was harder to convince and much harder to treat than the entire group of boys. Having difficulty to see at the distance even with her glasses, and not being able to see the blackboard or other things distinctly, caused her to be sullen. The child's eyestrain kept her from being happy as most children of her age are. She was reluctant to leave her glasses off after her first treatment as she felt she looked better with them. I asked her what difference it made whether she was better looking with or without her glasses as long as her eyesight improved with the treatment. Before treatment, her vision with the test card was 10/70 with each eye separately. After she had palmed a while, then swayed as she stood ten feet from the card, her vision improved to 10/50.

On her second visit, Anne's attitude had changed. She said that only one day had she worn her glasses in school since her first treatment, and that she was getting along very well without them. She practiced every day as I directed her, and palmed for more than ten or fifteen minutes at a time while someone read a favorite story to her. By having someone read to her, she was able to improve her mental pictures with her eyes closed, and her vision is now 10/10 by flashing one letter at a time. She is not entirely cured, but if she continues to keep up her enthusiasm to rival the boys who did so well at the start, I feel sure that Anne will soon be cured.

CASE REPORTS

By Elisabet D. Hansen

The following are case reports sent in by one of Dr. Bates' representatives, Elisabet D. Hansen, Chicago, Illinois.

Dear Dr. Bates:

It has been so interesting to watch the unfolding of a recent case, pronounced hopeless by ophthalmologists, that I am writing about it.

Dr. M. L. Cleveland, Palm Beach, Florida, came to Chicago on July 9, 1926, having been told that she had glaucoma in one eye, would be blind in three months, and more than that, the eye would have to be removed in the faint hope of saving the other. Her vision with glasses was 10/15 minus. Without glasses both eyes 10/100 minus, right 10/75 minus and left 10/100 minus. When she had done the long swing until she was fully relaxed, she palmed, listening to happy memories of snowy mountains, plains, forests, skies, etc.

After half an hour of this, she was asked to open her eyes and look at the test card, which she read to 10/50. You can easily imagine that enthusiasm had full sway. Handing me her glasses, she said she was through with them. It being a sunny day, I gave her the sun treatment for a short while with the sun glass and taught her the easy sun swing. This, she said, was delightfully soothing. July 10, the following day, her vision had improved to 10/40. There was a good reason for this. Dr. Cleveland has a wonderful imagination and quickly saw how to use it. We began with the flashing lesson, that is, with the perfect memory of a known letter with closed eyes, she was able to flash every letter on the 30-line. Then I gave her a diamond print card and noticed that she tried to read it and did not blink at all. For relaxation, I explained the value of blinking and imagining white spaces on the card swinging.

Our lessons were interrupted for a while—Dr. Cleveland had to attend a convention out West, but having already gained perfect confidence in the Bates system of Better Eyesight, she knew she was on the right track, and kept on with her exercises. When we met again on August 23, her vision had improved to 10/15 minus. Looking into the eye with the retinoscope, I saw that the dark shadow had disappeared almost entirely and the pupil that had been abnormal was now nearly normal in size. Moreover the hardness of the eyeball and terrible pain were gone. Continuing our lessons (thirteen in all) until she had to return to Florida, her progress was wonderful.

She was ingenious, using each lesson in a way that best suited her case, and between lessons practiced—in the house, on the porch, and in the park. In the latter she was able to read the 10-line at twenty-five feet, 25/10, and when she left Chicago she had perfect far vision and almost perfect near vision.

At this time Ms. W., an elderly lady, was brought to me. She had been blind for sixteen years. The ophthalmologists called it obstruction of the optic nerve. She had only perception of light—the right eye being a little better than the left.

We began the treatment by practicing the long swing and palming. Then, after imagining the big "C," she discerned it on the chart at about six inches distance as something dark and round. After palming again, she was able to get the two letters on the next line as two moving black spots. I ended this lesson by teaching the sun swing with closed eyelids. The next time she came, she told me she had swung the sun and palmed many times a day. We began our lesson with the sun glass treatment; palmed and swung the sun with closed eyes; more palming, and to her surprise she saw, with the card one foot instead of six inches away, the big "C" and the smaller "R" and "B" easily, and the still smaller letters down to the 20-line as spots. Corrections had to be made: when she became very interested, she narrowed her eyes in an effort to see more. As this was evidence of an attempt to see through strain, the habit [of squinting] had to be curbed at once.

After more palming and the memory and flashing exercises of the black period, she could make out bushy forms in the garden, saw that some were more compact than others, and as we were going down the walk at the end of the second lesson, she recognized by their shape some hollyhocks she was passing. Those were the first objects that she had been able to identify in all her years of blindness.

Following this great encouragement, the next striking improvement was seen through the retinoscope. Day by day the veins of the optic nerve took on a healthier color, and in a short time there was a contraction of the pupil in noticeable accommodation to light. After nine lessons, the eye, which had first failed her and which had been least able to discern light, is beginning to show the same improvement as has gone on so gratifyingly in the other, and with this encouragement the patient and her family are enthusiastically looking forward to renewed sight for this sixty-three-year-old woman, who has been blind since her forties.

Very cordially yours, Elisabet Hansen.

Better Eyesight
April 1927—Vol. XI, No. 10

DEMONSTRATE: PALMING

1. Palming improves the sight. When both eyes are closed and covered with one or both hands in such a way as to exclude all light, one does not see red, blue, green or any other color. In short, when the palming is successful one does not see anything but black, and when the eyes are opened, the vision is always improved.

2. An imperfect memory prevents perfect palming and the vision is lowered. Remember a letter "O" imperfectly, a letter "O" which has no white center and is covered by a gray cloud. It takes time; the effort is considerable and in spite of all that is done, the memory of the imperfect "O" is lost or forgotten for a time. The whole field is a shade of gray or of some other color, and when the hands are removed from the eyes, the vision is lowered.

3. When a perfect letter "O" is remembered, palming is practiced properly, continuously and easily and the sight is always benefited.

4. To fail to improve the sight by palming, or to palm imperfectly, is difficult. To fail requires a stare or a strain and is not easy. When an effort is made, the eyes and mind are staring, straining, or trying to see. When no effort is made, the palming becomes successful and the vision is benefited. Successful palming is not accomplished by doing things. Palming becomes successful by the things that are not done.

5. The longer you palm, the greater the benefit to your vision. Palm first for two minutes, then four minutes, six, etc., until you have palmed for fifteen. Notice the improvement gained in 15 minutes has been greater than that in four minutes.

PRESBYOPIA: ITS CAUSE AND CURE

By W. H. Bates, M.D.

Most people, when they reach the age of forty years or older, become unable to read or see things clearly at the near point, while their sight for distance is usually good. This is called presbyopia or middle-aged sight. It is sometimes, although infrequently, found in children.

While it is sometimes very difficult to cure presbyopia, it is, fortunately, very easy to prevent it. Oliver Wendell Holmes told us how to do it in *The Autocrat of the Breakfast Table*. [See July 1919 issue.—TRQ]

I remember an old man who said he was a hundred and six years old, who was quite blind for distant objects, and was unable to read an ordinary newspaper at one foot or farther. With the aid of eye education, his vision for distance soon became normal, and his vision for the near point also improved so that he could read diamond type at six inches without glasses.

The cause of presbyopia has been ascribed by most authorities to a hardening of the lens of the eye, so that the focus of the lens cannot be readily altered. This theory is incorrect. When the lens has been removed for cataract or some other reason, most cases have become able, by education, to read fine print at six inches or less without glasses.

Authorities on ophthalmology have always claimed that the focus of the eye was benefited by a change in the curvature of the lens. The evidence that the lens is not a factor in accommodation has only been recently proved. The eye changes its focus by a change in its length, brought about by the action of the muscles on the outside of the eyeball. In nearsightedness, the eyeball is squeezed by the external muscles and the optic axis is lengthened, i.e., the eyeball becomes [chronically] elongated. The human eye acts in the same way as a photographic camera acts. If a picture is taken at the near point, the bellows of the camera is lengthened in order to focus the near object, while to focus objects at the distance the bellows of the camera is shortened. When the eye is at rest, it has the form of a perfect sphere.

[The fact that many people past age 40, including Dr. Bates, eliminated their need for presbyopic glasses (along with the fact that many elderly people have normal sight with normal accommodation) is a great stumbling block for the orthodox. Either a rigid lens has returned to (or maintained) normal flexibility (and therefore normal lens accommodation), or the oblique muscles are accommodating the eyeball. Both of these positions are unacceptable to the orthodox. I am not aware of any other plausible mechanisms of accommodation offered by the orthodox.

If presbyopia is caused by a chronically tense ciliary muscle preventing the lens from accommodating, Dr. Bates' relaxation principles could explain how people have eliminated presbyopia, while one continues to subscribe to the Helmholtz lens theory of accommodation. It will be an interesting day when all the facts on accommodation and presbyopia are finally known.

In the meantime, it is unfortunate that the orthodox get stuck on this accommodation issue, "throw the baby out with the bath water," and thereby fail to appreciate the tremendous benefits available by relearning relaxed, correct vision habits.—TRQ]

Fundamental Facts

In studying the cause of presbyopia it is well to remember or to demonstrate some fundamental facts. In the first place, the printed page has more white exposed than it has black. One can look at the white spaces between the lines and hold the book very close to the eyes, four or five inches or more without any discomfort, but if one looks at a letter or part of a letter and tries to keep his mind fixed on that one part continuously, sooner or later the eyes become tired, the mind wanders, and the vision becomes imperfect. Looking at the white spaces and imagining them to be perfectly white, is a rest and can be accomplished more readily than improving the black letters by an effort.

When the white center of a letter "O" is seen gray, blurred and indistinct, one is seeing something that is not there. In other words, imperfect sight is never seen; it is only imagined. With perfect sight one may see the white center of the letter much whiter than it really is, or whiter than the rest of the card. By covering over the black part of the letter "O" with a screen and exposing only a part of the white center, one can demonstrate that the whiteness in the center of a letter "O" when seen perfectly, is not really seen, but imagined. Imagination of perfect sight is easier than imagination of imperfect sight. When one remembers a letter "O" perfectly, it is accomplished without effort, and it may be remembered more or less continuously, but if a letter "O" is imagined imperfectly without a white center, blurred, or cloudy, it prevents the letter from being seen, remembered or imagined clearly as an "O." To improve the memory or the imagination of an imperfect "O" requires time, a second or longer. To make an attempt to remember an imperfect "O" continuously is difficult, requires much trouble, causes pain in the eyes and head, and discomfort of various kinds in all the nerves of the body. The memory of imperfect sight is difficult, because it requires so much effort to maintain it. In spite of all the efforts that are made to remember imperfect sight, one soon demonstrates that the imperfect letter "O" will not be remembered continuously. It is the things that we stop doing that promote the memory of perfect sight. We do not need to practice something new nor learn by mental training how to do something that we have never done before. When a patient is convinced of these facts it is difficult to realize why he keeps on doing wrong, when using his eyes correctly is so much easier and brings renewed vision.

Fine Print

When people are able to read fine print with perfect sight at six inches or farther, the white spaces between the lines are seen or imagined whiter than the rest of the card. The ability to imagine the white spaces between the lines to be very white is accomplished by the memory of white snow, white starch or anything perfectly white, with the eyes closed for part of a minute. Some patients count thirty while remembering some white object or scene with the eyes closed. Then, when the eyes are opened for a second, the white spaces between the lines of black letters are imagined or seen much whiter than before. By alternately remembering something perfectly white with the eyes closed and opening them for a few seconds and flashing the spaces, the vision or the imagination of the white spaces improves. One needs to be careful not to make an effort or to regard the black letters. When the white spaces between the lines are imagined sufficiently white, or as white as they can be remembered with the eyes closed and with the eyes open, the black letters are read without effort or strain, or without the consciousness of regarding the black letters. Many people discover that they can imagine a thin white line where the bottom of the letters comes in contact with the white spaces. This thin line is very white, and the thinner it is imagined to be, the whiter it becomes.

This thin white line can be imagined much whiter than any other part of the page, and is more easily imagined or seen than any other part. When the vision of the thin white line is imperfect, the shifting is slow and imperfect and the vision for the letters is impaired. The memory or the imagination of the thin white line is usually so easy, so perfect and so continuous that everything regarded is seen with maximum vision. Patients with cataract who become able to imagine this thin white line perfectly, very soon become able to read the finest print without effort or strain, and the cataract always improves, or becomes less. Patients with hypermetropia, astigmatism, squint, diseases of the retina and optic nerve are benefited in every way by the memory or the imagination of the thin white line. Reading fine print with perfect sight benefits or improves all organic diseases of the eye.

The Universal Swing

There are a number of varieties of the optical swing which prevent, improve or cure presbyopia. Of these, perhaps the best one of all is called the universal swing. When one can practice the universal swing, and at the same time test the imagination of the thin white line or the white spaces between the lines, the presbyopia is usually very much benefited.

If you hold your finger about six inches from your eyes, by moving your head from side to side it is possible to imagine the finger to be moving in the opposite direction. This is the variable swing. While the eyes are moving in the opposite direction to the movement of the finger, all other objects can be imagined in the same way. Usually distant objects do not swing as much as the finger and may appear to be almost stationary. With the eyes closed, one can remember the finger moving from side to side and imagine that all objects to which the finger is connected, directly or indirectly, appear to move in the same direction, and the same distance as the finger moves, the only difference being that the eyes move with the finger and with everything else, while with the eyes open in the variable swing, the eyes always move in the opposite direction to the movement of the finger. One can improve the universal swing by remembering the movement of the finger with the eyes closed. This swing can be demonstrated more readily with the eyes closed than with the eyes open.

By holding the diamond type about six inches from your eyes and holding the thumb about an inch nearer the eyes, and about one-quarter of an inch to the left of one letter of the diamond type, one can demonstrate that when the head and eyes move from side to side, the thumb appears to move opposite, while the fine print appears to move with the movement of the head and eyes. [Double oppositional movement; yet without the thumb, *the fine print* appears to move opposite!—TRQ] At once, the fine print improves sufficiently to be read and the thin white line also becomes more perfectly seen or imagined.

Some patients are able to move the thumbnail more or less rapidly close to the bottom of the letters and read the fine print, perfectly continuously and rapidly. The thumbnail moving from side to side improves the imagination of the thin white line, and when the thin white line is imagined sufficiently white, the letters are flashed sufficiently black to be distinguished.

When the head and eyes move in a circular direction, the movement becomes continuous and the vision is also more continuous. The circular swing may be practiced with the head and eyes moving in the orbit of a large circle. When the movement of the head and eyes in a circular direction is shortened, the vision is further improved. However, one has to realize that in a short, circular swing, the movement stops readily, thereby lowering the vision. Patients should demonstrate that a short, circular swing, while being a greater benefit, may be unconsciously stopped, while the large circular swing is more apt to be continuous. When the vision becomes lowered while reading with the help of the circular swing, it is evidence that the circular swing has been unconsciously stopped.

Another cure of presbyopia is accomplished with the aid of the memory. When one can remember a color, letter or an object perfectly, presbyopia disappears and the vision becomes normal. Perfect memory is always accompanied by perfect relaxation with perfect sight.

STORIES FROM THE CLINIC

No. 86: Presbyopia

By Emily C. Lierman

I have recently had a few cases of presbyopia which were cured in a short time. One was a woman sixty-three years old who did fine sewing for her livelihood. She had worn glasses for more than thirty years and during the past two years her eye specialist found it difficult to fit her with glasses correctly. She had purchased her last pair the day before she came to me, and told me they made her so nervous and irritable that she could not possibly wear them more than half a day.

Her vision for the distance was normal, 15/15 with each eye separately. I gave her a small test card to hold, which has the Fundamentals by Dr. W. H. Bates on the opposite side, and asked her to read what she could on it. She held it at arm's length and said that she knew there was some kind of print on the card, but could not tell what it was. In despair she looked at me and said, "I fear you will have a hard time getting me to read this." I gave her the small booklet containing the microscopic type and also a small card with diamond type. I placed the booklet at the lower part of the Fundamentals card and the diamond type card in the center. She was told to hold these about twelve inches from her eyes and not to worry about reading the print. The patient looked at me in a blank sort of way wondering how it was possible to cure presbyopia in this manner. As she was optimistic, it was easy for me to treat her. She was willing to believe that I could do for her what had been done for others whom she knew had been cured by Dr. Bates. I told her to look at the small white spaces between the lines of print in the booklet, close both eyes and remember the white spaces. She could remember them white with her eyes closed. I then told her to open her eyes and again look at the white spaces. She said they appeared whiter than they had the first time. Again I told her to close her eyes and remember the white spaces and to open them in less than a second, look at the white spaces of the diamond type card, close her eyes and remember the white spaces; then for just a second to open her eyes and look at the white spaces of the Fundamentals card. I told her to keep this up while I was out of the room and left her to herself for almost a half-hour. Before leaving I warned her about trying to read the print, telling her that she was to flash only the white spaces. When I returned she looked at me very much frightened and said "What am I to do, I cannot help but tell you the truth, I can read this 'Fundamentals' card." I noticed that she held the Fundamentals card eight inches from her eyes instead of twelve. She read one sentence after another for me. After reading a sentence of the Fundamentals card she would shift to the white spaces of the blue booklet and then to the spaces of the small card and back again to the Fundamentals card. The treatment lasted about one hour. I told her to telephone me the next day and let me know if she had forgotten what I had directed her to do. She called, and said that she was able to read some of the Bible type as well as all of the print on the Fundamentals card. Having read my book before she came for treatment, she knew that staring produced much discomfort and realized that she should blink frequently. Her knowledge of the benefits of blinking helped her to be cured more quickly than the usual case of this kind. The last time that she telephoned she reported that her sewing was much easier to do. She has entirely discarded her glasses and promises never to wear them again.

The second patient was a man fifty-eight years old, a bank teller. He had heard of a bank president who had been cured by Dr. Bates. Then he obtained my book and Bates' book, *Perfect Sight Without Glasses,* from the public library. He understood the directions described in each book, but there were times when he was unsuccessful in getting good results, so he came to me for help.

His sight was tested for the distance and he read 15/30 with each eye separately, although he saw some of the letters double. He complained of headache and pain in the back of his eyes, especially while working. He was then directed to palm and to imagine that he was adding accounts. He said it caused more strain and discomfort in his head and eyes. He said that it would be impossible to palm during business hours. I told him that it would not be necessary, that there were other things that he could do to prevent his headaches and eyestrain. I taught him to blink and shift all day long like the normal eye does in order to keep the eyes relaxed and in good condition. He was told to remember something perfectly, easily and without effort. He said he could remember the ocean with the tide coming in and that every seventh wave was the largest. Knowing the game of football helped him to imagine the size, color and shape of the ball. All these little details which improved his memory helped to relax his mind while his eyes were closed.

After ten minutes, he was instructed to stand with his feet about one foot apart and sway his body to the right and then to the left. As the window was close by, I directed him to look off in the distance and notice objects moving with his body, eyes and head, while things up close seemed to move opposite. He said he was hoping I would let him do that for quite a while because the bad headache he had just before coming to me was disappearing.

Then I told him to keep up the swing, looking out of the window and then toward the test card. As soon as he saw a letter I told him to look away, keeping up the swing all the while. This time he read 15/10 with each eye separately. When I gave him the Fundamentals card to read, he could see only sentence No. 2. All the rest of the card was very much blurred to him. Again I directed him to stand and swing and notice distant objects moving with his eyes and body, while things close appeared to move opposite.

I then had him sit in a chair with his back to the sun and told him to remember the sway of the body with his eyes closed. In a short time he began to practice again with the Fundamentals card, and this time he read up to No. 8 by imagining the white spaces whiter than they really were. I watched him as he tried to read further and when he began to read the small type, he stopped the blinking unconsciously and stared at the print. I noticed that his forehead became wrinkled and that he squeezed his eyes almost shut to read. I stopped this and asked him to close his eyes quickly and tell me how he felt. He had produced a strain that caused his head and eyes to ache. I reminded him that by squeezing his eyes and staring and making an effort, a strain had been produced. While his eyes were covered with the palm of one hand, he remarked, "Now I realize what I must do all day long to see without straining." I told him that when patients found out for themselves that staring brings on tension and pain, they are cured much more quickly than others who do not realize this fact. He was cured in three visits.

My third case of presbyopia, which took the longest time to cure, was a music teacher forty-nine years old. It was very hard to convince her that I could benefit her. Her vision for the test card with each eye was normal, 15/15. When I gave her the Fundamentals card to read, she was quite positive that she would never read any of it without her glasses. I gave her a *Better Eyesight* magazine and told her to look at the title. She said that she could see it, but that the type was blurred as she held it at arm's length from her eyes.

She was told to close her eyes and palm with one hand and remember one of the letters of the test card that she had read at fifteen feet. Then, in less than a moment's time, I told her to remove her hand from her eyes and look at the white spaces of the Fundamentals card. She did this a few times and then began to smile. She said the print was beginning to clear up, but that it soon faded away and she became unable to read it again. When I told her to avoid looking at the type, she laughed. Immediately I became convinced that this was the way she read her sheet music. She looked directly at the notes and lowered her vision by staring. By closing her eyes and remembering white spaces, then opening them and looking at the white spaces, words began to clear up and she became a very different person. When she was successful in doing as I directed, she read up to No. 3 of the Fundamentals card. I saw her once a week for more than a month before she was able to read the entire Fundamentals card, eight inches from her eyes. She was told to place the small black test card on the piano near the sheet music and to frequently flash a letter of the card; then read her music. In this way she was cured. All patients cannot be treated in the same way, no matter what trouble they may have with their eyes. Eyestrain has a great deal to do with the mind and the Bates Method has surely proved it.

CASE REPORT

January 14, 1927
Mr. Robert C. Fager

Dear Sir:

In reply to your letter of the 11th concerning Dr. Bates' book *Perfect Sight Without Glasses,* I would like to say that after reading this book about five years ago and practicing the methods outlined in the book, I was able to lay aside my glasses which I had been wearing more or less for twenty-one years. I have not used my glasses since that time and have noted no bad effects; in fact, I have continued to feel better and gain in weight until I am now, at forty-two years old, better than I ever was.

I still have some slight astigmatism in my right eye, but feel that if I would really take the time and trouble to practice Dr. Bates' methods more thoroughly, I would easily overcome this difficulty.

When I used to wear glasses, I would get headaches in a few minutes time if I tried to read without them. Since learning Dr. Bates' exercises, I have had no trouble reading as long as I wanted to without any headaches.

If you have had no operation on your eyes, I feel sure that you can obtain normal vision if you will conscientiously practice the methods described in Dr. Bates' book.

Sincerely yours,
Wm. J. Dana,
Professor of Experimental Engineering, North Carolina State College of Agriculture and Engineering.

QUESTIONS AND ANSWERS

Q–1. In case of illness where one is unable to practice with the Snellen test card or stand up, what method is used?

A–1. Blink frequently and shift your eyes constantly from one point to another. Turn your head slightly from side to side on the pillow or close your eyes and think of something pleasant, something that you can remember perfectly and let your mind drift from one pleasant thought to another.

Q–2. The sun shining on the snow darkens and almost blinds my vision. What is this caused by, and how can I obtain relief?

A–2. This is caused by a strain and can be relieved by practicing blinking, shifting and central fixation all day long. Notice that stationary objects appear to move in the direction opposite to the movement of your head and eyes. Notice that the trees or other near objects move opposite, while the horizon or distant objects move with you.

Q–3. It is very hard for me to think in terms of black and white. Is there some other method which is just as beneficial?

A–3. Yes, letting your mind drift from one pleasant memory to another will accomplish the same results.

Q–4. Is it necessary to practice with the Snellen test card if you follow the method otherwise?

A–4. Yes, it is advisable to keep up your daily practice with the test card for at least a few moments. This will improve your memory and the memory must be improved in order to have the vision improve.

Better Eyesight
May 1927—Vol. XI, No. 11

DEMONSTRATE: SHORT SWAYING

A short, swaying movement improves the vision more than a long sway. Place the test card at a distance where only the large letter at the top of the card can be distinguished. This may be ten feet, farther or nearer. Stand with the feet about one foot apart and sway the body from side to side. When the body sways to the right, look to the right of the card. When the body sways to the left, look to the left of the card. Do not look at the Snellen test card. Sway the body from side to side and look to the right of the Snellen test card, and alternately to the left of it. Note that the test card appears to be moving. Increase the length of the sway and notice that the test card seems to move a longer distance from side to side. Observe the whiteness of the card and the blackness of the letters. Now shorten the sway, which, of course, shortens the movement of the card. The card appears whiter and the letters blacker when the movement of the card is short, than when the movement of the card is long.

MYOPIA

By W. H. Bates, M.D.

Myopia, or nearsightedness as it is commonly called, is caused by a strain to see at the distance.

In myopia, the eyes are habitually focused for a point about twelve inches or less. In high degrees of myopia, the eyes may be focused at less than twelve inches, ten inches, six inches, three inches or nearer to the eyes. Some patients can read the test card perfectly when they regard it close enough to the eyes. They may be able to read the diamond type when held two to three inches from the eyes. In low degrees of myopia, the vision may be almost as good as in the normal eye.

When the normal eye is at rest, there is no myopia. When the normal eye reads at twelve inches, with an effort or a strain, it becomes temporarily myopic. In order to produce myopia in the normal eye, it is necessary to strain or make an effort to see. In all cases, myopia is caused or is accompanied by an effort or a strain to see at the distance.

Many children, at ten years old, may have normal eyes, which remain normal until they begin to strain and make an effort to see at the distance. Such patients are cured of their myopia when they can regard the Snellen test card or other objects without any effort or strain.

It can be demonstrated, with the aid of the retinoscope, that myopic patients do not have myopia all the time. When regarding a blank surface, where there is nothing to be seen, or when the patient makes no effort to see, the retinoscope always demonstrates the absence of myopia. When, by treatment the myopic eye does not strain nor make an effort to see at the distance, the myopia becomes less or may disappear altogether.

The quickest cures of myopia are accomplished with the help of the memory, the imagination and central fixation.

Memory and Imagination

A perfect memory and perfect imagination cures myopia under favorable conditions. Patients who have a good memory of mental pictures have no myopia when the mental pictures are remembered or imagined perfectly. There are nearsighted people who, after a course of eye education, can look at a Snellen test card at ten feet or farther and remember or imagine the white part of the card perfectly white and the black letters perfectly black. When this is accomplished, the myopia improves.

When schoolchildren regard the blackboard, they often half-close their eyelids, or stare and strain to see and thus produce myopia. When they can remember a mental picture of some small letter, and remember it as well with the eyes open as with the eyes closed, normal vision and a temporary cure of their myopia is obtained. In myopia and other phases of imperfect sight, the white centers of all letters are imagined less white than the rest of the card. When the patient becomes able to imagine the white centers with a white background to be whiter than the rest of the card, the vision is improved and there is no myopia.

Central Fixation

When the vision of myopic patients is imperfect, it can always be demonstrated that the point regarded is not seen best, and other parts of a letter may be seen equally well or better. When the patient becomes able to remember or imagine one part of a letter or an object best, the myopia is lessened and the vision improves. When the strain is prevented, by shifting from one side of the letter to another, the letter appears to move from side to side. The vision may then become normal and the myopia disappears.

Universal Swing

The universal swing is of great value in the treatment of myopia and may be practiced as follows: Regard the Snellen test card at ten feet. Hold the forefinger of one hand about six inches to the front and to the side of one eye. The finger may be held at a nearer distance and good results obtained. Then move the head a short distance from side to side, without looking at the finger, and without trying to read the letters on the distant Snellen test card. Do not look directly at the finger, or the apparent movement becomes modified or stops. Now close the eyes and remember the finger as moving from side to side. If the hand and finger are placed in the lap, one may still be able to remember the moving finger. With the help of the imagination, one may realize that when the finger moves, the hand which is fastened to the finger also moves at the same speed and to the same extent. The same is true of the arm, the elbow, the shoulder, all moving with the finger.

The universal swing is characterized by the fact that one becomes able to imagine the eyes are moving with the finger when the eyes are closed, but when the eyes are opened, they usually move opposite to the movement of the finger.

When the eyes are open, one can note that by moving the head from side to side, near objects move opposite to the direction of the head and eyes, while distant objects may appear to move in the same direction as the head and eyes.

When one is regarding the Snellen test card, the letters of the card move with the head and eyes, and when the letters move, one can, of course, imagine the whole card to be moving with the head and eyes. Under these conditions, the eyes become more thoroughly relaxed with a consequent improvement in the vision and lessening of the myopia. When the universal swing is practiced correctly, the movement of the letters and the card is slow, short (about one-quarter of an inch), and easy.

One should practice the universal swing for a sufficient length of time to become able to imagine the letters of the Snellen test card moving in the same direction as do the head and eyes. It is impossible to imagine the Snellen test card moving with the head and eyes unless some nearer object moves opposite to the movement of the head and eyes.

A Test of the Imagination

There are a number of phenomena which always occur when the universal swing is practiced. With the back of one Snellen test card toward the patient and placed ten feet away from him, and with the face of the second towards him and placed at twelve feet, both cards can be so arranged that the patient can observe an open space between the two of about four or five inches in width.

When the patient moves the head and eyes to the left, the space between the two cards becomes less, and one can imagine the near card moving to the right, while the more distant card with its letters appears to move to the left.

When the head and eyes move to the right, the near card appears to move to the left, the space becomes larger between the two cards, and the patient can imagine the face of the more distant card moving to the right.

When the vision is normal and the head and eyes move from side to side, the near card moves opposite, while the more distant card moves in the same direction as the head and eyes.

When the vision is imperfect and the head and eyes are moved from side to side, the near card moves opposite, while the more distant card may also move opposite to the movement of the head and eyes, or it may stop or move in an irregular, jerky manner. When one letter of the distant card is seen imperfectly or when one side or part of a letter is imagined imperfectly, consciously or unconsciously, the movement of the more distant card is modified and very irregular.

When the imagination of a small part of an unknown letter is correct, the swing of the more distant card becomes normal, the card moves from side to side in the same direction as the head and eyes and moves slowly, easily, and continuously. By repetition, one may become able to imagine a part of an unknown letter with the eyes open nearly as well as with the eyes closed, and the imagination of an unknown letter may improve until the imagination becomes as good or better than the sight. The distant card always moves in the same direction as the movement of the head and eyes, when a part of an unknown letter is imagined perfectly. The reverse is also true, that when the distant card does not move with the head and eyes, the imagination of an unknown letter is imperfect.

The patient should learn to practice the universal swing not only indoors with the help of the Snellen test card, but it should also be practiced while walking or driving. Some people can demonstrate that all objects become clearer or more distinct by imagining them to move with the head and eyes. This result, however, cannot be obtained unless nearer objects appear to move opposite to the movement of the head and eyes.

When the universal swing is practiced, it is possible for patients with myopia to improve the vision to normal, and the myopia is no longer apparent. Many patients with myopia complain that the benefit obtained from palming, swinging, central fixation and other methods is only temporary. If by continued practice of these methods, however, the flashes of improved vision do not become more frequent and last longer, the universal swing is usually beneficial.

Some patients have difficulty in practicing the universal swing successfully. They are benefited in many cases by imagining the universal swing with the eyes closed for a longer time than with them open.

A Familiar Card

When patients practice reading a familiar test card a number of times daily, it is not very long before the letters become memorized. The criticism is made that patients do not see the letters, they only remember or imagine them. It is true that when the sight is perfect, the imagination as well as the memory is perfect. Practicing with the Snellen test card with the help of the memory and the imagination is a benefit. Myopia is always relieved or corrected with the aid of a perfect memory or a perfect imagination. Practicing with a familiar card is one of the quickest methods of curing myopia temporarily or permanently. The more perfectly the letters of the Snellen test card are remembered or imagined, the more completely is the myopia relieved.

Case History

A boy, eight years old, practiced with a familiar Snellen test card twice daily for six months. His mother was discouraged because she said that her son had learned the letters by heart and one could not tell whether he saw the letters correctly or just imagined them. A number of Snellen test cards which the boy had never seen before were used in testing his sight. Much to the surprise of his mother, he read the strange cards just as readily, if not more readily than he did the familiar card. This, of course, convinced his mother that his vision was normal for the strange test cards. She was very curious to know why.

With the aid of the retinoscope she was able to see the red reflex in the pupil and to imagine a cloud moving from side to side in the same direction as the retinoscope was moved. This always occurred when the patient had normal vision with the familiar or unfamiliar card. When he imagined the letters imperfectly, his mother demonstrated that the shadow moved in the opposite direction to the movement of the retinoscope. It was not difficult to convince her then that, when his vision for the familiar card was perfect, he had no myopia.

Many patients with myopia have been tested and in all cases when the memory was perfect, the sight was perfect. As a rule, schoolchildren who had good memories were more readily cured than other children. In most schools young children under twelve years old, who had myopia, were temporarily or permanently cured by the use of the familiar Snellen test card.

The Snellen Test Card

The Snellen test card, while it is of value as a test for the ability of the children to see, is of far greater usefulness as a means for improving the sight.

Acute myopia is usually cured by very simple treatment. Children under twelve years old who have never worn glasses are usually temporarily cured by alternately reading the Snellen test card and resting their eyes by palming.

I have found that in schools where the Snellen test card is visible continuously, the vision of the pupils is always improved and that the children in the higher grades acquire more perfect sight than they had when they first entered school. Most children demonstrate that while the Snellen test card improves the vision that it is also a benefit to the nervous system. It prevents and cures headaches, lessens fatigue, encourages the children to study, and increases the mental efficiency.

STORIES FROM THE CLINIC

No. 87: Cases of Myopia

By Emily C. Lierman

A woman, forty-six years old, who has had myopia as long as she can remember, placed herself under my care, but doubted that I could give her a permanent cure for nearsightedness.

About forty years ago, noticing that she stumbled over objects which were easily seen by others with good vision, her parents had her fitted with glasses. After having had her glasses changed about five times, she came to me for help. At the oculist's advice, she tried faithfully to wear the last pair of glasses continuously, for at least a week, and then returned to him. The glasses were much stronger than those she had previously worn and magnified everything to such an extent that it was impossible to go without them. Although the patient was skeptical about the Bates Method, she was desperate and willing to believe anything in order that she might be able to do without glasses. I feared that with that attitude she would not continue with the treatment, but I found that I was mistaken. She was very faithful in practicing what I directed her to do.

Now, after four months of treatment and advice, which was carried out religiously by the patient, she drives her car and reads signs, sometimes half a city block away, without glasses. This patient is not entirely cured, although for days at a time she reads 10/10 with the test card and holds her book for reading at normal distance.

In the beginning, it was hard to convince her that it was strain which produced her myopic condition. In treating myopic cases, Dr. Bates and I have proved that all cases of myopia cannot be treated in the same way. This patient's vision with the test card in December 1926, was the same in both eyes; namely, 10/70. The 70-line letters, however, were very much blurred. Palming helped temporarily, and her vision improved to 10/40 with the aid of blinking, swinging the body a short distance from left to right and flashing one letter of the test card with each sway of the body. I realized that this was not helping her enough and that she should progress more rapidly, so I experimented with other methods of treatment.

One day she came to me and told me that I was improving her mental condition. Knowing what good results Dr. Bates had had with the universal swing, I used that with my patient. I had her stand before a window and told her to swing from left to right as I was doing. A decided swing of the body from left to right made distant buildings, flagstaffs and other distant objects appear to move with her body, head and eyes. I encouraged her to keep looking off at the distance while she explained to me how the things at the near point appeared to move. With great surprise in her voice she said, "The window, curtains, shade cord, and other things nearby appear to move in the opposite direction." I continued swinging with the patient, encouraging her to keep it up for five or ten minutes. I watched her eyes closely to be sure that she was blinking. She noticed that I was watching her and made an unusual remark which I did not expect from her, because myopic patients usually stare without knowing it. She turned to me and said. "You are watching to see whether I blink or not. Don't worry about that, it feels more comfortable to blink while I am swinging." She also said that she noticed that her eyes felt less heavy while she kept up the swing and that the sun seemed to shine brighter than she had ordinarily noticed it at anytime. All the while she was talking she kept up the swing.

When I made a test of her vision again before her first treatment was over, her vision improved to 15/15. The patient was much excited and asked if this improved condition of her eyes would continue. I answered, "Yes, if you will remember every day to practice the universal swing frequently."

To vary the treatment for home practice, I gave her two small Fundamentals cards with the test letters on the opposite side. She was directed to place one card on her desk as she sat or stood about five feet from the card. The same kind of a card with the same letters was to be held in her hand. She was to begin with the largest letter, which is seen by the normal eye at fifty feet. Looking at the "C," to the right of it where the small opening is, closing her eyes and remembering the small opening and imagining the opening and center of the "C" whiter than the margin of the card, then looking at the card placed on her desk and shifting from the card in her hand to the other card, helped to improve her vision when practicing in another way failed. This practice helped her for awhile, but that which helped her most to bring about temporary normal vision was the practice of the universal swing.

The patient still reports her progress. After a short period of palming, which is practiced several times each day, she always does the universal swing and emphasizes the fact that it helps her more than anything else.

She told me that at first her husband had been afraid to ride with her after she had removed her glasses and had warned her not to attempt driving without putting them on. Now he no longer doubts her ability to see better without the use of glasses, and helps to give her the sun treatment every day with the sun glass, which I suggested might be of benefit during the treatment.

Recently I had an unfavorable report of the condition of her eyes. There had been no sun for a few days and she was depressed. I assured her that her depression would disappear when the sun shone again. Practicing the universal swing often, whenever she had the opportunity, relieved her of tension and strain and her vision became normal again.

Encouragement helped, and I believe that she will not need much further advice or instruction from me, because she drives her car with perfect ease. She sees the center of the road coming toward her from the distance and as it comes close, she enjoys seeing it pass under the car. Instead of suffering her usual headache after driving an automobile as she did when she wore her glasses, she feels better after driving. She said that when she learned to see things moving to avoid the stare, her focus for the distance was changed and she could not wear her glasses again even if she wanted to, because they no longer suited her.

Another case, a woman age forty-eight, had worn glasses for more than fourteen years for myopia and headaches. She feared the strong light of the sun because it caused great pain in her eyes. I could not encourage her to practice the Universal Swing until I had first placed her in the sun with her eyes closed, and focused the sun's rays on her closed eyelids with the sun glass. This gave her instant relief. She complained that at all times while she kept her eyes open, they felt tightened up. This was true with her glasses on as well as off. After the use of the sun glass for more than ten minutes I placed her before a window and instructed her to look at the distant houses and other objects. She said that everything appeared blurred to her and that it made her eyes ache all the more while swinging. I knew that she was not practicing it correctly, so I had her sit in a chair and directed her to keep her eyes closed for awhile. While conversing with her, I discovered that palming caused more tension and strain, so I did not encourage it.

The vision of this patient was 5/200 with the right eye and 5/50 with the left. When the patient covered her left eye, she stared fully a minute with her right eye in order to see the largest letter of the test card at five feet. Directing her to count two with her eyes closed, then opening her right eye just long enough to count one as she looked at the test card, then closing her eyes and counting two, the vision of her right eye improved to 5/50, the same as that of her left eye.

I then placed her in the sun again and used the sun glass on her closed eyelids for about ten minutes. The expression of her face was entirely changed. Her forehead, which was all lines from tension, became smooth and the corners of her mouth were drawn upward instead of downward.

After the sun treatment, we started the universal swing again while standing by an open window. Off in the distance, an American flag was waving gently with the breeze. She noticed that the flagstaff moved or appeared to move with the movement of her body, head and eyes. The window, shade-cord, curtains, and a chair placed directly in front of her, all seemed to move opposite. This swinging was kept up for fifteen minutes, and immediately afterward in a bright light she read the white letters on the black test card ten feet away. Her vision improved to 10/10 reading with both eyes.

I treated her every day for a week and when she left me on the last day, she said that she had found blinking a help and felt that she must blink to keep the eyes relaxed, but she believed as I did, that the universal swing was what really cured her.

She assured me that her friends would have to swing with her if she noticed at any time that they caused her to strain.

CASE REPORT

Hypermetropic Astigmatism

By Dr. H. M. Peppard

Last fall a young man presented himself to me for examination complaining of headache, nervousness, insomnia and eyestrain. He had previously had a nervous breakdown and said he felt as if he were going to have another. This statement was apparently correct if general appearances can be considered as an indication. The eyes were bulging with a dry, glassy appearance and the upper lid markedly retracted.

The eye examination revealed a very hard eyeball with 1.25 diopters of hyperopia with 2.50 diopters of astigmatism with the axis 180. Glasses had been worn but gave little relief. The visual acuity was 20/50 for both eyes and the same in each eye.

Treatment by the Bates Method was started on August 4. Palming, swinging, blinking, flashing and reading of diamond type was used. The flashing was especially beneficial.

On August 27, the eyes were again tested. Visual acuity was 20/15 for both eyes 20/15 in the right, and 20/20 in the left. The hyperopia or farsightedness was not present and the astigmatism was decreased to 1.00 diopter. A few more treatments relieved the remainder of the astigmatism and the vision improved to 20/15 in each eye.

With the improvement in vision, the general symptoms cleared up. He became able to sleep, was free from headaches and was not so nervous.

The eyes felt comfortable and his entire facial expression was changed from the relaxation around the eyes. The eyes no longer were starey, but bright and moist and the blinking frequent and easy. Six months later the eyes were in perfect condition and the patient no longer feared a nervous breakdown.

SIMULTANEOUS RETINOSCOPY

By W. H. Bates, M.D.

By simultaneous retinoscopy is meant the use of the retinoscope while the patient is using his eyes for distant or near vision.

In order to obtain accurate results by simultaneous

retinoscopy, a patient was seated in a chair which was placed about ten feet from the Snellen test card. To the right, to the left, and above the Snellen test card was a blank, dark gray surface. An examination was made with the retinoscope which was held about six feet from the eyes of the patient. While the patient was looking at a blank surface without trying to see and the retinoscope was used at the same time, it was demonstrated that there was no myopic refraction manifest. The eyes were normal and the patient was able to see with perfect sight.

When the patient moved his eyes quickly from side to side and no effort was made to see, it was demonstrated by simultaneous retinoscopy that no myopic refraction was produced. After shifting from one point to another, closing and opening the eyes and seeing the letters in flashes, the patient's vision improved. By repetition the flashes of improved vision became more frequent and lasted longer, until finally the patient became conscious of a permanent improvement.

Shifting has proved a very valuable method of improving the sight, not only in myopia, but also in all other eye troubles. When the eyes shift to the left, they are stationary for an appreciable length of time, before they can look to the right. When they are stationary, they may stare or strain sufficiently to lower the vision. In order to become myopic while shifting, it is necessary to strain sufficiently to change the shape of the eyeball.

Circular or elliptical shifting may be all that is necessary to prevent the eye from staring or making an effort. When the eyes shift to the left and move in the orbit of a circle or an ellipse, the movement is continuous, and the eyes do not have time to stop before they look to the right. Two areas may be regarded alternately. One part of the background above and to the right of the test card may be regarded with normal sight. Use this area as a point of departure which may be seen for part of a minute or longer. Then shift to the lower left-hand corner of the test card and quickly back again to the point of departure. This should be done in one second or less.

When regarding the plain background, the eyes are relaxed or at rest and have normal sight. Shift rapidly downwards to the lower left-hand corner of the card and back again to the upper area of the background. In this way shifting may be practiced with benefit. When one can regard the point of departure with normal vision, the eyes become normal temporarily in flashes.

A benefit to the sight comes in flashes at first, although simultaneous retinoscopy indicates that the eye may be, at the same time, continuously normal. The flashes become more and more frequent and continue for a longer time.

Better Eyesight
June 1927—Vol. XI, No. 12

DEMONSTRATE: WALKING

The eyes can be used correctly or incorrectly when walking.

Many people have complained that after walking a short distance slowly, easily and without any special effort, they become nervous, tired and their eyes feel the symptoms and consequences of strain. When they were taught the correct way to use their eyes while walking, the symptoms of fatigue or strain disappeared.

The facts can be demonstrated with the aid of a straight line on the floor or the seam in the carpet.

Stand with the right foot to the right of the line and the left foot to the left of the line. Now put your right foot forward and look to the left of the line. Then put your left foot forward and look to the right of the line. When you walk forward, look to the left of the line when your right foot moves forward. Look to the right of the line when your left foot moves forward. Note that it is difficult to do this longer than a few seconds without uncertainty, discomfort, pain, headache, dizziness or nausea.

Now practice the right method of walking and using the eyes. When the right foot moves forward, look to the right; and when the left foot moves forward, look to the left. Note that the straight line seems to sway in the direction opposite to the movement of the eyes and foot, i.e., when the eyes and foot move to the right, the line seems to move to the left. When the eyes and foot move to the left, the line seems to move to the right. Note that this is done easily, without any hesitation or discomfort.

When you walk, you can imagine that you are looking at the right foot as you step forward with that foot. When you step forward with the left foot, you can imagine that you are looking at your left foot. This can be done in a slow walk or quite rapidly while running straight ahead or in a circle.

ASTIGMATISM

By W. H. Bates, M.D.

The study of astigmatism is important because of its frequency and because so many serious diseases of the eye are preceded by astigmatism.

Definitions

[See definitions in the December 1926 issue.—TRQ]

Occurrence

Astigmatism occurs frequently and is usually combined with hypermetropia or myopia.

I have investigated the facts of the occurrence of astigmatism in newborn children. For the past one hundred years or more, atropine has been used to assist in measuring the astigmatism of the eye. It dilates the pupil and is supposed to paralyze the muscles which change the focus of the eyeball. While young babies were under observation, atropine, of sufficient strength to produce a maximum dilatation of the pupil, was accordingly used. Although the pupils became widely dilated, the ability of the eye to change its focus was not prevented by the atropine. With the aid of the retinoscope it was found that the form of the eyeball changed from hour to hour or from day to day. My observations showed that the children were born with normal eyes and had no astigmatism, but it was very commonly found to be present as early as a half-hour after birth. The degree and kind of astigmatism varied within very wide limits.

These cases were kept under observation and examined at intervals. In nearly all cases the eyes were normal and there was no astigmatism present when they had reached the age of about six years. After attending school a few years, astigmatism was frequently acquired. When those children who wore glasses for the correction of astigmatism were examined at the age of twelve years or older, it was found to be still present and increased as they grew older, necessitating stronger glasses. Those children who wore no glasses for the correction of astigmatism did not have it when they reached the age of twelve or older which, of course, suggested treatment. Whenever it was possible to remove the glasses of young children, the astigmatism invariably became less or disappeared altogether.

Symptoms

When a high degree of astigmatism is present, the vision is appreciably lowered. Usually when vertical lines are regarded, they may appear more distinct than horizontal lines, or the reverse may be true. This is, however, not a reliable test because patients with normal vision do not always see vertical or horizontal lines equally well.

Many patients with astigmatism complain of headaches and pain in various parts of the head and eyes. Some patients have said that when their eyes became tired or felt uncomfortable in any way, they could rest them by removing their glasses.

One elderly lady obtained a pair of glasses from an optician for the relief of astigmatism. After wearing them for a few days, she returned complaining that every morning, when she put her glasses on, the pain in her head increased very much, and that after wearing her glasses for a few hours, the pain was occasionally only partially relieved. The optician remonstrated and told her that she needed to wear her glasses several weeks before her eyes could get used to them. The patient then told him that she had come to have glasses fitted to her eyes, and not her eyes fitted to glasses.

An optician was wearing window-pane glasses for the relief of headaches, and said that glasses were a great help to him. His wife, however, informed her friends that his headaches were much more frequent while wearing the glasses than when he did not use them.

Cause

Astigmatism is caused by a mental strain or an effort to see, either consciously or unconsciously. Patients have demonstrated that astigmatism can be produced by staring or straining to see.

The normal eye with normal sight, normal memory or normal imagination has no astigmatism, but when the normal eye remembers or imagines imperfectly, the retinoscope demonstrates the presence of astigmatism.

Pain in the eyes and head can always be produced in the normal eye by straining or making an effort to see. Such headaches disappear promptly when relaxation methods are employed.

Treatment

Astigmatism is caused by a mental strain and can only be cured by complete relief of the strain. Glasses should not be prescribed because they increase mental strain which is accompanied by an increase in the degree of astigmatism.

To relieve astigmatism, it is necessary for the patient to practice those methods which rest the mind and eyes. Children, when asleep, may acquire in an hour or less a high degree of astigmatism, and the muscles of the face may show a great deal of tension or strain. If this manifest tension can be relieved or corrected altogether, the retinoscope demonstrates that the astigmatism has become less or has disappeared entirely. When astigmatism is present in young babies, it can be lessened by relaxation methods. The mother can rest the child by swinging it in her arms with a slow, short, easy swing. In children twelve years old and older, astigmatism is often acquired, and can be corrected very promptly by palming or swinging.

Adults suffering from various forms of astigmatism are benefited by practicing central fixation, by improving their memory and imagination and by other methods which secure relaxation.

FAVORABLE CONDITIONS

For the correction of astigmatism, we should consider favorable conditions which promote the best vision. Some patients with astigmatism, perhaps the majority, prefer the illumination to be bright. They can see better in the strong sunlight and the astigmatism becomes less than when the light is dim. Other patients with astigmatism see better, and the astigmatism becomes less or disappears, in a dim light, while it may be very much increased in a bright light.

The distance of the Snellen test card from the eyes is also important. A patient may, at twenty feet, read the card with normal vision, when the astigmatism is not so great. The same patient may read the Snellen test card at ten feet with normal vision and the astigmatism may become worse. Some of these cases are difficult to understand. One patient became worse when the eyes were tested at three feet, but when tested at fifteen feet, the patient read the last line of the Snellen test card and the astigmatism disappeared. Each individual case, in order to obtain the best results from relaxation methods, should be tested at a distance which is favorable.

CENTRAL FIXATION

The normal eye with normal sight sees with central fixation, i.e., it sees best where it is looking and not so clearly where it is not looking. The astigmatic eye sees with eccentric fixation, i.e., it sees best where it is not looking. It is important, therefore, that patients with astigmatism consciously practice central fixation until it becomes an unconscious habit.

For example, one may look at the notch at the top of the large letter "C" of the Snellen test card and observe that the notch is seen best, while all other parts of the letter are seen worse. When one looks at the bottom of the large letter and sees that part best, the top is not seen so clearly. With the use of the retinoscope, it can be observed that the astigmatism has become less or disappeared altogether when this is done correctly.

SHIFTING

The normal eye with normal sight is constantly shifting from one point to another and does not hold one point longer than a second. It may shift only a short distance, a quarter of an inch or less, and then back again to the point previously regarded. Patients with astigmatism stare or make an effort to see. When a letter or other object is regarded, they attempt to see the whole letter or object at once, or they may concentrate on one point for a continuous period of time, thereby increasing the astigmatism.

MEMORY AND IMAGINATION

The normal eye has no astigmatism when the memory and imagination are perfect. The memory of a perfect letter "O," with a white center imagined whiter than it really is, can be accomplished easily, promptly, continuously, without effort, pain, or fatigue. The memory of the same letter, with the white center covered over by a gray cloud which blurs it, requires a stare or a strain to see or to remember, and astigmatism is manifest. A letter may be remembered imperfectly for a few seconds, but this is difficult or impossible to do for an appreciable length of time. The gray blur constantly changes and always becomes worse or more blurred when the effort to see or remember increases.

A perfect memory can only be obtained when the sight is perfect. A large area of white can usually be remembered perfectly because it is seen perfectly. By regarding a white area alternately with the eyes open and closed, the memory is improved and the astigmatism is lessened.

When the memory is improved, the imagination usually improves. Since we can only imagine what we remember, in order to imagine letters or other objects clearly or perfectly, a good memory is necessary.

CASE REPORT

A girl, eight years old, had a high degree of astigmatism in each eye. The vision of the right eye was 5/200, one fortieth of normal, while that of the left eye was only 3/200 or one sixty-sixth of normal. The left eye habitually turned in—internal squint. The child was very bright and seemed to realize the value of central fixation almost from the beginning. By practicing central fixation and regarding the Snellen test card first at ten feet and later at twenty feet, the vision of each eye improved, so that in about a week the vision was normal in each eye and the left eye became straight permanently.

The patient's near vision was also tested. At ten inches, the usual reading distance for the normal eye, the patient by practice became able to imagine one part best of capital letters and, later on, of smaller letters. In about two weeks, she read diamond type at six inches by central fixation. The retinoscope indicated no astigmatism and no malformation of any kind of the eyeball. This young child acquired what may be called microscopic vision. In three weeks she became able to read very fine print with the paper in contact with the eyelashes of either eye, and very small objects were seen close to her eyes with the same clearness as they were seen with the aid of a microscope. For example, she could describe red blood corpuscles and white blood corpuscles mounted on a glass slide when held in contact with the eyelashes of either eye. This child was benefited or cured by the practice of central fixation. Although the results were very gratifying, the child received so much attention by exhibiting her ability to see, that I was very much relieved when the family left New York for a distant city taking the prodigy along with them.

Conical Cornea

The question has often been asked if relaxation treatment benefits conical cornea with its large amount of irregular astigmatism. The contraction of the superior and inferior oblique muscles squeezes the eyeball and increases the length of the optic axis. As a result of this pressure, the back part of the eyeball becomes thinner and bulges backwards with the production of irregular astigmatism. The scientific name for this bulging of the back of the eye is posterior staphyloma. Less frequently, the front part of the eye, the cornea, may bulge in the form of a conical mass and is accordingly termed *conical cornea*.

Since a strain causes the bulging of the back part or the front part of the eyeball, rest or relaxation of the strain should be and is followed by relief.

Conical cornea is a very painful, complicated disease of the eyes. The vision is always lowered and usually continues to grow worse from year to year. In the beginning, simple astigmatism with a clear cornea can usually be demonstrated in these cases. The amount of the astigmatism may be 2 diopters or less, and the impaired vision may be improved to the normal with a weak astigmatic glass. The bulging of the cornea increases slowly or rapidly and an ulcer appears near the center of the cornea where the parts are more severely inflamed. The astigmatism becomes the irregular type, in which glasses are not able to improve the poor vision to the normal.

A school teacher had been suffering from conical cornea in both eyes. Her vision was only 10/200 in each eye. With strong glasses for compound myopic astigmatism, her vision was improved to 10/50. For a number of years, she had worn glasses which had been made stronger from year to year. Each time that she was tested, stronger glasses were prescribed for the loss of vision during the preceding year. She suffered great pain which was not relieved by the strong glasses. By practicing palming, the variable and universal swings, the pain was completely relieved, and the vision improved to 10/40 without the use of glasses. The relaxation treatment improved her condition, so that she became able to see without glasses better than she had been able to see with them. It is important to realize that the relief from pain was accomplished in about half an hour of treatment and that the benefit was obtained after other methods had failed while she wore glasses.

The stare or strain to see has been demonstrated to be associated with all diseases of the eyes, and is the cause of all imperfect sight. When relaxation is obtained, the eyeball may at once become normal in form with normal sight. Anything that is done with an effort to improve the vision is wrong and always fails. The benefit is only temporary when the stare is only relieved temporarily, but it is always a permanent benefit when the eyestrain is continuously relieved.

STORIES FROM THE CLINIC

No. 88: Astigmatism

By Emily C. Lierman

During the holidays, a woman came to me for treatment and brought her prescription for glasses with her. She told me frankly that she was doubtful that I could cure the mixed astigmatism with which she had been troubled for so many years and which was getting worse from day to day. She was seventy years old and had worn glasses for reading and for distance for about twenty years. During the past few years she had suffered considerable pain in the back of her eyes. The pain was more intense on bright, sunshiny days, and because of the pain and discomfort caused by the light, she always wore a large hat as a protection from the sun and she frequently wore dark glasses.

The copy of her prescription for glasses showed that she had hypermetropia and mixed astigmatism. The vision of her right eye was better than that of the left for the distance, namely 10/50, but all the letters of the card were blurred. The vision of her left eye was 10/70. When she looked at me, she had no wrinkles in her forehead and her eyes were open in a natural way. When she looked at the test card, there immediately appeared more than a half dozen wrinkles in her forehead and her mouth became distorted as she tried to read the letters for me.

I directed her to palm her closed eyes and, instead of telling her to remember a letter of the test card, which is something I usually direct the patient to do while the eyes are closed and covered, I asked her if she had a flower garden. She answered, "Yes." I noticed how nervous she was and promptly proceeded to make her more comfortable by giving her a footstool, and a pillow to rest her elbows while palming. She said that she could easily remember the different flowers which she had planted herself and that it was always a pleasure to spend a great deal of her time in the garden watching the flowers grow. I asked her to name the different flowers and also to mention their colors.

We spent about five minutes' time in this way. Then I removed the footstool and cushion and had her stand as I taught her the universal swing. Swaying to the left, she got a glimpse of the tops of buildings from my office window. When she swayed to the right, she was told to glance at the test card on the wall ten feet away and to keep up the universal swing all the time. Her vision improved in less than ten minutes to 10/30. By reading one line of letters and then another as I directed her to do, swinging and blinking with each sway of the body, the vision of both eyes improved to 10/10. After one hour's treatment, the pain in her eyes had disappeared also.

She complained that she might not be able to do as well by herself at home, and was also doubtful whether her astigmatism could actually be cured. I then proceeded to make her sight worse by having her stare as she looked directly at one letter and then another. She soon complained that the pain in her eyes had returned. Many times I have heard Dr. Bates say, "If you know how to make your sight worse, you will then know how to improve it." It has always been a disagreeable task for me to have the patient demonstrate this, as I am sensitive to the pain and discomfort that the patient feels. It is only when a patient complains that she is not receiving much help or that she does not understand how her particular case can be cured, that I cause the patient to make her sight worse by doing the wrong thing. My patient soon discovered that staring and straining caused the pain to return and that it lowered her vision for the distance as well as for the near point.

I placed her by a window and directed her to swing with me as my body moved from right to left. Printed signs on the upper parts of buildings in the distance seemed blurred to her before she began to swing. By noticing that the buildings in the distance moved slightly with her, while the window and curtains up close moved rapidly opposite to the movement of her body, her pain and discomfort disappeared. She noticed also that her desire to see things better, which made her forget to blink, prevented her from improving her vision for the test card. Then she conscientiously kept up the blinking as she kept time with the sway of her body. This pleased her and she was satisfied with the treatment.

Ten days later her vision for the test card had improved to 15/10 with each eye, and the black letters on the white card were clear and distinct. I gave her a small Fundamentals card to hold in her hand. Immediately, she held the card off as far as her arm would reach. It was interesting to notice how the strain disappeared from her face when she drew the card farther away from her eyes. She was told to close her eyes and then draw the fine print card up to about six inches from her eyes. Then, when she opened her eyes and looked at the card, I held her hand in place so that she could not move it farther away. In an instant, she drew her head as far back as she could from the card. She said that looking at the letters of the card when it was held so close caused an instant pain in back of her eyes and made her feel nauseated.

I told her to quickly close her eyes and drop the card in her lap and forget about it. In trying so hard to please me, she had produced a terrible strain which made me almost as uncomfortable as it did her. I palmed with her as she again described her garden to me. While her eyes were closed, I placed a test card, which was fastened on a stand, five feet from where she was sitting. This card was black with white letters. When all else fails to improve the sight of the patient, this card is my greatest help.

I then told her to follow my finger as I pointed to the first letter of each line down to the bottom of the card. I pointed a half-inch below each letter and told her to look in the direction of my finger tip and not at the letter. Reading each letter clearly at five feet produced no strain whatever. As she mentioned each letter, she closed her eyes and remembered it.

Following my directions in this way, she became able to look at the white spaces of the small Fundamentals card which she again held in her hand at six inches from her eyes. By shifting and blinking from the small letter "o" of the test card at five feet to the white spaces of the small Fundamentals card, she read straight down to the finest print of the Fundamentals card, line No. 15. The change in her face was good to see because all signs of strain had cleared away.

She practiced at home for several weeks and then came to me again to hear what I had to say about her good sight. She was able to do without her glasses all the time and did not use them again. She wanted to take more treatment if I thought it was necessary.

I tested her eyes and at fifteen feet she read a strange card, which has small letters to be read with the normal eye at nine feet. This card she read with each eye separately and without any effort or strain, 15/9.

She told me that she had practiced faithfully every day for more than two hours altogether, and had done as I told her to, which was not to put her glasses on again. She practiced the universal swing almost an hour a day. She said that she enjoyed the universal swing so much that instead of counting to one hundred, which I told her was necessary to do in order to know that she was swinging enough for the improvement of her vision and the relief of strain, she practiced for twenty minutes at a time.

It only took me ten minutes to find out that she no longer needed help from me. I told her, however, that she could be sure of a relapse if at any time she punished her eyes by staring or by not blinking enough.

Palming and the universal swing helped her to rest her eyes and to see things moving all the time. This swing, with the help of the memory of the flowers in her garden, cured my patient.

Better Eyesight
July 1927—Vol. XII, No. 1

THE IMPERFECT SIGHT OF THE NORMAL EYE

By W. H. Bates, M.D.

People with normal eyes do not have normal sight all the time. It is only under favorable conditions that vision is continuously good or perfect. Some individuals may have normal sight at twenty feet, but not at a nearer or more distant point. Normal sight at twenty feet does not mean normal sight at ten feet, five feet, or nearer, or at twenty-five feet or farther. What may be favorable conditions for one person may not be favorable for everybody or for the same person at different times. Frequently imperfect sight may be found to a greater or lesser degree in cases of squint or strabismus, although the optic nerve, retina, and other parts of the eye may be normal. Such cases are suffering from eyestrain and are cured by relaxation treatment.

The amount of blindness produced by an unconscious or conscious strain is very variable. The amount of vision lost may be one-tenth of normal sight, or it may occasionally be six-tenths, or nine-tenths. I have found the vision to be lowered to no perception of light in eyes which had no organic changes in the retina, optic nerve, choroid or other parts of the eyeball. The pupil did not react to light by direct illumination. These cases were all cured by relaxation methods.

The imperfect sight of the normal eye is similar in its manifestations to *amblyopia ex anopsia* in which no organic changes are present to account for the poor vision. Not all cases of squint have imperfect sight of the eye which turns in or out habitually or continuously. Usually the eye with the poor vision is turned, but there are many exceptions; for example, the eye with good vision may be the one that is turned. Sometimes the vision may alternate and would then be good in the eye that is straight and poor in the eye which turns. After relaxation treatment has improved the sight of both eyes to normal, the eyes may become permanently straight, but it is always true that the patient can produce a relapse by a conscious or an unconscious effort, and as a result the vision in one or both eyes is always lowered.

A woman, age sixty, recently came to me for treatment. She had worn glasses for more than thirty years to improve her vision not only for the distance, but also for reading. Bifocals made her eyes feel worse and produced a greater amount of discomfort than any other glasses. Three years ago, the vision of the right eye was good and she could read a newspaper with the aid of her glasses. With the left eye she could not read even with glasses. Her vision for distant objects was imperfect and was not improved by glasses. Sometimes the right eye had good vision, while the vision of the left eye was much less. On other occasions the vision of the left eye was good, while that of the right eye was very imperfect. She had been to see a great many eye specialists for treatment, but none had been able to fit her properly with glasses for distance or for reading. All these eye specialists admitted that they did not know the cause of her imperfect sight. She was fitted with many pairs of eyeglasses, no two of which were alike.

Some doctors prescribed eyedrops, others internal medicines. With the hope of giving her relief from the agony of pain which she suffered, various serums were administered. Some eye specialists treated her for cataract, others for diseases of the retina, optic nerve and other parts of the interior of the eyeball.

She was suffering from eyestrain or a mental strain, which produced many different kinds of errors of refraction. When she strained her eyes, she produced a malformation of the eyeballs which caused imperfect sight. This condition had been temporarily improved by glasses. In a few days or a week, however, the glasses had caused her great discomfort and made her sight worse. I made a very careful ophthalmological examination, but found no disease in any part of the eye. Her eyes were normal, although the vision was imperfect.

The use of her memory and imagination helped to improve her vision. She committed to memory the various letters of the Snellen test card and with her eyes open, regarding each letter, her memory or imagination of the letters was good. When she closed her eyes, not only could she remember or imagine each letter perfectly black, but she also could remember the size of the letter, its location, its white center and the white halo which surrounded it. With her eyes closed, she could remember the whiteness of the spaces between the lines much better than she could imagine it with her eyes open. With the aid of the retinoscope, I observed that when she imagined normal vision with her eyes open, there was no myopia, hypermetropia, nor astigmatism present. When she suffered pain, however, the shape of the eyeball was changed and her vision always became worse. This patient demonstrated that the normal eye is always normal when the memory or imagination is good. When the memory or imagination is imperfect, the vision of the normal eye is always imperfect.

A Snellen test card with a large letter "C" at the top was placed about fifteen feet in front of her. To one side was placed another Snellen test card, with a large letter "L" at the top. She was unable to distinguish the large letter "L" with either eye, but she could read all the letters on the "C" card, including the bottom line, with the aid of her memory and imagination. With a little encouragement, she became able to imagine the large "L" blacker than the large "C," although she could not distinguish the "L." In a few minutes, when she imagined the "L" blacker than the big "C," she became able to distinguish it. By the same methods she became able with the help of her memory and imagination to imagine the smaller letters on the large "L" card as black as letters of the same size on the "C" card. By improving the blackness of the small letters on the large "L" card, and imagining them perfectly black alternately with her eyes open and closed, she was able to distinguish the small letters.

When this patient looked fixedly at, or centered her gaze upon, one part of a large letter at six inches, she found that it was difficult and it required an effort to keep her eyes open and to look intently at one point. She also found that by looking at other letters and trying to see them all at once, or by making an effort to see all the letters of one word simultaneously, her vision was lowered. When she was advised to look at the white spaces between the lines, she said that it was a rest and that the white spaces seemed whiter, and the black letters then seemed blacker.

After she had imagined the white spaces between the lines to be whiter than they really were, it was possible for her to imagine the thin white line. This line is imagined along the bottom of a line of letters where the black of the letters meets the white of the white space. She was not always sure that she looked at the white spaces, although she planned to do so. When she tried to read and felt pain or discomfort, she was unconsciously looking at the letters; but when she looked at the white spaces and succeeded in avoiding the letters, she felt no discomfort and she was able to read almost continuously without being conscious that she was looking at the letters. When she practiced relaxation methods, did not stare, did not strain nor try to see, her vision became normal.

A young man, age 18, desired to enter the Naval Academy at Annapolis. He had already passed a satisfactory physical and scholastic examination, but he had failed to pass the eye test. The vision of each eye was one-half of normal. By practicing the swing, and with the aid of his memory and imagination, his vision became 15/10, or better than normal. His great difficulty was that, although he read this test card with each eye with normal vision, 20/20, the day before his eye test he became so nervous just as soon as he met the eye doctor that he practically went blind.

The eye doctor was sorry and wished to help him as

much as possible and so referred him to me. I found, with the aid of the retinoscope, that the vision of each eye was normal when he looked at a blank wall without trying to see, but just as soon as he regarded the Snellen test card at twenty feet, he began to strain, his eyes became myopic, and his vision very imperfect.

It is seldom that one sees eyes as perfect as were the eyes of this young man. When his vision was good, the weakest glasses made his sight worse. The problem seemed to be to improve not only his eyes but his mental strain so that he would not lose the control of his eyes just by glancing at the Snellen test card.

A Snellen test card was placed at thirty feet, another card was placed almost directly in line at ten feet so that it covered the distant Snellen test card. When the patient swayed from side to side, the near card appeared to move in the direction opposite to the movement of his body, while the more distant card seemed to move with the movement of his body. When he moved to the right, the 10-line letters on the near card seemed to move opposite, while the 30-line letters on the distant card moved with the movement of his body. Later he obtained normal vision at twenty feet by the same method.

The following is a letter which I received from the patient:

June 16, 1927
Dear Dr. Bates:

I am happy to inform you that I passed my eye examination to the U. S. Naval Academy and I am now a member of the student body, a merry, meek "plebe."

Dr. Bates, I wish that there were some adequate way I could express my appreciation to you for your assistance and kind advice which not only has given me better eyesight, but has made possible a thing that I had long desired and which will equip me with a wonderful education and a wonderful career in life. In the absence of proper words and phrases, I will just say that you have my heartfelt thanks and the thanks and gratitude of my parents. I deeply enjoyed the work and I am now deeply enjoying my eyesight.

I have tried to apply your methods of relaxation to not only eyesight, but to every other organ of my body and to my different endeavors. The Naval Academy is perhaps as difficult a school from which to graduate as any in the United States, and it is by eliminating the unimportant and the wrong methods of doing that a fellow can stay here. I think that the difference between success and failure can be in the way an individual does his work. I have learned my lesson about the evils of concentration and strain, and I hope to apply my lesson.

If at any time it is in my power to render the least service to you, I will be very pleased to do it. Again I thank you and wish you the best of luck and success in the work you are doing.

Sincerely yours, —

STORIES FROM THE CLINIC

No. 89: Eyestrain

By Emily C. Lierman

A girl who had worn glasses for more than twenty years came to me to have her eyes tested after she had been to an oculist and had had her glasses changed. She complained of constant pain in her eyes. Her vision with each eye separately was 15/30, or one-half of normal vision. While reading the letters of the Snellen test card at fifteen feet, she did not blink until she began to read the letters on the line that should be read at thirty feet. Then her eyes began to water and she complained that they burned like fire.

I told her to sit down and close her eyes to rest them. I made her comfortable with a cushion for her elbows while palming, and a footstool to raise her feet from the floor. I asked her to remember something perfectly and then let her mind drift to something else. She was told that it was necessary to remember pleasant things; that otherwise her mind would be under a strain and her vision would not improve. Like many patients, she began to question me about what the mind had to do with the eyes. She was told that when the mind is under a strain, all other parts of the body are also under a strain. When the mind is relaxed, the eyes are also relaxed and things are seen without effort or strain. Mind strain is always associated with eyestrain. You cannot affect one without affecting the other.

While she was palming, the patient described many colors that came to her mind. She described their combinations in making beautiful paintings and fancy draperies. After palming for more than ten minutes, I told her to remove her hands from her eyes, to stand and sway her body from left to right. By glancing at only one letter of the test card at a time and then looking away, she read 15/10 or better than normal vision in ordinary daylight.

I tested her sight for the reading of fine print and she read it with perfect ease, first at four inches and then at ten inches. When I saw her again, she had discarded her glasses, her pain was gone, and her eyes no longer troubled her.

Glaucoma

A man, age fifty-nine, came to me recently to find out whether anything could be done to prevent blindness of his right eye. He had only perception of light in his left eye. In 1918, both eyes had been operated upon for glaucoma. The left eye had had no sight before the operation. The vision of the right eye with the test card was normal. After closing his eyes and palming for five minutes or longer, he noticed that objects about the room looked clearer. I placed him in a chair with his back to the light and gave him the booklet with microscopic type, a small diamond type card and a small Fundamentals card for practice. He held the booklet of microscopic type about ten inches from his eyes. Above this was placed the "Seven Truths of Normal Sight," by W. H. Bates in diamond type, and then above this the Fundamentals card, exposing sentences up to paragraph four which explains shifting.

I told the patient to look at any white space of the microscopic type, to close his eyes and remember it for an instant; then to open his eyes and look at a white space of the diamond type card. He was advised to quickly close his eyes again and remember the white space for an instant, then to open his eyes and look at the type of the Fundamentals card.

I encouraged him to shift, blink and remember the white spaces of the different types as he flashed them. Then, after closing his eyes for an instant, he became able to see the "F" of the word "Fundamentals" blacker than the rest of the word. I explained that this was called central fixation, and that seeing best where he was looking helped him to see the whole word more clearly. While he practiced in this way for ten or fifteen minutes, I watched him carefully so that he did not strain when looking at the fine type, and advised him to look only at the white spaces.

He read one sentence after another, stopping to mention a period, a semicolon or a colon. I explained that it was necessary for him to notice all little details, because it would improve his memory as well as his sight.

Remembering the white spaces or fine type, then of larger type, then of type a little larger than newspaper type, helped him to see type smaller than ordinary reading type. In an hour, after much encouragement, my patient read all the fifteen sentences of the Fundamentals card. He became very much excited because, while he had received help from others for distant vision, he had not been able to read such fine type for many years, even with glasses.

I then decided to attempt to improve the left eye in which he had no sight. One of the small Fundamentals cards has white letters on a black background and is an exact copy of a larger test card. After he had palmed for some time, I told him to be sure to keep his right eye covered, so that he could not see with it. Then I asked him to open his left eye and tell me if he could see what I was holding in my hand—about ten inches from his eyes. He answered, "I see everything dark with the exception of something that looks like a small white 'E' on the top of the black card." This was correct. He then became very much excited, and as a result of this strain, the vision left him.

I instructed him to practice all that he possibly could with the fine-print cards and also with the distant cards and to write me in a week's time. In his report he said, "Standing with my back to the window, the sky overcast with fog or clouds, I can see the 'T O Z' of the small test card at a distance of two feet, one letter at a time, with my left eye. I can also see the end of my thumb holding the card at the lower left corner. The sight of my left eye is almost as good at night, under a shaded lamp with an 80-watt light. You may be sure I am continuing the exercises daily, as you advised."

REPORTS

Editor's Note—*Edith Reid and Ian Jardine of Johannesburg, South Africa, who are qualified to improve defective vision by the Bates Method, have sent in the following reports of their respective cases.*

Report of Edith Reid

I had got to a stage where I had to wear glasses for all close work. My distant vision was poor and the light worried me terribly. The glare from the sun used to give me dreadful headaches so much so that when out sketching, I always wore two pairs of glasses, blue ones over my ordinary glasses. Even then I used to get home tired out with a horrible headache. My memory was shocking. When worried or excited, I used to almost forget my own name.

I had heard of Dr. Bates' method being practiced by Ms. Quail so I thought I would try and see if anything could be done for me. When tested I could read only 10/20 on the Snellen test card, and paragraph 2 on the small card. I was not able to see that there were any letters on the last line at all. It was proved that the trouble was all caused by strain. I was taught how to use my eyes without strain and to rest them by swinging and getting things to move everywhere.

I discarded my glasses, and at my second treatment I was able to read the entire test card at ten feet, 10/10. My near vision also improved. I was then taught to sun my eyes daily and to rest them by palming. Each day not only my sight but also my general health improved in every way.

One day I was travelling in the train with my husband and he came across a paragraph in the newspaper which he wanted me to read so he gave it to me saying, "Read that." I took the paper, never realizing what I was doing. When I had read about half of the paragraph, I realized that I was reading small print. I became very excited and shouted, "Goodness, I am able to read small print." I suppose people in the compartment must have thought that I was crazy, but it did not worry me. I felt only so very grateful that I wanted to tell everybody about Dr. Bates' wonderful method.

I was taught how to perfect my memory of a letter by looking at a letter and then remembering it with my eyes closed, and to remember something that was pleasant to me. This I found very difficult; but by this time I had absolute faith in the method, and so I practiced remembering mental pictures, at odd moments, all day long. After practicing this for several weeks, I found that I was able to palm and call up a picture of any place I had known and to paint a picture from memory.

Reading small print in an artificial light still bothered me, but I have been very fortunate to have been able to come to America and be treated by Dr. Bates himself. Now I am able to read diamond type and newspaper print by electric light.

I have had my glasses on only once since I was told to discard them. I was making a black velvet cushion at night and was afraid that I might strain my eyes, so I put my glasses on. I found everything looked misty, so I took them off and very carefully wiped them, but things were still misty. I then washed them but things continued to look misty, and only then did I realize that my eyes had become so well that the glasses were too strong for my improved vision. From the time I began wearing glasses my sight rapidly became worse, not only my near sight, but my distant vision as well. I always thought it wrong that when one reaches so-called "middle age," one's sight should fail. Now it has been proved that through this method one can live to be one hundred years old, not wear glasses and yet have perfect sight. It is impossible for me to express in words my deep gratitude to Dr. Bates for his discovery of the cure of imperfect sight without the use of glasses.

REPORT OF MR. IAN JARDINE

My dear Dr. Bates:

At the age of about eleven years I was completely blind for about five weeks during a severe illness. My vision slowly returned until about three months after, when it was apparently normal again.

A year after this, my eyes began to trouble me and glasses were prescribed. The prescription was made up wrongly, the left lens being placed before the right eye and vice versa. This was discovered only six months later on a re-examination because of continuous headaches. The next twelve years were a succession of examinations by the best eye specialists in South Africa, each one meaning stronger glasses with no relief of pain.

About eighteen months ago, I was assured by two prominent eye specialists in Johannesburg that I had an incurable eye disease and that nothing could possibly be done to save my sight, which they said would fail altogether in the near future. Unknown to me, my father had been told on my first examination that this disease was present in the eyes and would slowly spread, but so slowly that they did not expect blindness until the age of 50 or 60. My field of vision was so limited that I could see only what was immediately in front of me, and at night I was almost totally blind.

Faced with this cheerful outlook, I was granted a holiday during which time I heard of Dr. Bates' method of Eye Education being practiced by Ms. Quail of Capetown.

At the first lesson my glasses were removed and I was told that they were never to be put on again. This was a great shock as all the doctors had greatly stressed the fact that the glasses were to be left off only during sleep. Then I was taught the swing, in other words to see or imagine everything moving. The pain immediately disappeared, so that I walked home in the seventh heaven of delight led by Ms. Reid who helped me a great deal during the treatment. However, a day or two later, on the persuasion of well meaning friends, I wore my glasses. The old pain immediately returned, but I put up with it thinking that perhaps my eyes had to get used to the strong lenses again. Fortunately, next day was lesson day. Ms. Quail informed me that it was to be either glasses and no cure, or no glasses and a cure. As I had in the long run nothing to lose by leaving off the glasses, I determined never to have them near me again and to try out this new system quite fairly. Then I was shown how to sun my eyes by letting the rays of the sun fall on the closed eyelids, while moving the head gently from side to side. This seemed a strange thing to do, as previously I had worn blue glasses to shield the eyes from strong light.

By practicing the universal swing, i.e., imagining everything to be swinging gently from side to side, noticing the movement of all things when walking, pedestrians bobbing up and down, vehicles hurrying by, buildings and pavements gliding past as one moved forward—spending a good part of each day in the sun improved the vision so remarkably that three months after the first treatment, I was able to resume my profession, auditing, most times having to work under dim artificial light, but always without glasses and without discomfort.

However, I am afraid that during those three months I suffered many weak moments, becoming rather despondent and fearful at times when the sight did not seem so good as it was the day before, or when things still looked blurred; but I can look back on those unhappy days—real enough at the time—with a smile and without the least doubt for the future. My eyes are now entirely free from disease and the sight is normal.

QUESTIONS AND ANSWERS

Q–1a. How often should the sun glass be used? 1b. How long on the closed lids before using it on the eyeballs themselves? 1c. Can one use the sun glass on one's own eyes?

A–1a. Daily for two or three minutes. 1b. Usually for several weeks on the closed lids before using it on the eyeballs themselves, although the length of time varies with each individual case. 1c. Some people can, but it is rather difficult and awkward to do.

Q–2. My neck gets very cramped in the back and becomes very painful. Is there any way of relieving this?

A–2. Practice the long swing, variable swing and circular swing.

Q–3. Since I have taken off my glasses I find it almost impossible to not half close my eyes to see better.

A–3. Partly closing your eyes brings on a strain which increases your imperfect sight. Squinting is a bad thing to do because it injures your eyes.

Q–4. My vision after practice with the test card is good, but I cannot sustain it. What means can I use to have continuous vision?

A–4. Acquire a continuous habit of imagining stationary objects to be moving easily, until it becomes an unconscious habit.

Q–5. If I blink everything becomes blurred. How can I overcome this?

A–5. Practice blinking, slowly, easily, without a conscious effort as much as you possibly can.

Q–6. I have myopia and have been practicing your methods. At first, I had very good results, but I now seem to be at a standstill. How can I continue to progress?

A–6. There are three things which you can practice. One is blinking, one is palming, and one is the practice of the circular swing, that is, moving the head and eyes in the orbit of a circle.

Q–7. My eyes are so sensitive to light that it is impossible to use the sun treatment. In what way can I use it and avoid headaches and pain which it causes?

A–7. Sit in the sun with your eyes closed, allowing the sun to shine directly on your closed eyelids, as you move your head slowly from side to side.

Q–8. I have found blinking and shifting to be of great benefit to me but, although I have been practicing both for six months, it has not become a habit. I still have to practice both consciously. What means can I use to blink and shift normally?

A–8. Continue to consciously practice blinking and shifting until you acquire the unconscious habit. It is merely the substitution of a good habit for a bad one.

Q–9. Can one swing objects or letters by moving just the eyes, or must one always move the head or body?

A–9. It is easier to move the head and body with the eyes.

Better Eyesight
August 1927—Vol. XII, No. 2

SCHOOL NUMBER

DEMONSTRATE: GLASSES LOWER VISION

Stand fifteen feet from the Snellen test card and test the vision of each eye without glasses. Then test the vision of each eye with glasses on, after having worn them for half an hour or longer. Remove the glasses; test the vision again and compare the results. Note that the vision without glasses becomes better the longer the glasses are left off.

Test the eyes of a person who is very nearsighted. Remove the glasses and test the sight of each eye at five feet, nearer or farther, until the distance is found at which the vision is best without glasses. Now test the vision for five minutes at this distance, which is the optimum distance, or the distance at which the vision is best. For example, nearsighted people see best when the print is held a foot or nearer to the eyes. If the eyes see best at six inches, the optimum distance is six inches; but if the distance at which the eyes see best is thirty to forty inches, the optimum distance is then thirty or forty inches.

In nearsightedness, glasses always lower the vision at the optimum distance. The same is true in farsightedness or astigmatism. For example, a nearsighted person may have an optimum distance of six inches. If glasses are worn, the vision is never as good at six inches as it is without them. This demonstrates that glasses lower the vision at six inches, or the optimum distance in this case. In farsightedness without glasses, the optimum distance at which objects are seen best may be ten feet or farther. If glasses are worn to see at a near point, the vision without glasses at the optimum distance becomes worse.

THE PREVENTION OF IMPERFECT SIGHT IN SCHOOLCHILDREN

By W. H. Bates, M.D.

Eye education has been proved to be effective in preventing and improving defective vision in schoolchildren.

A negative proposition is one that cannot be proved. You cannot say that any methods recommended for benefiting the vision of schoolchildren prevent imperfect sight and the use of glasses, because the vision of the children might remain good if no measures were employed for their benefit. However, a positive proposition is something that can be proved to be true. For example, if the eyesight of schoolchildren is imperfect, eye education always improves the imperfect sight.

A Snellen test card was used for more than twenty years as a means of preventing and improving imperfect sight. This card was placed on the wall of the classroom. Every day, while sitting quietly in their seats, the children were encouraged to read the Snellen test card, with each eye separately, covering one eye in such a way as to avoid pressure on the eyeball. This required only a few minutes and did not interfere with the regular schoolwork. The results obtained from this simple practice were very gratifying.

In one high school, a teacher became interested in eye education and, with the consent of the principal, introduced the method into her own classes. She made it a rule not to treat a child unless he were willing to remove his glasses permanently. Besides curing children, she cured many teachers who were wearing glasses. Each teacher who had learned the method surreptitiously cured all the children in her classes who had imperfect sight. In this way an endless chain was formed. After a number of years, the method became known to the parents of the children and also to a number of physicians. As a result of this publicity, the teachers were asked to stop treating the children by the use of eye education. It is difficult to understand why eye education should be condemned when voice education is encouraged and teachers are appointed to educate children for the relief of stammering. Many teachers of voice culture have found that their pupils were suffering from nerve tension because of eyestrain. When the eyestrain was relieved, the nerve tension disappeared and the stammering was corrected.

Palming. Resting the eyes by palming is one of the best methods we have for obtaining relaxation and improved vision.

Many children suffer from headaches, eyestrain and fatigue. When the eyes are closed and covered with the palms of both hands, it is possible to obtain rest and relaxation of the nerves of the eyes and of the body generally, provided the palming is done properly. Palming is successful when all light is excluded and no light or colors are imagined. When a child with normal eyes and normal sight enters a dark closet, where all light is excluded, no light is seen or imagined. The same is true when the normal eye practices palming; no light is seen or imagined. Black is imagined easily, without strain; but any effort that is made to see black is wrong. Most children are fond of pleasant memories, and when they palm they usually think of pleasant things which help them to palm successfully. When schoolchildren learn by experience that palming is a benefit to their sight, headaches, nervousness, or other disagreeable symptoms, they will practice palming very frequently without being encouraged to do so.

Central Fixation. Those children, who have trouble in obtaining relaxation by palming, are benefited by practicing central fixation, which means seeing the point regarded best, and other parts not so clearly. For example, in remembering a pet dog, one child liked to think of his curly tail, then of his long silky ears, or of the black spots on his legs. When conditions are favorable, that is, when the light in a classroom is neither too bright nor too dim, eyestrain is less manifest. The children are more relaxed and become able to palm more successfully.

Swaying. Another method used is to have the children stand with their feet about one foot apart and sway the whole body from side to side. When this is practiced, the stare, strain or effort to see is prevented and the vision is always benefited.

Fine Print. When schoolchildren are able to read fine print at the distance from their eyes at which they see it best, the eyestrain is relieved as fine print cannot be read with an effort. The distance where fine print is seen best varies with people. All children should not be encouraged to see fine print at the same distance from their eyes.

Shifting. When the eyes are normal, they are completely at rest and when they are at rest, they are always moving, which prevents the stare or strain. When looking at an object, do not try to see all parts of that object equally well, at once. That is, when you look at the back of a chair, you see that part best, and the seat and legs not so clearly. But do not hold the point regarded longer than a second. Remember to blink as you shift rapidly to the seat and then to the legs of the chair, seeing each part best, in turn. When the eyes stare and an effort is made to see, the vision is always lowered.

Swinging. When the eyes move slowly or rapidly from side to side, stationary objects which are not regarded appear to move in the opposite direction. Like many things, the swing can be done wrongly as well as rightly. When done wrongly, the blackness of the letters and the whiteness of the spaces, between the lines of the Snellen test card, become imperfect. When the swing is imperfect, the vision also becomes imperfect. To be able to practice the swing perfectly is a great help to the sight of schoolchildren. The teacher can direct the children to stand beside their desks while swaying from side to side. The pupils can notice that the desks in front of them, the blackboard, and the Snellen test card are all moving in the direction opposite to the movement of their bodies. When the pupils look out of the window, the curtain cord and other parts of the window will appear to move in the opposite direction, while more distant objects, buildings, trees or mountains, will appear to move in the same direction as they sway. When walking straight ahead, children can notice that the floor appears to move towards them. If the children are conscious of the movement of the floor and other objects, the stare and strain is prevented, and the vision is always improved; but if the pupils do not notice the movement of objects when they, themselves, move, they are apt to strain and the vision is always lowered.

When pupils imagine the Snellen test card to be moving from side to side, the imagination of the black letters or of the white spaces is improved. If the head and eyes are moved an inch or less from side to side, the Snellen test card and the letters on it will also appear to move an inch or less. With the aid of the short swing, it is possible for the pupil to remember, imagine or see each and all the letters of the Snellen test card correctly and continuously, but if the letters do not move, an effort is soon manifest. The children then find that trying to see a letter, or part of a letter, stationary, requires a strain and is difficult. It seems strange, although it is true, that to fail to have perfect sight requires an effort and hard work. In other words, perfect sight can only come easily, and without effort, while imperfect sight is obtained with much discomfort and effort.

Blinking. The normal eye, with normal sight blinks frequently, easily and rapidly, without effort or strain. If children do not blink frequently, but stare and try to see things with the eyes open continuously, the vision is always impaired. At first the child should be reminded to blink consciously but it soon becomes an unconscious habit and the vision is improved.

Memory and Imagination. The scholarship of children is affected by their memory of mental pictures. Measures which have been practiced by many school teachers for the preservation or the improvement of memory are quite numerous. When children learn how to remember some things perfectly, the memory of other things is improved. With a perfect memory, it is also possible to have a perfect imagination. We see only what we think we see, or what we imagine. When the imagination is perfect, the sight is perfect and when the sight is perfect, the memory is perfect. These and other clinical observations have demonstrated the truth that sight is largely mental. Perfect sight or imperfect sight is due to the condition of the mind. When the mind is healthy and active, perfect memory can usually be demonstrated; but when the mind has lost its efficiency, the memory becomes impaired. The memory is benefited by those methods which bring rest and relaxation. With the eyes closed, the memory is usually better than it is with the eyes open.

After regarding a letter which is seen imperfectly at a distance of ten feet or nearer, the student can remember the same letter more perfectly by closing his eyes. When the child can remember a perfect letter at ten feet with the eyes open, he soon becomes able to see and remember the same letter at eleven feet, and can gradually increase the distance to fifteen or twenty feet. Practicing the sway, alternately with the eyes open and with the eyes closed, is a benefit to the memory and the sight, because when the eyes are moving, a stare, strain or effort to see is more or less prevented.

When a line of letters on a Snellen test card can be read easily, it is usually possible to read some of the letters on the line below. However, if this cannot be done, have the child come closer, until all the letters of the bottom line are seen at a distance of five or ten feet. When a child cannot read all the letters on the 10-line at ten feet, he may be able to remember or imagine all the letters of the 10-line, with the eyes closed, better than with them open. By alternately closing the eyes for part of a minute or longer, and then opening them for only a moment, the vision improves.

A child may be able to see the first letter on the bottom line of the card when he is told what the letter is. Although he may not know what the second or third letters are, he may be able to actually see them and other letters on the bottom line by improving the vision of the first letter so that it is imagined perfectly. When the memory and imagination of the first letter is quite perfect, or sufficiently perfect to be distinguished, the eye becomes normal and the other letters are really seen and not imagined.

A child, at some previous time, may have had an inflammation or disease of the eyeball, which caused his imperfect sight. For example, a scar, sufficiently thick to interfere materially with the vision, may have formed over the front part of the eyeball. A perfect memory or imagination of a letter with the eyes closed, always lessens the opacity, and the vision is always improved, at least temporarily. By repetition, the short periods of improved vision occur more frequently and last more continuously.

The imagination is very important, much more so than many of us believe. Some people think imagination is simply another word for illusion. However, it is possible to imagine correctly as well as to imagine incorrectly. Some people can imagine a truth perfectly, but react differently when they imagine things imperfectly.

A girl, twelve years old, had unusually good vision. She was able to read the 10-line of a strange card, which she had never seen before, at fifty feet, 50/10. She said that she could look directly at one letter of the 10-line and see it continuously, but when her eyes were observed while she was doing this, it was found that she shifted almost continuously.

Her memory was also unusually good, She was the only member of the party who could remember the names of the officers on the different steamers on which she had traveled to Europe. She remembered the numbers of her staterooms, as well as the numbers of the staterooms of the other members of the party. However, when she imagined all these things incorrectly, she felt decidedly uncomfortable, but when she remembered to imagined things perfectly, she felt no discomfort.

At school, her teachers considered her stupid because she disliked some of her studies and devoted no time to those lessons. Her poor scholarship disappointed her family very much. She was very unhappy and decided to prove what she could do. About a week before the examinations, she read through her Latin textbook and remembered it perfectly. She also read her other textbooks and remembered what they contained. She asked to be examined in all her subjects and much to the surprise of the teachers, she passed the examinations with unusually high honors.

SCHOOLCHILDREN

By Emily C. Lierman

Davey

Davey, eight years old, was very nearsighted, and the glasses he was wearing made him nervous and irritable. His father had been told about the Bates Method and what could be done to restore perfect sight without wearing glasses. Davey's father brought the boy to me, although he was skeptical and his mother was even more so. I could tell by the little boy's attitude toward me that the Bates Method had been much discussed in the home circle, and that I was considered a sort of mystic worker.

The first question Davey asked me was, "What are you going to do to me?" I answered, "I am not going to do anything to you, but I will try to do a whole lot for you. I will help you to get rid of your thick glasses that I am sure you don't like."

His answer was, "O, yes, I would like my glasses if I could see out of them. Father said that if you don't help me, he will try to find other glasses that will help."

I let the little fellow talk for a while because I thought it would help me to understand him better. I told him I was especially interested in children and that it was always my delight to give schoolchildren better sight. I said I would not interfere with him if glasses were what he wanted most. He said that he was afraid to play baseball or other games which might not only break his glasses, but perhaps hurt his eyes.

I tested his vision with his glasses on and found that at ten feet from the regulation test card he could see only black smudges on the white, but no letters. Then I placed the card six feet away. All he could see at that distance was the letter on the top of the card, seen normally at two hundred feet. I then had him take off his glasses to see what he could read without them. He could not see anything at all on the card. I asked him to follow me to the window and to look in the distance and tell me what he could see. To the right of me, about one hundred feet away, there was a sign. The letters of this sign appeared to be about three feet square. One word of the sign had four letters. The first letter was straight and the last was curved and had an opening to the right. I explained this to Davey, as I told him to look in the direction in which I was pointing, and then to a small card with fine print that I had given him to hold. I told him to read what he could of the fine print. He read it at two inches from his eyes. Under my direction, he alternately followed my finger as I pointed to the fine print and then to the building sign. He told me he could not see anything in the distance.

Davey felt very uncomfortable because of his poor sight and became rather restless. I told him to hold the fine print card closer, and not to read the print this time, but to look only at the white spaces between the sentences, and to blink often. He shifted from the white spaces of the fine print to the sign in the distance, watching my finger as I pointed, first to the near point and then to the distance. Suddenly, he got a flash of the first letter of the first word on the sign. This practice was continued for twenty minutes, and then we had a rest period. Davey sat comfortably in a chair and palmed his eyes. Children are very apt to become bored with anything that takes time and patience, and I know that Davey had little patience with anything regarding his eyes.

I asked him questions about his schoolwork and what subjects he liked best. He said he just loved arithmetic. I asked his father to give him an example to do while he palmed. The little fellow thought this was great fun, and without hesitation he gave his father the correct answer for each example. This gave Davey a rest period of fifteen minutes. His mother remarked that this was the first time she had ever noticed him sit quietly for so long a time.

Davey was then shown how to swing, by moving his body slowly from left to right, and getting only a glimpse of the letters on the card at six feet. When he looked longer than an instant at the card, he leaned forward and strained to see better, but failed each time. When he learned not to stare, but to shift and blink while he swayed, his vision improved to 6/50. We returned to the window. I told him to shift from the white spaces of the fine print, which I held close to his eyes, then to the distant sign, and he became able to read all of the sign without any difficulty.

Much had been accomplished in one treatment and both parents were grateful. Davey was given a card with instructions for home practice. He returned three days each week for further treatment. Every time he visited me, I placed the test card one foot farther away. Eight weeks after his first treatment, he read all of the test card letters at ten feet. This was accomplished by reading fine print close to his eyes, then swinging and shifting as he read one letter of the card at a time.

This boy has sent other schoolchildren to me as well as a school teacher with progressive myopia, who practiced faithfully until she was cured. Every week, she sent me a report about her eye treatment and the progress she made. Her pupils noticed that she had discarded her glasses, and after school hours she invited some of them who had trouble with their eyes to practice the Bates Method with her. In eight weeks' time her vision became normal, and all her pupils, with the exception of three, are improving their vision without the use of glasses.

ESTHER

Esther, age seven, first came to me in January 1927, to be relieved of squint. She had worn glasses since she was three years old for the relief of squint in the right eye. Her parents noticed, after she had worn glasses a short time, that she was more nervous than before. Later, they were much concerned because she acquired bad habits, such as holding her head to one side instead of straight, especially while studying and reading her school lessons. Her glasses were then changed. It was thought that wrong glasses had been prescribed because she still kept her head to one side as before, and her nervousness became more pronounced. The parents were told that in time the squint would be corrected if Esther wore her glasses all the time.

The squint continued to get worse instead of better, so the parents brought her to me. The vision of her right eye was 10/15, but in order to read the letters of the test card, she had to turn her head so that it almost rested on her right shoulder. Her left vision was 15/15 and she read the letters of the card in a normal position. I tested her right eye again, placing the card up close. She turned her head just as much to one side as she did when the card was placed ten feet away. I asked her mother to hold the child's head straight, and again told Esther to tell me what the letters were. I held the test card two feet away while she covered her left eye. She said everything was all dark and she could see nothing.

It did not take me long to find out that Esther was a bright child, and that she would willingly do anything for the benefit of her poor eye. She said to me, "It is too bad that my sister should have two good eyes and that I should have only one good one." I encouraged her to follow my directions closely and I told her if she continued to do so and practiced as often as she should at home, that we would then try to correct the vision of the poor eye.

I found her to be quite an artist. When her eyes were covered, I asked her if she could remember a drawing of some kind. "Oh, yes," she answered, "while my eyes are closed and covered I can imagine that I am drawing your picture."

I said, "All right, you keep on imagining that you are drawing my picture and later on I will let you sit at my desk and draw a picture of me." We talked about pleasant things for five or ten minutes while she had her eyes covered.

I then taught her to swing her body from left to right, glancing for only a second at the test card, and then looking away to her left. I purposely avoided having her swing to the right because she had the desire, while reading or trying to see more clearly, to always rest her head on the right shoulder. I drew her mother's attention to the fact that as she swung, both eyes moved in the same direction as her body was moving. When she stopped blinking, which I had encouraged her to do rhythmically with the swing, her right eye turned in and her head also turned to one side.

After she had practiced swinging for a little while, I noticed that she gaped a few times, which meant that she was straining. It is good for parents to notice this, in helping the child practice for the relief of squint, and to stop all practice with the exception of closing the eyes to rest them.

Esther palmed again for a little while and then I showed her some toy animals and asked her to name each one of them. She named each one correctly with the exception of the buffalo, so I did not use that one for her case. If a child under treatment for squint is asked to tell things in detail, the child must be familiar with the objects. While she again covered her eyes to rest them, I placed the animals on the floor five feet away from where she was sitting. I told her mother to touch each animal and have Esther name them. Out of eight animals, she named three incorrectly. They were among the last ones she tried to see. We then noticed that her head turned to one side in order to see them. All this time her left eye was covered.

Then I had Esther sit at my desk and asked her to draw my picture. The drawing was quite well done for a little girl of her age. She kept her head straight while drawing. When strain is relieved, the symptoms of imperfect sight are relieved also. She enjoyed drawing, therefore it did not produce a strain. When she was asked to read the test card letters, she strained in order to see them and the condition of her eyes became worse.

Esther was encouraged to do something that she liked at every treatment, such as writing figures from one to ten, or drawing a line without using a ruler. At the first attempt, the lines were very crooked and the figures not straight.

Swinging and palming, practiced several times daily, soon improved the right eye to normal. At the last visit, her head remained straight and the squint had entirely disappeared. The vision of her right eye became better than normal as far as reading the test card was concerned. She read the bottom line at twelve feet and seven inches. This line is read by the normal eye at nine feet. She did equally as well with the left eye which, of course, had normal vision in the beginning.

To be sure that the child was entirely relieved of squint, I told her to look at my right eye, then at my left eye, then to my chin and other parts of my face as I pointed with my finger to each part. She followed me with both eyes moving and as yet she has had no relapse.

A SCHOOL TEACHER'S REPORT

June 12, 1927

As a teacher of Speech Improvement I have found that some of the exercises that are used by Dr. Bates in the correction of poor vision are very helpful in the treatment of stammering. Those who stammer are invariably nervous, and the palming and swaying exercises calm the nerves and help the children to speak more quietly and slowly and therefore without stammering. In all cases where I have introduced the swaying in my stammering classes, the result has been a greater calmness both in reading and speaking and I believe that in this age of nerve tension, relaxation exercises are a boon even for children of school age.

Poor speech and poor sight often go together and it is a happy circumstance that Dr. Bates has devised exercises that will help both defects at the same time. An outstanding case of a child suffering both from defective speech and very poor eyesight was a little boy who was in one of my stammering classes. I asked him to read a sentence from the blackboard and he immediately bent his body way over to one side and stretched his neck as far forward as he could, straining to see the letters. I directed him to cover his eyes for a few minutes and then to sway for a while. He soon found that he could see much better and that he could read without stammering. He was very backward in reading and spelling. Although in the second year of school he did not even know the names of all the letters of the alphabet I believe that this was largely due to his poor vision and that the stammering came as he became aware of his inability to keep up with the rest of his class. During the short time that he was with me, his speech and sight greatly improved.

Posture is another thing that may be improved by the swaying exercise. Ordinarily, when you ask a child to stand in good posture he will place his feet close together like an Egyptian statue. In the sway, he is shown that by putting his feet apart he has a broader base for standing and more ease and comfort for moving. I hope that some day we may be able to bring all these beneficial exercises to all the children in the schools who need them.

Better Eyesight
September 1927—Vol. XII, No. 3

DEMONSTRATE: SUN TREATMENT

1. Sun treatment is an immediate benefit to many diseases of the eye.

Before the treatment, take a record of your best vision of the Snellen test card with both eyes together and each eye separately without glasses. Then sit in the sun with your eyes closed, slowly moving your head a short distance from side to side, and allowing the sun to shine directly on your closed eyelids. Forget about your eyes; just think of something pleasant and let your mind drift from one pleasant thought to another. Before opening your eyes, palm for a few minutes. Then test your vision of the test card and note the improvement. Get as much sun treatment as you possibly can—one, two, three or more hours daily.

When the sun is not shining, substitute a strong electric light. A 1,000-watt electric light is preferable, but requires special wiring. However, a 250-watt or 300-watt light can be used with benefit, and does not require special wiring. Sit about six inches from the light, or as near as you can without discomfort from the heat, allowing it to shine on your closed eyelids as in the sun treatment.

2. The strong light of the sun focused on the sclera, or white part of the eyeball, with the sun glass also improves the vision.

After the eyes have become accustomed to the sunlight with the eyes closed, focus the light of the sun on the closed eyelids with the sun glass. Move the glass rapidly from side to side while doing this for a few minutes. Then have the patient open his eyes and look as far down as possible, and in this way, the pupil is protected by the lower lid. Gently lift the upper lid so that only the white part of the eye is exposed, as the sun's rays fall directly upon this part of the eyeball. The sun glass may now be used on the white part of the eye for a few seconds, moving it quickly from side to side and in various directions. Notice that after the use of the sun glass, the vision is improved.

BLINDNESS I

By W. H. Bates, M.D.

When the normal eye has normal sight, it is constantly moving. When it has imperfect sight or is partially or completely blind, it is always seeing stationary objects or letters stationary, or is making an effort to do so. These two truths suggest the prevention or cure of blindness.

When adults, schoolchildren and others are taught to imagine stationary objects to be always moving, the vision always improves. To do the wrong thing, namely, to imagine or try to imagine all [stationary] objects stationary, very soon becomes associated with an effort or strain. Why is it a strain to have imperfect sight? Because it is impossible for the eyes or mind to concentrate. To regard a point continuously is difficult or impossible. Trying to do it, is trying to do the impossible; and trying to do the impossible is a strain. All cases of imperfect sight or blindness are caused by a strain. When the strain is relieved or corrected by closing the eyes and resting them, the vision always improves.

It can be demonstrated that blindness from conical cornea, ulceration and inflammation of the cornea can, in all cases, be made worse by straining or making an effort to see. This is a truth, and, therefore, has no exceptions.

Glaucoma

Glaucoma is a serious disease of the eyes. In most cases, the eyeball becomes hard and this hardness can be felt by pressing lightly on the closed eyelid with the fingers. For the relief of this hardness various operations have been performed to promote the escape of the fluids of the eyes. These operations have not always been satisfactory. Many cases of glaucoma have been relieved for a limited period of time, but sooner or later become totally blind. When blindness occurs, operations have usually failed to restore the sight.

Cause. The theory that the disease is caused by a hardening of the eyeball is incorrect, because we find cases of glaucoma in which the eyeball is not increased in hardness, and there are cases of hardening of the eyeball in which there is no glaucoma. The normal eye may be hardened temporarily by conscious eyestrain. The cause of glaucoma, in all cases, is eyestrain, and may be demonstrated as follows: When the normal eye has normal sight, it is not under a strain. When a letter or an object is remembered or imagined imperfectly, the eyeball at once becomes hard. Other symptoms of glaucoma may also be observed, namely, one may see rainbow colors around the flame of a lighted candle. Another symptom is the pulsation of one or more of the retinal arteries. In most cases, severe pain has been observed.

Patients with glaucoma usually suffer not only in ways already mentioned, but also from other symptoms just as severe and more difficult to describe. Glaucoma affects the nervous system and produces not only extreme depression but disturbances in all the nerves and organs of the body.

Treatment. When a person is suffering from glaucoma, the memory of perfect sight produces complete relaxation with a temporary cure of the glaucoma.

Too many cases of absolute glaucoma, totally blind with no perception of light, suffering an agony of pain with great tension or hardness of the eyeball, have been enucleated. Acute, absolute glaucoma may have no manifest organic changes in the eyes. When the eyestrain is relieved by palming, swinging and the use of a perfect memory or imagination, these cases have always obtained temporary relief at once and a permanent relief by the continuation of the relaxation treatment.

Cataract

[See the June 1926 issue.—TRQ]

Conical Cornea

In conical cornea, the front part of the eye bulges forward and forms a cone-shaped body. The apex of the cone usually becomes the seat of an ulcer, and sooner or later, the vision becomes very much impaired. In advanced cases, the patient suffers very much from pain. Various operations have been performed, but the results have always been unsatisfactory.

Cause. The cause of conical cornea is eyestrain. The fact has been demonstrated that those measures which cure eyestrain, palming, swinging, the variable swing, as described in paragraph No. 7 of the Fundamentals card, and the use of the memory and imagination—are a benefit or a cure of conical cornea.

Opacity of the Cornea

The cornea, when healthy, is perfectly transparent and does not interfere with the vision of the colored part of the eye, or pupil, but when the cornea becomes opaque, the opacity may be so dense that the color of the iris cannot be distinguished, and there is no perception of light.

Cause. Opacities of the cornea are said to be caused by infections, ulcers or some general disease, but there are many cases which are caused by eyestrain, because when the eyestrain is relieved by relaxation treatment the opacity of the cornea always improves and the vision becomes normal.

Treatment. One patient, forty years old, had been blind from birth. The corneas of both eyes were totally opaque, so that it was impossible to see the color of the iris. The patient was helpless on the street and required someone to lead him. Central fixation, the use of his memory and imagination, and other methods for the relief of eyestrain were practiced. The sun treatment was especially beneficial. The patient was taught to expose his closed eyelids to the sun for many hours daily.

At the end of a few months' treatment, he became able to recognize people on the street. He was taught the alphabet and the names of the figures. When his knowledge of the letters became perfect, he was able to read the Snellen test card, 20/20. He was also able to read fine print without glasses. After thirty-five years, his friends reported that his eyes were still normal.

Another case was that of a woman, age seventy-five, who had to be led into the office. She had suffered from inflammation of the cornea of both eyes for many years, and had frequent attacks of ulcers. From time to time, these ulcers would heal, but they always left a scar.

When the patient was first seen, a scar tissue involved the whole cornea, so that one could not distinguish the colored part of the eye. I believe that eyestrain was the only cause of the trouble because the sun treatment, palming and swinging, brought about an improvement so that the cornea became perfectly clear, and the vision of the patient for distant and near objects was normal.

THE BLINDNESS OF SQUINT OR AMBLYOPIA EX ANOPSIA

In cases of squint, the vision of the eye that turns either in or out is variable. In many cases, the squinting eye may have normal vision, but in the majority of cases, the vision may be very much lowered, and in rare cases, the squinting eye may be totally blind with no perception of light *[amblyopia ex anopsia]*.

Cause. There have been many theories proposed to account for the blindness of squint. I have found, however, that the cause of the blindness is due to eyestrain.

Treatment. The vision of these cases is benefited by relaxation methods—palming, swinging, and the use of the memory or the imagination. A letter may be imagined perfectly or imperfectly. When imagined imperfectly, the vision is always lowered. When imagined perfectly with the eyes open as well as with the eyes closed, the vision is always improved. By remembering or imagining a letter with the eyes closed for half a minute or longer, one becomes able to imagine a letter quite perfectly with the eyes open for a few seconds. Repeat.

Case History. In one case, a woman, about thirty years old, was totally blind in the right eye which turned in, although the eye itself was apparently normal. That is to say, there were no opacities in any part of the eye, and the retina and optic nerve were normal.

With both eyes open, the vision was 15/20. By practice, with the aid of her memory and imagination, the vision with both eyes soon became normal without glasses, 15/10. Coincident with the improvement of the vision of both eyes together, which meant an improvement in the vision of the left eye, the patient gradually became able to distinguish light in the right or blind eye. In less than two weeks, after daily treatment, the vision of the right eye became normal and the eyes straight.

It seems curious that so many articles have been published on *amblyopia* (dimsightedness) *ex anopsia* (from lack of education or use of eye) without going further and studying the results of the opposite of *ex anopsia,* relaxation methods of treatment.

BLINDNESS II

By Emily C. Lierman

On March 19,1927, a woman came to me who was affected with temporary blindness. She was not with me longer than five minutes when I noticed that she was under an intense mental and nervous strain. When I spoke to her, tears welled up in her eyes. Every part of her body was tense and the white parts of her eyes, i.e., the sclera, were bloodshot and she had no desire to keep them open in a natural way

She told me that she had had trouble with her eyes as long as she could remember. Blocks of blind spots were visible before her eyes at all times; blindness caused by strain. She said she always kept her glasses near her bed so that she could put them on first thing in the morning.

Her sight was better at night than in the daytime. The daylight caused her a great deal of discomfort and pain and most of the time she had a desire to keep her eyelids lowered. When she was wearing her glasses, she felt more depressed than when not wearing them. Her eyes itched and she had rubbed her eyelids until they had become sore. This caused her to be more nervous than ever. Long periods of daily sun treatment finally cured the itching of her eyelids.

When I tested her sight with the test card, her right vision was 15/20 but she strained very hard to see the letters, which gave her eyes the appearance of being closed. The vision of the left eye was 15/50 and it caused her pain when she read with it. I encouraged her to palm and while her eyes were closed, I asked her to talk about her loved ones at home. As she told me of some of their habits and how she loved them, I noticed her smile for the first time.

She was taught to stand with her feet one foot apart and sway her body from left to right; flashing the test card letters one at a time. I reminded her many times to blink her eyes in order to stop the stare, for she stared a great deal. When she finally learned how to blink while swaying, her vision improved to 15/15 with each eye separately.

I then had her sit in a chair with her back to the sunlight and gave her the Fundamentals card to hold. I asked her what she could read on it. She said she could not read any of the print at all on the card. I told her to shift from the white spaces of the microscopic type to the white spaces between the lines of the "Seven Truths of Normal Sight," which she held with the Fundamentals card, flashing only the white spaces and avoiding the reading of print. This practice was kept up for almost a half-hour and I then suggested that she notice the numbers at the beginning of each sentence of the Fundamentals card. Her attention was drawn to the period next to each number. She was told to notice the white spaces of the different sized type as she held it in her hand. Before her first treatment was over, she read the sentences from number one to number five.

At the beginning of her second treatment she said that the food placed before her at the table was beginning to look like food to her before she ate it. Before, she never knew what she was eating until she tasted it.

Sun treatment was kept up regularly every day. This improved her vision for the test card and fine print to normal. I handed her a newspaper and pointed to the smallest type that I could find on the front page. The smallest print was about the size of diamond type. She read this clearly for the first time in her life. During her second treatment, when she held the card in the sunlight, her vision improved for the Fundamentals card to No. 8.

After several treatments she told me that her friends were noticing how much younger she looked. The sclera of both eyes was clearing up and she was smiling most of the time. She became able to read all of the Fundamentals card at reading distance, ten or twelve inches from her eyes and sometimes closer. The blind spots and black spots that had appeared before her eyes for many years, also disappeared. She was told to remain in the sun for hours at a time, keeping her eyes closed while her head moved slowly from side to side. The sway of the body was advised and she did this a hundred times in the morning and a hundred times at night before retiring.

She told me how much better she slept at night since having had her first treatment. She said it had been many years since she had had a restful night's sleep. She enjoys walking fast on the street now, noticing stationary objects moving in the opposite direction as she walks. She reads numbers in the telephone book and other print that was not clear before. Since she has been cured, she is helping others and writes about her eyes continuing to be a blessing to her. This patient has proved again that faithful practice and patience brings about the much desired result—normal vision.

She describes her own case in the following way:

"Before I was treated by Ms. Lierman for the improvement of my sight, an American flag a short distance away looked to me like a dark piece of cloth hanging from a pole. Now I can clearly distinguish the colors—the red, the white, the blue, and I believe I could count each star if the flag would stay still long enough.

For many years the first thing I would do on awakening in the morning would be to look for my eyeglasses. I could not see or find anything without them. At the dinner table, I could not see a small fishbone on my plate in a poorly lighted room, much less other things that the normal eye sees without any effort. Now I can see the tiny crumbs, even though they may be as white as the color of my table cloth.

Along the street, whether I was walking or riding, I could not read signs as the normal eye does. After my second treatment all signs along the street and shop windows were easily seen by me. Before I started treatment, I could not see any objects moving at all. They all seemed to stand still. Now I can see all objects moving that are moving, and since I have learned how relaxing the sway of the body is, I can imagine stationary objects are moving as I sway. If I carried an umbrella or a purse on my arm, I would hold so tightly to these things that the effort caused pain in my hands and arms before I realized it. Now my arms and hands feel relaxed and I carry packages, an umbrella and other things without causing strain or effort. Things now come easily to me. Perhaps others who are troubled in this way would be glad to know how I was cured of this particular strain and tension caused by holding on tightly to things unnecessarily.

Ms. Lierman taught me how to place the palm of one hand gently, easily on the palm of the other hand. At first I did not do it gently enough for her and we practiced it together. My strain was so great, which she realized too, that I was willing to follow her in any suggestion that she made for my comfort and relief from strain. This helped me so much that I began to uncross my knees for more relaxation and rest. This helps more than one realizes and now since I know it does, I notice that nine out of ten people are under a tension most of the time because their knees are crossed.

For years I have been under constant strain and tension, which caused greater depression than anything else. Since I have taken the treatment and followed Ms. Lierman's suggestions for home treatment, I no longer feel depressed.

After my second treatment, I could thread a needle and I was not particular either as to the size of the eye of the needle. I believe this is worth reporting because for many years I had to have my glasses handy to thread a needle whether the eye was large or small; it made no difference.

Since I was treated, a friend of mine drew my attention to something away off in the sky. She pointed to this object and said, 'Look at that balloon in the distance!' I looked and said, 'No, it is a kite, I can see the tail clearly.' The kite became visible to my friend and she remarked how much better my eyes were since I had discarded glasses. I have much cause to be grateful for my renewed vision!"

QUESTIONS AND ANSWERS

Q–1a. Is memory and imagination the same? 1b. When we remember an object, do we have to visualize it?

A–1a. No. 1b. It is best when you remember an object to visualize it with the help of the imagination, but it is not always necessary to visualize it.

Q–2. When I try to imagine a black period, it blurs and I get all colors but black.

A–2. When you fail to imagine a black period, it means that you are making an effort to see black. It may help you to think of a black football that has been thrown into the ocean and is being carried farther and farther from shore. As it recedes in the distance, it becomes smaller and smaller until it seems only a small black speck or period.

Q–3. Why is it a rest to read fine print? I should think it would be a strain.

A–3. Fine print can be read perfectly only when the eyes are relaxed. If any effort is made, the print immediately blurs. It is, therefore, evident that the more fine print you are able to read, the more continuously relaxed your eyes are [due to centralization—TRQ].

Q–4. I am following your method for squint. While riding in an automobile or train, is it necessary for me to palm?

A–4. No. It is beneficial to observe the universal swing, that is, looking in the distance and noticing that everything on the horizon, the clouds, treetops, etc., seem to move in the same direction in which you are moving. Without looking directly at near objects, you are conscious of the fact that they seem to be moving past in the opposite direction. Remember to blink frequently, as the normal eye does.

PERFECT SIGHT

By W. H. Bates

If you learn the fundamental principles of perfect sight and will consciously keep them in mind your defective vision will disappear. The following discoveries were made by W. H. Bates, M.D., and his method is based on them. With it he has cured so-called incurable cases:

I. Many blind people are curable.

II. All errors of refraction are functional, therefore curable.

III. All defective vision is due to strain in some form.

You can demonstrate to your own satisfaction that strain lowers the vision. When you stare, you strain. Look fixedly at one object for five seconds or longer. What happens? The object blurs and finally disappears. Also, your eyes are made uncomfortable by this experiment. When you rest your eyes for a few moments the vision is improved and the discomfort relieved.

IV. Strain is relieved by relaxation.

To use your eyes correctly all day long, it is necessary that you:

1. Blink frequently. Staring is a strain and always lowers the vision.

2. Shift your glance constantly from one point to another, seeing the part regarded best and other parts not so clearly. That is, when you look at a chair, do not try to see the whole object at once; look first at the back of it, seeing that part best and other parts worse. Remember to blink as you quickly shift your glance from the back to the seat and legs, seeing each part best, in turn. This is central fixation.

3. Your head and eyes are moving all day long. Imagine that stationary objects are moving in the direction opposite to the movement of your head and eyes. When you walk about the room or on the street, notice that the floor or pavement seems to come toward you, while objects on either side appear to move in the direction opposite to the movement of your body.

[Section IV is an extraordinarily concise summary of the key habits and principles of perfect sight. This section, along with the last paragraph in "Routine Treatment" in the December 1927 issue, are the two most important writings I have ever found regarding natural eyesight improvement. These writings, which I found in a used bookstore in 1987, completely changed my perception, and my teaching, of the "Bates Method."

In essence, the Bates Method is not about "eye exercises"; rather, it is an educational process of literally *relearning to see*—in exactly the same relaxed, natural way we used our mind and body all day long, before strained vision habits interfered. It is this discovery and teaching that was the brilliance and courage of Dr. William H. Bates.—TRQ]

Better Eyesight
October 1927—Vol. XII, No. 4

SQUINT

By W. H. Bates, M.D.

Definition. When one or both eyes are habitually turned in toward the nose, the condition is called internal squint or convergent strabismus.

When the eyes turn out, it is called divergent squint. Sometimes one eye may be turned up, while the other remains straight or may be turned down. This has been termed vertical squint. Some cases of squint may be a combination of several kinds of squint, vertical convergent or vertical divergent.

Cause. The cause of squint is a mental strain. Internal squint is produced by a different strain from the one which turns the eyes out, upward or downward. Double vision is produced by a mental strain different from that which lowers the vision or causes fatigue, pain or dizziness. Normal eyes have been taught to consciously produce all kinds of squint at will. This requires an effort which is variable in its intensity.

The facts suggest that since squint in all its manifestations can be produced at will, it should be considered curable by eye education, and this has been demonstrated in all cases. It is a well-known fact that many persons, including children, can learn how to produce squint and become able to relieve permanently all the varied symptoms of squint. The success of the operative treatment of squint is very uncertain.

Treatment. Since squint is always caused by an effort or a strain to see, mental relaxation is a fundamental part of the successful treatment. This may explain why teaching the eyes to see better is a relaxation method, which promotes the cure of the squint. If the vision of each eye is about one-half of the normal, the right or the left eye may turn in. With an improvement in the vision of each eye to the normal, the eyes may become straight. If the good eye has a vision of 15/20, while that of the poorer eye is only 15/70, improving the vision of the good eye may also improve the vision of the eye that turns in and the eyes may become straighter.

In many cases of squint, double vision can be demonstrated. These cases are more readily cured than those cases of squint which do not see double. [Many, if not most, cases of squint have amblyopia and, therefore, monocular vision. See "Stereoscopic Vision" in *Relearning to See* for a detailed explanation.—TRQ] This fact suggests that all cases of squint should be taught how to produce double vision. When the patient regards a small light with both eyes open, it is possible to encourage him to see two lights with the aid of prisms, the blue glass over the eye with good sight, when the light seen by the good eye is very much blurred. If the person is unable to imagine two lights a short or long distance apart, palming frequently helps. By resting the eyes with the aid of palming, the separation of the two lights is changed. With the help of the swing and central fixation, the two images approach each other and may merge into one light.

Squint cases are materially benefited when they become able, by an effort, to imagine the double vision better with their eyes closed than with their eyes open. They are able to demonstrate with their eyes closed that the image seen by the right eye is to the right of the image seen by the left eye. This is called *homonymous diplopia.* By a little training or encouragement, they become able to imagine the two images closer together by relaxation methods.

When the image seen by the right eye is to the left of the other image, it is called crossed diplopia and, with few exceptions, divergent squint is present. With the eyes closed, a person with internal squint may imagine double vision with the images separated or close together. Or he may become able to imagine the images crossed, or the image seen with the right eye to be to the left of the other image; in other words, he may be able to produce divergent squint with the aid of his imagination. A number of people have been cured of internal squint by teaching them how to produce divergent squint.

Young children, two years old, have been cured of all forms of squint by swinging the whole body in a circular direction and swinging them strongly enough to lift their feet from the floor. While swinging, the hands of the child are held by the hands of the adult who is swinging the child. At the same time the child is encouraged to look upward as much as possible. The little patients always seem to enjoy this form of exercise. Games of all kinds have been practiced with much benefit to the squint in children.

One can obtain small toy animals of various sizes and colors. The names of the animals and their colors can be taught to the children. In the beginning they learn the names of the animals more readily when they are close, about two feet away. When the child recognizes each animal correctly at this distance, one can, by gradually placing each animal farther off, improve the vision for a greater distance. The more perfectly the child becomes able to see the animals, the less is the squint.

Teaching children with squint the names of the different colors at a near or greater distance is a benefit. In the beginning, the size of the colors may need to be large to help the memory, imagination or sight. As the sight improves, the child becomes able to distinguish the colors of very small objects. One may need to spend half an hour or longer daily for some weeks in order to improve the vision for colors to the maximum. Numbers and letters of the alphabet can also be taught to the child who has squint with benefit.

DOUBLE VISION

Not all children are conscious of seeing stationary objects multiplied. When they reach the age of six years or older, double vision, when it occurs, is usually very annoying. Adults with double vision and squint are usually more seriously disturbed than are young children.

One of the best remedies for double vision is palming for longer or shorter periods of time. It is well to remember that while double vision often requires the vision of each eye, one may have multiple images referred to each eye alone.

Any method of treatment which secures relaxation corrects the double vision and lessens the squint. Some patients are benefited by standing with the feet about one foot apart, the arms and hands hanging loosely at the sides, while they sway the body slowly, continuously, easily, from side to side. The swaying of the body from side to side lessens or prevents concentration or other efforts to see. Since double vision can be demonstrated to be caused by concentration or some other effort to see, the prevention of effort by the sway naturally lessens or corrects double vision. Should this not be sufficient to cure the squint, one may practice blinking, palming, or the memory or the imagination of perfect sight.

The Snellen test card may be useful in the cure of squint. While swaying from side to side, standing a few feet from the card, all stationary objects in the field of vision may appear to be moving in the opposite direction to the sway. More distant objects that have no background may appear to move in the same direction as the movement of the body. When practicing with a white card with black letters, the whiteness of the card improves in whiteness, while the blackness of the letters becomes darker and the vision improves.

THE TROPOMETER

The tropometer is an instrument invented by Dr. George T. Stevens of New York to measure the strength of the muscles of the outside of the eyeball. It is a very valuable instrument for some cases. For example, a patient, a young man of about twenty-three years old, came to me suffering from an alternate squint of a very high degree. I measured the strength of the muscles which turned the eyeball in. He had the maximum strength of these muscles. A free incision was made through both muscles and the result was negative. The eyes turned in as much as they had before the operation.

In order to increase the effect of the operation, I removed a quarter of an inch of the internal rectus muscle and then measured the effect produced with the aid of the tropometer. Much to my surprise, the tropometer measured little or no diminution of the strength of the internal rectus to turn the eyeballs in. I then proceeded more or less cautiously, alternately using the tropometer to measure what progress I was making.

When the tropometer indicated that the strength of the internal rectus was reduced to normal, functional tests demonstrated that both eyes were straight, with single vision. I exhibited the patient before the Ophthalmological Section of the New York Academy of Medicine. Every ophthalmologist, and there were many prominent men present, made the statement that the eyes would turn out within a very short time. Twenty years later, a large, heavy man came up to me after I had finished a lecture on the cure of the eyes at one of the public schools of New York. Although I did not recognize him, he was the same patient. He had had no relapse during all these years

Case Reports

About fifteen years ago, a southern lady came to me with her daughter, age ten. When she arrived at the office, she found a number of patients who had come to be cured of their bad eyesight without glasses. She was one of those nervous people who disliked above all things in this world to have to wait, especially in a doctor's office. When my secretary advised her not to wait, she took a firmer grip on the arms of her chair and resolved to see it through.

The child was suffering from well-marked alternate internal squint. Sometimes the right eye would turn in so far that the pupil was covered over by the inner corner of the lids. At other times, the child was observed to be afflicted with internal squint of the left eye. Her mother told me that they had been to several large cities, including the capitals of Europe, where she had hoped to obtain a cure for her daughter's squint.

The child was an avid reader and had read many books. Her memory was unusually good. She also had a very good imagination. She could read the 10-line of the Snellen test card at more than twenty feet in a good light, 20/10. When the light was poor and her vision was tested with the aid of a strange card, she was able to imagine correctly each of the four sides of any letter. For example, the letter "E" was the fourth letter on the fifth line of the test card. When the test card was placed thirty feet away in a poor light, she was unable to distinguish the letter as a whole.

After closing her eyes and covering them with the palms of both hands (palming), she imagined the left side of the "E" to be straight. When she imagined the left side of the "E" was curved or open, she strained. She imagined the top straight, and the bottom straight; and the right side open, which was, of course, correct. When any of the sides were imagined wrong, she always strained and was more or less uncomfortable.

She was then asked to imagine the fourth letter on the sixth line. She was still practicing palming. She was able to imagine the left side of the unknown letter to be straight, the top straight, the bottom open and the right side open. She imagined that the letter was an "F" and was correct.

She was then tested with diamond type at about ten feet from her eyes, a distance at which it was impossible for her to read the letters. She was then told to palm. While palming, she was asked to imagine the first letter of the fourth word, on the fifteenth line of the diamond type. With her eyes closed and covered she was able, without effort, by imagining each of the four sides correctly, to demonstrate a letter "M." She imagined this letter so perfectly that she was able also to imagine other letters of the same word correctly. The exercise of her imagination was continued for an hour during which time she imagined correctly a number of lines of the diamond type. The result was very gratifying because the squint disappeared in both eyes and the relief was manifest two days later.

The mother supervised the imagination of the fine print for half an hour daily for many days and weeks, with the result that at the end of six months, the child's eyes were still straight. The treatment was then discontinued, and at the end of five years, her eyes still remained straight.

A girl, age twenty-five, was afflicted with a complicated squint of various muscles of the eyeball of each eye. She habitually looked straight with the right eye, while the left eye turned down and out. When the right eye was covered, the left eye looked straight, and the right eye turned down and out. She had a vertical divergent squint in each eye. At times, she turned the left eye up and inward.

She was instructed to produce all forms of vertical, internal or external squint. With her eyes closed, she was directed to place her fingers lightly on the outside of the closed eyelids. With the help of her imagination, she became able to move the right eye in, while the left eye remained straight. When the left eye turned in, the right eye remained straight. She could produce every imaginable form of squint with her eyes closed, better than she could produce a squint with her eyes open. With her eyes open, she was able to do it in flashes or temporarily and later more continuously. It was interesting to observe how readily the patient could tell by the sense of touch whether the eye was looking in, out, down, up, or straight.

Many patients have been cured of internal squint by teaching them how to produce divergent squint, either with the eyes open or with the eyes closed. There were times when it was difficult for the patient to produce some forms of squint. With the aid of a small candle light, with the eyes open, the patient could imagine she saw two candle flames. The one seen by the right eye was to the right of the one seen by the left eye when one or both eyes turned in. By practice, she became able, with an effort, to increase the distance between the two candle flames. By lessening the effort, she became able to bring the two candle flames closer together, which was evidence that the squint required an effort and that a cure could be expected when the eyes were relaxed.

[Some people with squint have learned to force the squinting eye to look temporarily straight by strain and effort. This approach, of course, is not recommended, because the underlying strain is not removed.—TRQ]

There were times when her ability to produce internal squint with her eyes open was not always easy. With her eyes closed, her imagination of the two candle flames was better. With an effort, she was able to imagine the candle flame seen by the right eye to be to the left of the candle flame seen by the left eye. In other words, the two candle flames were crossed. With her eyes closed, she could imagine the crossed images farther apart, or she could bring them closer together by relaxation until they merged into one. Her ability to produce all kinds of squint helped her to do those things which were necessary to correct the squint. She devoted many hours to the production of vertical squint which enabled her to quickly correct divergent squint. When she became able to produce internal squint, it was not long before she was able to correct divergent squint.

When the patient began treatment, she was wearing glasses for the correction of imperfect sight. After her eyes became straight by eye education, her vision became normal without glasses. Because of her wonderful control of her eye muscles, very satisfactory photographs were obtained of her eyes.

[Dramatic photographs of the voluntary production of squint by one of Dr. Bates' patients are reproduced in "Stereoscopic Vision" of *Relearning to See,* p. 279.—TRQ]

STORIES FROM THE CLINIC

No. 90: Squint

By Emily C. Lierman

A young mother, who was much worried about the condition of her little boy's eyes, brought him to me for my candid opinion as to the cure of squint. When he was two years old, it was noticed that his left eye frequently turned in. At the age of three, when I first saw him, the right eye seemed to turn in more than the left. The mother had visited many eye specialists but none of them gave the child permanent relief.

I felt so sorry for the little fellow when he stood before me with his large rimmed spectacles. He tried to keep his head still while he looked up at me, but he could not. His head moved in a sort of semi-circle as he tried to see me more clearly through his glasses. I pretended not to understand what he said to me, and he really had a great deal to say.

I sat down and took him on my lap. Then I asked him to remove his glasses so that I could understand him better. "Glasses don't talk, do they?" he said. "No; but they make me stare like you do, and I also think they make me a little hard of hearing," I remarked, jokingly. He looked at his mother and quietly asked her to remove his glasses so that Ms. Lierman could hear him better.

I had no desire to have him take me seriously, nor did I want him to feel that he was going to be examined as he had been heretofore. I asked him his name. "Frank," he said, and then gave his full name and address and the date of his birthday, which I thought was bright for a child so young. He had spent many hours and days during the last year being examined and having drops put in his eyes. He asked me if I were going to put those drops in his eyes and said that if I were, he would run away.

I told him that I would not even touch his eyes with my hands. His mother and father were with him, and to prove to Frank that I really meant what I said, I asked both the mother and father to hold my hands, which they did. In the meantime, Frank slid off my lap, threw himself on the floor before me, kicked his heels in the air and wept with fear. His father apologized for his behavior, but I assured him that it was not necessary to make excuses for little Frank, because it was not unusual for children with squint to act that way.

"Yes," the father answered, "I noticed that you emphasize that in your book, *Stories from the Clinic."* Nothing could be done until the father threatened to take the boy from his position on the floor, and even then he kicked and screamed, begging at the same time to be left alone, saying that he wanted no drops and no examination of his eyes. I asked both parents to leave him entirely to me.

His mother took two packages of chewing gum from her handbag. One package she handed to me, while the other she held concealed in her hand. I never saw a child move as quickly as he did from the floor for that chewing gum. I said he could not have any of it until he stood on a chair, ten feet from a test card that I had placed on the wall opposite. This test card is the one we call the inverted "E" or the "pothook" card, and is used for young children and patients who cannot read or write. He willingly consented to do as I wished him to, and without further fuss he stood on the seat of the chair opposite the card.

At my suggestion, his mother stood twenty feet away from him and held a piece of wrapped gum in her hand for him to see. She asked him what the name of the gum was. The mother had previously told me that he could mention the name on the wrapper of the gum and could tell whether it was Beechnut or Wrigley. He said immediately that it was Beechnut. I watched his eyes as he looked at the gum and both were straight. I then told Frank to close his eyes and showed him how to palm. While his eyes were closed and covered, his mother replaced the Beechnut gum with the Wrigley.

Frank was then told to remove his hands from his eyes and look at the package his mother held up for him to see. He said, "Oh, I know that is Wrigley Spearmint gum." The mother then placed both hands behind her back and changed the gum from one hand to the other, then held up both hands for him to name the gum. He mentioned them correctly, saying that the right hand held the Wrigley and the left hand held the Beechnut. I drew his father's attention to the fact that when he shifted from her right hand to her left hand, noticing first the object which she held in one hand and then the object she held in the other hand, he blinked his eyes, and while swinging and blinking his eyes moved in unison. The father remarked how straight both eyes were during this exercise.

After his mother had promised that he could soon have the chewing gum, I told the little fellow to palm his eyes again. When he removed his hands from his eyes, his right eye turned in decidedly. I pointed at a letter "E" on the test card for him to see, and he leaned forward, straining hard to see how the letter "E" was pointing. He rubbed both eyes with his chubby hands and complained that he could not see anything.

I explained to his parents how unfamiliar objects seen at the distance caused the blindness of squint, while familiar objects seen at the same distance produced no tension, no strain, and therefore no blindness from squint. The inverted "E" card was unfamiliar to him and made him strain.

His mother noticed, among other test cards, one that was familiar to him, but the letters of the card had not been memorized by the child. I placed this familiar test card fifteen feet away and pointed to the 10-line of letters, or the line of letters that should be seen by the normal eye at ten feet, and he immediately strained to see them. His right eye turned in as it had before. I then placed the familiar test card ten feet away and directed Frank to close his eyes after he had seen each letter as I pointed to it. In this way, he read the 10-line letters with both eyes straight.

I placed a toy on the floor and told Frank to go and pick it up. He reached for the toy but missed it by a foot. By turning his head around in a sort of semicircle, he finally put his hand on the toy and picked it up. I spent almost a half-hour longer with him than I usually do with each patient, swinging him around as I held both his arms, and raising him slightly from the floor. He laughed with glee, enjoying every moment of the swing.

He was rather heavy for me to lift, so I asked his father to take my place. Frank thought this was a wonderful game and all the while his father swung him around from left to right, he looked up toward the ceiling and then to his father's face. All three of us noticed how straight both eyes were during this procedure. His parents were directed to practice this swing every day, always making a game of anything that was done for Frank's eyes. They were told to report to me, from time to time, how he was getting along.

Later, when I saw him again, I placed him fifteen feet from the test card. He knew the alphabet, as well as the numerals, so I used the card with unfamiliar letters. He covered his left eye and read with the right, and when I pointed to a "C," he said, "That is a broken 'O'." I began to smile, which disturbed him somewhat, and then asked him why he called it a broken "O." He said, "Anybody would know it wasn't broken if it didn't have an opening to the right side, and maybe grown-ups like to call it a 'C,' but I know it is a broken 'O'." When I pointed to a "G" and asked what it was, he said, "That is also a broken 'O,' only it's different." He read 15/10 with each eye separately, and with both eyes straight.

I had him stand by my window and asked him to look off in the distance and notice the letter signs on the tops of the buildings. In trying to see the letters correctly, he strained and both eyes turned in slightly, the right one more than the left. He demonstrated again that unfamiliar objects seen at the distance cause more strain. Every time Frank's eyes turned in as he tried to see, he would say that he could not see at all. When questioned about whether he saw black before his eyes, he answered, "No, but I just can't see." Immediately after a failure to see at the distance and while looking at unfamiliar objects, he would have a sort of nervous spasm, which his mother said was hysterics.

It has been some time since I have seen Frank, but I believe, or hope, that his mother has continued to help the little fellow. I always think of him when I look at the "C" of the test card, which he called the broken "O."

QUESTIONS AND ANSWERS

Q–1. When doing the swing, what does one move, the head or eyes?

A–1. One moves the eyes in the same direction as the head is moved.

Q–2. Does massaging benefit the eyes?

A–2. No, because it does not relieve the mental strain which caused the eye trouble.

Q–3. Is practicing under a strong electric light as beneficial as practicing in the sun?

A–3. If the sun is not shining, the strong electric light can be used with benefit, although more benefit is derived from direct sun treatment.

Q–4. Can one remember perfectly and see imperfectly?

A–4. It is impossible to remember perfectly and see imperfectly at the same time. Perfect sight can only be obtained with the aid of a perfect memory. When the memory is perfect, the mind is relaxed and the vision is normal. Imperfect memory requires a strain of the eyes which produces imperfect vision.

Better Eyesight
November 1927—Vol. XII, No. 5

TENSION

By W. H. Bates, M.D.

The tension of the muscles and nerves of the human eye is a very important subject for various reasons. Perhaps the most important of all is the fact that it occurs so frequently and so universally. When a person has nearsightedness, eye tension can always be demonstrated, because when the eye tension is relieved and corrected, the nearsightedness is cured. All persons who have astigmatism have eye tension. When the eye tension is relieved, the astigmatism disappears. Patients with cataract, diseases of the optic nerve or diseases of the retina are suffering from tension.

When the tension is relieved, the eye disease disappears.

In some cases, it is more difficult to relieve the tension than in others. No matter whether it is difficult or not, there can be no cure of the eye disease unless the tension is corrected. This tension, besides affecting the eyeball, is also manifest or can be demonstrated in any or in all parts of the body. A person who has glaucoma is under not only tension of the eyes, but a tension or an unusual contraction of the muscles of the arm, the hand, or all the muscles.

Tension of the internal muscles is always present when a patient has a disease of the chest, and it can be demonstrated that he is also suffering from tension not only of the chest, but also of other muscles and nerves in other parts of the body. There is a tension that contracts the bronchial tubes which interferes with the proper circulation of air into the lungs and out of the lungs. People with pneumonia, tuberculosis of the lungs, or tuberculosis of any part of the body are all suffering from eye tension, and when the eye tension is relieved, the tension in other parts of the body is also relieved. It is an interesting fact that all diseases of the eyes and all diseases of the body are generally associated with eye tension.

A very remarkable case of tension was that of an opera singer who suddenly lost her ability to sing. Specialists on the throat examined her very carefully and they were united in the statement that she had paralysis of the muscles on the left side of her larynx. In connection with this paralysis there was a tumor on the left vocal cord. Her symptoms of paralysis were caused by tension, because when the tension was relieved, the paralysis of the vocal cord was also relieved and cured. The tumor which had grown on the left vocal cord disappeared.

There are two things about this case which can be discussed; one is that the paralysis was caused by tension, and the other that the tumor of the vocal cord was also caused by tension. When we analyze her case and try to give an explanation of what the tension accomplished, we will probably say a good many things which are not so. It is exceedingly difficult, as I have said a great many times, to answer the question, "Why?"

We may have cases of eye diseases in which it is difficult to relieve the tension, but it may be easy to relieve the tension in the muscles of the stomach or in the various groups of muscles in the arm, or hand, and when such tension is relieved, that of the eye muscles is relieved, and in this way the disease of the eye, no matter what it may be, can always be relieved or cured. This is a very important fact, because when understood and practiced, some very severe forms of diseases of the eyes can thus be cured, and in no other way so well.

The question that comes up more prominently than any other is: "What can the patient do to bring about relaxation of any group of muscles?" A man, by the name of F. M. Alexander of London, England has accomplished a great deal in the cure of all kinds of diseases. He says that all diseases of the body are caused by tension. They can all be cured by the relaxation of the tension. He has offered many methods of bringing about relaxation in the most interesting, although seemingly incredible, way and the most successful is to bring about relaxation by having the patient state that it is desired.

For example, a patient sitting in a chair or lying down on the floor, whichever is easier, says, "I desire relaxation of the muscles of my neck so that my head can be lifted forwards and upwards." This is sometimes repeated one hundred to a thousand times. Mr. Alexander has always succeeded in having the patient bring about relaxation of the muscles of the neck by this method.

Mr. Alexander goes further and brings about relaxation of the muscles of the chest, both outside and inside, by having the patient say, "I wish my shoulder to relax and to move downwards and backwards. I wish my chest to relax and to move backwards. I wish my whole body to relax and move backwards. I wish my foot to move backwards without effort, without strain of any muscles of the body."

It has been a great shock to many orthodox physicians to observe the cures that Alexander has made. Epilepsy, considered by the medical profession to be incurable, has been cured by relaxation, without the use of any other form of treatment. Of course, rheumatism responds perhaps more quickly to relaxation than a great many other diseases, but there are cases of so-called rheumatism affecting the shoulder in which all parts of the joint become immovable.

One patient was afflicted with Parkinson's disease; all the joints of the body became so fastened together, so immovable, that the patient was unable to produce any voluntary movement of the hand or the arm. As time passed, the voluntary and the involuntary muscles gradually became useless from tension. Mr. Alexander had the patient relax those muscles which she could relax most readily. When this was done, the more difficult muscles became relaxed, until finally she was cured completely by the relaxation of tension.

Bier's Congestive Treatment

We may say that tension is a very important factor in the cause of most diseases of the body. A very instructive case was the following: About twenty years ago I came into my Clinic and found there a coal heaver whose face and hands and all parts of his body were covered with soot, or black particles of coal. His right eye was suffering from an ulcer of the front part. The case interested me very much and I took him in to see the surgeon in our department, a man who believed very strongly that an abscess in any part of the body is caused by germs, and when there is a collection of pus, it is the physician's duty to drain it and get rid of it.

I said to him, "Would you drain that pus?" He answered, "Certainly, a man would be crazy not to drain it." I then said, "Doctor, do you know that some patients in this condition who have had the pus drained have lost an eye, and oftentimes both eyes from sympathetic ophthalmia?" "I don't care, it ought to be drained," he said.

"Just watch me," I said. Without cleansing the patient's face or eyes, a pressure bandage was placed over his eye and tied so tightly that his face became much swollen. I told him that in two days, his eye would be cured. The surgeon said, "Impossible." I said, "Take a good look at him so that you will recognize him if you ever see him again." At the end of two days, the man came back, very much annoyed with me. He said that the bandage nearly killed him. "Take it off," I said.

He took it off and the pus had disappeared. The surgeon who saw it said that I had not cured him, that the man did not have an abscess to start with, that he had a perfectly healthy eye, and that anybody who said that the eye was full of pus two days before was wrong.

Strange as it may seem, the pressure bandage relieved the tension in the eye to a considerable degree, with a result that the pus in the anterior chamber was entirely absorbed. The eye recovered its health in forty-eight hours and the eyeball became very soft, because the tension was relieved.

It is well to demonstrate the results produced by tension. When the letter "O," for instance, is remembered imperfectly, the white center becomes a shade of gray and the black part of the letter becomes less black and often covered with a gray cloud. To remember an imperfect letter "O" requires an effort.

The demonstrations of these facts have repeatedly appeared in this magazine and should have suggested methods of treatment of the greatest value.

Many writers have stated that imperfect sight can be obtained without any difficulty. Usually, the contrary is the truth. Recently a girl was treated for nearsightedness. With some instruction, she became able to demonstrate that to see a letter "O" imperfectly for any length of time was difficult or impossible. She imagined the left-hand side of the letter "O" to be straight. I asked her how it felt. She answered, "It hurts."

Then I asked her to imagine that the right-hand side was open. She quickly said, "It hurts." Then I asked her what she meant by saying, "It hurts." "Well," she replied, "when I imagine a part of a letter wrong, my eyes feel uncomfortable and I don't like the feeling." I then said to her, "Can you imagine what this letter might be?" "Yes, I can imagine what it might be, but it hurts." Then I said, "Suppose you imagine it is an 'O,' what happens?" She smiled and said, "That doesn't hurt. It is an 'O'." I then pointed to a letter which came after the "O" and asked her if she could imagine what it was. She said, "Don't ask me, because it hurts."

I then asked her to close her eyes and remember the letter "O." She was able to do this without any discomfort. The next step was to have her look at the letter "O" on the card, remember it as well as she could with her eyes closed, and then imagine that she could see it. The memory and the imagination were repeated a number of times until she told me that the letter which came after the "O" was a "K."

I said to her, "Are you sure?" She answered, "No." "Why not?" "Because it hurts." "Can you imagine that the left-hand side is straight?" She answered, "Yes, and it doesn't hurt." "Can you imagine the top is straight?" "Yes," she answered, "and it doesn't hurt." "Can you imagine the bottom is straight?" She said, "Yes, and it doesn't hurt." "What is the letter?" I asked her. "The letter is 'E'," she said, "I am sure. Yes, I am positive that it is a letter 'E' because it doesn't hurt."

During this treatment, the patient's friends and relatives became interested. She had them all practice it and all of them were able to demonstrate that when they imagined the letters or parts of the letters correctly, there was no pain, and when a letter or part of a letter was imagined incorrectly, decided pain and symptoms of tension were produced.

STORIES FROM THE CLINIC

No. 91: Tension in Myopia

By Emily C. Lierman

Hildreth Lennox, age twenty-eight, came to me as a patient on May 2, 1927. She informed me that she had read *Perfect Sight Without Glasses,* and had studied it for about a year before coming to me. During that time she had discarded her glasses entirely after having worn them for fourteen years. Her vision was R.V. 15/200, blurred; L.V. 15/200, blurred.

When she read the card with both eyes, she could just about make out the 70-line, and the letters were more blurred than the 200-line letters. She enjoyed palming, so while she had her eyes covered, I asked her to remember anything that she could remember having seen without effort or strain and, if possible, to remember only pleasant things. She understood very readily that memory of unpleasant things caused more strain. Being a musician, she could remember her notes very well and also compositions that she enjoyed playing on the piano. She described to me, while her eyes were closed, how she had worked her way from Canada to Palo Alto, California, by giving concerts on the way.

After she had palmed for a while, I taught her the universal swing. This she did gracefully. She remembered to blink each time she swayed to the right. I have noticed that the myopic patient makes a hard task of blinking. A strain is produced then, and the vision does not improve except for an instant. Then I notice that the patient squints and squeezes the eyes almost shut. To avoid this, I have them swing just a little faster than usual. I find that the patient likes to blink in unison with the sway in one direction only, and not to the right and then to the left.

I test the sight of the patient with the white test card first—the one with the red and green lines. After the patient has palmed and has practiced the universal swing for a period of ten minutes or a little longer, I again test the sight of both eyes at fifteen feet.

I did this in Ms. Lennox's case and the vision improved to the 30-line, but all the letters of this line were seen double. The patient was again asked to palm and to describe to me what she remembered having seen from the train window on her way to the Coast. This helped her to relax so that when her test was made again—this time with the black test card with white letters—she read all of the black card at ten feet, as she covered her eyes for a part of a minute after flashing each letter. When she was told that she could not possibly stare if she covered her eyes after seeing one letter of the test card at a time, she never stopped smiling as she read one letter and then another of the test card in this way.

I did not have another patient until more than two hours later, so I spent more time with Ms. Lennox than I usually do with any patient. She did so well for me that I encouraged her to go right on regardless of the time. Again she covered her closed eyes and explained her mental pictures, and when she removed her hands from her eyes and then swayed her body, blinking as she swayed to the right, she flashed 10/10 of the black card and each letter was seen clearly.

To the right of her, also ten feet away, I had placed a test card on the wall. I directed her to blink as she moved her body to the right, and to flash a letter of the card that she could see without making an effort of any kind.

The memory of each of the letters seen helped her to read the black test card more easily. After she had finished reading the last letter of the 10-line, I was amazed to have her ask this question, "Ms. Lierman, I have not seen this card before, so I am not sure, but I see a figure '10' over the 10-line letters very plainly. Am I right?"

I became excited myself and answered, "Why, yes, but according to most of the eye specialists, it is impossible for you to see that figure '10' at ten feet. You should see that figure only at five feet with the normal eye, not at ten feet."

I find that myopic patients improve their sight and are cured more quickly by having them stand near a window and look off in the distance at large signs about a block away, or perhaps not quite so far. When the patient is able to see the large letters of the signs by blinking and shifting to a smaller sized letter of the test card, they soon become able to distinguish sign letters which they did not know were there at all when they were first asked to read the signs within their line of vision. Ms. Lennox could only see the large letter of a sign about half a city block away from my window. The smaller letters were blurred to her and she was not encouraged to try to read them.

On May 3, her second treatment, we stood at the window before test card practice, shifting to a large letter of a sign she had seen the day before. She became able, by blinking and shifting to the skyline, flashing a white cloud in a blue sky and then back to the sign letters, to read a sign which had letters, I should imagine, about a foot high. This sign was more than three city blocks away. The patient never stopped smiling and I was encouraged to help her more in this way.

The little blue booklet with Bible type was given to her. We used the page that has Psalm 119 on it, and which has more white spaces than either the Beatitudes or Psalm 23. Holding the fine type about six inches from her eyes, she was told not to read the type, but to look at the white spaces and remember them with the eyes closed. Alternately closing her eyes for a part of a minute and then opening them for a second, she read the small sign letters at more than three city blocks away.

When she looked at the fine print, which she did often, she asked me if she could read a sentence or two. At first she read the fine print, which was easy for her to do, at a little more than four inches from her eyes. I wanted to see how far off she could hold the type and still read it. At six inches the print was not clear and the white spaces were less white—they seemed gray to her.

I told her to look at the white clouds as they moved very slowly and gracefully in the beautiful blue sky above us. She said she could easily remember the cloud being very white and the sky a beautiful blue as she alternately opened and then closed her eyes. Each time she remarked that the white clouds could be remembered whiter and the blue sky bluer while her eyes were closed. While she was practicing this, I took hold of her right hand, which held the Bible print. I drew it twelve inches from her eyes. When I told her to look at the white spaces and not worry about the type at that distance, she smiled and remarked, "Why, I can read this fine print just as well at this distance." Memory, improved by imagining white clouds and a blue sky as well with her eyes open as with them closed, improved her myopia. Then we started the test card practice. She read a strange white test card with the black letters at 15/15 with each eye separately.

On May 4, when my patient came again, I noticed that her eyes looked tired. She said she feared that she had practiced too hard, or had made too great an effort to improve her imperfect vision. I told her she had no cause for worry and to just forget about it. We again practiced with microscopic print, shifting to the distant building signs more than three city blocks away, then back to reading a sentence of the microscopic type by looking at the white spaces instead of the print. She read smaller letters of the signs far away and her eyes were wide open. She also read another test card that she had not seen before, and at the normal distance, 15/15.

On May 5 she was all smiles and both eyes were wide open. She informed me that she had made a discovery. She said, "Do you know that I don't dare to stop blinking, because if I do, my eyes feel like hornets' nests. They sting. I can get relief only by blinking. I make it a habit now, to read smaller letters of words and signs on the housetops. I shift from the white line of my fine print booklet to distant signs that I see as I walk along the street or while riding in the trolley cars. Shifting from the near point to the distance always improves my eyestrain and relieves any tightness that comes for an instant when I stop doing the right thing. The moment that my eyes feel uncomfortable I find out, to my sorrow, that I have been unconsciously staring. I have learned that by shifting and blinking, I see all words move the least bit when I read, and I can now read book print for hours without any discomfort. I notice that when I sit at my piano and read my music, I can sit perfectly straight instead of leaning forward to see my notes. I feel proud that I can see just as well without leaning forward. I now read my notes easily at the right distance. I feared becoming round-shouldered from leaning over to see the notes. I noticed too that when I do not see things moving, my eyelids seem to close and I feel tired quickly."

On May 6, Ms. Lennox read No. 15, which is diamond sized type, with the Fundamentals card by Dr. W. H. Bates on the opposite side, at three feet, ten inches. I produced the small test card with the inverted "E's," and held it at a farther distance from where she was standing. She began: the universal swing, blinking always, and read the bottom line of the card at four feet, ten inches.

The normal eye can tell the direction in which the letters of the bottom line of the inverted "E's" are pointing, at two feet—not at four feet, ten inches—so her vision had improved to more than normal in five days. I saw the patient a week later and her vision was still the same. On her last visit she told me that she had been warned by an eye specialist in Canada never to leave off her glasses again or she would go blind.

She said, "You know how well I appreciate what you have done for me. I can now see my friends across the room better without my glasses than I could with them. Before I came to you for treatment, my friends at a tea found fault with me because I did not return their smiles when I looked at them from the other end of an ordinary-sized room. It was not so long ago that I could not read the 'Specials' on the menu card in a restaurant without my glasses. Now I can read clearly the print on my menu card that would be best for me not to read, such as French fried potatoes and other things that I enjoy, but which are not good for me."

CASE REPORT

By Anne Woessner

Editor's Note—*The following is a report of a case treated by Anne Woessner, West Nyack, New York. Ms. Woessner is one of Dr. Bates' representatives.*

Ada, age 24, from childhood has had hypermetropia combined with partial paralysis. Very strong glasses had been prescribed for her by a New York specialist. These glasses were shaped like two miniature searchlights, which together with the nosepiece and shafts resembled some fantastic bug.

Last February, the first time she came to me, she had left off her glasses. It was indeed pitiful to see her walk up the short path from the gate to the porch steps. Without her glasses she could only see a dim, blurred outline of people or objects two feet away.

Upon testing her sight, the four and one-half inch high "C" appeared a gray smudge at two feet. When handed a card printed with regulation reading type she saw only a blank. After palming a half-hour, she became able to read the 70-line at four feet. I then explained the importance of blinking, shifting and swinging, which she practiced for twenty minutes. This resulted in the reading of the 20-line at four feet, but blurred and gray in color.

She practiced faithfully at home the following week and started the next lesson with 4/40 quite clear. From this time on she improved steadily. The sun treatments became so soothing that she often dozed, much to our mutual amusement.

Her phenomenal memory greatly helped her to relax. She could relate many incidents which had happened in her childhood. Often I would read a story while she palmed, and while still palming she would repeat the story almost verbatim. This always helped. The large letters became clearer and the small type on the Fundamentals card seem to be very clear to her in spots.

With the practice of central fixation, memory of period and two to three hours of sunlight daily, she is now able to read newspaper type slowly and the diamond type on the back of Dr. Bates' professional card. The change in her appearance is as remarkable as that of her sight. She is now a true sunshine girl with large eyes of blue, cheeks and hair touched by the sun, and is smiling always. She fairly flies around her home. She phoned me specially one night recently to say that she had read the clock clear across the room.

There is still much to be done, however. She has had just fourteen treatments to date, and if she continues to practice so conscientiously she surely will be rewarded eventually with normal sight. In closing I wish to state that I am still holding her glasses which she handed me upon her second visit. She stated, "Don't ever want to see them again."

Better Eyesight *December 1927—Vol. XII, No. 6*

FAVORABLE CONDITIONS

The vision of the human eye is modified in many ways when the conditions are unfavorable to good sight. Unfavorable conditions may prevail when the light is not agreeable to the patient. Some patients require a very bright light and others get along much better in a poor light. Many cases are hypersensitive to the light and suffer from an intolerance for light which has been called *photophobia*.

While intolerance of light may be manifest in most cases from some diseases of the eyes, there are many cases in which the eye is apparently healthy and in which the photophobia may be extreme. The cure for this condition is to have the patient sit in the sun with his eyes closed, allowing the sun to shine on his closed eyelids as he moves his head from side to side.

There are patients with good sight whose vision is materially improved when used in a bright light, as well as those with good sight whose vision improves when the eyes are used in a dim light. The patient should practice with the test card in a bright as well as a dim light to accustom his eyes to all conditions.

The ability to perceive halos, or an increased whiteness, around letters is a favorable condition. By using a screen or a fenestrated card, it is possible for many patients to see an increased whiteness around a letter, which improves their vision for the letter. When a screen is not used, one may be able to imagine a white halo around the inner or outer edge of the black part of the "O." When a screen covers the black part of the letter "O," for instance, the white center becomes of the same whiteness as the rest of the white page, which proves that it is the contrast between the black and the white which enables one to imagine the white halos. The presence of the black improves the white; the presence of the white improves the black.

ROUTINE TREATMENT

By W. H. Bates, M.D.

Many doctors do not think well of treatment which has become continuously the same. I believe, however, that when routine treatment benefits a large number of patients, one is justified in practicing it in most cases. In the beginning, the writer very soon became impressed with the fact that there was something about routine treatment which had advantages over other forms of treatment. The particular advantage was speed; that is to say that by routine treatment it was often possible to cure many cases at the first visit. However, to obtain the best results, I have found it necessary to modify the routine from time to time or to make certain changes whenever improved methods of treatment were discovered. If a patient does not respond readily to a regular routine, it is evidence that this treatment is not for him and that he requires a different form of relaxation treatment.

When a person presents himself for treatment, a record is made of his name, address, date of birth, et cetera. If the patient is over fifty years old, one should be prepared to treat presbyopia; many persons over fifty years old are unable to read fine print at six inches without glasses.

The next procedure is to have the patient remove his glasses, if he is wearing them, and test the vision of each eye with the aid of the Snellen test card at fifteen or twenty feet. If none of the letters can be seen at this distance, the card is placed at eight feet, five feet or nearer and the vision tested at that distance. The eyes are then examined with the ophthalmoscope or retinoscope. (The ophthalmoscope is valuable in diagnosing cataract, opacities of the cornea and diseases of the interior of the eyeball. The retinoscope is used in diagnosing nearsightedness, farsightedness and astigmatism.)

Rest. The patient is then directed to either close his eyes or palm for half an hour, whichever is more comfortable for him. In palming, the patient closes both eyes and covers them with the palms of both hands in such a way as to exclude all light. To palm successfully, he should make no effort to remember, imagine or see black. If black cannot be seen perfectly, the patient is told to let the mind drift from one pleasant thought to another.

The Sway. After the patient has rested his eyes or palmed for half an hour, he is directed to stand before the Snellen test card, with his feet about one foot apart and then to open both eyes. He is then told to sway his body gently from side to side, while his vision is again tested with the card. While swaying from side to side, he is told how to imagine the Snellen test card to be moving. His attention is called to the fact that when his body, head and eyes move to the right, the Snellen test card moves to the left, and when he moves to the left, the Snellen test card appears to move to the right. The patient then is called upon to demonstrate that when his eyes move from side to side, that not only does the Snellen test card move from side to side, but that all the letters or figures on the Snellen test card move with the card. It is well to have the patient demonstrate also that when an effort is made to stop the movement of the letters, the letters become blurred or cannot be seen. The sway is beneficial in many ways because it lessens or prevents the stare, tension and strain.

Blinking. It can always be demonstrated that when a patient with imperfect sight looks intently at one point, keeping the eyes open constantly, or trying to do so, a strain of the eyes and all the nerves of the body is usually felt and the vision becomes imperfect. It is impossible to keep the eyes open continuously without blinking. Each time the eyes blink, a certain amount of rest is obtained and the vision is benefited. For this reason, the patient is instructed to blink frequently while swaying before the card, and at all other times.

Central Fixation. Central fixation is seeing best where one is looking and worst at all other points. When the patient is swaying before the card, he is told to see one part of a letter which he is regarding at a time and to see that part better than any other part; then to quickly shift his glance to another part, seeing that part best and other parts of the letter worse. The letter is seen much more readily in this way. The patient is reminded that the normal eye uses central fixation at all times.

Imagination. Another method is to improve the vision by a perfect imagination. If the patient is unable to see the letters on a certain line, he is told what the first letter is and is directed to close his eyes and imagine that letter as perfectly as he can, and then alternate by imagining it as perfectly as he can with his eyes open. When the letter is imagined perfectly enough, other letters on that line when regarded are seen and not imagined.

It is very evident that one cannot imagine unknown letters. Therefore, if the vision improves by the use of the imagination, unknown letters when regarded are seen and not imagined. It has been repeatedly demonstrated that an opacity of the cornea, which may be so dense that the pupil or iris are not seen, will clear up in some cases after the alternate imagination of a known letter or a known object is practiced with the eyes open and closed. When opacity of the lens is examined with the aid of the ophthalmoscope, the opacity becomes increased when the patient remembers imperfect sight. The memory of imperfect sight causes a contraction of the muscles on the outside of the eyeball, which in turn produces imperfect sight.

Memory. The pupil is told to remember a small letter "o" with a white center which is whiter than other letters on the Snellen test card. A small letter may be imagined much better than large letters of the Snellen test card. When the facts are analyzed, it is discovered that the reason small letters are imagined better than large ones is because a small letter has less of an area to be seen. It is easier for the eye to remember or imagine a small object than a large one. A perfect letter "o" can only be remembered when no effort is made; an imperfect letter "o," on the contrary, is difficult to remember. When a letter "o" is remembered very black with a very white center, the vision is benefited because no effort is made.

A great many nearsighted patients believe that they can remember or imagine an imperfect letter "o" much easier than a perfect letter "o." These people are encouraged to remember or imagine an imperfect letter "o," which helps them to understand and realize as thoroughly as possible that the memory or the imagination of imperfect sight is very difficult and requires a good deal of hard work, whereas the memory of perfect sight can only be accomplished easily without effort.

The Period. With the help of the imagination, alternating with the eyes open and closed, it is possible for many patients to remember or imagine they see a small black period. It may not necessarily be a black period but may have any color of the spectrum and be of any shape—round, square, triangular or irregular. It is impossible to remember or imagine a period that is stationary. It must always be remembered by central fixation and be moving. Some patients can imagine a period as small as it is printed in the newspaper. Unfortunately, it is difficult or impossible to teach all patients how to remember a period perfectly. The great value of the period is that when it is remembered perfectly, many serious diseases, such as opacities of the cornea, opacities of the lens, diseases of the retina and choroid, diseases of the optic nerve and blindness can all be relieved promptly.

Sun Treatment. An important part of the routine treatment is the use of the direct sunlight. The patient is told to sit in the sun with his eyes closed, moving his head a short distance from side to side, and allowing the sun to shine directly on his closed eyelids. He is instructed to forget about his eyes, to think of something pleasant and let his mind drift from one pleasant thought to another. Before opening his eyes, he palms for a few minutes. When the sun is not shining, a strong electric light (1000-watts) is substituted. The patient sits about six inches from the light, or as near as he can without discomfort from the heat, allowing it to shine on his closed eyelids as in the sun treatment.

Fine Print. If the patient has presbyopia, he is directed to practice with the fine print in the Fundamentals card in the following way: The card is held at first at the distance from his eyes at which he sees best. He is told not to look directly at the letters, but just at the white spaces between the lines and imagine that they are perfectly white—whiter than the margin. He is asked if he can imagine that there is a thin white line beneath each line of letters, and that it is whiter than the rest of the white spaces between the lines.

When this line is imagined perfectly white, the letters are read without effort or strain. If the patient cannot imagine the white line easily, he is told to close his eyes and think of a series of white objects; he may recall a white-washed fence, a snow drift, several pieces of white starch, or a pot of white paint. He is then directed to open his eyes again and look at the white spaces, imagining them to be as white as the white objects he remembered. He is told to close his eyes again and imagine that he has a pot of white paint and a fine pen and that he is drawing a thin white line beneath a line of print, then to open his eyes and imagine that he is drawing a thin white line beneath each line of letters on the Fundamentals card, as he moves his head from side to side. [Use a pretend "nose-pen"!—TRQ] He is told to blink as he shifts from one end of the line to the other, to occasionally look away and to close his eyes frequently for half a minute or so to rest them.

By practicing in this way, letters which could not be seen before appear black and distinct. As one's ability to read is improved, the card is brought closer and the patient is instructed to practice in this way until the entire card can be read at six inches from his eyes. If it is impossible for him to do this during his treatment at the office, he is directed to practice in this way every day at home. The patient is told that fine print cannot be read when an effort is made to see it and that it can only be read when the eyes are relaxed. For this reason, the reading of fine print is helpful in producing relaxation.

Instructions for Home Treatment

The most important fact is to impress upon the patient the necessity of discarding his glasses. If it is impossible or unnecessary for the patient to return at regular intervals for further treatment and supervision, he is given instructions for home practice to suit his individual case and is asked to report his progress or difficulties at frequent intervals.

The importance of practicing certain parts of the routine treatment at all times, such as blinking, central fixation, and imagining stationary objects to be moving opposite to the movement of the head and eyes, is stressed. The normal eye does these things unconsciously, and the imperfect eye must at first practice them consciously until they become an unconscious habit. [These are possibly the two most important sentences ever written about improving eyesight naturally. See also my comments at the end of the September 1927 issue.—TRQ]

PANSY LAND

By Emily C. Lierman

Once upon a time in a town near the Pacific Coast there lived a boy named George who suffered intensely from poor eyesight. One day he met a girl named Christine. The little boy had heard that Christine knew the great secret of good eyesight and begged her to tell him what he could do to cure his eyes. It did not take Christine long to teach George how to use his eyes right and keep from straining them. Christine soon found that George was not lonely like she was, for one day he brought Amy with him, the girl who made many children happy with her stories. She was beautiful to look at and had many friends. George and Amy were constant pals and helped to make Christine happy. Amy's eyes also became wonderfully bright through Christine's guidance and help, and everyone in Pansy Land wanted to know how this came about.

One day these three friends of Better Eyesight took a trip to the land of pansies. Before they were allowed to enter the gate, they had to seek admission from the doorkeeper. They waited until he went to see whether or not the pansies had gone to bed, as it was near closing time. He soon came back to them and told them to enter, that the pansies still had their eyes open and would welcome them. They walked a great distance and found that with the exception of narrow paths, everything was covered with miles and miles of pansies. There were yellow pansies with eyes as blue as the skies, brown and tan pansies with rose-colored eyes, and others dressed in all the colors of the rainbow. All of them were swaying with the gentle breeze and they were most beautiful to see.

Suddenly, a jolly gnome appeared before them. They noticed that his eyes were shining brightly and that he had the kindliest face of anybody they had ever seen. George knew him right away. He said, "This is Horatio the Great. It is he who first discovered how to cure people without glasses and help those who had pain and other troubles with their eyes." George also remarked that he had the biggest heart that anybody ever had, and was the best friend of poor children all over the world. Horatio the Great stood by, listening to these kind remarks but was too modest to make any reply. He just listened.

After George got through talking, the kindly gnome invited them to sit in his parlor, which was made of the loveliest pink mushrooms imaginable. He told them to place their palms over their eyes and not to think of anything bad or wrong and then to make a wish. They wished that they could be two very little girls and a very little boy again.

All of a sudden, there was a rumbling sound like thunder, and George, Amy, and Christine became very much frightened. The good gnome knew what had happened. He said, "Take down your hands and let me see how badly you have been frightened when there was nothing at all to be frightened about." He looked into their eyes and said, "Because you were frightened, you began to strain and your eyesight is now bad. You must be calm like I am, no matter how much trouble or worry you might have or how frightened you become. Don't you know that fear always affects good eyes and makes them bad?"

He then told them to again cover their eyes with the palms of their hands and he would tell them what caused their fright. He said, "You know I have many helpers in Pansy Land; some of them are my good gnomes. It was the good gnomes that you heard when they returned to their places on the roof of my palace. Don't be alarmed."

After this remark, there was no more fear and no more eyestrain. He then told them to remove their hands from their eyes. When they opened their eyes again he held in his hand a shining light, which was really a star on the end of a wand. With this he touched their eyelids and they were little children again.

When he touched the lonely little girl he said, "Now your name is Crystal because you will use the crystal glass with the help of the warm sunshine. You will cure children and grown-ups all over the world in time to come. You are ordered to finish your work here on the West Coast of this great big world where many people want you. You must be strong in your mind and heart and know that when your enemies want to hurt you, the good gnome, Horatio the Great, will always be standing by you and will keep you from harm. You must never be afraid."

Amy and George stood by listening with their eyes wide open, but blinking all the time to be sure that they would not strain and displease Horatio the Great.

The good gnome then touched little Amy with the shining star and said, "You will do greater things than you have ever done, now that you have better eyesight and no longer need glasses. You will go to many boys and girls and give them the sunlight with your sun glass. You will take away all pain and sorrow from those who suffer with eye trouble. Sometimes you will go alone, but most of the time little George will take you in his chariot so that you will not be weary in well doing." This pleased little George because he did not ever want to be separated from Amy, who had always made happiness and joy for him. Little Crystal knew in her heart how much they loved each other and this made her very happy.

The kindly gnome, Horatio the Great, then placed his wand with the shining star on the head of little George and said, "My book which tells you how to take care of people's eyes will help you to understand the work that you have to do. What you must enjoy is helping people with bad tummies and relieving eyestrain. I give you my special blessing because of the good work you have already done. You will take Crystal and Amy to your beautiful home in Marston Hills."

This made George very happy. His beautiful home has a frog pond in a lovely garden. In the pond lives one large frog. He has many friends who live near him all the time. Their names are Climbing Rose, American Beauty, Geranium, Calla Lily, Honey Suckle, and many others that would take much time to name.

This kindly frog is never thirsty and is ever ready to share with you the sparkling water that flows from his mouth. Even the frog has his work to do. In the pond directly under the throne on which the frog sits during the day, there lives a family by the name of Goldfish. Not so long ago the family increased in great numbers. They are lively and hungry all the time and Amy and George always feed them. All of the goldfish have perfect eyesight. The frog will tell you that at no time is eyestrain allowed in his kingdom. He has for his kindly assistant, Mary, who looks after things not only in the garden, but in the house that George built.

Horatio the Great led the procession to a little woodland which belonged to the pansies. Little Crystal noticed that a beautiful palm had been crushed on one side and many leaves were scattered on the grassy carpet. The two little girls and the little boy closed their eyes while the gnome told them the story of the crushed palm, and what had happened on that day. He told how the Queen of the fairies had been honored by all the fairies of Pansy Land. No disorder is ever allowed, because it causes much work and strain to those who are the caretakers, but on this special occasion when the Queen of the fairies that live all over the world had been given a reception, he made excuses for the fairies because of the disorder of the place.

From there he led them away to the center of the pansy bed that had the most colors. He told them to palm again and remember the color of any pansy they saw. While their eyes were closed and covered, the good gnome passed his wand with the shining star over the heads of the pansies. When Crystal, Amy and George opened their eyes, lo and behold, there was a beautiful fairy on the top of every pansy right before their eyes. What a beautiful sight it was and how happy these children were. The sun never shone more brightly; never in their lives did they smell more wonderful perfume. Immediately, there was a beautiful fairy dance and the more the children blinked, the more wonderful the fairies danced.

All good things must come to an end, for a little time at least, and soon the kindly gnome remarked that it was bedtime for the fairies and the pansies. Horatio the Great, with his kindly manner, led the way to the gate and gently bowed before the two little girls and the little boy, who honored him with their smiles and good wishes and said goodbye for awhile.

George remembered what he had promised the gnome, and placing little Amy and Crystal in his chariot, drove on to his home in the hills to the frog pond and the flowers.

Because of their happiness, the good gnome did not wish to change them into grown-ups again, so they will always be children and live happily ever after.

QUESTIONS AND ANSWERS

Q–1. Are movies harmful?

A–1. No. Quite the contrary.

Q–2. Trying to make things move gives me a headache. Palming gives me more relief. Why?

A–2. Making an effort to do a thing will not help you. When you are walking along the street, the street should appear to go in the opposite direction without effort on your part. Some people get more relief from palming, while swinging helps others more.

Q–3. Is it necessary to practice with the Snellen test card if you follow the method otherwise?

A–3. Yes, it is advisable to keep up your daily practice with the test card for at least a few moments. This will improve your memory and the memory must be improved to have the vision improve.

Better Eyesight

January 1928—Vol. XII, No. 7

EYESTRAIN DURING SLEEP

Many people complain that when they awaken in the morning, they are suffering from pain in their eyes or head. They often feel as weary as though they had been working hard all night long. Many of them do not recover from the pain and fatigue until after they have been up for an hour or longer. Their vision also may be found to be reduced to a very considerable degree. Some complain that they see illusions which are occasionally very slow in disappearing. One patient complained that the tiled floor of a bathroom had a very strange appearance; although the tiles were white, to him they appeared blue and red alternately. A feeling of strain was always present and did not subside until the illusion had disappeared. It seemed as though the eyes were under a strain during sleep, because when the eyes were examined with the ophthalmoscope while the patient was asleep, a strain could readily be observed.

Sometimes, as in the case of many children, other parts of the body may be under a strain during sleep. By an unconscious effort, the muscles of the face, arms and limbs may be distorted as may be muscles of different parts of the eyeball. In some cases, the strain produces accommodation or myopia, while in other cases hypermetropia or astigmatism are produced by this unconscious effort. These eyes frequently were found to be normal during the day.

Treatment to prevent eyestrain during sleep is not always successful. Some patients obtain most relief by practicing the long swing one hundred times or more just before retiring and the same number of times in the morning immediately after awakening. Other patients find that palming for twenty minutes before retiring is a help, and frequently the palms are left in place with benefit after the patients have lost consciousness.

GLAUCOMA

By W. H. Bates, M.D.

Glaucoma is a serious disease of the eyes which some years ago was considered incurable when chronic. In most cases, the eyeball was usually too hard and this is the symptom which more than any other was the strongest evidence we had that the eye was suffering from glaucoma.

The field of vision was contracted on the nasal side and the pupil was usually more or less dilated; the cornea was not as sensitive as the normal eye. Sometimes the *anesthesia,* or that condition in which the cornea is not sensitive to the touch of a blunt pointed instrument, was quite marked. One characteristic symptom was the apparent appearance of colors around the flame of a candle or some other similar light.

Glaucoma is a disease of adult life and seldom occurs in children. Its uncertainty is unusual. For example, a person with normal eyes and normal sight may retire feeling perfectly comfortable. Sometime in the middle of the night, he may be awakened by a very intense pain, with total permanent blindness in both eyes from glaucoma. In a limited number of cases, pain may be absent, although the vision may be partially lowered. The sudden onset may not occur, but one or both eyes may slowly, without pain and after a long time, a year or longer, become totally blind.

In the *American Encyclopedia of Ophthalmology,* the article on glaucoma consists of 170 pages of solid type, describing facts connected with the symptoms, cause and treatment of glaucoma. These facts are so numerous that the writer did not have to repeat himself. He emphasized how little ophthalmologists actually knew about glaucoma. It is evident that many theories cannot all be true.

One authority claimed that the cause of glaucoma was connected with a loss of the iris angle (that part of the eye which is located at the outer part of the iris) when a formation of new tissue, resembling scar tissue, formed in the iris angle and acted as a sort of plug preventing the proper circulation of fluids of the eyeball, when there was less fluid in the front part of the eyeball than is found in the front part of the normal eye. Many cases were benefited by an *iridectomy,* an operation in which a portion of the iris is removed. This theory went the way of some of the others when numerous exceptions were observed.

Another authority claimed that dilation of the pupil was an important factor in the cause of glaucoma. However, many cases were found in which the pupil was contracted as much, and in many cases more, than in the normal eye.

The results of the various methods of treatment which were suggested and practiced have been so disappointing that we hesitate to foretell what may happen after many of them have been practiced.

It was a very welcome discovery made by my assistant, Ms. Lierman, that the relief of eyestrain always lessens tension, relieves pain and improves the vision. The discovery that relaxation methods cured glaucoma suggested that the cause was due to eyestrain. Experimental work proved this to be true. All methods of treatment which promote relaxation always benefit glaucoma. When the vision is good, a stare or strain or an effort made to see brings on an attack of glaucoma. It is a difficult thing consciously to produce glaucoma by an effort to see. It is much easier to relax and benefit glaucoma. The writer has always felt great satisfaction in convincing patients that in order to have glaucoma and blindness, they had to go to a lot of trouble, work hard, and strain in order to produce it, but to benefit glaucoma was easy and required no effort whatever.

TREATMENT

By seeing one part of a letter best and all the rest of the letter not so well (central fixation), the letters of the Snellen test card appear improved to the maximum. Sometimes one has trouble in imagining central fixation of all the letters. On a card at fifteen feet, a patient with glaucoma could not imagine the letter "F" by central fixation, but the figure "6" of the same size and at the same distance was imagined by central fixation quite readily. The patient became able to imagine a period on the top of the figure "6" and the rest of the letter appeared worse. Usually, however, when looking at the letter "F," a period could not be imagined on any part of it. Sometimes, however, after the figure "6" was seen by central fixation, the patient could, by alternately shifting from the "6" to the "F," imagine the latter also by central fixation. I might say that there were times when the figure "6" was an optimum and the letter "F" a pessimum. Then, there were other occasions when the figure "6" was not an optimum and the symptoms of glaucoma were variable, changing, increasing, and diminishing. It is well to remember this truth, because when the patient found which letter was an optimum, or could be seen by central fixation, he was enabled to improve his vision for other letters, together with simultaneous improvement in the glaucoma.

Some of the best methods of producing relaxation are the practice of the long swing, the variable swing, the sway, palming and sun treatment. There are some people who cannot practice a certain swing correctly until after weeks of instruction. They are full of excuses and are quite ready to find fault with the method rather than with their own lack of practicing properly. (The above-mentioned methods have been described from time to time in previous issues of the magazine.)

Glaucoma may be produced solely by the memory of imperfect sight. If a person with normal eyes and normal vision presses lightly on the eyeballs through the closed eyelids and remembers or imagines a letter "O" with a gray, blurred outline very imperfect, the eyeball can be felt to increase in hardness. When the patient remembers a letter "O" perfectly, the hardness of the eyeball disappears and the eyes become normal as they were before. These experiments are offered as proof that the memory of imperfect sight is a strain which may produce glaucoma, and the memory of perfect sight a relaxation, which will relieve glaucoma.

One patient with acute glaucoma together with cataract could not distinguish 10/200, or the large "C" at the top of the Snellen test card. By looking at a light off to one side and flashing 10/200 alternately, the vision improved almost immediately to 10/30. She was able to remember the light when regarding the Snellen test card for a few seconds only. By alternately looking at the light and regarding the Snellen test card, her memory for the light improved, while her memory for the letters of the Snellen test card also improved.

She seemed to need supervision, because when practicing by herself, she did not flash the letters or look at them for a moment only. She stared at the light and the Snellen test card and instead of her vision improving, it became worse and it required encouragement to induce the patient to flash letters or other objects.

The memory was also improved by the practice of central fixation. When she looked at the first letter of a line of letters on the Snellen test card, she saw the other letters on the same line not so well; the memory of letters and other objects seen by central fixation became very much better in a short time. The patient's memory was also improved by the imagination of the halos, that is, when she regarded a white center of a letter "O" and imagined that she saw it whiter than the rest of the card, her memory and the halos also improved.

Case Reports

1. A woman, fifty years old, was suffering from retinitis pigmentosa, incipient cataract and chronic glaucoma. After daily treatment for six months, the vision was improved from 10/200 to normal. Palming, shifting and swinging gave the best results. She acquired the habit of imagining stationary objects to be constantly moving. The objects in her rooms—the furniture, window shades, the rugs, the ceiling, in fact all stationary objects seen—could be imagined to be moving whenever she moved her head and eyes. When she was out of doors, she imagined the sidewalk to be coming towards her, or if she looked to one side that the buildings or other objects were moving in the opposite direction.

Another method which helped her was to stand before a window and imagine the curtain cord to be moving in the opposite direction as she swayed her body from side to side, while a building in the distance appeared to be moving in the same direction as the movement of her body.

It was very interesting to observe that the pigment spots of the retinitis pigmentosa were disappearing from view; the symptoms of glaucoma also disappeared gradually. When she remembered perfect sight, one could with the ophthalmoscope see the cataract immediately becoming less. When she remembered imperfect sight, the cataract became very opaque. Besides obtaining normal sight for the distance, she became able to read diamond type at six inches without glasses.

In the beginning of the treatment, the left eye was the better eye. However, the left eye was treated for more than six months before normal vision was obtained, while the vision of the right eye improved from 10/200 to 20/20 after only one week of treatment.

This patient was very grateful for the benefit she received and could not understand why many of the ophthalmologists whom she had consulted previously did not refer her to me. Her constant question was, "If these other doctors could not cure me, why did they not send me to the Doctor who could?"

2. A physician had been in the habit of attending a gymnasium and after he had finished with his exercises he usually bathed in the pool. The exercise and the bathing seemed to agree with him perfectly and although he had been taking these baths almost daily, no injury to his eyes could be detected. One night he was awakened by a severe pain in both eyes, which stopped only after the use of morphine. In the morning he was practically blind.

The doctor whom he consulted said that he was suffering from glaucoma and iritis. The iris was inflamed and the pupil opaque from the presence of inflammatory exudation. The eyeballs were very hard. This severe inflammation continued for more than six months. Accidentally, he heard of my method and came to see me, very hopeful. He told me that he had had my book read to him and that he had felt decidedly encouraged.

Upon examining him, I found the eyeballs very hard, his field of vision contracted more on the nasal side than elsewhere; the pupils of both eyes contracted and his sight reduced to 1/200. He asked me if I thought that his eyes had been infected or if he had injured his eyes by striking the water when he dove into it. I told him that I did not believe that had anything to do with it, and that his trouble was brought on by mental strain.

The patient was advised to practice at home those measures which had already improved his sight while he was at my office, palming, swinging and sun treatment. At his second visit, a few days later, he was further encouraged. The redness of the white part of the eyes had entirely disappeared. The pupil was no longer contracted but was dilated to the same extent as is found in most normal eyes.

He was much pleased that the sun treatment had been of marked benefit. He said that he had read in many eye books that persons suffering from iritis should protect their eyes from the injurious effects of the light by wearing dark glasses. He also said that he was convinced that the sunlight and other forms of light were a benefit to his iritis and not an injury.

His condition continued to improve and in a few days he was able to read the large type of a newspaper without discomfort. I said to him, "Why don't you read the small type?" He answered that he was afraid he would strain his eyes. My answer to this was to hand him a card on which was printed some sentences of diamond type. He was able, much to his surprise, to read the diamond type at about six inches. This amused him so much that one could hear him laughing almost a block away. He compared his ability to read fine type with his ability to read the large type of a newspaper and found that the diamond type was easier. He said, "Why is it that I see the diamond type easier than I do the large print?" I replied that it was because in order to read the diamond type, his mind had to be relaxed. If he strained, he could not read it. If he could not read it, he strained. He was advised to read as much diamond type as he had time for.

The patient was encouraged to keep up the treatment until a complete cure was obtained.

A CASE OF ABSOLUTE GLAUCOMA

By Emily C. Lierman

A man, age 68, with absolute glaucoma was brought to me by his physician, who was quite sure that the Bates Method could do nothing to restore his sight. This man had had three operations on both eyes; the first operation was performed in the year 1924. He had no perception of light in the right eye and could see but very little with his left eye, not more than 1/200. The doctor who brought him was the most skeptical person I have ever come in contact with. His manner in regard to the method was almost insulting, and I resented his attitude very much. I had a conversation with him over the telephone previous to the appointment which was made with his patient. He was to give me an hour with this man and if at the end of that time I could improve the patient's sight, even a particle, he would believe that Dr. Bates was right when he claimed that glaucoma was curable by his method.

I never felt more determined in my life to do the best that was in me for this patient. Before the hour of his appointment, I sent him my book, *Stories from the Clinic,* by special messenger and asked him to read what I had written about the relief of strain in glaucoma.

When the doctor entered my office with his patient, one could see by his face that he was ready to prove that his patient would receive no benefit in his sight. I was in a fighting mood myself and my eyes, I feel sure, told him of my determination to prove that he was wrong and I was right. I informed the doctor immediately that even though his patient was a wealthy man, I would not accept a fee at this time, but if the patient received further treatment from me or from Dr. Bates, he would have to pay a bonus in advance besides the regular fee for the hard work which would be before us. As I look back upon that day and hour which I spent with his patient, I realize how hard I worked.

The right eye, as I have said, had no sight at all because the retina was almost destroyed and there were other complications caused by the operations. Because of this, it was not necessary for my patient to cover his right eye while the left eye was being tested.

I produced the white test card with black letters, as the patient sat by a window with the sunlight shining on the whole card. I watched to see what effect the strong light reflected on the card would produce. Immediately the patient drew back, as if the strong light hurt his sight. I was pleased to note this, as I knew then that the patient was sensitive to the strong light which, of course, was in my favor, because sun treatment would overcome this sensitiveness and probably improve the vision. The doctor made no comment. At one foot from his eyes, the patient could flash the 200-line letter "C" as he moved the card slowly from left to right before his eyes. [The original text is "2 line"; this is likely an error since there are two references in this report to the patient beginning with 1/200 vision, and next he improves his vision to the 100-line. There are additional clarifications of line numbers below.—TRQ] More than that, he could not see without a great deal of effort. Then I changed the card and replaced it with the black test card with white letters, placing the card in his hand as I had the white card. I directed the patient to keep the card moving slowly from side to side and to blink as he moved the card. By doing this, he flashed the 100-line letters, one at a time. Occasionally, I glanced at the doctor's face to see whether he was pleased or not. He might have been a sphinx for the lack of interest which he showed.

My next plan was to have the patient palm, which I told him how to do, and while he was palming I asked him to tell me what interests he had in life. He said he was a banker, so I advised him to remember figures on banknotes as well as he could; also to remember other things in regard to the work which he was most interested in. I avoided any unpleasant conversation regarding his eye trouble, which he unconsciously referred to from time to time.

I explained to him that his poor sight worried him more than he realized, but if he believed in what I was trying to do for him, he would not feel so hopeless in time to come. Jokingly, and half in earnest, I remarked, "You must have a better attitude of mind than your doctor has at the present time," which brought for the first time a smile to the face of the doctor. The patient said he was willing to believe that I could help him and I know that he meant it.

While the patient was palming, I placed the large black test card with white letters upon a test card stand, which I arranged five feet from where the patient was sitting, and in an ordinary light. Again I looked at the doctor, but he made no sign of being in doubt or otherwise. This would have been discouraging, I know, to most of our students, but I have had so much experience with people like him that I paid no more attention to him than if he were not in the room. It was the only way for me to keep from either weeping or gnashing my teeth.

After the patient had palmed for more than ten minutes and had removed his hands from his eyes, I asked him to stand. As I held both his arms at the elbow, I asked him to sway from side to side with me. Of his own accord the patient remarked with a smile how relaxing it was to sway his body, and that he enjoyed doing it. At first he did not recognize the card where I had placed it, and I myself did not mention to him what I had done while he was palming. I told him that he was to keep up the swing of his body until he discovered the test card and was able to read some of the letters. I also informed him that he was not to try hard to see any letter, but to keep up the sway.

Anyone interested in our work can imagine how happy I was to hear him say, "I think the middle letter of the third line is an 'O'." Before I allowed him to go any further, I told him to sit down again and palm. I felt that the palming had had as much to do with the improvement in his sight as did the swinging of his body. While the patient was palming, I told him to remember anything which was pleasant, that it did not matter much what it was. Some patients enjoy remembering a sunset, or a white cloud in a blue sky. I reminded him of these things and also told him that it was necessary for him to shift from one thing to another and not to concentrate on any one thing.

While he palmed, he said that he had had a bad habit for years of concentrating or trying to concentrate, which he thought was beneficial, but now realized that this produced more strain and discomfort. It was nice to hear the patient explain these little things to me, because it proved to the doctor who brought him that he was anxious to help me in what I was trying to do for him. This time the patient palmed for about fifteen minutes and then we started the standing sway of the body, having him blink regularly as he did before. This time he read every letter of the 50-line, seeing one letter at a time and looking away quickly to avoid staring. [The original text is "5 line"; Emily is referring to the 50-line, which begins with the number "5."—TRQ] A great feeling of satisfaction came over me as I saw that the doctor was watching the patient closely. Nothing was said, however, because we both felt the need of silence at this time.

The patient began to strain unconsciously to read the next line of letters, but I avoided having him read any further until he had again rested his eyes by palming. This time it was not necessary for me to again remind him to use his memory, for he immediately mentioned how white the letters looked on the black background when he did not look at the card longer than a fraction of a second. I said that it was a good thing for him to alternately remember the black margin of the card and then remember the white letters as he saw them, or if he possibly could, without an effort, to imagine the letters whiter than he really saw them. After he had rested his eyes in this way for ten minutes or longer I placed him in the sun, and with my sun glass I focused the strong rays on his closed eyelids. Some patients draw away when they first receive the sun treatment, but this patient enjoyed the strong light of the sun from the start, which made it easier for me to treat him.

After the sun treatment he again read the test card at the same distance, and this time he read all of the 30-line. [The original text, "3 line," refers to the 30-line, which begins with the number "3." This patient's final improvement in this lesson results in a vision of "1/6 of normal," which agrees with the improvement to 5/30 vision.—TRQ] The patient turned to me and thanked me for my efforts and for what I had done for him. He also told me that he would try to do without the strong magnifying glass which he had been using for a few years to help him in his work. I explained how dangerous it was for him to continue the use of the magnifying glass even though it helped him to see things better at the time. As this patient had never heard of the Bates Method before, I am not sure that he realized the importance of what I explained to him. I really helped him and improved his vision from 1/200 to 1/6 of normal in one hour's time under unfavorable conditions, for which he was grateful.

As the time for the treatment was over, I had to let the patient go, but I had satisfied the skeptical doctor who not only fought me with his mind, but also tried to prove to me that Dr. Bates' statements were false when he claimed to relieve tension in glaucoma and also improve the sight when other methods had failed.

QUESTIONS AND ANSWERS

Q–1. I have a high degree of myopia. Approximately how long will it take to obtain a cure by your method?

A–1. It is impossible to say, as people vary so in their response to the treatment.

Q–2. How often should one with imperfect sight palm during the day and for how long?

A–2. Palming should be done as often as possible during the day, ten times at least, for five, ten, fifteen minutes or longer at a time. Some people obtain more benefit from short periods than from longer periods.

Better Eyesight
February 1928—Vol. XII, No. 8

THE THUMB MOVEMENT

Rest the hand against an immovable surface. Place the ball of the thumb lightly in contact with the forefinger. Now move the end of the thumb in a circle of about one-quarter of an inch in diameter. When the thumb moves in one direction, the forefinger should appear to move in the opposite direction, although in reality it is stationary.

While watching the movement of the thumb, remember imperfect sight. At once, the thumb movement becomes irregular or may stop altogether. Demonstrate that any effort, no matter how slight, to see, remember or imagine, interferes with the movement of the thumb. The thumb is so sensitive to an effort or strain that the slightest effort is at once recorded by the motion.

While watching the movement of the thumb, remember perfect sight. Notice that the movement of the thumb is slow, short, continuous, and restful—with relaxation of all parts of the body.

Many patients have been successfully treated for pain, fatigue, and dizziness with the help of the thumb movement, after other treatment had failed. Some patients with severe pain complain that when they forget to practice the movement of the thumb, the pain comes back.

Not only have patients suffering from pain and symptoms of fatigue been relieved, but an equal number have been relieved of imperfect sight by the correct practice of the thumb movement.

FACT AND FANCY

By W. H. Bates, M.D.

The attention of the editor was called to a copy of the *British Medical Journal* of October 8, 1927, p. 641, in which my discoveries on the cure of imperfect sight without glasses were adversely criticized. The following is the article in question:

> "There are some who deny that the world is round, and some who still believe in the mystery of Joanna Southcott's boxes, so that it is not altogether a matter of surprise that there are others who deny the facts of physiology and of experience. There is a book before us, written by one W. H. Bates, M.D., which for boldness of denial and strangeness of assertion rivals the others. The title of the book is *The Cure of Imperfect Sight by Treatment Without Glasses,* but that on the cover is *Perfect Sight Without Glasses.* The author would have us throw away our useful glasses, and beguile ourselves into the belief that we see better without them. Trial shows that we do not and that his alleged treatment is no more than a beguilement that does not stand the test of experience. To practice judgment of what is seen is one thing, to see that same thing better is another. To 'palm' the eyes—otherwise make use of familiar and refreshing massage—is one thing; to alter anatomical defect another. But then this author denies anatomical facts and alleges that all errors of refraction are merely functional. Strangely enough he admits the use of glasses for patients who have no lenses as the result of cataract operation but denies the use of the lens in accommodation, despite the evidence of Purkinje's figures, which he has heard of, for he reproduces the classical picture in his pages. His cult extends to the assertion of the value of small print, even that which is so small that it cannot be read: 'Those who cannot read such type may be benefited simply by looking at it.' Excessive light, he alleges, is not injurious, but actually beneficial; . . . Reading in bed is 'beneficial rather than injurious'—perhaps when the print is not seen! But, strangely, black has its virtues: 'It is possible to perform surgical operation without anesthetics when the patient is able to remember black perfectly.' Perhaps the author got somewhere near a truth in a sentence in the last paragraph of this book: 'The fact is that, except in rare cases, man is not a reasoning being.'
>
> We met one of this cult recently; a parent had been summoned to attend a certain place owing to his persistent refusal to provide his child with glasses for school use. The child had myopia of 3 D; without glasses vision was 1/60, with glasses 6/6. The child appreciated the value of the glasses, but the father would not allow them to be worn, alleging other treatment. But the recalcitrant parent wore glasses himself for an equal degree of myopia. It seems a pity good paper should be wasted on such a book, or that our columns should give space to its notice. But there have been inquiries and so this review."

"There are some who deny that the world is round" and we hold such misguided ignorant people more or less in contempt, because they appear to ignore the learning of other people who are very highly respected for their scientific knowledge. It so happened that an ignorant man said to me, "Doctor, do you know that they found out that the world was not round?" I answered, "No, I had always believed that it was round." "Well," he said, "my boy came home from school one day and told me that the earth was flattened at the poles," and then he showed me his son's geography. The book stated very clearly that the shape of the earth is not a perfect sphere, but because it is flattened at the poles, it is an oblate spheroid. Since then I have not learned that the man was persecuted who called the earth an oblate spheroid and published the facts in a book which was used as a text by schoolchildren all over the world.

Reference has been made to Joanna Southcott by my worthy critic, and he probably suggests that I am no better than she. I looked up the history of Joanna Southcott and found that she was a domestic servant born in Devonshire, England. She joined the Methodist Church in 1790 and in 1792 announced herself a prophetess giving forth revelations. At one time she sold 6,400 sealed packages or boxes warranted to secure salvation to the purchasers. She prophesied that she would give birth to Shilo or the Prince of Peace on a certain day, but failed to do so.

I deny that I ever attempted to beguile anybody into an error. When a patient comes to me wearing glasses, I usually test his vision without glasses and tell him that the treatment consists of eye education for the purpose of improving his sight so that he can, without glasses, see as well as, or better than he can with them. It never occurred to me that any of my patients would call this beguilement. The word, however, is a good one and may be useful in the future as a substitute for the word imagination. My practice is built up by the recommendation of patients whom I have cured without glasses.

If my critic had read the chapter on palming more carefully, he would not have made the mistake of calling it massage.

I have been criticized for denying an anatomical fact. I do not deny that in myopia, the eyeball as well as the optic axis is elongated; that in hypermetropia it is lessened; that in astigmatism its form may be modified, or that in presbyopia glasses improve the vision. My book describes how errors of refraction are curable and have been cured by eye education. The cause is an effort or strain. When this effort or strain is corrected, all errors of refraction disappear and the patient becomes able to see as well, if not better, without glasses than he formerly did with them.

When a patient with normal eyes and normal sight regards a blank surface and makes an effort to see, an error of refraction can always be produced and demonstrated with the aid of a retinoscope. When a patient with imperfect sight looks at a blank surface without trying to see, the retinoscope demonstrates that the error of refraction has disappeared temporarily or more permanently. It is a fact that it is possible to teach patients who have progressive myopia of 16 diopters how to cure their myopia by relaxation. What is true of myopia is also true of hypermetropia, astigmatism and presbyopia.

Although some years ago I usually prescribed glasses for the benefit of the sight after cataract extraction, I do not do so at the present time. With the aid of eye education, such patients become able to read diamond type without glasses at six inches or nearer to their eyes or eighteen inches or farther. These facts are offered as evidence that the lens is not a factor in accommodation, because the eye can change its focus within wide limits after the lens has been removed.

[If the eye changes its focus without a lens, then the lens is *not essential* for accommodation.—TRQ]

In my investigations, the figures of Purkinje were studied. For some years, I tried to obtain a perfect image, reflected from the front part of the lens, which was sufficiently clear and distinct to be photographed or measured accurately. The pictures I obtained were very much blurred and one could draw wrong conclusions from their behavior during accommodation, as well as imaginary ones which "proved" a great many theories. In short, one may say that as a result of studying these blurred Purkinje figures, almost any explanation of how accommodation was brought about might be imagined erroneously. Helmholtz was not satisfied with the pictures he obtained by photography, and his illustrations of the behavior of the images of Purkinje were usually in the form of diagrams, which I do not consider good evidence of the truth of his conclusions. My book has described the work of Helmholtz in this field and I would respectfully offer that to the reader's consideration for criticism.

About a year ago, a friend living in England attended a meeting of one of the optometric societies. The speaker of the evening considered the cause of accommodation. He obtained photographs of the reflection of the image from the front part of the lens before and after accommodation. I was very glad to receive these photographs, but was very much disappointed when some experts who were taking movies for me pointed out that the photographs of the optometrists were retouched.

While working in a physiological laboratory, the director suggested that I repeat the experiments of Helmholtz on accommodation, with the end in view of finding out how he made his mistakes. This seemed a very difficult problem to solve. After some years of hard work I became able to obtain photographs of images reflected from the front part of the lens both before and after accommodation. These images were clear and distinct and furthermore I learned how to arrange an apparatus by which an observer could see a clear image reflected from the cornea, iris, the front part of the lens, the front part of the sclera and from the different parts of the outside of the eyeball. There was no change in the image reflected from the front part of the lens during accommodation.

The director of the laboratory was able to demonstrate with his own eyes, with the aid of this apparatus, the truth that the lens is not a factor in accommodation.

The great trouble with the physiology of the eye is that most of us feel that after a man like Helmholtz finishes a job, it is not possible that he has made any mistakes. I believe that he has made a monumental blunder and I do not hesitate to say so. Helmholtz was a great man and he helped things along very well, but his *Physiological Optics* has almost spoiled everything else that he wrote. Someone has said that the pupils of Helmholtz were thoroughly convinced that the lens is the only factor in accommodation, while he himself was more conservative. In short, he published a statement to the effect that he did not prove that the lens was the only factor in accommodation.

[For someone who wanted to convince the orthodox that Helmholtz had erred on such an important topic, Dr. Bates should have been able to give a better answer to the question "What is the function of the ciliary muscle?" than "I do not know" (February 1922 issue); similarly he answers, "If the lens is not a factor in accommodation, what is its purpose?" with the highly implausible "The lens is for protective purposes, just as fat is a protection to the bones of the body." (September 1928 issue).

An ophthalmologist friend of mine told me that modern research, using highly sophisticated equipment, indicates that the front side of the lens changes its curvature during accommodation.

Still, many questions regarding the lens and accommodation remain: If modern research is correct, was Dr. Bates' experimental setup not sensitive enough to detect a change in the lens' curvature? Is presbyopia due to a chronically tense ciliary muscle preventing the lens from accommodating? Is the lens necessary for accommodation after it becomes rigid? Can the ciliary muscle change the lens' curvature for reasons other than accommodation, e.g. light intensity, like the iris muscle?—TRQ]

My critic says, "His cult extends to the assertion of the value of small print, even that which is so small that it cannot be read, 'those who cannot read such type may be benefited simply by looking at it'." People with imperfect sight are benefited by looking at fine print provided no effort or strain is made. I recommend this treatment to my critic if he is suffering from presbyopia.

"Reading in bed is beneficial, rather than injurious." Reading in bed without effort is a benefit. If one makes an effort while reading, it is an injury.

It is a fact that it is possible to perform a surgical operation without anesthetics when the patient is able to remember black. I have repeatedly operated on the eyes and other parts of the body painlessly when black was remembered perfectly. [Surgical operations have also been performed without anesthetics using acupuncture.—TRQ]

The patient whom my critic mentioned who wore glasses for myopia and denied the same practice to his son is certainly open to criticism.

I do not see why my critic has published so much against me without a proper scientific investigation and without conclusive evidence that I am wrong. If John Doe says that myopia is incurable, before accepting this as true, we would like to know what his evidence might be. In my book are published many facts which are of sufficient importance, I believe, to be investigated. My critic has said very little about the evidence which has been offered there by me to prove that my statements of the truth are correct.

Just today a patient came to me with a diagnosis of chronic glaucoma and told me that the best doctors in this country had advised an operation at once. In my experience, chronic glaucoma does not respond favorably to any operation. This patient was treated by relaxation or rest and obtained normal vision, without glasses, for the distance and became able to read fine print, diamond type (Jaeger No. 1) at six inches. She was very grateful for the relaxation obtained and was overjoyed to find that an operation was unnecessary. This case is suggestive and the temporary or permanent cure which she obtained in one visit was a fact that no amount of contradiction can modify or lessen.

Children less than three years old, too young to learn the letters of the alphabet, have been cured of squint by practicing the swing. Let the mother or father or some member of the family with whom the child associates give the child confidence. They should take hold of both hands of the patient and swing him around and around until his feet are lifted from the floor. The child enjoys this immensely after he has practiced it for a few times. Frequent swinging of the child for a few minutes during the day usually cures squint, divergent, convergent, or vertical—at first temporarily and later on more continuously or permanently. It does not require an ophthalmologist to observe the benefit.

Children less than a year old who are suffering from tension with many forms of eye disease, are relieved of their tension by rocking them in the arms of the mother and by the use of an old-fashioned cradle. I believe that the eyes of children are more frequently diseased at the present time than they were when the cradle was used. It should be emphasized that motion is a benefit, not only to children but also to adults.

All through my book are reports of cases in which patients have been blind from one or more of the numerous diseases of the eyes. They were all benefited by the relaxation treatment. When they recovered and became able to see without glasses, no amount of criticism without facts could shake these persons' faith in my methods.

INDIVIDUAL TREATMENT

By Emily C. Lierman

During my year's experience treating patients in the West, I came in contact with a number of patients who were treated, but not benefited, by those who did not properly understand the method. I finally stopped counting the number of patients who came to me for the relief of presbyopia, cataract, glaucoma and other troubles. I shall try to describe the worst case among all these patients who appealed to me for the relief of pain, so that the readers of our magazine and others will know the truth about things.

One or two so-called doctors or specialists were directly responsible for the pitiful condition of this patient. There was so much wrong with this man that I hardly knew where to begin. This was his story, related before I tested his vision with the test card:

Up to the time he was twenty-five years old (he was now 51) he had good sight for the near point as well as for the distance, but soon after that he found difficulty in reading ordinary type unless he used a strong light. He decided to wear glasses for reading only and got along with them for a short time. Then his eyes began to smart and pain when he was out in the sun and his sight for the distance became very blurred. He suffered with headaches almost every day for a while and finally was advised to have his glasses changed. Two pairs of glasses were prescribed for him by one eye specialist, one pair for reading and the other for his distant vision.

He said he was faithful to the doctors who from time to time had given him eyeglasses, as he wore them constantly every day for some years. He finally discarded glasses altogether because he found no relief from pain. After obtaining Dr. Bates' book, *Perfect Sight Without Glasses,* and receiving some benefit from what he practiced, he decided to try the complete treatment. He went to a doctor whom he understood gave the Bates treatment, although at this time he was not informed so by the doctor. He had to pay a sum of money in advance for a course of treatment which ended in the spring of the year. By that time his condition was worse than it was in the beginning.

He was told that if he would take another course of treatment, he would surely be cured, and as an inducement he was told of special summer rates of which he ought to take advantage. What a tale for the ears of Dr. Bates!

The patient, however, submitted to another course of treatment, hoping to be benefited. After another month of this treatment, with his condition of health getting worse every day, he found out for the first time that the treatment was not the Bates Method. He questioned the assistants who helped in the treatment if Dr. Bates used all the apparatus and eye muscle exercises that were given him there and he was told by the doctor that the treatment was his own discovery and not the Bates Method. What a pity that he had not been informed of this in the beginning!

On July 20 of the same year this patient came to me and the nervous twitch of his shoulders as he talked made me nervous too. It took just one hour for the patient to explain to me what I have written about him. He not only stuttered, but some words were so long drawn out that it took considerable time. He did not blink, but stared all the while he was talking. However, when he finally did blink consciously or unconsciously, I noticed that the nervous twitch of his shoulders subsided.

The patient emphasized the fact that as far as seeing ordinarily, his vision was not bad. The treatment which he had previously received was not a benefit but an injury to his nervous condition.

Before I tested his sight with the test card, I made him promise to help me because at that time I did not know whether or not I could do anything for him. His vision with the test card was normal, 15/10 with the right eye and 15/15 with the left, but the letters were a little blurred. I directed him to palm, which he knew how to do, but I noticed while he was palming that his shoulders twitched continuously all the while he had his eyes covered. After palming for about ten minutes or a little less, the 15-line of letters still looked blurred to him with the left eye, showing that the palming had not benefited him.

I told him to stand and sway his body from side to side and to observe that the Snellen test card and other distant objects were moving opposite to the sway. While swinging with his right eye covered, he again read the 15-line and then the 10-line letters, without any blurring.

I then tested his vision at the near point with the fine print on the Fundamentals card. At first, he held the card about six inches from his eyes, as I directed him, but drew his head back some distance as though he had been struck. This happens very often while testing a patient for the reading of fine print. I directed the patient to hold the card twelve inches away instead. He was able to read No. 3, or the third sentence from the top of the card, which has good-sized type. He said that the words were blurred. As he tried to read the fourth sentence on the card, his shoulders began to twitch again, as they did while he palmed, so I did not encourage him to go any further.

I saw from the beginning that I would have a problem to solve, so I decided to study his case until the next time I treated him. The directions I gave him for home practice were very simple. He was glad to know that what he was called upon to do by himself was simple; he was directed to stand, with his feet one foot apart, and to sway his body with a long, slow, easy swing, not noticing anything that came in his line of vision. He was told not to worry about what line of letters he was able to read on the test card, but to be sure not to try to improve his vision by making any sort of an effort.

He was to remember to glance only at the white spaces dividing each letter on the card and to place himself at least a foot farther away from the card each day. While walking in the street, he was to hold his chin up and look ahead instead of looking down at the pavement, which had been his habit for many years. He was to imagine in this way that he saw the pavement coming towards him as he walked. Automobiles and other vehicles which were not moving but were against the curb were to be imagined to be moving opposite as he looked to the right or left while walking.

Eight days later he came for a second treatment. I used a large card which he had not seen before and placed him eighteen feet away from it. As he swayed, shifting from the test card to a picture on the wall and then back again to the test card, he was able to tell me which way the inverted "E's" were pointing on the line, which is usually seen by the normal eye at ten feet. The letters were quite clear to him.

I find that with difficult cases it is good to introduce palming in some way or another. When this patient closed his eyes and placed his one hand or both hands over his eyes, the twitch was very noticeable. If I asked him a question while his eyes were covered, he stuttered even more than he did when he was staring at me. This surely was a problem for me to solve and I will say that I worried a great deal about him. I did not want to fail him as others had. The thing for me to do was to undo the harm that was done to him.

The sun was shining brightly in the window of my office, so I placed him in a comfortable chair and arranged his head so that the sun shone directly on his closed eyelids. The sun is much brighter in the West than it is here in the East and it also has a great deal of healing power. Of course, I expected that the sun would be a great factor in the cure of this patient. I kept him in the sun fully a half-hour and then when I placed him in the shade afterward, I told him still to keep his eyes closed for a little while. I did this purposely to get him accustomed to the darkness as well as the bright light while his eyes were closed.

I placed myself in a chair directly opposite him and held the small test card, black with white letters, in my hand. Then I told him to open his eyes and to read one letter at a time and immediately afterward to close his eyes to rest them. While he did this, his shoulders were perfectly still and he mentioned each letter without dragging his words as he did before. He flashed the letters on the line which is marked "5" as I was sitting about five feet away from him. I considered that very good.

I told him to sit in the sun again and with his chin raised and eyes closed, he sat perfectly still for another ten minutes. After that he was able to read the line of letters of the small black card which is marked "4" and each letter was clear to him as he read, with his body perfectly still and relaxed.

Then I spoke to him about palming. I explained that it was not necessary for him to keep his hands over his eyes any length of time, but to try what I have called "instant palming." He was to hold his hand cupped about a foot away from his eyes and as he drew it toward his face he was to gradually close his eyes and keep them closed as the cupped hand touched his forehead. This worked splendidly. As he kept his hand over his eyes only for a part of a minute, he did not cause any strain as he did before, and he enjoyed doing this because as he explained it, he felt free from strain and tension. It was good to see the patient smile and to listen to his speech of gratitude which I enjoyed and understood very well.

After the treatment was over, I told him not to try palming at all by himself until I saw him again. Sun treatment was advised and he was to get as much of it as he possibly could, always allowing the sun to shine on his closed eyelids, which was best for him. He was told again to imagine stationary objects moving when he moved his body and to remember to blink frequently. I also explained to him that the thumb movement (see "The Thumb Movement" of this issue), which Dr. Bates discovered some time ago, was a benefit in cases where it was difficult to have a patient relax while trying to improve his sight.

One week later he came again for another treatment. He had a tale of woe for me; the sum and substance of his failure in home treatment was that he tried too hard. To begin with, he blinked too fast, which is as bad as not blinking at all. When patients acquire the habit of blinking too fast, they are very apt to stare while they blink. Some of my work with him had to be done over again because he had tried too hard by himself. He had forgotten something that I had asked him to do, and that was to telephone me every day and let me know how he was getting along. It only takes a few minutes to write a short letter or go to a telephone and explain the failures or the success in home practice. Because this patient failed to do as he was told, much of what I had already told him had to be repeated over and over.

I made the next treatment as simple as possible and he spent most of the hour shifting to the white spaces of the large test card and then to the white spaces of the small test card that he held in his hand. Shifting from the near point, where letters were easily seen, to the distant card brought about a relaxed state of mind and body and we proceeded once more with other things which were to help him permanently. In order to avoid blinking too fast, I told him to again place his hand "cup fashion" about a foot from his eyes. This time he was not to touch his face with his hand but to draw the hand in as though he were going to touch his face. As the hand moved toward him, he was to close his eyelids gently and in this way as he again drew his hand away, he opened and closed his eyes, keeping time with the hand as he moved it backwards and forwards. As the hand was drawn away from his face he opened his eyes easily and not too quickly.

I had emphasized that he must not snap his eyes shut or open them too quickly. He practiced this until he became tired, which was more than ten minutes each time, and then he would sway as a diversion. This new way of teaching him to blink without blinking too fast helped him to keep his eyes open for part of a minute, while closing them took only part of a second. This helped him to blink one blink at a time instead of blinking rapidly with a nervous twitch which caused more strain. In order to improve his vision and lessen his strain and tension I had to give him treatment just opposite to the usual way in which patients are benefited.

He came again one week later for his last treatment, at which time he read the whole of the Fundamentals card, reading No. 15, which is fine diamond type at less than twelve inches holding the card in the shade. In the sun he was able to read it at less than eight inches. He no longer dragged his words as he had in the beginning when I first treated him, and only at rare intervals did I notice his shoulders move with a twitch when he forgot to blink as he was talking to me.

On July 20, 1927, he came to me for his first treatment in a pathetic condition. On August 25, about a month later, he was a different man entirely, having no more discomfort or pain in his eyes.

Better Eyesight
March 1928—Vol. XII, No. 9

FIRST VISIT CURES

The word "cures" is used advisedly. It is a fact that some people have been cured of myopia in one visit, after relaxation of the nerves of the eyes and other parts of the body was obtained.

Suppose the patient is nearsighted and can only see the big letter "C" at fifteen feet, a vision of 15/200. Let the patient walk up close to the card until he can read the bottom line. The distance may be three feet, five feet or farther. The first letter on the bottom line may be the letter "F." With the eyes open, it is possible for the patient to imagine the letter "F" quite perfectly, but with the eyes closed he is more easily able to remember and imagine he sees the letter "F" much better.

Palming is a great help when remembering or imagining the letter "F" with the eyes closed. By alternately imagining the letter "F" with the eyes open and remembering or imagining it better with the eyes closed, the memory, the imagination, and finally the vision for the letter "F" are very much improved.

If the patient becomes able to see the letter "F" at three feet or to imagine he sees it quite perfectly, he should be encouraged to walk back and increase the distance between the eyes and the letter "F" about one foot. When the patient becomes able to imagine the letter "F" at four feet, he should go back another foot, alternately imagining it with his eyes open and remembering it much better with his eyes closed. By gradually increasing the distance of the eyes from the letter "F," all patients who practiced this method obtained normal vision temporarily at the first visit.

The length of time required to obtain a permanent cure is variable. Some patients with not more than one or two diopters of myopia may require many weeks or months of daily treatment before they are permanently cured, while others with a higher degree of myopia sometimes obtain a cure in a much shorter time.

THE PERIOD

By W. H. Bates, M.D.

Of all the methods employed in obtaining normal vision, the memory and the imagination of the small black, white or any color period is among the best. The period may be an optimum for some persons who can obtain relaxation with its aid after other methods fail.

When the period is seen perfectly, it is not stationary but moves in various directions with a slow, short, easy swing. It is a fundamental fact that a period is seen best when it appears to move a distance of about its own diameter. When the period has a slow, short, easy swing, the eye is at rest and when it is at rest it is always moving to prevent concentration, trying to see and other efforts to improve the vision.

It has been demonstrated that when the vision is good, any effort, no matter how slight, always impairs or lowers it. When this truth is demonstrated, it follows that normal vision cannot be obtained when an effort is employed. When a period is seen, remembered or imagined perfectly, central fixation is manifest or the period is not seen in all parts equally well. When the eyes of the patient move a short distance to the right of the period, the period should appear to the left of where he is looking. When he looks to the left of a period, it should appear to be to the right of where he is looking, and the left side of the period is seen best while all other parts are seen worse.

Many patients complain that they find it difficult or impossible to remember a mental picture of a period. They say that the period is blurred or indistinguishable. To them the larger letters are apparently clearer than small print or a period. It is difficult to make some patients understand that the large letters may have blurred outlines of a fraction of an inch or more if an effort is made, and the letter may still be distinguishable, whereas any effort to remember the period perfectly will cause a blur which is sufficient to make the small period indistinguishable. With perfect sight, no blur is seen, and the eyes are at rest.

When a patient has perfect sight, it is usually continuous. One may see a large letter quite perfectly and by covering over one-half of it the uncovered half is just as black as the whole and may be remembered, imagined or seen as black as the whole letter. Then if a small area is blocked off, with the help of a screen, one-quarter, one-eighth, one-tenth—any part in fact is just as black as the entire letter.

If the patient holds his forefinger six inches in front of his face and moves his head and eyes from side to side, it is possible, without looking at the finger, to easily imagine that the finger is moving in the opposite direction to the movement of the head and eyes. This is called the *variable swing,* because the amplitude of the swing varies within wide limits. At six inches from the face, the amplitude may be three or four inches, while a similar object held at five feet or farther will have a very short swing—so short that it is not always apparent. A small period, likewise, at six inches may appear to move within an amplitude of several inches, while at ten feet it may appear to move less than one-half of its diameter. At times, the movement may be so short that it cannot be distinguished at ten feet, although it is present. Since a short swing improves the vision more than a long swing, the benefit of the short swing of the period at the distance is manifest.

The vision of a perfectly black period may be used to improve the vision of large letters or other objects. By practice, one becomes able to remember or imagine a perfect period at all times and in all places when desired. An imaginary period, when placed on the top or some other part of a large letter, improves the vision of the letter.

The memory of a perfect period is a benefit to other conditions than the sight. When the eyes are tired, the perfect memory of a period at once brings a feeling of perfect rest. Symptoms of various diseases of the eye have been relieved at once by the memory of a perfect period.

It has been published more or less frequently that the memory of a period brings quick relief to pain. A man may have a broken arm which is ordinarily very painful, but the perfect memory of a period always relieves the pain so that he is not conscious of the broken arm. One may suffer considerable discomfort or pain in a dentist's chair. The memory of a perfect period brings instant relief. It is impossible for a patient to suffer pain while his teeth are being treated, provided he is able, in spite of his surroundings, to remember a perfectly black period. A severe cough is usually relieved very promptly by the memory of a perfectly black period after other methods have failed.

There are many diseases which cause a great deal of suffering in which the memory of a perfectly black period has brought relief. A most interesting case was that of a nervous woman who complained that she suffered from a variety of symptoms. She could not imagine the cause which produced the symptoms of her trouble.

She said to me, "Doctor, I am a great sufferer with pain, fever, loss of appetite and from one thing in particular which I am unable to describe." I remonstrated with her and said, "How can you expect me to treat you unless I know what is the matter with you?" She answered, "That is what many other doctors tell me."

This case interested me very much and I said to her, "Your unknown disease is causing you much suffering, but I can promise you complete relief, provided you are able to remember a period which is perfectly black."

She said that she didn't think that she could do so because her memory was not good, and so I spent a great deal of time with her trying to improve her memory and imagination of black, white, blue and other colors. I had her look at a black letter and imagine one part best and the rest of the letter worse.

Under my instruction she became able to see quite perfectly a letter "O" which was about one-quarter of an inch in diameter, and to see it quite perfectly if it were near enough to her eyes. With the aid of a screen, she became able to see one-half of the "O" as well as the whole of it. By further use of the screen, the part of the "O" which she saw best became very small, until it was reduced to the size of a small period. This seemed to help.

Then I gave her a rubber ball and told her to go down to the seashore, near which she lived, when the tide was going out, and throw the ball in the water and watch it recede from the shore. She was also directed to note that the ball appeared smaller as it gradually floated out to sea.

When the relief came she at once telegraphed the glad tidings to me. At once I telegraphed back to her to practice with a rubber ball in the same way each day until her memory of the ball floating out to sea and appearing to be the size of a small black period was perfect. After her memory of the rubber ball becoming the size of a period became perfect, she found that she could obtain a mental picture of the small black period without using a rubber ball. She believed that she had been cured of her unknown malady.

About twenty years ago I had been walking through Central Park and decided to sit down on a bench to rest. A well-dressed man and woman came along and sat down on the same bench. The woman was very much excited and talked very rapidly in Italian to the man. Finally the man turned to me and said:

"Do you know Dr. Bates? We are looking for his office because it is very important that my brother sing tonight in the opera. My brother's voice failed and we at once consulted a doctor on the throat who said that my brother's throat was paralyzed and that nothing could be done. We have just heard that Dr. Bates helped another opera singer by giving him instant relief after his voice had failed."

I asked the man where his brother was. He replied that he was at his hotel. I then confessed to him that I was Dr. Bates and said that I would be very glad to help his brother. I told him that I was well-acquainted with the people at the opera house, having been the attending physician there for several years and that they would vouch for me.

The man at once called a cab. I asked him if he were going to the opera house first, but he replied that it was not necessary, that he believed that I was Dr. Bates. When we reached the hotel, we went to the singer's room at once. The man spoke a few words in Italian to the singer who was lying on a bed. He smiled and opened his mouth wide so that I could see his throat, which seemed to be very large. I requested the man to tell him that it was not necessary for him to keep his mouth open.

There was a piano in the room with a great deal of music lying around. I had the patient sit down at the piano while I examined some of the music. One sheet that I picked up was full of complicated music. I asked the lady to let me have her breast-pin for a moment and with the aid of the pointed pin I touched a small black dot which came after one of the notes. Then I turned to the man and asked him to have the singer sing that note.

The singer looked at the note and laughed. I walked up to him and pounded him on the back and said with a laugh, "It's funny, isn't it?" He replied, "Yes, it's very funny." I said, "Sing it." He did sing it. They were all very much overcome and could not express their gratitude enough. They thought that it was the blow on the back which I had given the singer which had restored his voice, or that my finger had a magic touch when I pointed out that particular note of music. They did not know, and I never told them, that he was suffering from paralysis of one or both vocal cords due to mental strain. When he looked at the music and saw the little black dot perfectly black, his mental strain was relieved and his voice came back.

THE STORY OF JACQUELINE SHERMAN AND HOW SHE WAS BENEFITED

By Emily C. Lierman

The story of Jacqueline Sherman and how she was benefited in a very short time is well worth writing about. She came to me with her mother in January 1927, at the age of seven, and was recommended by a colonel of the United States Army. After he had cured himself of presbyopia and pain caused by eyestrain, he sent many patients to Dr. Bates and to me.

Because of the great distance from Dr. Bates' office, the Colonel was unable to visit the Doctor personally and therefore obtained his knowledge of the method from the Doctor's book. Being an Army officer, it was necessary for him to have good sight and, as glasses were objectionable to him, he had to do something to improve his defective vision. After practicing the methods described in *Perfect Sight Without Glasses,* he became able to read book type and also newspaper type without the use of glasses, and then he began to boast about it. Jacqueline's father, also an Army officer, became interested in the Bates Method through him.

Jacqueline was wearing very heavy glasses, which she had worn for more than six months. She had difficulty to keep from staring or squinting through them in order to see any distance at all. At fifteen feet, her vision was 15/30 with glasses, proving that glasses did not improve her sight very much if at all. Without them, her vision with the right eye was 15/200 blurred, and with the left eye 15/50 blurred.

Although she read up to the 50-line with her left eye, while her right eye was covered, she strained hard to read and twisted her head from left to right in such a way that her mother called her attention to it and asked her to keep her head still, if possible. I was glad to have her mother present in order to see this, because I felt that she would be of help to Jacqueline in her treatment at home. Her mother told me that she saw the child but once a week, as she attended a school some distance from her home. For this reason, she needed her mother's encouragement as well as mine to practice enough to keep up her interest in the method for bettering her eyesight after she had left my office.

Jacqueline had a wonderful memory and it was not hard for me to help her while her eyes were closed, which I had her do after the test. She palmed for more than five minutes while I was talking to her mother, and as I noticed her becoming uneasy or restless, I encouraged her to keep her eyes closed and covered while I asked her a few questions. I asked her if she could imagine that she was writing her name with pen and ink on a sheet of white paper. She said she could do that quite easily. I directed her to spell her whole name and then imagine each letter, and to place an imaginary period at the end of her name. I asked her next to forget about her name and remember the period, which she was able to do, and then she remarked, "The period seems to move, it doesn't stand still." Immediately after that I told her to open her eyes and to read the card with each eye separately. Her vision in that short time improved to 15/30 and she remarked how clear the letters were.

She was asked to palm again and to describe things which she had seen while her eyes were closed. She told me the different colors of dresses which she had worn recently and she very readily described each one in detail. This time she palmed for about ten minutes or longer and when she again read the card her vision with each eye separately had improved to 15/10. Her mother and I noticed that the squinting had stopped and that her eyes were open in a natural way. I gave her test cards and other material necessary for her to practice with and explained to the mother that it was necessary for her to supervise the practice at school and at home if the child wished to be relieved of her eyestrain.

Jacqueline could not come to see me for some time after that and it was on July 19 of the same year that I saw her again. She had a great deal to tell me and it was good to listen to her explain how the one treatment I had given her had benefited her sufficiently to forget that she had ever put on glasses. It was only when she became excited while explaining things or telling something of great interest to her that she forgot to blink. Then something happened which frightened the mother but which caused me no concern whatever, because this happens very often to children. When she was excited or talked fast and forgot to blink, the pupils of both eyes became very large. This, however, had no effect upon her vision whatever, as her mother soon found out.

I asked the child if she had been faithful in the directions I had given her, which included the reading of microscopic print which is much finer than diamond type. She immediately produced some of the fine type I had given her at her first visit and placed herself by a window with her back to the sun. In this way the sun shone directly on the card and she read the fine type without any effort at six inches. She said that she never forgot to practice with fine print almost every day since I had seen her.

I then placed an unfamiliar test card fifteen feet from where she was sitting and asked her to read the card for me. She read every letter on that card with each eye separately and without squinting or straining. Her mother wanted to be sure that her vision for farther distances had improved, so I placed her by my window and told her to look off at a distance at a sign which was about 400 feet away. From the window the letters on this sign seemed to be about the same size as the letters on the last line of the card she had just read. She held the card with microscopic type in her hand, and as she shifted from the white spaces of this type, holding it close to her eyes, to the distant sign, she read every word of the sign without a mistake. Her mother exclaimed that such a thing would have been impossible before she had had her first treatment.

We chose another sign at less than 400 feet away. To prove to her mother and to Jacqueline herself that staring and straining always lowered the vision. I told her to stop blinking for a fraction of a second and to look at the print instead of the white spaces and then to look off at the distant sign we had picked out for her to read. She immediately turned away with a strained expression on her face and with a great deal of squinting. She objected strongly to doing the wrong thing, as she explained it.

I gave her a little sun treatment with her eyes closed, using my sun glass steadily for about five minutes. I next directed her again to shift from the white spaces of the nearby fine type to this sign less than 400 feet away, and to frequently shift from the nearby white spaces to the spaces between the letters of the sign; she read every part of the sign perfectly.

It does not require a great deal of intelligence to do what Jacqueline did, nor does it mean that the patient has to be young to accomplish as much as she did. She merely followed my directions and asked no questions as to whether the vision would continue to improve. She accepted everything I said or directed her to do as a positive means of benefiting her sight. Her mother's silence during the treatment helped me greatly in benefiting the child. It so often happens during a treatment that the parent or guardian will interfere or ask questions regarding the progress that the child is making, and this, of course, does not help the child nor me.

At the time I was treating Jacqueline, I also had a boy under treatment for myopia. He was twelve years old, almost twice as old as the little girl. Every time the boy came, his mother worried me all through the hour of treatment and because of the mother's interference it took me twice the length of time to cure him. I am not speaking against this mother; I am only stating a fact. Both mothers were equally fond of their children, but mothers often make the mistake of fussing when it is quite unnecessary.

Jacqueline was again brought to me by her mother four days later as a sort of a checkup. I repeated to her over and over again that staring lowered the vision and that blinking always improved her ability to see without tension or strain. Every card that I had for testing was used so that her mother could see for herself that her child had really improved. She did well with the memory of the period whenever it was introduced during each treatment, so I decided that it would be a good plan to teach her mother how to apply the treatment at any time in the future when it seemed necessary.

The mother was directed to tell her to palm and imagine that a sheet of white writing paper was placed in her lap; then to imagine that she was making a small black period, just large enough so that she could imagine it as a small black spot. She did this without any difficulty. Her mother reminded her that she must imagine that the period was moving, so we spoke of the pendulum of a large clock which moves slowly from side to side, and I instructed the child to imagine that her body was moving just that way. She kept up this movement as she sat perfectly relaxed in her chair and then she was asked to imagine that the period was moving opposite to the movement of her body. Jacqueline enjoyed this very much.

Before she opened her eyes, I placed myself six feet away from her and held in my hand the small Fundamentals test card with the inverted "E's." The bottom line of this card is seen with the normal eye at two feet. In the presence of the mother who wanted to be doubly sure that her child was not memorizing instead of actually reading, I placed this small card upside down. In this way, the letters pointed directly opposite from the way in which they point when right side up.

When the girl opened her eyes after the period practice, she said that the "E's" looked perfectly clear to her up to the fourth from the top line which, of course, would be the fourth from the bottom line when the card was right side up. She could see the separation between each letter "E" on the other lines but not very clearly. Purposely, I had my hand over the three upper lines, but suddenly I removed my hand. Jacqueline leaned forward in her chair unconsciously, and as she did so, she began squinting her eyes. Her mother checked her before I had a chance to do so, which pleased me.

She closed her eyes for an instant, remembering the swinging period and then opened her eyes and looked toward the card held in my hand. Immediately she exclaimed, "If I remember the swinging period as I look at the card, I can imagine that the first letter "E" on the bottom line is turned the right way." Her mother came close to the card to see whether the child had made a mistake; she had not. Her mother asked if it were possible that the child could see so small a letter at such a distance when less than a year ago, she had been so terribly myopic. By alternately closing her eyes and opening them, looking at the white spaces between each letter "E," she could tell in which direction each letter on the top line was pointing. When she closed her eyes for a fraction of a second, she had relaxed enough with the memory of the moving period to see each letter "E" perfectly without tension or strain.

At her last visit to me, the final test was made. This was on August 1, 1927. As I stood ten feet away from her, I held in my hand a popular magazine with ordinary sized type. She did not know the name of the magazine, nor did she have any idea of what I was going to do. I was standing in a good light and her mother was sitting where she could watch us both. I placed my finger at the beginning of a sentence at the top of a certain page. I told her to watch my finger as I passed it below the sentence and told her not to pay any attention to my finger, but to see the thin white line which separated this sentence from the one below. This was done in a flash and then she closed her eyes again.

I asked her to imagine what the second word of that sentence might be. While her eyes were still closed, she said that it appeared to be a word with three letters and that the first letter appeared to be straight. She said that she could imagine that the word might be "was," which was correct. Her mother said that it was almost impossible for her to see that word so far away, but when she again mentioned words correctly as I passed my finger along the page of that magazine, her mother was convinced that Jacqueline's vision had really improved to more than normal average vision.

Jacqueline was what I call an unusual case, but I feel that any child of her age can do as much if not more than she did. This case recalled to my mind something which I had heard Dr. Bates say many times, "There is no limit to vision."

CASE REPORT

By W. B. MacCracken, M.D.

Editor's Note—*We believe that the following letter recently received by Ms. Lierman will interest our readers. It is from W. B. MacCracken, M.D., Berkeley, California, who has been very successful in applying the Bates Method to his patients. We would recommend him to anyone living in his vicinity who desires treatment by this method.*

February 24, 1928.
Dear Ms. Lierman:

Perhaps you have once or twice wondered why I have not written you anything about the Bates work that I am doing here. I trust you have. There are several reasons why so many long weeks have elapsed and I have not made any report. Tonight I am going to have a little talk with you. And I feel sure I will get to the ear of Dr. Bates himself through you.

First, to put it briefly, I can do some of this work very well. I know this because I have had some very fine success. The reverse side is that nobody wants to have their eyes cured this way. This does not mean that I am discouraged in the least. The ripples are getting a little larger. Last Monday night I had four beginners—two who were about to put on glasses and two who have worn them for several years. It is very encouraging to see evidence accumulating to prove that this little small whisper is beginning to be heard in the din of this wilderness of eyesight moderns.

On January 9, a Mr. S. came to me, 66 years old, with a cataract in each eye. One had been operated on several months before, and that eye was distinctly worse. He had spent $300 in two years. His last experience was $47 for a pair of glasses that were useless. He came on Monday morning, and could not read his watch without glasses, nor see the "C" of the small card, and on Saturday morning of that week he read the bottom line of Fundamentals—so much was his "vision benefited" in one week. In one month he had read in one day, without glasses, five pages of the Sunday newspaper, and another day twenty-one pages of a book, and could read big signs two hundred feet away. At the house of a patient of mine he read half a column of a newspaper.

A few days after that, he simply broke an appointment and went off and bought another pair of glasses. A Ms. Chandler, an old graduate nurse who is helping me with this work, found out from his wife that he decided it would take too long by this method to see without glasses. I believe he got into a mental complex, the crisis of his last few years of misery, and could not realize that another four weeks would probably have had him back at work.

On Saturday last, a Ms. Kinley came ten miles to me. She is eighty-four and has a cataract in each eye. When I took her glasses off, she could not walk around freely, and could not read the "C." In a little while she read four lines. Palming and the sun glass. On Thursday, five days later, she came again on the trolley, and reported that she had not put her glasses on since I placed them in her bag myself, and that she had done all her housework and her marketing and her sight was very much improved. She is a keen, strong woman at eighty-four, and I am hopeful that her earnestness and courage are going to make a better ending than I had with Mr. S. who was only 66.

You once suggested that I get some clinical work. This was actually promised me in the City Clinic.

I am always mentioning the work to my patients and my friends, and I am more determined than ever to go to New York for a proper training as soon as it is possible.

You may be very sure that I will be more than pleased to hear from you at any time, and I hope that when I write again it will be to tell you that I can set the date when I can start for New York.

With kindest personal regards for Dr. Bates, as well as for yourself. Yours most sincerely,

W. B. MacCracken, M.D.

[Later Dr. MacCracken obtained training from Dr. Bates. He self-published two books: *Use Your Own Eyes* in 1937 and *Normal Sight Without Glasses* in 1945.—TRQ]

Better Eyesight
April 1928—Vol. XII, No. 10

BRAIN TENSION

The brain has many nerves. Part of these nerves are called ganglion cells and originate in some particular part of the brain. Each has a function of its own. They are connected with other ganglion cells and, with the aid of nerve fibres, are connected with others located in various parts of the brain as well as in the spinal cord, the eye, the ear, the nerves of smell, taste, and the nerves of touch. The function of each ganglion cell of the brain is different from that of all others. When the ganglion cells are healthy, they function in a normal manner.

The retina of the eye contains numerous ganglion cells which regulate special things such as normal vision, normal memory, normal imagination and they do this with a control more or less accurate of other ganglion cells of the whole body. The retina has a similar structure to parts of the brain. It is connected to the brain by the optic nerve.

Many nerves from the ganglion cells of the retina carry conscious and unconscious control of other ganglion cells which are connected to other parts of the body.

When the ganglion cells are diseased or at fault, the functions of all parts of the body are not normally maintained. In all cases of imperfect sight, it has been repeatedly demonstrated that the ganglion cells and nerves of the brain are under a strain. When this strain is corrected by treatment, the functions of the ganglion and other cells become normal. The importance of the mental treatment cannot be overestimated.

A study of the facts has demonstrated that a disease of some ganglion in any part of the body occurs in a similar ganglion in the brain.

Brain tension of one or more nerves always means disease of these nerve ganglia. Treatment of the mind with the aid of the sight, memory and imagination has cured many cases of imperfect sight without other treatment.

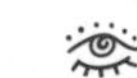

CATARACT

By W. H. Bates, M.D.

Some years ago a professor of anatomy was exhibiting the effect of pressure on the enucleated eyeballs of a dead cow and some other animals. At a distance of about twenty feet from the eye, the audience observed that the pupil was perfectly clear. Immediately after the eyeball was squeezed by the fingers of the professor, the area of the pupil became at once completely opaque from the production of a cataract. Then when the pressure on the eyeball was lessened, the cataract at once disappeared and the eyeball became normal. Again squeezing the eyeball, a cataract was produced as before. And again the cataract disappeared when the pressure was lessened. The experiment was repeated a number of times with the result that the pressure on the eyeball always produced a cataract, which was relieved by reducing the pressure.

There are two oblique and four straight or recti muscles on the outside of the eyeball.

The superior and inferior oblique pressing on the eyeball at the same time have always been followed by lengthening of the eyeball. The four straight muscles on the outside of the eyeball shorten the globe or eyeball by their contraction. In animals the eyeball has been shortened experimentally by operations on each of the four straight muscles, which increased the pressure temporarily. These operations were performed after death. Similar operations on the two oblique muscles at the same time produced pressure and increased hardness of the eyeball with cataract following.

Patients suffering from cataract have increased the hardness of the eyeball, at the same time increasing the density of the cataract. While the cataract is being observed with the aid of the ophthalmoscope, it can be seen to change in size or density when the patient consciously or voluntarily increases or diminishes the hardness of the eyeball with the aid of the memory or the imagination.

When a word, a letter, part of a letter, or other object is remembered perfectly with the eyes closed or open, the cataract can be seen by the observer to become less. But if the memory of letters, colors or other objects is imperfect, the cataract always is seen by the observer to become worse. A great many cases of senile and other forms of cataract have been temporarily improved and this improvement has become more complete and more permanent by the practice of a perfect memory.

A perfect memory usually becomes manifest when the patient practices the optical swing. However, the cataract always becomes worse when the optical swing or the perfect memory is not practiced. To keep the eyeball hard by practicing an imperfect memory is difficult and requires effort. The practice of an imperfect memory is tiresome and requires constant attention of the patient. In others it can be demonstrated that the formation of cataract in elderly people requires hard work and is exceedingly difficult.

A perfect memory is easy. It is quick, continuous and beneficial. Patients with a perfect memory have consciously or unconsciously a perfect optical swing. They are able to remember, to imagine letters, colors and other objects continuously without any strain or fatigue. These cases are favorable and recover from cataract after they demonstrate that a perfect memory is beneficial.

The study of cataract has occupied the attention of eye doctors for many hundreds of years. It occurs very frequently in India, China, Japan and among people of the highest intelligence, as well as among those whose intelligence is of the lowest order. Some cases appear without apparent cause. It may increase rapidly or slowly and continuously until the vision is completely lost.

Of all organic diseases of the eye which have received medical attention, measures of relief by operation or by the use of eyedrops have usually, in a large number of cases, been unsatisfactory. Cases have been operated upon in which a temporary cure was obtained. However, in too many of these cases the good vision obtained soon after the operation did not remain good. In some of these cases and without apparent cause, inflammation of the interior parts of the eye developed and was followed by serious loss of vision.

Some cases of cataract are found in the eyes of children soon after birth, sometimes in one eye, less frequently in both. The cataract which occurs in children is softer than in the eyes of adults and is more readily benefited by operation than in the eyes of adults. In some cases of cataract in children, the front part of the lens becomes opaque. Such a cataract is called an anterior polar cataract. Often, after the lens has been punctured, it becomes absorbed and good vision is obtained. In other cases an opacity forms on the back part of the lens which increases until the lens becomes entirely opaque. Here again repeated puncturing of the lens is followed by a total opacity of the lens and its complete absorption. In a third variety of cataract in children, an opacity of the lens forms in one or more layers of the lens which is usually absorbed after repeated punctures of the lens are made with a sharp needle. This operation has been called "needling of the lens."

When cataract occurs in adults of forty years or older it is called senile cataract. In adults, the operation of needling the lens is not so successful in being followed by absorption of the lens. In some cases, if not in a large number, better results are obtained by removing the whole lens by one or more operations. There are many diseases of the eyes, such as inflammations of the iris and choroid, which are believed to produce cataract. The removal of the lens is usually very difficult without injuring the iris, choroid and retina.

In cataract the crystalline lens becomes opaque, and being opaque it interferes very seriously with the vision. To obtain good vision, eye doctors were usually able to improve the sight by the removal of the opaque lens. After the lens was removed, the vision was materially improved by the use of strong glasses which rarely improved the sight to normal.

I have studied the physiology of the eye and I have repeatedly published the fact that it is much better to cure the opacity of the lens so that the patient could have normal vision with a normal eye rather than to relieve the blindness by the removal of the lens. Curing rheumatism of the hand by an operation which removes the hand is not the best treatment. Likewise rheumatism of the big toe is not considered a proper case for amputation. Medical or simple treatment without an operation will usually result in a cure. I do believe in operations when necessary or where medical treatment fails to correct the trouble. However, removing the lens from the eye does not cure cataract of the lens nor does it prevent cataract from forming in the other eye.

Since cataract or opacity of the lens is caused by tension, relaxation should cure or prevent the trouble. If relaxation fails to cure cataract we should consider this fact an evidence that tension is not the cause of cataract. Relaxation can be obtained with the aid of memory, imagination and sight. If the eye of a child is injured by a blow and a cataract forms early or late in life, it has always been demonstrated that the eye with cataract is under a tension.

Treatment which brings about relaxation always cures the cataract after a considerable amount of treatment which may require several months or longer. Among the many methods of treatment, the amount of relaxation necessary to be followed by a cure is a perfect memory, perfect imagination and the benefit obtained by sun treatment. Central fixation has in some cases cured all forms of cataract—senile cataract, soft cataract in children, cataract caused by sugar in the blood and other poisons.

It is found that when patients sit facing the sun with both eyes closed and move the head a short distance from side to side, they can stand the strong light of the sun for longer periods of time than they can with the eyes open.

When the sun is not shining, a strong electric light is a good substitute.

Much quicker improvement in the sight can be obtained with the proper use of the sun glass. The patient is directed to look down while facing the sun and to do this continuously without effort or strain. The operator lifts the upper lid with the thumb of one hand. When the white part or sclera of the eyeball is exposed to view, he quickly concentrates or focuses the strong light of the sun on the sclera, moving it continuously and only for an instant at a time.

A CASE OF CATARACT

By Emily C. Lierman

There was a time when I thought that all cases of cataract could be treated and benefited by one and the same method. I know now that this cannot be done for many reasons. Age has nothing to do with treatment for the cure of cataract, because I have had patients over eighty years old who responded much quicker and became well much sooner than younger patients who were troubled the same way.

I was treating a woman with cataract who was seventy-seven years old, at the same time that I was treating another woman, age sixty-two. Both women had the same amount of vision with the test card, and neither one could read newspaper or book type. Yet the elder of the two was benefited and the cataract of both eyes had entirely disappeared, while I was still working hard with the younger patient who was becoming irritable, rebellious and most discouraged because of the increased length of time required to benefit her.

Neither of us was at fault as far as my good judgment goes because she was faithful in what I directed her to do when I was not with her. While I was treating her I had to remember constantly that there was a man named Job who was severely tried, according to the Old Testament of the *Bible*. However, my dear patient did not know of my endurance because I kept smiling always. She was very nervous and had cause to be. Money was no object to her, but a great disappointment had come into her life. So great was it, in fact, that all who knew her thought she was losing her mind. For this reason, my heart went out to this patient who suffered mentally because of her wayward son.

During the hour, or I should say two hours of her treatment, because I could never accomplish anything much in less time, she would mention the name of her boy who, although he was of age and married, was still her little boy. Her room, which was cheerful and sunny, had pictures of him all over the walls. Some of them were baby pictures and there were others taken at the ages of sixteen and twenty-one and when he graduated from college. I noticed particularly that when she looked at his baby pictures her face would show signs of tenderness and relaxation. But when she looked at the pictures of his later years she would close her eyes and her face would become wrinkled with age and tension.

For days after I had noticed this. I studied her case and planned a different way of treating her. All my spare moments were spent in thinking out the best way to relieve her strain which prevented a permanent benefit.

Weeks grew into months before I finally conquered the wrong, or really helped her to overcome her disappointment and nervousness. In seven months' time with treatment several times every week, never less than three treatments each week, she finally became able to read every test card, even to the 10-line letters, at fifteen feet, 15/10.

She had been a great reader, and could read a whole book in less than two hours when she was much younger. Therefore it was a terrible disappointment to her when her sight failed and she had to forego that pleasure. Occasionally a neighbor or a friend would visit her and read her favorite books aloud to her. Now at the end of seven months' treatment of her eyes she was convinced that I had told her the truth; that she would become able to read again without the aid of glasses.

Neighbors and friends were invited to call so that they could see with their own eyes what she was able to do. These friends knew how she had doubted me. They doubted me too, except one who was at one time a patient of Dr. Bates. This friend had not called because she was too far away, but she had written to my patient. What she wrote gave my patient enough faith and confidence in me to start the treatment, although she doubted me. She told me so in plain English. She was not the only patient who doubted me at the beginning of the treatment and who later on believed in me completely.

When the vision of this patient became normal for distant sight, she soon was able to read the finest print readily without glasses. I had not tested her ability to read fine print because I feared the bad effect of disappointment if she failed to read it. My experience with other and similar patients encouraged me to believe that if I could improve her distant vision to the normal, that she would soon become able to read the fine print, "diamond type," without the aid of glasses.

I felt that it was useless for me to test her ability to read fine print from our usual test cards, so I asked her if she had some book in her possession containing small print, and she answered me by pointing to a large dictionary fastened to a stand in a sunny corner of her room.

Before I asked her to go near the dictionary, I said, "I have had patients with your trouble who became able to read the small print of the dictionary by placing a small card with much finer print in the neighborhood of the small letters of the dictionary." As I watched her closely while saying this and noticed her frown, I said quickly, "Of course, I do not expect you to do this just now."

This remark worked something like a magnet, for she at once hurried to the dictionary and with the aid of the small card which she received from me and which contained fine print or diamond type, she read occasional words of the dictionary, much to her delight.

There were times during the months which followed when she had relapses which caused depression, but after she had removed some of the pictures of her son from the walls of her room, the conversation while I was with her was more about herself and the improvement in her eyes. In the beginning her distant vision with the test card was 10/30 with the right eye and 10/50 with the left. At the end of her treatment her sight was better in each eye than the average normal eye.

During the last treatment, I spent the day with her, and she read for me a large part of a book in which the print was very small. She announced with a great deal of pleasure that for years she had been unable to read this book, with or without her glasses. The cataract in both eyes was very materially improved. Only the lower inner part of the pupil had a trace of the cataract in each eye.

The principal part of the treatment given this woman was the sun treatment. While I was with her, I applied the sun glass. When I was not with her she was able to use the sun glass with benefit or just the same as I used it. Because she was of a nervous temperament, I always focused the sunlight on the outside of her closed eyelids.

QUESTIONS AND ANSWERS

Q–1a. Is it all right to palm while lying down? 1b. Is it better to sit or stand while doing so? 1c. If the arms get tired is it all right to rest the elbows on a desk or something like that while palming? 1d. Or is it best to hold the elbows up free from all support?

A–1a. It is all right to palm while lying down. 1b. Palming should not be done while one is standing. 1c. The elbows should rest on a desk or table or on a cushion placed in the lap. 1d. One should be in as comfortable a position as possible while palming in order to obtain the most benefit.

CASE REPORT

By Edith Reid

Editor's Note—*The following is a report of a case treated by Edith Reid, one of Dr. Bates' representatives, who is now practicing in Johannesburg, South Africa.*

Many times I have been asked, "Is it really possible to cure cataract by Dr. Bates' method without an operation?" I can prove that it is. One morning in January during our very hot weather a lady called to see me. Upon being told that as I was leaving town very shortly I could not see her, she became very much upset and declared that she would go blind, as she had cataract. As soon as I heard it was cataract I had her shown into the room knowing that if she was not taught the Bates Method she would become worse if left until I returned some months later. This lady made her living by teaching singing.

When tested, she read the 50-line at ten feet from the test card; then her vision blurred as she began to strain terribly. She was taught to palm and rest her eyes. Hers was a bright, sunny nature and she was very happy at finding such an easy simple way of resting her poor, tired eyes.

She was told to discard her glasses, but she declared that would be very difficult as she had worn them for thirty-seven years. However, she said that she would be plucky and try. She was asked to come again the following day, which she did. She was all smiles and said that she was sure she was better as her eyes felt moist and so rested.

She was taught the swing and was told to swing and palm all day long if possible. She had a journey of about two hours on the train every morning to come into the city to teach, so she was told to look out of the windows and see everything moving, and when talking to friends to be sure to close her eyes often, so as to keep herself from staring.

Every morning for the next eight days she came to my rooms to get the sun glass treatment and rest for at least an hour before starting her teaching. She was always bright and cheerful and came every day saying how much better she was.

On the ninth morning she was tested and she was able to read the test card 15/10 and diamond type print at twelve inches. She became very much excited and told of how she had been told by an eye specialist that she had cataract and that she would go totally blind and then they would operate. She was also told never to take off her glasses. When asked how she found time to practice, she answered, "I work with my eyes all day long. When I play the accompaniments for my pupils I swing, and then when I speak to them I close my eyes."

She is now able to read the newspapers and any small print with perfect comfort. She says her friends come to see her teach as they had never known her without glasses. She is most grateful to Dr. Bates.

Better Eyesight
May 1928—Vol. XII, No. 11

COLOR BLINDNESS

Some people are unable to distinguish red from blue or other colors. Many doctors explain color blindness to be due to something wrong with the retina, optic nerve or brain. They believe that organic changes in the retina are the principal cause. But this is not always true because in some cases cures occur without any apparent change in the retina.

I have found that color blindness occurs in a great many cases in an eye apparently normal. There are, however, a number of individuals who can be demonstrated to have color blindness as a result of a disease of the retina caused by mental strain. These cases cannot be cured, however, until the disease of the retina is cured.

Some patients with color blindness are sensitive to a bright light. On the other hand, there are patients with color blindness who are more comfortable in a bright light. These patients are usually relieved by the practice of sun treatment, central fixation, palming, the long swing, or any other method which brings about relaxation.

One patient had a normal perception for colors at three feet and at ten feet. But at a nearer point than three feet she was color blind, the color blindness being most marked at three inches. At a distance greater than ten feet the color blindness was evident. After her eyestrain was relieved by relaxation her color blindness disappeared.

People who have been born color blind as well as those who have acquired color blindness have all been cured by the practice of relaxation methods.

THE STARE

By W. H. Bates, M.D.

Much can be written about the stare. In the first place, when a patient stares, an effort is always made to hold the eyes still without moving them. It is impossible to hold the eyes perfectly still. Trying to do the impossible always requires a strain. This strain can be demonstrated to be a mental strain which affects all the nerves of the body as well as the eye. With a mental strain, the memory and imagination become imperfect and imperfect sight results. Pain, fatigue or dizziness are acquired or made worse. With relaxation of all the nerves, the sense of touch is improved, but with the stare or other efforts to see the sense of touch is lost while the sense of pain is increased.

Glaucoma, acute or chronic, has been consciously produced by the stare. The fundamental symptoms of glaucoma may be present with or without increased hardness of the eyeball, contraction of the nasal field, or glaucomatous excavation of the optic nerve. In glaucoma the blood vessels of the retina appear to be arranged in the form of a right angle just as they dip down into the nerve. The whole papilla where the optic nerve enters the back part of the eye is white instead of pink. Changes which are seen in the optic nerve are organic. The contracted field may be considered to be functional because there are many cases which recover and the field becomes clear.

This suggested that in glaucoma the patient be recommended to alternately stare and relax. When he is staring and trying to improve the vision by an effort, all the symptoms of glaucoma may be increased. If the stare is the cause of glaucoma, relaxation should always lessen the severity of the symptoms.

There are some patients who have been using the stare for a sufficient length of time to acquire the habit without being conscious that an effort was being made. Each individual case may require individual treatment in order that the patient may become, by practice, conscious of the stare when the vision is lowered. Of course, if the stare increases the glaucoma, by stopping the stare we would expect the eye to improve. If it does not improve, the patient is still staring, whether he knows it or not. Sometimes by increasing the distance of the test card from the eyes while the patient is staring, he often becomes able to demonstrate that the stare is present when the vision becomes worse.

Many adults past middle life unconsciously stare and produce glaucoma. By practice they become conscious of the stare. While the stare, when it is strong enough and sufficiently prolonged, usually increases the hardness of the eyeball, in the matter of treatment the great problem is to suggest measures which will enable the patient to demonstrate that the stare is the cause of increased tension of the eyeball in glaucoma.

Absolute glaucoma is a serious disease and the stare can become so great that a large amount of pain and total blindness will be produced. The pain may be so severe that many ophthalmologists feel justified in removing the eyeball to bring relief. While many cases of absolute glaucoma obtained much relief from pain after the removal of the eyeball, there were too many cases which still had severe trouble, even after such an operation. A strain which produces absolute glaucoma is really a mental strain and not a local one entirely.

Trigeminal neuralgia is also a very serious eye trouble. Many operations have been performed for its relief, most of which were failures. Some patients have had nearly all of the fifth nerve with its branches removed in order to relieve the pain. There are many patients who have not obtained permanent relief from pain after various methods of orthodox treatment were employed. In the severest cases the branches of the fifth nerve at their origin in the gasserian ganglion in the brain have been removed, as well as the ganglia, without any permanent benefit whatever. I have discovered that the stare was the cause of the brain tension and that when the stare was relieved, all the symptoms of trigeminal neuralgia were relieved or cured and the vision became normal.

Conical cornea has for many years been considered incurable. A great many operations have been performed in which a small part of the cornea was removed with the expectation that when it healed, the conical shape of the cornea would be corrected and the vision would thereby be improved. These operations were usually a disappointment. Conical cornea has been treated by relaxation methods and with great success.

When the forefinger of one hand is held about six inches to one side of the face and about six inches straight ahead, the patient, by moving the head and eyes from side to side slowly or rapidly, can imagine the movement of the finger from side to side. This movement of the finger is called the variable swing and is specific for the benefit of all cases of conical cornea. It owes its value to the fact that when the finger appears to move, the injurious stare is prevented. The length of time necessary to improve the vision with the help of the variable swing usually is not very long.

Iritis occurs quite frequently. The cause has heretofore been ascribed to syphilis, rheumatism, or some other constitutional disease. Chronic cases are seldom cured until after months of persistent treatment. Pain in acute iritis may be very severe and the vision is usually lowered. While treating patients in one of the out-patient departments of a city hospital, one of them applied for treatment of iritis which had produced so much blindness that he required an attendant to help him. The eyeball was very red, the pupil contracted, and the vision very imperfect. He suffered very much from photophobia or sensitiveness to light and kept his eyes covered most of the time.

I turned him over to my assistant with directions to obtain relaxation by palming, swinging or the memory of perfect sight. A half-hour later the patient disturbed the Clinic by laughing frequently because the symptoms of iritis had almost entirely disappeared. He walked about the place, telling anyone who would listen to him about his prompt recovery. This patient was able to increase the symptoms of iritis by the stare and lessen them by relaxation.

It may not be generally known that the stare is the cause of corneal astigmatism. With the aid of the ophthalmometer most cases of corneal astigmatism can be diagnosed and measured. The ability of some people to produce corneal astigmatism is interesting. Some years ago a house surgeon in one of our largest hospitals acquired considerable notoriety or fame by his ability to produce temporarily a considerable amount of corneal astigmatism by staring at the opening tube of the ophthalmometer. He spent many hours experimenting on his eyes and he had become able not only to produce astigmatism at an angle of 90 degrees but also at an angle of 180 degrees. It required many months of constant practice before he became able, with the aid of the stare, to produce astigmatism with an oblique axis. Although he enjoyed the experimental work, which had for its object the cure of corneal astigmatism, so many doctors criticized him adversely that he stopped.

It was believed at one time by many physicians that myopia was caused by straining to see at the near point. Experiments to produce nearsightedness by an effort to see at the near point were failures. All the men, and there were many, who tried to produce nearsightedness or to lengthen the eyeball by efforts to see at the near point and so produce myopia, found instead the opposite condition, hypermetropia, with a shortening of the eyeball. The stare can produce a different kind of strain in each case and therefore cause a different eye defect or disease.

Some years ago a friend of mine called to see me and to learn about my experiments. I said to him, "Doctor, would you like to see a case of cataract produced and cured?" I took him into a dark room where one of my patients, a woman about seventy years old was seated. After he had seen her he recognized her as one of his former patients. He told me in a low voice that arrangements had been made for taking her into a hospital and operating upon her eye.

I gave him an ophthalmoscope with a plus 18 convex glass which produced a very much enlarged image of the cataract. I asked the doctor if he could see the cataract, and he replied that the area of the pupil was completely filled with the cataract and that there was no red reflex. He said that he believed that one would be justified in operating for its removal.

"Before we do that," I said, "suppose we look at the lens again." So we looked at the lens again with the ophthalmoscope and again he showed me that it was a proper case for operation.

"Well," I said, "suppose we keep looking at the cataract for a few minutes." I asked the patient if she had a good memory for flowers. She replied that she had. I asked her what flower she could remember best. She answered, "I believe I can remember a yellow chrysanthemum better than any other flower." I then said to the doctor, "How is the cataract?" "Why," he said, "it has disappeared." He was evidently very much puzzled.

I then asked the patient if she could remember my first name. She answered, "No." I said. "Suppose you try." She immediately began to stare and the upper part of the lens became opaque and all the muscles of her face were under a strain.

We investigated this case for half an hour or longer and came to the conclusion that the memory of perfect sight was a cure for cataract and the memory of imperfect sight, which is usually associated with a stare, the cause of cataract.

The relief of eyestrain or the stare has benefited so many heretofore considered incurable cases that the conclusions made should be investigated. If it is true that the stare can cause so much pain or suffering, it is a breach of medical ethics for any doctor to deprive a man or women of relief by the use of such simple successful methods of treatment.

STARING RELIEVED BY TREATMENT

By Emily C. Lierman

A woman who had been suffering from pain and imperfect sight was sent to me for treatment. She suffered more at business than at any other time and glasses did not help her much. Having charge of a tea room she was continually greeting patrons and placing them at tables. At times she seemed to have no trouble at all with her eyes and was able to read any part of the menu to patrons who asked her to do so, without using her glasses which she wore most of the time. She had worn glasses off and on for four years and disliked them exceedingly because they did not become her. Shortly before coming to me, she was told by an eye specialist that she would have to wear bifocals. She was ready then to try most anything rather than wear them.

Her vision for the test card was 15/20 in both eyes, but with fine print and ordinary type she did not do so well. I began treating her by having her palm and while her eyes were closed and covered, I explained that some patients were not helped by palming, but if that were so in her case we would try something else. She had a good memory for objects and people's faces but her memory for names was not so good.

I asked her to describe to me all the sections of the tea room that she could remember. In this way, her memory and imagination would improve for other things which were not remembered or imagined so well. She described in detail how the tables were arranged and the design of the table silver. She could not remember the pattern of the tablecloths and napkins, although when she purchased the table linens she purposely selected a certain pattern because it appealed to her. This worried her, but I explained that after she had learned how to relax under unfavorable conditions she would be able to remember such details. I directed her to keep her eyes closed for more than half an hour, at times keeping perfectly still without speaking to me.

I watch patients very closely while they are palming to see whether they are in a comfortable position, and if not I try to arrange it so. I find that when the knees are crossed, the position soon brings on an unconscious strain; therefore I direct the patient to keep the knees uncrossed. Then I arrange the feet so that they are comfortably placed either on the floor or on a footstool or hassock. The patient is usually most comfortable in an armchair and if the arms of the chair are not upholstered, I place a cushion under one elbow in such a way that the patient is most comfortable. This brings the patient in a position leaning over to the right side or to the left, so I try to have the patient change the position while relaxing by reversing the cushion to the opposite arm of the chair. With children I manage a little differently, especially when not tall enough to rest their feet on a footstool.

The test card which I used for this patient had an extra line of letters smaller than the 10-line letters, which are read by the normal eye at ten feet. After this woman had palmed sufficiently, I removed the footstool and while her eyes were still closed I told her to stand up and to start swaying her body slowly with an easy sway of the body from left to right. Then I told her to open her eyes and look from one edge of the Snellen test card to the other and to tell me what the letters were as I pointed toward them. She read every letter of the test card with each eye separately without any difficulty whatever.

The patient was so excited over her sudden improvement in sight and the relaxation which she felt of her whole body, that she thought one lesson was all that would be necessary for her. I thought that the improvement during her first treatment was only temporary and told her so. However, I was willing to give the patient the benefit of the doubt and told her that if her vision remained normal and she felt no more strain or discomfort that it surely would not be necessary for her to take another lesson.

Early the next morning my telephone rang and it was she, explaining her discomfort and strain and begging me to see her again. I was surprised that the change came so soon. I thought that she would have at least a few days of relaxation and freedom from strain, but she had been at a bridge party after seeing me and something had happened to her during the course of the evening which brought her quickly to me the next day.

I feared that it would worry her if she could not do so well during her second treatment with the large Snellen test card, so we worked together with another part of the method. This time we used fine print. I sat directly in front of her as she looked at the little card with fine print, but it was pitiful to see her staring at it, trying to read.

Staring is such a common thing and most people stare unconsciously at times. A great many people stare unconsciously most of the time and cause much or all of the discomfort which soon brings on chronic trouble with the eyes and sometimes causes blindness. If school teachers were instructed to remind pupils at intervals during the daily sessions of the permanent punishment to their eyes as the result of staring, it would be avoided in time and less eyeglasses would be prescribed for schoolchildren.

People do not wait until they are physically tired out before they sit or lie down to rest, but most people do not know what to do about their eyes when they are mentally tired. In some cases just closing the eyes frequently for a second or two is all that is necessary to retain good vision for life. This I know to be true because my grandmother, who lived until she was 79 years old, did not wear glasses at all until she was over 70 years old and then they were not fitted by an oculist, but were purchased at the price of ten cents from a solicitor who came to her door. She used them only when threading a fine needle. Without glasses, she could see fine stitches while sewing, whether the thread was black or white. What I particularly remember was that she blinked her eyes often, which I thought at the time was a mistake or an affliction, but since I have become Dr. Bates' assistant, I know that she was doing the natural thing.

If all mothers would watch their babies as they begin

to notice things and avoid any possible stare by just attracting the baby's attention to various things instead of just one thing, I believe that a great deal of squint could be avoided, as well as other eye troubles. Of course there are squint cases which have been brought on through illness or injury of some kind, but even these cases can be eventually cured by teaching the patient how to shift and blink and avoid the stare.

I informed this patient that her principal trouble was staring and that I noticed it more on her second visit than I did at the first. She was told to close her eyes and while they were closed to remember a white cloud or a piece of white cloth, such as her handkerchief which was in her lap at the time, then to open her eyes and instead of looking directly at the fine black print she was to look at the white spaces and then close her eyes again and imagine them as white as her handkerchief.

She said she could remember a white cloud much better while her eyes were closed. While looking at her handkerchief she could see it perfectly white, but when she closed her eyes the memory of the white handkerchief was not so good. She said the whiteness became sort of gray or a soiled white which made her uncomfortable while her eyes were closed. This proves again that Dr. Bates is right in saying that an imperfect memory of anything brings on strain and imperfect sight.

At first she could not do so well with the white spaces of fine print as she held the card six or eight inches from her eyes. We tried the other extreme then by placing the card close to her forehead, too close for her to read the fine print even if she had no trouble with her eyes.

She was directed to move the card slowly, slightly touching her forehead over the bridge of her nose and opening her eyes with the slow movement of the card and closing them again. In this way she got flashes of the white spaces, and as she closed her eyes the memory of the white spaces improved so that when she drew the card away finally, after practicing this method for ten or fifteen minutes she could read the fine print at six inches as well as she could at twelve inches. Again she became excited as she did the day before and felt that at last she had grasped the idea of avoiding the stare and that she would not need to come again.

Two days later she telephoned me for another treatment, saying that she could not retain the good sight that she had while practicing with me. When she came for her third treatment, I tested her sight with the large test card, using various cards that I had. She did very well with the two cards she had read at her first visit, but with the strange cards her vision was the same as it was during her first visit, 15/20.

I decided to try a different method of treatment by having her imagine that my room was her tea room. A desk and small table with a few chairs were imagined to be tables at which she was to place imaginary patrons who were coming toward her. She told me that it was customary for her to have a napkin in her hand which served sometimes to wipe the top of a glass or to rearrange a plate on the table. I gave her a towel to hold which served as a napkin and told her to shift from the napkin to the imaginary table, and in this way she learned how to shift and blink as she would have to do to retain her relaxation while at work in the tea room. She remembered this lesson very well and did her work in the tea room better for a few days.

When I saw her again, which was in less than a week's time, she said that she got along splendidly in the mornings, but in the afternoon after she had been busy for part of the day, she felt a strain coming on as usual, which caused a great deal of tension at the back of her head.

The method that we used that day at her fourth visit was used again at her last visit, the fifth treatment, when she did so well that I thought it unnecessary for her to come again. There were several pictures hanging on the wall of my room distributed in different places. I told her to imagine that she was in her stockroom where canned goods were stored. She explained how there were rows of canned tomatoes, which had the picture of a red tomato on the label. Then there were other shelves arranged with cans of peas, which, of course, were green. There were shelves in another section of the room with canned vegetables, with various colored labels.

I told her to stand in the center of the room and to sway her body from left to right, blinking as she swayed and shifted from the canned peas to the canned tomatoes and other canned goods with various colored labels. She remarked that if she could keep up that good feeling of relaxation and freedom from tension and strain while she was practicing in the stockroom of her establishment, she would be amply repaid for the time she spent with me.

Her report over the telephone a few days later was favorable. She said that she had taken her car with friends and had driven many miles over a mountain trail, and if it had not been for her ability to blink and shift, she could not possibly have avoided an accident which would have thrown her car over the cliffs. I had told her to occasionally shift from the speedometer to the center of the road ahead and vice versa. I told her to remind herself continuously that it was not necessary to hold on very tight to the steering wheel but to hold it loosely, which meant relaxation.

She said that her storeroom, she believed, was responsible for the absence of strain and tension late in the afternoon when before she had seen me there was not a day that she was free from pain in the back of her head. She wore a fancy white apron during business hours, but always in the little pocket of her apron rested the small test card and a small fine print card which she would use when she had the opportunity to do so, practicing shifting from the white spaces of the fine type to sections of the room, which helped her to see things clearly and without strain.

I hope this article will be of benefit to those who do close work in offices, as well as people who do similar work to that of my patient.

CASE REPORT

By Helen Kupferburger.

As is generally known, fevers of all kinds are apt, if not treated with the utmost care, to result in defective eyesight, hearing and many other troubles, and it was at the age of six years, after severe scarlet fever, that my eyes became weak and subsequently developed a convergent squint. In order to check this defect, it was found necessary to harness me to a pair of huge unsightly spectacles with the usual thick corrective lenses. As a result of this drastic treatment my eyes weakened still more, becoming myopic and astigmatic, although the squint had certainly improved but only at the cost of producing the other complications, for exceptionally strong lenses were used to this end.

[When strained, eye muscles do not become "weak"; they become tense. It is important for the student to understand this, since *relaxation* is the key to normal sight.—TRQ]

I continued to pay periodic visits to the best available eye specialists in Johannesburg and Capetown, South Africa, all of whom at first encouraged me into the belief that eventually I would be able to discard them. Later however, I received no such encouragement, but instead was warned that blindness could result if I went without them at any time. I reached the age of 26 years without having received any benefit from the wearing of glasses. In fact even more technical terms were introduced into the condition of my eyes and I had come to the conclusion that nothing could be done for them, and that I would always wear glasses, and that continuous headaches were my lot. Such a dreadful state of mind for any one to get into!

Imagine my joy when at a tea party (they have their uses after all) I heard Dr. W. H. Bates' name and methods of treatment mentioned for the first time; that was in 1926, and of course anything to do with the eyes attracted my attention at once. At that time a Ms. Reid and Mr. Jardine, both students of Dr. Bates, had been carrying out exceptionally good work with the Bates Method. I immediately consulted with them, overlooking entirely the fact that at that time I had a great deal of work to do which would require the use of my eyes. The first thing I was told to do was to remove my glasses and not to wear them again, and my implicit obedience in this regard surprised even myself, for since then I have never returned to my glasses. To Ms. Reid and Mr. Jardine I am forever grateful for what they did.

I think what caused me to put such faith in Dr. Bates and his methods was the fact that I had been going to eye specialists for some twenty years, and instead of my eyes being benefited, they became steadily worse, which fact coincided with one of his observations.

I carried out the various exercises prescribed, under somewhat difficult circumstances, my entire day being consumed with office work. However, this did not deter me, for I did the modified sway while sitting at the typewriter, got into the habit of blinking. I palmed my eyes in between, for at this time my eyes were being called upon to do work which they had never done before. It was indeed a hard and uncomfortable period through which I was passing. In addition to all the relaxation exercises, I did physical exercises to keep me generally fit, and this helped greatly.

After three weeks, quite by accident I began to realize the value of relaxation, for up until then I was undergoing too much of a strain; from this time on I steadily improved. Of course I realized that after having worn glasses for twenty years I couldn't expect to be cured immediately and that it would be only by hard work and patience that eventually my eyes would be normal.

I became absorbed in this treatment and felt that a great deal could still be learned. The fact that my own eyes were not yet normal urged me to learn more of the methods of treatment by this wonderful system. When in London, I received more benefit from Mr. Price, another student of Dr. Bates to whom I am very grateful.

I feel that if all the followers of Dr. Bates, and there are many, would cooperate and perhaps pool the knowledge acquired by experience, we could help this treatment to spread throughout the world. What a benefit this would be to humanity at large!

Better Eyesight
June 1928—Vol. XII, No. 12

SUBJECTIVE CONJUNCTIVITIS

By subjective conjunctivitis is meant that the conjunctiva is inflamed without the evidence of disease. Many people with subjective conjunctivitis will complain of a foreign body in the eye and yet careful search with the use of a good light and a strong magnifying glass will reveal no foreign body present. Some people with subjective conjunctivitis complain that they have granulated lids and that they suffer from time to time from the presence of little pimples on the inside of the eyelids and the pain that they suffer is out of proportion to the cause that they give to it. Among the many symptoms of subjective conjunctivitis may be a flow of tears from very slight irritants. However, the tear ducts, with the aid of which the tears are drained from the eye, are usually open in these cases and they are sufficiently open to receive a solution of boric acid which may be injected through the tear duct into the nose. This shows that the tear duct is open normally, and therefore can drain the tears from the eyes.

Dr. C. R. Agnew, at one time professor of ophthalmology at Columbia University, gave many lectures on subjective conjunctivitis in 1885 and 1886. The treatment which he advocated was dry massage of the whole body and I can testify that it was an excellent remedy. However, the treatment which I found was the greatest benefit was the aqueous extract of the suprarenal capsule, or adrenalin, the properties of which I discovered, using one drop in each eye three times a day.

Many cases were benefited by the sun treatment, by central fixation and by the practice of the swing.

SWINGING

By W. H. Bates, M.D.

The muscles on the outside of the normal eye are at rest when the sight is normal. Any contraction of one or more of these muscles by pressure, by operation or by electrical stimulation always produces an error of refraction. The removal of the crystalline lens may be done without changing the form of the eyeball.

The normal eye has normal sight when it is at rest. It is at rest, or relaxed, when it is moving to prevent the stare, strain, or effort to see. When the patient becomes aware that his eye troubles are always caused by one of these three, all of which are difficult, he becomes able easily to maintain the swinging of all objects.

Shifting or moving the eyes from side to side with a similar movement of the head improves the sight when done properly. It can be done wrong when the eyes move in a different direction to the movement of the head. In some cases, when turning the head to the right, the eyes may turn in the opposite direction, for example, at the same time. Cases have been observed where one or both eyes appear stationary while the head may be moving.

One patient complained that when he planned to move his eyes with the movement of his head that he was not conscious that his eyes were moving as desired or that the eyes were moving and not stationary.

In some cases the eyes would move irregularly and unconsciously a longer or a shorter distance than the movements of the head. When one or more of the patient's fingers were pressed lightly on the closed eyelids, the eyes could be felt to move rapidly, slowly, or in any direction.

The eyes may move to the right while the head moves opposite, or to the left. Swaying the head and body a long distance to the right or left may be accompanied by an apparent movement of stationary objects in the opposite or in the same direction. Stationary objects with a prominent background move opposite, while objects partly covered may appear to move in the same direction.

Some people have difficulty in practicing the swing successfully. They cannot imagine any stationary object to be moving no matter how much swinging is practiced. They usually complain that they cannot imagine stationary letters or other objects to be moving when they move their head or eyes. They feel absolutely certain that the stationary object is always stationary and cannot be expected to move when the body sways from side to side in a long or short movement.

It is absolutely necessary that all persons with imperfect sight should become able to imagine stationary objects to be moving. When an effort is made to imagine stationary objects to be stationary, the eyes become fixed or stare at the letter or other object and make an effort which always fails. A very successful method of teaching nervous people how to imagine stationary objects to be moving is as follows:

The Snellen test card is fastened to a support about fifteen feet away from the patient. When the patient looks at a point about three feet to the right of the test card, the card is to the left of the point regarded, and advances farther to the left when the point regarded is moved to the right. When the patient is directed to regard a point to the left of the Snellen test card, the card moves to the right side of the point regarded.

The greater the shift from one point to another, the wider becomes the swing. By repetition, the patient becomes able to realize that whenever a point regarded is to the right of the card that the card and all other objects are to the left of the point regarded. When the eyes move to one side of the card, the card moves to the opposite side and this movement of the card can always be demonstrated by insisting that the patient imagine the Snellen test card moves to the left every time the eyes move to a point to the right.

This method is always a truth without any exceptions because no matter how much the patient may insist that he is right, he has to acknowledge that when he looks to the right, the Snellen test card moves to the left, and this movement is so decided that it very soon becomes impossible for the patient to fail to imagine stationary objects to be moving whenever the eyes move from right to left, from left to right, or in any other direction. This demonstration may be made very convincing with a little time and patience. There are so many of these patients who have difficulty in imagining stationary objects to be moving when the eyes move from side to side or in other directions that the swing should be practiced.

[See previous issues for descriptions of the Long, Variable, and Universal Swings.—TRQ]

Circular Swing. There is one objection to the universal swing and that is that at the end of the count to the right or left, the patient in some cases stares. This stoppage of the swing may be corrected by the practice of the circular swing, when all objects are imagined to move continuously in a circular direction. The circular swing may be remembered with the eyes closed and differs from the other swings in that the finger, Snellen test card, or other objects appear to move in a circular direction. In the circular swing, the head and eyes are moved in a circular direction. [The best swing is the modern Infinity Swing; see *Relearning to See* for a description.—TRQ]

Square Swing. In the square swing, the head and eyes are moved in a horizontal line from one side to the other and then downward, across, upward, and across, without a stop being made in any part of the swing. Many patients can practice a square swing when they find it difficult or impossible to practice a circular swing. Either the circular or square swing may be practiced with the eyes open or closed.

Not all persons can practice any particular kind of a swing successfully with the eyes open, but with the eyes closed, with the help of the memory and the imagination, almost any swing can be practiced with benefit. It is interesting to observe that swinging the head and eyes a long distance from side to side is more easily accomplished than a short movement, although a short swing when practiced properly is more beneficial.

Case Reports

Some years ago, a patient came to me suffering from progressive myopia with well-marked imperfect sight. The patient was unable to practice central fixation, to remember, imagine or see perfectly. The square swing, with the relaxation that it brought about, corrected this patient's troubles.

A patient who was born blind was treated several years ago. He had the symptoms of chronic glaucoma, partial atrophy of the optic nerve and progressive myopia. He was unable to imagine stationary objects to be moving when he moved his head and eyes from side to side or in other directions. He had great difficulty in consciously controlling the movements of his eyes. When he desired to look to the right both eyes would at once look to the left and the movement was very irregular.

He was also troubled with nystagmus. Sometimes the nystagmus was very regular, but usually both eyes moved jerkily from side to side. He was unable to hold either eye stationary. The eyes appeared very small because the margins of the upper and lower lids were close together; it seemed as though the lids were partially paralyzed.

When he was asked to move his eyes consciously, he soon became fatigued and found it difficult and at times impossible to move his eyes at all. When pressing down his upper lid, while I was determining the hardness of the eyeball, I was surprised to notice that the pressure of the forefinger on the eyeball stopped the nystagmus and enabled him to move his eyes in various directions, which he had not been able to do before.

When the right eye looked twenty feet to the right of

the Snellen test card, the card appeared to be to the left of where he was looking. When he looked as far to the left, the Snellen test card was about twenty feet to the right of where he was looking. By practicing the long swing alternately, he acquired, after a few weeks, a great deal of conscious control of the movement of the eyes. Later, after the movement of his eyes became more easy and continuous without effort or strain, the eyes seemed to become more widely open. By continued practice his other symptoms gradually disappeared.

A girl, age ten, came to my office with her father. He desired that I examine the child and find out if her sight was normal or not. I tested her sight and she read the bottom line at ten feet. When I asked her if the last letter on the bottom line could be a letter "O," she answered that it could not be a letter "O," because it was a figure "6."

I said, "All right, is the figure '6' stationary or does it move?' She breathed deeply because it was a new experience for her to imagine stationary objects to be moving. After a while she said, "Yes, the figure '6' moves about its own diameter from side to side." I said to her, "Can you stop the swing?" Almost before I asked the question, she looked away from the card. "Why did you do that?" I asked. She replied, "When I tried to stop the swing, it gave me a headache; I lost the figure '6,' the whole card was blurred and I didn't like it." Thus I demonstrated that normal sight cannot be maintained without a continuous, slow, short, easy swing of all stationary objects regarded. To stop the short swing requires a conscious or an unconscious effort, which in turn may produce discomfort and pain in the eyes or head.

One patient was suffering from chronic glaucoma, cataract, progressive myopia and chronic iritis. One eye was totally blind and was unable to locate a strong light in any part of the field. The other eye had vision from one side only, the temporal field. This patient received most benefit from the long swing; other methods of treatment seemed to be of no benefit.

One of the most difficult patients to relieve was a patient who had been injured in one eye, so that sympathetic ophthalmia appeared after some years. The vision in the right eye was perception of light only; the left eye had been enucleated, but the operation had not been performed sufficiently early to be of much benefit. The eyeball was soft, like mush, showing that the ciliary body had been very much diseased. This patient learned the universal swing at the first visit. With the help of this swing, the hardness of the eyeball increased and his vision became better. The benefit which he received from this particular swing was the only benefit that amounted to anything.

MYOPIA AND PRESBYOPIA RELIEVED BY TREATMENT

By Emily C. Lierman

A woman, age 51, whose vision had been impaired for a good many years, thought that she would try the Bates treatment and see if she could in time discard her undesirable glasses. When I tested her eyes, her vision was 15/70 with the right eye and 15/200 with the left. When I first meet a person I have an unconscious habit of looking at the eyes and I noticed particularly that this woman seldom blinked. She had worn glasses for twenty years, but recently she had worn them only at the theater, movies and in places where the light was dim.

She complained of floating specks which at times seemed to her like miniature airplanes or tiny round white circles with gray centers. She boasted about being able to multiply these imaginary things floating before her eyes and to see them just as clearly with her eyes closed as she could with them open. It is hard to even imagine how terribly she strained in order to bring about such a condition.

She told me that previous to her coming to me she had visited an eye specialist who examined her eyes thoroughly and who told her that he could see no condition of her eyes that would cause floating specks, and that the retinas of her eyes were perfectly clear. He diagnosed her case as progressive myopia and then gave her a stronger pair of glasses than she had been accustomed to wearing. It was because of these stronger lenses and the discomfort that she experienced in trying to get accustomed to the wearing of them that prompted her to come to me.

The black card with white letters was used in testing the sight of my patient. While she was resting her eyes by palming, I placed the test card ten feet from her eyes instead of fifteen just to see how much more she could read at a nearer distance. After a short period of palming, I asked her to read the card again and her vision had improved to 10/50. I was glad to see this improvement even though it was slight. However, I thought that it might have been her right eye which was reading the 50-line, even though she was reading the card with both eyes.

I wanted to be sure that improvement had been made, so I asked her to cover her right eye and read the card again with the left. She read up to the 50-line just the same, which I thought was a good improvement in so short a time. I told her how other patients had improved by practicing many times a day at home and that if she would follow my directions and come to see me for a few lessons that she would make steady progress.

A few days later she came again and I noticed that she had acquired the habit of blinking. This was encouraging because it is not often that patients who have only had one treatment can remember to keep up this good habit which is done unconsciously by people who have no trouble with their eyes. I did not mention this to the patient because I was afraid to make her conscious of the fact and again unconsciously get into her bad habit of staring. However, I made note of this in my record and the last time I saw her I drew her attention to it, which pleased her.

During her first treatment I did not make any special effort to relieve her trouble with the floating specks, nor did either one of us mention it. Before I tested her sight at her second treatment, she said she had something to tell me. She noticed for the first time that in trying to increase the number of floating specks which she formerly was able to do, she had produced a terrific pain in both eyes and so she stopped doing it.

At my patient's second treatment I used the black test card and I gave her a card with diamond type to hold near her eyes. I gave her the usual advice, saying that she was not to try to read the print but only to look at the white spaces between the lines of fine type. Closing the eyes often and remembering the white spaces helped her to see the letters of the distant card, seeing one letter at a time and then looking to the white spaces of the fine type. She read 10/40 with each eye separately, seeing each letter clear and white. She remarked that the whiter the letters appeared to her, the more black became the background of the card.

At her first treatment I noticed that the sclera or white parts of both her eyes were bloodshot and looked as though she did not get enough sleep. I wrote this in my record of her case, but I said nothing about it to her. At this, her second visit, I noticed that the patient's eyes looked clear and the white parts were as white as my own eyes.

I placed her before a mirror and told her to blink and to look at her right eye and then at her left. This helped her to see that her eyes were moving while she blinked. It was then that she remarked how white the white parts of her eyes were. I enjoy treating a patient like her because there is a great deal of satisfaction in having the patient know that there has been an improvement in so short a time. She told me that her husband had read to her for one whole hour while she was palming or just keeping her eyes closed and resting her arms on her lap or on the arms of her chair.

I gave her more advice about what she was to practice at home and then two days later I saw her again. This time I asked her to hold the fine print as close as she could read it and to read what she saw on the little card.

During her first treatment, I did not ask her to read the fine print because I thought she would have no trouble in reading it. I was much surprised to hear her say that she could not read it.

I was out of town treating patients at this time and, as I was away from Dr. Bates, I was not allowed by the medical authorities to use a retinoscope or an ophthalmoscope, or to do any examining of the eyes of any kind. I was perfectly willing to abide by the law and was told particularly by Dr. Bates himself to do so. Therefore, I could not determine just what was wrong and why, when she was myopic, she could not read fine type as most myopic patients can. However, that did not worry me in the least because all the articles comprising my book were reports of cases treated by me during more than nine years when I did not at any time use any apparatus in the treatment or in the cure of these cases. I did, however, use a sun glass.

This patient was sitting near a window with her back to the sun. I asked her to stand up while I turned the chair the opposite way and told her to keep her eyes closed as she sat in the sun while I used the sun glass on her closed eyelids. I timed this treatment and gave her exactly eight minutes of the sun, focusing the sun glass on the closed eyelids, at the same time advising the patient not to open her eyes even for a second. Then I pulled down the shade to shut out the sunlight and immediately after opening her eyes she became able to read all of the fine print. And this with just that one treatment with the sunlight. After that she gave her eyes sun treatment many times a day and remained in the sunshine as much as possible, discarding her parasol which she usually carried with her and also leaving off her hat whenever it was possible.

All patients do not have the advantages which this patient had, I know. Yet patients are cured who have no chance to take sun treatment during the day except at their lunch hour. Patients who have found it impossible to get any sun treatment during the day have been successfully treated and cured of their imperfect sight by the use of a strong electric light.

While I was away from Dr. Bates, doing his work at the seashore and in other places, it was astounding to see so many people wearing dark glasses called "sunglasses" to protect their eyes from the glare of the sun. What a mistake it is to wear these glasses, even though so many specialists advise such a procedure! One cannot always wear them; therefore it is best for the human eye to get accustomed to all kinds of light without protection of any kind.

During the time I was treating this patient, while she was rapidly improving at each lesson, I had the great pleasure of meeting a noted criminologist who was very nearsighted. He had difficulty in seeing things clearly while driving his car and doing other necessary things which required good sight, unless he wore his strong glasses. This man mentioned the case of his brother, who had read Dr. Bates' book, *Perfect Sight Without Glasses,* and practiced the methods advised.

He said that every day he practiced in the hot sun in the desert where all he could see was sand, distant mountains and the sky; he would close his eyes and allow the sun to shine on his closed eyelids, then open his eyes and look off at the distant mountains, alternately shifting from the saddle of his horse to the distant mountains. He was not only cured of his imperfect sight.... He also noticed, being an expert in the different breeds of horses, that those which had blinders put on them acquired cataract, or could not see as well as horses who were free from any encumbrance as far as their eyes were concerned. After reading Dr. Bates' book he wrote to his brother and said that if the strong light of the sun was not injurious to an animal, why should it be injurious to the human eye? He was convinced that imperfect sight was caused by strain or an injury and if there were any sight at all that it could be improved by natural methods and not by the use of glasses.

To go back to my patient. She came for four days in succession for treatments, being encouraged at the progress she had made. At each treatment she improved, reading another line of the test card by first reading the fine print as close as she could get it to her eyes. Shifting from a blank wall to the test card while she was standing and swaying her body slowly from side to side also helped in the improvement of her sight for the distance.

Each day I varied the treatment. One day I placed her by a window and had her shift from the fine print up close to her eyes to the distant signs which I called to her attention, and to tops of houses and other buildings. An American flag waved in the distance and shifting from the flag to the flagstaff helped her to see the staff more clearly, and by keeping up the constant sway of the body, blinking easily but steadily all the while, she became able to see the harbor in the distance and also the boats which were moored near the shore. She told me that this was the first time in her life that she could ever see at such a distance.

She was the means of changing the mind of a skeptical husband who thought that the Bates treatment was a myth or something like it. However, he decided that if palming and swinging was a good thing for his wife and could make her so much more contented in her home duties than she was before, that perhaps it would help him to be a more agreeable person in his office as well as in his home. With just a few suggestions from me, my patient treated him successfully at home, and her last report was that he was reading his newspaper and book type without the use of his glasses.

I realized more and more that if Dr. Bates could live until the end of time that it would be his cured patients who would advertise him in the right and only way. Times without number there have been magazine and newspaper writers as well as authors of books who were cured after being treated by Dr. Bates who offered to advertise him in the way that they thought best.

Many years ago, without realizing that it would harm him, Dr. Bates allowed these grateful patients to advertise him in their own way. They unintentionally caused him much worry and concern with the medical profession. The only way to make Dr. Bates' work known to the world is to have his cured patients talk about the benefit they received and in that way help others who are suffering from defective vision.

During the last treatment I gave my patient, she read the various test cards, 15/15, with the exception of the black card with white letters, which she was able to read 15/10. Also, the floating specks had entirely disappeared after her third treatment. This case was very interesting because it is seldom that one has presbyopia and myopia simultaneously.

To carry out treatment successfully, I try to be careful to vary the method of treatment at each lesson. I find it true also that if I try out things by myself, without the help of Dr. Bates or his suggestions in the matter, that I fail sooner or later. Our students will benefit greatly by doing the same thing always. If the student is in doubt as to whether he or she can cure a difficult case, it is always best to write or come directly to headquarters and find out what is wrong. It is Dr. Bates' desire always to help the students to cure any case which may be difficult.

Better Eyesight
July 1928—Vol. XIII, No. 1

DARK GLASSES ARE INJURIOUS

He was a very intelligent chauffeur, and very polite and popular with most people. I enjoyed listening to his experiences in driving various types of cars.

One day we were driving to the seashore. The sun was very bright and the reflection of the light from the sun on the water was very strong and made most of the occupants of the car very uncomfortable. Personally I enjoyed the strong light of the sun. The chauffeur did not wear glasses for the protection of his eyes from the sun or dust and I asked him if he had ever worn them. He very promptly answered me by saying that he had worn them at one time, but discontinued wearing them because he found that after wearing them for a few days, his eyes became more sensitive to the light than they were before. He said he could not understand why it was that when he wore glasses to protect his eyes from the dust he accumulated more foreign bodies in his eyes than ever before. This seemed strange to the people in the car and they asked him to explain. It was decided that when the dust got into the eyes, the glasses prevented the dust from going out.

The eyes need the light of the sun. When the sun's rays are excluded from the eyes by dark glasses, the eyes become very sensitive to the sun when the glasses are removed.

FUNDAMENTALS

By W. H. Bates, M.D.

Central Fixation. When the vision is best where the eyes are looking, and worse where the eyes are not looking, central fixation is evident. Central fixation when properly used is a relaxation and a benefit. It is interesting to observe that one cannot have perfect sight without central fixation. One should not strain and make an effort to obtain central fixation of a letter or any object, as by so doing, imperfect sight is very soon apparent. The normal eye shifts unconsciously from one part of an object to another, seeing the part regarded best and other parts worse, and the eye with imperfect sight must acquire this habit by practicing it consciously until it becomes an unconscious habit.

Favorable Conditions. There are many ways in which the vision may be improved by having the conditions or the environment favorable. There are many facts to be considered when discussing the most favorable conditions for the improvement of the sight without glasses. Some people see better in a bright light, while others see better in a dim light. The distance of print from the eyes where seen best also varies with different people.

It is natural to suppose that to secure relaxation or rest, the hours of sleep should be increased. While this may be perfectly true, it is difficult to harmonize the fact that increasing the hours of sleep does not always promote relaxation or rest of the eyes. Many people will retire with their eyes feeling perfectly comfortable, yet they may be awakened during the night by severe pain in their eyes. During sleep, eyestrain may be so severe or continuous that no rest is obtained for the nerves of the eyes or other parts of the body. (As I have stated in previous issues of this magazine, I have examined the eyes of patients with a retinoscope while they were asleep and have found the eyes to be under a great strain. Sleep, therefore, is not always a favorable condition for the improvement of the eyesight.)

The optimum distance or the distance at which the vision is at its best is widely variable. Some people may have normal vision at twenty feet but not at fifteen feet. Others are able to read fine print better at twelve inches than at six inches. By practice one can improve the vision so that it will be normal under all conditions.

Shifting and Swinging. When shifting is done properly it is practiced easily without effort or strain. When one shifts from a point to the left to a point to the right, the swing produced is continuous, regular, and promotes relaxation. It is possible to shift with the eyes closed with as much benefit as with the eyes open. There are some people who cannot shift with the eyes open without a strain and yet they can shift or swing or imagine perfect sight with the eyes closed.

Whenever the head and eyes are moved from side to side, one should imagine that stationary objects are moving in the opposite direction. This should be practiced at all times until the habit is obtained. (The various swings are described in earlier issues of this magazine.)

Memory and Imagination. A perfect memory is a great benefit in obtaining perfect relaxation of the eyes as well as all the nerves of the body. One cannot remember a letter or other object perfectly unless it has been seen perfectly. When the memory is perfect, the imagination may also be perfect. Some people with a good imagination find it easier to imagine a letter or other object perfectly when they do not expend an effort in trying to see it. Knowing what the letter is, with the aid of the imagination, one becomes able to imagine that it is seen perfectly.

It is well to keep in mind that many patients believe that they see large letters perfectly when they do not and they can be tested by bringing the card up close to the eyes. The vision should be just as good at fifteen feet as it is at one foot. By improving the memory and imagination one improves the vision.

Rest. Rest or relaxation of the nerves of the eyes, mind and all other parts of the body is necessary before perfect vision can be obtained. When the nerves of the body are at rest, it is possible to remember, imagine or see all letters or other objects perfectly. It is not possible to remember, imagine, or see anything without perfect relaxation. Perfect relaxation or rest comes without effort. When the mind is at rest, any effort to improve the memory, imagination or sight is wrong. When the eye is at rest, it is perfectly passive. The eye at rest is never stationary, it is always moving. This seems a contradictory statement to make, but it is a fact which does not permit of any explanation.

[When the eye is at rest, *what* we see is left-brain: conscious, active, centralized on details; *how* we see is right-brain: receptive, subconscious, automatic, habitual, and—most importantly—relaxed.—TRQ]

Palming. One of the best methods of obtaining relaxation is by palming. There is more than one way of palming. One very good way, however, is to cup both hands, press the sides of the palms together, and place the two hands over the closed eyes and in front of the nose. When done properly, all light is excluded, one sees black perfectly and relaxation is obtained.

Blinking. When the normal eye is at rest, the eyelids are continually closing and opening. Blinking may be done so rapidly that it does not become conspicuous. Movies have demonstrated that the normal eye may open and close, or blink, five times or more in one second. The habit of blinking may be acquired by remembering to blink at frequent intervals. All patients with 15 diopters or more of myopia may blink five times or more in one second when the eye becomes normal and myopic alternately five times in one second. There are no exceptions to this truth.

Mental Pictures. The mind is capable of imagining all kinds of mental pictures. When the mind is at rest and the memory and imagination are perfect, all kinds of mental pictures are produced. When the mind is under a strain, the memory and imagination are imperfect and mental pictures are indistinct and cannot be remembered for any length of time. Central fixation when properly imagined is very helpful. With its aid a perfect mental picture may be obtained easily. When a mental picture is remembered easily and perfectly, the vision is benefited.

It is a fundamental truth that when one letter of the Snellen test card is seen perfectly, all the letters of the Snellen test card can be seen perfectly. When the sight is perfect, a letter is remembered, imagined or seen as well with the eyes open as when the eyes are closed. The vision of one letter of the Snellen test card can be improved with the eyes open by practicing the memory or the perfect imagination of the same letter alternately with the eyes closed. Whatever is done to improve the memory of one letter is a great benefit, because all the other letters are improved at the same time. This truth can be demonstrated in all cases. There are no exceptions.

One patient who visited me recently was a girl of about fifteen years old who announced that she would have to be cured that day because her parents would not allow her to spend any more time. By teaching her the fundamentals, this girl became able to improve her memory, imagination, and sight until she could read all the letters on the test card perfectly. By remembering the first letter of each line perfectly, by imagining it perfectly, she became able to see it perfectly because with the help of the retinoscope she demonstrated that when she imagined the first letter on each line perfectly that her nearsightedness was cured temporarily. When the first letter of each line was seen perfectly, not only was the letter seen without any error of refraction, but she was able to read all the strange letters on each line with normal sight. She did not imagine the other letters; she actually saw them.

Usually when persons have become able to read a familiar Snellen test card with normal vision and to read it continuously, they are able to read a strange card and to read it just as perfectly as the familiar card.

A knowledge of the fundamentals which can be demonstrated during the process of the formation of cataract has suggested successful treatment. The most important fundamental to consider is that cataract always disappears when the memory or imagination are perfect.

Many cases of opacity of the cornea which have been preceded by diseases or ulceration are benefited or cured by an intelligent use of the fundamentals. The law of fundamentals has proved the fact that an imperfect memory will cause an opacity of the cornea. It is not too much to believe that conical cornea is caused by eyestrain. If this were true we would naturally expect that when the eyestrain was relieved that the conical cornea would be benefited. It is a good thing to know that "this is the truth."

Acute or chronic glaucoma in which increased tension is present has always been relieved by practicing the fundamentals as described above.

In the normal eye the tension of the eyeball is always normal. Tension can be increased by an imperfect memory and the tension can be lessened or corrected completely by the practice of a perfect memory, perfect imagination, and a perfect optical swing.

The encouraging thing about the fundamentals is that they are always true without any exceptions, that they always suggest successful treatment and that they always explain the cause of imperfect sight.

PRESBYOPIA AND DOUBLE VISION RELIEVED BY TREATMENT

An Artist Suffering From Presbyopia

By Emily C. Lierman

An artist, age 61, who had for many years painted portraits of people who are well known in the West, suddenly became unable to go on with a painting which was almost completed. Before I tested his vision with the test card or asked him any questions at all, he told me his story. As a boy, he began to paint landscapes and ships of all description and when his parents found that he was especially interested in painting, they encouraged him to make it a special study in school. Before he was twenty years old he painted heads of young children, and the expressions of the faces as he painted them were so lifelike that older and more experienced artists were anxious to have him do work for them. Later in life he came from England to California and there he has become well known because of his work.

I became acquainted with him through a cured patient of Dr. Bates who had some painting done by this artist. She had noticed that he was straining his eyes to see at the near point and that at times the work was not satisfactory to himself. He got into the bad habit of using a magnifying glass for the fine details of a certain painting he was doing. He told me that he had been seriously thinking about giving up the work that he loved so much, but his wife objected strongly to this because it made him melancholy and despondent.

He had worn glasses for twenty years and the four latter years he had tried bifocals which were unsatisfactory. His oculist failed to help his double vision which interfered greatly with his work; he would see two brushes instead of one, and two objects where there was but one. Having become well known among the artists in the colony where he lived, it was not easy for him to decide what was best for him to do.

His eye test was, R.V. 15/40, L.V. 15/20. When he read the letters of the test card with his right eye, all of the letters appeared double—the large letters appeared double as well as the smaller ones. When he read with his left eye all the letters were clear.

I began treating him by improving the vision of both eyes together until he became able to read 15/15. Then we began to work with the right eye while the left eye was covered with a black patch. Palming helped him a great deal, so while he was under treatment he was encouraged to keep his eyes closed and covered with the palms of his hands for half an hour or longer each time. I again tested his right eye with the test card. The double vision still continued, even though the vision had improved in that eye.

I directed him to palm for a longer time and to get a mental picture of a painting he had been working on recently. I improved his vision during his first treatment to 15/10 with the right eye as well as with the left and the double vision temporarily disappeared. Mental pictures of the work that he loved to do relaxed his mind and he himself realized that it was the strain that produced the double vision and that he had been using his right eye more than the left.

How many people are there in this world who know that they are really using their eyes correctly? I fear that there are many who do the same as my patient did in unconsciously using one eye more than the other; that is to say, he strained more with one eye than he did with the other.

If I can make myself more clear to those who are interested in this article by explaining how double vision can be produced consciously, as well as unconsciously, I should like to do so as follows: If one will press the lower lid of the eye with the forefinger, while both eyes are open, one can immediately produce two objects where there is only one. The harder the pressure against the lower lid, the farther away the one object moves from the other.

I believe that it is a good thing to practice this consciously where one is troubled with double vision. When the double vision becomes worse consciously, one is very apt to become able to cure this error sooner than is expected. One can imagine how my patient must have strained his right eye in order to produce the double vision constantly, not only while he was at work but at all times while he was awake.

I had a pair of discarded glasses in my office which were left by a cured patient who gave them to me as a souvenir. I used a paper to cover the lens of the left eye and removed the glass entirely from the right. In this way my patient was able to practice for a length of time with the right eye without having to use his hand to keep the other eye covered.

I placed a large test card on the back of a chair which I located about a foot away from the patient's eyes. I then gave him a small test card to hold in his hand. The letters of the small test card were similar to those on the card which was on the chair. The patient was directed to look at a letter of the test card in his hand and then shift to the same letter on the card a foot away. By doing this he avoided staring. When shifting is done correctly, not only is the vision improved, but one is relieved of strain in all other parts of the body. The patient practiced the above for more than half an hour with the result that during the next half-hour we were able to improve his distant vision and he did not see double.

I was not so sure about the patient being able to continue the treatment at home by himself, so I advised him to come again a week later. When I saw him again, he said that he had noticed a decided improvement in distant objects while driving his car and also for near work such as reading his correspondence, but when he tried to do a little painting he did not find the shifting so easy, and because of that he could not avoid the double vision at that time. I was pleased to hear that he had improved to some extent and that it was only left for me to solve his problem of avoiding double vision while at his work.

During this lesson I described a way to shift from a letter that he was writing to a small test card which was placed on the desk to the left of him. He glanced at any letter that came within his line of vision, remembered the letter, and looking back to his pen and paper he was able to continue writing for a while without knowing that he had eyes. But going back to the work, which meant fine details and getting them accurate, had caused the same kind of strain which produced double vision.

I had him try the following: I tore a test card in half and by making a hole in it made it similar to a palette. He held the card in his hand, blank side up, and on it were placed letters and numerals in different places. He was told to imagine that the numeral which was placed in the upper right-hand corner of the card was a certain color to be used for the painting. He was to place the right hand under the numeral and then point to the card with his right hand. Then again he placed his finger on a letter which was placed on the lower left-hand corner of the card and then shifted to a card about a foot away, always pointing to the duplicate of the letter on the card in his hand.

While practicing in the above way he did not once complain of double vision, so he was advised to try this method at home and to write me within a few days, giving me a report of the progress he was making. He could not wait a few days, so he wired the next day telling me that he was successful in shifting from the palette and paint that he was using to the canvas and to do it in an easy way, without effort or strain and by doing so, for the first time in a long while he did not see double while at work.

I helped him a great deal by advising him by mail. For a while I did not hear from him and finally one day I received a telephone message from him. He was at the home of one of the subjects whose portrait he was painting XE "painting" . This man was seated in a wing chair with his one arm placed over the side of the chair. My patient stated that his vision blurred as he tried to finish the details of this painting. The harder he tried to relax and to remember some of the things I had told him to do, the worse his vision became.

I asked him to start swaying his body slightly from side to side and to imagine that the telephone was moving in the opposite direction to the way in which his body was moving. He said that he could do that very well and that when he blinked while he was swaying it was restful. I told him to keep this up for about five minutes or longer and then to go back to his subject, and imagine that he was moving his body from side to side as he did while he was talking to me over the telephone.

I told him that I would be in my office for the rest of the day, but the arrangement was made that if he had no more trouble in completing this painting that I would not hear from him again that day. He did not call again. Sometime later he wrote me a letter, telling me that for the first time he had noticed that some of our test cards had imperfections which he explained to me in detail. Dr. Bates and I had noticed the mistakes in the printing of some of the cards, but it was seldom that the patients had noticed these small defects. It pleased me very much that his sight should improve to such an extent that he was able to detect these mistakes.

Another method which I used during his treatment has also helped others in their particular line of work. I gave him a small test card with the Fundamentals on the reverse side and asked him to hold it where he could see the print best. He said that he could not see it well at any distance, but if he held the card at arm's length, he could read the Fundamentals up to No. 6 without the sentence appearing double to him. He thought he had made a fine discovery when he found that he could read to sentence No. 3 by squeezing his eyelids together. I gave him a hand mirror and asked him to look at himself while he squeezed his lids together, and asked him if he thought it would look well for him to go through life reading in that way.

The strange part of it was that he did not squint very long while he was looking in the hand mirror because, he said, he did not like the expression of his face.

I placed him at my desk with the hand mirror in front of him, about two feet away. I gave him the Fundamentals card to hold and told him to shift from the white spaces of the type to the mirror and to look at his eyes each time he looked in that direction. He said that shifting from the narrow white spaces of the Fundamentals card to the mirror helped to avoid the double vision at that time, so I told him to practice it. By alternately palming and shifting from the microscopic type to the Fundamentals card type, he became able to read No. 15, the finest print on the card at six inches without double vision.

Better Eyesight
August 1928—Vol. XIII, No. 2

SCHOOL NUMBER

SUGGESTIONS

It is recommended by the editor of this magazine that every family should obtain a Snellen test card and place it on the wall of some room where it can be seen and read every day by all the members of the family. Not only does the daily reading of the card help the sight of children, but it is a benefit to the eyes of adults as well.

It is a well-known fact that when many people arrive at the age of forty or fifty years, they find that their vision for reading or sewing is lowered. These people believe that they must put on glasses to prevent eyestrain, cataract, glaucoma, et cetera. Daily practice with the Snellen test card, together with the reading of fine print close to the eyes will overcome their difficulty. Reading fine print close to the eyes, contrary to the belief of many ophthalmologists, is a benefit to the eyes of both children and adults.

SCHOOLCHILDREN I

By W. H. Bates, M.D.

About fifteen years ago, before the medical society of Greater New York, I read a paper on the prevention and cure of imperfect sight in schoolchildren, illustrated with stereopticon pictures. Physicians who attended were very much interested in what I had to say. In the course of my reading I mentioned that most books on ophthalmology have published the statement that nearsightedness was made worse by an effort or strain to read at less than six inches or to read in a dim light. I went on to say that a careful study of the facts demonstrated that much reading in a dim light at the near point will not produce nearsightedness in schoolchildren, but will produce the opposite condition, farsightedness. A great many members rose up immediately to disprove this statement. They were unable favorably to impress those present because not one of them had investigated the subject. They admitted that they condemned such statements because most German physicians and many French, Italian and others had, like them, condemned the methods employed from hearsay and not from actual investigation or experience.

It was a rule of the society that every paper should not require more than twenty inches for its reading. After more than half an hour had passed I asked the president of the society how much more time I could have for finishing my paper. He answered that as much time would be allowed for finishing the paper as was necessary. The answer was so encouraging that nearly two hours elapsed before I was finished. The meeting was then thrown open for discussion and many of the ophthalmologists present publicly stated that nearsightedness, farsightedness, astigmatism, cataract, glaucoma and many other eye diseases could not be cured by operation or by the use of drops or other local eye treatment.

Those present asked many questions and the answers satisfied some and annoyed others. One question was asked which would have required some hours before it could be answered intelligently. It was as follows, "What percentage of cases of myopia in schoolchildren can be cured or prevented without treatment?" I answered that statistics were misleading. Someone has said that one can prove anything by statistics, but I disagree with him.

About midnight, the janitor appeared on the scene and whispered in the ear of the president a message which must have been annoying from the way the president acted when he received it. The president then said that the paper was so valuable that its discussion must not be curtailed, and if the janitor expected the society to adjourn, the members would go downstairs to one of the large rooms which was not occupied. It seemed to me as though all the members passed on to the new room.

A few weeks later another paper on myopia was read by invitation before the medical society of the County of New York. Among other things, I said that if it could be demonstrated that one child of the Public Schools of the City of New York did not produce or acquire myopia by an effort to see at the distance that I was wrong about the whole matter. The Board of Education heard of this statement and became interested. They sent for me to appear before them. I visited the Board of Education and told them about my investigations and offered to introduce the method in the schools for the prevention of myopia in schoolchildren. Some of the members of the Board themselves demonstrated that when they made an effort to see at the distance that the sight became less from the production of myopia, and that rest lessened the myopia. Much to my surprise it was voted that my method should be given a trial in the public schools of the City of New York.

Soon afterwards I called on the principal of one of the schools and asked for an opportunity to prove that I was right. The principal listened to my story and when I had finished said to me, "Come with me and we will try to prove whether you are right or wrong."

She invited me to one of the schoolrooms where a number of the children were suffering from eyestrain or were wearing glasses. When their glasses were removed their vision was imperfect. While their glasses were removed they were asked to sit with their eyes closed. At the end of fifteen minutes the sight was tested and all were found to have improved sight. Some had even obtained normal vision. The principal then said to me, "Remain here, Doctor, until I return."

She then went to one of the other classrooms. In a little while she returned smiling. She said, "Doctor, you are right; rest of the eyes does improve the imperfect sight of myopia. I am pleased to inform you that I was able to cure about a dozen children just by having them close their eyes and resting them for some minutes. I would like to have you meet some of my teachers and explain your method to them for their benefit." I found out later that she treated these children privately herself so that she could be sure that magic was not used.

In the beginning it was demonstrated that the memory played an important part in the cause, prevention and cure of imperfect sight in schoolchildren. It was also observed that improving the imagination enabled the children to improve their sight. They soon learned that they could only see what they imagined and that they could imagine what they remembered, and remember only what they saw.

A number of children were found wearing glasses who were backward in their studies and complained of attacks of headache and pain in their eyes; they were restless and took very little interest in their studies. After eye education was practiced, not only did the vision improve but the mentality as well.

Teachers in other cities also used my method of eye education in their classrooms. A teacher in the West devoted considerable time to teaching children how to remember, how to imagine, and how to see by using their eyes without effort or strain. She taught them how to palm until their eyes were rested. She had the whole class stand up and sway from side to side and imagine stationary objects to be moving.

Her efforts to improve the imagination of the children were most interesting. One method was to have the child close the eyes and draw some fantastic and unusual figures of people, animals and other objects while the eyes were closed. Some of these drawings were so valuable and interesting that they were used by older patients to improve their imagination. Many weary hours of work were relieved by having the children practice relaxation methods. In time the children enjoyed these relaxation methods and practiced them at recess.

One child who was able to improve his sight very promptly enjoyed teaching other children how to improve their sight.

The Superintendent of the Public Schools in North Bergen, New Jersey, published in this magazine in August 1925, a report of the result of the adoption of my methods in his schools. In many of the schools were children 16 years old in the same class as other children much younger. One very important result of the practice of relaxation methods in his schools was that children suffering from retardation were materially benefited or cured so that their teachers were able to place them in the classes in which they belonged according to their years.

After my methods were practiced in the Public Schools of New York for several years with great benefit, some physicians interested in eye work believed that the eyes of the children were not benefited by eye education and through their recommendation the practice of my method was stopped. I cannot understand why the Board of Education was willing to abandon methods which were practiced by teachers who were much pleased with the results obtained, in favor of methods which had failed to bring about any material benefit.

SCHOOLCHILDREN II

By Emily C. Lierman

During the spring of last year I had a class of boys under treatment. There were twelve in this group and each one had to be treated individually in order to improve his vision permanently. Two of them were brothers. The younger of the two, age nine, had normal vision in the right eye or 10/10 and he read all the various test cards I had without effort or strain. The vision in his left eye was also 10/10 but while reading the cards, while his right eye was covered, he held his head to one side and strained to see each letter. When he read the letters with both eyes together his left eye turned in considerably. His mother, who had been treated by me, was much concerned about the possibility of this condition becoming worse.

While he kept his right eye covered, I placed him fifteen feet from the cards and at this distance, with some effort, he read 15/30 and he complained that the letters were blurred. Palming seemed to help and I noticed that while his eyes were closed he sat quietly in his chair. At other times he was nervous and never still for a moment.

While he was palming, I talked about animals and their habits, how they moved about without any effort on their part—especially how the deer, cow, and even the bulky elephant could move about without any effort. Blinking their eyes was something they knew nothing about, yet they blinked all the time which helped them to keep relaxed always. The deer only strained and showed signs of fear when danger was near. The cow not only blinks but chews a cud and this keeps her busy and at the same time relaxed. The elephant sways his body when he is quiet and relaxed. Even when he walks his head and body move up and down. Elephants live many years longer as a rule than any human being and I sometimes wonder if they would live so long if they suffered eyestrain like human beings.

My boy patient listened as I explained all this to him and it certainly helped. I only saw him four times and during his last treatment his left eye remained straight just like the right and his vision with each eye improved to 20/10. He practiced faithfully every day for more than two hours, alternately swinging, palming, and consciously blinking his eyes as he looked from the first letter to the last letter of a line on his test card. At other times while swaying his body from left to right he would look at a picture on the wall to the right and then to another on the left wall, always blinking, keeping time with the swaying of his body.

His elder brother had no trouble in reading his books or seeing letters or figures on the blackboard at school, but when he joined his schoolmates at baseball, basketball or any other game, including golf, his eyes pained him so much that he began squinting his eyes continuously while he was in the sun and he sometimes became blinded by the sun for a half-hour or longer. This, of course, alarmed his parents.

This boy needed sun treatment and as I was teaching this class of boys in the evening, I used electric light for the treatment instead. A 350-watt electric light was adjusted to a floor lamp which was arranged without a shade so that with the sun glass I could focus the light directly on his closed eyelids. Previous to placing the bulb in position, I had directed the boy to keep his eyes closed so that he would not know what I was going to do next. If he had watched me adjusting the light he would have strained as he faced it. I explained to him that if he would keep his eyes closed I would give him some light treatment which would be of benefit not only to his eyes but in other ways.

Before I gave him the light treatment he told me how difficult it was for him to read in the sunlight or with an ordinary electric light without squinting and wrinkling his forehead and distorting his face. I placed a book near him, which was given to him after the light treatment, and we had good results instantaneously. There were others in the room besides my class of boys who were interested in this particular case. They watched closely as the boy held the book eight inches from his eyes and read distinctly without any signs of effort or strain.

The boy's mother made an appointment with me for the next day and an hour's treatment was given him in the bright sunlight. Two treatments were all that were necessary to give him permanent relief and he had no more discomfort or signs of strain or tension while he played basketball or baseball with the rest of the boys.

Another one of this group had irritated eyelids, the appearance of which was worse than the discomfort or pain that the boy experienced. He blinked more rapidly than the normal eye does unconsciously. Sun treatment was given to him also. When the mother saw that he had obtained a noticeable amount of relief from the first treatment, she purchased a sun glass and under my supervision she learned how to use the glass on his closed eyelids, and in this way all he needed was the one treatment.

The rest of the boys in my class were soon relieved of their eyestrain, which was due to straining while reading at the near point and trying hard to see objects at the distance. By shifting from the white space between two lines of microscopic type and looking at a test card placed ten feet from where they were sitting and then at a test card placed twenty feet away, they were relieved during the one treatment. It was not easy to make them understand that it was not a game that I was playing, but I became as one of them because it is the only way that I can be successful in my work. It is always good while treating boys of their age to be interested in their work or in those things which interest them especially.

As I explained in previous articles it does not take long for a boy who is interested in baseball to obtain normal vision if it is only nearsightedness or farsightedness which troubles him. While they are palming they can always imagine the size of a baseball and the color of it. They can always imagine that they are pitching the ball and that they are running to first, second and third base. In this way their minds become relaxed during the palming period or while their eyes are closed without being covered with the palms of their hands. This method always improves their vision for the test card and for big type.

With girls who are of school age, I find out, while they have their eyes closed and covered, what special study they like best. If it is arithmetic, for example, I have them give me an example and purposely I make a mistake in answering, which they correct. In their minds they are doing the example correctly and their minds become relaxed because there is no cause for strain. I have tried having a child do an example when arithmetic is not a favorite study with her, and I have not at any time found such a child who could get the answer correctly within a reasonable length of time because I produced mind strain, which in turn produced eyestrain and imperfect vision. This demonstrates that Dr. Bates is again right in saying that when the mind is under a strain, the eyes cannot have normal vision.

CASE REPORT: A BLIND SOLDIER

By Joseph Ouimet

To begin my story, it is necessary that we go back to the year 1917. At this time, from all cities of the United States, men in the prime of life were leaving for Europe, some never to return but to remain on the battlefields of France as a testimony of the heroism and sacrifice of a nation who willingly sent millions of soldiers to fight for a principle.

I was one of the many who, from the shadows of night to daylight, was converted from a peaceful citizen to a war soldier and who received the baptism of fire on French soil. There I slept in muddy trenches, suffered hunger and cold, fought in defense of my life. One afternoon while repelling a counter-attack, I was enveloped in a cloud of poison gases. Tears came to my eyes, which were inflamed to such an extent that I was unable to distinguish the objects which were located two feet in front of me. In despair, I rubbed my eyes with my hands and almost crazy with pain I started to run without knowing where, until I stumbled and fell, a blow mercifully relieving me of all pain and making me lose consciousness.

Upon regaining my senses, I found myself in a hospital bed, where started many tedious and ineffective treatments designed to bring me out of the world of darkness to which the poison gases had doomed me. Days, like a long endless night, passed in the hospital, during which my eyes endeavored to form images and visions of things that in former times were so pleasing to my eyes. Only within my soul and as memories, such images took shape as though it were a new irony of life looking with delight at my loneliness and showing me the treasures that I had lost.

One day the doctor under whose care I was, being tired of making trials and seeing that his efforts were in vain, gave me up as incurable. When I was so informed, when the doctor's words shattered the only rays of hope that I still had, it seemed as though the world was sinking from under my feet. It seemed as though the world had come to an end as far as I was concerned; I had no further hopes or ambitions, but resigned myself to my fate and to wait for death to visit me as soon as possible so that I might take my trip to the infinite.

I thus returned to my native land, discouraged at heart, without being able to see anything, not even the ocean that was murmuring under me, nor the sun that shone upon my body, nor the faces of my comrades who happily commented about the proximity to their happy homes. When the boat sirens, the jubilant screams of my comrades; when the distant voices of the multitude who were anxiously awaiting the arrival of the steamer, made me aware of our arrival at the port of debarkation, I experienced the most bitter moments of my life, especially when, at the dock, with eyes filled with tears I embraced my dear beloved ones, holding them strongly in my arms, so as to behold with my sense of feeling those whom my eyes could not see.

Then, little by little, by resigning to my fate I was able to drive out bitterness from my soul, until one day I was told about the Clinic of Dr. W. H. Bates, which I visited for the purpose of simply trying out one more cure but without having hopes of any kind. A few days after visiting the Clinic and without receiving any other treatment but sun baths and relaxation treatment under the electric light, I observed a rare change. It seemed to me as though the darkness were becoming less dense and at times it seemed to me that I could see small objects which would appear from time to time to disappear again rapidly, until one day a miracle took place.

A ray of light penetrated my eyes; it was like a shadow which I could distinguish vaguely in the shape of a bundle without being able to determine exactly what it was. Although I could see so very little, my soul was filled with joy. From then on I dismissed from my mind all lack of confidence, and practicing faithfully the methods recommended, the bundles that my eyes vaguely could make out gradually took a shape of reality until I was able to distinguish objects in their true form. Once again a return to life after having been for several years in the worst of all human jails and now that my sufferings have come to an end almost entirely. I am in a very good position to appreciate this treasure that God has given us so that we may behold the infinite wonders of his creation.

I wish that my knowledge were more extensive so as to describe in detail the methods that Dr. Bates employs in his Clinic so as to bring about similar miracles, details which although very simple, inasmuch as the methods are not tedious nor difficult, involve certain technicalities which only through the lips of a man of science can be made sufficiently clear for the layman to understand in all its details. It is not the technician who is writing these few lines but a grateful person who desires to pay with the only available means for a good service.

The results in my case I do not hesitate to call miraculous, in view of the fact that I had been considered as incurable by other doctors who, by using antiquated methods, made me lose time and money, and endure years of suffering. In view of these circumstances, any praise that I may give Dr. Bates will not be enough and, if I have refrained from using more appealing terms in my narrative, it is because I would not want my sincerity and good faith to be doubted in any way. Should it be necessary, I have not only one witness but several, as well as friends, acquaintances and persons of reliability who have known me for a long time and who would not hesitate to corroborate every word of my statement.

Today my satisfaction is complete on account of being almost entirely cured, and I think that in this world there must be many unfortunate ones who, not being as fortunate as I, have been unable to obtain relief from such a terrible malady. How much would I like to have this message reach their hands! Were I one of the sons of fortune who from birth has been showered with wealth, I would be glad to devote part of my money so that everyone who may have any eye affliction may receive these good tidings, but inasmuch as my limited resources do not permit me this pleasure, I hope that these few lines will serve as a sincere testimony of one who is very thankful for the services obtained in the Clinic of Dr. Bates.

[See "Christmas—1927" in the December 1928 issue for more on this case.—TRQ]

Better Eyesight
September 1928—Vol. XIII, No. 3

EYESTRAIN DURING SLEEP

The eyes of all people with imperfect sight are under a strain. This is a truth. Most people believe that during sleep the eyes are at rest and that it is impossible to strain the eyes while sound asleep. This, however, is not true. Persons who have good sight in the daytime under favorable conditions may strain their eyes during sleep. Many people awake in the morning suffering pain in the eyes or head. Often the eyes are very much fatigued and have a feeling of discomfort. There may be also a feeling of nervous tension from the eyestrain, or there may be a feeling as of sand in the eyes. At times all parts of the eye may be suffering from inflammation. The vision is sometimes lowered for several hours whereupon it begins to improve until it becomes as good as it was before the person retired the night before. Many people become alarmed and seek the services of some eye doctor. Usually the doctor or doctors consulted prescribe glasses which very rarely give more than imperfect or temporary relief.

There are various methods of correcting eyestrain occurring during sleep. Palming is very helpful even when practiced for a short time. A half an hour is often sufficient to relieve most if not all of the symptoms. In some cases the long swing, practiced before retiring, is sufficient to bring about temporary or permanent benefit. Blinking and shifting are also helpful. Good results have been obtained by practicing a perfect memory or imagination of one small letter of the Snellen test card alternately with the eyes open and closed. A number of patients were benefited and usually cured by remembering pleasant things perfectly.

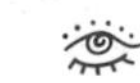

AVIATORS' EYES

By W. H. Bates, M.D.

Aviation is becoming more popular than ever before. The writer has treated many aviators who had, within a few months, acquired trouble with their eyes which made it dangerous for them to continue to fly. During the war a Major, an aviator in the Army, consulted me about his eyes. His principle trouble was dizziness. He was wearing glasses for the correction of a slight astigmatism. The glasses did not relieve the dizziness. At this time a large number of aviators had been killed by falls.

The history of this aviator was very interesting and valuable. He was positive that a number of years previously when he began to practice flying that his sight was normal—20/20 with each eye or with both. After a few years he noticed that his sight was impaired and that he had attacks of dizziness which did not last long in the beginning. These attacks of dizziness would come without warning while he was flying about one thousand or more feet above the ground. While he was conscious of the dizziness, he noted that his airplane started to fall and continued falling until the dizziness stopped. It was some months before he realized that with every attack of dizziness the machine fell a greater distance and he feared that these spells would ultimately cause his death.

Like most Army and Navy men, the Major did as he was told and was cured by me. This is the way it was done. I tested his eyes with the ophthalmoscope and retinoscope and found no disease of his eyes. The retinoscope revealed a small amount of astigmatism in each eye. His vision for the test card was 20/30. When he closed his eyes and rested them, the astigmatism became less and his sight for the test card became normal—20/20. This was accomplished in about an hour. The improvement was only temporary, however, and he was given advice for treatment at home. A large test card was given him with directions to read it with each eye separately at twenty feet. He was directed to rest his eyes often by closing them. It was suggested to him that he look at one letter which he remembered better with his eyes closed than he imagined or saw it with his eyes open. By repetition, his vision for the known letter improved and his sight for unknown letters and other objects improved until his vision became 25/10. He was under treatment for about a month and he was seen at irregular intervals during that time. Since that time I have not heard from him personally.

Other aviators have been benefited by the same treatment. There is a right way and there is a wrong way to use the eyes when controlling an airplane. The time required to do the wrong thing is just as long as the time required to do the right thing. The aviator can also demonstrate that an imperfect memory, imagination or sight is more difficult than a perfect memory, imagination or sight.

For example, a small letter "o" can be remembered imperfectly on one of the lines of small letters of the Snellen test card, but a stare or strain to see it with a white center as white as snow may require much effort, time and trouble. The imperfect whiteness of the letter soon disappears while its blackness turns to a shade of dark or light gray, all covered by a blurred cloud. The concentration, the effort to see, brings on discomfort, fatigue, pain, dizziness and other nervous symptoms which are all difficult to remember, imagine or feel. The memory, imagination or sight can only be demonstrated easily when exercised without strain. The successful pilot when at his best is always doing the right thing.

When riding in a fast moving train, the telegraph poles, although fastened to the ground, appear to move in the opposite direction. But any effort to stop this movement brings on a strain which may cause much pain, dizziness, fatigue or other nervous discomfort. The Major, who recognized the bad effects of dizziness from imperfect sight, believed that the dizziness, if sufficient, could cause fatal accidents when flying. He became able consciously to produce dizziness by eyestrain or by an effort to improve his vision.

He was taught to imagine the floor to be moving when he walked about his rooms. Swaying his head and eyes from side to side enabled him to imagine the floor to be always moving. When he steered his plane to the right, all objects seen appeared to move to the left. When he moved to the left all objects seen appeared to move to the right. He was able to lengthen the apparent movement of stationary objects. The wider the movement, the less was the sight improved, while a shorter movement of his eyes or head was followed by a greater improvement.

It was difficult for him to demonstrate that perfect sight can only be obtained by rest and prevented by an effort. But when he had learned that it was a truth without an exception he soon became able to demonstrate the facts. He was encouraged to improve his vision by using various or all parts of his machine as objects for testing and improving his sight. The more successful he was in improving his memory for objects, the better was his vision. We can only remember perfectly what we see perfectly; we can only imagine perfectly what we remember perfectly; we can only see perfectly what we imagine perfectly.

The time required for a cure varies with individuals. The eyes of some aviators may be under a greater strain than that of others.

The aviator should demonstrate that shifting the eyes or moving the eyes from one small part of his plane to other objects is restful and that his sight is always improved by resting his eyes. Blinking or closing the eyes and opening them quickly is also a rest. He should also demonstrate that closing the eyes for a few seconds or longer and then opening them for a shorter time is a benefit to the sight. Palming or covering the closed eyes with the palm of one or both hands when done right always improves the vision. Blinking, shifting, or palming can be practiced before entering the plane and so accidents may often be avoided.

While attacks of dizziness are a frequent cause of accidents, many of them fatal, there are numerous other causes which are just as serious or important. Many fliers of airplanes seldom have accidents. What is the secret of their success? It is due to their control at all times in all places. Control of what? The answer is: Control of the mind, control of the eyes and of all the nerves generally.

When the efficiency of the mind is at its maximum, it is at rest. Nothing is done consciously or unconsciously. It was a shock to the writer to discover with the aid of the retinoscope that the greatest strain of the body occurred during sleep. Strain is always accompanied by a loss of mental control when things go wrong. Accidents, fatal accidents, always mean a loss of mental control. The fact should be demonstrated. It should also be demonstrated that it is more difficult to fail than to succeed.

"Lindy" [Charles Lindbergh] could not have crossed the Atlantic Ocean, a 3,000 mile journey, by making a constant effort to obtain nervous control. The effort would have caused fatigue, and no man can have control of his nerves by using some form of effort. Dizziness is caused by prolonged effort and no man could fly very far when dizzy. The eyesight of even the best of us would become imperfect in a few minutes or less. Now let me ask how many of the best aviators could be efficient if their sight should become imperfect?

Control is necessary. How can it be obtained? Very easily. First demonstrate that doing the wrong thing—like staring, straining or making an effort to remember, imagine or see requires an effort, while resting the eyes or mind is easy and requires no effort.

It is a common experience for many people to fail to remember a person's name. An effort to remember it always fails, but if they rest their minds by thinking of something else the name comes to them without their volition. A perfect memory can be obtained by practice. Perfect mental control comes or is manifest when the memory is perfect.

Practice is important and very necessary. One may see and remember familiar or well-known objects with the eyes open, but better with the eyes closed. By alternating, the memory with the eyes open improves until it becomes as good as with the eyes closed. This means mental control of the mind, eyes, and all the nerves of the body.

The imagination can also be improved by practice. For example, if a well-known or familiar letter of a sign or print on a card can be imagined more clearly than it really is, the vision of all parts of the letter is improved as well as the vision for other objects which were not seen before. Imagining the letter alternately with the eyes open and closed is a benefit to the imagination and the memory as well as to the sight. The aviator can improve his control by improving his memory, imagination, and sight, while flying. It is not necessary for him to practice on letters or other objects several miles away. He can practice successfully, more or less continuously, on the face of his compass or some other part of his machine. Finally he should remember that perfect control can only be obtained by rest and not by any effort whatever.

TEST CARD PRACTICE

By Emily C. Lierman

[Reproductions of the test cards mentioned in this article are located in the appendices. There are duplicates of the small test cards, as recommended.—TRQ]

My experiences with schoolchildren and with people who are advanced in years has proved to me that daily test card practice is the quickest way to completely relieve eyestrain and imperfect sight. It is the custom always to give a patient a large test card with a small pocket size test card for home practice. Patients are encouraged to write for more help if needed further to improve their vision if they no longer come to the office for treatment. There is not a day goes by but that a patient will report that he did not have time to practice reading the test card for the improvement of his sight.

This is a natural thing, because most of us have more plans made for the day than we have time to carry out. For that reason we find the miniature test card very valuable. The card is just large enough to be placed in a dress or coat pocket. It is not necessary to spend any extra time at home in practicing with this card if the patient has a journey before him in going to or from business. Riding in trains, taxicabs, the subway or surface car will give the patient time enough to improve the vision by practicing with the little card, even if it is only for ten minutes at a time.

If one is riding in the subway, either sitting or standing, one can use the small test card by holding it about six or eight inches away and shifting from a letter of the card to a sign directly opposite. If the print of a sign looks blurred, the print will soon clear up if one practices shifting and blinking from the letter of the card up close to the letter of the sign.

Many people whom I have helped in this way have enjoyed practicing with the signs and small test card because by the time they arrived at their destination their eyestrain was entirely relieved. It is so much easier then to use the memory for objects seen without effort or strain. One can remember part of the sign which was seen in the subway, and if during the course of the day there should be a strong desire on the patient's part to put on glasses again, all he has to do is to close his eyes for part of a minute and remember that sign. Instantaneous relief sometimes follows and this encourages the patient to practice.

Children like the small test card with numerals. The numbers are distributed so that wherever the eye glances there is always some number which can be seen perfectly within a normal distance from the eyes. Children, as a rule, are not satisfied until the card can be read normally with each eye separately. Over each line of numerals there is a small number indicating at which distance the normal eye should read it. Schoolchildren who have never been to the office or seen Dr. Bates or myself have been able to improve their imperfect sight to normal by the daily use of this small card.

Sometimes children do need encouragement from their parents or from their school teachers, because they forget just as grown folks do when a thing should be done for their benefit. I have been asked this question many times, "How about younger children who cannot read or write?" For them we have a card called the "pothook" card which contains inverted "E's." It does not take long for a two-year-old to be taught how to say which way the "E's" are pointing. Children soon learn how to say whether the "E's" are pointing up, down, left or right. By shifting from one "E" to the other, they notice the white spaces between the lines of "E's." Unconsciously they notice that the black letter "E's" become blacker or appear to, which is a good thing for the sight.

The "pothook" test card is also used for sailors who have difficulty in reading flag signals at sea. Many midshipman from Annapolis are at the present time using this card for the benefit of their sight.

There is a small black card with white letters for those who are partially blind, which is of great benefit to them. Such a patient is placed with his back to the sunlight and while the sun is shining on the black card, the white letters appear more clear and white and by closing the eyes often, avoiding the stare, the vision is not only improved, but if there is any pain or discomfort it soon disappears. The patient is advised to hold the card up close to the eyes and while the card is moved slightly from side to side about an inch or two, relief soon comes. The patient is then advised to hold the card a little farther away day by day.

Patients to whom the large test card beginning with the letter "C" is given at the first visit find the pocket size test card, which is a duplicate of the large one, a great help. They shift from the small card, which is held in the hand, to the large card which is placed ten, fifteen, or twenty feet away.

The patient looks at a letter of the small card, closes the eyes to rest them for part of a minute and then looks at the card in the distance and sees the same letter on the same line, which in most cases becomes clear and easy to see without strain.

For those who do close work, more than one small test card is used. During work hours two cards can be placed on the desk, for instance, or near to their work. One is placed to the left and the other to the right at an even distance of about two or three feet, or a little closer. The shifting, which is done rapidly and only takes a second to do, is done by first shifting from the work to the card at the left, back to the work, over to the card on the right and back to the work.

The patient soon notices that the small letters which were not seen clearly appear distinct. There are times when patients become discouraged because the sight does not appear to improve as rapidly as they expect. Sometimes the vision even becomes lower, which is discouraging. If those patients who have been to Dr. Bates can get in touch with him and explain just where the difficulty lies, the advice that will be given is sometimes all that is necessary.

I hesitate to mention my book to the subscribers of our magazine, but I always mention it to my patients. In it I have described as carefully as I could how important it is for patients to continue practicing after they have seen the Doctor. It is written so that everyone with eye trouble will find an article which will apply to his case. Those who have Dr. Bates' book find my book of additional help, and it is because of this that I mention it at this time. At the time the articles for my book were written, I had some blind and partially blind patients, an account of whose cases can be found in my book. Since the book has been written I have had further experience in treating difficult cases, which I try to explain in each number of the magazine.

[As mentioned earlier, all of the stories from Emily's *Stories from the Clinic* are contained in these *Better Eyesight* magazines.—TRQ]

I have found that practice with microscopic type is most helpful in nearsightedness. The patient holds the fine print as close as he can, looking at the white spaces between the black lines of type while blinking and then looking out of a window, for example, or at a distant corner of the room.

As I have said in this magazine before, all cases cannot be treated alike. There may be in one room at the same time ten or more cases of myopia, cataract, glaucoma or any other disease of the eye, and yet perhaps only one of the group would respond to one kind of treatment. It takes just as much time in a great many cases to cure a simple case of imperfect sight as it does a more serious eye trouble, and yet it does not require a college education to be able to be cured of imperfect sight by the Bates Method.

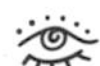

QUESTIONS AND ANSWERS

Q–1. Should one imagine a thin white line along the top of a word or sentence or just at the bottom?

A–1. If you can imagine it at the top as easily as you can at the bottom, do so, otherwise imagine it only at the bottom.

Q–2. If the lens is not a factor in accommodation, what is its purpose?

A–2. The lens is for protective purposes, just as fat is a protection to the bones of the body. [?—TRQ]

Q–3. If strain is the cause of imperfect sight, why are not all affected in the same way? Why is it that some have myopia, others astigmatism, etc.?

A–3. Different people react in different ways to strain. Some have mind strain, some nerve strain, some physical strain, etc. All these tend to cause various ailments. One's temperament also has a great deal to do with it. [A more complete answer to this question includes right-brain/left-brain factors. See "Brains and Vision" in *Relearning to See*.—TRQ]

Q–4. Can one blink too quickly and too often?

A–4. The normal eye blinks quickly, easily and frequently. Blinking can be done correctly or incorrectly. Some people, when they are told to blink, squeeze their eyes shut, or close them too slowly and then open them spasmodically, which is wrong. When the normal eye blinks, things are seen continuously.

Better Eyesight
October 1928—Vol. XIII, No. 4

NO GLASSES FOR QUICK RESULTS

The first and best thing that all patients should do after their first treatment, or before, is to discard their glasses. It is not always an easy thing to do but it is best for the patient and for the teacher. It is true that at one time I did not encourage patients to learn the treatment unless they discarded their glasses permanently. But since I have studied more about my method and have encouraged some of my Clinic patients to wear their glasses at times while under treatment, I find that some of them obtained a cure but it required double the amount of time that was required to cure those who discarded their glasses permanently. During the treatment when the glasses are worn temporarily, even for a short time, the vision sometimes becomes worse and in most cases a relapse is produced. It is much more difficult to regain the lost ground than ever before, and sometimes causes much discomfort.

Glasses for the correction of myopia do not fit the eyes all the time. To obtain good vision with glasses an effort is required to make the eyes change their focus to have the same error of refraction as the glasses correct. When the vision is benefited most perfectly by glasses it is necessary for the eyes to change frequently. To learn the amount of myopia in the eyes by trying different glasses to find the glass which continuously improves the vision best is usually difficult because the amount of the myopia changes so frequently. To change the amount of myopia requires an effort. Some people complain that no glasses fit their eyes permanently. These cases are benefited by discarding their glasses for a longer or a shorter period while being treated. Patients who require good sight to earn a living and find it difficult to discard their glasses while under treatment have been able to make slow or rapid progress in the cure of their imperfect sight by wearing their glasses only when it was absolutely necessary.

[Today, most students use reduced-prescription glasses as an intermediate solution. This is covered thoroughly in *Relearning to See*.—TRQ]

NYSTAGMUS

By W. H. Bates, M.D.

When the eyes move conspicuously from side to side, regularly or continuously, the condition is called nystagmus. These movements occur so frequently in connection with serious diseases of the eyes that the presence of this symptom is an indication that the cure of the eye disease will usually require much time and attention. So seldom are eye diseases with nystagmus cured that many physicians believe that most cases with nystagmus are incurable. I have found that many of these so-called incurable cases will recover by treatment.

We have observed that many eyes with imperfect sight do not have nystagmus but acquire it at almost any age.

It has been produced repeatedly by a conscious stare or effort to see. It has been relieved by conscious relaxation with the aid of palming. When the patient is reminded that the stare or an effort to see is injurious, he becomes better able to lessen or relieve the eyestrain which is usually very harmful. Patients with nystagmus have less control of the movements of their eyes and for this reason require more supervision and help before they become able to use their eyes properly without strain.

All patients with nystagmus cannot be treated in the same way because I have not found two alike. The treatment which is helpful in one case may not be of any benefit to any other. One patient, a woman age twenty-five, who was born with a very bad case of nystagmus and who also had mixed astigmatism, with retinitis pigmentosa, was under my observation at different times for a number of years. In the beginning her vision without glasses was 10/200 in each eye. She obtained a vision of 10/70 in each eye with the aid of the glasses which corrected her mixed astigmatism. Without glasses her vision improved to the normal temporarily with the aid of palming, shifting, and swinging. She also became able to read without glasses. The nystagmus was also benefited at the same time. The patient was encouraged and practiced the relaxation exercises more continuously.

In her case, palming was the most beneficial treatment of her eyes, both for the nystagmus and vision. This may have been due to the fact that when she palmed with both eyes closed, she was able to remember black letters on a white card more perfectly with her eyes closed than with her eyes open. She was also able to remember or imagine white letters on a black card better with her eyes closed than with her eyes open. When she remembered letters perfectly, her eyes became relaxed and her vision for trees, flowers, the colors of the spectrum, red, green and blue as well as other objects and other colors was perfect without any effort or strain whatever. Her memory seemed perfect to her because she could remember letters and other objects as well at twenty feet or farther as she could at two feet or nearer. Palming helped her to remember things better. The longer she palmed, the better became her memory. With an improved memory her sight became much improved and the nystagmus became less. The palming improved her memory of the notes of her music. Many of the black notes had a white center which she remembered better by the aid of palming.

It is important to mention that the sun treatment also lessened the nystagmus and improved the sight because the eyes became relaxed. This improved her sight and lessened the nystagmus. In the beginning the sun treatment was not so beneficial as it became later, after palming. The sun treatment was employed with the aid of a strong magnifying glass which focused the light of the sun on the outside of the upper lids, the glass being moved rapidly from side to side for short periods of time. For several weeks this treatment was given daily when ever there was sun, and the nystagmus and vision decidedly improved.

(There have been cases of nystagmus treated which failed to improve by the sun treatment. Other methods were then employed.)

With the improvement of the nystagmus, this patient's vision for distant objects and her ability to read also improved. The inflammation of the retina at the same time improved remarkably. In the beginning of her treatment a large part of the retina of both eyes was covered with black pigment spots. The ophthalmoscope was used each time she came. It was noted that these black specks became less numerous and finally disappeared. The fields of each eye were improved and the night blindness from which she suffered became less.

Her visits to the office were very irregular and uncertain, with the result that the improvement which she obtained during this time was not continuous. She earned her living as a music teacher. When she neglected to practice the treatment which I recommended to correct the tension, stare, and strain, her vision became worse and she lost her occupation. Having to depend upon her family for support was embarrassing to her. She came again for treatment after an absence of over a year. She told me that she was ready to come at regular intervals whenever I advised her to come.

While she was away she had a relapse but did not lose all the improvement that she had gained; there was an improvement in the nystagmus, but it was not rapid or conspicuous. This patient was examined with the aid of a movie camera. She was able to lessen the movement of her eyes and was able to show on the screen how it was done. When these pictures were taken by an expert, the doctors who were invited to be present testified that when the nystagmus became less or disappeared and the vision improved, it was because the stare, strain, or effort to see was corrected. What I have been unable to prove in my publications, the movie screen proves.

My patient gradually and steadily improved until she became able to see well enough to resume her work. Her vision for distant and near objects improved so that she could see better without glasses than she had formerly seen with them.

While the movie work was in progress, this patient offered her services to show how the nystagmus could be produced by an effort. The condition of her eyes was so much improved that I doubted that she had the ability or the courage to strain or produce the amount of tension necessary to show her nystagmus condition on the screen. While the camera was running I was amazed to see the nystagmus return. I thought that I had met my Waterloo. Now that I had improved a case that I had at one time deemed impossible to help, I feared that in order for her to strain sufficiently to cause the nystagmus to return would be a calamity. My fears were relieved when the camera again registered a picture of her while she remembered perfect sight by reciting for me all the letters of the Snellen test card which she had committed to memory.

This picture showed plainly no evidence of effort or strain and the nystagmus had stopped. Later the patient told me about the pain and discomfort she suffered in order to produce the nystagmus for the picture. Her sacrifice was worthwhile because others since then have been benefited.

Some patients with nystagmus do not know that they have it. The first step in their cure is to teach them to feel the eyes move when the closed upper lids are lightly touched with the finger tips.

One day some years ago a boy about twelve years old came to my office. He was ushered in by his mother, a middle-aged woman who just pointed to his eyes, and then sat down and waited. The patient had nystagmus. His vision was about one-half of the normal. With the ophthalmoscope no disease of the retina, optic nerve or any other part of the eyes could be found. The nystagmus was variable. He was able to lessen it until his vision improved very much and even became normal, 20/20 for short periods of time. By straining to see, the nystagmus became worse and his vision less. His mother became more interested. Her eyes were full of questions but she remained silent.

I asked the boy, "Can you move your eyes more rapidly?" "Yes," he answered. Then he was asked, "How is your sight?" "Very poor," he replied, "and growing worse." "Can you stop the movement of your eyes." He answered, "Yes." "How do you do it?" "I do not know," was the reply.

He was told to palm or to cover his closed eyes with the palms of his hands. He said this felt restful and when he opened his eyes his vision was improved and the nystagmus had stopped. For some minutes he was able to demonstrate that he could stop the nystagmus and that his sight for a short time was better. He was also able to produce or increase the nystagmus by making an effort to try to see. All this time his mother watched the proceedings. By the way she acted one could read her mind. The nodding of her head, the frequent moistening of her lips, the satisfied look in her face showed that she believed that the boy produced the nystagmus consciously for his own amusement, which was the truth. It was not necessary for me to explain. She now understood what was the matter with him and she also knew what to do. After thanking me she grabbed the boy's arm none too gently and disappeared from my office quicker than she came in.

CASE REPORTS

By Emily A. Bates (formerly Emily C. Lierman)

It is encouraging to meet people who have become able to discard their glasses by the benefit they obtained just from reading Dr. Bates' book. There are those also who write to us and complain that they have not received any benefit whatever after reading it. But the latter are in the minority.

Sometimes I feel that I would have been one of the complaining kind if I had not been fortunate enough to meet Dr. Bates before his book was written. I agree with some people that parts of his book are too technical for the layman to understand. But the principal part of his book is not technical and is so carefully written that even schoolchildren have been benefited and cured by practicing the methods recommended. While I was in California I met a number of children who came to see me for one visit only and brought Dr. Bates' book with them. Dr. Bates himself would have felt honored if he could have seen so many of his books so worn out that the pages had to be pasted together again, while others were very much soiled from handling.

These children wanted to be sure that their relief from eyestrain was complete. I appointed the oldest one to test the sight of each eye of all the pupils. According to the tests made, the vision of all the pupils was normal with the Snellen test card and other objects. They all read correctly the captions on the movie screen thirty feet away. A question was asked as to whether the movies caused more or less eyestrain and I replied that the facts were quite the contrary, but that one must become accustomed to the strong light of the sun. Most children out West are accustomed to the sun and for that reason there are fewer children wearing glasses than the children of city schools here in the East. Doctors and instructors from various schools came to learn the Bates Method so that they could teach others how to use their eyes correctly.

A young woman came to me for the relief of her eyestrain. While visiting in New York, one of the professors of the University of Southern California had been treated and cured of presbyopia by Dr. Bates. This woman was one of the professor's students at the University and he recommended her to come to me for treatment. She had myopia, or nearsightedness, and at times suffered a great deal of pain, especially at night after her studies were over. It was impossible for her to read at night no matter how strong an electric light was used. The stronger the light was, the more discomfort she had in her eyes. This made her unhappy because she was a lover of books. The temptation was very strong to obtain suitable glasses so that she could enjoy reading her books at night, when the instructor advised her to try the Bates Method for the relief of her eyestrain.

I began treating her by placing her fifteen feet from the test card which was fastened to a stand. With much straining on her part she read the 70-line with her right eye and only saw the largest letter on the card, which is called the 200-line letter, with her left eye. I immediately decided to draw the test card up to ten feet, where she would not strain so hard to see. Again she read the letters, reading with the right eye and then with the left. Her facial expression became more natural, less strained, and without her telling me so, I knew that she felt more like going on with the treatment.

Her disposition was directly opposite to that of her friend and classmate who came with her. Her friend was so determined not to wear glasses that there was no doubt at all in her mind about receiving some benefit from me. But not so with my patient. She was willing enough to have me try to help her, but she did not have much faith in me. I was not Dr. Bates and that made a difference with her. She felt that I could not possibly understand her case. She told me later that I had read her mind correctly but was glad that she tried and won out.

At ten feet she read the 40-line with her right eye with the evidence of strain decidedly less. With her left eye she read one letter correctly of the 100-line, or the second line from the top of the card, which is an "R." The other letter on that line is a "B" which she thought was an "R" also. I did not correct her but told her to close her eyes and forget about the test. I asked her about the subject she was most interested in at college and she seemed eager to tell me about it. She was studying art and the correct combination of colors for interior decorating. Some patients, when asked to close their eyes and remember something perfectly cannot do so without help from the Doctor or instructor. This patient did so immediately. She did not have her eyes closed for more than ten minutes when she became able to read the whole test card as well with the right eye as with the left at ten feet.

The memory of colors, describing them to me while her eyes were closed, was all she needed to give her relaxation of mind and body and temporarily improve her sight to normal. I told her to close her eyes again and describe her ideas of colors for different rooms of a home she had in mind. While she was doing this I again placed the test card fifteen feet away and with both eyes she read 15/20. She complained of a sharp pain over both eyes, the pain being more over the left eye.

I placed her chair in the sun and while her eyes were closed I used the sun glass very rapidly for five minutes on her closed eyelids. This not only relieved her pain but it improved her sight to 15/10. She read microscopic type just as well in an ordinary light as she did in the sunlight. Because she had been nearsighted it was not difficult for her to read it. She was told to read the fine type several times every day after sitting in the sun with her eyes closed.

Having worn a green shield over her eyes while in her classroom every day for two years, it was not easy for her to take the sun treatment. However, the results she obtained during her first treatment encouraged her to continue the practice. She purchased a sun glass and I taught her friend how to use it on her eyes. My patient in turn also learned how to give the sun treatment which not only benefited her friend but also others at the University. My patient returned for two more treatments a month apart and after that she reported over the telephone to me that she had had no relapse to imperfect sight.

Better Eyesight
November 1928—Vol. XIII, No. 5

PRACTICE TIME

A large number of people have bought the book *Perfect Sight Without Glasses* but do not derive as much benefit from it as they should because they do not know how long they should practice.

Rest. The eyes are rested in various ways. One of the best methods is to close the eyes for half an hour after testing the sight. This usually improves the vision.

Palming. With the eyes closed and covered with the palms of both hands, the vision is usually benefited. The patient should do this five minutes hourly.

Shifting. The patient looks from one side of the room to the other, alternately resting the eyes. This may be done three times daily for half an hour at a time. The head should move with the eyes and the patient should blink.

Swinging. When the shifting is slow, stationary objects appear to move from side to side. This should be observed whenever the head and eyes move.

Long Swing. Nearly all persons should practice the long swing one hundred times daily.

Memory. When the vision is perfect, it is impossible for the memory to be imperfect. One can improve the memory by alternately remembering a letter with the eyes open and closed. This should be practiced for half an hour twice daily.

Imagination. It has been frequently demonstrated and published in this magazine that the vision is only what we imagine it to be. Imagination should be practiced whenever the vision is tested. Imagine a known letter with the eyes open and with the eyes closed. This should be practiced for ten minutes twice daily.

Repetition. When one method is found which improves the vision more than any other method, it should be practiced until the vision is continuously improved.

HYPERMETROPIA

By W. H. Bates, M.D.

Hypermetropia is the opposite of myopia. The optic axis is shortened instead of being elongated as in myopia.

Most writers attach very little importance to hypermetropia. They publish that the hypermetropic eye is usually congenital and not acquired. Risley examined many eyes with hypermetropia. He believed that hypermetropia caused headache, pain, fatigue, and other symptoms to a greater degree than did myopia. Many statistics showed that in the eyes of schoolchildren about 80 percent had hypermetropia, about 10 percent had myopia, and about 10 percent had good eyes. It is well that the objections to hypermetropia should be studied and published. It is more necessary to relieve the symptoms of hypermetropia than those of myopia if for no other reason than the fact that hypermetropia is more injurious to the eyes.

The old methods recommended for hypermetropic eyes are insufficient to obtain the best vision, and to relieve or cure pain, fatigue, dizziness, double vision or other nervous troubles. Hypermetropia of low degree is quite often as difficult to improve without glasses as many cases of hypermetropia of a high degree.

What are the limits of improved or cured vision in most cases of hypermetropia? There is no limit. A hypermetropia of 15 D or 30 D can obtain as good sight by relaxation treatment as a hypermetropia of 1 D or less. Such claims are open to criticism. They can all be demonstrated by different operations on different cases.

In the early days of scientific medicine the facts connected with the changes that might take place in the hypermetropic eye were studied and they might have been a benefit if the facts were understood, but these men did not realize the importance of many truths which they demonstrated. In those days, as in our own, science was not governed by ordinary rules. For example, Donders published in his book the claims of some ophthalmologists that hypermetropia was not curable because they had never seen any such cases cured. Yet most eye doctors in the early days reported the truth correctly.

After extraction of cataract, the amount of hypermetropia is about 10 D. In most cases they admitted that the hypermetropia became less without any treatment, and that the eye, after extraction of cataract, had been observed to become normal without any hypermetropia, when the patients were able to not only obtain perfect sight for the distance but also were able to read fine print or diamond type at six inches from their eyes without any difficulty.

One doctor stated the changes which took place in eyes which had considerable hypermetropia. It is difficult to understand why it is that this doctor published that an effort to see always increased the amount of hypermetropia and for that reason no treatment could be expected to help these cases. One physician, whose scientific attainments were unusual, published statements like this, "I have never cured hypermetropia and because I have never cured hypermetropia nobody else can." Another so-called authority, after testing results obtained from massage of the muscles of the eyelids, could see no benefit from this treatment. He was asked by a friend, "Are you still using massage?" He answered, "Yes." Then his friend said, "Does it do any good?" The doctor answered, "No." "Why do you do it then?" "Because there is nothing else to do."

An effort always increased the hypermetropia and makes the sight worse. This is a fact so universally true that it is unfortunate that the physicians who found that a strain was bad did not try the opposite of strain—relaxation. Those people who become able to read at a distance of less than twelve inches are unable to read by an effort. With a vision lowered by hypermetropia at twenty feet or farther it is very easy to demonstrate that a strain to see by concentration or some other effort always increases the hypermetropia. A strain to see at the near point produces hypermetropia, while a strain to see at the distance produces myopia.

Rest when properly employed cures all forms of imperfect sight. The great difficulty is that all people are not able to rest their eyes properly.

It has been found that the tendency of most people is to concentrate or stare. Concentration or an effort to concentrate is a strain which produces almost all cases of imperfect sight. When one letter of the Snellen test card is regarded continuously, or a part of one letter of the Snellen test card is regarded, imperfect sight is produced. Trying to keep the eye immovable causes imperfect sight. The normal eye when it is at rest is always moving and sight becomes imperfect when an effort is made to imagine the letters or other objects stationary. It is not possible to keep the eye stationary without an effort. It is impossible to move the eye and keep it under a strain at the same time.

If the patient stands with his feet about one foot apart and sways the body, head, and eyes from side to side, it is possible to obtain a movement of the eyes which is a rest to the eyes and a benefit to the vision. When the sight is good continuously, the movement of the eyes is slow, short, easy, and continuous. When things are seen wrong or when the vision does not immediately improve, one can, by touching the upper lid with the forefinger lightly, feel all kinds of movements of the lid muscles and this movement affects the eye itself. The proper movement which is beneficial can only be obtained when stationary objects are imagined to be moving.

Some patients obtain benefit from moving the eyes in a circular direction because when the eyes move continuously, there is no stoppage of the swing and no opportunity to stare.

For years it has been observed that many cases of hypermetropia changed to myopia. The number of theories as to how this was brought about were numerous and not one of them would stand criticism for any length of time. One of the most important theories that was published was by Risley, who mentioned that a large number of cases of hypermetropia became changed to mixed astigmatism in which one meridian of the eyeball was more fixed than any of the others. This astigmatism was changed at first into mixed astigmatism. Later on it became a refraction of myopia. It was a very attractive theory which lost its value when it was found that no one case was observed continuously until the hypermetropia became changed to mixed astigmatism and finally myopia.

One day the physician in charge of the physiological laboratory made a tour of inspection. He asked for information or for statistics of the experimental work that was performed on a rabbit to find the cause of accommodation. He desired to know why results of experimental work on the rabbits which were 100 percent successful were not offered for publication before. He was told that these had not been published because there had not been a failure. A few days later a failure came. Electrical stimulation did not produce myopia in the rabbit with hypermetropia. Here was the failure that we had been waiting for. There was much excitement when we failed to obtain myopic refraction. However, it was found that the rabbit was born without any inferior oblique. When the function of the inferior oblique was obtained with the use of sutures, with the aid of the retinoscope myopic refraction was obtained as readily as in eyes which had nothing wrong. The director told us that when his experiments were 60 percent of the truth that they could be considered a contribution to the science of medicine and should be consequently published. The director was told about the failure and he agreed with us that the publication of the failure was a very necessary thing to do. It might have ended here perhaps but it was believed that the 100 percent of successful operations were worthy of investigation, but so far as is known no one else has performed similar experiments to determine the truth of thc results claimed.

There are some facts which ought to be emphasized. In the first place, hypermetropia is the most frequent cause of discomfort, pain, or imperfect sight. The medical men of the last century tried to prevent the harm done by hypermetropia just as they are still trying to prevent the harm that comes from nearsightedness or myopia. The younger men of today are not encouraged to work in this field when some of the authorities can stand up and say, "If I fail no one else can succeed; I know all there is to know about the eye."

There are a number of people at the present time who are studying hypermetropia, but it is not being studied as much as it should be. I believe that every school, public and private, should devote a short time frequently to the prevention and cure of imperfect sight. I am very much opposed to the practice of most ophthalmologists who fit each patient with imperfect sight with glasses which are not indicated.

For some years I have found that a large number of cases of myopia were suffering from hypermetropia which produced disagreeable symptoms. It is really surprising that so many cases of hypermetropia have been neglected. They are more readily cured than the myopic cases, but when a man at the head of a medical department of the schools tells me that it is useless to treat hypermetropia because he failed, it means that he will do all that he possibly can to injure or to interfere with the methods practiced by other men.

When studying the works of Donders forty-five years ago I was very much impressed when he gave the histories of quite a number of patients who had been cured of hypermetropia and other errors of refraction by one or more operations and by other treatment. This was an encouragement to me to keep on studying the facts which occurred in hypermetropia. I wish to state here that I feel very grateful to Donders for the many things which he taught me. That which pleased me the most and benefited me more than anything else that I learned from other doctors was his claim that there were some cases of hypermetropia and other errors of refraction which could be cured by treatment. I am sure that he did not know how voluminous were the writings on the use of glasses or the importance of wearing glasses which were written under his name. It seemed as though there were many articles on the cure of hypermetropia which were not written by him.

Hypermetropia is curable. Being curable it can also be produced, increased, diminished, or modified. If it were not curable it would be difficult or impossible to do this.

The cure of hypermetropia is very simple. When one practices in the right way, a cure is always brought about. It takes no more time to practice in the right way than the wrong way. Hypermetropia is cured by rest, and cannot be benefited by an effort. When one regards near objects or parts of a letter at the near point, hypermetropia is always increased. Practice with fine print is one of the best methods of relieving hypermetropia.

HYPERMETROPIA

By Emily A. Bates

A woman, age 63, who had been wearing glasses for twenty years decided to try the Bates Method and do without them. She called to see me for treatment while I was in the West and asked me when she first came if I would examine her eyes with the ophthalmoscope. As I was working by myself I was not permitted to use any instruments to examine the eyes, so I did my work just the same and cured my patients without examining the eyes. Some patients were advised to see an eye specialist who took care of cases where examinations were needed. This patient had had eye tests made several times by eye specialists and opticians, so I knew pretty well what her trouble was without the retinoscope or ophthalmoscope to help me.

Many cases like hers have come to me both in Clinic and in private practice and with a few exceptions I am usually right after I have tested the patient with the Snellen test card. When this patient gave me a history of her case, she told me that in the beginning when she first put on glasses, her vision for the distance was not bad, but her sight for reading and sewing was poor and her glasses only helped her for a while. Eyedrops and massage treatment were given her for the relief of eyestrain and headaches, but after a year of this treatment she had her glasses changed on the advice of her doctor. Her sight was tested again and she was told that her distance vision was impaired. Then she was advised to wear bifocals or to have two pairs of glasses with her at all times. She tried bifocals because she thought it would be much easier wearing only one pair of glasses, but she could not become accustomed to them so she tried two separate pairs of glasses.

As I listened to her explaining all this to me in her mild, soft way of talking, I could imagine how much discomfort she endured without saying very much about it, and I could well imagine how anxious she was to get rid of her glasses altogether after having tried as faithfully as she had for more than twenty years. The last glasses which were given her for close work helped her to see better at the near point, but the strain and headaches came on periodically just the same. She tried massaging the eyes, thinking that this might help. She also went to Europe and tried different climates thinking that the change of air would be of benefit to her, but the pain in the back of her neck and in back of her eyes kept on just the same and at times became worse.

She obtained Dr. Bates' book and studied it according to the advice given for her particular case. She was able to do without her glasses for the near point, but as her sight for the distance still troubled her a great deal she did not know how to go on by herself.

I began treating her by the palming method after I had tested her vision for the test card. Her vision in both eyes was the same, 10/30. When I placed the test card twenty feet away all the letters were blurred and she also had double vision when she tried to read the smaller letters.

She had traveled a great deal and liked to talk, so while she was palming, I encouraged her to tell me about a recent trip she had taken, and the memory of things which she had seen as she described them to me helped to improve her vision to 15/10 or better than normal with each eye separately. Before I tried another method I wanted to find out what caused her vision to be lowered at times and also what caused her pain and discomfort. During the course of a short conversation with her she told me of a very unpleasant experience she had had with someone whom she loved and who greatly disappointed her. I encouraged this conversation, not so much to get information from her but to have her talk about this unpleasant thing which was interesting to her but not to me because I did not know the person under discussion. The patient palmed for ten minutes and I timed her especially to find out whether her vision would be the same for the test card after she had explained her unpleasant experience while her eyes were covered. I kept the test card at the same distance as I had before and when I told her to remove her hands from her eyes and to look at the test card and read it again, she said that with the exception of the three upper lines of letters all the rest of the card was blurred.

I knew immediately that speaking of or thinking about unpleasant things was the cause of a great deal of strain. I did not tell her so right away but she was eager to explain that this was the way her vision was a great deal of the time. It was lowered at times when she suffered discomfort and pain; then at other times her vision was good without any sign of strain. She did not realize that while she was palming and explaining about her unpleasant experiences that the thought of what she was telling me caused all her trouble or a great part of it. When I finally explained it to her, she believed that I was right. I did not have her close her eyes again during her first treatment, but I placed her by the window where the sun was shining and I gave her the sun treatment while her eyes were closed, using the sun glass on her upper eyelids.

After this treatment, I told her to sway her body slightly with a short sway from side to side, glancing at the test card in my room and then as she swayed toward the window to look at a distant sign about two city squares away. At this distance she read a sign which was painted on the side of a large building. She saw all the letters clearly and read them without any hesitation whatever. This seemed a revelation to her because it was something she could not do for many years without her glasses. She kept up the sway as I directed her, but at times I had to encourage her not to stare as she looked at the test card while she swayed toward it.

She asked me to explain to her why the test card looked more clear to her at times only, so I told her to do the wrong thing, stare at the letters, for instance, as she looked at the card about ten feet away from her eyes. I also told her to look off at the distance as she looked out of the window and to stare at the distant sign which she read so easily just a few minutes before. She did this for only a few seconds when she promptly closed her eyes and asked for more sun treatment to relieve her pain. She was directed to practice parts of the method which helped her most, but only the method of treatment which I had given her and to do it as faithfully as she could every day until she was able to return for another treatment.

After a week of silence she telephoned me and notified me that she desired another treatment. She found out that she could not get along very well by herself with the treatment, so I gave her a special treatment each day for the next two weeks. Then she was asked to telephone me from time to time. Her reports were encouraging. She could read ordinary type and also fine type at the near point and she had no more trouble with her distance vision.

The year before she had come to me for treatment, she had given up in despair the driving of her car. She feared an accident when her vision would fail her for the distance and did not expect to drive her car again without having someone near to help her in time of trouble. She now drove many miles every day, she told me, and never forgot what I had advised her to do while she was driving, which was to shift from the speedometer to the center of the road and notice how the distant road in front of her car came toward her and finally rolled, as it were, under her car. Then again to shift from the speedometer to the center of the road ahead of her and to notice the same thing again and again. I explained to her that the roadside to her left and to her right would appear to move toward her and then move away from her if she would keep up the blinking and the shifting from the near point to the distance.

She called one day while I was out of town and told my secretary that she was helping others with the treatment of their eyes. She was a person who spent a great deal of time with poor people. The children near where she lived were fond of her and it was through them that she was able to benefit those who needed help. She purchased from my secretary enough material to help the young as well as the old folks. She purchased many sun glasses and taught mothers how to use the glass on the eyes of their children. This helped greatly in improving the sight of children, both for reading book type and also reading letters on the blackboard. She purchased test cards and took them to the Old Folks Home and those who believed that she could help them did as she directed them to do. She did a great deal of good work in helping elderly people to read book type and their newspapers without the use of glasses.

When I saw my patient again I gave her advice for helping various cases of imperfect sight and I was surprised to hear that she had benefited an old lady who had had cataract for many years and whose sight was failing fast. The vision of one of her eyes was nearly gone and the other eye was becoming almost as bad when my patient came to her and helped her. This old lady in time became able to take care of the more unfortunate ones in the home and to help in arranging personal things in their tiny rooms. This is indeed charitable work and much of it goes on in many places. If all patients who are benefited as this patient was would just help one other person with imperfect sight who cannot afford the treatment or who cannot find their way clear to visit an instructor of the Bates Method, much more work could be accomplished.

Better Eyesight
December 1928—Vol. XIII, No. 6

PRACTICE METHODS

Many people have asked for help in choosing the best method of treatment for their particular eye trouble. A woman age sixty complained that she had never been free of pain; pain was very decided in her eyes and head. She also had continuous pain in nearly all the nerves of the body. The long swing when practiced 100 times gave her great relief from pain. The relief was continuous without any relapse. At the same time a second woman of about the same age complained of a similar pain which, like the first patient, she had had almost continuously. She was also relieved by practicing the long swing. The long swing was practiced by other people with a satisfactory result.

It seemed that the swing was indicated for pain; it seemed to bring about better results than any other treatment. Later on, however, some patients applied for relief from pain which was not benefited by the long swing. Evidently one kind of treatment was not beneficial in every case. A man suffering from trifacial neuralgia which caused great agony in all parts of the head was not relieved at all by the long swing. Palming seemed to be more successful in bringing about relief. Furthermore, there were patients who did not obtain benefit after half an hour of palming who did obtain complete relief after palming for several hours.

Patients with cataract recovered quite promptly when some special method was tried.

The experience obtained by the use of relaxation methods in the cure of obstinate eye troubles has proved that what was good for one patient was not necessarily a benefit to other patients suffering from the same trouble, and that various methods must be tried in each case in order to determine which is the most beneficial for each particular case.

MYOPIA

By W. H. Bates, M.D.

Myopia, or nearsightedness, is usually acquired. In myopia the vision for distant objects is much less than for objects at the reading distance. Rest of the eyes and mind is the cure for myopia. Any effort to improve the vision always fails. How can people with myopia be conscious of a strain? This is a very important question. When methods are practiced in the wrong way or practiced unsuccessfully, a strain or effort to see better can usually be felt, demonstrated, or realized by touching the tips of the fingers lightly to the closed eyelids of one or both eyes.

Quite frequently it is difficult for people with imperfect sight to believe that perfect sight requires no effort and that any effort to improve the sight is wrong. It has been so habitual to strain, and the habit of straining to improve the sight, the memory, or the imagination, has been practiced so long that it requires much time and patience to stop.

Recently a schoolboy, age twelve, boasted that he could stare at one letter of a test card with his eyes wide open without blinking or closing them and for a longer time than most children could stare. He also produced a greater amount of myopia than other scholars of his school.

Mr. Priestly Smith says, "To prevent myopia we must prevent young people from using their eyes too closely and too long on near objects. This principle was established long since by the labors of Donders, Arlt, and others, and has been practically developed by Cohn and other reformers of school hygiene."

It is not true that myopia is caused by too much use of the eyes at a near point. On the contrary, near use of the eyes in a poor light lessens myopia. This fact has been demonstrated frequently with the aid of the retinoscope, while the eyes were being used too closely for long periods of time on near objects. It is difficult to understand how or why so many eminent ophthalmologists like Priestly Smith, Donders, Arlt, Cohn, and others should have neglected the aid of simultaneous retinoscopy in solving this problem.

It was a great disappointment to find in schools that although the desks and seats were mathematically correct, myopia was not prevented any more than before. In some schools iron braces adjusted to the head and face prevented the scholars from leaning forward when doing their schoolwork. Myopia was not prevented. One eye doctor, who was convinced that the braces were useless, continued to use them because he said that he did not know what else to do.

In order to measure the brightness of the light of the schoolroom the light was regulated by a photometer, invented by Professor L. W. Weber. He also invented an instrument called the stereogoniometer to measure quickly the amount of light from parts of the visible sky. Professor H. Cohn recommended that much money be devoted to the building of better schoolhouses and also recommended that the schoolrooms be properly lighted. It was a great disappointment. No more myopia was acquired in a poorly lighted schoolroom than in a well-lighted one. A great deal more might be written describing the failures of these scientific men, who finally had to admit that they had not discovered how to prevent myopia from being acquired by schoolchildren.

The treatment of myopia which I have found best is as follows: The vision of each eye is tested and the patient is then directed to sit with the eyes closed and covered with the palms of each hand in such a way as to avoid pressure on the eyeball. At the end of half an hour or longer, the patient is directed to stand with the feet about one foot apart and sway from side to side as he reads the Snellen test card at five or ten feet. When the myopia is more than 5 D, the patient may make better progress by practicing at a lesser distance than ten feet—five feet or nearer.

Some cases obtain a decided improvement in their vision in the course of about fifteen minutes. Other cases require additional methods. One of the best methods is to have the patient look directly, for five seconds, while blinking frequently, at one letter of the Snellen test card which has been committed to memory. When the eyes are closed, the memory of a known letter is usually better than when the eyes are open. By alternately regarding a letter, closing the eyes and remembering it better than with the eyes open, the vision of this letter will improve in most cases.

Those persons with a high degree of nearsightedness may not improve until the memory or the imagination of one known letter has improved to a considerable degree. It is interesting to demonstrate that the more perfectly a letter is remembered or imagined, the better becomes the sight. When a letter is remembered or imagined as well with the eyes open as with the eyes closed, a maximum amount of improvement in the vision is obtained.

Some cases are benefited after other methods have failed by teaching the patients how to make their sight worse by staring, straining, or making an effort to see. When the cause of the imperfect sight of myopia becomes known, the vision oftentimes improves to a considerable degree. When myopic patients learn by actual demonstration the cause of their trouble, it makes it possible for them to improve their sight.

Some children with myopia may be unable to stand bright light. Many doctors prescribe dark glasses for the benefit of such cases. In my experience, the wearing of dark glasses or the use of other methods to reduce the glare of strong daylight or artificial light is an injury rather than a benefit. One of the best methods to relieve or prevent the intolerance of all kinds of light is to encourage the individual to become accustomed to strong light. A convex glass of about 18 D is very useful in these cases. One way to use the glass is to have the patient look far downwards while the instructor lifts the upper lid of the eyeball with the help of the thumb. This procedure exposes a considerable amount of the sclera. The strong light of the sun is now focused on the white sclera for only short periods of time to prevent the heat produced by the strong glass from causing discomfort.

This ends the routine treatment.

For low degrees of myopia the results are usually very good. Imperfect sight without glasses has been temporarily or more permanently cured in a few visits.

One of the best treatments for a high degree of myopia is suggested by a few truths. All cases of myopia are temporarily cured by looking at a blank wall without trying to see. The retinoscope used at the same time has always demonstrated in flashes or for short periods of time that myopia was never continuous. When the best vision of fine print is obtained exactly at ten inches, the retinoscope always demonstrates under favorable conditions that the eye is not at this time myopic. But if an effort is made to see better by a strain the retinoscope demonstrates flashes of myopia. It should be emphasized that the strain which produces myopia is different from the strain which tends to produce other causes of imperfect sight.

When the memory or imagination is perfect, the retinoscope used at the same time demonstrates that myopia is absent. When a letter or other object is remembered or imagined imperfectly the sight is always imperfect and the retinoscope demonstrates that myopia has been produced.

Shifting the attention from one point to another point may be done in such a way as to rest the eyes by lessening or preventing strain. Staring or shifting with an effort always produces myopia. Moving the head and eyes from side to side produces an apparent movement of stationary letters or other objects. A complete rest of the eyes with improved vision may be obtained in this way or it may be done wrong with consequent bad results.

One of the best methods of obtaining complete relaxation of the eyes and mind is to move the ball of the thumb lightly against the ball of the forefinger in a circular direction in which the circle has a diameter of less than one-quarter of an inch. Just moving the thumb in this direction does not always succeed unless one can count one, three, five, or more odd numbers, when the motion is downwards, and an even number when the thumb moves upwards. A great amount of relaxation is always obtained by practicing the movement of the thumb against the ball of the forefinger. It is not necessary for the patient to watch the movement of the thumb in order to keep up the practice.

Many patients complain that when walking about the house, walking up and down stairs or when they are lying down, the movement of the thumb is not kept up continuously. Relaxation may be obtained by practicing the memory of the movement of the thumb and forefinger. Dizziness which is caused by strain of the eyes and mind has been relieved most successfully, continuously, or perfectly when an incentive is used. For example, many patients with symptoms of eyestrain, pain, or fatigue were encouraged to practice the movement of the thumb when it was found that at those times when the thumb was stationary, the symptoms of eyestrain became permanent or disagreeable. One patient found that when he walked up a steep flight of stairs that the movement of the thumb was forgotten. When he again practiced the movement of the thumb, all the symptoms of discomfort caused by eyestrain disappeared.

A patient told me that at one time a prominent physician of New York made a diagnosis of walking pneumonia and said that if he did not retire or go to bed and obtain complete relaxation or rest, he would most surely die. To have pneumonia at that time and to have to go to bed would have been a great inconvenience because he had many things to look after, and so he practiced the thumb and finger movement. After practicing it awhile, to his delight and the astonishment of his friends, all the symptoms of pneumonia disappeared and did not return. Having a case of walking pneumonia was a great incentive to him to practice this movement of the thumb and obtain just as much rest at his work as he would have obtained if he had gone to bed.

Another patient with a case of walking pneumonia was also suffering from a high degree of progressive myopia. The movement of the thumb, besides acting as a cure for the pneumonia, was also a great benefit to the progressive myopia from which this patient was suffering. On many occasions, while walking along the street, he would notice that the movement of the thumb had stopped—he had forgotten about it. After a while he became able to remember it almost continuously with great benefit to his progressive myopia as well as the pneumonia.

Another patient was suffering from heart disease, angina pectoris. His eyes bothered him very much and he was very much pleased to note that when the movement of the thumb had improved his heart trouble, the myopia from which he was suffering also improved. It was a problem for him to find out how to keep up this relaxation of the nerves continuously. By practicing the movement of the thumb continuously he acquired the conscious habit. Later the conscious habit became an unconscious one with benefit to his eyes and heart.

Myopia has many complications. In some cases detachment of the retina may occur suddenly without warning. Cataract, glaucoma, and other serious diseases of the eyes are often found as a complication in myopia. In glaucoma the eyeball becomes increased in hardness. The practice of relaxation methods usually relieves tension and brings about relief.

Conical cornea is a form of myopia which causes much pain and loss of vision. The cause of conical cornea is a strain or an effort to see. It can be cured by practicing the long swing or other methods of resting the eyes.

Inflammation of the iris, retina, or choroid is always benefited by the same treatment which improves or cures myopia.

The cause of myopia in schoolchildren has been discovered. Its cure is now known, and I believe that in time no child will be found wearing glasses.

CHRISTMAS—1927

By Emily A. Bates

Our office surely was a busy place last December and a large number of poor people were made happy at Christmas. There were not very many patients in our Clinic at that time, but each patient was invited to come to the Tree and bring his or her whole family along. One blind patient, a young man, who before the World War had good sight, was so grateful for the help he had received that he wanted to give and give. He had the spirit all right and even though his pockets were empty and he could not give in that way, he gave in the best way he could.

His way was to bring other blind patients from the Blind Men's Home to Dr. Bates. It never dawned on him that there was a limit to the poor souls the Doctor could treat while he was taking care of his regular practice. No one in the office had courage enough to stop him, and so they came. His enthusiasm was so great that he himself worked more earnestly than ever in his own case. Later on he wrote an interesting article in the August 1928 issue about himself and the help that he received from Dr. Bates.

After many months of steady treatment, which was given him without any charge, he became able to see again. Sightless eyes, made so by the ravages of war, again saw light after several years of darkness and no hope. Other physicians who had examined him said his sight was destroyed. This was not true, for if it were, even Dr. Bates with all his knowledge of the human eye could not have given him his sight again.

He had been gassed during the war and many operations had to be performed. All of one lung was removed. It is true that his case seemed hopeless. Operations and treatment of all kinds failed to help. The constant strain he was under, which was brought about by shell-shock and much suffering, caused depression, which could only be relieved by morphine and other drugs. After he was treated for a short time by Dr. Bates, he stopped this bad habit, but it had to be done gradually. It was pathetic to watch him struggling to do the right thing. In trying to stop using drugs he acquired the habit of smoking many cigarettes every day. In some way he was well-supplied with them all the time and preferred to smoke rather than eat. One day I talked with him for a long time and he finally promised me to smoke a smaller number of cigarettes each day. The poor fellow tried hard and won out.

His vision at the present time is 10/10. He can read diamond type at less than six inches; if the occasion warrants it, he is able to read diamond type at two inches.

The light and heat of the sun was a great factor in bringing about a better condition of his eyes, and the added sun glass treatment, focusing the sun's rays upon the eye as the lids were raised, and also using the sun glass on the closed eyelids, was a given every time he came. When there was no sun a strong light called a Thermo-lite was used for hours at a time and then the test card practice was begun. Little by little each day the blood circulation of the eyes became better and the nystagmus condition from which he was suffering also improved. For the first time the eyes looked healthy to the observer and the pupil of each eye, instead of being very small, became almost natural size. This was not accomplished in a day but in a few years time.

Many times we are asked why some patients are cured and others not. The only answer is that if the patient will practice as earnestly and as often as the Doctor advises and does not become discouraged, a better condition of the eyes and vision occurs in time. The question "How long does it take?" is asked many times. This young man of whom I write had no such question to ask. He came with the hope of getting some relief but he was not quite sure before the treatments were started. He was willing to wait, although it was hard on him and meant patience and labor on the Doctor's part. This patient had to be led when he first came to us and now he leads others who are afflicted!

I think I would know what to do with a million dollars if I had it. I would hire competent people to make a house to house canvass in the different districts of the poor of my city and I would reach the needy ones in that way. Anyway, there were a few made happy with what was contributed by Dr. Bates and those who have given to the Christmas fund. And I must not forget to extend my thanks to those who have again made it possible for us to make the poor of our Clinic and others happy this Christmas time.

Better Eyesight
January 1929—Vol. XIII, No. 7

TIME FOR PRACTICE

So many people with imperfect sight say that they have not the time to practice relaxation methods, as their time is taken up at business or in the performance of other duties. I always tell such people, however, that they have just as much time to use their eyes correctly as incorrectly.

They can imagine stationary objects to be moving opposite whenever they move their head and eyes. When the head and eyes move to the left, stationary objects should appear to move to the right, and vice versa.

They can remember to blink their eyes in the same way that the normal eye blinks unconsciously, which is frequently, rapidly, continuously, without any effort or strain, until by conscious practice, it will eventually become an unconscious habit, and one that will be of benefit to the patient.

They can remember to shift or look from one point to another continuously. When practicing shifting, it is well to move the head in the same direction as the eyes move. If the head moves to the right, the eyes should move to the right. If the head moves to the left, the eyes should move to the left. By practicing in this way, relaxation is often obtained very quickly, but if the eyes are moved to the right and at the same time the head is moved to the left, a strain on the nerves of the eyes and the nerves of the body in general is produced.

ASTIGMATISM

By W. H. Bates, M.D.

Astigmatism occurs in nearly all cases of imperfect sight for which glasses are employed to improve the vision. It is so often observed in many eyes soon after birth that many writers have stated that it is congenital and not acquired. The majority of statistics, however, show that astigmatism is usually acquired. As a general rule we may say that it always is a complication of myopia and less often of hypermetropia. In nine-tenths of the cases, the astigmatism is due to a malformation of the cornea. Some writers have published accounts of cases of astigmatism produced by organic changes in the eyeball without necessarily producing corneal astigmatism.

Astigmatism frequently is recognized to be always changing. Without interference or treatment the astigmatism may increase to a considerable degree or it may become less and even disappear altogether.

The vision in most cases of astigmatism can be improved by the use of proper glasses. However, there are some forms of astigmatism in which no glasses can be found to correct the error. In regular astigmatism, two meridians of the cornea are at right angles to each other. Astigmatism often follows inflammation of the cornea. After the inflammations and ulcerations of the cornea have healed, they may leave behind scar tissue, which by its irregular contraction produces irregular astigmatism. In such cases, glasses seldom or never improve the vision, but it has been helped by relaxation methods.

When astigmatism is present, eyestrain is usually manifest. It should be more widely published that regular astigmatism, although not benefited by proper glasses, has been improved or cured by the practice of central fixation. A perfect memory for letters and other objects is a cure for astigmatism.

Conical cornea is usually acquired. In the beginning, the astigmatism which is produced or acquired is slight. After some years, however, the conical cornea will increase to a considerable degree. The astigmatism is so irregular that no operations on the cornea to correct this malformation have succeeded. The pain caused by conical cornea may become so severe that some physicians have recommended that the eye be removed. The treatment of conical cornea with the aid of central fixation has relieved pain in many of these cases. It is not right to ignore central fixation as a cure for conical cornea. Many eye doctors have condemned the treatment without a proper investigation.

Patients who suffered from conical cornea have consulted numerous physicians to obtain relief. These physicians too often informed the patients that there was no relief known to medical science to lessen pain in severe cases and improve the vision in conical cornea. Some of these unfortunates, after obtaining the opinion of prominent physicians, have been cured by central fixation and then returned to the specialists who had previously given them a bad prognosis. In some cases I have heard that these physicians were so annoyed by the report of the cured patient that the interview was not always a pleasant experience.

The results obtained in the treatment of astigmatism of all kinds, without glasses, and by the methods I have recommended, have been very gratifying.

Some cases of irregular astigmatism suffer an unusual amount of pain in ordinary daylight. After the eyes become accustomed to the sunlight or other forms of light, the astigmatism becomes less when measured with the help of the ophthalmoscope, retinoscope, or the ophthalmometer. No matter how sensitive the eyes may be to different forms of light, gradual exposure of the eyes to the same degrees of light has benefited the patient.

In the beginning of treatment the strength of the light used should be less than will be used later on, after the eyes have become more accustomed to the strong light. It is an interesting fact that eyes which have normal vision without astigmatism seem able to stand a strong light reflected into the eyes much better than can patients whose eyes are imperfect or who have a considerable amount of astigmatism.

The treatment of astigmatism is a matter of importance because for many years no methods of treatment were at all successful. One of the most successful methods of treating astigmatism is to encourage the patient to remember, imagine, or see letters of the test card perfectly. The patients are encouraged to commit the card to memory. When letters or other objects are memorized perfectly, the astigmatism always becomes less until it disappears altogether. This is a truth to which there are no exceptions and suggests a method of treatment which should always prevent or cure imperfect sight produced by astigmatism.

With the consent of the principal of a large school in New York City, I placed a Snellen test card in all the rooms of the school. The principal asked me how I could prevent the pupils from memorizing the card. She was told that it was planned to encourage the pupils to memorize the card because letters on the Snellen test card could be remembered, imagined, or seen best after they were memorized. She was also told that the teachers could help materially in the prevention or cure of astigmatism.

The principal shrugged her shoulders and said that she would not be a party to any such foolish plan and that she would not allow any of her pupils to use the Snellen test card for any purpose whatever. She told some of her friends, however, that she was going to put the card up and encourage the children to memorize it and then prove that she knew more than the Doctor—namely that the Snellen test card memorized was of no benefit whatever in curing astigmatism. She also admitted that she did not know the first thing about astigmatism and did not want to know anything about it.

At the end of three months I called on the principal again. A friendly teacher told me that my enemy was gloating over the prospect of finding out how little most doctors knew about the eye. She seemed very glad to see me and shook hands and smiled and said that they were all ready to test the sight with the Snellen test card and find out how much good had been done by its use.

First she examined the sight of all the children and compared it with a record that she had made previously. She was not satisfied with the result and asked another teacher to test the sight of the children and report. Quite a number of teachers were present at this second examination as well as at the first and the number of visitors increased until there were more teachers than there were pupils. Everyone was anxious to know the result of the trial.

It was a shock to all the teachers who tested the sight of the children to find that the vision of every pupil had improved and many children wearing quite strong glasses for the improvement of astigmatism had read the card perfectly without glasses. My enemy was not satisfied; she thought there must have been something peculiar in my cards so she obtained some strange cards from other teachers and it did not add anything to her peace of mind to find that the vision of the children tested with the strange card was much better than when my card was used.

Some patients with astigmatism complain that when they first awaken in the morning their eyes are under a much greater strain than in the afternoon. When such cases are examined with the aid of the retinoscope during sleep, they are found to be suffering from a great strain. The strain is not always apparent; the patient does not always know when it is present. Children are sometimes great sufferers from eyestrain during sleep. Many others have been advised to watch their children during sleep and if they believe the child is straining his eyes, the child should be awakened and taken out of bed. The mother can tell that the child is suffering from eyestrain if the eyelids twitch and if different parts of the body twitch. The mother should then have the child practice the long swing for a few minutes or longer.

One man came to me suffering great pain almost constantly, which was not relieved by the use of glasses for the improvement of his astigmatism. He was told about how eyestrain during sleep can produce astigmatism, and of the symptoms of astigmatism which were pain, fatigue, and dizziness, and also how much benefit is obtained by practicing relaxation methods more or less frequently during the night.

He had no one to call him during the night, so he gave orders to a clerk in a nearby hotel that he should be called by telephone every two hours during the night. When he was awakened he would practice relaxation methods. The relief was considerable and there were mornings when he testified that he was rested and had no symptoms of eyestrain at all. It was a great comfort to him to get rid of his headaches and the agony of pain which he described as being in his eyes and had been there many years.

One patient, a boy about twelve years old, memorized the Snellen test card so that he could read the whole card of fifty-three letters in less than ten seconds. It was discovered that with the improvement in his memory, his vision for a strange card was also improved and his astigmatism became less and finally disappeared entirely.

Many people are unable to stare for any length of time because staring is painful, disagreeable, and produces fatigue. However, a boy ten years old had practiced this staring and had acquired much skill; he was able to outstare any boy or girl in his classroom. He then went to other classes and challenged each boy and girl in those classes to a contest to find out which one could outstare the other. In order to excite their antagonism he called them names, so they stood around him and attempted to outstare him, but he, being in good practice, came out the winner.

The boy's teacher noticed that after some of these staring contests, his eyes became quite inflamed, and his vision was unusually poor. His parents took him to a competent eye doctor who discovered that when he stared he produced a considerable amount of astigmatism. The doctor wanted to put glasses on him but the boy objected; he did not want glasses on because that wouldn't be fair to the others. The doctor said that if he did not get well he would have to wear glasses, so the boy made up his mind to stop staring.

Anyone who can stare and strain to an unusual degree is able to relax the strain. It is interesting to demonstrate with the aid of the retinoscope that staring may produce a very high degree of astigmatism, but always after the staring is stopped the vision improves very much and the astigmatism becomes less. In short, it is more difficult to produce astigmatism than it is to cure it.

A man, age sixty, suffering from astigmatism, had great difficulty in practicing central fixation, shifting, swinging, and the long swing. After four visits to my office he said that he had obtained no relief from his depression, his headaches, or other symptoms of astigmatism. He was advised to sit in the waiting room and try to do nothing whatever. At the end of this time his vision was tested and found to be normal. He was unable to practice relaxation methods because he made too great an effort, but when he did nothing and made no effort, his vision improved.

CHRONIC IRITIS RELIEVED BY TREATMENT

By Emily A. Bates

In Santa Monica, California, there lives a grateful patient who was cured of iritis and nearsightedness by the Bates Method during my stay in the West. He held a responsible position in one of the large banks there and he needed his sight most of all at his work. Two years previous to the time I saw him, he suffered an attack of iritis which caused much pain and discomfort most of the time. The usual drugs were used to relieve the pain but at times even these gave little relief. At the advice of some eye specialists he put on dark glasses and these enabled him to go out in the bright sunlight, something which he could not otherwise have done. Most patients who suffer from iritis cannot open their eyes at all while they are in a bright light. Dark glasses relieved the pain somewhat but they did not cure his trouble. He obtained Dr. Bates' book, *Perfect Sight Without Glasses,* and tried to apply the method by himself and then later came to me.

I wanted to be sure about the diagnosis which had to be made before I started treating him, so I sent him to an eye specialist who was taking care of my diagnostic cases. After my patient had called on this specialist for an examination of his eyes, he returned to me with the statement from the physician. It was purely a case of chronic iritis and the doctor was interested to see how the patient would get along under my care.

In March 1927, the patient paid his first visit for treatment and he came alone. His vision for the test card with the right eye was 15/40, and with the left 15/50.

The letters were blurred and indistinct and he lowered his head considerably while trying to read. When he was directed by me to hold his head straight while reading the card, his eyes closed tightly and he did not have the ability to keep them open long enough to read even one letter at a time.

I handed him the Fundamentals card and he said that at no distance, as he held the card farthest away from him and as near to his eyes as he could get it, could he read any of the type. After closing his eyes again for a short period of time he read No. 3 as he moved his body from side to side while sitting comfortably in a chair. By shifting from the white spaces on the card of the microscopic type that I gave him to the white spaces of the diamond type and then to the white spaces of the Fundamentals card, he read as far as No. 5 of the Fundamentals card.

I had a case similar to his about four years ago, a case in which it ordinarily takes from four to six weeks to cure the pain alone. This patient was entirely relieved of pain, and her sight, which formerly was not normal, became so at the same time the iritis was cured, which was inside of two weeks. She had an acute attack of iritis before I saw her, which lasted for several months. A physician friend of Dr. Bates and myself saw this case while she was under treatment and while she was still suffering intense pain. When he examined her, at my suggestion, his opinion was that she could not possibly be cured within six or eight weeks at least. After she was cured the case was reported to this doctor who was amazed at what had been done for her. This case came to my mind instantly when the patient mentioned above visited me.

I noticed that he did not sit quietly while he was palming and thought that he was not getting any benefit in that way, but when I suggested it to him, he said that he liked to keep his eyes closed but that covering his eyes with the palms of his hands seemed to bother him. He was encouraged then to keep his eyes closed for a period of half an hour while I was planning a regular routine of treatment for him.

Before he opened his eyes to read the card again, I asked him to describe parts of his daily work at the bank. It was interesting to hear him describe the difference between the notes that passed through his hands. He explained to me how a counterfeit bill is discovered by examining it carefully.

Because of the pain he had been suffering for a long time I refrained from joking in any way, which I sometimes do if the patient is agreeable. There usually comes to my mind some funny incident which occurred while treating someone and I like, if possible, to change the subject from pain to something else, especially while the patient is palming.

This patient, however, did not make me feel that way in the beginning because of his reserved manner and also because of his pain. It was quite unexpected then to have him answer me in a funny way and tell me of something which he could remember most of all and which was constantly before him while he was at work. He said it was a nice, shiny thing with a black hole at one end and he made me laugh when he said it was a revolver, which was only introduced on rare occasions when there were suspicious people a little too close to him. This was something new to me and I had not expected it. His hearty laugh was most relaxing not only to him but to me also.

I told him that my sight was apparently normal but I feared that if I came in close contact with his revolver as I came near his window, I was sure that I would become myopic or acquire a cataract or something else. As quick as a flash I asked if he had any pain and as quickly he answered me saying "No, I haven't any discomfort whatever just now."

Immediately he was told to open his eyes and to read the card, which he did without squeezing his eyelids together as he did before. His vision improved to 15/10 and he said that the letters were clear. I am anxious for those who read this not to misunderstand me. He was not cured by any means nor was his vision permanently relieved right at this time. His vision improved and his discomfort and pain were relieved because his mind was relaxed. I thought this was a good beginning for the first treatment and told him so. He agreed with me and promised to practice as I directed him to do until I could see him again.

Financial difficulties prevented him from coming to me every day, which he should have done and which would have made the cure of his eyes permanent in a much shorter time. I surprised him the next day by telephoning him and offering to help him over the telephone. I happened to call him at a busy time, so the discussion was short and took less than ten minutes of his time and mine. He wrote me a letter in a week's time telling me how much good I did him in those few moments.

As he talked to me at that time he stood before his telephone which was fastened to the wall. Just before I called him he had had an attack of pain and explained that all the window shades in the room where he was had to be drawn because the light caused so much pain. My advice was to place himself before a bright electric light as close as he could stand the heat and, with his eyes closed, move his head slowly from side to side in order that all parts of the eyes would receive the benefit from the light and heat.

I held the receiver while he did this and he soon came back to the telephone to tell me that the pain had gone and that he had raised the shades and was able to look out into the bright light from one of the windows without feeling any pain. I advised him to write down immediately the things that helped him most and to practice these things, no matter how short a time he had each day. I told him to sway his body from side to side as he held the receiver and was talking to me and to blink his eyes with the movement of his body. This gave him some relief also. From time to time I advised him by letter and also by telephone.

In May of the same year my patient came again and this time he brought his wife, asking for permission to have her watch the treatment so that she could help him at home. I was glad that he brought her because I knew when I saw her that she would be a great help to us both. The instructions I gave her at this second visit were carried out by her and by the patient during the summer months while they were vacationing in the mountains. Toward the end of the summer, they both came to visit me and the condition of my patient's eyes as well as the expression on his face indicated no more trouble. I tested his sight for fine print and he read the Fundamentals card, by W. H. Bates, M.D., through to the end, holding the card slightly farther than six inches from his eyes. His vision for the distance was also normal, 15/15 with each eye separately.

His wife had told me that at times he suffered agonies of pain during the night after he had slept for a few hours. As long as she could remember, she said, he had never slept quietly all through the night. He was troubled with nightmares and he also had insomnia for many years, and at such times he would sit up for hours and smoke his pipe in order to while away the time until daybreak. For quite a few years, Dr. Bates has been benefiting patients by having them do the long swing 100 times early in the morning and 100 times just before retiring. I remembered this and advised my patient to try it and let me know in a week's time whether he had any success with the swing or not.

Three days later I received a message over the telephone saying that since his last visit to me he had faithfully practiced the long swing 100 times in the morning and 100 times at night as I have advised. The results were good. He slept all through the night without waking up and without tossing about as he had been doing for so long a time. His wife remained awake purposely to watch the results and at other times, being a light sleeper, she would wake up to find her husband in the same position as he had placed himself before going to sleep.

My patient purchased a sun glass from me and I directed his wife how to use it on his closed eyelids as he sat in the warm sunshine on his patio. In the beginning, when I first used the glass upon his closed eyelids he resented the treatment very much and the strain he was under while the sun glass was being used caused a considerable amount of tearing of the eyes. The patient feared the outcome of such treatment, but while the condition was made worse temporarily for a short period of time, it proved to be the best treatment in permanently curing his trouble.

Every day he became more accustomed to the sun glass treatment and all during the summer while he was on his vacation, the sun treatment was given more frequently each day. A tent was used so that his body as well as his eyes could receive the sunshine. This proved to be a benefit to his general health as well. When he returned at the end of the summer, I was much surprised to see a change in the expression of his face. The sclera or the white part of each eye was as clear as mine and his eyes were wide open in a natural way.

He told me of the different things he tried each day for relaxation of the eyes and mind. His wife would read to him while his eyes were closed and he would construct mental pictures of what she was reading. At other times he would run and race with his pet dog, who could run much faster than he could and the dog would get quite a distance away from him. However, the wagging tail that he could see above the tall grass would always help him to find his pet and to run again with him. He said the wagging tail of the dog helped him to see things move opposite to the sway of his head and eyes. He said he had not realized how much of a strain he had caused his wife, who was at one time a carefree girl with a jolly disposition, but through his suffering had become a very serious person.

The gratitude of both my patient and his loyal wife was most profound and they have since then proved loyal friends to Better Eyesight. Many patients have come through them for treatment.

Better Eyesight
February 1929—Vol. XIII, No. 8

CORRESPONDENCE TREATMENT

Many letters are received from people in various parts of the world who find it impossible to come to New York and who believe that something might be done for them by correspondence treatment. I do not advocate correspondence treatment as a general rule, as the results are uncertain. There is always the possibility that the patient will not practice correctly the things which he is told to do.

If a patient has had one treatment at my office or at the office of one of my representatives, it is possible to treat that patient more intelligently through correspondence.

Some years ago a gentleman living a thousand miles from New York called and asked if anything could be done through correspondence for his wife who was bedridden and suffering with an agony of pain in her eyes. He described all her symptoms to me and gave me her last prescription for glasses. He was told that if he would take the treatment in my office, and so learn how to treat his wife, it would be possible for him to aid her intelligently when he went home. He did this and after taking several treatments, returned. He wrote me later saying that his wife was almost cured.

When my book, *Perfect Sight Without Glasses,* is read carefully, those things which are not understood may be cleared up by intelligent questions, which I am always pleased to answer. I do not consider this as regular correspondence treatment.

SQUINT

By W. H. Bates, M.D.

In squint, the right or left eye may turn in toward the nose while the other eye may be continuously straight. When the straight eye is covered with a screen, the squinting eye usually becomes straight temporarily. There are several types of squint, one of which is called divergent squint, in which one or both eyes may be turned out to a greater or lesser degree. In another type, vertical squint, either eye may be turned upwards [or downwards] while the other remains straight. In rare cases both eyes may be turned above the horizontal meridian, or the eyes may be turned below the horizontal meridian. Squint is usually acquired soon after birth, but a great many children do not squint until they are three or four years old or older. Rare cases will acquire squint when past fifty years old.

The eye which turns in different directions habitually usually has imperfect sight which is not always corrected by glasses. The vision of the squinting eye when imperfect is called amblyopia. Amblyopia means blindness without any cause which can be seen or described by the attending physician. The best treatment is to get rid of the strain which is always present. One of the early writers on squint, its treatment and cure, said that the blindness of squint was a condition in which neither the patient nor the doctor could see anything wrong with the eye.

Amblyopia is a condition of imperfect sight in which the retina, the optic nerve, and other parts of the eye show no organic change. The blindness of the squinting eye may be so great that the patient may not be able to see even daylight. These cases may develop absolute blindness with no perception of light and yet have been cured by treatment by doing away with the strain. It should be emphasized that eyestrain has been frequently found in all kinds of squint and this eyestrain is sufficient to lower the vision until even light perception is lost.

Eyestrain, which is a mental phenomenon, is capable of producing in the eyes organic changes which are sufficient to cause total blindness. By relieving the eyestrain the vision always improves until it may become normal. The men who for years have published in books or in various periodicals that the blindness of squint cannot be cured should investigate the facts by the aid of modern scientific methods, which prove that the blindness of squint is not very difficult to cure.

In searching through the literature for facts I found some very peculiar statements. One very prominent ophthalmologist published in a medical journal the statement that the blindness of squint could not be cured. In the very next sentence, he gave the history of a patient born blind with amblyopia, squint, and cataract who obtained perfect sight by treatment. The patient was forty years old. The cataract in both eyes was operated upon successfully. The patient had never seen letters and could not read a newspaper, even with small size headlines. He could see flowers of different colors but he did not know the names of any of them. He was taught the names of familiar objects that he saw and in a very short time his eyesight seemed to be normal.

The eye surgeon called attention to the fact that the imperfect sight was improved to the normal by treatment of the eyestrain. The surgeon described how the cataract was removed and how the patient became able to read by being taught by school teachers who discovered the difference in the vision of each eye. The eye which habitually turned in had very imperfect sight. The vision of one eye and later both eyes improved to the normal by eye education which relieved or cured the eyestrain. Some of the readers of this doctor's article asked him embarrassing questions and he finally stated that he now believed amblyopia could be cured by eye education. He had unconsciously practiced my method. The amblyopic eye was blind from eyestrain and vision was restored after the eyestrain was relieved by relaxation treatment.

To obtain improved vision with the good eye covered, one patient wore a patch over the eye which was straight, while the vision of the squinting eye was benefited by eye education. At the end of a few months it was found that the eye which formerly had looked straight was now turned in. At periodic intervals the right eye became straight while the left eye turned in [alternating strabismus]. After covering the good eye with a screen, the vision of the other eye became straight. It required several months before both eyes became straight at the same time and each had good vision.

In the cure of squint without operation it is important that the instructor become able to practice a few fundamentals in order that the patient may be more readily taught to do the same. In all cases of squint, double vision should be imagined at three feet, ten feet, twenty feet or farther. It often requires considerable practice before the teacher can produce double vision. The best possible vision should be obtained in each eye before much is attempted to cure the squint.

Most children can see or imagine double vision by practicing with a lighted candle or other object. In some cases two candles are imagined five feet apart when one is practicing with a candle at twenty feet. By closing the eyes and resting them, it is possible for the patient to demonstrate that two objects appear to be five feet apart by the use of the memory. Images five feet apart can be imagined to be either more or less separated.

The eyes of most people are capable of remembering, imagining, or apparently seeing two images one foot apart at twenty feet. If the objects are on the same level they can usually be controlled much better than when one is higher than the other. In a case of convergent squint it is quite easy to imagine the two objects as they should be imagined; the image of the right eye should be to the right, the image of the left eye should be to the left. When the two images are on separate levels it is well to practice so as to attain the two images on the same level. This makes it easier to control the two images in other directions.

By alternately regarding the images without effort or strain, they will approach each other until they touch, overlap or become fused into one object. Then more practice should be done with the object of obtaining control of the location. By some forms of effort the image of the right eye may be forced to the left while the image of the left eye may be forced to the right. This should be practiced for half an hour or longer, forcing the images seen by each eye to appear crossed. At first the images are not controlled; they may cross and separate a wide distance, three feet, or even six feet.

It is well to practice the production and control of the crossed images in cases of convergent squint in which the image of the squinting eye does not always reach a position on the opposite side of the image seen by the right eye. It is interesting to observe how quickly two images can be made to cross, to approach each other, to touch, and to merge into each other and form one. By practicing the production of crossed images a considerable time each day, the crossed images become consciously, habitually, or permanently merged when a cure is obtained.

A girl, age fourteen, had vision of the right eye of 3/200 while that of the left eye was 20/10. When she was two years old the tendon of the muscle which turned the right eye inwards was cut. The result was variable. Sometimes the eye turned in as before, but there were periods when the right eye was straight. Relaxation methods were employed daily with success and the squint became less when the vision improved.

The method which helped the most was to improve the vision of the amblyopic eye by remembering or imagining perfect sight of one letter of 20/10 with the eyes alternately closed and open. The vision of the right eye improved until it became 20/10. The patient was also encouraged to imagine fine print six inches from the right eye. When she succeeded in improving her vision for twenty feet and later her ability to read fine print at six inches, the squint disappeared. Both eyes focused on one point at the same time.

Central fixation, or seeing best a letter or other object regarded while all other points are seen worse, is a successful method of curing squint and improving the sight in cases of squint.

A very remarkable patient, a girl age eight, was treated more than fifteen years ago. The vision of the right eye was

2/200 while that of the left eye was 10/200. The right eye turned in most of the time. The vision of the left eye was improved without glasses by alternately resting the eyes.

An attempt was made to teach her how to see best where she was looking. She very soon acquired the ability to practice central fixation when the larger letters were regarded. The child became much interested when she realized that her eyes felt better while the vision and squint improved. She practiced central fixation on smaller letters and other objects. The strain which was manifest by the contortions of the muscles of her eyes, face, and other parts of her body disappeared. Her voice became more musical with the improvement of her vision and the subsidence of the squint.

It was remarkable how well she became able to practice central fixation on very small letters and other objects. She would hold a glass slide on which a small drop of blood was mounted and claim that she saw the red cells, the white cells, and other minute particles with her right eye while the glass slide was pressed against her eyelashes. She was able to read each letter and period in photographic reductions of the Bible, by central fixation.

Many people have complained that they could not see black or imagine a black period for an appreciable length of time. This patient, when palming, stated that black was seen and that with the aid of central fixation even the smallest black periods were seen but they were always moving a distance nearly equal to the width of the period. An effort to see always failed. By central fixation, distant objects were seen as far off as it was possible to imagine them.

This patient was able to produce at will, consciously and continuously, internal squint of the right eye with the left eye straight or could keep the right eye straight while the left eye turned in.

DON'T BE AFRAID

By Emily A. Bates

I have heard many patients who came for first treatment say "I am afraid." This remark is usually made when we suggest that the patient should stop wearing glasses immediately in order to receive a permanent benefit. I have known of patients who only had a minor defect of vision who were uncomfortable at work unless they wore their glasses. Those who have worn glasses for just a few years and received little or no benefit while wearing them would go to many doctors with the hope that they would obtain the proper eyeglasses which would relieve them of their tension and pain.

Most of our cases are chronic and they appeal to Dr. Bates or to me to help them when all others have failed. I hope to be able to reach such cases through this article, and if what I am trying to explain will be of just a little help, it will be worthwhile.

A patient came to us recently who had traveled three thousand miles to see the Doctor, but when he was told that he could not possibly be helped unless he removed his glasses at once and did not wear them again, he became panic stricken and wept. The Doctor is at a loss sometimes when such things happen and he usually appeals to me for assistance. Encouragement is not always enough for a stranger who comes to us not feeling at all sure that he is in the right place, even if he has been well recommended. He wants facts and he wants to meet others who have gone through the same ordeal that he is expected to go through.

Fortunately there was a patient in the next room who overheard the conversation I had with this man. He came to the door of our room and asked if he might talk to this patient and tell him of his own experiences. He explained how he had traveled many miles to see what Dr. Bates could do for him. He had worn glasses many years and they helped him for some time, but even with glasses on his vision became worse for the near point. He did not need glasses at all for the distance but at the near point he was unable to distinguish large objects clearly enough to know what they were.

When our new patient first met Dr. Bates, who in his quiet way started right in to treat him, there was a fear in his heart that he had perhaps made a mistake in coming. He wanted things explained to him. He was afraid that sooner or later his vision, even for the distance, would become impaired and that in time blindness would surely overcome him. He was afraid. The older patient explained to this man how Dr. Bates had kept him for two hours in his office during the first visit and how, after he left the office, he was able temporarily to read finer print than newspaper or book type. He wanted to save time and expense and did not come again for several days, which was a big mistake, and he realized that it was.

He could not practice so well at home by himself and he became discouraged and put on his glasses again. When he called for another appointment he had to go right back to where he started from. He had wasted two precious hours and the fee besides because he had been afraid. During the second treatment, however, he was able to read finer print with less difficulty that he had during his first treatment. This encouraged him very much. This time he made no promises to the Doctor that he would not wear his glasses, but he was determined that he would not. He explained to our new patient how some days he could not practice as successfully as he could on previous days, but he kept right on remembering what the Doctor had directed him to do and he did it. Two weeks of daily treatment have given him almost normal vision. All he needs now is a little more knowledge of what he has to do when a relapse comes and then he will be rid of glasses for all time. This talk with the other patient helped Dr. Bates to manage his new case more easily and with more confidence in the Doctor, I feel sure that the patient will win out.

Not long ago I had a patient who came from Chicago to be relieved of a swelling eyelid condition and a burning of the eyes whenever she read for an hour or longer, or when she did a little sewing of any kind. Even threading a needle was painful to her with her glasses on. She had received treatment from one of our students in Chicago with some benefit. She assured us that her lack of complete success was not the student's fault, but her own in not understanding just what to do first for the relief of pain and discomfort.

After Dr. Bates had examined her eyes with the ophthalmoscope he found that her condition was mostly mental; she strained hard to see the print of the book or newspaper she was reading.

All proof readers or those who are obliged to read in a poor light can read without strain if they do not stare at the print. Public speakers often make mistakes in reading to an audience, even if they have beforehand studied the subject of their paper so well that they could almost say it by heart. They become unable to memorize and become mixed up in what they are saying or reading because they unconsciously stare at the print in order to read it, mostly because they are afraid they may make a mistake.

A few months ago a mother brought her daughter from high school where they had noticed that she was squeezing her eyes almost shut in order to see the writing on the blackboard. It is unusual to see a young girl sixteen years old with many wrinkles in her forehead. It was so noticeable to others that she was soon made unhappy because of this. The authorities at the school that she attends notified the mother that her eyes must be examined for glasses. Neither her grandparents nor her mother or father had ever worn glasses and it was a shock to the mother to think that the daughter would have to wear them. The girl became depressed and unhappy and felt, as did her mother, that there must be some way in which to relieve her trouble so that she would not have to wear glasses.

As Dr. Bates has so little time to explain the reason why, he often calls upon me to do the talking if it is necessary, or even when it is not necessary. I thought I had convinced the mother that her daughter would not have any more trouble with her eyes if she would learn to do what we had told her, and that if she would practice every day the treatment we would outline for her while at school and in her home, she would enjoy good sight and not need her glasses. I was much surprised when the mother answered me like this:

"How can you possibly understand the discomfort that patients have who need glasses or who ought to wear them when you have never had imperfect sight yourself?"

[Emily A. Bates' own improvement follows; see also "Discarding Glasses Not Injurious" in the September 1929 issue.—TRQ]

I forgot myself and laughed at the remark and then I explained to the mother how for thirteen years I had worn glasses to do my work. When it was first noticed that my eyes were not functioning correctly and that I was making mistakes in my work, which was matching colors and combining them, my employer suggested that I should be examined for glasses. He explained to me that the mistakes were minor ones but that from day to day I would perhaps make more serious mistakes and I would lose my position.

That was a shock to me, and immediately I went to the New York Eye and Ear Infirmary, where I was placed in a dark room after drops had been applied in each eye. I explained to this mother how I had been forgotten and left in that dark room much longer than was necessary and it seemed hours to me. The thoughts that went through my mind were mostly fearful ones. I was afraid that my eyes were going back on me. The doctors at the infirmary did not explain a thing to me before they gave me the drops.

The eyeglasses which were fitted for my eyes suited me very well for two years and then my eyes began to trouble me more than ever and the glasses had to be changed. I did not go in the Eye Infirmary the second time but I went to an optometrist who had the most elaborate apparatus I ever saw for examining the eyes. After an hour of much fussing on his part I was given glasses which did not at first suit my eyes. I tried them for two weeks or a little longer, I believe, and then I went back to him and complained that they did not suit my eyes.

"Oh," said he, "'you must get accustomed to the glasses; your eyes will sooner or later be adjusted to them."

Receiving no further encouragement or help, I tried again for a short time, always afraid when I was crossing the street that I would have an accident, because before I reached the curb I thought I was there and would step up. At other times I reached the curb sooner than I thought I would and I stumbled a few times and almost fell.

I returned to the optometrist and demanded a different lens which he gave me and this I wore until I came to Dr. Bates as a patient nineteen years ago. I was skeptical, too, just as some of our patients are when they first come to us for help. That is why I try to understand a new patient and to give him the encouragement and advice that he needs as soon as it is possible to do so.

What a blessing it was for me to meet Dr. Bates and to be relieved entirely of my eye trouble in six weeks' time. When Dr. Bates first examined my eyes, the letters of the test card up to the 30-line were clear and black. The next three lines I could not distinguish clearly, and every letter had a tail which bothered me very much. He did not spend very much time with me because he said I was an easy case to cure and advised me what to do at home.

I did exactly as some of our patients do now. I did the wrong thing, but one thing I did not do was to put my glasses on again. I put them back in their case and placed them in the back of my bureau drawer where they remained until sometime later when I displayed them to my friends very much as I would an antique or a curiosity.

Some of my friends did not like to see me without glasses and told me so. I did not look so well without them, they said. Others said I would surely make my eyesight worse by not wearing them, while still others said that I may have been able to do without glasses at any time, and that perhaps I did not have to wear them. Of course, these remarks were not always encouraging, but just the same I believed in Dr. Bates and was determined to win out. After the fourth treatment I had more confidence in the Doctor and I made progress from then on, although there were days when I had sudden relapses and became somewhat discouraged. He often said this to me, "If you are not afraid, you will obtain normal vision, but fear makes you strain; don't forget that."

This mother was grateful for what I had told her of my experience and we began to treat her daughter with unusual success during her first visit. She went back to school and returned in a few weeks' time for more treatment and the first thing I noticed was that the wrinkles had vanished. Various test cards were given her so that she would not tire of the practice at school and at home. A few months after her first visit to us she was pronounced cured. Her vision, which in the beginning was about half of the normal, and her sight for the near point had both improved to normal. It did not matter to her what size type she was asked to read or how close she held it. She could read it just as well at any distance. With the familiar test card and strange cards she became able to read 15/10 with each eye. She wrote us a letter of gratitude which encouraged us greatly.

What applies to the eyes also applies to the mind and other parts of the body. Fear causes great suffering and often impairs the mind permanently. Relaxation and rest of the mind can only be obtained when we stop making an effort. With more faith in those who are trying to help us, whether it is mentally, physically, spiritually, or otherwise, we help to remove all fear of what might happen to us. It is not the thing that has happened that causes one to be afraid, but it is the unknown that frightens us.

Better Eyesight
March 1929—Vol. XIII, No. 9

THE PERIOD

Many people have difficulty in obtaining a mental picture of a small black period. They may try to see it by an effort which always fails. They may persist in their efforts to see or remember it, paying little or no attention to their failures or the cause of their failures. As long as they continue to strain by trying to see, they will always fail; the period becomes more indistinct.

A small black period is very readily seen. There is no letter, no figure, no object of any kind which can be obtained more easily. Demonstrate that an effort to see a small black period by staring, concentrating, or trying to see, always makes it worse. Rest, relaxation, the swing, shifting, are all a great help. Practice with a large black letter. Imagine that the upper right corner has a small black period. Do the same with other parts of the large letter. This practice will enable you to understand central fixation, seeing best where you are looking. Central fixation can always be demonstrated when the sight is good. When the sight is poor or imperfect, central fixation is absent.

The benefits which can be obtained from the use of the period are very numerous. A perfect memory can only be obtained when the sight is perfect. A perfect imagination can only be obtained when the sight and the memory are perfect. The period is the smallest letter or other object which is perfect or becomes perfect by perfect memory or perfect imagination.

SYMPATHETIC OPHTHALMIA

By W. H. Bates, M.D.

I have been asked by the readers of this magazine what "sympathetic ophthalmia" really is. Many definitions of sympathetic ophthalmia have been given in my book and other publications. I will try, if I can, to explain it again in still simpler language. In sympathetic ophthalmia, the eyeball is soft when pressed lightly by the fingers of the attending physician. It is a serious symptom and unless it is corrected by treatment is followed by loss of sight. The reduced tension of the eyeball is usually due to an inflammation of the ciliary body—cyclitis—with loss of function.

The function of the ciliary body is to supply fluids to the inside of the eyeball. When its function is modified, lessened, with less fluid excreted, the tension or hardness of the eyeball naturally becomes less. It is also a truth that when the ciliary body supplies more fluid to the inside of the eyeball than usual, the tension of the eyeball is increased with the symptoms of glaucoma. In sympathetic ophthalmia, the activity of the glands of the ciliary body may be variable. For example, the increased tension of the eyeball may be due to an increased amount of fluid secreted by the ciliary body, while in other cases the amount of fluid secreted may be less than normal and the eyeball may be softer than it should be. The stimuli which regulate the activity of the ciliary body are variable. The mind controls the symptoms of strain.

When one eye is injured by a blow or by a foreign body lodged inside the globe, the other eye, from sympathy, becomes inflamed and diseased with loss of vision.

After the foreign body is removed one naturally expects benefit or complete recovery of both eyes. This rarely occurs. In a large percentage of cases the injured eye may heal and regain good vision, while the other eye may acquire a severe inflammation and become blind. When there is a doubt in the mind of the attending physician whether to remove the foreign body or not, the opinion of the patient may be valuable. If an eye containing a foreign body is removed, it is less dangerous to the other eye, which may heal more quickly. It is well to keep in mind that it is dangerous to practice a waiting policy because one or both eyes may be lost from neglect. If the patient travels long distances he is likely to have trouble with one or both eyes. Soldiers, sailors, engineers, conductors, forest rangers, or others occupied without supervision may be attacked at times or in places where no help can be obtained promptly. These people, for their own safety, are justified in having the eye with its foreign body immediately removed. It is far better to have the use of one eye than to be blinded in both.

For more than forty years I have been an eye surgeon and have removed injured eyes which contained foreign bodies which were not removable by an operation. It is only within recent years that I have been unable to operate because of a serious tubercular inflammation of my right elbow. Therefore when such cases come to me, I immediately refer them to other eye surgeons for proper surgical treatment.

In many cases, patients with sympathetic ophthalmia are usually affected periodically—not continuously. Sometimes the affected eye will have relapses quite frequently. The prevention of relapses is often very difficult. A continuous memory of the optical swing can be demonstrated to be of great benefit.

One of the most difficult conditions to relieve is cyclitis in which the affected eye has become soft. In these cases the ciliary body has atrophied, which is followed by loss of the fluids of the eye. It is difficult, very difficult, in such cases, even with conditions most favorable, to bring about a sufficient amount of relaxation to promote a continuous flow of the normal fluids of the eye.

HYPERMETROPIA

By Emily A. Bates

Two cases of hypermetropia were being treated by me at the same time, and both had to be treated in a different way to obtain permanent benefit. The patients were man and wife and both were over fifty years old. Such cases as these sometimes require many hours of study in order to relieve the symptoms of imperfect sight. These patients had trouble in reading at the near point and both suffered a great deal of pain which glasses did not relieve.

The man had worn glasses many years and for a time they helped him in his work. He had always been employed in some piano factory and did good work until he became ill with Bright's disease. After he returned to his work again, he found that his eyesight was impaired. His eyes were examined by an eye specialist of good standing and he was told that the Bright's disease had affected his eyesight. After some treatment by this doctor who instilled some eyedrops, his sight was improved. Some years later he had a relapse and he called on another doctor who prescribed glasses. These glasses did not do him any good. He was examined by another doctor who prescribed glasses that helped him for some time, when he noticed the sclera or white parts of his eyes were bloodshot. He thought it was just a cold that had settled in his eyes but later the redness in his eyes increased and the watery condition alarmed him, so he came to me.

I tested his sight with the test cards and found the vision of each eye was impaired. His vision was 15/40 with each eye and he stared at every letter that he read.

His wife who was with him drew his attention to this fact of which he was previously ignorant. The patient noticed that while he was reading, the watery condition increased. His sight was first tested with a white card with black letters and later with a black card with white letters. He read equally well with both cards, but the black card was more comfortable, so this one was given him to practice with at home.

We have small test cards which are similar to the large ones, for the benefit of patients who are very nearsighted or have diseases of the eyes which prevent them from reading the large card at the distance. I gave him one of these small black cards with white letters, which was exactly the same as the larger card on the wall fifteen feet away, to hold in his hand. By reading the two cards alternately, his vision improved to 15/20; the redness of the white parts of his eyes was decidedly less and the patient volunteered the statement that he had not felt so comfortable in a long time. I wanted to see if he could do as well with fine print and all he could read was sentence No. 2 of the Fundamentals card. By closing his eyes frequently and remembering the white spaces between the lines of type, he became able to read No. 5 in less than fifteen minutes' time. I gave him the sun treatment using my sun glass rapidly on his closed eyelids and advised his wife to do the same thing every day for him and to be sure that he did not open his eyes while the treatment was being given.

A month later the sclera or white parts of the eyes were no longer bloodshot and his vision for the black test card was 10/10. He boasted about his being able to read all of the fine print of the Fundamentals card but he remarked, "Oh, that was nothing at all; I became able to read that fine print in less than a day."

His wife, who also had hypermetropia, told me that at times with her glasses on she could see at a distance with no discomfort or pain, but at other times distant objects were very much blurred and seemed more distorted the more she tried to correct the trouble. For instance, a flagpole less than two hundred feet away would wriggle like a snake and there would appear to be two instead of one. She always used glasses while sewing and if the material had stripes or checks, the pattern appeared to come up toward her eyes, which frightened her and made her uncomfortable. She tried a new pair of glasses—bifocals—but she could not become accustomed to wearing them. She then decided to come to me for help.

When the examination was made, cataract was seen in her right eye and I told her about it, but quickly explained how it would disappear by the treatment I would give her. It was a shock to her, no doubt, to learn that she had a cataract but she wanted to know the truth and I could not conceal it. Her vision when tested was 6/200 with the right eye and 10/200 with the left and all the letters were blurred.

Palming helped her, and with her good memory for colors and works of art while palming, the vision with her right eye which had cataract improved temporarily to 10/100 in less than an hour and her left eye to 10/40. The dear woman did not worry about the cataract after that. When she found that her sight could be improved in such a short time she did not need much encouragement to practice. She did as I told her to do and in four months' time she had no sign of a cataract. She could see distant objects clearly at all times if she practiced shifting from an object near by to the distance, remembering always to blink her eyes, which she had failed to do before she began treatment.

If she had any trouble in threading a needle she would hold the needle where there was a background, close her eyes for part of a minute, remembering a small letter "o" while her eyes were closed and this would help her to thread the needle without delay or trouble.

The oculist who gave her the bifocals had been an old friend for years and he doubted very much that the Bates Method could give her a permanent relief because he knew she had incipient cataract of her right eye but feared to tell her about it. He believes now that the Bates Method cured her. I hope in the near future he will become a student of Dr. Bates and stop prescribing eyeglasses, especially for those who do not like to wear them.

CASE REPORTS

By Edith Reid

Editor's Note—*The following are reports of cases treated by Edith Reid and Ian Jardine, Dr. Bates' representatives in Johannesburg, South Africa.*

Squint is a very ugly disfigurement, especially when seen behind glasses. A girl of eighteen had been given glasses when she was three on account of a squint in the left eye. At eighteen the eye was straight, but she was almost totally blind in that eye and suffered from severe headaches. After a few weeks' practice of the Bates Method her headaches were relieved and the sight of the bad eye was about one-half of normal.

Most cases of squint are caused by strain and if the strain can be removed, the squint will disappear. A little boy of six, who had worn glasses for three years and was told that when he was eight he would have to be operated on to have the eye straightened, was able to picture with his eyes closed a white cloud drifting across a blue sky. When he opened his eyes, still remembering this mental picture, his eyes were straight. Having his eyes open and imagining that his dog was in the room with him immediately straightened the squint. He has now reached the stage where he can make his eyes straight at will. He is reminded to do so, both at home and at school, as soon as the eye turns, with the result that after five months his eye is straight practically all day. His was a very bad squint, the one eye being hardly visible and with glasses the vision was 10/15. Today he reads 20/10 easily without glasses and with eyes straight.

Another little fellow of four who was also threatened with an operation for squint and who had worn glasses for some time had his eyes straightened temporarily by having his head moved from side to side. His mother, who followed the whole proceedings, nearly had hysterics when I took her son's head between my hands and moved it from side to side. When I stopped, his eyes were straight for nearly five minutes, but he strained again and the right eye ran in almost under his nose. Again I moved his head and again the eyes were straight. The mother was most amused and excited to see his eye being apparently shaken straight just as one would with a doll's eye which had gotten out of place. After this had been repeated a few times I asked him more jokingly than seriously what he would do at home to straighten his eye when it went crooked. "I'll do this," he said, moving his head from side to side, and sure enough the eyes were straight again. This was kept up at home and now the little chap squints only occasionally when he is very tired or angry.

It is rather wonderful to think that so small a thing as moving the head from side to side could straighten a crossed eye when so many eye specialists were able to suggest only glasses or an operation.

A man thirty-eight years old, whose eyes and health were in a very bad way, visited us on the 21st of October 1927. He told us that he had been under chloroform 21 times and had had a series of injections for his eyes lasting 18 months; these at the instigation of three eye specialists in South Africa. As a result of the injections, he was compelled to go to bed every day at 12 o'clock, tired out, and every weekend was also spent in bed. He received no benefit. His eyes were so bad that even glasses could not be given him. The right eye, slightly crossed, was blind with cataract and the left eye had been bad all his life. The doctors said that the optic nerve was diseased. His test showed 10/70 and No. 4 on the Fundamentals card.

He was a printer by trade and had to have everything read to him. Also, he took on an average of two aspirin tablets every day to try to relieve his constant headaches. He was taught to palm, swing, and to sun his eyes, all of which he has practiced regularly ever since. He was told to blink all day long and to keep his eyes moving, never to stare or look hard at anything, and when he himself moved to notice the apparent movement of the stationary objects about him. All this he has practiced most assiduously with the result that on February 6, 1928, he was able to read books for himself, sometimes even the newspaper, and was able to do all his own work without the aid of a "reader." With his blind eye he read the big "C" of the card one foot away.

Today he rides a bicycle about the city, plays tennis, and is able to thoroughly enjoy himself because of his better health and freedom from headaches. He is a strong upholder of Dr. Bates' method and never tires of telling others of the wonderful results he has obtained in his own case. His wife and two children have also benefited by the help he was able to give them.

After reading the above, the patient asked if he might add something and if he might attach his signature to it. This is what he wrote:

"The left eye has been bad from the age of about seven years and I was under the best men in Melbourne, Australia, on and off until the age of 18 years, and they all told me nothing could be done for the left eye, the one I now read with. I have read the above and every word is true. I can never thank Ms. Reid and Mr. Jardine for what they have done for me, and are still doing. I have hardly had a headache for the last twelve months and I no longer take aspirin. My average weight is now 150 pounds; before coming here it used to be 130-135 pounds.

Yours with thanks for the Bates Method.

(Signed) Geo. H. Bowden."

One day in January a little boy was led to the office by his mother. He had pink eyes, white hair, a very white face, and even his lips were pale. Both eyes had squint. He was almost blind and had severe nystagmus. His mother was heartbroken and told of how she had worked her passage from South Africa to London so as to see what could be done for the little chap. Specialists had declared his case hopeless and had said that nothing could possibly be done.

She also took him to several hospitals, always hoping that he would be able to find some doctor who could offer a little hope, but every doctor who looked at the little fellow pronounced his case hopeless. She had to come back to South Africa as it was her home and her husband was there. She returned feeling thoroughly sad and miserable. She was told of Dr. Bates' method by a friend who had benefited greatly by it, so she came, hoping something could be done for her son. We immediately taught him how to sun his eyes and asked his mother to see that it was done two or three times daily. He was also shown how to rest his eyes by palming. He was a very bright, intelligent child which made it very easy to teach him; he understood and appeared to grasp all we said to him. Both mother and child left the office very happy and full of hope. He was not able to read, so he was given a book of pictures of animals.

At his next visit, which was three days later, he came in with the book under his arm and declared that he was feeling much better and that he was going to get quite well. After that he was brought every day to get the sun glass treatment and each day there was a marked improvement in the eyes. They were turning from pink to blue; the blue came in patches which each day appeared to be spreading until the eyes became a beautiful blue. He was being taught his alphabet so that he was able to practice with the Snellen test card which proved that his sight was improving wonderfully. The squint and the nystagmus had also improved very much.

Better Eyesight
April 1929—Vol. XIII, No. 10

BLINKING

Blinking is one of the best methods that may be employed to obtain relaxation or rest. When rest is obtained by blinking the vision is improved, not only for one letter or part of one letter, but for all the letters of a page which may be seen some parts best, other parts not so well. This is called central fixation and one cannot see anything clearly without it. In order to maintain central fixation there should be continuous opening and closing of the eyes by blinking which makes it easier for the vision to improve. When the eye discontinues to blink, it usually stares, strains, and tries to see. Blinking is beneficial only when practiced in the right way.

What is the right way? The question may be answered almost as briefly as it is asked. Blinking when done properly is slow, short, and easy. One may open and close the eyes an innumerable number of times in one second, and do so unconsciously.

Lord Macaulay was able to read a page of print in one second, and blinked for every letter. In order to read perfectly he had to see each side of every letter by central fixation. We know that he acquired or had a perfect memory because it was only with a perfect memory that he could recite the pages of any book which he had read many years before.

A casual observer would not be able to determine the number of times Lord Macaulay blinked, as it was done so quickly and easily without any effort on his part. While most of us will not be able to blink without effort as frequently as Lord Macaulay did, it is well to practice his methods as well as we can. Those with imperfect sight who do not blink sufficiently should watch someone with normal eyes blink unconsciously and then imitate him.

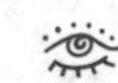

ILLUSIONS

By W. H. Bates, M.D.

Many people who know little or nothing about physiological optics have the habit of criticizing adversely anyone who has the courage, or who is foolish enough, to announce discoveries which do not meet with the favor of people who theorize. In order to bring about quick and lasting cures of myopia, hypermetropia, astigmatism, and many other causes of imperfect sight, one needs to know a great deal about illusions.

Many years ago a student of the eye, a man of great authority, after studying the illusions of perfect sight and comparing these illusions with those of imperfect sight, was very much upset because the more facts he obtained, the greater became the illusions. He finally made the statement that "seeing is deceiving." By this he meant that no one could understand the physiology of the eye without going to a great deal of trouble to prove that somebody else was deceiving the scientific world. He admitted that he was very much discouraged himself by the large number of illusions which were imagined or seen. To correct most diseases of the eyes it is absolutely necessary that one should learn by repeated experimental work something about illusions. Unfortunately for the rest of us, this man was persecuted by his friends to such an extent that it ceased to be a joke and became a matter of great importance. It was hard for him even with all his "backbone," which was considerable, to keep on studying illusions when these studies were so very unpopular.

It may be a shock to some people who have not studied the illusions of vision to find that imperfect sight is difficult. In fact it is so difficult that the majority of people in this world dodge the illusions of imperfect sight because these illusions are usually so disagreeable or painful. Perfect sight can only be obtained easily without staring or straining to see. When the eye is normal, any effort to improve it always makes it worse.

It has been proven over and over again that with perfect sight the eyes are completely at rest. The movement that they always have is necessary in order to prevent the stare and other efforts to see which are difficult, painful, disagreeable, and cause fatigue. But when the eye with normal sight is permitted to move sufficiently to prevent the stare or the strain, the head and eyes do not make any effort. To make an effort requires that the eye should be kept stationary. When the eye stares, it is always stationary; when the eye stares, it is always trying to be immovable unconsciously. The stare is only possible when a mental effort is made, consciously or unconsciously, to imagine that everything is stationary.

The normal movements of the eyes are passive. As soon as they become active and the eye is made to move by a strain, or stare, then the movement of the eye is no longer passive, it is active and it is this active movement of the eyes done consciously or even unconsciously which causes so much trouble.

This question is often asked, "What is the evidence that the normal eye is permitted to stare and strain unconsciously?" This is the answer. Many people can stare or strain as much during sleep as when they are awake. If the active strain is practiced, a patient may awake in the morning with pain in the eyes, head or in other parts of the body or they may feel a sense of great fatigue. The vision is always worse. When the passive movement of the eyes occurs, the movement may be imagined passively. The active movement requires the stare, strain, or an effort to remember, imagine, or see. This can often be recognized in myopia. The retinoscope is a great help in discovering the active swinging of the eyes. When the patient is asleep and straining the eyes unconsciously, the stare or strain is recognized with the aid of the retinoscope.

Negative Afterimages. When a person with good sight regards a white Snellen test card which has black letters and does so with his eyes open, he may see the truth that the white card appears white and the black letters appear black. When the eyes are closed an illusion is sometimes evident: the white card when remembered appears black and the black letters appear white. This illusion is promptly corrected with the aid of central fixation. One patient, a teacher of mental science, was able to see a white pillow perfectly white with his eyes open, but when he closed his eyes an illusion was seen or imagined at once—the white pillow appeared to turn into a black one. This was a great surprise to the professor. The illusion was prevented when the eyes were closed, remembering or imagining each part in turn of the pillow best. He was then recommended to see two corners at the same time. The illusion returned, but it required a strain in order to bring it back.

The patient's memory was improved by practicing central fixation with the eyes closed, seeing, imagining, or remembering one corner of a pillow at a time best and the rest of it worse. It was all done so quickly that the patient was not able quickly to remember, imagine, or see by central fixation. When he became able to produce the illusion or to prevent the illusion, his memory, imagination, and sight were very much improved.

He had worn glasses for the relief of headache for more than fifty years. It was a new and pleasant sensation for him to discard his glasses without suffering, as he had previously, with frightful headaches. The correction of various illusions of the sight are one of the best methods we have for the cure of imperfect sight without the use of glasses. If we correct the illusion, the eyesight may be improved.

One time I happened to be in the office of a well-known professor of astronomy. With me was a high schoolgirl, one of my patients, who wanted to learn something about astronomy. The professor asked us what we would like to see and with the naked eye I looked up toward the center of the sky where one could see the moon about the size of a nickel. I spoke to the professor and told him that I had so often seen the moon appear as big as a house and instead of being a dull gray it was usually a fiery red. I told him that I would be very much obliged if he would explain to me why the moon looked so much larger on the horizon than it did overhead. The professor said that there was a change in the density of the atmosphere when the moon was viewed low down on the horizon, which was entirely different from the air overhead. This, of course, is an illusion, not of imperfect sight, but of perfect sight, caused by conditions over which we have no control.

A man interested in the illusions of imperfect sight reported the following facts. One morning when he entered the bathroom he was surprised to observe that the tiles composing the floor had changed their colors. All the blue tiles had become pink and all the pink tiles had changed to blue. The illusion was very vivid. "What can I do" he asked, "to prevent this illusion, because it is maintained with a strain or effort to see which lowers my vision?" He was advised to practice central fixation which prevented or relieved the illusion very promptly.

Illusions are not harmless, as many people may think. They are always one cause of pain with imperfect sight. It is interesting to observe that when an illusion causes imperfect sight it also causes the stare, strain to see, or an imperfect memory (imagination) with poor vision. Illusions which are beneficial do not cause pain, dizziness, fatigue, or any discomfort whatever. Beneficial illusions always improve the sight. For example: The thin white line below the bottom of a line of letters is an illusion because there is no white line there. When it can be imagined, the vision is improved and this illusion is so important, even necessary, that one cannot read small letters or the newspaper unless the thin white line is imagined. The thin white line helps to improve the imagination of the black letters so that they can be read in a dim light.

The same man described the illusions he had when a headache bothered him in the morning soon after opening his eyes. In one illusion there seemed to be a thin white transparent curtain floating up to the ceiling and then slowly dropping downwards toward the bed. It surprised him very much to observe that when the illusion of the floating curtain was manifestly at its height that the headaches became worse and a severe pain was felt in his eyes, head, and in other parts of the body. The illusion lasted about fifteen minutes and slowly disappeared. In this case also, central fixation was a great help in correcting or preventing the illusion.

A well-known surgeon of the city of New York came to me for treatment of illusions. He had so many of them that the available space of this magazine is too small to describe them all. Among his many illusions was the fact that at irregular intervals while walking along the street, he would suddenly become totally blind and unable to see the light of the sun. The blindness would continue for about a minute, usually less. The frequency of these attacks increased.

In the beginning he had three or four in a week, but after some months he had a partial or complete attack of blindness more frequently. The attacks made him very despondent; he was afraid that he might have one in the midst of a surgical operation.

While he was being treated, an illusion of double vision became almost constant and interfered very much with his vision for the Snellen test card. The illusions of double vision were corrected by teaching him how consciously to produce them rapidly and in any form. That is to say, he could imagine two lights, one directly above the other, at an angle of 90 degrees, or when he strained sufficiently the two lights would be seen on a horizontal plane. With the help of the stare, strain, or trying to see better, he saw the two images at an angle of 45 degrees, 60 degrees, or 75 degrees. In short, he became able, after some instruction, to produce double images close together or double images farther apart and at any angle he desired. During the many months of treatment he demonstrated without knowing himself that he was able to produce illusions at will. Furthermore, he was able to produce illusions which lowered his vision and illusions which improved his sight. To produce double images, one above the other, he looked at a light about ten feet away and strained to see a small letter just below it at an angle of 90 degrees. To obtain double vision at an angle of 90 degrees required an effort.

I called this doctor's attention to the fact that in order to produce an illusion of letters of the Snellen test card or to produce double vision required a stare or strain. I asked him this question, "Would you like to learn how to produce double vision of the Snellen test card?" He answered, "I do not see how you can do it, but the matter is so interesting I am willing that you should produce or show me how to produce double vision." He was taught how to produce double vision consciously and this pleased him very much.

He finally came to me less frequently than every day. Eventually he became able, with the help of central fixation and other methods, to obtain his previous normal vision. When war was declared between Germany and France he enlisted in the medical department of the French Army; he never had a single relapse; he knew the cause of his double vision and how it was produced and was therefore able to avoid it.

MENTAL STRAIN

By Emily A. Bates

Children who are nearsighted are suffering from a mental strain. Children who are crossed eye are also suffering from mental strain. Eyes that have been injured, as by a foreign body entering the inside of the eyeball, even after it has been removed, may be responsible for a mental strain. This strain is different from that caused by nearsightedness or crossed eyes.

Mental strain is only evident in these cases when symptoms are present. Children who are nearsighted are not always conscious of it. Therefore, at such times mental strain and the myopic condition are less, and the retinoscope has proved this in every case examined by Dr. Bates. What is true of children is also true of adults. After an attack of whooping-cough or fever, such as measles, scarlet fever, diphtheria, malaria, hay fever, or other conditions, some patients have acquired crossed eye. Sometimes the right eye turns in while the left eye is straight, or the reverse may be observed. The eye which turns in usually has imperfect sight, while the eye which is straight may have normal vision for distant objects and for near objects. These cases can always be benefited. Strain, which is evident in cases of crossed eyes may be relieved but never cured by wearing eyeglasses. All such cases under my observation have proved this to be true. Some patients have told me that they feel a sense of relief when they remove their glasses. It is the mental strain that is relieved and not the eyestrain.

When a child is placed under my care for the cure of squint, or crossed eyes, before I test the sight I hold a short conversation with the child to find out his mental attitude. It helps me to treat the child successfully and it helps my young patient to become acquainted with me. It is always best to have the guardian or parent in the room during the treatment given the child so that they can help in the home treatment, but sometimes I wish that I could be alone with my patient. I can do better work. This desire only comes when an anxious mother continually nags her child to do as I wish. Repeating to my patient that he or she must be good, must sit still, or must do as I say, is only a waste of time and does not help.

Some children troubled with crossed eyes have very sensitive minds and constant or frequent nagging or scolding only causes more mental strain. While I was assisting Dr. Bates at the Harlem Hospital Clinic I was able to study the child mind. I found in cases of squint or crossed eyes, which is the same thing, that children who were fortunate enough to have parents who loved them and helped them were cured of this trouble much quicker than those who were less fortunate. Sometimes I would send for the school teacher when a case was hard for me to benefit and with her help at school, encouraging the child to practice with the test card with the aid of palming and the long swing, in due time the eyes would become perfectly straight and the vision normal.

In the early days of our work together, we gave test cards away to our Clinic patients so that they would surely practice at home or at school or elsewhere. For the child of the Clinic there was no alternative. They could not afford glasses; they must be cured without. A short while ago a little woman came to our office and with her was a girl twelve years old who was just a head taller than the woman. She asked to see me and when she stood before me she smilingly asked if I didn't remember her. This question is asked of me quite often by patients I have not seen for a few years and I do not always remember. When she smiled and spoke in her usual slow way, I recognized her. I said, "Of course, I remember you and this big girl is Ruth whom I treated for crossed eye at the hospital Clinic nine years ago."

She apologized for taking up my time but said that Ruth was anxious to see me again because she had forgotten how I looked and she did want me to see how straight her eyes were. Indeed I was glad to see my little patient all grown up and I like to boast of my work being so well done. The mother also deserves credit for the cure of Ruth's eyes. Every day before the school hour the child practiced reading the test card letters with her mother to help her if she made a mistake. Immediately after school she practiced again. When her test cards became soiled she sent for new ones. Her efforts and mine were all worthwhile because Ruth can read all letters of any test card with either eye.

There is always a mental strain while glasses are worn. Sometimes patients are not conscious of it until they are informed that their glasses must be changed for a stronger pair. During the absence of Dr. Bates, I have been called upon to take care of his practice. At such a time I remember a patient placing on my desk four pairs of glasses which she wore at different times of the day. One pair was worn while she was reading or sewing, another pair for the movies or theatre, another pair, amber colored, to wear in the bright sunlight, and the strongest pair she was advised to wear early in the morning at which time she suffered most pain and discomfort. She did not realize that she strained during sleep, which explained the pain and discomfort she had in the morning. I did not help her until after I had corrected the mental strain. After that it did not take me long to give her normal vision. The patient helped me by following my directions, practicing at home and elsewhere those things which helped her the most.

For many years she had avoided the bright sunlight, so during her first treatment I placed her near a window where the sun was shining. While her eyes were closed and shaded with the palm of her hand, I led her to the window. I used my sun glass, focusing it quickly on her closed eyelids, first on one eye and then on the other. Sometimes this treatment when it is first given causes a tearing of the eyes which is only temporary, but this patient had no such trouble. She enjoyed it so much that she asked for more of it. When there was no sun, a strong electric light was used with benefit. After the patient had had a few treatments, her vision improved for the near point and for the distance. After she had been doing well for some days she suddenly had a relapse and her vision was lowered. I asked her if she had put on her glasses again and she admitted that she had done so. In her case this was the worst thing she could do. It retarded her cure and made my task more difficult. I felt keenly her mental strain and proved without a doubt that imperfect sight is contagious, for I suffered with her mentally. Long ago, Dr. Bates trained my mind so that I would not lose patience with those who were under treatment for their eyes, but just the same neither he nor I are immune to their suffering or mental strain. We give each other the same treatment we give our patients sometimes when the day is almost done, so that we can enjoy the remainder of the day without any strain or discomfort. It requires only a few minutes to relieve the mind of strain when you know how to do it.

QUESTIONS AND ANSWERS

Q–1. Which is the best method of obtaining relaxation?

A–1. The object of all the methods I recommend is relaxation. Some patients obtain more benefit from the practice of one method than another.

Q–2. Should I think only of a black period when palming? Should I imagine my body swaying and the period moving?

A–2. If it requires an effort for you to think of a period, you should not try to do so. It is just as beneficial to let your mind drift from one pleasant thought to another. When one remembers a period, it should be imagined to be moving from side to side.

Q–3. Should one always imagine stationary objects to be moving in the opposite direction?

A–3. When one is riding in a train, one should imagine that telegraph poles and other stationary objects are moving in the opposite direction. When one is walking on the street, he can imagine when looking down, that the pavement is coming toward him; when he looks to the right or left, he can imagine that objects on either side are moving opposite. The object of this is to avoid the stare.

Q–4. How much time should I devote to palming each day?

A–4. The more time one devotes to palming, the quicker will results be obtained, provided one practices correctly. Palming should be practiced for five, ten, fifteen minutes or longer at a time. Some patients obtain more benefits from practicing palming for short periods of time at more frequent intervals.

Better Eyesight
May 1929—Vol. XIII, No. 11

SHIFTING

When the normal eye has normal sight it is at rest and when it is at rest it is always moving or shifting. Shifting may be done consciously with improvement in the vision, or it may be done unconsciously with impaired vision.

Shifting can be practiced correctly and incorrectly. A wrong way to shift is to turn the head to the right while the eyes are turned to the left, or to turn the head to the left while the eyes are turned to the right.

To improve imperfect sight by shifting, it is well to move the head and eyes so far away that the first letter or object imagined is too far away to be seen at all clearly. Shifting from small letters to large letters alternately may be a greater benefit than shifting from one small letter to another small letter. Quite frequently the vision is decidedly improved by shifting continuously from one side of a small letter to the other side, while the letter is imagined to be moving in the opposite direction. When the shifting is slow, short, and easy, the best results in the improvement in the vision are obtained. Any attempt to stop the shifting always lowers the vision. The letter or other object which appeared to move is usually shifting a short distance—one-half or one-quarter of an inch. It is not possible to imagine any particular letter or other object stationary for a longer time than one minute.

While the patient is seated, benefit can be obtained from shifting, but even more benefit can be obtained when the shifting is practiced while the patient is standing and moving the head and shoulders, in fact the whole body, a very short distance from side to side. Shifting the whole body makes it easier to shift a short distance and may explain why this method is best.

TREATMENT

By W. H. Bates, M.D.

Vision is largely associated with the activity of the mind. The memory, imagination, must be nearly perfect for the vision to be nearly perfect. When the memory is imperfect, the imagination and sight are always imperfect. There are no exceptions.

In myopia, or nearsightedness, the eyeball is elongated. Myopia can be produced by a stare, concentration, or an effort to see distant objects. When all objects are regarded with an effort to see more than two parts perfectly at the same time, myopia is always produced. To do the wrong thing, a strain or effort is made. The greater the strain, the more imperfect becomes the vision. To do the wrong thing requires much trouble, hard work, and a useless effort. The production of myopia is not easy. Rather it is difficult. This truth, when demonstrated by the patient, is important. It demonstrates the cause of myopia and when the cause of myopia is known, treatment can usually be suggested which helps in the cure.

The production of improved or perfect sight is easy. Rest or the absence of strain is helpful in obtaining normal vision.

When the sight is normal, the eye is at rest. Any effort to improve the sight is wrong, always fails, and the vision soon becomes less. Perfect sight is easy and is not benefited by strong efforts to improve the sight. Myopia is cured by the efforts which are not made, rather than by strong efforts to see. Most people with myopia are not conscious of the stare, strain, or effort. Persons with normal sight are often able successfully to demonstrate the existence of strain in myopia and to suggest successful methods of treatment for the prevention of strain.

One method of treatment has been practiced consciously, continuously, and successfully, namely, "Make the sight worse by a strong effort to stare." The imperfect sight of myopia does not come easily by staring. When it does come, the patient feels a manifest strain in his head and all his nerves. By alternately producing the stare consciously and unconsciously he realizes the harm it can produce. He becomes acquainted with the stare. By practice, he becomes able to produce it to any extent and at all times.

Imperfect sight is difficult while normal or improved sight is easy and enables most people with myopia to obtain a cure in a very short time. It should be known that high degrees of myopia are not always easy to produce. It is a truth that quick cures of myopia can only be obtained by persons who have the ability to make the myopia worse.

Some statistics on the production of myopia in schoolchildren and others show that 10 percent of the population are myopic, 80 percent have imperfect sight from other causes, and 10 percent have normal sight. Some statistics state that 50 percent of the population of China and about the same percentage in Japan have acquired myopia by improper use of their eyes. What is improper use of the eyes, and what is known of the cause of myopia in these countries? They are a book-reading people to such a slight extent that we need not consider the use of books in the daily life of the Chinese. No one can say that the Chinese have acquired imperfect sight from reading. The characters of the books that they do possess are very large compared to our print and that used in other countries. Many writers have stated that fine print is a strain on the eyesight and is the cause of myopia; the Chinese use very large print and there is no nation in the world that has so much myopia! Large print instead of being a rest to the eyes is a great strain.

Some years ago, a prominent ophthalmologist of Cleveland was told to introduce in the public schools books printed in very large type. After a short time, the teachers complained to the authorities that the large print hurt the eyes of the children and increased the production of myopia and made so much trouble that they requested that the new books be discarded and books with finer print be used again. This is offered as evidence that myopia does not result from the reading of fine print. Fine print, instead of being the cause of nearsightedness, is the best preventative that one can use.

The Snellen test card can be used in various ways to improve the vision. The best distance of the card from the patient is variable. Some patients with a high degree of myopia will improve more when the card is read at a short distance, five feet or less. Other patients prefer to have the test card at a greater distance from their eyes and they improve their vision more when they practice with the card at a long distance off—twenty-five, thirty, or, forty feet. The optimum distance of the card from the patient is the distance at which the best results are obtained. To imagine the card to be moving when held in front of the patient, who at the same time sways from side to side, is usually beneficial. After a little practice, when the patient sways from side to side, the card may be imagined to be moving about four to six inches from side to side. If the card seems to sway a very short distance or not at all, it usually means that the patient is staring, straining, or trying to see.

One should avoid looking directly at the Snellen test card, because then the movement of the card becomes uncertain or disappears altogether. A long movement of the card from side to side can be shortened with an improvement in the vision. When the patient stands with the feet about one foot apart and sways from side to side, without looking directly at the card, the letters may be seen to move in the same or in the opposite direction.

Sometimes practice with the card will be followed by double or multiple vision, due to the fact that the patient stares, strains, and makes an effort to see the letters. For example, one patient saw one line of letters multiplied two or three times. This would not have occurred if the patient had imagined the card moving slightly from side to side, and had not tried to see the letters. Palming, when practiced successfully, has relieved many cases of double vision.

Some patients, when they palm, see flashes of light and all the colors of the spectrum without at any time seeing black. It is strange to hear patients complain of the numerous objects they remember or imagine when they palm. Thinking of pleasant things has helped some people to palm more successfully. The memory of imperfect sight is a strain and should not be practiced when palming. The length of time that patients can palm with benefit is widely variable. Some patients have gone to sleep while palming and when they awakened in the morning they were still palming, with their hand covering their eyes with the result that their vision was very much improved. Others obtain more benefit from palming for short periods of time at frequent intervals.

If one can imagine a thin white line below letters of the test card or beneath a line of fine print it is very helpful. This thin white line is only imagined, it is not seen, because the line is not really there. It is valuable in the treatment and cure of presbyopia, hypermetropia, astigmatism and many cases of myopia. It is well to imagine it in the right way. The wrong way is to try to imagine the thin white line and the black letters at the same time. This is a strain which always blurs the black letters and prevents the thin white line from being imagined.

Many patients complain that they have difficulty in imagining the thin white line. To overcome this, one should imagine it just below some word or collection of words which are known. The line is then readily imagined and it can be imagined extending from one side of the page to the other, and wherever it becomes manifest the vision is always improved.

It is well for each patient to test his ability to concentrate on one point of a large letter or of a small letter. In less than a minute the patient suffers fatigue, pain, imperfect sight. When concentration causes trouble, common sense would suggest that the concentration be avoided.

Most cases of imperfect sight are cured by relaxation—relaxation of the mind, relaxation of the nerves of the head and of all other parts of the body. The importance of the control of relaxation is very great because most diseases of the eyes are caused by the stare or strain, and cannot be cured until the stare or strain is relieved.

Case Report

A man, age 51, had worn glasses for hypermetropia and for reading for 20 years. Without glasses his vision at fifteen feet was 15/200. He was told to imagine a thin white line between the white spaces of the Fundamentals card. In about five minutes the patient became able to remember or imagine a thin white line when regarding the white spaces between the lines of black letters. By repetition and some patience he became able to read diamond type at six inches. After this was accomplished his vision for distance became normal and he read the bottom line without trouble at fifteen feet, 15/10.

EYE INJURIES

By Emily A. Bates

It is not always easy to treat a case where the sight has become impaired through an accident or injury to the eye. I have in mind particularly two patients who came to me recently and who at one time had had normal vision.

One was a young man, 23 years old, who had been to several doctors for treatment during a period of ten years, and as he explained his case to me I realized how despondent he was, fearing that he would go blind completely. He was thirteen years old when he was taken on a long automobile trip at which time the accident occurred. Being far away from civilization it was some time before he was able to receive medical aid, and during that time his vision became very poor in both eyes. Some of the occupants of the car were instantly killed. He was found pinned under the overturned car some days after the accident, and after he had recovered consciousness he found that he could not see well. His head had been cut very badly and the doctors feared that internal injuries in his head and other parts of his body would prove fatal, and for a time it was thought that he would lose his mind as well as his sight. When he came to me, there was a scar on his forehead directly over each eye, but otherwise he showed no outward signs of injury.

He had received a different kind of treatment from every doctor who had treated him with the result that he did not go blind entirely. He got along very well with the aid of glasses for a time and then cataract began to form in each eye. An operation was advised but the boy refused to submit to this. Friends cared for him and helped him with his education but his sight was too poor to aid him in doing any kind of work which would require the use of his eyes. He stopped going to doctors for help because each one who had treated him advised an operation for the removal of cataract, with the exception of the last doctor who had given him medical treatment. This doctor knows Dr. Bates very well and has from time to time cured headaches and other pain by the Bates Method, although he is not an eye specialist.

At the advice of this doctor the boy came to me for treatment while I was in the West. The cataract could easily be seen by the naked eye but there was a small spot about the size of the head of a pin in the retina which was clear. Not being allowed to use my retinoscope in California in the absence of a doctor, I asked him to bring me a written statement from a specialist who had given him a thorough examination of his eyes. He replied that he had already been to one and explained that the doctor had said that there was no hope of his ever regaining his sight. He gave me a written report from a few of the doctors who had examined him and each one had given him a different diagnosis, but all of them said there was no hope of his ever seeing again unless he submitted to an operation, which would probably be useless.

Sometimes I have to spend a considerable amount of time convincing a patient that I can really help him if he can have enough confidence in what I am able to do, but this young man did not need any explanation for I seemed to be his last hope. He did not ask me for an opinion, but just came at the advice of his family physician. He felt that I really could help him if there were any chance at all.

I placed a large test card five feet from his eyes. I thought I would use the black card with white letters first, because this card seems easier for the partially blind patient, or those patients who have diseases of the eye, such as glaucoma, atrophy of the optic nerve, and so forth. Before I placed the card in position at five feet I had told him to close his eyes to rest them because all the while he had been in my presence, he stared hard to see me and seldom blinked his eyes. I placed the test card with the blank side of the test card facing him. There was only a plain white surface to look at and I was hoping that he would see it as it really was. When he opened his eyes at my suggestion, he was waiting for me to tell him what to do while he looked at the blank side of this card. I asked him if he could see any letters on the card and he said, "No, it seems like a blank white paper."

I was pleased that he saw the card as it really was, without my telling him. I told him to close his eyes immediately and while his eyes were closed, I turned the card right side up. I told him to open his eyes and tell me what he saw. He was able to read three lines of the test card immediately. I encouraged him then and told him that if he were willing to sacrifice his time that I surely would give him my time to help him to improve the little vision he had.

After he palmed and improved his memory by reciting history, which was his favorite subject at school, he read the card again for me, and this time his vision improved to 5/30. I gave him a test card to practice with at home and told him to report to me in a few days' time.

Seven months later he came again for treatment. His eyes looked much better and his face showed signs of relaxation which were absent at his first visit. I tested his sight again with the same black card with white letters and his vision had improved to 5/20. He reported that he had practiced two hours in the morning and two hours in the evening every day since his first visit. He remembered what I had said to him about blinking his eyes consciously all the time in order to avoid the stare which made the cataract worse.

I placed him by a window and told him to look across the street where there was a large sign with letters that looked to be about three feet in height. He said he could not read any signs from the window. I gave him a fine print card to hold in his hand and he looked at the white spaces below the lines of black type that were on the small card. I told him to look at the white spaces, and then to close his eyes and to imagine the white whiter than he saw it on the card. He did this alternately for about five minutes and when he looked out of the window to where this large sign was, he began to see the letters one by one by quickly looking away after seeing each letter as I directed him, and taking the sun treatment as he stood by the window, which I thought would help him. Without giving him notice, I told him to turn round with his back to the light and to look at the test card which was five feet away, and he read another line of the test card at 5/15.

I gave him the Fundamentals card to read, but all he could see was sentence No. 1 and the words "Fundamentals by W. H. Bates, M.D." All the rest of the card was a blur to him. He knew there were words on the card, but he could not distinguish them.

Not far away from any office there was a public park where he would sit for hours at a time to take sun treatment. The warmth of the western sun is the most healing thing in the world in cases where the sun is helpful. I can prove it by this particular case, because the next time my patient came, he was able to read the whole of the Fundamentals card up to sentence No. 15 which is in diamond type. He did not read it immediately as one with normal sight would have done, but with many hours of patience on my part and, with the aid of the sun glass treatment in between times he finally read it. Sometime later he came for another treatment and this time he read the microscopic type I gave him, which is a reproduction of that contained in the small Bible. He read this type at nine inches from his eyes. I then tested his sight for the large test card and his vision had improved to 7/20, and later 7/15 by palming and the long swing.

He left the West for other parts and I did not see him again but I received a letter sometime later, saying that he was still practicing with the test card and also with the fine type every day. After that, however, I lost track of him. There is not much satisfaction in treating a case like that unless we can cure it, but I hope that wherever he is that he is still keeping up with the Bates treatment and receiving benefit. At any rate, I was very much encouraged to know that the Bates Method helped when all else failed and that I was able to improve his vision instead of saying as others had said to him that there was no more hope.

The other case which was interesting to me was a young man, twenty years old, who had started to wear glasses at the age of ten years. He had been playing with some boys near a building that was being torn down and without realizing it the boys were playing near a section of a wall which was about to come down. It finally did tumble down and buried them under a mass of debris. The boy's glasses were broken and the right eye was severely injured, having been cut by the broken glass.

His father was a physician and he took him to various eye specialists in the hope that the left eye could be saved. For some time the left eye was discharging and he almost lost the sight of it. With medical treatment and care the discharge ceased and apparently there seemed to be nothing wrong with his left eye. He strained terribly in daylight, but at night he had very little trouble in seeing things. Since the accident he had acquired the habit of turning his head to one side and squeezing the lids of his right eye together tightly in order to see with the left.

Before I tested his sight with the test card he told me that there was a dead nerve in the left eye which was caused by the injury to the right eye—at least he was told by the eye specialists that this was so. After the accident he said that he had had an attack of malaria, and then keratitis settled in both eyes. At the age of fifteen he suffered a great deal of pain in his right eye and was treated for iritis.

After listening to all he had to say, I tested his sight. He could only see the large letter "C" of the test card at six inches from his right eye. Everything else was a blank to him. His vision with the left eye was 15/20 and all the letters were clear and black. In order to read with the left eye, he turned his head to one side. I told him to palm and reminded him that he must not remove his hands from his eyes while I was talking to him. I told him that no matter what the diagnosis was or how bad his sight was that he could at least see something on the test card with his right eye and that I did not believe that there was anything radically wrong with his left eye. If there were, he could not have seen the 20-line letters of the card at fifteen feet.

I gave him some sun treatment after he had palmed a little while and then told him to palm again before I tested his sight the second time. I felt that it was necessary for him to close his eyes and palm after being in the bright sunlight.

This poor fellow had quite a story to tell me and I had a strong desire to become better acquainted with him and help him in other ways besides improving his sight. He was not a nice looking boy and neither was he clean. He did not wear a coat or vest and he had no hat with him when he came. His shoes were soiled and much worn and he looked as though he had not received much affection or care for a long time. He was short in his answers and when he looked at me, he would just look for a moment and then look away. I told him that I believed that he was far away from his home, but that he was not the only one, and that I was three thousand miles away from my home too.

While he was palming, I noticed a tear drop on the front of his shirt and then I encouraged him to tell me all about everything that was on his mind. I told him I wanted to be his friend if he would let me. He told me that he was sad and lonely too and that his family no longer cared about him. He said that it was his own fault, of course, but a strict father whose confidence he never had made it hard for him to live at home. He said that he did not know what was the matter with him, but that he could never hold a job for any length of time. He knew there was something wrong with him but he did not know how to become better and he had no one to guide him.

I asked him if he had a home somewhere and he said "Yes." He said that a distant relative had befriended him and given him a place to sleep. What I had to say to him that day helped, I know, because the next time he came his shoes were cleaned, his top shirt had been washed and ironed and his face and hands were clean.

We became friends after that and up to the last week of my stay in the West, I helped him with his sight and in other ways. As his vision improved he obtained a position in an office which paid him a fair salary. Every day he arose early in the morning to practice with the test card and before retiring at night he practiced again. During the day he remembered what I had advised him to do with the small pocket test card and microscopic type.

He practiced the long swing and palming which always helped to improve his sight, and on the last day I saw him his right eye had improved to the 50-line of the test card as he held the card at two feet from his eyes. His left eye improved to 12/10 which is more than normal vision.

Better Eyesight
June 1929—Vol. XIII, No. 12

CATARACT

By W. H. Bates, M.D.

Sinbad the sailor told many stories of his voyages which have pleased some adults and many children. I wish to maintain that some of his experiences were true while many were not. On one of his voyages, when sailing in the tropics, a violent storm struck the ship and he was wrecked on the shores of an island in the Pacific Ocean. As usual, most of the sailors were drowned, but Sinbad lived to return home and tell of the wonders he had seen.

It was related by him that the island was frequented by goats who were blind for a variable length of time. After a few days or weeks many of them recovered their sight, being cured in some way by a thorn bush which had large thorns. Sinbad watched them closely and discovered that each goat pushed each blind eye directly onto one of these thorns. After a few efforts the goat became able to see. How was it accomplished?

The cause of the blindness was the presence of an opaque body behind the pupil. This opaque body is a cataract. There are numerous operations for the cure of cataract but all are planned to move it to one side, above or below the optic axis so that the pupil appears perfectly clear and permits good sight. Eye doctors during the period when Sinbad flourished had no other cure for cataract except an operation such as the goat performed on his own eyes. It was done so easily, so quickly, and in most cases so successfully that many quacks or irregular practitioners who did not understand it failed to remove the cataract properly and the sight was not improved.

Sinbad wrote a very clear account of how the goats got rid of their cataracts. He told how a goat would, in his blindness, move his head and eyes about different parts of the thorn bush until he was able to push one of the thorns into his center of sight and push the opaque cataract out of the way.

Sinbad wrote a great deal about the failures. He described how in many of the goats which operated upon itself, foul matter would form and destroy one or both eyes. But when the goat did things right, the eyes healed without any bad symptoms whatever. Sinbad's operation for the cure of cataract was described so long ago that there are still many doctors who claim that as they had never heard of Sinbad's operation there never was such a person as Sinbad.

Modern physicians believe that the thorn is not the best instrument to use to remove the cataract in elderly people. Various and numerous operations have been recommended and practiced with good results.

An opacity of the crystalline lens which is sufficiently opaque to interfere with the vision is called a *cataract*. There are two kinds of cataract—hard and soft. The hard cataract occurs usually in adults. An operation for its removal is usually advised for an improvement in the sight. When the operation is done properly, the vision is usually permanently improved. After the operation is completed without accidents, strong glasses are prescribed, which increase the vision. Two pairs of strong glasses are used by the patient. One pair is to improve distant vision, while a second pair with much stronger glasses may be necessary for reading, sewing, or other close work.

Soft cataract occurs usually in children or in adults at the age of 45 or younger. One operation is called "needling," in which a needle or very sharp knife penetrates a small part of the lens. A slight opacity of the lens may be seen for several days or longer, which usually causes no discomfort. It is customary to wait a few days or longer until the opacity made by the operation has disappeared. The operation is then repeated as before. By alternating in this way, the opacity of the lens becomes less after each needling until the cataract has disappeared altogether. The patient uses two pairs of glasses just the same as after the operation for the removal of a hard cataract.

Who were the earliest physicians? Who were the best doctors to cure the blindness of cataract? Barbers at an early date always bled their patients to cure any disease. Their motto was to bleed the patient until he was cured.

If the first bleeding failed it was considered good practice to bleed him some more. George Washington met his death at the hands of the barbers from too much bleeding. In the treatment of cataract in modern times we do things which are not always considered to be proper. At one of the best eye hospitals in this country patients suffering from severe pain and loss of sight have been bled from the temples and elsewhere and lost much blood that I considered unnecessary. While bleeding has apparently in some cases been a general benefit, this method of treatment is seldom indicated in a large number of patients.

Cataract occurs in a small percentage of persons with imperfect sight. One and the same method of treatment for all cases of cataract is not advised. It has been demonstrated and frequently published in this magazine that the cause of the opacity in the lens is a strain, a stare, an effort to see. When the strain is removed by relaxation methods, the cataract disappears and good or perfect sight is obtained without an operation of any kind. This being true, the removal of the cataract by some sort of an operation is the same as it would be to amputate the foot to cure rheumatism of the big toe.

People with cataract in one or both eyes may suffer from rheumatism, diabetes, bladder trouble, or other serious diseases which make it impossible for them to travel on land or water. Headache is sometimes continuous and of great severity. These patients may become bedridden and unable to walk without distress. The heart is often inflamed to such an extent that the slightest exertion brings on severe symptoms.

Some years ago a very intelligent Spaniard called to see me in reference to treatment of his wife who was a very sick woman and had been bedridden for many years. Her vision was very poor. She was unable to count her fingers when held in front of her face at a distance of two feet or more. The husband was told that it would be better for his wife to be cured of cataract while she was at home, as the trip to New York would probably cause her so much discomfort that it would be very difficult to cure or improve her cataract by treatment. I told him that it would be possible for him to learn relaxation methods and have his wife practice them under his supervision. The fact that he himself had good sight would enable him to treat her more successfully than someone who had poor sight. He accepted my suggestion and told me that he would faithfully carry out any treatment which I might suggest.

The first thing I had him do was to read the Snellen test card at fifteen feet with each eye separately. Then he was directed to stand with his feet about one foot apart and to sway from side to side, while facing the Snellen test card. He learned how to do this very quickly. His attention was called to the fact that when the Snellen test card appeared to move in the opposite direction to the movement of his head, eyes and body, that the white card appeared whiter than it really was. The black letters also appeared much blacker and more distinct than when he did not practice the sway. He was then told to close his eyes and by opening and shutting them alternately, his vision improved. With his eyes closed he was able to imagine a small letter just as black as a large one and to imagine it better with his eyes closed than with his eyes open. When he imagined a small letter at the beginning of a line of letters perfectly black or as black as the larger letters, his vision improved to better than the average sight.

I examined his eyes with the retinoscope and found that the memory of imperfect sight caused the area of the pupil to appear blurred. When he strained or made an effort to improve his sight, the area of the pupil became very cloudy, the eyeballs became hard and the vision worse—a condition similar to that which occurs in cataract. This man was told that with his good sight he could at will increase the hardness of his good eyeballs more readily and lower his vision more readily than his wife who had cataract.

It is a truth that persons with normal eyes can produce imperfect sight at will to a greater degree than when the sight is imperfect from cataract. A large number of patients with cataract have been examined with the retinoscope at the same time that a strain is made to improve the sight. In all cases without exception the cataract became worse by an effort to see and the vision was still further lowered. Many persons with normal eyes were also examined at the same time. An effort to see better lowered the vision to a greater extent than occurred with the patients suffering from cataract.

It should be emphasized that a stare or strain is the principal cause of cataract. The retinoscope demonstrates that when an effort is made the cataract becomes worse. When the patient remembered or imagined letters or other objects the cloudiness and imperfect sight disappeared. An important point is the readiness with which an eye with good sight is able to produce imperfect sight while one with imperfect sight has great difficulty in straining sufficiently to increase it.

The husband was very much pleased because it seemed to him that there would be more difficulty in teaching his wife how to increase her cataract than to lessen or cure it. In due time I received a very grateful letter from him; he was much pleased to inform me that his wife had cured her cataract by my methods and after the cataract was cured, she became able to leave her bed. (She had been bedridden because of fear of walking about because of her poor eyesight.) The method was a benefit not only to her eyes but to her general health as well.

We have received many letters of inquiry from patients who have cataract who ask the questions: Can people eighty years old be benefited? Which are the best methods of helping cataract? These questions were answered by the results of treatment in a man who was 106 years old. He came to the Clinic with cataract so far advanced in each eye that he was unable, even with strong glasses, to read ordinary type. He was treated by rest of his eyes with the aid of shifting, swinging, memory, and imagination. After the first visit, he became able to read large print without glasses. His vision rapidly improved so that after some weeks of treatment the cataract had disappeared and his vision for distance became normal. It was interesting to watch his cataract disappear while he was forming mental pictures of the white spaces between the lines of black letters.

Many patients with cataract who knew about this old man asked me how it was that he was cured in so short a time while many younger patients were not cured so quickly. The word obedience suggests that the reason this patient obtained so prompt and permanent a cure was because of his ability to obtain perfect relaxation of his eyes and mind as well as all the nerves of his body. For example, when he was told to close his eyes and keep them closed until told to open them, he did this thoroughly and well. Too many of my cataract patients do not practice central fixation as obediently as did my elderly patient.

So many people with cataract, when they close their eyes, feel that they are doing what they were told and cannot understand why they obtain so little benefit. Closing the eyes is not always followed by relaxation and rest. In short, there are many patients with cataract who strain their eyes more when they are closed than they do when they regard letters and objects with their eyes open. These patients are directed to practice the universal swing, the long swing, the variable swing and other methods of obtaining relaxation. One of the best methods of lessening cataract is to encourage the patient to regard a blank wall of one color. When the eyes are examined at the same time, it is usually found that the cataract has become less because the eye is not straining to see any one particular object.

Some cases of cataract acquire the ability to read without glasses very fine print held a few inches from the face. When such patients are recommended to read the fine print many hours daily, the cataract becomes less and the vision improves. The practice of regarding fine print or other small objects is one of the best methods of curing cataract.

ITCHING OF THE EYELIDS

By Emily A. Bates

Itching of the eyelids is sometimes a difficult thing to relieve. When a patient is troubled that way, Dr. Bates usually prescribes a salve and eyewash or eyedrops to relieve the condition. Usually such applications help, but there are times when a patient is troubled for a long period without much or any relief.

A middle-aged woman came to me in a highly nervous state and told me that she had been to several doctors, but they could only give her temporary relief. The doctors had given her exactly the same prescription that Dr. Bates usually prescribes for such a condition. Before coming to me as a last resort, she tried wearing dark glasses, thinking that she would find relief that way. Wearing the dark glasses indoors only aggravated her trouble, but while she was in the sunshine she felt relief most of the time.

She was a business woman and managed a summer hotel which kept her indoors most of the day. She was called upon at times to do some bookkeeping and after she had worn the dark glasses for a while, she discovered that she could no longer see at the near point. The last doctor whom she had called upon diagnosed her case as presbyopia, but he did not say what had caused it. He told her that at her age she had to expect a change in the condition of her eyes. He advised her to wear the glasses he prescribed for her only when it was absolutely necessary, and if that would not help to come and see me.

I had benefited the wife of this doctor and I am greatly disappointed that I did not have an opportunity to meet him before I left the West where I was taking care of patients. I tested the patient's vision for the distance and she read 15/15 with much effort and squinting of her eyes. She squinted her eyes most of the time in order to see without discomfort. I gave her the Fundamentals card to read. The type on this card starts with larger than ordinary reading type and ends with diamond type, which is much finer than ordinary type. She held this card at arm's length and then drew back her head as far as she could in order to read the diamond type on the card. She could not understand how I could bring back her sight to the normal by our method of eye training. Before she came to me she believed that proper glasses would eventually relieve her of all her trouble, but that she would have to wear glasses at all times as long as she lived.

After a doctor friend of mine had examined her eyes and diagnosed her case as presbyopia caused by strain, he asked me to examine her eyes with his retinoscope and verify his statement. The itching and burning of her eyelids had nothing to do with her sight. Sun treatment sometimes instantly relieves itching of the eyelids and also does more sometimes than medicine applied to the eyes. I placed my patient in the sun and while her eyes were closed I focused the strong light of the sun on her closed eyelids with the aid of the sun glass.

Immediately after I used the sun glass I placed my hand before her closed eyelids to shade her eyes from the sun. Then I placed myself between my patient and the direct rays of the sunlight and asked her to open her eyes. She began to blink in a natural way as she looked at me and remarked how differently everything looked about her. She sighed with a sense of relief and asked me to do it again.

The second time I applied the sun glass she could stand the strong rays of the sun for about a minute and then I again placed myself between the sunlight and my patient's eyes. Again I told her to open her eyes and look at me, but this time I held the Fundamentals card before her, about twelve inches from her eyes. She read No. 3 or the third sentence on the card and then her eyelids began to itch again. The sun treatment was repeated for an hour, while she alternately read the Fundamentals card and she read two more sentences without noticing that she was gradually reading smaller type.

The patient was pleased with her first treatment and came daily for a week and each time her vision improved for the near point and the itching and burning of the eyelids became less.

We seldom advise patients about the amount of water that they drink or the kind of food that they eat, but this patient had brought up the subject herself. My experience for many years with Clinic patients has taught me much about the mistakes people make in eating the wrong food and not drinking sufficient water. I feel quite sure that my patient's assistance and intelligence about eating unseasoned foods and drinking a large quantity of water every day helped to cure the irritation and discomfort of her eyes.

I did not cure this patient in a week's time but at the end of one week's treatment, after I had seen her for the last time, the presbyopia was entirely cured and she read microscopic type in bright sunlight as well as she could read ordinary type at six inches from her eyes. When reading microscopic type, she had to have a strong, artificial light, or place herself directly in the sunlight in order to read it. By looking at the white spaces of the diamond type, which is a little larger than microscopic type, she became able to see the white spaces between the lines of microscopic type and in this way, she was able to read it.

Like most people who have trouble with their eyes, she seldom blinked, which she thought was an affliction instead of a natural thing to do. While I did not like the discomfort that staring caused me, I purposely stared or blinked less frequently than I ordinarily do as she stood before me. It helped her to understand how necessary it was to blink often and to do it continuously, in order to form the unconscious habit of blinking, when she no longer had trouble with her eyes. She noticed that when I blinked my eyes that the eyes moved slightly and when she began to practice this, she said that the burning of her eyes and itching became less. She made a mask from a large linen handkerchief and only exposed her eyes when she placed herself in the sun. She would sit in the sunshine for an hour at a time each day while her eyes troubled her. At the end of seven days, giving her daily treatment, her trouble disappeared entirely.

On the seventh day, I returned the dark glasses which she had placed in my possession so that she would not be tempted at any time to wear them while under treatment. I asked her to put them on while she was sitting in the sun and tell me how she felt with them on. She said it seemed as though the world had become dark, without any sunlight. While she was talking to me, the discomfort she felt while the glasses were on was such that she threw them off quickly and said she did not want to use them again.

There comes to my mind a Clinic case which I would like to report now. A woman who seemed fairly well dressed brought her little boy to the Clinic and as he appeared before me, I noticed how shabbily he was dressed. His hair looked as though it had not been combed for many days and from the appearance of his little hands it seemed to me that soap was almost an unknown thing to him. The poor little fellow was about eight years old or perhaps younger.

While I was giving my attention to some of the children who were having their eyes tested with the test cards, he came close to me and watched every move I made. His mother was holding his hand and as he moved closer to me, she drew him away none too gently. A thought passed through my mind instantly that surely this was not his mother. He looked so shabby and dirty and she looked just the opposite. Dr. Bates placed him in the little dark room where all the patients had their eyes examined and after he had finished examining the little fellow's eyes, he called my attention to the condition of his eyelids, which I had not noticed before.

His eyesight was normal. There was nothing wrong with the retina, but the cornea and sclera or the white parts of his eyes were much inflamed. The eyelids of both eyes were much mattered. Dr. Bates asked him what his greatest trouble was and he said his eyes itched all the time and even at night the itching prevented him from sleeping. Dr. Bates questioned the little boy's mother and asked her how long he had had this trouble. She said she had noticed him rubbing his eyes for a few weeks or longer, but did not pay any attention to it until his school teachers sent him home to be examined by the Doctor.

We placed him in a good light and as the Doctor focused his magnifying glass on the eyelids, he drew back suddenly and asked me not to touch the boy's eyes. On a slip of paper, the Doctor wrote the word "parasites." The mother became enraged when the Doctor diagnosed the case as such. My heart went out to the little fellow. Dr. Bates advised the mother not to have anyone else use his towel or washcloth and he directed her further to use an eyewash he prescribed and a salve to be applied afterward and to come regularly every Clinic day until he was rid of his trouble.

Apparently the directions for his treatment at home meant time and attention which she did not care to give for the little fellow. Before we realized what had happened, the mother had left the Clinic and we did not see her or her little boy again. We reported this case to someone in authority at the Clinic who was to send a social worker to the home of the little boy. What became of the case we could never find out, but for the sake of any child who may be afflicted or become afflicted as this little boy was, I decided to tell about this case so that mothers of public schoolchildren who might possibly read this article will know what to do to help their children.

If the mother cannot afford to visit a physician at his office, she can always find a competent one at any eye clinic and receive treatment with permanent benefit. Sometimes through no fault of the mother or child, a thing like this happens and it seems out of nowhere that this contagious thing strikes even the cleanest and well cared for children. The itching in this condition is terrific. If the trouble is noticed and looked after in time, it can be easily cured by treatment. As Dr. Bates explained this condition to me, he said that he did not believe that he nor any doctor can tell where such things originate. We do know, however, that cleanliness helps to eliminate the trouble.

Better Eyesight
July 1929—Vol. XIV, No. 1

MENTAL PICTURES

With imperfect sight, a mental picture of one known letter of the Snellen test card is seldom or never remembered, imagined, or seen perfectly when regarded with the eyes open. By closing the eyes, the same mental picture may be imagined more perfectly. By alternately imagining the known letter as well as possible with the eyes open and then remembering it better with the eyes closed, the imagination improves the vision and unknown letters are seen with the eyes open.

The improvement of the vision is due to a lessening of the organic changes in the eye. When the imperfect sight is caused by opacities of the cornea, a mental picture imagined clearly lessens or cures the disease of the cornea. A large number of cases of cataract in which the lens is more or less opaque have been benefited or cured by the imagination of mental pictures. Nearly all organic changes in the eyeball which lower the vision have been improved to some extent in a few minutes; by devoting a sufficient amount of time, all organic changes in the eyeball, no matter what the cause may be, are benefited or cured by a perfect imagination of a letter, a tree, a flower, or anything which is remembered perfectly.

I do not know of any method of obtaining relaxation or perfect sight which is as efficient and certain as the imagination of mental pictures. It should be emphasized that a good or perfect imagination of mental pictures has in all cases brought about a measure of improvement which is convincing that the imagination is capable of relieving organic changes in the eye more quickly, more thoroughly, and more permanently than any other method.

"THROW AWAY YOUR GLASSES"

By W. H. Bates, M.D.

Editor's Note—*The following is a reprint from an article which appeared in* Hearst's International, *September 1923, which is being republished in* Better Eyesight *at the suggestion of some of our readers.*

More than thirty years ago, not knowing any better and being guided by the practice of other eye doctors, I recommended patients with imperfect sight throw away their eyes and see with their glasses. Since that time I have made some discoveries which have enabled me to cure people without the use of glasses. The slogan now is, "Throw away your glasses and see with your eyes."

We are rapidly becoming a "four-eyed" nation. The enthusiasm of the eye doctors is putting glasses on many people who do not need them. Just as soon as we go to the doctor and complain about our eyes or some nervous trouble with our minds and our heads, the stomach or something else, the doctor prescribes glasses. Fifty years ago the number of persons wearing glasses was very much smaller than it is now. Human nature is such that when one person gets glasses, we believe everybody else should do as we do and wear glasses. When prominent people set the fashion, the rank and file feel that they must do the same. It is a matter of record in this country with a population of one hundred and ten million or more, that all persons over forty years old, according to the old theories, should wear glasses.

Some eye specialists have gone so far as to say that all children attending school should wear glasses either to relieve imperfect sight or to prevent their eyes from failing. This matter was considered by the Board of Education of the City of New York in 1912 and much pressure was brought to bear to have it done. I was the only physician that went before the Board of Education and recommended a method of treatment which had cured and prevented imperfect sight in schoolchildren without the use of glasses.

The craze for glasses has even included nursing babies. It is all wrong, and the evidence has been accumulating through the years that imperfect sight is curable without glasses. Most of us should have an interest in the welfare of every child and get busy and investigate the facts. The medical profession has neglected its duty. They have done noble work in the study and prevention of yellow fever and other conditions, but when it comes to the eyes the doctors can only recommend glasses. My investigations have demonstrated many facts of practical importance.

In the first place, all children under twelve years old with imperfect sight can be cured without glasses. This is a challenge. If there is one child who cannot be cured by my treatment I am wrong about the whole thing. There is no exception and when a proposition has no exception we call it a truth.

The teachers in the public schools have succeeded by practicing my suggestions with the children, reading the Snellen test card with each eye as well as they can every day, devoting in most cases only a few minutes daily. Those children whose sight is already normal only need to read with normal sight, one minute or less, every day to prevent eyestrain and imperfect sight.

One day I visited a classroom and I said to the teacher, "Can you pick out the children who have imperfect sight?" She selected a number of children that she thought had imperfect sight. In every case her selection was made because of the way the children used their eyes. Some of them squinted, some of them strained in other ways.

I tested the sight of these children and found it imperfect. Then I suggested to the teacher that she ask the children to use their eyes without strain, without making any efforts to see. I said, "You will find out how well they can see when they use their eyes easily, without effort."

Much to her surprise they all read the card with normal vision. Some of these children were wearing glasses. When they removed their glasses at first, their sight was imperfect but after resting their eyes by closing them for five minutes or longer their vision became very much improved. In one classroom the teacher found that all her children had imperfect sight; but by showing them how to rest their eyes, by avoiding the strain, and by closing them, the vision of all of them was improved and all obtained perfect sight except one. I learned that this one also obtained perfect sight a few weeks later.

In all my enthusiasm I felt that it was not proper for me to interfere with children who were under the care of a physician and while wearing the glasses he prescribed. Of course, I could not be blamed if the children lost their glasses and got well without them.

It should be emphasized that teachers wearing glasses have a larger percentage of pupils with imperfect sight than have the teachers whose sight is normal and who do not wear glasses. Why is this? The facts are that children, being naturally great imitators, not only consciously or unconsciously practice the strained look of the eyes of the teachers with imperfect sight, but also the strain of all the nerves of the body. For the benefit of the schoolchildren, no teacher wearing glasses or who has imperfect sight should have charge of children in any public or private school.

Parents wearing glasses are under a nervous strain almost continuously. It can be demonstrated in all cases that the children's eyes tend to strain and that the sight becomes imperfect because most children, if not all, imitate consciously or unconsciously the nervous strain of their parents. The future of our country is in the hands of the children and I believe that we should all make any sacrifice which can be made for their welfare.

It was demonstrated that all persons I tested wearing glasses were curable without glasses. I have demonstrated this fact, that the eyes of all nearsighted persons become normal while looking at a distant blank wall without trying to see. The same is true in all other cases, in farsightedness, in astigmatism; there are no exceptions.

It can always be demonstrated that when the normal eye with normal sight makes an effort to see at the distance, the eye becomes nearsighted; again, no exceptions. When the normal eye strains to see at the near point, the eye tends to become farsighted.

The strain in astigmatism can always be demonstrated. One can, by will, produce in the normal eye any kind of imperfect sight by the necessary strain. The normal eye is always at rest and nothing is done in order to see. If anything is done it is always wrong and always produces imperfect sight. This suggests treatment and prevention. Treatment can only succeed when perfect rest is obtained.

Every physician wearing glasses, like every child, every man, every woman, has to strain to make his eyes fit the glasses. In every case this fact can be demonstrated. Surely the leaders in this movement for the benefit of the eyes of the schoolchildren can be or ought to be the medical profession, and I feel that we are lax in our duty when we neglect to study and practice these methods which cure imperfect sight without the aid of glasses.

Imperfect sight is usually contagious. Actors on the stage do not feel the need of glasses. Fancy some operatic star going through a performance wearing strong glasses. The strain would spoil the music.

Many people are afraid of the light. They protect their eyes with dark glasses when they go to the seashore; they use umbrellas and sunshades; in tropical countries special kinds of hats are popular, hats which are supposed to prevent the bad effects of the sun.

Bookkeepers and people who work by artificial light wear contrivances of all kinds to shade their eyes from the artificial light. Is sunlight injurious? It is not. Of course after remaining in a dark room and suddenly going out into the bright sunlight one feels the change, and if one is at all nervous the effect of the light on the eyes is magnified—exaggerated. Some people believe it injures the eyes to read in the bright sunlight with the sun shining on the page. They complain that the light dazzles their eyes.

I know a farmer who for fifteen years had never been able to do work out in the sun. He complained that the light blinded him and so he remained in a dark room most of the time and was not as happy as he might have been. He had a large family and in their sympathy they believed as he did and all the time cautioned him to protect his eyes. If someone opened the door suddenly and let in the daylight, there was a great rush to close the door and protect the gentleman from the light.

He came to me with his eyes well wrapped up and protected from any light striking his eyes. I darkened the room and had him look down, and when he looked far down I lifted the upper lid and focused a strong light on the white part of his eye—first the artificial light and then the strong light of the sun.

The effect was miraculous. He smiled and walked around the room, looked out the window, put on his hat, walked down the street, and came back feeling first rate. Ever afterwards he enjoyed the light instead of suffering from it. All he needed was a little encouragement. Focusing the strong light on his eyes with the aid of the sun glass and doing it right caused him no pain or discomfort whatever.

I know a white man who lives in Borneo, an island in the tropics. This man goes around without a hat. He told me that the natives did not wear hats and had no discomfort from the sun and what was good enough for the natives was good enough for him, and it certainly worked. He has lived there thirty years or more and the sun does not do him any harm. Did he ever suffer sunstroke? No. Did anybody else ever suffer sunstroke in Borneo? There is no record. Out in the Canadian northwest in the summer time the sun is very strong and the crops mature in a few months. They raise fine wheat there. Do you hear of anybody being sunstruck working in the wheat fields?

In New York City the papers publish records of sunstroke from time to time during the hot weather. I have been called to attend such cases. Quite a number of people living in tenement houses have been ill during the very hot weather and I am quite sure that many years ago I believed that I was treating cases of sunstroke. It is very peculiar but many of these cases never saw the sun and most of them had a breath that we in the days of prohibition might envy.

I do not believe any baseball player or any tennis player, in spite of his strenuous exercise on bright sunshiny days, has ever suffered from any bad effect of the sun. Most tennis players do not even wear a cap to protect their eyes from the sun and you have to have good eyesight to play a good game of tennis. The light of the sun often shines directly into their eyes when they serve the ball and the experts are able to drive the ball quite accurately in spite of the sun.

Many years ago I listened to the older and the wiser men who treat the eye and they complained that something ought to be done to prevent children from playing out in the sun without any hats on. We are more liberal now and treat tuberculosis in children by exposing not only the head and eyes but their whole bodies naked to the sun and I understand it is a very successful treatment. Miners who seldom see the sun always have disease of their eyes. All people who wear dark glasses and avoid the bright sunlight have trouble with their eyes.

I had a patient once who spent two years in a hospital here in New York many years ago, occupied a dark room, had her eyes bandaged with a black cloth so that not a ray of light could possibly enter her eyes, and at the end of her treatment left the hospital worse than she was before. Her vision, which had been one-tenth of the normal with glasses, became normal without glasses after sun treatment.

Some scientists in Boston experimented on the eyes of rabbits. They focused the strong light of the sun directly into the eyes and then examined the retina with a microscope and much to their surprise found nothing wrong. They tried strong electric arc lights and found that the retina was not injured. They used every known light on the eyes of these animals and in no case did the light ever cause an injury.

Concentration

For many years it had been drummed into my mind by my teachers when I first went to school and later by my professors in college, that in order to accomplish things and to make a success of life, one should practice concentration. Recently in New York I received an advertisement from a man who delivers popular lectures, which was an invitation to attend a lecture with the title "Concentration: The Keynote to Success." About the same time one of my patients suffered very much from imperfect sight. The patient bought a book of 500 pages on concentration. He bought the book to improve his memory and his sight.

For many years from time to time patients from the faculties of Columbia, Yale, Harvard, Princeton, Cornell, and other colleges come to me for treatment of their eyes. They all say that not only are they unable to use their eyes for any length of time but that they are also ill in a great many other ways, physically, mentally, their nerves all shot to pieces. They complain that they have lost the power to concentrate.

By investigating the facts I find that invariably they have been teaching concentration. It does me a great deal of good personally to get square with them because these are the people who cause so much imperfect sight. It can be shown that all persons with imperfect sight are trying to concentrate. I have repeatedly published and described the evidence which proves conclusively that concentration of the eyes is impossible.

Trying to do the impossible is a strain, an awful strain, and the worst strain that the eyes can experience. So many people have a theory that concentration is a help and if we could all concentrate we would all be much better off. The trouble is that concentration is a theory and not a fact. If you try to concentrate your mind on a part of a large letter of the Snellen test card at ten feet or twenty feet it can be demonstrated that the effort fails and the vision becomes imperfect.

The same is true of the memory and of the imagination. The dictionary says concentration is an effort to keep your mind fixed on a point. I have tested a great many people and not one was ever able to accomplish it for any length of time, and the result is always bad for the eyes, the memory, the imagination, the nerves of the body generally. If the professors of concentration were wise they would avoid trying to practice it. It is only in that way that they can avoid trouble.

Treatment

If you have imperfect sight and desire to obtain normal vision without glasses, I suggest that you keep in mind a few facts. In the first place, the normal eye does not have normal sight all the time, so if you have relapses in the beginning do not be discouraged. First test your sight with each eye with a Snellen test card at twenty feet, then close your eyes and rest them. Cover them with one or both hands in such a way as to shut out all the light and do this for at least an hour, then open your eyes for a moment and again test your sight with both eyes at the same time.

Your vision should be temporarily improved if you have rested your eyes. If your vision is not improved it means that you have been remembering or imagining things imperfectly and under a strain. With the eyes closed and covered at rest, with your mind at rest, you should not see anything at all—all should be black. If you see colors—red, green, blue, or flashes of light—you are not resting your eyes but you are straining them.

Some people when they close their eyes let their minds drift and think of things which are pleasant to remember, things which come into their minds without their volition and which are remembered quickly, easily, and perfectly. Some patients have great difficulty in improving their sight by closing their eyes and trying to rest them. If you fail, get someone with perfect sight to demonstrate that resting the eyes is a help and who can show you how to do it.

When persons with normal eyes have normal sight they suffer no pain, discomfort, headaches, or fatigue. When a person with imperfect sight closes the eyes and rests them successfully the eye becomes normal for the time being. When such a person looks at the distance and remembers some letter, some color, or some object perfectly, the eyes are normal and the vision is perfect. This is a very remarkable fact; it has been tested in thousands of cases and one can always demonstrate that it is true.

One of the quickest and most satisfactory ways of improving the sight is with a perfect imagination. The normal eye at twenty feet imagines it sees a small letter of the same size as it does at one foot. The eye with imperfect sight on the contrary usually sees a letter at twenty feet larger than it really is.

The normal eye imagines the white of a Snellen test card at twenty feet, ten feet, as white as it is at one foot. The eye with imperfect sight sees the whiteness of the card less white or as a shade of gray.

The white centers of the letters are imagined by the normal eye to be whiter than other parts of the card, while the eye with imperfect sight imagines the white centers of the letters to be less white than the margin of the card. Persons with imperfect sight have been cured very quickly by demonstrating these facts to them and encouraging them to imagine the letters in the same way as the normal eye imagines them.

When reading small print in a newspaper or in a book the normal eye is able to imagine the white spaces between the lines whiter than they really are. The whiter the spaces are imagined, the blacker the letters appear and the more distinct do they become.

Persons with imperfect sight imagine the white spaces between the lines of fine print that they are endeavoring to read, to be as white as the margin of the page. Persons with imperfect sight do not become able to read fine print until they become able to imagine the white spaces between the lines of letters to be whiter than they really are.

When people with normal vision have normal sight they are always able to see one letter best or one part of a letter better than all the rest. It is impossible to see a whole letter at one time perfectly. One has to imagine different parts best. Persons with imperfect sight, when they regard a line of letters that they do not read, discover that they do not see best one part of the line of letters, but rather they see most of the line a pale gray with no separation between the letters.

By central fixation is meant the ability to see best where you are looking. When one sees a small letter clearly or perfectly it can be demonstrated that while the whole letter is seen at one time, one sees or imagines one part best at a time. The normal eye, when it has normal vision, is seeing an illusion and sees one letter of a line best or one part of one letter best at a time.

We do not see illusions; they are imagined. Central fixation is a truth to which there are no exceptions and yet it is all imagination. The more perfect the imagination, the more perfect the sight, and the more perfect is central fixation.

It is interesting to realize that the truth about vision in all its manifestations does not obey the laws of physiology, the laws of optics, the laws of mathematics, and to try to explain in some plausible way, why or how all these things are so, is a waste of time, because I do not believe anybody can explain the various manifestations of the imagination.

Most people have an imagination that is good enough to cure them if they would only use it. What we see is only what we think we see or what we imagine we see. When we imagine correctly we see correctly; when we imagine imperfectly we see imperfectly. People with imperfect sight have difficulty in imagining that they see perfectly at twenty feet the same letter that they do at one foot or less.

It can be demonstrated that when one remembers a letter perfectly one cannot at the same time remember some other letter imperfectly. The same is true of the imagination and of the vision. This fact is of the greatest importance in the treatment of imperfect sight without glasses. If one can remember perfectly a mental picture of some letter at all times, in all places, the imagination and vision for all letters regarded are also perfect.

One can improve the memory by alternately remembering a letter with the eyes closed for part of a minute or longer and then opening the eyes and remembering the same letter for a fraction of a second. Unfortunately it is true that many people with imperfect sight are unable to remember or imagine mental pictures perfectly. The treatment of these cases is complicated.

One patient when he looked at a white pillow saw it without any difficulty. He thought he saw it all at once. When he closed his eyes he could not remember a mental picture of the pillow.

With his eyes open I called his attention to the fact that he did not see the whole pillow equally white at the same time, but that his eyes shifted from one corner that he saw best to another corner or to another part of the pillow and that he successively imagined one small part of the pillow best. With his eyes open he could not see two corners of the pillow best at the same time. He had to see it by central fixation, one part best, in order to see it perfectly. I suggested that when he closed his eyes he remember the pillow in the same way, one corner at a time or one small area best at a time.

He immediately for the first time in his life obtained a mental picture of the pillow. Afterwards he became able to remember or imagine a mental picture of the pillow with his eyes closed by practicing the same methods. He became able to imagine mental pictures of one letter at a time. Always he found that he could not remember the whole letter at once. The strain was evident and made it impossible. By alternately remembering a mental picture of a letter with his eyes closed and remembering the same picture with his eyes open for a short fraction of a second, he became able to remember the mental picture of a letter when looking at a blank wall where there was nothing to see, just as well as he could with his eyes closed.

It required many hours of practice before he could remember the letter perfectly when looking anywhere near the Snellen test card, because he could not remember one letter perfectly and imagine one letter on the Snellen test card imperfectly without losing the mental picture. In other words he could not imagine one thing perfectly and something else imperfectly at the same time.

After a patient has become able, under favorable conditions, to imagine mental pictures as well with the eyes open as with the eyes closed, his cure can be obtained in a reasonable length of time. One patient, for example, could not see the largest letter on the Snellen test card at more than three feet, but by practicing the memory of the mental picture of a letter alternately with his eyes closed and with his eyes open he was permanently cured in a few weeks.

In the beginning, even with strong glasses, the vision that he obtained was one-tenth of the normal, but with the help of the mental pictures he became able to read without glasses at twenty feet the 10-line on the Snellen test card, 20/10. Schoolchildren who have never worn glasses, under twelve years old, can easily be cured by their teachers in two weeks or less.

It is very important that all patients who desire to be cured of imperfect sight should discard their glasses and never put them on again for any emergencies. It is not well to use opera glasses. Going without glasses has at least one benefit: it acts as an incentive to the patient to practice the right methods in order to obtain all the sight that seems possible.

Prevention of Myopia in Schoolchildren

About fifteen years ago I introduced my method for the prevention of myopia in schoolchildren in a number of the schools in the city of New York. In one year I studied the records of twenty thousand children who had been tested before and after the treatment. To prove a negative proposition, to prove that something does not occur because something else is done, is a difficult or impossible proposition. When I recommended my treatment for the schoolchildren I claimed that every child who used the method properly would see better and that no matter how poor the sight might be or how long the sight had been imperfect the vision would be improved always.

I made the statement that if there were one exception my method was only a working hypothesis at best or a theory, and that I was wrong about everything I said. Since all the children who used the method had their sight improved, it is evident that imperfect sight from myopia was prevented in those children at that time.

I have published from time to time reports on results of my method for the prevention of myopia in schoolchildren. These reports are on file in the New York Academy of Medicine and can be consulted by anybody.

In 1912 I read a paper on this subject before the New York County Medical Association in which I made the statement that every child with normal eyes and normal sight who strains to see at the distance becomes temporarily or more continuously nearsighted. There are no exceptions.

If one competent ophthalmologist can prove that I am wrong about one case, I am wrong about all the statements I have made about myopia. This experiment can be performed in the doctor's office or at his clinic and the facts determined with the aid of a retinoscope, an instrument used for measuring the amount of nearsightedness which may be present in the eye.

There were present at this meeting a large number of prominent eye doctors of the city of New York. They knew that I was going to make this statement and issue this challenge because I sent a copy of my paper to these gentlemen two weeks before I read it. It would have been very easy for any of them to have tested the matter and determined whether I was right or wrong, but when the Chairperson of the Society called on them to discuss my paper they declined to say anything about it or to publicly deny it.

I have the records of many persons who threw away their glasses and now have perfect sight with normal eyes.

They did it.

Everybody can do it.

YOU can do it.

Better Eyesight
August 1929—Vol. XIV, No. 2

SCHOOL NUMBER

SCHOOLCHILDREN I

By W. H. Bates, M.D.

Imperfect sight is found in the eyes of most schoolchildren of the United States, Canada, France, and other countries. In Germany a great deal has been done to lessen this evil among schoolchildren and it is well known that the statistics of imperfect sight in schoolchildren in Germany have proved that the numerous methods recommended for the prevention or cure of imperfect sight have been failures. It is estimated that in the city of New York, one-tenth or more of the children are wearing glasses. All attempts to benefit the eyes of schoolchildren so that they will not need glasses have been suppressed by the Board of Education and the Board of Health. Many principals of large schools have encouraged to the best of their ability the work that can be done to cure or prevent imperfect sight in schoolchildren. It is difficult to understand why there should be so much opposition to this work.

In 1912 all school teachers were encouraged in some of the larger schools to recommend and practice any methods which promised prevention or cure. One of the opponents of the prevention of imperfect sight in schoolchildren made the statement that it is impossible to prove a negative proposition and therefore a negative proposition cannot be proved. A positive proposition is one in which a cure can be obtained by treatment. When the methods employed do not cure imperfect sight without glasses, one cannot expect the same methods to prevent imperfect sight. A positive proposition suggests methods that cure; a negative proposition does not suggest successful treatment and does not prevent imperfect sight. Measures that cure also prevent; methods that do not cure cannot be expected to prevent.

In some cities it was believed by many that the cause of imperfect sight in schoolchildren was the use of small print in the textbooks. When schools were permitted to use only large print for the children, eyestrain, headaches and other troubles became more numerous than when small print was employed; repeated trials of books in which large print was used always failed to prevent discomfort. Just as many children wore glasses after the use of textbooks with large print as when the books were printed in small print. Even the school authorities and the Board of Health were finally convinced that large print was more injurious to the eyes of schoolchildren than was the small print which had previously been used continuously. Evidently, the cause of imperfect sight in schoolchildren was not connected in any way with the size of print used in textbooks.

It has been generally believed also that the imperfect light of schoolrooms is the cause of imperfect sight in schoolchildren. In some cases there seemed to be too much light, while in other cases it was believed that there was not enough light. I have studied the connection of the amount of light to the cause of imperfect sight. After many years of observation, I became convinced that the amount of light has nothing whatever to do with the cause of myopia, hypermetropia, astigmatism, or other cases of imperfect sight in schoolchildren. Many children with high degrees of myopia and other causes of imperfect sight have been permanently cured by practicing the reading of microscopic type, with changing powers of illumination. It is an error to claim that light has anything to do with the production of imperfect sight. Children with progressive myopia have been benefited or cured by eye education when a poor light or a bright light was used.

In Germany and in other parts of Europe, as well as in this country, the problem of the cause of imperfect sight in schoolchildren has received a great deal of attention. For example, in the year 1882, the minister of public education in France convoked a committee which investigated very thoroughly the light in schoolrooms. The committee dwelt especially upon the point that as the most essential light was that which shone directly from the sky upon the scholars, every scholar should be in a position to see a piece of the sky corresponding in size to a window space of at least 30 centimeters (about 12 inches) long, measured from the upper edge of the glass of the upper window.

There is a large library of books describing the necessity of the proper amount of light, as measured with scientific instruments, each instrument being different in some particular from every other instrument for measuring the light. These studies and the injurious or the beneficial effects of light will now have to be modified, as I have found that the light has nothing to do with the cause of imperfect sight and that any measures adopted to change, lessen or increase the light are usually a waste of time and effort. [Full-spectrum light has been proven beneficial to one's health. See the chapter "Light" in *Relearning to See.*—TRQ]

I have proved that any effort or strain to improve the vision always lowers the vision. Straining the eyes to see at long distances always produces nearsightedness. When efforts were made to see at the near point continuously, the eyes became farsighted. It can be demonstrated that the normal eye with normal sight becomes imperfect by a strain to see. When the eyes are relaxed, the vision always becomes normal. One of the best methods for children to practice in order to produce relaxation is that in which the body is swayed from side to side. This prevents strain, because the eyes are kept in motion and the stare is avoided. When the eyes stare, an effort has to be made to prevent the eyes from moving.

It is a rest to the eye to shift from one point to another point. When done easily, without effort, the eyes are rested, the vision improves, and the stare is prevented. Swinging was first used to rest the eyes and it was not expected that the movement of the eyes slowly and continuously would be followed by any other benefits. It was demonstrated, however, that all children who practiced the method, besides relaxing their eyes also obtained relaxation in all parts of their body.

It is a fact—a truth—that rest improves the sight and relieves or cures many diseases of the eyes. Those children who do not practice the sway correctly are not benefited. The most common mistake that is made is to turn the head to one side and turn the eyes in the opposite direction while swaying. In many cases the strain is so terrific that it is followed by much pain or discomfort, and imperfect sight.

I have found that a great many children strain while they are asleep; this I have discovered by the use of the ophthalmoscope, without necessarily awakening the child. Those children who strain during sleep are often very nervous while awake and suffer from headaches and pain in the eyes and other parts of the body. Practicing the swing properly just before retiring at night fifty to one hundred times is beneficial. Some children will palm until they go to sleep. This produces relaxation which may last through the night and bring relief. This method of prevention may be practiced by young children at the age of four as well as by older children.

The writer wishes to recommend a method for the cure or prevention of imperfect sight in schoolchildren which has been used successfully. A Snellen test card is placed permanently on the wall of a classroom in a place where it can be read at all times by the children. All the children's eyes were tested at ten feet each day, first with both eyes together and then with each eye separately. All the teachers who practiced the methods reported that every child who used the method regularly was benefited to a greater or lesser degree. Not only was the sight improved but also headaches, pains, and other nervous symptoms were relieved. One of the greatest benefits of the method was that it cured retardation. The mentality of children who had been backward in their studies was improved so that they were able to keep up with the work along with the other children.

SCHOOLCHILDREN II

By Emily A. Bates

The number of schoolchildren who were successfully treated during the past year by Dr. Bates, Ms. Hayes, our assistant, and myself, far exceeds that of the year before. Our records show that the Bates Method is becoming better known all over the world.

Children with imperfect sight who come to us for treatment and who have never worn glasses are very easily cured. Some need only one treatment while others need one or two weeks of daily treatment before the sight is brought back to normal. Some cases of high myopia or hypermetropia need personal supervision for even a longer time, especially when eyeglasses have been worn. During the last year I have had quite a number of schoolchildren under my care and up to date not one of them has failed me. According to my records and reports by letter, every one of them has had permanent benefit.

June and Donald are brother and sister. A former patient of Dr. Bates met their mother and told her what Dr. Bates had done for her and for her children. Then she came to us. They came on June 14, 1929, and each of them was examined by Dr. Bates. Donald, eleven years old, had mixed astigmatism with myopia. Two years ago he put on glasses for the first time, and from the time he put them on, his mother noticed that he acquired the habit of lowering his head to look at anything he wanted to see at close range. While lowering his head, his eyes were looking upward. This caused constant strain. The mother noticed that Donald did not do this when he removed his glasses at night. She also noticed that he was less nervous without his glasses than he was while wearing them. From time to time during the two years in which he wore his glasses, he was taken to different eye specialists, to find out if he was wearing the wrong glasses, which was thought to be the reason why he held his head in an unnatural position. The doctors who examined him told her that he would outgrow this habit in time and that the glasses were quite right for him.

The vision of both eyes was the same, 15/30 minus, which meant that Donald could only read some of the letters of the 30-line of the test card. Even with the largest letter of the card, which is seen by the normal eye at 200 feet, he strained to see. After his eyes were tested with the test card and Dr. Bates had examined him, we proceeded in the usual way of testing his eyes with the various test cards at ten feet. He was eager to see what could really be done for him so that he could get rid of his horrid glasses. I asked him if he enjoyed football, swimming, horseback riding, and baseball. He said there was no need in going any further about what kind of sports he liked most. He said he liked them all, but that his glasses hindered him from participating in such fun for fear of having an accident, which would cause him to lose his sight. When a boy talks like that, it doesn't take very long for him to respond to the treatment and to carry out the instructions necessary to restore his sight to the normal.

I explained to Donald how mental pictures help when the eyes are closed, and that if he could remember something perfectly, while he was resting his eyes, such as a letter of the test card, a rainbow with its many colors, a beautiful sunset, or his cravat with stripes of colors, which could be remembered while his eyes were closed, or any object which is pleasant to the eyesight, he would no doubt be able to read the test card better when he again opened his eyes.

He followed my suggestion carefully in looking at a letter of the test card, then closing his eyes and drawing the outline with his finger while his eyes were closed. I asked him if he could remember the shade of the letter. The letter was black and the background was white. He said that he could remember the letter was a perfect black by first imagining that the background was as white as snow or as white as a white cloud. He said he could feel the movement of his eyes as he outlined the letter with his finger. Donald enjoyed the fun, as he called it, outlining letters while his eyes were closed and then occasionally looking at the card to read a few more letters.

His sister, who was sitting outside of the room, but could hear everything that was said, was a little doubtful about what could be done for her eyes. The mother was in the room watching everything that was going on and taking notes so that she would know how to take care of Donald's treatment at home. Patiently, Donald worked with me, resting his eyes by closing them frequently when I told him to, and outlining the last letter he saw on the test card each time he rested. As the sun was not shining in the room where he was being treated, a Thermo-lite was used, which he seemed to like very much. The light and heat helped in the improvement of his vision and also helped him to look at the card, without lowering his head.

As his mother watched the steady improvement in his sight, she could not suppress her enthusiasm and gratitude. Occasionally, she would remark to her boy, "Think of it, Donald, you will not need glasses ever again." Gradually, I placed the test card farther and farther away and in an hour's time, he read 10/15 with each eye. I placed him comfortably in a chair, telling him not to open his eyes, but to take the light treatment until he felt uncomfortable, and then to shut off the light and still keep his eyes closed while I treated his sister, June.

June is nine years old and had worn glasses for a year or more. She had trouble in keeping her eyes open normally without her glasses and closed them almost entirely in order to see. She preferred to do this rather than to wear her glasses. She also had myopia, about the same degree as her brother. When I placed her before the test card, ten feet away, she strained to see the letters and did not blink as I pointed to the largest letters of the test card. She could read the first three lines by squeezing her eyes together, but the letters looked blurred to her. By closing her eyes often, following the treatment I gave her brother, imagining the white background of the card whiter than it really was and imagining the black letters blacker, outlining letters with her forefinger as she mentioned them, her vision with each eye improved to 10/30. It took about an hour to improve her vision to 10/10, but gradually as she read one line after another, alternately closing her eyes to rest them and receiving the Thermo-lite treatment frequently at short intervals, she became able to read with her eyes open in a normal way. I told her to sit with her eyes closed for a while and to remember familiar objects as I had advised Donald to do.

Then I returned to Donald to give him more help. I placed the test card thirteen feet away and by receiving a little light treatment, at intervals, with the light about ten feet away from him so that the rays was not too strong for his eyes or the heat too great, he became able to read the smallest letters of the test card without any strain or discomfort. The long swing was added to the latter part of his treatment, swaying and looking at a blank wall where there was nothing to see and then to the test card, reading one letter at a time and then swaying again to the blank wall.

Then June followed her brother in the treatment, doing just as well as he did with the reading of the test card letters at 13 feet, 13/10. This is more than the normal distance.

Both children expressed their gratitude to me for the help that had been given them and then they insisted that Dr. Bates be called away from his work to come to them for his share of praise. They wanted to shake hands with the great man who could do so much good for schoolchildren.

I was very tired that morning and did not feel physically fit to look after the work that had to be done. After Donald and his sister June had spent more than two hours with me, I was relieved of all fatigue and discomfort for the rest of the day. I had a good reason to be happy and to feel that something good had been done, because I had helped two children obtain normal sight in one treatment. After the children had left, their mother promised to write to us for further help if further help was necessary. She was not to communicate with us unnecessarily if the children retained their normal vision. Up to date, we have not heard from the mother.

Paul was another boy who came for treatment about the same time. His father telephoned before sending his son, telling me that the school authorities had insisted very strongly that he get glasses for Paul, but the father refused to submit to such a thing, until he was sure that nothing else could be done. Paul had never worn glasses and when they were suggested to him, if Dr. Bates could not help him, he wept bitter tears and at times was disobedient, which sometimes called for punishment.

Paul came with a written statement from his mother, saying that at the age of five years he was taken ill with measles and after that sties appeared at intervals, causing an almost constant inflammation of the eyelids. Because Paul had played with a child who was supposed to have an incurable eye trouble, Paul's mother feared that he had acquired this incurable disease also. His eyelids were itchy most of the time and at the advice of an eye doctor a solution of boric acid was used and a medicine called mecca was also applied. Paul found some relief from the use of these applications, but the sties appeared just the same and he noticed that the letters on the blackboard at school became less distinct at such times.

In 1928 he had scarlet fever, and pink eye began three months previous to his visit to me. Paul's vision with each eye was 10/10 but he strained to see as he read the smaller letters of the test card. The sun was shining through the windows in the room where I was treating him. I placed him in the sun with his eyes closed and used the sun glass rapidly on the edge of his eyelids as well as on the upper and lower lids. This was about midday, and the sun was rather hot so I had to use the glass very rapidly in order to avoid any discomfort or burning of the lids. His elder brother who came with him remarked how well the eyelids looked after the sun treatment. This was accomplished in less than an hour's time.

After the sun treatment, I placed the test card at ten feet. He read the smallest letters without any effort or strain. Again I placed him in the sun and taught his elder brother how to use the sun glass while I was occupied with something else. We had to keep Paul busy while he was resting this way because he was restless and being a perfectly normal healthy boy did not like being quiet. He told me a funny tale and then in turn I told him one and in this way we passed the time away. Finally after another half-hour of sun treatment, Paul read all the tests cards with different letters at fifteen feet from his eyes without any trouble whatever, 15/10.

The irritation of the eyelids had disappeared and the itching had stopped, but Paul was told that this might be only a temporary relief and that he would have to take a good deal of sun treatment before he was finally rid of his trouble. He promised to take all the sun treatment he could possibly get by placing himself in the sun, and raising his head so that the sun could shine on his closed eyelids. He was given a test card to practice with daily and to use to show his mother how far away he could read it while blinking and swaying his body from side to side to avoid the stare.

Paul and his brother promised to notify Dr. Bates if he needed further help, or if he had any further discomfort with his eyes. Two weeks later, his elder brother came to report that apparently Paul was cured in one treatment because no further complaints came from the school about his having to wear glasses nor did the irritation of the eyelids reappear.

CASE REPORTS: SCHOOLCHILDREN

By Katherine Hayes

Since it has been my privilege to assist Ms. Bates in Clinic work, I have come in contact with a number of interesting cases, especially among children of school age. I have found that children as a rule respond much more readily to treatment than adults and I believe the reason is because they have a natural aversion to the wearing of glasses and are willing to learn how to improve their vision without them. I think this is especially true of children from ten to fourteen years old who have some definite reason for wanting to discard their glasses.

About six months ago, a little girl came to the Clinic for treatment. I noticed that she kept looking down and did not raise her eyes once. When this girl's turn came for treatment, her mother gave me an account of her case. She was eleven years old and had been wearing glasses off and on for squint for five years. When she was six she had an attack of whooping-cough which caused her left eye to turn in. The vision in that eye was also impaired. They had been to several eye doctors, most of whom had advised an operation, but her mother was unwilling to have the child submit to this. After her mother had finished, the little girl came over to me and said in a confidential tone, without raising her eyes, "You know, people say that I would be quite a little beauty if it weren't for my crossed eye. I hate glasses because they make me homely and I only wear them once in a while. Someday I want to be an actress on the stage or in the movies and I know they won't take me if I am crossed eye. Can my eye ever be made straight again?" I told her I thought it could if she would do what she was instructed to do at home and come regularly to the Clinic.

I tested her sight and found that in the right eye it was 15/10 or better than normal, while in the left eye it was 15/50. I showed her how to palm, which she did for fifteen minutes. I then told her to remove her hands from her eyes. For a moment, her eye was straight. I tested her vision again and found that by having her sway and blink as she read the card, her vision improved to 15/30. I told her to practice palming every day as many times as possible for five minutes at a time, to practice the long swing 100 times morning and night, and to remember to blink her eyes frequently.

When she came again, two weeks later, her vision was still 15/30, which indicated that she had been faithful in her practice work. I also noticed that her eye was not quite as crossed as it had been. She came regularly for about four months and the last time she came her vision in the left eye had improved to normal and her eye was perfectly straight. Little Elsie was very happy. I told her that even though her vision was normal and her eye straight, she should remember to rest her eyes occasionally, in order to avoid any strain which might lower her vision and cause a return of the squint. I have not seen or heard from her since, but I am sure that her vanity, if nothing else, will encourage her to take good care of her eyes.

About the same time, a boy of thirteen came for treatment. He was wearing glasses which he had been using for three years. His dislike of glasses was not prompted by vanity as in little Elsie's case, but because he liked all sorts of sports and could not engage in any of them because of his "old glasses" as he called them. "Gee," he said, "if I didn't have to wear those things, I'd be happy."

After testing his vision, I found that he had quite a high degree of myopia. His vision was 15/70 with both eyes. Palming seemed to make him restless, so I told him to just close his eyes and sit back comfortably in the chair. After twenty minutes, he was directed to stand up and look out the window, then to start swaying from side to side as he blinked his eyes. After practicing this for five minutes, I again tested his vision, and found that it had improved to 15/40. I told him to leave his glasses off and gave him instructions to follow at home.

When he came again, his vision was not quite 15/50. He said that he had had a bad cold and was not able to practice. I gave him light treatment for about twenty minutes, after which his vision improved to 15/30 minus. I told him to get a great deal of sun treatment at home, letting the sun shine on his closed eyelids as he moved his head slowly from side to side. When he came again, his vision had improved to 15/20 minus. He continued to improve steadily and when he came the last time, which was about a month ago, his vision was normal in both eyes. Needless to say he was a happy boy, and incidentally, as he was leaving the office he said that he thought Dr. Bates was the most wonderful man in the whole world, with the exception of his own father.

Better Eyesight
September 1929—Vol. XIV, No. 3

THE COLON

While the colon is a valuable punctuation mark, it has a very unusual and better use in helping the memory, imagination, and sight. Medium-sized or small letters at the distance are improved promptly by the proper use of the colon. While the eyes are closed or open, the top period should be imagined best while the lower period is more or less blurred and not seen so well. In a few moments it is well to shift and imagine the lower period best while the upper period is imagined not so well. Common sense makes it evident that one period cannot be imagined best unless there is some other period or other object which is seen worse. The smallest colon that can be imagined is usually the one that is imagined more readily than a larger colon.

When palming, swinging, etc., cannot be practiced sufficiently well to obtain improvement in the eyesight, the memory or imagination of the small colon, one part best, can usually be practiced with benefit. To remember or imagine a colon perfectly requires constant shifting. When the colon is remembered or imagined perfectly, and this cannot be done by any effort or strain, the sight is always improved and the memory and imagination are also improved. It is interesting to note that the smaller the colon, the blacker and better can one remember, imagine, or see one period of it, with benefit to the sight. One may feel that the memory of a very small colon should be more difficult than the memory of a large one, but strange to say it can be demonstrated in most cases that the very small colon is remembered best. If the movement of the colon is absent, the sight is always imperfect. In other words, it requires a stare, strain, and effort to make the colon stop its apparent motion.

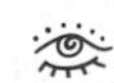

RETINITIS PIGMENTOSA

By W. H. Bates, M.D.

There are many cases of imperfect sight which are congenital. That is, people are born with different diseases of the eye. Retinitis pigmentosa is usually congenital. The condition is easily recognized in most cases with the aid of the ophthalmoscope. In all cases, the retina is covered more or less completely with black areas. These black areas are about 1/30 of an inch in diameter. They are very irregular in size and shape. In severe cases of retinitis pigmentosa, the retina may be covered so thickly by these black specks that the retina cannot be seen.

Most cases give a history of poor sight from birth. At first, only a small number of black spots are visible, but after the child is twelve years old or older, the number of these spots increases gradually. At the same time that these spots are increasing, there are serious changes taking place in the back part of the eye. The optic nerve becomes atrophied, but the atrophy does not increase sufficiently to produce complete blindness. The middle coat of the eyeball, the choroid, is inflamed and produces floating spots in the vitreous (one of the fluids in the back part of eye.)

All cases of retinitis pigmentosa acquire cataract before they are thirty years old. There are exceptions to this rule, however. Some patients acquire retinitis pigmentosa after they are fifty years old or older. One characteristic of retinitis pigmentosa is that the vision is always changing, sometimes for the better, sometimes for the worse. One very common symptom that is usually present is night blindness. Treatment for the cure of the night blindness helps retinitis pigmentosa. In some cases myopia is present and it is of a kind which is difficult to cure.

It is a prevailing belief that retinitis pigmentosa is incurable and that when it becomes manifest in its early stages, the condition goes on increasing and the blindness becomes more decided. Usually, the blindness does not become permanent. One case of retinitis pigmentosa with myopia was observed. The patient left town and was not seen again for more than six months. She then came into the office to report. Her first words were that her eyes were better.

A physician was calling on me at the same time, and he was asked, "Would you like to see a case of retinitis pigmentosa?" He replied that he would.

Before the doctor used the ophthalmoscope, I examined the eye myself. I examined the right eye first and found that the nasal side of the retina was not diseased. There were no black pigment spots anywhere to be seen on the nasal side. Somewhat disturbed, I examined more carefully the temporal side of the retina and again I was disappointed because there were no black spots there. After a long and tedious search for the black spots, I had to confess to my friend that the patient had recovered from the retinitis pigmentosa and accomplished it unconsciously without practicing relaxation methods. The doctor could not resist looking at me incredulously. I am quite sure he thought I was not telling the truth. The atrophy of the optic nerve had also disappeared and with its disappearance circulation of the nerve was restored. The size and appearance of the nerve were normal. The patient became able to read 20/20 without any trouble. It is very interesting to observe in most cases of retinitis pigmentosa how much damage can be done to the retina while the vision remains good.

Many physicians believe that night blindness cannot be cured. The majority of these cases in my practice have usually recovered and obtained not only normal vision, but they have become able to see better than the average. All patients who were suffering from chronic retinitis pigmentosa had changes in the optic nerve which were very characteristic. In the first place the blood vessels were smaller than in the normal eye and the veins just as small if not smaller than the arteries which emerged from the center of the optic nerve. In most cases the middle coat of the eyeball becomes inflamed and usually much black material is found in the vitreous. There are well-marked changes which take place in the crystalline lens. The back part of the lens becomes cloudy and this cloudiness moves forward toward the center of the lens and clouds all parts of it so that the vision is lowered by the opacity of the lens as well as by the more serious changes which occur behind the lens.

A patient sixty years old came to me for treatment. She said that the doctors told her that she had retinitis pigmentosa and that she could not be cured. Within the last few months her doctor had told her that a cataract had formed. Her vision was zero in the right eye, which had cataract. The vision of the left eye was about one-third of the normal and was not improved by glasses. She had a well-marked case of retinitis pigmentosa in which the retina of the left eye was apparently covered almost completely by the pigment spots. In some parts of the retina over an area of more than double the diameter of the optic nerve, the retina could not be seen. The patient was very anxious to have me do what I could for her sight. She said that her husband was a business man and had occasion to travel all over the United States, Canada, and Europe. He frequently took her with him, and whenever they came to a large town where some prominent ophthalmologist had his office, she would consult him about her eyes.

I found that the back part of the crystalline lens was covered by a faint opacity which was sufficient to lessen her vision. The patient was given a Snellen test card to practice with for the good eye. In twenty-four hours the vision of the right eye had improved from no perception of light to the ability to read some of the large letters of the Snellen test card at five feet. Improvement in the vision of the left eye was manifest. The great improvement in so short a time in the vision of the right eye was unusual.

The treatment which improved the vision of this patient was palming, swinging, and reading very fine print. This patient gave evidence that retinitis pigmentosa is caused by a strain or an effort to see. The fact that retinitis pigmentosa in the eyes of this patient was so promptly relieved, benefited, or cured was evidence that the disease was caused by strain.

The clinical reports of other cases of retinitis pigmentosa confirm the fact that strain or an effort to see produces retinitis pigmentosa. The efforts which are practiced by the patient can be demonstrated in every case. When the patient makes an effort to improve the vision, it can be demonstrated in every case that the cause of the eye trouble is always due to this effort and the cure of the disease is always obtained by relaxation methods.

I have found that among the methods of relaxation which secure the best results are the memory or the imagination of perfect sight. If the memory or the imagination is imperfect, the disease is not completely relieved or benefited. When one letter of the Snellen test card is seen perfectly, it can be remembered or imagined perfectly. There is no procedure which yields better results in the cure of this eye trouble than the memory of part of a letter, which the patient can demonstrate. It is very interesting to observe that in these cases the memory and imagination are capable of bringing about the absorption or the disappearance of organic conditions. This makes it possible for this treatment to accomplish results readily, quickly, when all other treatment is of no avail.

For example, a girl fifteen years old had suffered from retinitis pigmentosa from birth. The disease was rapidly progressing and it did not seem that any relief would be obtained by any form of treatment; the patient was simultaneously suffering from progressive myopia. Relaxation treatment, the correct use of her memory, and imagination improved the progressive myopia and much to the delight of the patient, the retinitis pigmentosa improved at the same time and continued to improve until all traces of the disease were absent and she was permanently cured.

It seems to be one of the peculiarities of the disease that it is variable. Oftentimes it gets better for a short time when all of a sudden, overnight perhaps, the disease will return with all its accustomed forms of black pigment spots, atrophy of the optic nerve, diminished circulation, and incipient cataract.

Retinitis pigmentosa has been observed in cases of glaucoma, chronic cases which progressed with more or less rapidity until almost total blindness was observed. In other cases, different parts of the choroid would be destroyed, and there would be loss of vision in these areas.

The vision of children ten years old, suffering from this disease, has been remarkably improved by swinging the child in a circular direction several times daily repeated for many weeks. This promotes relaxation. It is a mistake to dispose of cradles, rocking chairs, and other methods of promoting the swing. The long swing, (described several times in this magazine) is a very efficient method of obtaining relaxation. Many people object that children have not sufficient intelligence to practice the swing successfully. On the contrary, children ten years old or under can practice the long swing as successfully as many adults. It is a treatment that the patient enjoys to a decided extent. Games of all kinds should also be encouraged. It is well to protect the child from adults and others who make the child nervous. Nervousness always causes strain. Laughter and good times are relaxing. The kindergarten is a good place for all children at an early age, because relaxation methods of the best kind are taught there.

Before closing, reference should be made to a girl fourteen years old who cured herself of retinitis pigmentosa by playing games and engaging in sports that she enjoyed. In the summer time she enjoyed swimming and diving from very great heights; in the winter time she practiced skating, devoting long periods of time to this sport. Besides the relaxation methods which I have described, it is worth the trouble to teach children who have so-called incurable diseases how to enjoy themselves for long periods of time both winter and summer. Their eyes as well as their bodies are kept in motion while playing games or engaging in sports which relieve the stare and strain that cause imperfect sight. It is so much more efficient and better than drugs.

DISCARDING GLASSES NOT INJURIOUS

By Emily A. Bates

The most difficult thing for a patient to do is to discard glasses immediately. When a patient comes to us, recommended by his physician or oculist, we have no difficulty in this respect, even though he has worn glasses for many years. But when a patient comes for treatment at the suggestion of a friend or someone who has been benefited by the Bates Method, there is sometimes a doubt in the patient's mind as to whether it is a mistake or injurious for him to stop wearing his glasses immediately after having worn them for a long time.

[Emily A. Bates' own improvement follows; see also "Don't Be Afraid" in the February 1929 issue.—TRQ]

Nineteen years ago I came to Dr. Bates as a patient. Headaches, nausea, and continuous pain in the back of my neck made me irritable and nervous, and sometimes I was not a very agreeable person to have about. A neighbor of my little mother first told me about Dr. Bates and how he had cured her five children of imperfect sight and other ailments.

I felt quite comfortable at times with the glasses I wore and because they helped me to see better I wore them almost constantly. As I explained in a previous article, I had worn glasses a little more than thirteen years, and during that time I had them changed three times. The last glasses I wore did not help me when I first put them on. The oculist informed me that I would have to wear them for a few weeks until I became accustomed to them. They were much stronger glasses than those I had worn previously and for that reason the oculist told me my eyes would adjust themselves to the glasses in time.

This must have been the case because after a while I got along nicely with them for a few hours every day, but toward the end of almost every day the nausea and discomfort became a regular occurrence. When I visited Dr. Bates for the first time I did not know that the glasses I was wearing were the cause of my pain and discomfort. In fact I did not altogether believe that Dr. Bates was right in the diagnosis he had made of my case. I put my glasses away as he suggested, but the very next day I was ready to complain about my usual headache and other pains. However I did not have anything to complain about. But I neglected some of my daily duties about my home to practice what the Doctor told me to do.

I soon found out that blinking often made me feel easier—that things about the house looked clearer to me when I blinked. I liked that, so I kept it up all day. Dr. Bates noticed during my treatment that I did not breathe regularly and advised me to do so. I made it a practice to blink as I inhaled and exhaled so one thing reminded me to do the other. As I looked into a mirror I noticed as I blinked that my eyes moved slightly, which gave me a sense of relaxation I did not have while wearing my glasses. Dr. Bates explained in his book and in other articles that he has written that when eyestrain is relieved, strain in all parts of the body is also relieved. Dr. Bates advised me to close my eyes to rest them, which always improved my vision for the test card.

The second day I wanted very much to put on my glasses again because I woke up that morning with a terrific headache. I was almost sure that Dr. Bates was wrong about the whole thing. I telephoned to him and argued the matter with him. I was much surprised to have him tell me that I might have strained my eyes during sleep. How absurd this seemed to me, but he was right about this and I will explain how I found it out for myself and how I relieved the strain by doing exactly as he advised me.

I placed my alarm clock on a chair beside my bed and set the alarm to ring two hours after I had fallen asleep. If I had a dream during those two hours of sleep, I had a pad and pencil near me to write down what I could remember of my dream. Some of our *Better Eyesight* readers will say that this was a waste of time and may even laugh at such a procedure during the night. Later on I was glad I did this because I was entirely cured of nightmares which caused me many times to apologize for waking up members of my family with screams or causing other disturbances which were sometimes a great worry to those near me.

I practiced the long swing for five minutes or longer every night and morning in addition to other things that Dr. Bates advised me to do during the night.

Children are more ready to discard their glasses than are adults and for that reason there are more children cured without glasses than adults, and in a shorter time. Some patients who come to us for treatment have been wearing eyeglasses that are very weak in power and yet they say they cannot possibly do without them. Doing without glasses a little longer each day is a good way to begin. If one has been wearing glasses for a long time, it is much easier for the patient to gradually do without them, if he is not under treatment for the removal of glasses.

A man, age 57, who had astigmatism in both eyes, was afraid to leave off his glasses after the first treatment. He had worn glasses for thirty-six years, having had them changed several times during this period. At the age of 21, he paid his first visit to an oculist who told him that the compound hypermetropic astigmatism which he had would get worse if he did not wear his glasses steadily. He obeyed the oculist and in a year's time he had the glasses changed. The first few years he did not notice much discomfort while wearing the glasses, but later on if he did not remove the glasses occasionally and close his eyes to rest them, he would feel so tired that even at his work he would fall asleep.

He was examined by a good specialist who was recommended by his family physician, thinking that perhaps he might have had an attack of sleeping sickness. After chemical tests were made it was found that all the organs of his body were perfectly normal, and the doctor suggested that perhaps he might be wearing the wrong glasses. Then he became interested in the Bates Method and came for treatment. I asked him to read the test card with his glasses on and he read 10/40. Without glasses he could not see anything on the test card clearly at ten feet, so I placed the cards at seven feet. At seven feet he could only read up to the 50-line letters of the test card.

He liked palming very much and kept his eyes closed for a considerable length of time while I was talking to his family physician, who came with the patient to see what could be done for him. I told my patient while he was palming that a good memory usually helped, but not to remember anything disagreeable while palming. He liked outdoor sports and was a good golf player, so I told him to imagine the golf ball as he sent it across the field and to imagine that it went into the cup. After he had rested his eyes in this way it was amusing to hear him tell us that he had had a good game of golf while his eyes were closed. Evidently this helped because his vision improved to 7/15, although all the letters on the 15-line were not entirely clear to him. When he strained to see some of the letters they became blurred and distorted and he read them incorrectly. After he had palmed his eyes again for a shorter period, he read all the letters of the 15-line clearly and without any hesitation whatever.

I gave him the Fundamentals card to read and told him to hold it at the usual reading distance. He said all the print was blurred and he could not see anything but the word "Fundamentals" at the top of the card after he had closed his eyes for a few seconds. I told him to hold the Fundamentals card in his left hand while in his right hand he held the small card with diamond type. I directed him to look first at the white spaces of the small card in his right hand and then turn his head and look at the Fundamentals card and not to try to read the letters. While he was doing this I told him to draw the Fundamentals card a little farther away, about twelve inches from his eyes. By alternately closing his eyes to rest them, imagining the white spaces between the lines of type, and then looking at the beginning of each sentence, he read down to sentence No. 6.

I told him to look directly at the print and see what happened. He immediately closed his eyes and said that the print blurred and that it made him uncomfortable. For almost an hour he practiced looking from the white spaces between the lines of fine print to the white spaces between the lines of larger print of the Fundamentals card and before he left the office that day, he read all of the Fundamentals card at six inches as well as at twelve inches. He telephoned a few days later and said that he felt no discomfort although he had discarded his glasses. There were times, however, when he did have a strong desire to put them on again. Advice by mail helped, and in a year's time his vision became normal.

Having so little fear about removing his glasses after having worn them so many years was proof enough that it could be done. It requires will power and also confidence in the instructor or doctor who is teaching the patient to see without glasses.

While some patients are cured quickly, there are patients who do not do so well and keep practicing sometimes for a year or longer without obtaining a cure. This is because the method has not been practiced properly at home or the advice given by the Doctor has not been carried out completely. I have been assisting Dr. Bates long enough to know that glasses can be discarded permanently no matter how long they have been worn.

Better Eyesight
October 1929—Vol. XIV, No. 4

MENTAL ACTIVITY

By W. H. Bates, M.D.

It is a truth that activities of the mind under favorable conditions accomplish many things. As an example, let us consider the following case. A man, age 30, employed in a distant city as a helper in a library, was treated about 15 years ago. He called to see me at about seven o'clock in the evening and remained with me for more than two hours. The patient was born with cataracts in both eyes. He also had amblyopia from birth. Some months previous to his visit, the cataract in both eyes had been removed. The vision of the right eye was very poor and not corrected by glasses. The vision of the left eye was worse than that of the right and also was not improved by glasses.

The treatment which was prescribed was to rest both eyes by closing them. His attention was also called to a known letter of the Snellen test card, a letter which he imagined better with his eyes closed than with his eyes open. When a known letter was regarded by central fixation, the vision improved. It did not take longer than half an hour to improve the right eye in this way, at first in flashes and then more continuously later.

At first he was able to flash the letters of the Snellen test card when he had momentary glimpses of the known letter very much improved. It did not take long before, much to my surprise, he was able to read all the letters on the lowest line at 10 feet, 10/10. The vision of the left eye improved much more slowly, but after continual practice the vision of this eye became normal.

The eye which obtains improved sight by the aid of the memory and imagination very soon obtains improved vision for all the letters. It was demonstrated in this case and in others that the memory and the imagination of a known letter is a cure for myopia, hypermetropia, astigmatism, cataract, glaucoma, atrophy of the optic nerve, and other diseases of the eye.

With the aid of the retinoscope it has been demonstrated that the memory and the imagination are capable of improving the vision of these cases of refraction until the functional element is relieved. It is interesting to observe that these patients become able to see as well without glasses as they had previously seen with them.

Congenital cataract, traumatic cataract, and simple cataract have all been promptly cured with the aid of the imagination when it became as good with the eyes open as with the eyes closed. When one letter, a part of one letter, a period, a comma, or a semicolon, is imagined as well with the eyes open as with the eyes closed, there follows almost immediately a temporary cure of imperfect sight. To understand how this can occur, one should demonstrate how imperfect sight is produced by an effort. It is a truth that the memory of imperfect sight has produced myopia, hypermetropia, and the increased tension of the eye in glaucoma. Schoolchildren acquire myopia by a strain to see better. Some forms of concentration produce an inflammation of the retina similar to the imperfect sight of *amblyopia ex anopsia.* This must be a truth because it suggests proper treatment for amblyopia; namely, rest of the eyes.

Amblyopia is very frequently associated with imperfect sight, an imperfect field which may be irregular in its outline. For many years amblyopia has been considered by authorities to be incurable, but these cases have been studied in recent years so that now most authorities believe that amblyopia is usually curable. It is a fact that some individuals with *amblyopia ex anopsia* recover without treatment. It seems reasonable to believe, if a number of patients recover spontaneously, that the treatment suggested to achieve this result would be successful in obtaining a cure. Normal eyes have been observed to acquire amblyopia, which was increased by an effort or a strain to see. By the practice of relaxation methods the amblyopia is usually benefited or cured.

There are diseases of the choroid which for many years have been understood to be incurable. The fact that a strain or effort to see may produce choroiditis suggests that relaxation methods should be practiced in order to obtain a cure. Cases of this type are too often neglected because they have not been sufficiently studied. The proper kind of mental activity benefits and cures functional or organic diseases of the eye. Some patients suffering from choroiditis obtain benefit quickly, while others take a longer time.

A man, age 25, complained of many disagreeable symptoms. With both eyes open his vision at fifteen feet was one-third of the normal. He suffered very much pain. Treatment relieved this pain and made it possible for him to read at the near point. At ten feet he read the bottom line of the test card with his right eye, a vision of 10/10. With the left eye at ten feet he read the 50-line. In a poor light his vision for distance and for the near point was much below the normal with either eye. When he covered the closed eyelid of the right eye with the palm of his hand, he saw a field of green which continued to be evident for part of a minute. When the eyelids of the left eye were covered with the palm of his hand, he imagined the whole field to be red, changing to yellow and orange. When he produced these colors in his closed eyelids he complained of headache, dizziness, and considerable pain in both eyes.

Some months previous each eye had started to turn in at different times. A stare, strain, or effort to see better increased the squint of the left eye. When the left eye was covered, an effort to see produced a squint of the right eye, which turned in. An operation, which was a failure, was performed on the left eye by a prominent ophthalmologist. Shortly after the operation the left eye turned out almost continuously.

The patient was nervous. His mind planned very unusual things which lowered the vision of the right eye when he stood six feet from the card. When he regarded the Snellen card at six feet and a half, only half a foot farther off, his vision became much worse. When he regarded a letter at seven feet that he remembered or imagined, the vision of the right eye became normal for a few minutes. When the illumination of the Snellen test card was imperfect, his vision became very poor.

At a distance of ten feet, in ordinary daylight, his vision became normal. At twelve feet the vision of the right eye was reduced to one-fourth of the normal. Most of the time the vision of the left eye was imperfect at a near distance, five feet or farther. He was able to read fine print at ten inches from his eyes. At twelve inches he could remember or imagine diamond type, which he read quite readily, but at the same distance, he was unable to read print which was five times as large as diamond type. Such cases are rare. After resting his eyes by palming for long periods of time—one hour, two hours, or longer—the vision of the right eye was improved to the normal for a few hours, but the vision of the left eye was improved to 1/20 of the normal for a few minutes only. Under favorable conditions the vision of the left eye was decidedly improved. When the light was quite bright the vision of the left eye improved, while the vision of the right eye became worse. At twelve inches or farther, he was unable to read any of the print.

It was interesting to study his mind while the left eye was reading the Snellen test card at different distances. There were times when he could straighten the left eye when the Snellen test card was placed at five feet or ten feet. This ability to straighten the left eye was very changeable. With the right eye covered, the left eye read one-half of the Snellen test card at five feet. Later the large letters of the Snellen test card were distinguished at 20 feet, while strange to say, his vision at five feet or ten feet was very poor. At about the same time he could read the Snellen test card with normal vision with the left eye at twelve inches.

It was difficult to explain or to find out why it was that there were periods of time when the vision at the middle distance was poor and why the vision at 20 feet was good. Sometimes the vision at the middle distance would be almost entirely absent. It was difficult or impossible for me on many occasions to understand the idiosyncrasies of this man's vision. Another important fact was that the patient himself could improve his vision for any distance desired by some activity of his mind which was neither a strain or a relaxation. This patient, like other and similar cases, was bothered by a large blind area which interfered seriously with his sight. There were times when he was able to increase the blind area while there were other occasions when the area lessened its size.

The activity of this man's mind was very uncertain, and neither he nor his friends could prophesy what was going to happen next. He discontinued coming to me before he was entirely cured and I have not heard from him since.

Glaucoma is a very serious, treacherous disease of the eyes. The principal symptoms are hardness of the eyeball and a contracted field with imperfect sight. By prescribing rest or relaxation of the eyes all cases of acute glaucoma have been benefited.

Recently a number of patients were seen suffering from a mild form of glaucoma. Usually the field was contracted on the nasal side, but there were periods of time when the contracted field was on the temporal side. One patient could consciously manipulate the size, form, and location of the blind area of the field. A large letter, which would appear about three inches in diameter when regarded by an eye with normal sight, would seem to some cases of glaucoma to be only an inch or less in diameter. The large letter which was seen by the normal eye to be a dark shade of black would appear to some patients as brown, lavender, yellow, or fiery red when regarded at fifteen feet or farther. At twelve inches the letters of the Snellen test card might have almost any color.

The letters might appear to be single, double or more numerous [multiple images]. Every other line of letters would appear to consist of a number of letters instead of being seen properly one at a time. The mental strain to accomplish this consciously was not understood. As a matter of common sense, one would expect that if one line of letters was seen double, all the lines of letters should be seen double. Sometimes the letters of one line would be apparently one above the other. Sometimes the double images appeared to be slanting. The ways that the patient mentioned he was able to have imperfect sight were very numerous. One of the peculiarities of his case was that he was able to see small letters more clearly than large letters. The different ways that he could see imperfectly with the left eye were not duplicated with the right eye.

Another patient, a girl with a very high degree of nearsightedness, had difficulty in finding a way which would produce some improvement in her sight. After spending a good many months in studying the problem and in trying various methods, she became able with the aid of a rectangular swing, a swing which was accomplished by moving one hand in a rectangular direction, to obtain benefit. A finger of one hand was moved in such a way that she appeared to be drawing a rectangle, three feet by one foot. The patient was very much thrilled to find that the improved vision occurred at the same time that she produced the rectangular swing.

Some patients improved their vision by practicing the vertical swing; others, by practicing the oblique swing or horizontal swing, obtained an improvement in the sight. The more the facts were investigated, the greater became the evidence that it is a mental strain which lowers the vision and not a local strain of the eye itself. In all cases of imperfect sight a mental strain can always be recognized. When this strain is relaxed, the vision always improves.

In the treatment of imperfect sight by eye education, the results should be obtained very promptly. One soon becomes able to remember many other ordinary objects besides the letters of the Snellen test card. When the memory becomes as good with the eyes open as with the eyes closed, the mental strain disappears and the vision becomes normal. This suggests that by practicing with the Snellen test card at a near point—three, five, or ten feet—the memory will become more nearly normal. Patients with high degrees of myopia have been cured very promptly, perfectly, and continuously by the memory of perfect sight.

It is very important that mental activity be understood, because imperfect sight is not possible without a mental strain. When a patient with very imperfect sight is benefited or cured by relaxation methods he is very much inclined to say that he does not see the letters on the Snellen test card—that he just remembers or imagines them. The mind of the patient with imperfect sight will always imagine things wrong, although the patient may not be conscious of this fact. For example, he may see a large letter "E" at fifteen feet, and make the statement that it is not a letter "E," but that it is a letter "O." The patient may argue about that for some time. When he is told that it is a letter "E," he says that it can't be a letter "E," that it must be something else.

In short, most patients are more apt to miscall large letters than to miscall small letters. Sometimes the letter "E" is not imagined or seen until the letter is brought a foot or two away. Then when the letter becomes known by regarding it at the near point, it may gradually be taken farther away and still be seen as a letter "E." The next day when the "E" is regarded, it may not be seen, although it is known to be an "E." It may be necessary to place the letter "E" closer to the patient again before it is recognized.

I have repeatedly stated that it is usual for patients to see a known letter better with the eyes closed than with the eyes open. In the treatment of such cases one should realize that the number of ingenious methods employed to make the sight worse are sometimes very remarkable. If the patient knows what is wrong with his eyes, the knowledge is a great help in obtaining a cure. Some patients have been told a number of times that when they know what is the matter with their eyes or their sight that they are more readily cured. By repetition, the vision of most people has been permanently cured.

There are many ways of securing relaxation, but the best one of all is the simplest. The perfect memory of a house or a chair is a great help, but one obtains still greater assistance by the memory of a very small part of a chair. The smaller the object, the more perfectly can it be remembered, imagined, or seen. After the patient becomes convinced that he is suffering from a mental trouble as well as an eye trouble, progress toward a complete recovery in a very short time is obtained. Patients with a high degree of myopia have been cured by the memory of one-half of a large letter, but others have been cured more quickly by the memory of a smaller area. Large letters are not seen, remembered, or imagined as well as small periods.

PRESBYOPIA

By Emily A. Bates

Presbyopia is middle age or old-age sight. When people who are troubled with presbyopia try to read fine print at the near point, or even try to read ordinary type at the reading distance and fail, they usually put on eyeglasses to correct their trouble. If the wrong eyeglasses are prescribed there is sure to be trouble ahead. When eyeglasses do not fit right or the wrong glasses are worn, the patient usually suffers from headache or he tires sooner than a person with normal sight.

People who have myopia or nearsightedness sometimes obtain normal vision just by removing their glasses and not wearing them again. Reports of such cases come to us from time to time. Those who have acquired presbyopia, however, and have worn glasses for a considerable length of time do not find it so easy to do without glasses, either for reading or doing fine work at close range. Such cases need supervision in order to bring back their sight to normal.

I had a patient over 60 years old who wore glasses for 25 years for the correction of presbyopia. She was told by an eye specialist who fitted her with glasses that in time she might be able to do without her glasses and that if she lived long enough she would have what is called "second sight." Instead of this happening, her vision gradually became worse and her bifocals had to be changed three times during the 25 years. She gradually became deaf in her left ear and could only hear a loud noise like an automobile horn or a whistle if the sound was near. There was a swelling below her lower lids and her forehead was wrinkled much like that of an older person. When she did not have her glasses on, the wrinkles became more numerous as she tried to see at the near point.

Her vision when first tested was 15/20 with each eye. Resting her eyes by keeping them closed for over a half an hour improved her vision to 15/10. The long swing, counting up to 100 as she swayed from side to side, caused the wrinkles of her forehead to disappear temporarily and her eyes looked more natural than they did when she first came to me. I placed her before a long mirror and asked her to sway backwards and forwards with me, as she put her right foot out about a foot farther than the left. I told her as she swayed before the long mirror to look down to the tip of her shoe, and as she swayed backward to look in the mirror at the top of her head. She said that she could feel the strain leaving her, so she kept that up for a considerable length of time, alternately placing the left foot out farther than the right and vice versa.

Occasionally she would make a mistake and not look at the tip of her shoe as she swayed forward and when she swayed backward she seemed to forget to look at the top of her head. I had to watch her almost constantly to keep her swaying properly so that she would keep up the relaxation that caused her discomfort to become less. She came to me daily for a week and at the end of that time she noticed that the baggy condition under the lower lids was considerably reduced. She had spent three hours each week at the masseur and had received all sorts of facial massage and treatment to help her get rid of her wrinkles and the baggy condition of her eyelids. Now, in one week's time with daily treatment, spending a little over an hour each day with me, she found that the Bates Method was doing something that she had not expected.

When I tested her vision for fine print, she held the little Fundamentals card with graduated type at arm's length. She could see the figure "1" for sentence No. 1 and the figure "2" for sentence No. 2. She could see that there was black print on the rest of the card, but she could not make out words or sentences. Neither could she imagine that the sentences were divided by white spaces. I made her comfortable in an arm chair and told her to keep her eyes closed—palming if she cared to but at no time was she to open her eyes until I told her to.

The memory and the imagination always help the sight when things are remembered or imagined perfectly. I explained to her that in order to imagine something it would have to be seen first. To imagine something which is explained to her, but which has not been seen, would cause her to have an imperfect imagination.

This patient traveled a great deal but when she was at home she attended to a beautiful garden of flowers which beautified a section of her home overlooking a lovely spot on the Pacific coast. She mentioned an orchid in the bud and how beautiful it seemed to her when it was in full bloom. She mentioned the different flowers which needed her daily attention to help them grow from the seed to the flower in full bloom. In this way she remembered the seed as she planted it, then the little green speck as it appeared above the dark soil, then later with the warmth of the sunshine and fresh water that she gave the little flower each day, she saw the little plant grow into a living thing lovely to look at. She had a perfect imagination and memory for plants and flowers and as she explained these things to me, her mind became relaxed and when she opened her eyes to read the Fundamentals card, which I had placed twelve inches from her eyes instead of arm's length, she read all of sentence No. 8.

She made only one mistake when she first began to read sentence No. 8 and saw the word "Variable" as "Vegetable." She knew immediately that she had seen the word wrong, that it must be something in connection with the swing, and that it could not be a "Vegetable." I told her to place her finger directly below sentence No. 8 and told her to shift slowly from the white spaces above sentence No. 8 to the sentence below, directing her all the time to blink as she shifted this short distance. She did this faithfully as I directed her to do and then she read sentence after sentence to sentence No. 15 which she read without any trouble. She became hysterical as she finished reading this little card and her gratitude was most profound.

To be sure that she would practice properly while she was away from me, I told her to hold the Fundamentals card again at arm's length and to look at the sentences without blinking or shifting. Immediately the whole card became blurred and she could not read at all. She asked me not to have her do that again because it gave her pain and discomfort in her eyes. It was necessary for me to have her do this, however, because she would have done this same thing without knowing it. Again I had her close her eyes, using her memory and imagination and before she opened her eyes again I held the Fundamentals card six inches from her eyes instead of twelve inches as we did before. Holding the card in my own hand she did not realize how close it was to her closed eyes. When she opened her eyes and read all the sentences of the Fundamentals card, she did not realize that I was holding the card so close to her eyes. We measured the distance to be accurate about it and when she found out how much she had improved she was quite sure that she understood the method enough to go on by herself.

I saw her recently for the first time in about two years and her ability to read at the near point has not changed during that time. I asked her if she had stopped practicing after she found that her vision had become normal again and her answer was "No, indeed, I have been very careful to give my eyes enough time for practice every day since I came to you for treatment." This is another proof that if patients carry on the work by themselves after they no longer receive personal attention, that the vision does not go back to where it was before the Bates Method was first practiced.

Another patient, age 58, first put on glasses at the age of 30 for the relief of headaches. At her first visit she had with her the four pairs of glasses which she had worn from the time she had first started to wear glasses. She gave me her history, explaining that she looked at figures all day long, being a bookkeeper and accountant for a large corporation. She said that the first glasses she wore gave her instant relief from pain until one day about a year later she received a shock which caused her great sorrow. She had lost a member of her family whom she loved dearly and this caused a great deal of depression. Feeling that her glasses needed to be changed, she called on her oculist who gave her another pair. She did not wear them constantly because they did not give her much relief or help in her work. Again she had them changed with better results this time and she got along very nicely with these glasses until shortly before she came to me to be relieved of eyeglasses altogether.

When Dr. Bates examined the first pair of glasses she had worn, he said that they were plain window glass. I explained to my patient that apparently the mental effect which the glasses gave her when she put them on was what helped her, and not the glasses themselves. When she received the nervous shock which caused depression and sadness in her life, she undoubtedly strained her eyes, which caused imperfect sight.

The second pair of glasses, not suiting her properly, probably made the condition of her eyes worse. At any rate, when Dr. Bates examined her eyes, he said that she had mixed astigmatism with presbyopia. I am sorry that there are not more eye specialists who find it a mistake to exchange eyeglasses for stronger ones for those who come to them for relief of their eye trouble. In this particular case eyeglasses did not help and the patient was grateful to her friends who recommended Dr. Bates and his treatment for the relief of eyestrain.

With the right eye her vision was 15/40, but none of the letters were clear or distinct. Her left eye had normal vision, 15/15, and she saw all the letters clearly. Palming and mental pictures also helped this patient and she found the long swing most helpful in obtaining relaxation of the mind and body before starting out to her work each day. I improved her right eye to 15/15 in less than an hour's time which, of course, was only a temporary improvement. I did not have much trouble in teaching her to read fine print and to see figures by shifting and noticing the white spaces between lines of type and figures.

She needed only one treatment with instruction for home practice to restore her sight to normal. She corresponded with me regularly several times a month, just sending reports of the progress she made or the difficulty she had in practicing certain things before she started out to business in the morning and before retiring at night. She was told to return for another treatment if she found it necessary, but apparently she did not need it because I did not see her again.

The most important thing for people who have presbyopia or astigmatism or any other trouble which causes imperfect sight is to avoid looking at reading type or at anything, in fact, without shifting or blinking, which is something the normal eye does frequently all day long.

Better Eyesight
November 1929—Vol. XIV, No. 5

IMPROVE YOUR SIGHT

When convenient, practice the long swing. Stand with the feet about one foot apart, turn the body to the right, at the same time lifting the heel of the left foot. The head and eyes move with the body. Now place the left heel on the floor, turn the body to the left, raising the heel of the right foot. Alternate.

Rest your eyes continually by blinking. The normal eye blinks irregularly but continuously. When convenient, practice blinking in the following way: Count irregularly and blink for each count. By consciously blinking correctly, it will in time become an unconscious habit.

When the mind is awake it is thinking of many things. One can remember things perfectly or imagine things perfectly, which is a rest to the eyes, mind, and the body generally. The memory of imperfect sight should be avoided because it is a strain and lowers the vision.

Read the Snellen test card at 20 feet with each eye separately, twice daily or more often when convenient. Imagine the white spaces in letters to be whiter than the rest of the card. Do this alternately with the eyes closed and opened. Plan to imagine the white spaces in letters just as white, in looking at the Snellen test card, as can be accomplished with the eyes closed.

Whenever convenient, close your eyes for a few minutes and rest them.

AMBLYOPIA

By W. H. Bates, M.D.

When the sight is poor and cannot be improved promptly by glasses, the cause is usually due to amblyopia. The word amblyopia means blindness. In amblyopia the vision is less in the region of the center of sight. One cannot have imperfect sight without having at the same time a measure of poor vision in which all parts of the field are involved. It seems curious that it is possible for the most sensitive part of the retina [the fovea centralis] to become blind while other [peripheral] parts of the retina have considerable vision—better, in fact, than the vision obtained by the activity of the center of sight.

Some cases of amblyopia cannot count fingers. Many others have no perception of light and yet, strange to say, the advanced cases can oftentimes be cured just as quickly as other cases in which the vision is only slightly lowered. Some cases of amblyopia may have poor vision at a distance of fifteen or twenty feet, a similar reduced vision at six inches or less, but at ten feet the vision may be nearly normal.

In most cases of amblyopia the field of vision is usually very small. Sometimes the letters regarded at fifteen feet appear to be blood red while other letters regarded at three feet may seem to be brown or to have a tint of green or some other color. The perception of colors varies greatly at different distances. Red may look like green when the card is regarded at fifteen feet or farther; yellow may give one the appearance of blue.

For many years color blindness has usually been considered incurable, but since amblyopia and color blindness are usually found together, the treatment which helps or improves the sight without glasses also benefits the color blindness. The reverse is also true; when color blindness is benefited the amblyopia becomes less.

Since it is a truth that staring, concentration, causes imperfect sight, any treatment which relieves strain should always improve the sight or improve the vision in amblyopia and color blindness. A great many lives have been lost as a result of acquired color blindness. A patient with imperfect sight was brought to my office by his family physician with a history of having run into another automobile while driving his own car. When I tested his vision with the Snellen test card, I found it to be normal.

The patient was very much upset and said in his defense to me, "Doctor, I never saw that automobile." A good deal of time was spent in demonstrating that the patient had acquired amblyopia which was so complete that he really did not see the other car, but the blindness had lasted for such a short time that it was not an easy matter to prove that he had an attack of temporary blindness or an attack of amblyopia.

This phenomena has occurred very often to locomotive engineers who would state after an accident that they had suddenly gone blind for a short time and when they were blind they did not see the danger signals.

There are other occasions when these attacks of amblyopia with color blindness have interfered with the work of some artists. A portrait painter gave a history of attacks of temporary blindness while at his work. Sometimes after devoting considerable time to his work he found that he had to do it all over again because of the attacks of amblyopia and color blindness.

In another case a well-known surgeon suffered from attacks of blindness at irregular periods. The blindness was complete so that he had no perception of light. The attacks of blindness worried him very much because he was afraid, while performing an important or dangerous surgical operation, that in the midst of it would come an attack of sudden blindness which would tend to interfere seriously with his work.

The neurologists whom the surgeon consulted all told him that he was threatened with insanity and that unless he took a long rest he might unexpectedly find himself blind and insane. Every ophthalmologist whom he consulted gave him a different pair of glasses to wear, none of which gave him any relief. He not only suffered from attacks of blindness but he was also bothered by illusions of sight.

He said nothing about the amblyopia at his first visit, but told me that he called to have something done for his eyes. He had many symptoms of discomfort and he would be very much obliged to me if I would cure him. While examining his eyes with the ophthalmoscope and seeking to find some treatment which would improve his vision, I discovered that he was suffering from amblyopia. Then he was told that the reason that his sight failed and that he had attacks of double vision was because of this amblyopia. Then began a great battle. The doctor knew a great deal about physiological optics and would not encourage me to treat him until he was convinced that I was right and he was wrong.

When he was in his office he said that where he knew there was only one light, he saw two, three, or four lights. The images in some cases were arranged one above the other and the distances between them varied within very wide limits. He said, however, that the principal illusion that he suffered from was that it seemed to him that his hands and feet were double, sometimes more than double. The size of the double images varied; sometimes one image was four or five times as large as the other. In some cases the double images were arranged one above the other, while in other cases they were arranged in an oblique direction. When he looked at a Snellen test card hanging up in my office, the bottom lines were double and the color of each line of letters appeared different. With the aid of central fixation this illusion disappeared and did not return.

To satisfy the surgeon I made repeated examinations

of his eyes with the aid of the ophthalmoscope and each time I reported that his eyes were all right and that there was nothing in either of his eyes which could explain the illusions from which he suffered. They did not come from any malformation of the interior of the eyeball but were imagined. He was very much impressed when I told him how to produce illusions of sight consciously whenever he so desired. He discovered that it was necessary to strain in order to do this and knowing the cause of his trouble made it easier for him to relieve it by doing away with the strain.

This doctor went through the World War and when he returned he came to my office and thanked me for what I had done for him. He said that he had not had a single attack of temporary blindness from the stare or strain of amblyopia, because knowing the cause of his trouble he was able to prevent it.

The great mistake that has been made for the last one hundred years or more was in ignoring amblyopia. It was astonishing to find the number of doctors who did not believe that amblyopia was of great importance. Time after time patients with amblyopia were treated in my office with success by relaxation methods. Some doctors stated very strongly that amblyopia was congenital and emphasized the matter so strongly, so continuously that most other doctors hesitated to treat amblyopia at all, but were very glad to turn such cases over to someone else.

AMBLYOPIA AND SCHOOLCHILDREN

By Emily A. Bates

As Dr. Bates' article in this issue is on amblyopia, I thought that it would be a good opportunity for me to tell about some interesting cases which I have taken care of.

In 1912 when I first began assisting Dr. Bates in his experimental work in the Physiological Laboratory of the College of Physicians and Surgeons in New York I had no idea that there was so much to be learned about the cure of imperfect sight without glasses. As I became more acquainted with the Doctor's work, the desire to learn more grew stronger. Each day I helped him. Watching the Doctor in his experiments with animals (these experiments were always performed immediately after the death of the animals) was most interesting and often students in the Physiological Laboratory who were doing their experimental work would stop long enough to watch Dr. Bates doing his work and making new discoveries.

I felt very proud then to stand by his side after our work at the office was finished, taking an hour before Clinic time and an hour after the Clinic session was over. There were times when our work together seemed almost too strenuous for me, and many times I felt as though I could not go on another day. Before I offered my assistance there were doctors who tried to keep on in assisting the Doctor until his experimental work was accomplished, but in due time, one by one, they had to give up, because they could not spare enough time away from their offices and for other reasons.

Dr. Bates has always been a great reader and has studied every book written by prominent eye specialists. He always found time enough to try other ideas and experiments even while he was doing his own work. While other doctors were away for the summer months enjoying a rest away from their work, Dr. Bates, who did not at that time believe in vacations, would sometimes be the only physician doing any experimental work at the laboratory. Occasionally Professor Lee, who in his heart believed in Dr. Bates' work and respected his ability to do what other doctors failed to accomplish, would come into the room to watch the experimental work going on.

Having had the opportunity of being with Dr. Bates during his experimental days, I was able to understand how something could be wrong with the eyesight of schoolchildren when apparently there was no organic change in the retina. I made a special study all by myself of the cure of the eyes of schoolchildren and this is what I found:

Usually children of the poor have very little or no idea of schoolwork before they enter the schoolroom. When it comes time for the mother to take her child to the public school, usually the mother does not know what is in the heart or the mind of that child. He has been accustomed to a little play each day in the streets and at other times was happy and familiar in the surroundings of the little place called home. Usually children are shy when visitors call; some become irritable for no reason whatever and are sometimes punished for that. The mother does not realize that strain of the mind is produced because the child either likes or dislikes the visitor. House pets such as dogs or cats which are accustomed to the members of the household usually run away and hide when a visitor calls. It doesn't require much to cause mind strain, and when there is strain of the mind there is always eyestrain.

When a child is brought into a large school he feels as though he is in another world. The child meets children who seem different from those with whom he has been acquainted. He meets a teacher who tries her best to become acquainted with him and doesn't always succeed. He sees his mother leaving him to the care of those whom he has never met before. All these things have to be overcome, and this is not readily done in every case.

After a while the tests begin. Children soon have to

read the writing on the blackboard. When this cannot be accomplished by the pupil it is understood that the child has imperfect sight and needs glasses. Eye tests are made with the aid of the Snellen test card and it is found that the vision is not normal. (Even the sound of the voice of the person who tests the vision has a mental effect on the child.) Then the mother receives a note saying that the child needs to be fitted for glasses.

In some schools this is still going on, but in others it is not. I found many schools using the Bates Method without calling it so. Schools in New Jersey have used the Bates Method successfully for many years, and while it has been stopped by the authorities as a daily routine, there have been a large number of children benefited by the use of the Snellen test card. In the larger cities of the United States as well as in Germany, South Africa, Great Britain, Switzerland, and Spain, the Bates Method is being carried on.

A great deal of eyestrain could be prevented if children were told what to do before they begin their studies. Amblyopia could be prevented by explaining to the child how necessary it is not to stare in order to see better. Blinking irregularly but often is something that is done universally by people who have no trouble with their eyes. Animals in the same way blink their eyes often, although they themselves are not conscious of it, as far as we know. When blinking is done right, the eyes move and it is seldom that amblyopia is observed in people who practice this.

In the October issue of the magazine *Good Housekeeping,* there is an article entitled "A New Job for the Public Schools," by Elizabeth Frazer. Her illustration of the children studying at their desks shows mental strain as well as eyestrain. In the article the following appears, "What is the matter with these children? What causes them to fail in school? What can be done to help them? Progressive educators are beginning to ask these questions and want to help to prevent failures."

I can tell them how, for I have been with schoolchildren a good many years and have helped them along just by improving their eyesight to normal. All schoolchildren who are unruly should have their sight tested every day with the Snellen test card. I can prove, if I am given a chance with a group of such children, that every one has eyestrain. I can prove that when eyestrain is entirely relieved by resting the eyes, the mentality of such children is improved. Not only does the child benefit by the Bates Method of relieving eyestrain, but the mother is relieved of a great problem and the teacher is able to teach with less mental strain for her. I am ready for an interview at any time and I shall greet with pleasure anyone who is interested enough to let me help in improving the defective eyesight of schoolchildren.

During the nine years of Clinic work which was done by Dr. Bates and myself at the Harlem Hospital here in New York City, many such cases as Elizabeth Frazer describes came to us to be fitted for glasses. In my book, *Stories from the Clinic,* I wrote about a case of squint or crossed eyes. [See the case of Francisco in the September 1921 issue.—TRQ]

A boy, age fifteen, was brought to my attention through a patient who was treated and cured by Dr. Bates. This former patient was Ms. H. D. Messick of Cleveland, Ohio, who has done a great deal of charity work in relieving eyestrain in schoolchildren among the poorer classes. She heard of this boy whose left eye was almost blind and whose vision for the right eye was 10/30. The best eye specialist in the Midwest pronounced the left eye incurable and advised him never to be without glasses for fear of going absolutely blind in the other eye. The eye which was almost blind was examined with the ophthalmoscope and nothing could be found wrong with the retina or optic nerve or any other part of the eye, yet he could not see out of that eye.

This is amblyopia or blindness without any apparent cause. The patient does not know what is wrong; neither does the doctor, yet the patient cannot see. This boy had for many years tried to improve his ability as an artist by drawing pictures of ships, but he always drew them imperfectly because he could not see them perfectly. When this boy, who was well acquainted with the Doctor's cured patient, found out what had been done for her he promised to do anything he was advised to do if he could receive help as she did. If only he would not go blind in the one eye, he said, he wouldn't mind it much having one blind eye, and the great specialist who had pronounced his apparent blindness incurable had no hope whatever for that eye.

With such thoughts in his mind I first began to treat him. When he noticed how quickly the vision improved in the blind eye, he went to work with the Bates Method as no other boy under my supervision has done since. He improved steadily, sending me reports regularly until the vision of the poor eye was normal. This was due to the help and encouragement he received from Ms. Messick. The teachers in school knew that he had worn glasses and when he returned to school without them, they attempted to persuade him to wear them, but he wouldn't and he said that they were thrilled to notice the improvement not only in his eyesight, but in all the class work that he did under their supervision. He sent me a picture of a ship which he had drawn, after his vision became normal. "It is as perfect as any drawing could be," Dr. Bates exclaimed after he had examined it.

What was done for one boy can be done for other boys who need help as Elizabeth Frazer has explained so well in her article.

Better Eyesight
December 1929—Vol. XIV, No. 6

HYPERMETROPIA

By W. H. Bates, M.D.

The importance of hypermetropia cannot be overestimated. It is sometimes acquired soon after birth, or it may be manifest at ten, twenty, thirty, or forty years old. Eighty percent of eye troubles are caused by hypermetropia, while nearsightedness occurs in ten percent. There are only ten percent of normal eyes. These figures are startling. The majority of persons at the age of forty-five or over acquire hypermetropia, and it is of the utmost importance that such cases be carefully studied.

Nearly everyone has the symptoms of hypermetropia. When the sight is good for distant vision, that does not necessarily mean that the sight is also good for reading at a near point of ten or twelve inches. Too often such cases are not treated seriously. Poor sight for reading (hypermetropia) is usually corrected by the use of reading glasses, while vision at all other distances is neglected.

In middle age, serious eye diseases are caused by hypermetropia. Among the most common are glaucoma, cataract, and diseases of the optic nerve and retina. In the early stages of these serious diseases, they are more readily curable than after they become chronic and more serious because the vision is only slightly affected and the treatment which cures hypermetropia is the treatment which prevents serious eye diseases. Cataract and glaucoma are now being prevented or cured by treatment which cures hypermetropia. It should be emphasized that early treatment of hypermetropia yields quicker, more continuous results than later treatment.

Eye physicians or ophthalmologists have almost universally believed that absolute glaucoma is not curable by any form of treatment. It has been demonstrated that glaucoma is caused by strain—the strain of hypermetropia. When this strain is relieved or corrected, glaucoma usually improves. This treatment is more successful than operation or eyedrops. It is only in the last ten years that it was discovered that glaucoma is caused by a strain which produces hypermetropia and that when this strain is relieved the glaucoma improves. I think it is a mistake to condemn this simple method of relieving the hypermetropia, which also relieves glaucoma. The eyestrain which produces hypermetropia also produces cataract.

It has been repeatedly demonstrated that in all diseases of the eyes which cause imperfect sight, the eye is under a strain and when this strain is removed all diseases of the eye are benefited. Patients with atrophy of the optic nerve have good sight when eyestrain is not present. For example, a patient came from Austria for treatment of amblyopia which was so advanced that the vision in one eye was only perception of light and in the other eye it was one-half of normal. She had consulted many physicians who advised operation for the cure of the total blindness. She was given the hypermetropia treatment daily for about two weeks, at the end of which time the vision was normal in both eyes. Surely if hypermetropia treatment can be so beneficial, more physicians ought to know about it. There have been numerous similar cases. It can be demonstrated that atrophy of the optic nerve can be caused by the eyestrain of hypermetropia. Palming, swinging, and central fixation have always improved the sight temporarily or permanently. It is interesting to prove that such a disease as atrophy of the optic nerve can be benefited by the treatment which relieves hypermetropia.

Patients suffering from squint are benefited by hypermetropia treatment. Patients with hypermetropia not only strain to produce squint with one or both eyes turned in, but they also strain to correct the imperfect sight which is caused by the squint. This fact should be more widely known, because even at this time many physicians believe that the poor sight caused by hypermetropia is incurable.

What is the lowest degree of hypermetropia that can be produced is a question that has been asked. The answer is that there is no limit, not only to the low degree of hypermetropia, but there is no limit to the high degrees. In other words, by an effort hypermetropia of 30 diopters or more can be produced and, by treatment, perfect vision can be obtained just as readily.

In studying the production of high or low degrees of hypermetropia it is interesting to discover the conclusions of well-known ophthalmologists. One prominent doctor was asked this question: Is hypermetropia curable? He replied that it was not curable. He was then asked, "Why do you claim that no one can cure hypermetropia?" He answered, "I know that it cannot be cured because I was unable to succeed, and if I cannot succeed no one else can."

Massage of the eyelids has been recommended for the cure of hypermetropia. Another doctor claimed that he was able to cure a majority of the cases of hypermetropia, and that if the patient was not cured by massage, no other doctor in the world could succeed. Other physicians, however, did not believe that massage was a cure for hypermetropia.

Since hypermetropia is so common and produces so many different kinds of eye trouble—imperfect sight, pain, dizziness, and other nervous symptoms to a greater extent than do other errors of refraction—it is well to understand as much as we can of the occurrence, symptoms, prevention, and cure of hypermetropia.

The best methods of preventing hypermetropia are the sway, reading fine print such as diamond type, palming occasionally, and imagining stationary objects to be moving when the eyes move in the opposite direction. The last one of these methods is not always easy to practice. Some cases are very obstinate without any known reason. They may try for days, without success, to imagine stationary objects to be moving. The cause of failure is usually due to concentration, staring, looking fixedly at stationary objects, and efforts to try to see.

When success is not attained, hold the finger about six inches from the chin while looking at distant objects and move the head and eyes from side to side, taking care not to look directly at the finger. When this movement of the head and eyes is practiced easily, continuously, the finger appears to move. This method is called the variable swing and most people have no trouble whatever in imagining the finger moving. The length of the movement of the finger is much wider than stationary objects regarded at ten, twenty, or forty feet or farther.

Another case of failure occurs when the patient turns the head to the right and simultaneously turns the eyes to the left. It is a very painful experience. When one fails to obtain movement of stationary objects with the variable swing, he suffers much pain, dizziness, and other nervous symptoms.

Hypermetropia may be prevented by many other methods. The memory or the imagination of perfect sight prevents hypermetropia in the normal eye. The memory of imperfect sight is very difficult and the memory or imagination of perfect sight is easy.

In the city of Chicago a school teacher developed a method of treating children which prevented hypermetropia from being acquired. She had charge of about fifty or more children at the age when fatigue is common. As a result, all the teachers in the Chicago school allowed their children to rest for a time at frequent intervals about every half an hour in two. They were taught relaxation methods, although they were all under ten years old. It was astonishing to observe how much they could remember, how much they could imagine, and how much their activities were improved with benefit to their eyes. Sometimes the usual exercises in the classroom would be stopped and the children would be taught how to palm successfully and while palming to improve their imagination. They were taught to draw pictures which they copied from the blackboard twenty feet away. After some months, the hypermetropia was improved—and finally entirely cured.

A school teacher in Long Island was treated by me for compound hypermetropic astigmatism. By the use of relaxation methods the hypermetropia and astigmatism were corrected and the patient obtained normal vision. The hypermetropia was prevented from increasing by curing it. The patient was very much pleased with the results and told the principal of her school that because hypermetropia was curable, it was also preventable. A negative proposition cannot be the truth. Hypermetropia could be prevented when it was found possible to cure it.

A number of teachers became interested and all those wearing glasses for hypermetropia were cured either by palming or swinging or by the memory of fine print. The principal was much pleased and placed a Snellen test card in all the classrooms with directions that it should be read by all the teachers and pupils who were afflicted with hypermetropia. The first patient cured of hypermetropia was to continue the work.

Since she could not treat patients in the classrooms, she decided to treat them outside the school building. She made an arrangement with the teachers who wished treatment that she would teach them how to use their eyes properly and prevent or cure hypermetropia. She made arrangements with them all that after a teacher was cured, she would agree to teach, cure, or prevent some other teacher from acquiring hypermetropia. So much interest was shown by the teachers in this school building that it made an endless chain and a great many teachers and schoolchildren were cured of hypermetropia.

For many years it has been believed that retardation is incurable. It seemed wrong that children, fifteen or sixteen years old and older should be kept in the grades with children ten years old or under. These children did not like to study. Many of them complained of severe headaches and other discomforts. Truancy was common. After retardation was cured by relaxation methods, most of the children started in and worked hard with their studies, with the result that many of them graduated into the rapid advancement classes.

I was told by many principals that imperfect sight was never found in the rapid advancement classes. Nearly all cases of retardation were suffering from hypermetropia. It was demonstrated that patients suffering from imperfect sight from any cause were also suffering from retardation. The teachers who devoted an hour or more every day to the cure of hypermetropia discovered much to their surprise that almost every disease of the eye and nervous system was benefited or cured by treatment which cured hypermetropia.

In one year, 20,000 pupils suffered from pain, headache, loss of memory, imperfect sight from hypermetropia. In one year after, 80 percent of the 20,000 children who were suffering from headaches and other nervous troubles all recovered after the hypermetropia was cured.

Better Eyesight
January 1930—Vol. XIV, No. 7

ASTIGMATISM

By W. H. Bates, M.D.

In all cases of astigmatism one meridian of the cornea is more convex or less convex than all the other meridians. One definition of astigmatism is that the astigmatic eye is not able to focus the light from an object down to a point. There are many authorities who claim that astigmatism is always congenital or that people with astigmatism were born with it. However, recent work on astigmatism has demonstrated that it is always acquired and never congenital. Young children, babies, when examined with the retinoscope soon after birth usually have astigmatism which is acquired by a strain or effort to see. When the child's eye is at rest no astigmatism is manifest, but when the child's eye or the child's mind is under a strain, astigmatism is always present.

Schoolchildren are often nervous and when the nervousness is considerable, a large amount of astigmatism may be produced by a strain of the eyes or mind. When rest is secured the astigmatism in schoolchildren promptly disappears. Rest of the eyes is not always obtained readily. Closing the eyes, palming with the help of a nearly perfect memory of some letter or other object, secures a considerable amount of rest. The more perfect the memory the greater is the rest or relaxation. Rest of the eyes and mind is also obtained after the child practices central fixation or seeing best where the eyes were looking. However, it is necessary to practice central fixation without a conscious effort. When the eye is fixed on a point, it is oftentimes very easy to make an effort and the effort, even when slight, is capable of lowering the vision when astigmatism is present.

There are many conditions which are favorable in securing relaxation or rest. Some people see better when the illumination is unusually good, whereupon the astigmatism immediately becomes less. There are other people who cannot stand even a moderate amount of light and their astigmatism is less when the light is poor. The distance of the print from the eyes when seen best also varies with people. In some cases letters or other objects are seen well at twenty feet or farther and not so well at twelve inches. One patient had a vision of 20/30 plus. The large black letters of the Snellen test card appeared blood red, but at one-half or one-quarter of the distance the astigmatism was worse or increased. In other patients the color of the black letters was a shade of brown or yellow or green at a distance of fifteen feet, while the black letters never appeared black, but corrected the astigmatism when the distance was less than ten feet.

The facts observed on the production of astigmatism were modified by shifting. One patient looking directly at the first letter of a line of letters had no astigmatism at six feet. The patient was told that he would be asked to look at the last letter of the Snellen test card and he was able to do this, but before his eyes looked from the first letter to the last letter on the same line the astigmatism became very decided. Shifting from one letter to another at ten feet produced astigmatism. Astigmatism was temporary and by alternately shifting from the top period of the colon to the bottom period of the colon his vision improved. When he tried to see all parts of the colon simultaneously a strain resulted and a severe headache annoyed the patient very much. He found fault and said that he came to have his headaches cured, not to have them made worse.

To increase astigmatism is a very difficult thing. It requires much effort and with that effort to increase the astigmatism and to make the sight worse the patient complains that it is more difficult to increase the astigmatism and make the sight worse than it is to lessen the astigmatism and make the sight better. After many methods have been tried with much strain, it can be demonstrated that the production of a large amount of astigmatism is difficult. To lessen the astigmatism and improve the sight to normal is easy and can only be accomplished without effort.

The successful treatment and the cure of astigmatism without glasses is generally accompanied by so much strain that it is not always easy to make progress. It is very easy, however, to demonstrate that astigmatism is caused by a stare or strain and that rest or relaxation of the eyes will bring about a cure of astigmatism. The memory of familiar objects with the eyes closed is a great help in obtaining relaxation and lessening the amount of astigmatism. After the astigmatism is lessened by treatment, greater benefit can often be obtained by having the patient close his eyes and remember letters, music, and other mental pictures. Perfect memory means more perfect sight because the greater the relaxation the quicker does the astigmatism disappear. It often happens that patients with astigmatism find it difficult to obtain relaxation because they try to see too much of any one object at once and try to see letters, left side best, top best, bottom best, right side best. The mere act of seeing one side of a letter at a time makes it easier to imagine the vision of each part of a letter.

One patient, when examined with the retinoscope, had a high degree of astigmatism. When he looked at the left side of some letter he could imagine the left side was straight, curved, or open. He imagined it straight with his eyes open and more or less clear; with his eyes closed the left side of the letter was remembered or imagined straight; the top was also imagined straight; the bottom was also imagined straight; and with the eyes open the left side, top, and bottom were imagined correctly. By alternately regarding each side of the letter with the eyes open and imagining these sides much better with the eyes closed, each side was imagined correctly. The patient was told to close his eyes and think of a letter, the left side straight, the top straight, the bottom straight, right side open. "What can you imagine the letter to be," he was asked. He answered, "It is an 'E'." The patient was drilled on a number of other letters with success. He was convinced that the imagination of one part of the letter improved the relaxation and enabled the patient to ignore the blurred outline of the letter regarded.

When the imagination improves the vision improves. One can at will plan to imagine a letter with the left side more or less straight and do it successfully after a number of times. Many failures occur because patients try to imagine the unknown letter by a strain. One of the most difficult cases to cure by relaxation methods responded favorably when his attention was called to the fact that he could, when the astigmatism was corrected, see a part of a letter better than a number of small letters. The letter was so imperfect that he could not distinguish the size, the color, or the form. By explaining to him that he could see these blurred letters, one part of the letter at a time much better than he could see the whole of the letter at once, he soon became able to see the letters perfectly in this way. When a pointer was placed in the neighborhood of the letter, the vision for that one letter was improved more than for other letters of the same size and color. He could not see the left-hand side correctly with his eyes open or closed. He was asked if he could imagine how the left side of the unknown letter would look if it had no blur. The imagination improved and with the improvement in the imagination the sight improved.

Some time ago there was printed in this magazine a description of a method of curing astigmatism which is far superior to all other methods. The patient was advised that there were white spaces between the lines of black letters and that these white spaces became whiter by alternately imagining them as white as possible with the eyes closed and then with the eyes open. The attention of the patient was called to the fact that one could imagine the bottoms of the letters resting upon the upper part of the white spaces, and when the letters were read a thin white line could be imagined going across the card from left to right. This thin white line was improved by the imagination of the line with the eyes alternately open and closed. When the imagination was successful in improving the thin white line, the black letters were imagined blacker and could usually be distinguished very quickly; but when the imagination of the white spaces was less perfect, the black letters could not usually be normally seen. In other words, the improvement in the vision for the black letters depended primarily upon the improvement of the whiteness of the thin white line. Of the two, the thin white line was more important because one can imagine the whiteness of the thin white line much whiter relatively than the imagination can picture the blackness of the black letters.

Letters are frequently received by me, containing this very important question, "How can I remember black? It is impossible for me to remember black." One person wrote from the Midwest that he could not remember or imagine black by central fixation. Whenever he tried he always failed and a number of friends of his also tried and they believed that it was impossible to remember or imagine a period that was anywhere near black. The man who complained had a high degree of astigmatism. This astigmatism was corrected by relaxation methods. His vision improved rapidly. By alternately practicing with his eyes open and with his eyes closed, his memory, his vision, and his imagination soon became normal.

Many people who try to see one period of a colon blacker than the other fail. If the patient can demonstrate that the cause of failure is a strain he soon learns that his failure is due entirely to strain. This strain is a mental strain. Many people fail because they lose their sight, memory, and imagination by an effort. It is a benefit to people with imperfect sight to demonstrate that the cause is always an effort or trying to see. It is astonishing to know that the memory of imperfect sight is so difficult and that it requires considerable time and patience to help a patient realize the facts. Most people believe that to do wrong is easy and are very much surprised when someone tells them the contrary, and still more surprised when the facts are demonstrated.

Children eight years old or younger have repeatedly demonstrated that imperfect sight, imperfect memory, and imperfect imagination are difficult.

When the largest letter of the Snellen test card is regarded, the blackness and clearness of it are so much better that people erroneously believe that the imagination of a large letter is much easier than the imagination of one-half of the letter. When one-half of a letter is covered, some people can imagine successfully that one-half of the largest letter on the card is just as black, clear, and distinct as the same letter very much smaller. By continued practice the size of the letter or other object can be reduced to an area as small as the eye of a needle.

On one occasion a child ten years old was brought to my office with normal eyes. The vision was tested and found to be normal. Her father asked her, "Can you tell that the largest letter on the test card is blacker than the very small letters?" The child intelligently declared that the large letter was not blacker or clearer than the smaller letters. She could also make an effort sufficient to produce a considerable amount of astigmatism. Having normal vision, her control over her imagination was much better than that of patients with imperfect sight. The father then asked his daughter how she explained that she could see the small letters better than large ones. She replied that the reason she saw small letters better than large ones was because there was not so much to see.

Having good sight the child could very readily produce a considerable amount of astigmatism by an effort of which she was conscious. Her father had much less control over his eyes than his daughter had. He could regard the card with good vision but his daughter could strain much more and produce a higher degree of astigmatism measured with the aid of the ophthalmometer. She was also able to imagine, when she saw a small letter at fifteen feet, that it was moving.

She was asked if she could stop the movement and when she did so a larger amount of astigmatism was demonstrated in her eyes than in those of her father. She was very much annoyed when she produced astigmatism because she said it gave her great pain. His central fixation was not so good as hers. It was difficult for him to imagine the top period of a colon best and the bottom worse or to imagine the bottom best and the top worse. He invariably saw both at the same time nearly equally well, while the daughter always saw one period at a time, the upper or lower, best.

A boy came to me to obtain glasses for the correction of astigmatism in each eye. With the right eye his vision was 10/20 or one-half of the normal, but with the other eye he saw four times as much and the astigmatism was four times as great as in the other eye. This boy, when he covered over both closed eyes with the palm of one or both hands, instead of seeing black, saw everything else but black—gray, green, blue, yellow, and other colors and his efforts to obtain black did not readily succeed. When he imagined imperfect sight he did not see black. When he imagined perfect sight and remembered perfectly the things which he had seen the astigmatism disappeared and he was able to remember, imagine, or see perfect black.

Many facts of considerable value were observed. When the boy imagined a large object while palming, his astigmatism was slight when he opened his eyes, but when he remembered letters or other objects with imperfect sight with the left eye open his vision became worse. Perfect imagination enabled him to produce a greater amount of astigmatism than he was able to do when the vision was poor. When the right eye had more perfect imagination he became able to imagine more perfect vision and in addition he could imagine sight that was more imperfect. With a good imagination he had more perfect sight and at the same time remembered or imagined a greater degree of astigmatism than when his sight was poor. He demonstrated that when his mind was more under his control, he could remember or imagine a larger amount of astigmatism. When his sight was good, the mental control of his vision was improved. When his eyes were closed he could remember or imagine more perfect black than he could remember or imagine when his eyes were open. He demonstrated that he could produce a larger amount of astigmatism or a lesser amount of astigmatism as he desired because, his mind being under his control, he could remember things or imagine things better than he could when his mind was not under his control. The retinoscope was a great help in controlling the astigmatism. With its aid the amount of the astigmatism could be determined.

TWO CASES OF MYOPIA

By Emily A. Bates

A little girl, age seven, came to Dr. Bates for the first time for treatment. She had a high degree of myopia with astigmatism and had worn glasses for a few years. According to her mother's statement she was a very nervous child due to eyestrain. The vision in each eye was 15/40 minus. The usual treatment was given the child, first having her close her eyes to rest them. Then with the aid of the long swing, the variable swing, and the sway of the body, which was a rest to her, her vision improved to 15/20 minus. Dr. Bates explained to the mother that it would be necessary for her to have daily treatment for at least two weeks in order to bring about a satisfactory improvement in her sight. The mother explained that she was taking a long trip with her family and could not at that time remain longer than a day.

On her way west she stopped at a place where we had a competent student who treated the child successfully and gave her a temporary improvement in her sight as Dr. Bates did. The mother then went west where her child was placed under the care of a person who has only a slight knowledge of what the Bates Method really is. As the result of the improper treatment given this child, in one year's time her vision was lowered from 15/40 to 15/100 in each eye. Dr. Bates was much concerned about the lowering of her vision and found out that diathermy and other appliances were given as treatment for the relief of eyestrain. The treatment produced more strain and the myopia became worse. When such patients return to Dr. Bates they are extremely hard to treat and if I can possibly help it I try to dodge such cases unless I am promised a reasonable length of time in which to benefit the patient.

After the Doctor saw the child again, Katherine Hayes, our secretary and assistant, was directed to treat the child, which she did with satisfactory results. On October 19, the day the patient returned for more help, her vision was 15/100. On October 22 her vision had improved to 15/15.

On September 12, 1929, the mother returned again with her child for more treatment. It was found that the vision in both eyes was the same and by practice she improved to 15/10. During her absence between September 12 and October 26, her vision gradually became better because the mother had kept in constant communication with Dr. Bates. The advice which she received for home treatment for her child helped. With but a few exceptions results are usually obtained if the mother keeps up the constant practice for her child every day.

On September 14, the mother again left for her home in the west and again returned early in December for a checkup. It was found that Betty had carried out the instructions given her for daily practice at home, or wherever she might be, with the result that she no longer made an effort to read the letters of the various test cards placed before her, which was something she always did and had to be reminded constantly not to do. She found out all by herself that the harder she tried to read the letters of the cards, the more her vision blurred. Shifting from a near object to the test card as she was reading avoided any effort to see better. When she noticed that the black letters of the white test card became blacker if she did not look too long at them, she enjoyed the treatment much more. The card which she had moved near her was placed at ten feet and she began to strain her eyes to see, causing a frown and a wrinkling of her forehead, which the mother herself corrected before I had a chance to do so myself. I know that the mother's efforts to help me with the child brought about a better vision which remained with her most of the time.

The next day Betty did better, improving two lines on a strange test card. On a sign about fifty feet to the left of our office windows were letters which she could not read distinctly at first, but during the treatment she became able to read all of the sign letters which were much smaller at the bottom of the sign than at the top. Shifting from this sign to the test card in the room again improved her vision for another line, namely 10/15.

The next day, having sunshine in the room, we gave her the sun treatment for about twenty minutes. Small test card letters, seen by the normal eye at four feet, she was able to read nine inches farther away by shifting from the white spaces to the type. Then all the test cards which were used in our office were placed at a distance of fifteen feet and she read each one of them through to the bottom line without a mistake, 15/10. Her mother and I decided to test her memory for these various test card letters by having her close her eyes and read from memory. She was able to do this successfully with two of the test cards but she had not memorized the others, even though she had practiced with them while she was in our office. This proved to the mother that the memory of the known letters with her eyes closed helped her to read all the other test cards when her eyes were open and to read them at more than the normal distance. The nervous twitch of her body which was in evidence always toward the end of her treatment and during her last few treatments had entirely disappeared. I believe that Betty is entirely cured now.

Betty's brother Bobby, age twelve, had never worn glasses although he has for many years had myopia or nearsightedness. His vision in the right eye was 10/50 and with some help from me he was able to read some of the 10-line letters of the card with his left eye. He explained that the bottom line of the test card looked as though each line had a tail to it, and that all the "P's" looked like "T's" and the "F" much like a "P," only distorted. He could not raise his head sufficiently to read the test card but always while reading he would lower his head so that his chin almost touched his chest. This produced a strain which Bobby did not at first believe was the cause of his trouble. He thought that it was perfectly right for him to lower his head in order to see better.

I did something to Bobby which I rarely care to do with most patients, although it is a good demonstration to the patient that strain causes the lowering of sight. Dr. Bates is successful in having patients demonstrate for themselves that producing discomfort from straining helps them to overcome the trouble. In most cases I have hesitated to try this because it affects me personally and causes me to strain so that sometimes I cannot go on with the treatment. Bobby was so enthusiastic about wanting to be cured that he was perfectly willing to have me demonstrate anything that he did which was wrong so that he could cure it.

Bobby had the mind of a boy sixteen or seventeen years old instead of a boy of twelve, and he carried out my instructions very much like our West Point cadets or the boys who are ready to enter Annapolis. We have had many from both academies and so far we have not found one of them difficult to treat no matter how severe their eyestrain might be. Dr. Bates thinks that discipline and knowing what it means to pay attention makes this type of patient easy to treat and to benefit. I think little Bobby is headed for either one of these places, for he spoke about it every time he came.

He was encouraged to do the long swing, not paying any attention to stationary objects in the room. Occasionally I had to remind him to keep his chin up like a soldier, which always spurred him on. I believe that his sister being in the room and watching his treatment helped me in treating him also. She looks upon him very much like a hero and is proud of everything good that he does. Just a little sound of approval from her made him show off a wee bit, which made it amusing to me. His vision improved in less than a half-hour's time to 12/10, reading with both eyes together at first. Having no sunshine while treating him I gave him the Thermo-lite for half an hour. Then I tested his right eye, having his left eye covered, and found that he had improved to 10/15 from 10/50 in less than one hour's time and not once had he lowered his head to read better.

The next day we had sunshine and while Bobby resented the strong light of the sun at first as the sun glass was used on his closed eyelids, he soon became accustomed to it and liked it, asking for more. After the sunlight treatment the vision of the right eye improved that day to 10/10. The next day we did some mental arithmetic while he was taking the sun treatment and found that that was not so good. Trying two things at one time was not helpful to Bobby. The sun glass was then used and after half an hour of sun treatment he palmed and then we did some mental arithmetic. He visualized the numerals as they were given to him and as quickly as I mentioned the figures he gave the answers correctly, not once making a mistake. Again his right eye was tested with a strange card and his vision had improved to 12/10.

I drew his attention then to the sign outside of our window and then to a more distant sign about five hundred feet away and he became able to read all of the sign at that distance with both eyes together. Then I turned him around, facing another strange test card and he read the bottom line, the smallest letters of the card, at fourteen feet two inches, 14/10.

This boy, before coming to me, had had diathermy and other treatment, which perhaps improved his vision temporarily but did not last. He explained to me that the electric treatment which was given him for the improvement of myopia caused a nervous affliction of the body. The advice given Bobby to keep up the good vision obtained through our treatment was to play ball, watch the ball as he threw it to the other player and then blink and sway a little bit as the ball was thrown back to him. I gave him a little demonstration of this in the office, which he enjoyed. I told him to play other games where only two objects were used, one a ball and the other a goal or certain point where the ball should be thrown. The old fashioned horseshoe game is not only relaxing but it gives the patient an opportunity to practice shifting.

Better Eyesight
February 1930—Vol. XIV, No. 8

THE SWAY

By W. H. Bates, M.D.

When one imagines stationary objects to be moving in the same or opposite direction to the movement of the head or eyes when both heels are resting on the floor, it is called the sway. When both heels are lifted from the floor it is not called the sway, but the swing. The apparent movement of stationary objects may be horizontal, vertical, or at any angle. The sway is a very valuable thing to use because it promotes relaxation or rest much better than many other methods. In fact, so general is this conclusion that I always try to have every patient practice the sway immediately upon starting treatment.

The sway may be practiced rapidly or slowly and with a wide or a narrow motion. When the sway is practiced, distant objects are covered more or less completely, which explains why rest is obtained. When the sway is used properly, all stationary objects regarded appear to be moving. Whether the sway is short or long, if practiced properly, the vision is usually improved after other methods have failed.

Patients suffering from insomnia are much benefited by the sway. They soon become able to sleep at night and a maximum amount of rest is obtained. Most people with imperfect sight have a constant strain and tension of nearly all the muscles of the body. The nerves are also under a strain and their efficiency is frequently lost. By practicing the sway properly, fatigue is relieved as well as pain, dizziness, and other symptoms. The sway always brings about a relief from the effort of trying to see, staring, or concentration.

The normal eye needs relaxation or rest; it does not always have normal sight. When it is at rest it always has normal sight. Things which are done by the patient to improve the sight do not always succeed. There are many ways of improving the sight by the sway, provided it is practiced correctly. I remember a patient who came to me about ten years ago, who went to London to obtain relief from a severe and constant pain in her eyes and head. She could obtain no relief in London and was advised to come to me. When I saw her, she was in a pitiful condition from the constant pain which was often present every hour during the day and at night. Many people suffer from pain unconsciously during the night and the characteristic symptom is pain the first thing in the morning as soon as the patient becomes conscious.

This patient had eccentric fixation simultaneously practiced unconsciously most of the time when the patient was conscious. She was examined and shown that when she practiced the sway with her eyes moving in one direction and her head in the opposite direction, the result was a very bad strain which was very painful. This is another illustration of the fact that many things which can be practiced properly can also be practiced improperly. I do not know of a pain which is more severe than that which happens when the eyes are moved in one direction while the body moves in the opposite direction. This method of practicing the sway is to be condemned because of its bad results in producing pain and other symptoms. When this patient practiced the sway properly, her pain disappeared.

A physician wrote to me about his ten-year-old son. The vision of the left eye was good, but the vision of the right eye was very poor because the center of sight was gone. As a result of an injury his central vision was lost and one could see that the retina was destroyed, forming a disk of about one-quarter of the size of the papilla of the optic nerve. When examined with the ophthalmoscope it was found that the center of sight had been destroyed over an area of one-eighth of the size of the papilla of the optic nerve. The boy was treated for about six months and much to my surprise his vision improved and became normal in the injured eye by the practice of the sway without any other treatment.

A third patient was treated for central scatoma. The vision of the left eye was normal but that of the right eye was very poor. The principal cause of her defective sight in the right eye was inflammation of the retina and choroid. She had called on many physicians and most of them told her very positively that she would become blind in the right eye and later on blind in the left eye. When she came to see me she was almost frantic with apprehension and with tears in her eyes she begged me to help her. I was having very good results with the sway and knowing very well that the sway could do her no injury I did not hesitate in having her practice it. In two weeks she was cured and had perfect sight in each eye.

About fifteen years ago an elderly woman was ushered into my office. It seems that she had traveled all over the country consulting prominent ophthalmologists, but had had no success in obtaining relief. She gave a history of constant pain, constant fatigue, inability to sleep at night, and many other symptoms which she could not describe. She told me that if she could only find out what was wrong with her, she might by some possibility obtain relief. She had so many and varied symptoms of discomfort that she could not discover the cause of her trouble. Every doctor who examined her admitted that he did not know what was wrong. Her sight for distant vision was good, and although over fifty years old she had no presbyopia and could read diamond type at six inches rapidly, easily, without discomfort. In fact there were times when she could read all night without fatigue, but suffered from some discomfort that she could not describe. In other words she did not know what was the matter with herself.

Blindness was expected by some doctors in the course of two or three years. Some other doctors believed that she could live for only one year without becoming totally blind. I told the lady that I did not know what was the matter with her either, but I believed that she could be cured even without any diagnosis being made or without discovering the cause of her trouble. Then I said to the lady, "Place your finger about opposite the lower part of the chin and then move your head and eyes from side to side. When you do it properly, you can imagine the finger to be moving and there will come to you a relief from all the various troubles from which you suffer." She started to do as I suggested and by watching her very closely it was quite easy to keep her head and eyes moving as they should. This sway was a great relief to all the troubles of which the patient complained and it gave complete relief to many discomforts from which she had suffered.

A woman from Washington came for treatment of disease and blindness of the central part of the right eye. The left eye was nearly normal, with good vision. She had been told that the right eye was inflamed to such an extent that it was probable that it would require a long time, many months, before the symptoms were relieved. When she moved her head and eyes a short distance from side to side, the test card five feet away and other stationary objects appeared to move in the opposite direction. But when her right eye moved to the left while her head was moved in the opposite direction, pain and imperfect sight were produced. The sway was practiced daily and in a few weeks her vision became normal in both eyes.

WHY PATIENTS FAIL

By Emily A. Bates

On page 15 of my book *Stories from the Clinic,* I have suggestions which if read by patients would help them to do the right thing while taking treatment for their eyes. [All of Emily's "Suggestions" are in the June 1930 issue.—TRQ] Suggestion No. 1 reads as follows, "If the vision of the patient is improved under the care of the doctor, and the patient neglects to practice when he leaves the office what he is told to do at home, the treatment has been of no benefit whatever. The improved vision was only temporary. Faithful practice permanently improves the sight to normal." This does not mean one must work hours at a time practicing the advice given for the improvement of sight, but it does mean that he should devote as much time as possible to practice and not make hard work of it.

We have repeated in a great number of articles that it only takes a minute to test the sight with a test card and if the patient practices a few minutes in the morning, it will help a great deal during the day. If at any time during the day a strain is produced for some reason or another, the memory of one of the test card letters which was seen perfectly usually relieves all symptoms of strain and discomfort. Sometimes relief is only for a minute or two, but if the patient can remind himself to do this several times a day, the improved vision remains for a long time. Even with errors of refraction and organic diseases, the symptoms are lessened by the memory of a known letter or a known object seen clearly.

Most people, even those who have no trouble with their eyes, feel relieved from strain and discomfort of other parts of the body by the memory of some pleasant scenery or beautiful colors which are remembered without effort. There are certain shades of color which do produce mental strain and at the same time cause a lowering of the vision. Green, no matter what shade of green it may be, is usually a rest and relaxation to the mind and eyes. Personally I can relax immediately if I am suffering from mental strain, which is frequently the case, by thinking of a Nile green shade or any object of that color.

Perhaps I can make myself understood better by telling about a case of hypermetropia in a woman, fifty-one years old, whose sight was poor for the near point as well as for the distance. She suffered from a great deal of pain and discomfort in her eyes at times. I tested her sight for colors, using different shades of yarn which I held exposed to her view at a point about ten feet from her eyes. She wore a light colored dress which had the combined shades of brown, tan, and yellow. She mentioned the different shades of yarn as I held them up for her to see and when I placed before her a shade of black yarn, she said, "Isn't it funny that I don't care for black especially."

Here was a problem. For years the Doctor had helped patients by the memory of black, usually remembered by the patient with his eyes closed. For some time we had made good progress in benefiting patients' eyes by having them remember colors with their eyes closed and imagining one period blacker than another and then vice versa. I had planned to treat this woman in this way, using a colon as an object. I immediately removed that thought from my mind and planned to help her in some other way. Some of our test cards have red and green lines which are sometimes a great help in improving the patient's vision for the smaller letters at a distance of ten feet or farther. Testing her with these cards and improving her sight with the memory of the green colored line not only helped the patient's eyes, but also relieved the symptoms of pain and discomfort that she had had for some time.

At this patient's second treatment she gave me a report of the progress she had made while practicing at home. She enjoyed drawing, which I advised her to continue to do, and then for pastime while she was practicing she used different colored crayons for the drawings. She brought the drawings with her, and we thought they were beautifully done. At her second visit she wore a black gown, and all through her treatment I had to listen patiently for twenty minutes to her account of the sadness she had had through her life, of the care that some of the members of her family were to her, and of how hard it was for her to remain cheerful.

I tested her sight and found it about the same as it was before I treated her in the beginning. I made the room unusually bright by using the Thermo-lite as well as the ceiling lights which we have in our office. I then started testing her sight for colors at fifteen feet, using the yarns again and while it took a little longer to have her mention the colors correctly, I did succeed finally in making her forget about her family troubles and worries. I wanted to be sure that I was right about the change of temperament because of her black gown, so I mentioned it to her and told her to remember black while palming. Instead of being quiet she talked incessantly of her pain and the operations that she had had from time to time and the only way I could quiet her was to tell her that I had several of them myself but that I did not worry about them any longer. I asked her if she had read Irvin Cobb's book on operations and told her some of the funny stories which were in his little book. She soon found out that I did not care to discuss operations.

What I want to explain at this point is that color has a great deal to do with mind strain. I believe that people are much happier now that brighter color combinations are being used in our homes.

Some time ago I had a patient over sixty years old who had double vision almost all the time. Large objects were seen single but small objects were always seen double. Test card reading was not easy for this patient so I had to conceal every letter on the test card with the exception of one. After he mentioned that one correctly it was covered over and another letter was exposed to view. If he looked at a card longer than a fraction of a second without turning his head either to the right or to the left, he would always see the letter double. Shifting quickly from a letter to the blank wall on either side of our room helped him to see the letter single and not double when he looked at it again. He was told to do the long shift when he practiced with the card and to shift only an inch or two to the right or to the left whenever he was looking at anything else either up close or at the distance.

This patient did not come regularly for treatment, but he came off and on for about a year, when he was finally cured of his double vision. A variety of flowers which were growing near his home helped when he was outdoors where he practiced the sway of the body, moving from left to right and always remembering to blink. As he did this he saw the flowers as they were, instead of seeing them double which had been his trouble for many years.

At the present time we have a little child taking treatment for blindness in one eye. Both eyes have cataract, but the left eye also has scar tissue in the cornea. Apparently there was not any sight in the left eye because there was no red reflex seen when the ophthalmoscope was used. Toys of different colors were placed before her and as she mentioned the names of each of the animals they were placed on the floor at a distance of five feet or farther. At this distance she sometimes made a mistake in naming the animal. The harder she tried to see the toy at the distance, the more blind she became.

I taught her the long swing, having her shorten the swing to a short sway of the body and advising her to blink as she swayed. She then became able to name the animals correctly as they were placed a few feet farther, but only when she mentioned the color of the toy first. Just by blinking as she swayed she remembered for part of a minute the color of the animal she was asked to mention. When she was not reminded to blink or to keep up the sway she made an error in naming the animal.

It is good to have someone in the room while such patients are under treatment, especially if they are to help the patient away from our office. They can understand very readily why some patients fail when they stare even for only a fraction of a second. It is necessary constantly to remind the patient that in order to bring about a permanent benefit, he must not fail to do as he is advised when away from the office.

Failure to remember a color with the eyes closed lowers the vision and causes the sight to become imperfect. Failure to take time enough to practice or to read the chart every day is a mistake and causes failure. Daily practice counts, no matter how little time one has. After all, the Bates

Method is eye education. To miss one day in the cure of the eyes when they need attention for the improvement of sight is much like failure to study a certain lesson each day in school, or to attend to any work which requires daily study or practice. In most cases when improvement is made in the sight by a teacher of eye education it is only a temporary one, but it is enough to encourage the patient to keep on with the practice until the sight becomes normal. Patients who are cured in one visit are those who can retain the relaxation and rest which is the foundation of the method.

Eye diseases such as atrophy of the optic nerve, iritis, glaucoma, and cataract, are always benefited when the patient does not neglect to practice every day. The sight of patients who suffer from organic diseases is usually very poor. All organic diseases become less when the sight improves by relaxation and rest.

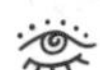

CASE REPORT

By Dr. Rath

Editor's Note—*We believe that the following letter will prove of interest to our readers. Dr. Rath of Jackson, Michigan has recently completed a course of instruction and, as the following report of a case indicates, he is already doing splendid work.*

Dear Dr. and Ms. Bates:

It just occurred to me that you might be interested to know how I am coming on with the little boy that had so many doctors. We call him "the little boy of the forty doctors." His name is Stanley and when Stanley's father first came to me he had just about given up hope. He remarked that Stanley lived in a world all his own. He did not play much with other boys because he could not see. Stanley spent most of his time with his mother when not in school. The school physician placed Stanley in the "Eye Saving School." They use great large letters in all their books.

Stanley's father was not satisfied with his last doctor and really did not know what to do. He talked to the superintendent at the factory where he works about it and he sent him to us for advice. Having just returned, full of inspiration, I told him to bring the boy down and let me look at him. He has now been to see me just ten times. He is now reading the bottom line on the "C" chart, the white card with black letters, 10/10 vision, and the bottom line on the little hand chart. He does not do this very rapidly, but he is doing it. I wish you could see him do the "long swing." He does this with a grace that is charming.

The last time they came, his mother told me that Stanley's complexion had actually changed since he began the "Bates System." The neighbors are noticing the great change in the lad, and the mother and father want to send him to the regular school. I don't know how we will come out in this respect as they likely will not believe he can see well enough. I had him bring with him a book that they use in the regular school, and he reads it without the least difficulty. He plays with the other boys, and he tells me, in playing ball, he not only sees it but be can hit it too.

Every time Stanley comes to see me he is just a little better. When I first saw him he was downcast; now he is happy and buoyant.

I am doing wonderfully well with the "Bates System" and if it were not for making a tedious and long letter I would write you more.

With best wishes, Sincerely, John A. Rath.

P. S.—I neglected to state that when Stanley was first brought to me he was seeing all colors of the rainbow, especially green. This has all ceased.

NOTICE

Dr. Bates, as well as the Central Fixation Publishing Company, has been receiving a number of letters recently from people who have been unsuccessfully treated by practitioners who have not taken Dr. Bates' course of instruction and do not understand the Bates Method thoroughly.

Dr. Bates gives a course of instruction to doctors, teachers, nurses and others who wish to practice his method professionally. At the end of the course the student receives a certificate authorizing him to help others by the Bates Method. Those wishing further particulars may obtain them by writing direct to Dr. Bates.

[See Appendix E, "Becoming a Natural Eyesight Improvement Teacher."—TRQ]

We wish to inform our subscribers that the *Better Eyesight* magazine will be discontinued after the June 1930 issue. This will enable Dr. Bates and Ms. Bates to devote more time to the writing of new books on treatment alone for which there has been a very great demand during the past year.

[I am not aware of any *new* books that were published by Dr. W. H. Bates or Emily A. Bates. In 1940, *Perfect Sight Without Glasses* was revised by Emily A. Bates and published as *Better Eyesight Without Glasses*. Almost all of the original pictures and illustrations were removed.—TRQ]

Better Eyesight
March 1930—Vol. XIV, No. 9

CASES OF SQUINT IN THE CLINIC

By Emily A. Bates

Among the numerous letters we receive from correspondents there was one which drew my attention. Reports of cases are usually from those who have myopia or presbyopia. Cases of squint are less numerous. Most of the patients who have been treated for this trouble have been children whose ages ranged from two years to sixteen years and sometimes up to eighteen.

The older ones are usually high schoolboys. There are just as many cases of squint among girls of school age as there are among boys, but those who have come to me for treatment were mostly boys.

The letter which caught my attention was from a man about 40 years old who had squint of the left eye. This eye also had myopia and the other eye was farsighted. The man did not mention this in his letter, but explained how difficult it was for him to do his work under constant strain because of his eye trouble. He had subscribed to the *Better Eyesight* magazine and after reading the reports of squint cases, he mustered up courage enough to write and ask for help. To begin with he had very little money to pay for treatment and yet he did not wish to be a charity case. He had lost his wife when his two sons were quite young. Because of his affliction he had no desire to have a housekeeper in his home to take care of himself and his children. His boys were sent out to board but they were dissatisfied and this worried him. This worry caused still more mental strain to the poor man.

When he first wrote for help we could not admit him into our Clinic at the Harlem Hospital because patients who lived outside of the hospital district were not admitted there. We gave him a little help for a while and in each letter he wrote he sent a grateful message for the help we were giving him.

We gave this patient an appointment for office treatment, and with our help he was able to go on with his work and do it more easily and with less strain. Being employed every day and living about forty miles outside of New York City, he could come but once a week. Anyone who understands the treatment of squint cases will realize how difficult it is to make progress with a patient under these conditions. He was a temperamental type and most sensitive because of his eye trouble. For years he had avoided looking at people's faces and when I first met him his voice trembled when he answered my questions. I knew that mental strain was his main trouble.

I decided that the first thing to do was to speak to him in as low and gentle a voice as possible and see what effect that would have upon him. It was easier to speak to him with my eyes closed, and while my eyes were closed I asked him to close his. I noticed that having our eyes closed while we talked had a soothing effect upon him because his voice sounded more relaxed and he was pleased because I spent enough time with him to listen to his troubles and the difficulties he had in taking time to practice with his eyes.

His vision for fine print is now normal at six inches, although it was much impaired when he first came for treatment. His vision for the distance improved but only at times did he have normal vision. Other cases of squint have been treated at the Clinic but none received the care that he did because it was not required. The mental strain that he had almost constantly was the principal trouble and a stumbling block in the path of permanent benefit within a reasonable time.

In the beginning of the treatment, when I pointed to a letter of the test card at ten feet he would see it, and if he forgot to blink regularly or stared at the letter it would disappear entirely and the test card was immediately a blank to him. The methods for treating him were varied from time to time because it was necessary on account of his mental condition. His vision first improved but then he seemed to lose ground and he stayed away from the Clinic for a while. When he again returned he could not talk to me for quite a while nor could I treat him until he had finished weeping, which was an unusual sight to see at the Clinic.

It is marvelous the fortitude and the splendid way in which some of our Clinic folks go about the cure of their eyes. They have so little time to spend for themselves and yet they find the necessary time, even though it is early in the morning and late at night, to practice as they are directed to do. Patients at the Harlem Hospital Clinic have an advantage over patients in our Clinic because they may be seen and treated three days each week, but this poor man had to wait until Saturday before he could come and then there were times when his work prevented him from keeping even these weekly appointments. The day he wept he told me that he had contemplated suicide and was about to do so when he remembered my voice and what I said to him at one time, which was that even though his eyes was crossed, others did not notice it as much as he was conscious of it himself. He also remembered what I said about being a coward and not being brave enough to face life as he had to face it, and that there were others who were less fortunate than he was.

I hope that those who have taken up the Bates Method and are practicing it seriously will have an extra amount of consideration for a man like that. His condition could not be reached or improved until he was relieved of tension and strain. After that was accomplished he improved steadily; he still comes for treatment occasionally. He can now read diamond type at six inches with his left eye and right eye separately and can read the 15-line of the test card with the left eye at ten feet, 15/10. Only at times is the squint noticeable.

Another squint case which we had lately was that of a little girl age eight. She seemed to respond right from the start just for the sake of a smile. When I first became acquainted with her, she looked like a very serious little person who seldom smiled. When I greeted her with a smile and said that I could easily help her condition if she would cooperate with me, she settled herself comfortably in the large arm chair where I placed her and after I had tested her sight for the distance and told her that closing her eyes to rest them was a benefit to her, she obeyed me. Her vision when tested on November 24 was 15/10 in the right eye and 15/100 in the left eye, the eye with squint. By practicing the sway and blinking, her vision improved to 15/20 in the left eye the first day, a temporary improvement.

A doctor who was especially interested in this case wrote me a letter asking me if I would see what I could do for her. In his letter he told me that glasses did not help or improve the squint and that her duties at school were a great punishment to her because she could not see the blackboard. While treating her in the beginning I used but one test card which was a black one with white letters. Closing her eyes, remembering her best doll, and explaining to me how it was dressed improved her vision considerably for the smaller letters of the card. Shifting while she was seated in her chair, looking first at a blank wall and then at the test card also helped to improve her vision, and as her father looked on he commented upon how straight the eye was as she shifted from the wall to the test card.

Purposely I had her stare to see the letters of the card without shifting and immediately her eye turned in as it had when I first tested her sight. Her father was given directions on how to take care of her eyes at home and she got along very nicely when all of a sudden our little girl stayed away and we did not see her for some time. She had retained the better vision she had shown upon her previous treatment and she again took up her eye work very seriously when she returned. Her sister, who is a few years older than she, came with her from time to time and learned how to help Elizabeth at home. A record was kept, not as regularly as we had wished, but it was enough to convince us that she was doing her part at home. The last time she came she read all of the card at normal distance 10/10 and both eyes were straight during the time she read the card.

When such cases are under treatment we cannot emphasize too strongly that using the poor eye or the eye with squint for a period of time each day while the good eye is covered with a patch is a benefit to the poor eye and lessens the squint. I know children do not like to wear a patch, because no one cares to have the eye with good sight covered while the eye under treatment is called upon to see everything for a length of time. At first the patch should be worn for five minutes each day and then the time gradually increased until the patient is able to wear the patch all day long. Every morning and night the test cards should be read with both eyes together and then with the poor eye alone, having the good eye covered.

I do not know of anything which helps more than the long swing, which can be practiced fifty or one hundred times by the patient each morning and night. After the long swing I usually have the patient shorten the swing so that he is able to read one letter at a time of the test card and then sway the body to the left or to the right, whichever is found to be best for the patient. If the right eye turns in, it is best to sway to the right and then to the test card which is placed directly in front of the patient. In this way both eyes move at the same time in the same direction and there is no squint visible while the swing and the reading of the test card is going on. When the squint is again noticeable while reading the card and practicing the half swing, it is best to draw the card up a little closer where the patient has less strain while reading. The squint will then be less and the patient can practice better without any discomfort.

The reason why some cases of squint take longer than others is because the patient does not practice enough at home every day.

One cannot encourage the patient enough to blink often, do the long swing morning and night as Dr. Bates advises often in his articles in this magazine, and if possible to do the long swing 100 times at least twice daily. While the long swing is being practiced, both eyes move together and at such times both eyes are straight. Every day one should notice how long the eye remains straight during treatment. If the eyes remain straight for just a few minutes longer from day to day, the improvement will soon be noticed by the patient and this will encourage him to do more practicing.

Better Eyesight
April 1930—Vol. XIV, No. 10

SUGGESTIONS FOR MYOPIC PATIENTS

By Emily A. Bates

In the morning when you awaken, before getting out of bed, sit up and palm. Memory helps. While palming, the memory of a flower or of the color of it, of a white cloud with the sun shining behind it, of the blue of the sky, or of any pleasant thing that you can remember perfectly, something that you have seen perfectly, helps. If nothing else can be remembered you can imagine part of the test card and when you imagine some of the letters with your eyes closed and imagine the form of each letter, not trying to remember any particular letter any length of time, because that is a strain, your mind will be relaxed when you get out of bed.

After arising, practice the sway. Always blink while swaying. After the sway do the long swing; let your head and eyes alone, allow your body to do the moving. Pay no attention to stationary objects which appear to be moving as you swing. After practicing the long swing, keep up the blinking while dressing, but do not blink fast. The eyes move gently with every blink and that is a rest. You will notice that heretofore you have stared.

If the test cards can be used for practice before going to business, so much the better. Place the "C" card to the right of you, a little more than arm's length away. Place the black card to the left of you, also a little more than arm's length away. Then place the number card to the left six feet away, and the inverted "E" card to the right of you six feet away. Now start the sway. Pay no attention to anything, but just keep looking right ahead of you at the wall. Blink and keep up the sway. Notice that all cards appear to be moving opposite to the movement of your body. Blink. Never stop blinking, still noticing that the cards move opposite to the movement of the sway. Do not sway too fast; take it easy. Better vision comes without effort. Notice that when things become too blurred that you are staring, that you have forgotten to blink.

When it is noticed that the cards appear to be moving opposite to the movement of the body, then start the long swing, flashing a letter of the "C" card as you swing to the right, then noticing a letter on a line of the black card as you swing to the left. Be sure to move your body and not only your head and eyes. Don't forget to blink. Then, while keeping up the long swing, flash a numeral on the number card to the left and then as you swing to the right, flash an inverted "E" on any line of that card. Every day see if you can flash a smaller numeral on one of the lower lines of the number card as well as an "E" pointing either to the right, left, up, or down on one of the lower lines of the "E" card.

The improvement in your vision all depends upon the time that you have to practice in the above way.

If sun treatment can be given to the closed eyelids by placing yourself in the sun, raising your head, and letting the sun shine on the closed eyelids for five minutes or longer, it will help to improve the vision when doing the long swing.

If palming is irksome, just sit comfortably and close the eyes, remembering something pleasant every time the eyes are being rested in this way.

Alternate practicing with the distant cards by placing yourself at a desk. When writing for practice always place your small black card to the right or to the left of your desk and after writing a sentence or two, raise your head and look over to the card at any letter that you see easily without straining. It helps to close the eyes immediately afterward, remembering that letter. Write a few more sentences, again glancing at the card after raising your head in the direction of the letters and not trying hard to see any particular letter.

When large test cards are not used for practice, place two small cards on the window sill if possible and while swaying shift from one card to the other.

Better Eyesight
May 1930—Vol. XIV, No. 11

TEST CARD PRACTICE

By Emily A. Bates

Editor's Note—*The following is taken from Ms. Bates' book,* Stories from the Clinic. *Although the majority of our subscribers have Ms. Bates' book, we believe that these suggestions can always be re-read with benefit.*

1. Every home should have a test card.

2. It is best to place the card permanently on the wall in a good light.

3. Each member of the family or household should read the card every day.

4. It takes only a minute to test the sight with the card. If you spend five minutes in the morning practicing, it will be a great help during the day.

5. Place yourself ten feet from the card and read as far as you can without effort or strain. Over each line of letters are small figures indicating the distance at which the normal eye can read them. Over the big "C" at the top of the card is the figure "200." The big "C," therefore, should be read by the normal eye at a distance of two hundred feet. If you can read this line at ten feet, your vision would be 10/200. The numerator of the fraction is always the distance of the card from the eyes. The denominator always denotes the number of the line read. If you can only read the line marked "40" at ten feet, the vision is 10/40.

6. If you can only see the fifth line, for example, notice that the last letter on that line is an "R." Now close your eyes, cover them with the palms of the hands and remember the "R." If you will remember that the left side is straight, the right side partly curved, and the bottom open, you will get a good mental picture of the "R" with your eyes closed. This mental picture will help you to see the letter directly underneath the "R," which is a "T."

7. Shifting is good to stop the stare. If you stare at the letter "T," you will notice that all the letters on that line begin to blur. It is beneficial to close your eyes quickly after you see the "T," open them, and shift to the first figure on that line, which is a "3." Then close your eyes and remember the "3." You will become able to read all the letters on that line by closing your eyes for each letter.

8. Keep a record of each test in order to note your progress from day to day.

9. When you become able to read the bottom line with each eye at ten feet; your vision is normal for the distance, 10/10.

10. The distance of the Snellen test card from the patient is a matter of considerable importance. However, some patients improve more rapidly when the card is placed fifteen or twenty feet away, while others fail to get any benefit with the card at this distance. In some cases the best results are obtained when the card is as close as one foot. Others with poor vision may not improve when the card is placed at ten feet or farther, or at one foot or less, but do much better when the card is placed at a middle distance, at about eight feet. Some patients may not improve their vision at all at ten feet, but at one foot. While some patients are benefited by practicing with the card daily, always at the same distance, there are others who seem to be benefited when the distance of the card from the patient is changed daily.

Better Eyesight
June 1930—Vol. XIV, No. 12

SUGGESTIONS

By Emily A. Bates

1. If the vision of the patient is improved under the care of the doctor, and the patient neglects to practice, when he leaves the office, what he is told to do at home, the treatment has been of no benefit whatever. The improved vision was only temporary. Faithful practice permanently improves the sight to normal.

2. If the patient conscientiously practices the methods, as advised by the Doctor, his vision always improves. This applies to patients with errors of refraction, as well as organic diseases.

3. For cases of squint we find that the long swing is beneficial to adults and to children.

4. When a patient suffers with cataract, palming is usually the best method of treatment, and should be practiced many times every day.

5. All patients with imperfect sight unconsciously stare, and should be reminded by those who are near to them to blink often. To stare is to strain. Strain is the cause of imperfect sight.

The following rules will be found helpful if faithfully observed:

6. While sitting, do not look up without raising your chin. Always turn your head in the direction in which you look. Blink often.

7. Do not make an effort to see things more clearly. If you let your eyes alone, things will clear up by themselves.

8. Do not look at anything longer than a fraction of a second without shifting.

9. While reading, do not think about your eyes, but let your mind and imagination rule.

10. When you are conscious of your eyes while looking at objects at any time, it causes discomfort and lessens your vision.

11. It is very important that you learn how to imagine stationary objects to be moving.

12. Palming is a help, and I suggest that you palm for a few minutes many times during the day, at least ten times. At night just before retiring, it is well to palm for half an hour or longer.

GLOSSARY

Some of the definitions in this glossary are simple and incomplete. For example, there are many other types of astigmatism than the type described here. In some cases, alternative definitions are given. Most of the vision problems in this glossary have been reported improved or completely eliminated by Bates Method re-education.

(Bates) = Indicates comments by William H. Bates, M.D.
(Lierman) = by Emily C. Lierman

3-D VISION: A right-brain quality of depth perception obtained through relaxed vision habits and by removing corrective lenses; not the same as STEREOSCOPIC VISION.

ACCOMMODATION: The process of changing focus from distance to near vision; due to increased curvature of the front side of the LENS by the action of the CILIARY MUSCLE (orthodox); due to the two OBLIQUE EYE MUSCLES contracting and elongating the eyeball (Bates).

AGGRAVATION PHASE: See HEALING CRISIS.

AMBLYOPIA EX ANOPSIA: Literally "dimsightedness due to lack of use," without disease; partial suppression of vision in one eye; usually affects the central visual acuity; almost always present in STRABISMUS, e.g. crossed eye, because if the picture from the strabismic eye remains "switched on" in the brain, the person would likely experience DOUBLE IMAGES; also common in an eye that has significantly less vision than the other eye; sometimes the amblyopic eye "switches on" and sees better instantaneously when the other eye is covered or closed. See also SQUINT (STRABISMUS).

ANESTHESIA: "A condition in which the CORNEA is not sensitive to the touch of a blunt pointed instrument" (Bates).

ANGINA PECTORIS: A type of heart disease.

APHAKIA: An eye in which the crystalline LENS has been removed or is absent.

APHASIA: A total or partial loss of the ability to understand or use words; usually caused by an injury or brain disease.

APHONIA: Loss of voice; usually due to an organic or functional disorder.

AQUEOUS HUMOR: Clear liquid produced by the CILIARY BODY, filling the aqueous chamber—the front chamber of the eye between the LENS/IRIS and CORNEA.

ASTHENOPIA: Eyestrain; often accompanied by headaches and dizziness.

ASTIGMATISM: An imperfect curvature of the eyeball, CORNEA, or LENS; oval or lopsided eyeball from the front point of view (MYOPIC and HYPERMETROPIC eyes are round from the front point of view); in an eye with only ASTIGMATISM: nearsighted along one axis (light rays focus in front of the RETINA), while farsighted along another axis (light rays focus in back of the retina); DIOPTERS cylinder (D. C.) indicates the amount of astigmatism; cylindrical "+" or "-" lenses; axis indicates the angle (not the amount) of astigmatism, in degrees; significant fluctuations, within minutes, possible, especially with the axis; can create two or more MULTIPLE IMAGES (in one eye), shadows, distortion of an object's shape; can be produced by uneven tension and contraction of the external eye muscles.

ATAXIA: Total or partial inability to coordinate voluntary muscular (primarily) body movements.

ATROPHY: "Wasting away," usually due to disuse, lack of circulation, or insufficient nutrition.

ATROPHY OF THE OPTIC NERVE: Also called optic atrophy; a disease of the OPTIC NERVE; often diminished light and form perception, or complete blindness; "can be caused by the eyestrain of HYPERMETROPIA" (Bates).

ATROPINE: An alkaloid drug used to dilate the PUPIL; also used to paralyze the CILIARY MUSCLE and thus, by preventing any change of curvature in the LENS, bringing out "latent HYPERMETROPIA" and getting rid of "apparent myopia" (Bates).

AXIS: The angle, or orientation, in degrees, of ASTIGMATISM.

BATES METHOD: An educational program created by ophthalmologist William H. Bates, M.D., in which natural, correct vision habits—based on relaxation of the mind and body—are taught; optional self-healing activities and games are often included to accelerate integration and self-healing; commonly misunderstood as only "eye exercises"—even by many "Bates Method" teachers.

BIFOCALS, TRIFOCALS, MULTIFOCALS, PROGRESSIVE LENSES: Lenses that have different amounts of correction from top (distance vision) to bottom (near "reading" vision); for MYOPIA the top portion of the lens has a higher (minus) prescription; for HYPERMETROPIA or PRESBYOPIA the bottom portion has a higher (plus) prescription.

BLINKING: The natural, frequent, soft, quick opening and closing of the eyelids; an essential, key vision habit necessary for normal sight; serves many important functions; see Chapter 14, "The Third Habit—Blinking," in *Relearning to See*.

BODY SWING: Movement of the body from left to right to encourage SHIFTING and OPPOSITIONAL MOVEMENT, and especially to prevent STARING; the short body swing is approximately one-quarter of an inch from side to side.

BRIGHT'S DISEASE: A type of kidney disease with albumin in the urine.

CATARACT: Literally "waterfall"; opacity of the crystalline LENS (or its enclosing LENS CAPSULE); partial or complete opacities with corresponding vision loss; many different types; can be produced in a cow's eye by applying pressure around the eyeball; pupil often appears light gray. "Cataract has been produced in normal eyes by the MEMORY or the IMAGINATION of imperfect sight. The MEMORY of imperfect sight produces a strain of the outside muscles of the eyeball, which is accompanied by a contraction of these muscles, and cataract is produced" (Bates).

CENTRAL FIXATION: also called centralization; the normal mental vision habit of seeing best a small point in the center of the VISUAL FIELD; an essential key to normal sight; the CONES in the FOVEA CENTRALIS (and MACULA) of the RETINA dictate that only the center point of the picture can be seen clearly at any one moment; RODS, which pick up PERIPHERAL VISION, can register only 20/400 vision—at best—and are, therefore, incapable of clarity perception; a person with NORMAL VISION naturally "centralizes," or keeps the primary visual attention in the center of the picture; central fixation is learned automatically and subconsciously after birth; people with better than 20/20 vision centralize into a very tiny area; central fixation does *not* mean ignoring or "switching off" the PERIPHERAL VISION. "Shift your glance constantly from one point to another, seeing the part regarded best and other parts not so clearly" (Bates); see Dr. Bates' chair example in "Perfect Sight" in the September 1927 issue; see also ECCENTRIC FIXATION, which is the opposite of central fixation.

CENTRALIZATION: See CENTRAL FIXATION.

CHALAZION TUMOR: A swelling of one of the glands of the eyelids; cyst.

CHLOROFORM: A general anesthetic.

CHOROID: The middle coat of the eye containing blood vessels that supply the eye, especially the RETINA, with nutrients.

CHOROIDITIS: Inflammation of the CHOROID.

CILIARY BODY: A highly vascularized, enlarged continuation of the CHOROID that contains the CILIARY PROCESS and the circular and meridional-radial CILIARY MUSCLES and that encircles the LENS.

CILIARY MUSCLE: Actually two muscles within the CILIARY BODY: the circular and meridional-radial; credited with ACCOMMODATION by producing greater and lesser curvature on the front side of the LENS (orthodox); "I do not account for the presence of the ciliary muscle" (Bates).

CILIARY PROCESS: A part of the CILIARY BODY that produces AQUEOUS HUMOR.

CIRCULAR SWING (OR SHIFTING): The head and eyes move in the orbit of a circle to prevent staring; the shorter the diameter of the orbit, the better—as long as staring is avoided. See also INFINITY SWING.

COLOR BLINDNESS: Diminished color perception; usually one or two of the three types of CONES (red, green, and blue) are not functioning normally, resulting in a deficiency of some, but usually not all, color perception.

CONCAVE LENSE: See DIOPTERS SPHERICAL.

CONES: The light receptors located in the central part of the RETINA; highest concentration is in the FOVEA CENTRALIS; high concentration is in the MACULA LUTEA; register sharp acuity and color; the high concentration of cones in the fovea centralis is the reason CENTRAL FIXATION is necessary to see clearly; contrast to RODS; there are at least three types of cones: one that registers primary red, one for green, and the third for blue.

CONGENITAL: Occurring at or before birth.

CONJUNCTIVA: A thin, transparent membrane that extends along the inner surfaces of both eyelids, over the front portion of the SCLERA, and over the CORNEA.

CONJUNCTIVITIS: Inflammation of the CONJUNCTIVA.

CONICAL CORNEA: also called keratoconus; "anterior staphyloma, or bulging, of the front of the eyeball, similar to the posterior staphyloma which so often occurs in MYOPIA" (Bates); sometimes associated with ASTIGMATISM.

CONUS: A condition of the CHOROID in which the neighborhood of the OPTIC NERVE is destroyed, exposing the SCLERA, forming a crescent and later a complete circle around the OPTIC DISC.

CONVERGENCE, NORMAL: The normal alignment of the two eyes so that they are both directed to the same point at the same time; if the point of interest is straight ahead, the left eye rotates to the right and the right eye rotates to the left, so that the light rays from that point arrive at the FOVEA CENTRALIS in each eye; absence of normal convergence is called SQUINT (STRABISMUS).

CONVEX LENSE: See DIOPTERS SPHERICAL.

CORNEA: The transparent, front part of the eyeball; accounts for 80% of the REFRACTION needed to focus light rays onto the RETINA (the LENS accounts for the remaining 20%); a continuation of the SCLERA.

CROSSED EYE: Also called esophoria and esotropia; one or both eyes turns in excessively toward the nose;

many types and degrees; a common type of SQUINT (STRABISMUS).

CYCLITIS: An inflammation of the CILIARY BODY.

CYCLOPLEGICS: Drugs used to paralyze the CILIARY MUSCLE.

D. C.: See DIOPTERS CYLINDER.

D. S.: See DIOPTERS SPHERICAL.

DETACHED RETINA: A tearing or detachment of the RETINA away from the CHOROID; common with prolonged, high degrees of MYOPIA.

DIAMOND TYPE: 4-point type; one of the smallest sizes of type used in printing; helps to improve the vision if it is read every day, if relaxed vision habits are used, due to the necessity of CENTRALIZATION.

DIATHERMY: A medical treatment in which heat is produced in the tissues beneath the skin by a high-frequency electrical current.

DIFFUSION: See ECCENTRIC FIXATION.

DIMSIGHTEDNESS: SEE AMBLYOPIA.

DIOPTERS CYLINDER: ABBREVIATED "D. C."; THE AMOUNT OF CORRECTION IN A LENSE MADE FOR ASTIGMATISM. Diopters Cylinder always has an AXIS associated with it.

DIOPTERS SPHERICAL: Abbreviated "D. S."; the amount of correction in a concave lense made for MYOPIA if preceded by an minus (–) sign, or in a convex lense made for HYPERMETROPIA and PRESBYOPIA if preceded by a plus (+) sign.

DIPLOPIA: Seeing two images of one object; often present in SQUINT (STRABISMUS) if AMBLYOPIA is absent; contrast with MULTIPLE IMAGES.

DOUBLE IMAGES: SEE DIPLOPIA and MULTIPLE IMAGES.

DRIFTING SWING: Imagining drifting in a boat down a river while constantly SHIFTING the attention from one point to another.

DROOPING OF EYELIDS: Same as PTOSIS.

DRY EYE SYNDROME: Adacrya; a deficiency or absence of tears; can lead to infection, burning, poor sight, scar tissue in the LACRIMAL GLANDS, OPACITY of CORNEA, and PHOTOPHOBIA; often caused by insufficient BLINKING.

ECCENTRIC FIXATION: Attempting to see, or seeing, best (but not clearly) with the PERIPHERAL VISION; diffusion; "spreading out" the visual attention into the peripheral parts of the VISUAL FIELD; taking the primary visual attention away from the center; attempting to see all parts of the visual field equally clear; attempting the impossible: to see peripheral parts of the visual field—picked up primarily by the RODS—as clear as the center part; the rods that pick up "unclear" peripheral vision are designed to perceive movement and extremely low levels of light (the CONES in the FOVEA CENTRALIS are incapable of extremely low-level light perception); the opposite of normal CENTRAL FIXATION; oftentimes associated with the harmful habits of STARING and straining to see; normal central fixation can be lost by suppression of the sensitivity of the cones in the fovea (Bates); generally, the greater the eccentric fixation, the worse the vision; eccentric fixation is a strain and always lowers vision.

ELLIPTICAL SWING: The head and eyes move in the orbit of an ellipse to prevent STARING; the shorter the diameter of the orbit, the better—as long as staring is avoided. See also INFINITY SWING.

EMMETROPIA: A normal, spherical eyeball. See also MYOPIA and HYPERMETROPIA.

ENEMA: Cleaning the large colon, often by water inserted into the rectum; (colonics, using pressurized water, clean the colon more thoroughly).

ENUCLEATION: Removal of the LENS from the eye.

ERROR OF REFRACTION: Light rays do not focus on the RETINA, e.g. MYOPIA, HYPERMETROPIA, and ASTIGMATISM.

ERUCTATION: Belching.

ESERINE: A drug used to contract the PUPIL.

EYEGROUND: The physical condition of the RETINA, CHOROID, and OPTIC DISK.

EYELIDS, DROOPING OF THE: Same as PTOSIS.

FACIAL NEURALGIA: See TIC DOULOUREUX.

FARSIGHTEDNESS: See HYPERMETROPIA and PRESBYOPIA.

FIELD, VISUAL: The area of sight; central, nasal, temporal, etc.; various parts of the visual field can be lost due to disease or injury.

FINE PRINT: SMALL, 7-point type.

FLASHING: Closing the eyes while imagining or remembering a letter on an eyechart as perfectly as possible until a greater feeling of rest or relaxation is obtained; then opening the eyes for only a short moment to "flash" the letter to see it more clearly; the eyes are immediately closed when the letter is seen more clearly to prevent straining to see it better, and to avoid possibly seeing the letter less clearly; then the process is repeated; with practice, the eyes remain open for longer periods of time while maintaining improved vision; objects other than letters on the eyechart can be used.

FLOATING SPECKS: Also called *muscae volitantes,* "flying flies", vitreous floaters, "spots before the eyes"; usually small debris floating randomly in the eye; may be due to early fetal blood vessels in the center (VITREOUS HUMOR) of the eye; can also be due to accidents to, or diseases of, the eye; common type tends to be ignored by the mind when a person has correct vision habits.

FOVEA CENTRALIS: The small "central pit" in the middle of the RETINA that contains, by far, the highest concentration of CONES; located in the center of the MACULA LUTEA; the only part of the retina that perceives sharp detail; the anatomical basis for CENTRAL FIXATION; the "central pit" allows light rays to reach the cones with less interference; there are no blood vessels in the top layers of the retina to supply nutrients to the foveal cones; foveal cones are supplied with nutrients only from the CHOROID.

FUNDAMENTALS CARD: A small card made up of different size type which starts large at the top and graduates down to fine reading type at the bottom of the card; designed by Dr. Bates; contains a summary of the principles and habits of normal sight; for a more complete description of the "Fundamentals," see the July 1928 issue; see also Appendix F, "Snellen Eyechart and Test Cards."

FUSION: The normal merging of the two images received from the two eyes in the brain at the point of central fixation.

GANGLION CELLS: A central group of nerve cells from which impulses are transmitted.

GLAUCOMA: A serious eye disease often associated with increased intraocular pressure and a hard eyeball; can lead to blindness; often severe pain; OPTIC DISC often depressed, causing damage to the OPTIC NERVE; may be caused by a constriction of the IRIS preventing normal drainage through Schlemm's canal.

GOITER: An enlargement of the thyroid gland, usually with a swelling in the lower front part of the neck.

GRANULATED EYELIDS: Tiny bulges or pimples on the inside of the eyelids.

GRIPPE: An earlier term for influenza.

HALO: The normal appearance of exaggerated whiteness around letters or just underneath a sentence; usually not noticed consciously; an illusion (Bates); halos tend to be suppressed with STARING and other incorrect vision habits.

HEALING CRISIS: Usually a relatively short period of healing discomfort "earned" by improving health naturally; symptoms similar, if not identical, to those in the past (known as a REVERSAL PROCESS); often mistaken for symptoms of a recurring illness and "becoming sick again"; Hering's Law of Cure: True healing occurs from within out (digestive tract out to skin), from above down (head to feet), and in the reverse order the diseases have developed.

HYPERMETROPIA: Also called hyperopia (modern) and farsightedness (common); a foreshortened eyeball in which light rays from near objects focus in back of the RETINA, resulting in blurred near vision; caused by abnormal contraction of the four RECTI MUSCLES (Bates); the opposite of MYOPIA; near vision is more blurred than the distance vision; convex "+" lenses used for correction; Dr. Bates considered the term "farsighted" a misnomer because even the far vision can be lowered; associated with right-brain-dominant people who acquire strained vision habits, especially with near objects; according to Dr. Bates, hypermetropia is the same as PRESBYOPIA because he did not believe the LENS plays a role in ACCOMMODATION. "In middle age, serious eye diseases are caused by hypermetropia. Among the most common are GLAUCOMA, CATARACT, and diseases of the OPTIC NERVE and RETINA." (Bates).

HYPEROPIA: See HYPERMETROPIA.

IMAGINATION: The ability to see, or to think of seeing, letters or other objects when the eyes are closed as well as they can be seen with the eyes open; used to improve eyesight since "it is impossible to relax and imagine a letter perfectly and at the same time strain and see it imperfectly" (Bates); a primary method used by Dr. Bates to teach correct vision habits; see also MEMORY.

INFINITY SWING: The head and eyes are moved in the shape of an infinity sign (a sideways Figure 8), counterclockwise on the left side and clockwise on the right side; while not mentioned by Dr. Bates, it is the best type of SWING; see full description of the "Infinity Swing" in *Relearning to See*.

IRIDECTOMY: Removal of part of the IRIS by surgery.

IRIS: A colored, circular muscle located in front of the lens; controls the amount of light entering the eye by expansion and contraction, increasing and decreasing the size of the PUPIL; used in iridology as a diagnostic tool for determining imbalances in the body.

IRITIS: An inflammation of the IRIS.

KERATITIS: Inflammation of the CORNEA.

KERATOCONUS: See CONICAL CORNEA.

LACHRIMAL GLANDS: Almond-size, sponge-like glands located above the eyes that supply necessary tears through the pumping action of BLINKING.

LAZY-EYE: See AMBLYOPIA.

LENS: The crystalline double-convex lens that lies between the IRIS and the VITREOUS HUMOR; accommodates to see near objects clearly (orthodox view); accounts for 20% of the refraction necessary to focus light rays onto the retina. (The CORNEA accounts for the remaining 80%.) Dr. Bates did not attribute any function to the lens.

LENS CAPSULE: A thin, transparent membrane that contains the LENS; connected to the CILIARY BODY by suspensory ligaments.

LIGHT TREATMENT: A type of SUN TREATMENT.

LONG SWING: Swinging the head, eyes, and body to the

left while lifting the right heel, and to the right while lifting the left heel; the purpose is to prevent the STARING habit and to notice consciously the illusion of OPPOSITIONAL MOVEMENT of stationary objects; usually precedes the SHORT SWING, which is more beneficial in the longterm.

MACULA LUTEA: A small, yellowish area with a high concentration of CONES in the center of the RETINA; the FOVEA CENTRALIS is located in the center of the macula lutea.

MACULAR DEGENERATION: Degeneration of the cells in the MACULA LUTEA, especially the CONES; can lead to loss of sharp acuity since the peripheral RODS are incapable of sharp acuity; United States currently (2000) has the highest rate of macular degeneration. See also FOVEA CENTRALIS.

MEMORY: The ability to recall letters or other objects when the eyes are closed as well as they can be seen with the eyes open (Bates); it is suggested that myopes notice a perfectly clear letter or object up close, and then close the eyes and remember that letter or object perfectly clear in the distance; farsights and presbyopes do the opposite; astigmatics do both; used by Dr. Bates as a primary method of improving sight; see also IMAGINATION.

MICROSCOPIC TYPE: Extremely small type, smaller than FINE PRINT; used to encourage CENTRAL FIXATION; a benefit to sight as long as straining is avoided.

MINION: Type size smaller than diamond type.

MONTESSORI SYSTEM: A method of child education with emphasis on interest, senses, and guidance instead of rigid control.

MULTIFOCAL LENSES: See BIFOCALS.

MULTIPLE IMAGES: Two or more, usually overlapping, partial or shadowy images seen with one or both eyes; common with ASTIGMATISM; experienced by many people while improving sight from blurred to clear images; often confused with DIPLOPIA in STRABISMUS.

MUSCAE VOLITANTES: See FLOATING SPECKS.

MYOPIA: Also called nearsightedness and shortsightedness; an elongated eyeball with light rays from far objects focussing in front of the RETINA, resulting in blurred distance vision; the opposite of HYPERMETROPIA; concave "-" lenses used for correction; caused by abnormal contraction of the two OBLIQUE MUSCLES (Bates); associated with left-brain-dominant people who acquire strained vision habits, especially with far objects; sometimes associated with GLAUCOMA and DETACHED RETINA, especially in prolonged, high degrees of myopia.

MYOTICS: Drugs that contract the pupil and thus stretch "the iris, believed to draw the latter away from the 'filtration angle' and allow the excess of fluid to escape. They are commonly employed for the purpose of giving temporary relief in glaucoma" (Bates).

NATUROPATHY: A system of treating diseases without surgery and drugs; often combines many different modalities of natural healing, including nutrition, herbs, homeopathy, colonics, sunshine, iridology, etc.

NEARSIGHTEDNESS: See MYOPIA.

NEURALGIA: Pain along a nerve or its area of distribution. See also TIC DOULOUREUX.

NEURASTHENIA: A type of neurosis resulting from emotional conflicts; symptoms of anxiety, irritability, fatigue, weakness; oftentimes with localized pain without any apparent cause.

NORMAL CONVERGENCE: See CONVERGENCE, NORMAL.

NORMAL SWING: The natural, short, easy swing or shift of the eyes and head.

NORMAL VISION (NORMAL SIGHT): "Perfect sight at all distances. The SNELLEN TEST CARD is the standard for testing the vision. When the 10-line of the card can be read at ten feet or farther, and FINE PRINT can be read at six inches or less, one has normal vision" (Lierman); includes NORMAL CONVERGENCE.

NYSTAGMUS: A rapid, sometimes large, jerky vibration or oscillation of the eye, usually from side to side; could be considered an intermediate stage between NORMAL CONVERGENCE and SQUINT (STRABISMUS); caused by alternate tension and relaxation of an external eye muscle, usually a lateral or medial RECTUS MUSCLE. Compare with SACCADIC VIBRATIONS.

O. D.: *Oculus dexter;* right eye.

O. S.: *Oculus sinister;* left eye.

OBLIQUE MUSCLES: Two (of six) external eye muscles that wrap partially over the top (superior) and bottom (inferior) of the eye, forming a belt around the eyeball; they can contract abnormally tight, elongating the eyeball in MYOPIA and in various types of ASTIGMATISM; they are the muscles of ACCOMMODATION according to Dr. Bates—contracting to elongate the eyeball to focus near objects clearly.

OBLIQUE SWING: Swinging the eyes and head in an oblique direction to prevent STARING.

OCULIST: An earlier term for OPHTHALMOLOGIST.

OPACITY: Non-transparency of LENS, LENS CAPSULE, or CORNEA; see also CATARACT.

OPHTHALMIA: SEVERE INFLAMMATION OF THE CONJUNCTIVA or eyeball.

OPHTHALMOLOGIST: A medical doctor trained in the structure, functions, and diseases of the eye; compare with OPTICIAN and OPTOMETRIST.

OPHTHALMOSCOPE: "An instrument for viewing the interior of the eye. When the OPTIC NERVE is observed with the ophthalmoscope, movements can be noted that are not apparent when only the exterior of the eye is regarded"; it is "valuable in diagnosing CATARACT, OPACITIES of the CORNEA and diseases of the interior of the eyeball" (Bates).

OPPOSITIONAL MOVEMENT: The essential illusion that stationary objects naturally appear to move in the opposite direction of the movement of the eyes and head; usually occurs subconsciously and automatically while a person is moving; often noticed consciously when improving eyesight; a "visual massage" all day long; the opposite of the type of STARING in which one tries to make stationary objects appear fixed or locked.

OPTIC ATROPHY: See ATROPHY OF THE OPTIC NERVE.

OPTIC DISC: The area where the OPTIC NERVE connects to the back of the eyeball; an area of the retina where there are no CONES or RODS; creates a small "blind spot," approximately 15° toward the temple side, when only one eye is used.

OPTIC NERVE: A large nerve that connects the eye to the brain.

OPTIC NEURITIS: Inflammation and possibly degeneration of the OPTIC NERVE.

OPTICAL SWING: "When a person of normal sight regards one letter of the SNELLEN TEST CARD with NORMAL VISION, the letter appears to move about a quarter of an inch or less from side to side, continuously and slowly, a little more rapidly than a movement each second" (Bates); prevents STARING.

OPTICIAN: A person who prepares and dispenses corrective lenses; compare with OPTOMETRIST and OPHTHALMOLOGIST.

OPTIMUM SWING: "The swing which gives the best results under different conditions" (Bates).

OPTIMUMS: Any object, memory, thought, or action that creates better vision habits and, therefore, better sight.

OPTOMETRIST: A specialist trained in examining and measuring the eyes, especially for the purpose of prescribing and dispensing corrective lenses; often examines the eye for disease; compare with OPTICIAN and OPHTHALMOLOGIST.

OSTEOPATHY: A medical system that (classically) emphasizes physical manipulation of the musculo-skeletal system.

PALMING: Covering the eyes with the palms with the fingers resting on the forehead and the lower part of the hand resting lightly on the cheekbones, without touching the eyes; usually the eyelids are closed while thinking or remembering pleasant images or letters perfectly; often used during FLASHING; a primary method of eye-mind relaxation.

PAPILLA: The nipple-like area of the OPTIC DISC.

PEARL TYPE: 5-point type.

PERFECT SIGHT: See NORMAL VISION.

PERFECT SWING: See NORMAL SWING.

PERIPHERAL VISION: All of the visual field except the central, MACULA/FOVEA area; seen primarily with RODS.

PESSIMUMS: Any object, memory, thought, or action that creates worse vision habits, resulting in less clear vision.

PHOTOPHOBIA: Over-sensitivity to light; often painful; common when BLINKING is not normal; tends to increase with the use of sunglasses; many people have reported a lessening of photophobia after taking the Chinese herb Ming Mu Ti Huang Wan (also called Ming Mu Di Huang Wan).

PILOCARPINE: An alkaloid drug used to contract the PUPIL.

PINK EYE: See CONJUNCTIVITIS.

POLYURIA: Excessive urination, often with diseases.

POTHOOK CARD: "Test card which has a letter 'E' printed with the opening pointing up or down, in or out. The test letter is made of different sizes similar to other SNELLEN TEST CARDS. It is usually employed to test the vision of children or adults who do not know the alphabet. The smallest 'E' which the patient recognizes 'pointing' in the true direction measures the amount of sight" (Lierman). See also Appendix F, "Snellen Eyechart and Test Cards," and Index.

PRESBYOPIA: "Old-age sight" (orthodox); imperfect near vision; distant vision may or may not be clear; due to hardening of the LENS preventing ACCOMMODATION (orthodox); since Dr. Bates believed the lens does not accommodate, he believed "presbyopia" was HYPERMETROPIA occurring in middle age; Dr. Bates and many Bates Method students have eliminated their need for presbyopic reading glasses by relearning correct vision habits; many elderly people do not become presbyopic.

PRISM LENSES: Lenses that change light rays in a parallel direction (rather than bringing them to a focal point, like a convex lense; used to correct for SQUINT (STRABISMUS).

PROGRESSIVE LENSES: See BIFOCALS.

PTOSIS: A drooping of the eyelid.

PUPIL: The opening in the center of the IRIS that allows light rays to enter the eye and reach the RETINA.

PURKINJE IMAGES: Reflection of images from the CORNEA and front and back sides of the RETINA; used in experiments to observe possible changes in the curvature in the LENS during ACCOMMODATION.

RECTI MUSCLES: Four (of six) external eye muscles: top (superior), bottom (inferior), outer (lateral), and inner (medial); contract to turn the eyes in various directions; contract abnormally tight and shorten the eyeball in

HYPERMETROPIA and in various types of ASTIGMATISM (Bates).

RED REFLEX: The reflection of red light from the blood-rich CHOROID; absent or partially absent in some diseases of the eye, e.g. CATARACT and corneal OPACITIES.

REFRACTION: The bending of light rays through a lense; see also ERROR OF REFRACTION.

RETINA: A paper-thin, semi-transparent membrane containing CONES and RODS with their supporting structures; the third, inner coat of the eye.

RETINITIS: Inflammation of the RETINA.

RETINITIS PIGMENTOSA: "A disease of the interior of the eye, in which small areas of the RETINA and other parts of the eye are destroyed. They are replaced by small black pigment patches" (Bates).

RETINOSCOPE: An "exceedingly useful instrument" that can measure the REFRACTION of the eye, including MYOPIA, HYPERMETROPIA, and ASTIGMATISM; can be used to study sight in many "real life" situations; not typically used by the orthodox; a key to Dr. Bates' research proving that strain can cause ERRORS OF REFRACTION and that relaxation is the foundation for NORMAL VISION; see also "Simultaneous Retinoscopy" in the October 1919 issue.

REVERSAL PROCESS: The brief return of similar, if not identical, symptoms that occurred when a disease or injury was suppressed in the past; an indication of true healing.

RODS: The light receptors in the peripheral parts of the RETINA; designed for movements, gray and black and white contrasts, and the ability to pick up very low levels of light; acuity is very low—20/400; the harmful attempt to see the PERIPHERAL VISION clearly, or equal to or better than the central vision, is called ECCENTRIC FIXATION; contrast with CONES.

SACCADIC VIBRATIONS: Normal, small vibrations of the eye; approximately seventy vibrations per second; usually not noticeable; compare with NYSTAGMUS.

SCATOMA: Also called scotoma (modern); dark area or gap in the VISUAL FIELD, often due to disease of or injury to the RETINA or CHOROID.

SCLERA: The outer, protective layer of the eye; "the white of the eyes."

SCLEROTOMY: Surgical incision into the SCLERA.

SCOTOMA: See SCATOMA.

SHIFTING: Also SKETCHING; moving the sight constantly from one point of an object to another; avoids the harmful STARING habit; "both the eyes and head are moving all day long" and "the point regarded changes rapidly and continuously" (Bates).

SHORT SWING: To imagine things are moving in the opposite direction a quarter of an inch or less; eyelids can be open or closed; essentially the same as the SWAY; prevents STARING.

SHORTSIGHTEDNESS: See MYOPIA.

SIMULTANEOUS RETINOSCOPY: SEE "SIMULTANEOUS RETINOSCOPY" IN THE OCTOBER 1919 ISSUE AND RETINOSCOPE.

SKETCHING: A modern way of teaching SHIFTING, using a pretend nose-pencil, as described in *Relearning to See*.

SNELLEN EYECHART: "The Snellen test card is a chart showing letters of graduated sizes, with numbers indicating the distance in feet at which each line should be read by the normal eye. Originally designed by Snellen for the purpose of testing the eye, it is admirably adapted for use in eye education. The numerator of the fraction indicates the distance of the test card from the pupil; the denominator denotes the line read as designated by the figures printed above the middle of each line of the Snellen test card" (Bates). "The Snellen test card has letters or other objects printed in varying sizes. The smallest letter or picture seen clearly on the card is a measure of the vision" (Lierman). Examples: 200-line read at 20 feet = 20/200, or 1/10th normal sight; 200-line read at 5 feet = 5/200 or 1/40th normal sight; 50-line read at 10 feet = 10/50, or 1/5th normal sight; 10-line read at 20 feet = 20/10, or twice normal sight. 20/20 vision can read a 3/8" letter at 20 feet; in the beginning, the large Snellen test card can be placed closer than 20 feet, moving it out farther as vision improves for myopes; the human eye is capable of much better than 20/20; many Bates students have achieved better than 20/20 vision. It is helpful to consider the ratio: if less than "1," the sight is below normal; if "1," the sight is normal at the distance tested; if greater than "1," the sight is better than normal; near vision is measured at 14 inches; 3-point type size is "14/14," "20/20," or normal near vision; see also Chapter 3, "Understanding Lenses and Prescriptions," and Chapter 22, "Reading—For All Ages," in *Relearning to See*.

SQUARE SWING: Shifting from one corner of a square to another corner, to prevent STARING. [The INFINITY SWING is better.—TRQ]

SQUINT (STRABISMUS): Squint is an earlier term; strabismus is used to avoid confusion with "SQUINTING," which usually refers to a narrowing of the eyelids; "a condition of the eyes in which both eyes do not regard one point at the same time" (Bates); caused by abnormal contraction of external eye muscles, especially one or more RECTI MUSCLES; PRISM LENSES used to correct; many different types: CROSSED EYE/esophoria/esotropia (eye turns inward), WALL EYE/exophoria/exotropia (turns outward), upward vertical/hyperphoria/hypertropia (turns upward), downward vertical/hypophoria/hypotropia (turns downward); squint can alternate between the two eyes or occur simultaneously; squint often causes AMBLYOPIA; see the dramatic sequence of pictures of a squint case in *Relearning to See* or *Perfect Sight Without Glasses;* surgery often unsuccessful, and often only cosmetic if squinting eye remains straight; a strabismic eye can have 20/20 sight; most people with strabismus need specific directions from a Bates teacher.

SQUINTING: An abnormal tightening and partial narrowing of the eyelids, usually to see artificially more clearly by creating a pinhole effect; a harmful vision habit; straining to see; also a common habit in PHOTOPHOBIA.

ST. VITUS' DANCE: A nervous system disorder involving involuntary muscular contractions causing jerky, irregular movements.

STAPHYLOMA: Bulging, as in CONICAL CORNEA.

STARING: When a person is not moving both the head and the eyes and is not centralizing; the worst type of staring is the "spaced out" type in which the eyelids are open but the person is mostly unaware of the surrounding objects; locking fixedly on a stationary object; movement without CENTRAL FIXATION; central fixation without head and eye movement; not BLINKING normally; straining to see; SQUINTING; often occurs while worrying, fatigued, bored, or during an illness or injury; all types are harmful. "Staring is a strain and always lowers vision" (Bates).

STEREOSCOPIC VISION: NORMAL VISION with both eyes used together with NORMAL CONVERGENCE, aiding in depth perception.

STIES: Small, inflamed swelling of glands in the eyelids.

STRABISMUS: Same as SQUINT.

SUN GLASS: Magnifying lense used in SUN TREATMENT.

SUN TREATMENT: Also called Light Treatment. 1. Sunning: the eyelids are closed while moving the head across the sun (preferred) or other bright light; begin with low levels of light if necessary; 2. using a sun glass (a high-power magnifying lense) to focus light rays onto the SCLERA while using rapid movements; both types of sun treatment were used by Dr. Bates with many, if not most, patients; *never* look directly into the sun with open eyelids.

SUNNING: A type of SUN TREATMENT.

SWAY: See SHORT SWING.

SWINGS: Movement of the body, including the eyes and the head, in a particular way to encourage natural SHIFTING and OPPOSITIONAL MOVEMENT and especially to prevent STARING; the various swings can be done with either open or closed eyelids; see specific type: LONG, SHORT, OPTICAL, BODY, CIRCULAR, ELLIPTICAL, OBLIQUE, VERTICAL, DRIFTING, INFINITY, etc.

SYMPATHETIC OPHTHALMIA: A normal eye acquiring vision problems, even blindness, "sympathetically" due to an injury or disease of the other eye; can occur long after the original injury or disease.

TEAR GLANDS: See LACHRIMAL GLANDS.

TEST CARD: See SNELLEN EYECHART.

THIN WHITE LINE: The result of the combination of the HALOS appearing around the individual letters along the baseline of a sentence.

TIC DOULOUREUX: Same as trigeminal, facial, or trifacial neuralgia; periodic, intensely painful contraction of the facial muscles.

TRIFOCAL LENSES: See BIFOCALS.

TRIGEMINAL NEURALGIA: See TIC DOULOUREUX.

TROPOMETER: "An instrument invented by Dr. George T. Stevens of New York to measure the strength of the muscles of the outside of the eyeball" (Bates).

UNIVERSAL SWING: Noticing that *all* stationary objects appear to move in the opposite direction of the head and eye movements.

VARIABLE SWING: Noticing while SWINGING that a near object, e.g. a finger held still six inches in front of and six inches to the side of the head, seems to have a longer OPPOSITIONAL MOVEMENT than an object farther away.

VERTICAL SWING: Swinging the head and eyes up and down while observing the illusion of stationary objects moving down and up, respectively.

VERTIGO: Dizziness with a sense of objects whirling around.

VICTROLA: A phonograph or record player.

VISUAL FIELD: See FIELD, VISUAL.

VISUAL PURPLE: A chemical change in the RETINA that allows the RODS the ability to pick up very low levels of light.

VITREOUS HUMOR: A clear, jelly-like fluid filling the majority of the volume of the eye (the vitreous chamber) between the LENS/IRIS and RETINA.

WALL EYE: Also called exophoria and exotropia; a type of SQUINT (STRABISMUS) in which usually one eye turns abnormally outward toward the temple while the other eye remains normal (straight); caused by an abnormal tension of the lateral muscle.

APPENDIX A: BIBLIOGRAPHY

Vision

Agarwal, J. *Yoga of Perfect Sight*. Pondicherry, India: Sri Aurobindo Ashram Press, 1979.

Agarwal, J., and Mrs. T. *Care of the Eyes*. Madras, India: Gnanodaya Press, 1978.

Agarwal, R. S. *Mind and Vision*. Pondicherry, India: Sri Aurobindo Ashram Press, 1935. Based on Bates' 1920 book *Perfect Sight Without Glasses*. An ophthalmologist teaching the Bates Method.

American Optical. *The Human Eye*. Southbridge, Massachusetts: American Optical Corporation, 1972.

Banker, Deborah E. *Self-Help Vision Care*. Malibu, California: World Care, 1994. A holistic approach to improving vision naturally.

Bates, William H. *Perfect Sight Without Glasses*. New York: Central Fixation Publishing Co., 1920. Ophthalmologist who created an educational program for improving eyesight naturally. Difficult to find. (See following.)

—. *Rechts Sehen Ohne Brille*. Verlag von Paul Schrecker, Grimma I. SA., 1931. German translation of *Perfect Sight Without Glasses* by Elsbeth Friedrichs.

—. *The Bates Method for Better Eyesight Without Glasses*. New York: Henry Holt & Co., 1940. Parts of Bates' 1920 *Perfect Sight Without Glasses* have been eliminated in this edition revised by Bates' wife Emily after his death.

—. *Better Eyesight*. New York: Central Fixation Co., July 1919–April 1930 (or later.) A monthly magazine "Devoted to the Prevention of Imperfect Sight Without Glasses." Edited by Bates, these magazines contain a multitude of case histories of improved vision; articles contributed by other Natural Vision teachers, including at least one other ophthalmologist and several medical doctors. Originals are difficult to find.

Benjamin, Harry. *Better Sight Without Glasses*. New York: Thorsons/HarperCollins, 1984.

Corbett, Margaret D. *Help Yourself to Better Sight*. North Hollywood, California: Wilshire Book Co., 1949. Corbett trained with Bates in 1930 to become a Natural Vision teacher. She trained many teachers on the West coast.

—. *How to Improve Your Eyes*. Los Angeles: Willing Publishing Company, 1938.

—. *How to Improve Your Sight*. New York: Bonanza Books, 1953.

David, Thomas H. *Improve Your Vision with Television!* Los Angeles, California: DeVorss & Co., 1951. This chiropractor studied with Bates in 1925, and then added vision improvement education to his chiropractic work. The booklet is brief, and is very difficult to find.

Downer, John. *Supersense: Perception in the Animal World*. New York: Henry Holt and Company, 1988.

Dudderidge, Mary. "New Light Upon Our Eyes: An Investigation Which May Result in Normal Vision for All, Without Glasses," in *Scientific American*. January 12, 1918.

Forrest, Elliot B. *Stress and Vision*. Santa Ana, California: Optometric Extension Program Foundation, 1988.

Frisby, John P. *Seeing: Illusion, Brain and Mind*. Oxford: Oxford University Press, 1979.

Gesell, Arnold, Francis L. Ilg, and Glenna E. Bullis. *Vision: Its Development in Infant and Child*. New York: Paul B. Hoeber, Inc., 1949. A classic.

Goodrich, Janet. *Natural Vision Improvement*. Berkeley, California: Celestial Arts, 1985. Book contains proof of natural vision improvement, verified by an optometrist, an ophthalmologist and a researcher. A modern Bates book with lots of good information.

Gottlieb, Raymond L. "Neuropsychology of Myopia," in *Journal of Optometric Vision Development*. Vol. 13, No. 1, March 1982, pp. 3–27. An optometrist who teaches natural vision improvement.

Gregg, James R., and Gordon G. Heath. *The Eye and Sight*. Boston: D. C. Heath and Company, 1964.

Gregory, R. L. *Eye and Brain: The Psychology of Seeing*. New York: McGraw-Hill Co., 1966.

—. *The Intelligent Eye*. New York: McGraw-Hill Co., 1970.

Grossinger, Richard. "Bates Method" in *Planet Medicine: Modalities*. Berkeley, California: North Atlantic Books, 1995. Natural vision student and publisher of North Atlantic Books.

Grow, Gerald. "Improving Eyesight: The Bates Method," in *The Holistic Health Handbook*. Edward Bauman, Armand Brint, Lorin Piper, and Pamela Amelia Wright, eds. Berkeley, California: And/Or Press, 1978.

Gruman, Harris. *New Ways to Better Sight*. New York: Hermitage House, 1950.

Hackett, Clara A., and Lawrence Galton. *Relax and See*. London: Faber and Faber, Limited, 1957. Difficult to find.

Hahn, Joan Elma. *Eyes and Seeing*. New York: Atheneum, 1981.

Hughes, Barbara. *Twelve Weeks To Better Vision*. New York: Pinnacle Books, Inc., 1981.

Huxley, Aldous. *The Art of Seeing*. New York: Harper & Brothers Publishers, 1942; republished by Berkeley, California: Creative Arts Book Co, 1982. Widely available and highly recommended. Huxley, author of *Brave New World,* published this book after taking lessons from Margaret Corbett and improving his vision. Huxley attempts to "correlate the methods of visual education with the findings of modern psychology and critical philosophy."

Kahn, Fritz. "The Eye," in *Man in Structure and Function, Vol. II.* New York: Alfred A. Knopf, 1943. Exceptional description of the eye and vision for the lay person.

Kavner, Richard S. *Your Child's Vision: A Parent's Guide to Seeing, Growing, and Developing.* New York: Fireside/Simon & Schuster, 1985.

—, and Dusky, Lorraine. *Total Vision.* New York: A & W Publishers, Inc., 1978.

Kelley, Charles R. "Psychological Factors In Myopia" in *Journal of American Optometric Association,* 33(6): 833–837, 1967.

Kennebeck, Joseph J. *Why Eyeglasses are Harmful for Children and Young People.* New York: Vantage Press, 1969. An optometrist. Difficult to find.

Kessel, Richard G., and Randy H. Kardon. *Tissues and Organs: a text-atlas of scanning electron microscopy.* New York: W. H. Freeman and Company, 1979. Contains excellent high-magnification images of the eye.

Leviton, Richard. *Seven Steps to Better Vision: Easy, Practical and Natural Techniques That Will Improve Your Eyesight.* Brookline, Massachusetts: EastWest/Natural Health Books, 1992.

Liberman, Jacob. *Take Off Your Glasses and See.* New York: Crown Publishers, Inc., 1995. An optometrist who improved his eyesight naturally and eliminated his need for compensating lenses.

Lierman, Emily C. *Stories from the Clinic.* New York: Central Fixation Publishing Co., 1926. Later her name changed to Emily A. Bates. Essentially, all of the stories in *Stories from the Clinic* are contained in the *Better Eyesight* magazines. See Appendix B: Excerpts from *Stories from the Clinic* for more information.

Life, The Editors of, and text by Richard Carington. *The Mammals.* New York: Time Incorporated, 1963.

MacCracken, W. B. *Normal Sight Without Glasses.* Berkeley, California: Published by the author, 1945. Difficult to find.

—. *Use Your Own Eyes.* Berkeley, California: Published by the author, 1937. A medical doctor who trained with Bates, and taught natural vision improvement in Berkeley. Excellent, but difficult to find.

MacFadyen, Ralph J. *See Without Glasses: The Correction of Eye Strain and the Science of Sight.* New York: Grosset & Dunlap Publishers, 1948. Difficult to find.

Markert, Christopher. *Seeing Well Again Without Your Glasses.* C. W. Daniel Co., 1981.

Mueller, Conrad G., and Mae Rudolph and the Editors of Time-Life Books. *Light and Vision.* New York: Time-Life Books, 1966. Excellent.

Murphy, Pat, ed. *The Eye.* San Francisco: The Exploratorium, 1985.

—. "In the Darkness," in *Exploring.* San Francisco: The Exploratorium, 1993.

Murphy, Wendy, and the Editors of Time-Life Books. *Touch, Taste, Smell, Sight and Hearing.* Alexandria, Virginia: Time-Life Books, Inc., 1982.

Peppard, Harold M. *Sight Without Glasses.* Garden City, New York: Garden City Books, 1940.

Peterson, Roger Tory, and the Editors of Life. *The Birds.* New York: Time, Inc., 1963.

Price, C. S. *The Improvement of Sight by Natural Methods.* London: Chapman & Hall Limited, 1934.

Quackenbush, Thomas R. *Relearning to See: Improve Your Eyesight—Naturally!* Berkeley, California: North Atlantic Books, 1997, 1999. The second edition is in paperback. The title of the first, hardbound edition was *Relearning to See.* A 521-page, fully illustrated textbook on the Bates Method and Natural Eyesight Improvement by a professional Bates Method teacher for over seventeen years.

Rahn, Joan E. *Eyes and Seeing.* New York: R. R. Donnelley & Sons, Inc., 1981.

Raskin, Edith L. *Watchers, Pursuers and Masqueraders: Animals and Their Vision.* New York: McGraw-Hill Book Company, 1964.

Raskin, Ellen. *Nothing Ever Happens on My Block.* New York: Macmillan Publishing Co., 1966. For children.

Rodale, J. I. *The Natural Way to Better Eyesight.* New York: Pyramid Books, 1968.

Rosanes-Berrett, Marilyn B. *Do You Really Need Glasses?* Barrytown, New York: Pulse/Station Hill Press, 1990.

Rotte, Joanna, and Koji Yamamoto. *A Holistic Guide to Healing the Eyesight.* Japan Publications, 1986.

Samuels, Mike, and Samuels, Nancy. *Seeing With the Mind's Eye.* New York: Random House, 1975.

Schlossberg, Leon, and George D. Zuidema. *The Johns Hopkins Atlas of Human Functional Anatomy.* Baltimore: The Johns Hopkins University Press, 1972.

Scholl, Lisette. *Visionetics: The Holistic Way to Better Eyesight.* New York: Doubleday & Company, Inc., 1978.

Seiderman, Arthur S., and Steven E. Marcus. *20/20 Is Not Enough.* New York: Alfred A. Knopf, 1989.

Sinclair, Sandra. *How Animals See.* New York: Facts on File Publications, 1985. Filled with extraordinary color pictures and excellent descriptions of many different types of eyes. Difficult to find. Currently out of print.

Sutton-Vane, S. *The Story of the Eyes*. New York: The Viking Press, Inc., 1958. Difficult to find.

Tobe, John H. *Cataract, Glaucoma and Other Eye Disorders*. St. Catharines, Ontario: published by the author(?), 1973.

Wertenbaker, Lael, and the Editors of U.S. News Books. *The Eye: Window to the World*. Washington, D. C.: U.S. News Books, 1981. Excellent.

Windolph, Michael. *Do You Really Need Eyeglasses?* New York: Cornerstone Library, 1976. Difficult to find.

Yarbus, Alfred L. *Eye Movements and Vision*. New York: Plenum Press, 1967.

Other Recommended Reading

Bauman, Edward, Armand Brint, Lorin Piper, and Pamela Amelia Wright, eds. *The Holistic Health Handbook*. Berkeley, California: And/Or Press, 1978.

—. *The Holistic Lifebook Handbook*. Berkeley, California: And/Or Press, 1981.

Becker, Robert O. *Cross Currents: The Perils of Electromagnetic Pollution, The Promise of Electromedicine*. Los Angeles: Jeremy P. Tarcher, Inc., 1990.

Bertherat, Therese, and Carol Bernstein. *The Body Has Its Reasons: Self-Awareness Through Conscious Movement*. Rochester, Vermont: Healing Arts Press, 1989.

Biermann, June, and Barbara Toohey. *The Woman's Holistic Headache Relief Book*. Los Angeles: J. P. Tarcher, Inc., 1979.

Bricklin, Mark. *The Practical Encyclopedia of Natural Healing*. Emmaus, Pennsylvania: Rodale Press, 1976.

Brecher, Edward M., and Editors of Consumer Reports. *Licit and Illicit Drugs*. Boston: Little, Brown and Company, 1972.

Carter-Scott, Chérie. *Negaholics: How to Overcome Negativity and Turn Your Life Around*, New York: Ballantine Books, 1989. Excellent.

—. *The New Species*. New York: Coleman Graphics, Inc., 1980.

Chopra, Deepak. *Quantum Healing*. New York: Bantam, 1989.

Coulter, Harris L. *Divided Legacy, A History of the Schism in Medical Thought, Vol. I: The Patterns Emerge: Hippocrates to Paracelsus*. Washington, DC: Weehawken Book Company, 1975.

—. *Divided Legacy, Vol. II: The Origins of Modern Western Medicine: J. B. Van Helmont to Claude Bernard*. Berkeley, California: North Atlantic Books, 1977.

—. *Divided Legacy, Vol. III: The Conflict Between Homeopathy and the American Medical Association: Science and Ethics in American Medicine 1800–1914*. Berkeley, California: North Atlantic Books, 1982.

—. *Divided Legacy, Vol. IV: Twentieth Century Medicine, The Bacteriological Era*. Berkeley, California: North Atlantic Books, 1994.

—. *Homeopathic Science and Modern Medicine: The Physics of Healing with Microdoses*. Berkeley, California: North Atlantic Books, 1981.

Crouch, Tammy, and Michael Madden. *Carpal Tunnel Syndrome and Overuse Injuries*. Berkeley, California: North Atlantic Books, 1992.

Dennison, Paul E. *Switching-On*. Ventura, California: Edu-Kinesthetics, Inc., 1981. Excellent.

—, and Gail E. Dennison. *Brain Gym*. Ventura, California: Edu-Kinesthetics, Inc., 1986. Many practical activities.

—, and Gail E. Hargrove. *Personalized Whole Brain Integration*. Ventura, California: Edu-Kinesthetics, Inc., 1985. Excellent.

—, and Gail Hargrove. *E-K for Kids*. Ventura, California: Edu-Kinesthetics, Inc., 1985. Many practical activities for children.

Diamond, John. *Your Body Doesn't Lie*. New York: Warner Books, 1979.

Dufty, William. *Sugar Blues*. New York: Warner Books, 1975. You may give up white sugar after reading this book.

Edwards, Betty. *Drawing on the Right Side of the Brain*. Los Angeles: Tarcher, Inc., 1979.

Elben. *Vaccination Condemned*. Los Angeles: Better Life Research, 1981.

Ferguson, Marilyn, ed. *Brain/Mind Bulletin*. Los Angeles: Interface Press. Periodical.

Gelb, Harold, and Paula M. Siegel. *Killing Pain Without Prescription*. New York: Harper & Row, 1980.

Glendinning, Chellis. *My Name is Chellis, & I'm in Recovery from Western Civilization*. Boston: Shambhala Publications, 1994.

Grossinger, Richard. *Planet Medicine: Modalities*. Berkeley, California: North Atlantic Books, 1995.

—. *Planet Medicine: Origins*. Berkeley, California: North Atlantic Books, 1995.

Hall, Dorothy. *Iridology. Personality and Health Analysis Through the Iris*. Melbourne, Australia: Nelson, 1980.

Harrison, John. *Love Your Disease: It's Keeping You Healthy*. Sydney: Angus & Robertson Publishers, 1984.

Hayfield, Robin. *Homeopathy for Common Ailments*. Berkeley, California: Frog, Ltd., and Homeopathic Educational Services, 1993.

Huggins, Hal A. *It's All In Your Head: The Link Between Mercury Amalgams and Illness*. Garden City Park, New York: Avery Publishing Group, Inc., 1993.

Hunter, Beatrice T. *Consumer Beware: Your Food and What's Being Done to It*. New York: Simon & Schuster, 1971.

Jensen, Bernard. *The Doctor-Patient Handbook*. Escondido, California: Bernard Jensen Enterprises, 1976. Excellent discussion about nutrition, iridology, detoxification, the healing crisis, and reversal processes.

—. *The Science and Practice of Iridology*. Escondido, California: Bernard Jensen, 1981.

—. *Tissue Cleansing through Bowel Management*. Escondido, California: Bernard Jensen, 1981.

Kime, Zane R. *Sunlight Could Save Your Life*. Penryn, California: World Health Publications, 1980.

Léboyér, Frederick. *The Art of Breathing*. Longmead, England: Element Books Ltd., 1985. Breathing for childbirth.

Liberman, Jacob. *Light: Medicine of the Future*. Santa Fe: Bear & Co., 1991. A must-read book; covers the impact of natural and artificial light on the mind, body, and emotions.

Lowen, Alexander. *Bioenergetics*. New York: Penguin Books, Inc., 1976.

Mendelsohn, Robert S. *Confessions of a Medical Heretic* (Chicago, Illinois: Contemporary Books, Inc., 1979). Uses a Church/Faith/Sacraments analogy for discussing the problems of modern medicine.

Miller, Neil. *Vaccines: Are They Really Safe and Effective?—A Parent's Guide to Childhood Shots*. Santa Fe, New Mexico: New Atlantean Press, 1993.

Morrison, Douglas. *Body Electronics Fundamentals*. Cannon Beach, Oregon: Health Hope Publishing House, 1993. Outstanding iridology, nutritional, and other advanced healing methods. This book is scheduled to be revised and reprinted with a new title by North Atlantic Books in 2000.

Ott, John N. *Health & Light*. New York: Simon & Schuster, 1973. A classic.

—. *Light, Radiation, and You: How to Stay Healthy*. New York: Simon & Schuster, 1982.

Panos, Maesimund B., and Jane Heimlich. *Homeopathic Medicine at Home*. New York: G. P. Putnam's Sons, 1980. Natural remedies for everyday ailments and minor injuries. My favorite "practical" homeopathy book.

Peck, M. Scott, *The Road Less Traveled*. New York: Simon and Schuster, 1978.

Pelletier, Kenneth R. *Holistic Medicine: From Stress to Optimum Health*. New York: Dell Publishing Co., Inc., 1979.

—. *Mind as Healer, Mind as Slayer: A Holistic Approach to Preventing Stress Disorders*. New York: Dell Publishing Co., Inc., 1977.

Pitchford, Paul. *Healing with Whole Foods*. Berkeley, California: North Atlantic Books, 1993.

Reubin, David, M.D. *Everything You Always Wanted to Know About Nutrition*. Boston: G. K. Hall & Co., 1979.

Ribot, T. *The Psychology of Attention*. Chicago: The Open Court Publishing Company, 1890. The New York: The Marcel Rodd Company, 1946 edition contains a foreword by Bates teacher Margaret D. Corbett.

Robertson, Laurel, Carol Flinders, and Bronwen Godfrey. *Laurel's Kitchen*. New York: Nilgiri Press, 1976.

Rosen, Marion, and Sue Brenner. *The Rosen Method of Movement*. Berkeley, California: North Atlantic Books, 1991.

Schmidt, Michael A., and Lendon H. Smith and Keith W. Sehnert. *Beyond Antibiotics: 50 (or so) Ways to Boost Immunity and Avoid Antibiotics*. Berkeley, California: North Atlantic Books, 1993.

Selby, Hans. *Stress Without Distress*. New York: Signet, 1975.

Smith, G. Kent. *Homeopathy: Medicine for Today's Living*. Glendale, California: (private printing?), 1978.

Turner, James S. *The Chemical Feast*. New York: The Colonial Press, 1970.

Ullman, Dana. *Homeopathy: Medicine for the 21st Century*. Berkeley, California: North Atlantic Books, 1988.

Vithoulkas, George. *A New Model for Health and Disease*. Berkeley, California: Health and Habitat and North Atlantic Books, 1991. Read this book!

—.*Homeopathy, Medicine of the New Man*. New York: Arco Publishing, Inc., 1979.

—. *The Science of Homeopathy*. New York: Grove Press, 1980. The single most important book I have read on health and healing.

Wigmore, Ann. *The Wheatgrass Book*. Wayne, New Jersey: Avery Publishing Group, Inc. 1985.

Wurtman, Richard J. "The Effects of Light on the Human Body," in *Scientific American*, July 1975, Vol. 233, No. 1, pp. 68–77. Excellent.

Zi, Nancy. *The Art of Breathing*. Berkeley, California: Frog, Ltd., 2000.

APPENDIX B: EXCERPTS FROM *STORIES FROM THE CLINIC*

Below are a few excerpts from Emily C. Lierman's (later Emily A. Bates) 1926 *Stories from the Clinic*. All of the stories from Emily's book, with minor changes, are contained in the *Better Eyesight* magazines.

STORIES FROM THE CLINIC

By Emily C. Lierman

TO THE CHILDREN OF THE CLINIC
AND TO
W. H. BATES, M.D.,
THIS BOOK IS DEDICATED

PREFACE

The articles comprising this book were first published in the monthly magazine *Better Eyesight* during a period of five years.

Various eye defects are described in simple and intelligible language, so that those who are interested may follow the practical instructions and improve their own vision, or that of others.

The stories are drawn from my clinical experience in the cure of imperfect sight by treatment without glasses. I have been Dr. Bates' assistant for eleven years, and they were years of a great education in the knowledge of the eye, in health, and in disease.

To Dr. W. H. Bates, the discoverer of the method, I am indebted for his encouragement and help.

EMILY C. LIERMAN.

INTRODUCTION

I feel honored in being asked to write an introduction to this excellent book, *Stories from the Clinic*, by Emily C. Lierman.

The stories have come directly from Ms. Lierman's experience, and consequently are of intrinsic value. The patients, their symptoms of imperfect sight, and the treatment are all described in language which is so clear that anyone can understand.

For more than nine years Ms. Lierman was my assistant in the out-patient department of the Harlem Hospital. She showed a great deal of understanding in treating the patients, adapting my method to each individual case. The cures she obtained were of the greatest value. She was particularly interested in the schoolchildren, and was so kind and patient with them that they all loved her. Her cures of imperfect sight without glasses were numerous. The way she treated the patients and the results obtained were a contribution to the practice of ophthalmology. For example, an old lady with absolute glaucoma in one eye, totally blind with no perception of light, visited the clinic to obtain relief from an agony of pain. Many doctors had previously advised the removal of one or both eyes, which has been for many years considered by regular physicians to be good practice. It has also been taught that no operation or treatment can cure the blindness resulting from absolute glaucoma. Ms. Lierman was told that it was a hopeless case, but was asked to try to relieve the pain. She immediately treated the woman, and much to my surprise not only relieved the pain, but also improved the eye until the patient became able to see at the distance, and to read fine print without glasses.

Of course, her work attracted attention and criticism. A prominent physician was sent one day to investigate. We told him the facts and a number of patients were treated for his benefit. He was very much interested in an elderly colored woman with cataract. This patient became able to read diamond type from six to fourteen inches from her eyes without glasses. The doctor, himself, was wearing glasses for distant vision and a stronger pair for reading. Ms. Lierman treated him, also, with much benefit. From his personal experience and from his observation of the treatment of the patients by Ms. Lierman, he was convinced that the method was one of great value. He had been sent to condemn, and remained to praise.

W. H. BATES, M.D.

SUN TREATMENT

Most ophthalmologists prescribe dark glasses to nearly all of their patients who suffer from the brightness of light. This practice, in my opinion, has been overdone. I remember one patient who was in the hospital for two years in a dark room, with both eyes bandaged with a dark binding day and night continuously. When she left the hospital she was in a very pitiable condition. She was practically blind in the bright sunlight. She went to a great many clinics and eye doctors and all they did for her was to give her stronger dark glasses. In time these dark glasses did not give her any relief. Instead of being helpful to her weak eyes, the glasses had the effect of making them more sensitive to the light than they had ever been before. It has been my experience that all persons who wear dark glasses sooner or later develop very serious inflammation of their eyes. The human eye needs the light in order to maintain its efficiency. The use of eye-shades and protections of all kinds from the light is very injurious to the eyes.

Sunlight is as necessary to normal eyes as is rest and relaxation. If it is possible, start the day by exposing the eyes to the sun—just a few minutes at a time will help. Get accustomed to the strong light of the sun by letting it shine on your closed eyelids.... It is good to move the head slightly from side to side while doing this, in order to prevent straining. One cannot get too much sun treatment.

APPENDIX C: BIOGRAPHICAL SKETCH OF WILLIAM H. BATES, M.D.

• 1860
Born in Newark, New Jersey, on December 23, 1860, son of Charles and Amelia Bates.

• 1881
Graduated with a B.S. in Agriculture from Cornell University.

• 1885
Graduated with his medical degree from the College of Physicians and Surgeons, Columbia University. Initially directed his attention to all organs of the head. Practiced orthodox medicine for several years in New York City.

• 1886
Operated in many hospitals; clinical assistant at Manhattan Eye and Ear Hospital; attending physician at Bellevue Hospital, Northwestern Dispensary, and Harlem Hospital.

• 1886–1896
Assistant surgeon at the New York Eye Infirmary, Northwestern Dispensary, and Harlem Hospital.

• 1886–1891
Instructor of ophthalmology at the New York Post-Graduate Medical School and Hospital. Successful and well-respected eye surgeon.
Taught medical students how to improve their nearsightedness.
Expelled from the faculty.

• 1886–1902
Research at the Pathology Laboratory of Dr. Pruden at the College of Physicians and Surgeons, Columbia University.

• May 16, 1886
Report on his discovery of the astringent and haemostatic properties of the aqueous extract of the suprarenal gland, later commercialized as adrenaline, published in the *New York Medical Journal*.

• 1896
Resigned his hospital appointments for several years of experimental work.

• 1903
Licensed to practice medicine in Grand Forks, North Dakota.

• 1910
Elected president of the Grand Forks district Medical Society.

• 1910
Returned to New York City as attending physician in Harlem Hospital.

• 1912
Research at Physiological Laboratory of the College of Physicians and Surgeons. Assisted by Emily C. Lierman (later Emily A. Bates).

• 1919–1930
Published *Better Eyesight* monthly magazine.

• 1920
Published his book *Perfect Sight Without Glasses*.

• 1928
Married Emily Ackerman Lierman, his assistant and partner in experimental research on eyesight from 1911 to 1928.

• 1931
Died at age 70 at his residence in New York City on July 10, 1931, during a black flu epidemic.

The following letter was written by Emily A. Bates "To the Editor of *The New York Times*." The article is entitled "Carrying On Dr. Bates' Work," published on July 18, 1931, p. 12:

> I wish to express my gratitude to R. R. A. for the fine tribute he paid my husband, William H. Bates, M.D., in his letter in *The New York Times* of July 16. What he said was true. I myself have had the honor and the privilege of assisting the doctor in his research work during a period of six years at the Physiological Laboratory of the College of Physicians and Surgeons in New York City, also working by his side for nine consecutive years at the clinic of the Harlem Hospital. I have also had the privilege of instructing students in his method of [reversing] imperfect sight without the use of glasses. I am now going on with the work, which he left for me to do, in an educational way. There is a Bates Academy in Johannesburg, South Africa, where students of Dr. Bates are doing his work, and we have representatives in Germany, England, and in various cities throughout the United States. Emily A. Bates. New York, July 16, 1931.

"July 16" in the first sentence is likely a typographical error because the date R. R. A.'s letter appeared in *The New York Times* was July 15.

APPENDIX D: FINDING A NATURAL EYESIGHT IMPROVEMENT TEACHER AND CONTACTING THE NATURAL VISION CENTER SF (NVCSF)

Note: The Natural Vision Center SF has recently relocated to Ashland, Oregon. Please visit our website at www.NVCSF.com for the latest information.

NVCSF now stands for Natural Vision Center for Sight Freedom.

NVCSF maintains a list of Natural Eyesight Improvement teachers from around the world. To request the name of a Natural Eyesight Improvement teacher in your area, please send a self-addressed, stamped envelope, including your name, address, and phone number, to:

NVCSF
P. O. Box 986
Ashland, OR 97520 USA

Natural Eyesight Improvement Phone Consulting is often available from Tom Quackenbush or teacher trained by NVCSF.

For more information, please contact us at the above address, or:

Office: (541) 512-2525
Fax: (541) 512-2626
E-mail: RELRN2SEE@NVCSF.com.

More information, including how to order *Relearning to See* and *Better Eyesight,* can be found on our website at www.NVCSF.com.

APPENDIX E: BECOMING A NATURAL EYESIGHT IMPROVEMENT TEACHER

Note: The Natural Vision Center SF (NVCSF) has recently relocated to Ashland, Oregon. Please visit our website at www.NVCSF.com for the latest information.

NVCSF now stands for Natural Vision Center for Sight Freedom.

NVCSF has been training Natural Eyesight Improvement Teachers for over a decade. The Teacher Trainee does not need to have clear vision to become a Natural Eyesight Improvement Teacher. If you already have clarity, you will simply be teaching others the correct vision habits you already have—and the ones your students want to relearn.

Natural Eyesight Improvement Teachers who teach children to improve their sight are especially needed.

Read feedback from NVCSF Teacher Training graduates on our website at www.NVCSF.com.

For more information regarding the NVCSF's Certified Natural Eyesight Improvement Teacher Training Program, please contact us by any of the following means:

NVCSF
P.O. Box 986
Ashland, OR 97520 USA

Office: (541) 512-2525
Fax: (541) 512-2626
E-mail: RELRN2SEE@NVCSF.com

You can find more information on our website at www.NVCSF.com.

APPENDIX F: SNELLEN EYECHART AND TEST CARDS

Instructions for using the large Distance Snellen Eyechart and the small Snellen test cards can be found in the following *Better Eyesight* magazines:

• August 1919, "How to Use the Snellen Test Card for the Prevention and Cure of Imperfect Sight in Children"
• August 1923, "The Snellen Test Card"
• April 1924, "Distance of the Snellen Test Card"
• September 1928, "Test Card Practice"
• May 1930, "Test Card Practice"

The eyechart and test cards can be mounted on cardboard.

The number above each row on the eyechart and test cards indicates the distance, in feet, at which that row can be read by the normal, 20/20, eye.

The small "C" Test Card is a reduced version of the large Distance Snellen Eyechart.

Additional information on eyecharts can be found in Chapter 3, "Understanding Lenses and Prescriptions," in *Relearning to See*.

The "Fundamentals" test card was printed on the back of the original small Snellen test cards.

DISTANCE SNELLEN EYECHART

Assemble the Distance Snellen Eyechart as indicated on the next page.

To assemble the Distance Snellen Eyechart, cut along the six dashed lines on the next three pages. Then, align the bottom edge of the first page, ab, with the top edge of the second page, a'b'. Tape them together. Similarly, align the bottom edge of the second page, cd, with the top edge of the third page, c'd'. Tape them together. The chart can then be mounted onto cardboard.

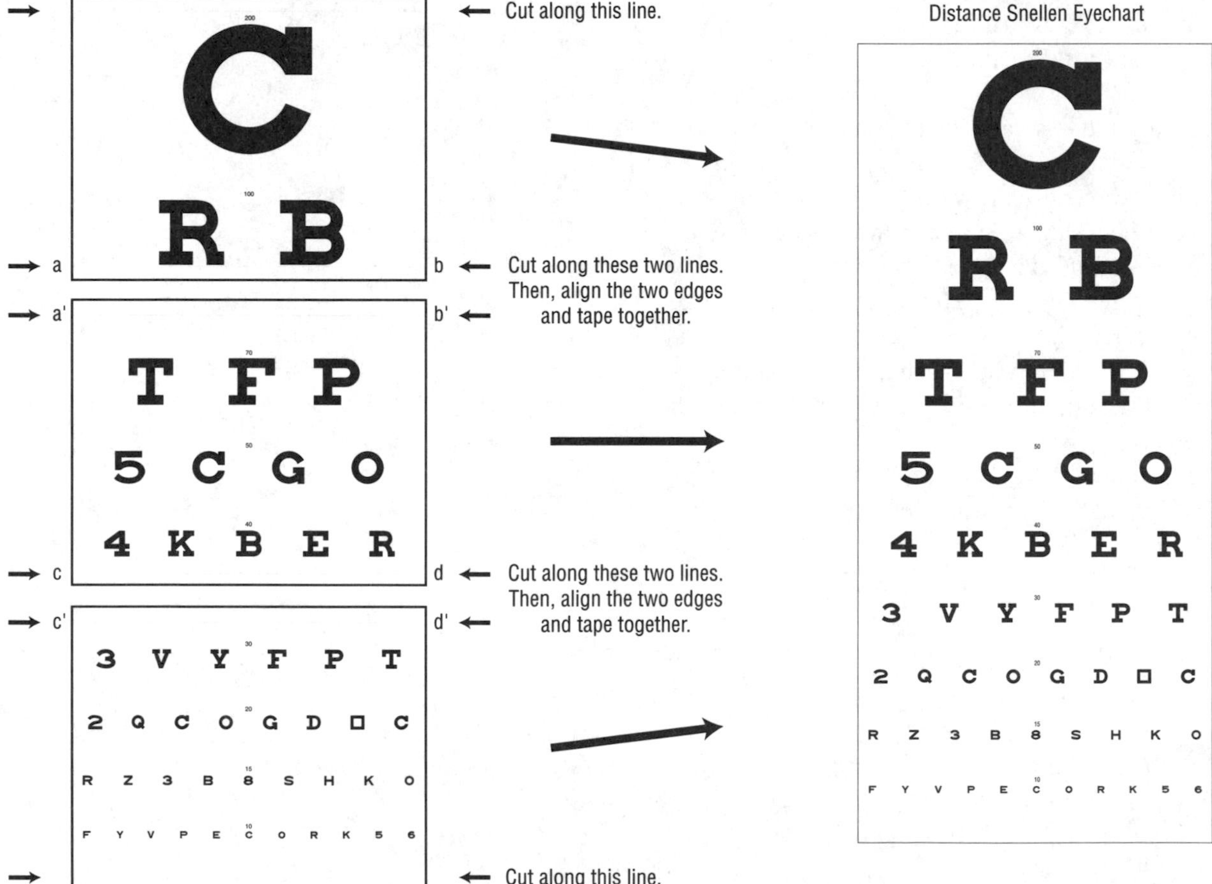

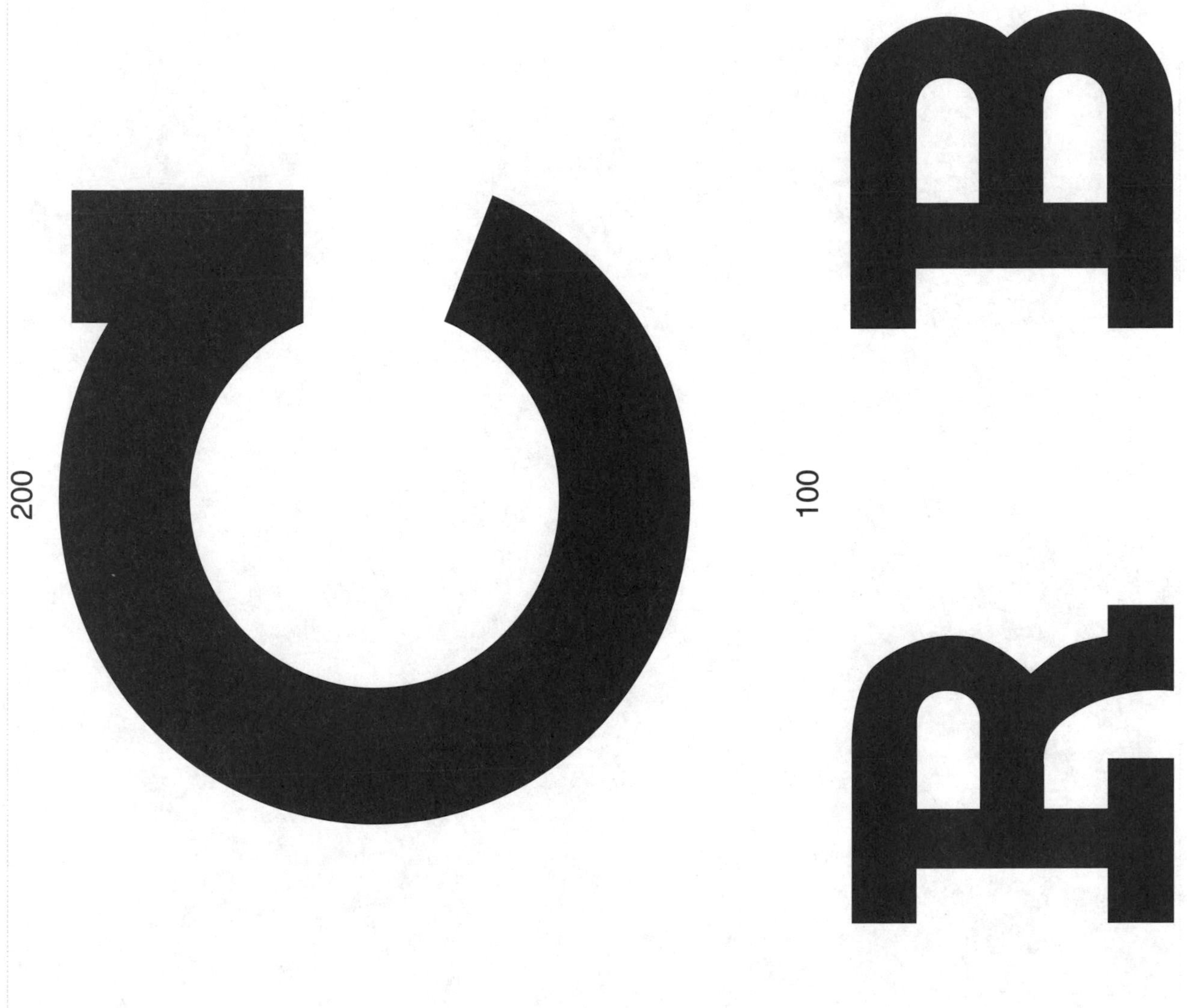
200
C
100
R B

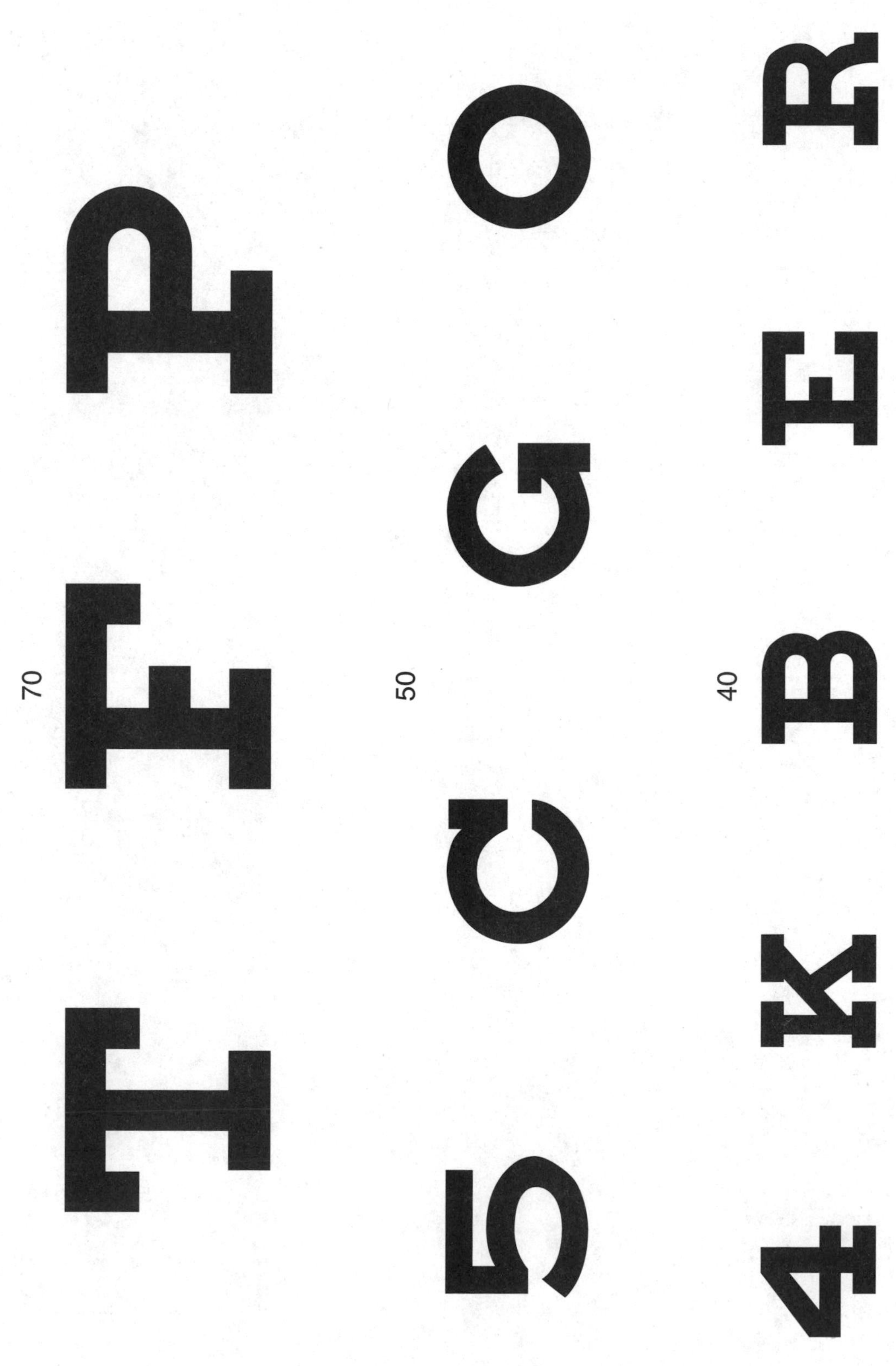
70
T F P
50
5 C G O
40
4 K B E R

c' d'

30

3 V Y F P T

20

2 Q C O G D □ C

15

R Z 3 B 8 S H K O

10

F Y V P E C O R K 5 6

"C" TEST CARDS

Shift alternately from a letter on the small "C" Test Card to the same letter on the Distance Snellen Eyechart.

The next page has reversed type cards.

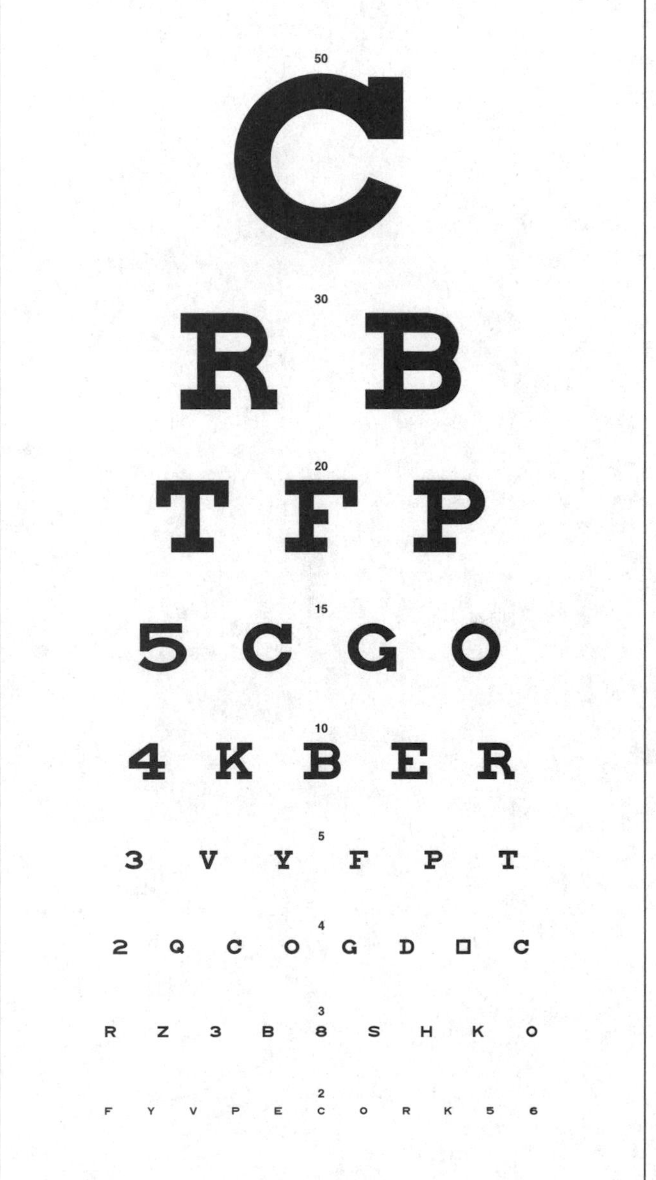

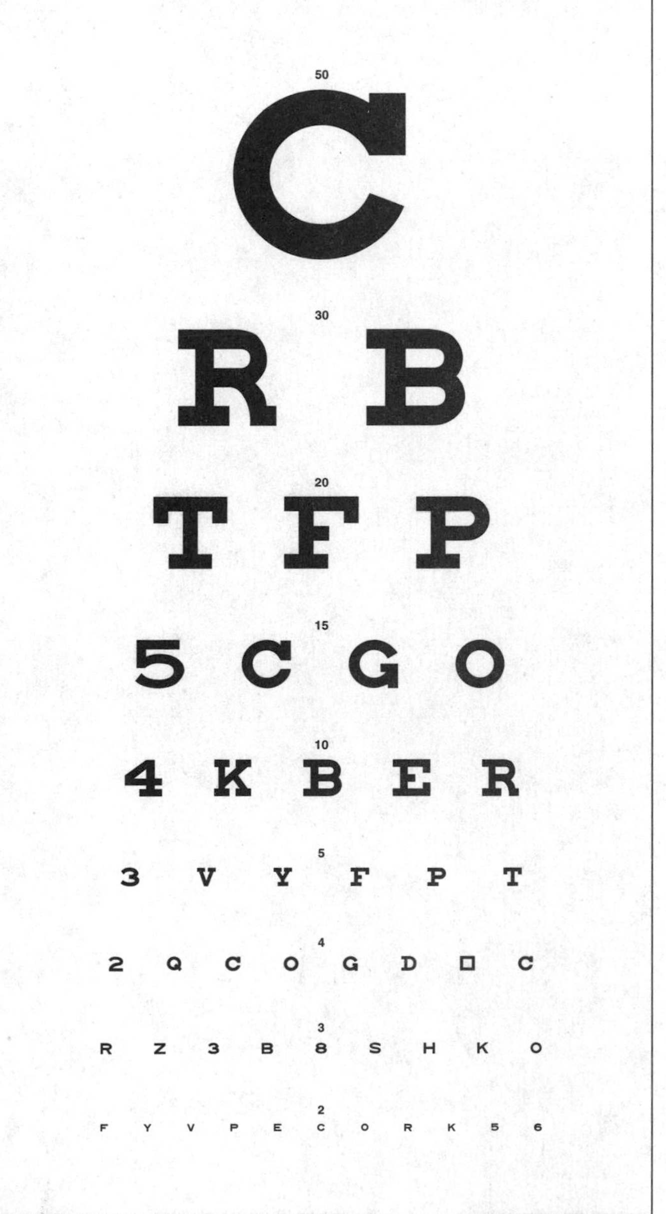

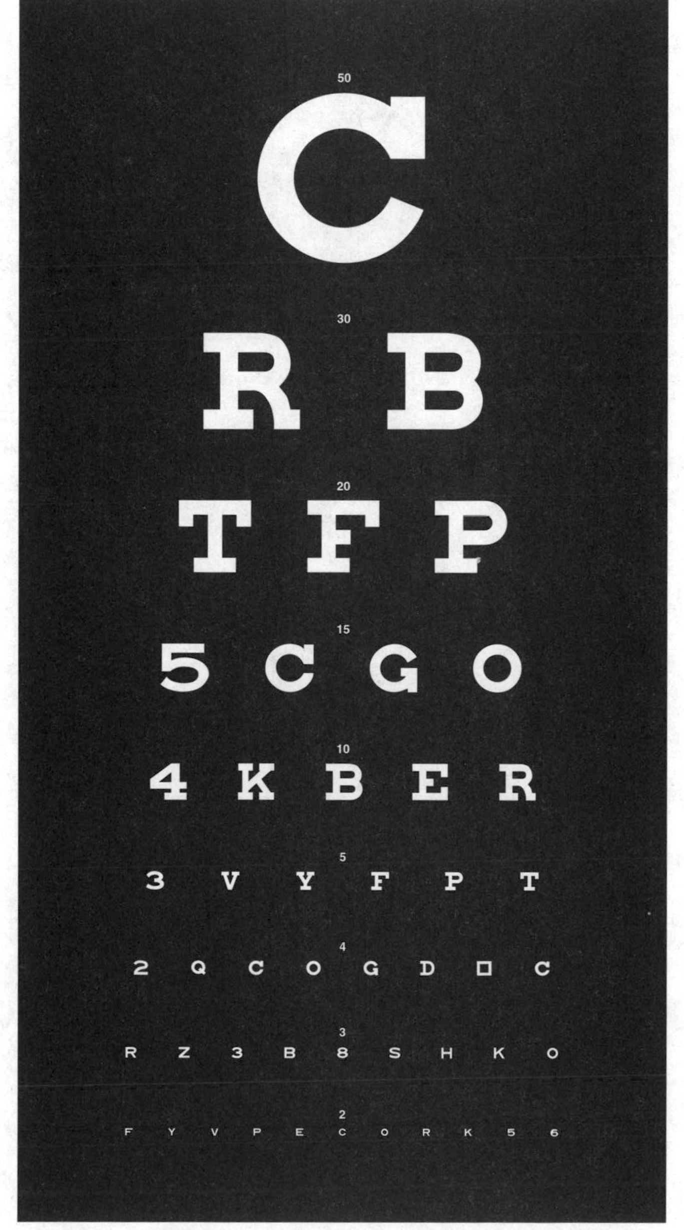
50
C
30
R B
20
T F P
15
5 C G O
10
4 K B E R
5
3 V Y F P T
4
2 Q C O G D □ C
3
R Z 3 B 8 S H K O
2
F Y V P E C O R K 5 6

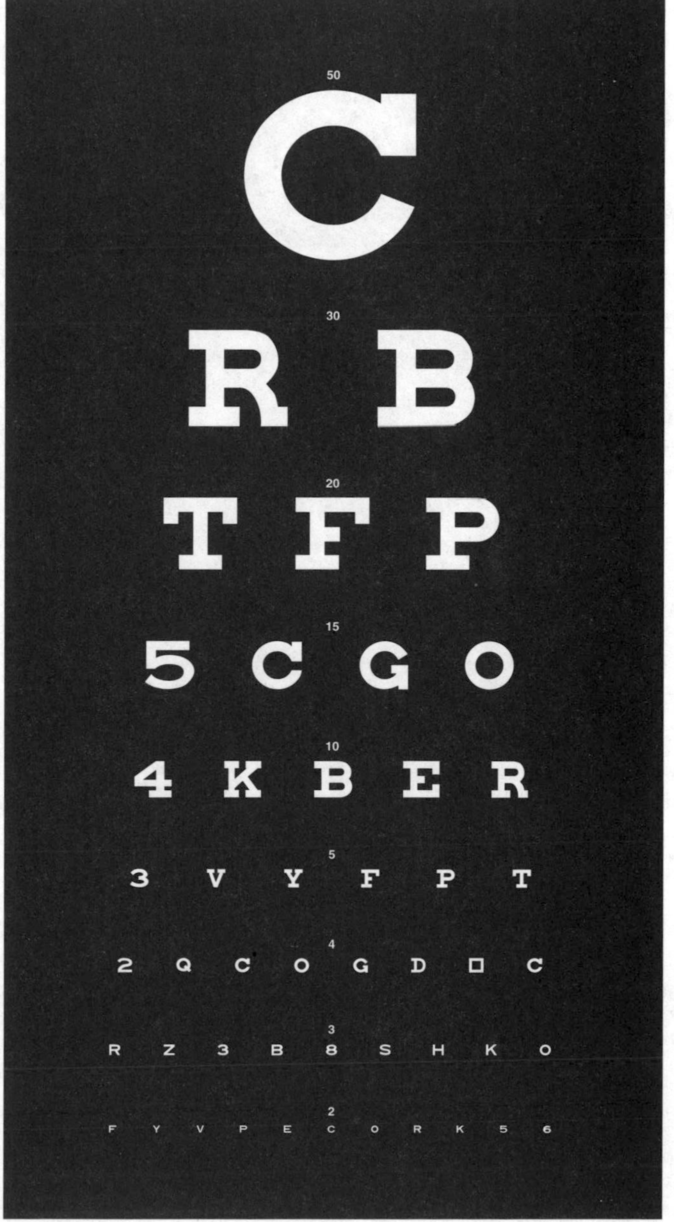
50
C
30
R B
20
T F P
15
5 C G O
10
4 K B E R
5
3 V Y F P T
4
2 Q C O G D □ C
3
R Z 3 B 8 S H K O
2
F Y V P E C O R K 5 6

"E" TEST CARDS

The next page has reversed type cards.

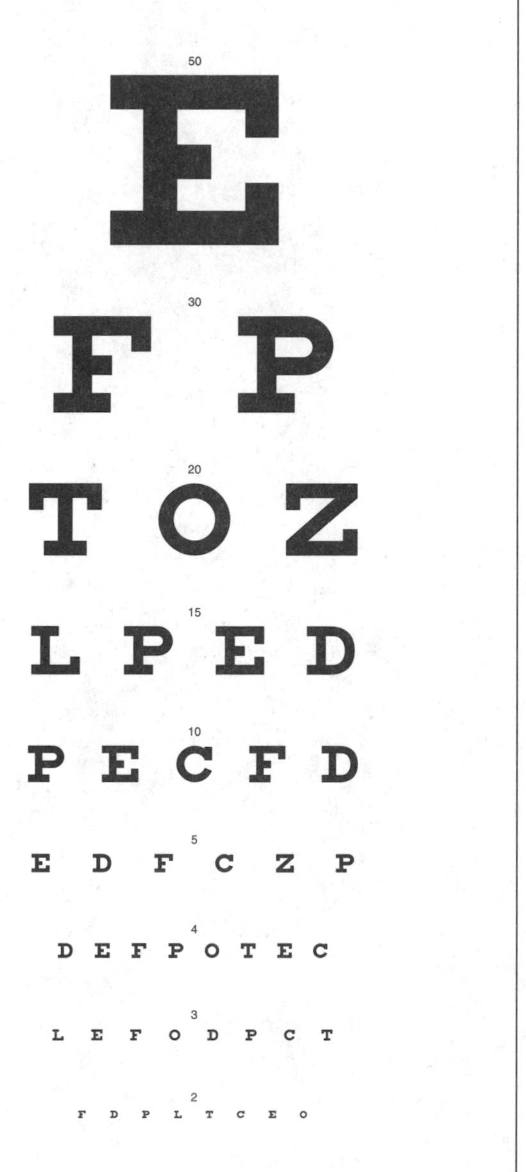

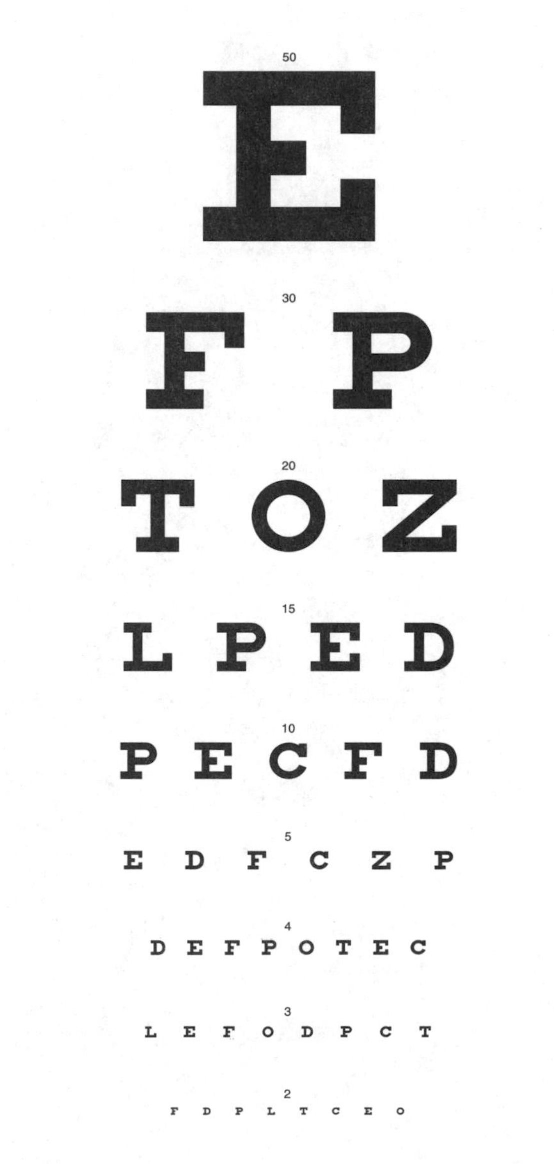

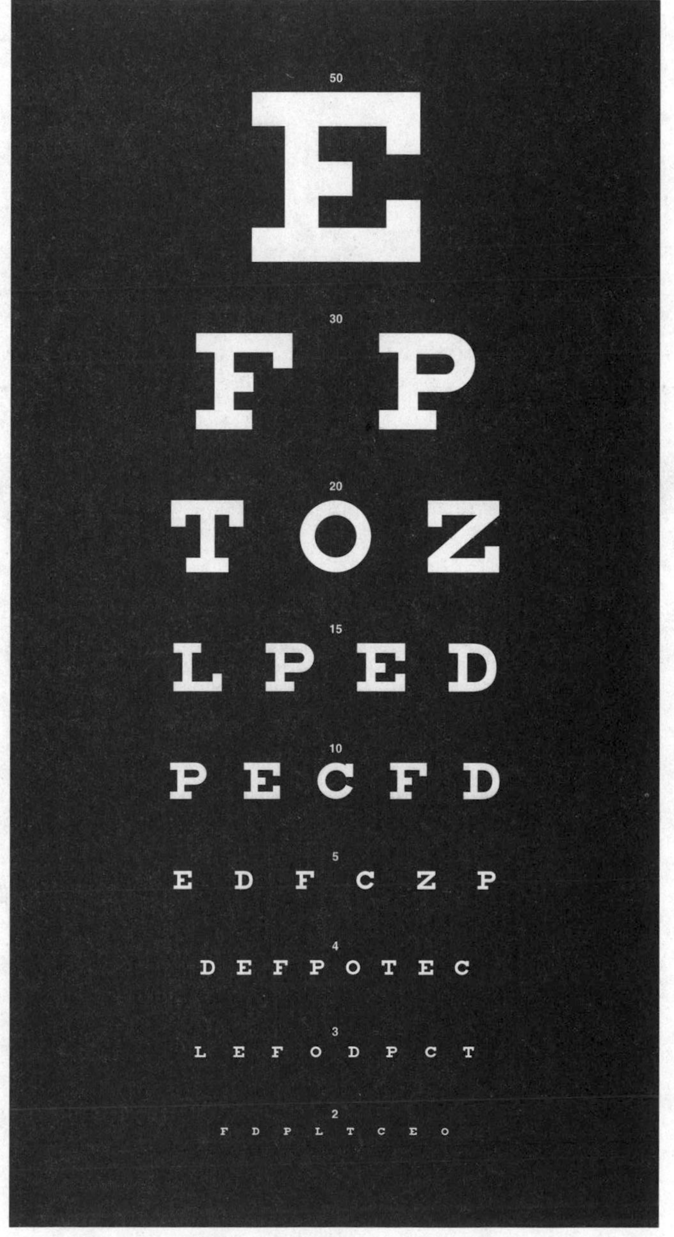
50
E
30
F P
20
T O Z
15
L P E D
10
P E C F D
5
E D F C Z P
4
D E F P O T E C
3
L E F O D P C T
2
F D P L T C E O

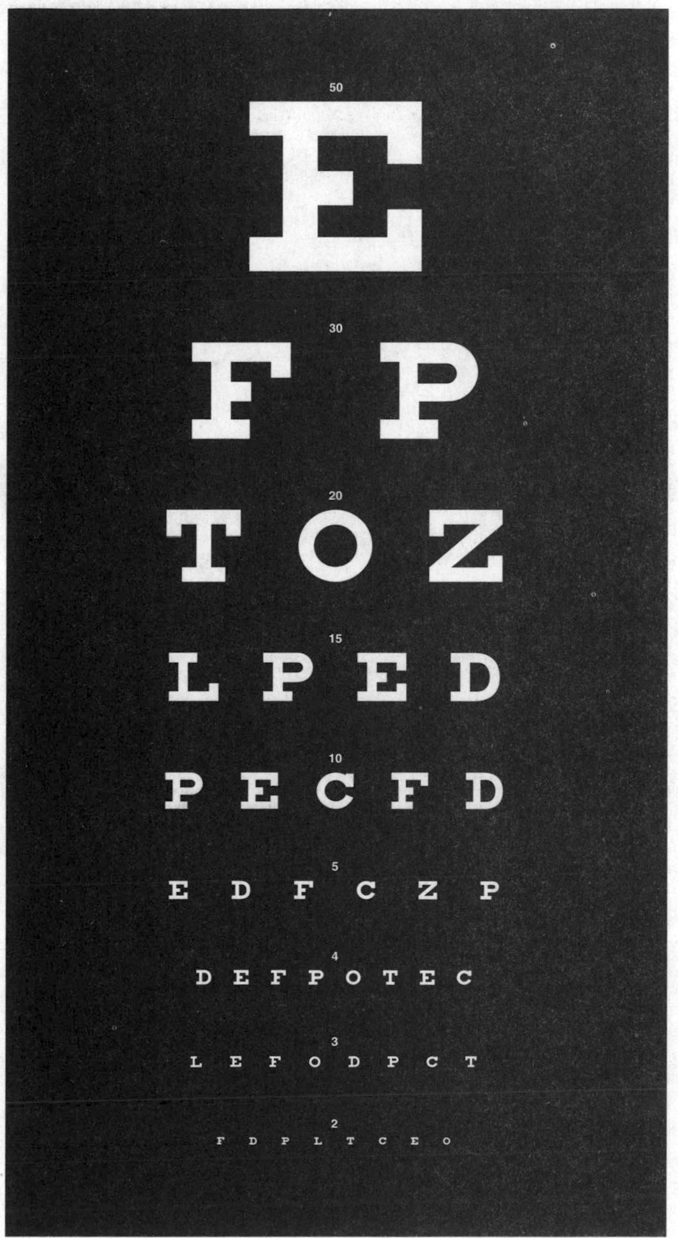
50
E
30
F P
20
T O Z
15
L P E D
10
P E C F D
5
E D F C Z P
4
D E F P O T E C
3
L E F O D P C T
2
F D P L T C E O

NUMERALS TEST CARDS

The next page has reversed type cards.

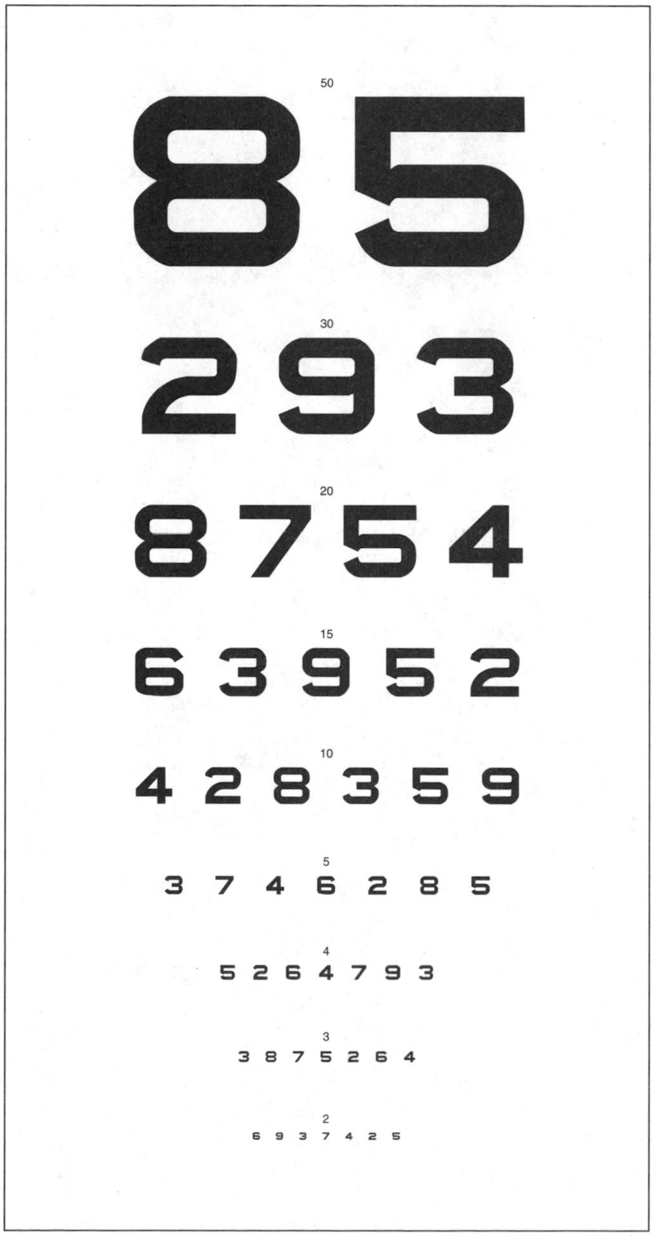

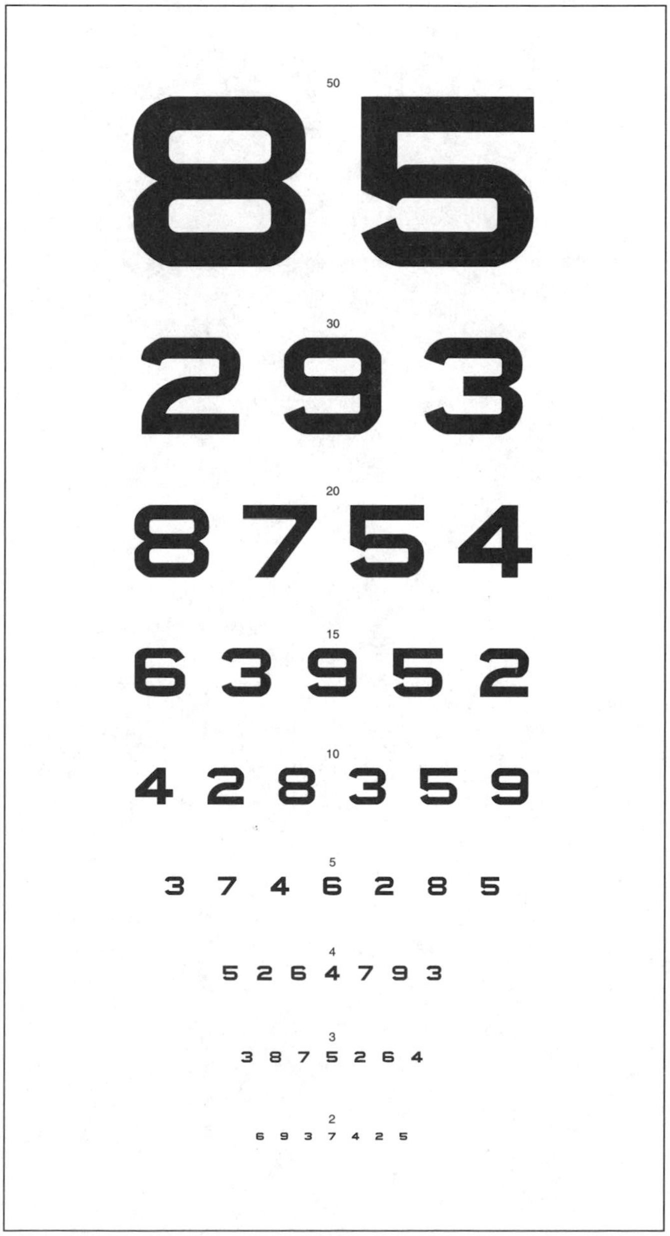

50
85
30
293
20
8754
15
63952
10
428359
5
3746285
4
5264793
3
3875264
2
6937425

50
85
30
293
20
8754
15
63952
10
428359
5
3746285
4
5264793
3
3875264
2
6937425

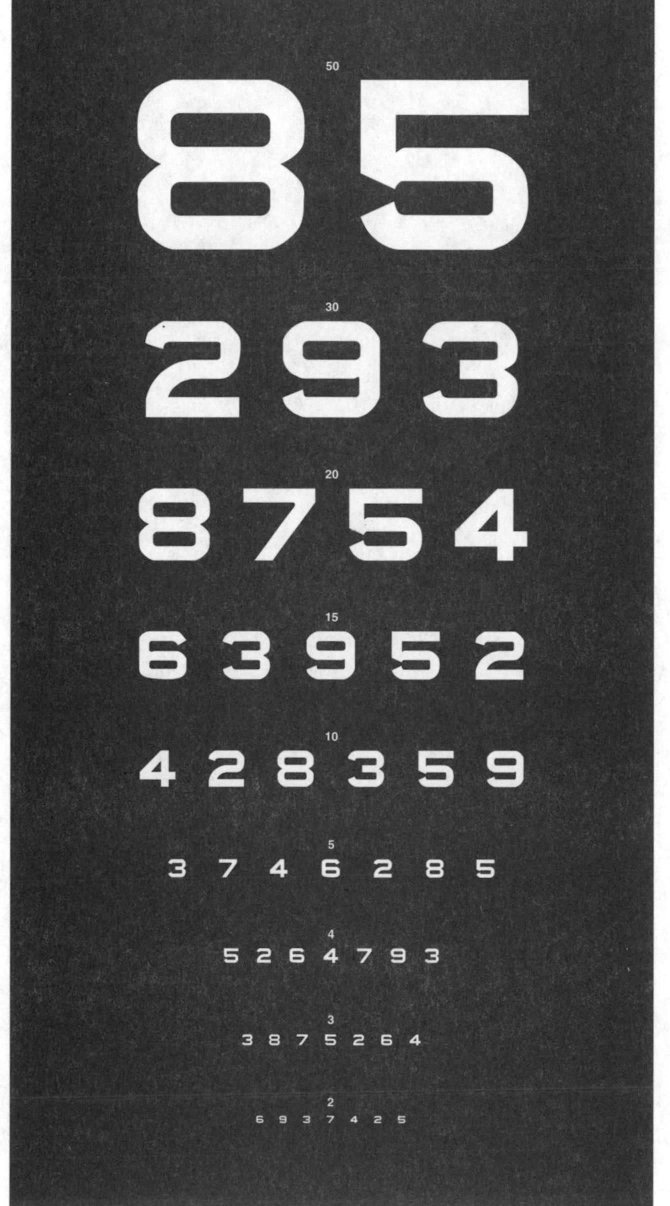

50
8 5
30
2 9 3
20
8 7 5 4
15
6 3 9 5 2
10
4 2 8 3 5 9
5
3 7 4 6 2 8 5
4
5 2 6 4 7 9 3
3
3 8 7 5 2 6 4
2
6 9 3 7 4 2 5

POTHOOKS TEST CARDS

The Pothooks Test Card is usually used with children who do not know letters and numerals.

The next page has reversed type cards.

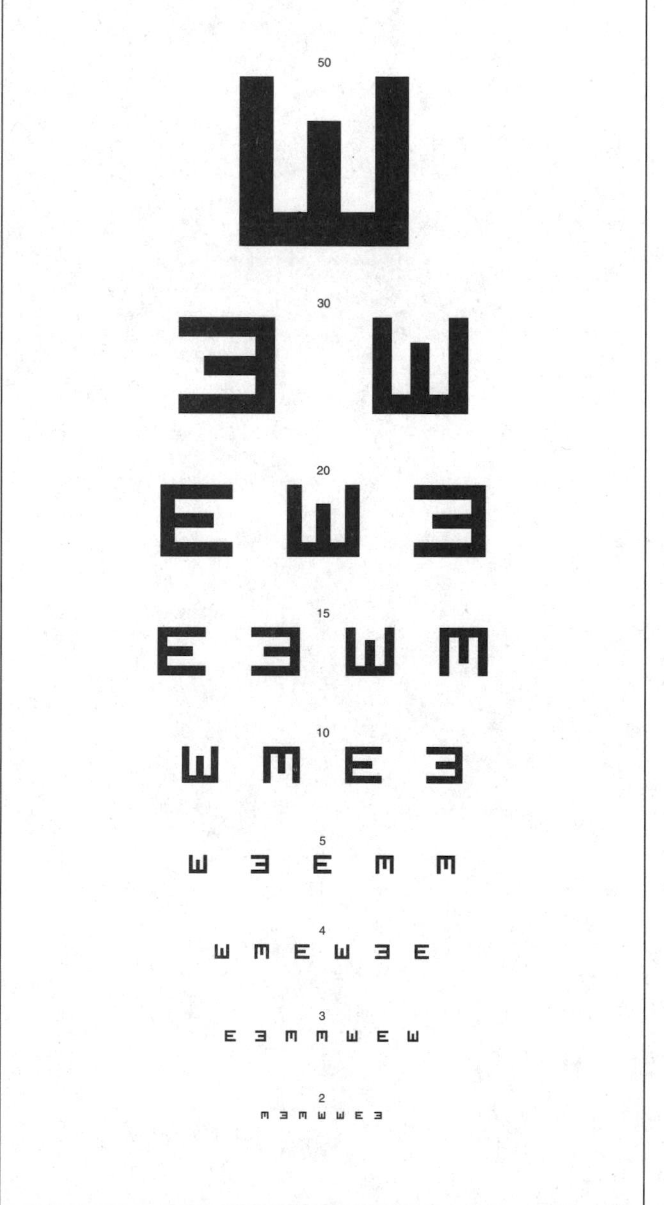

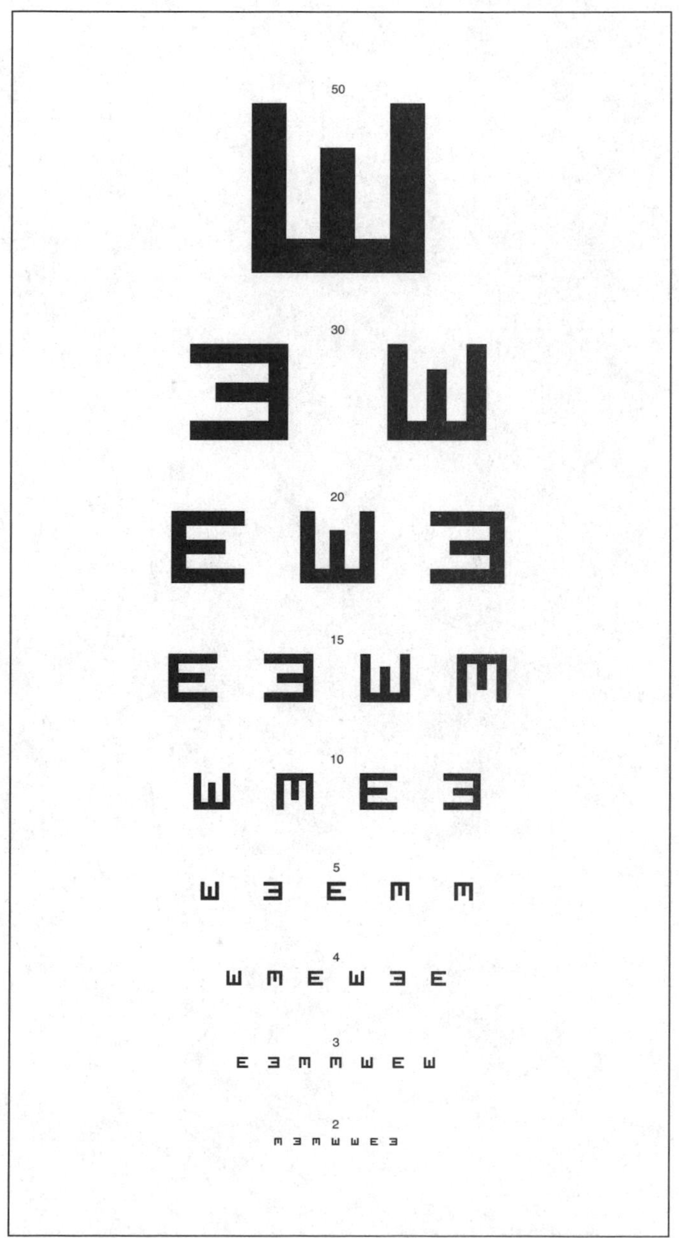

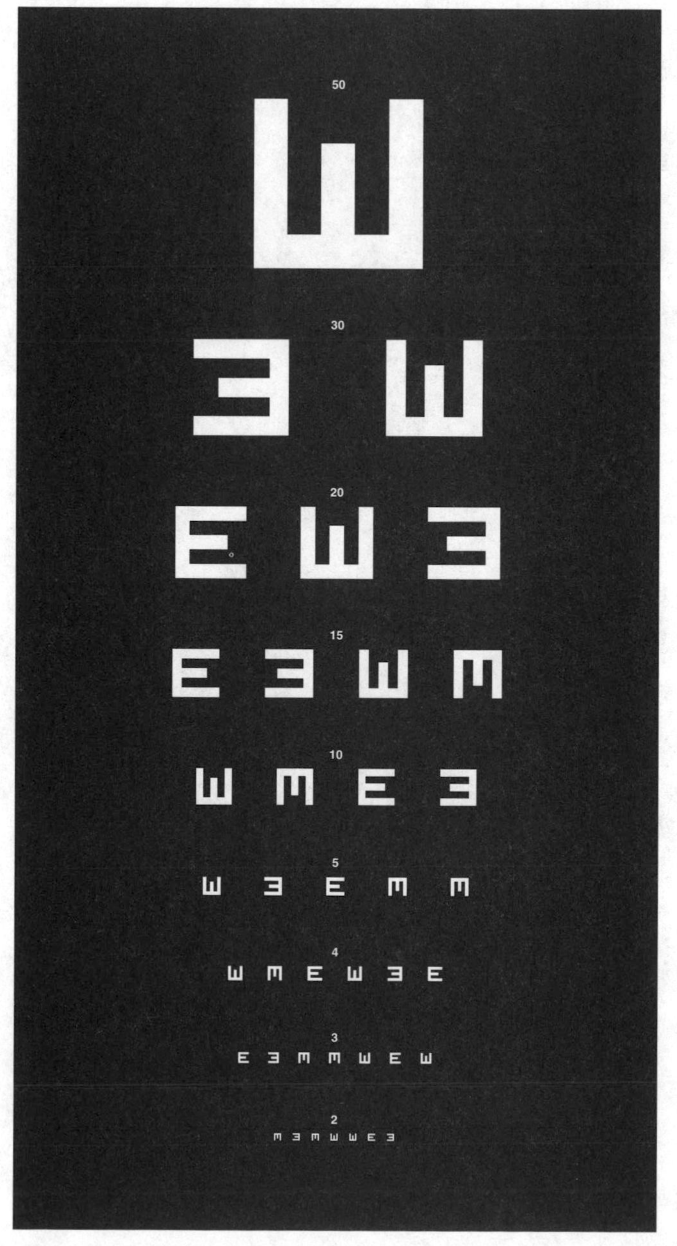

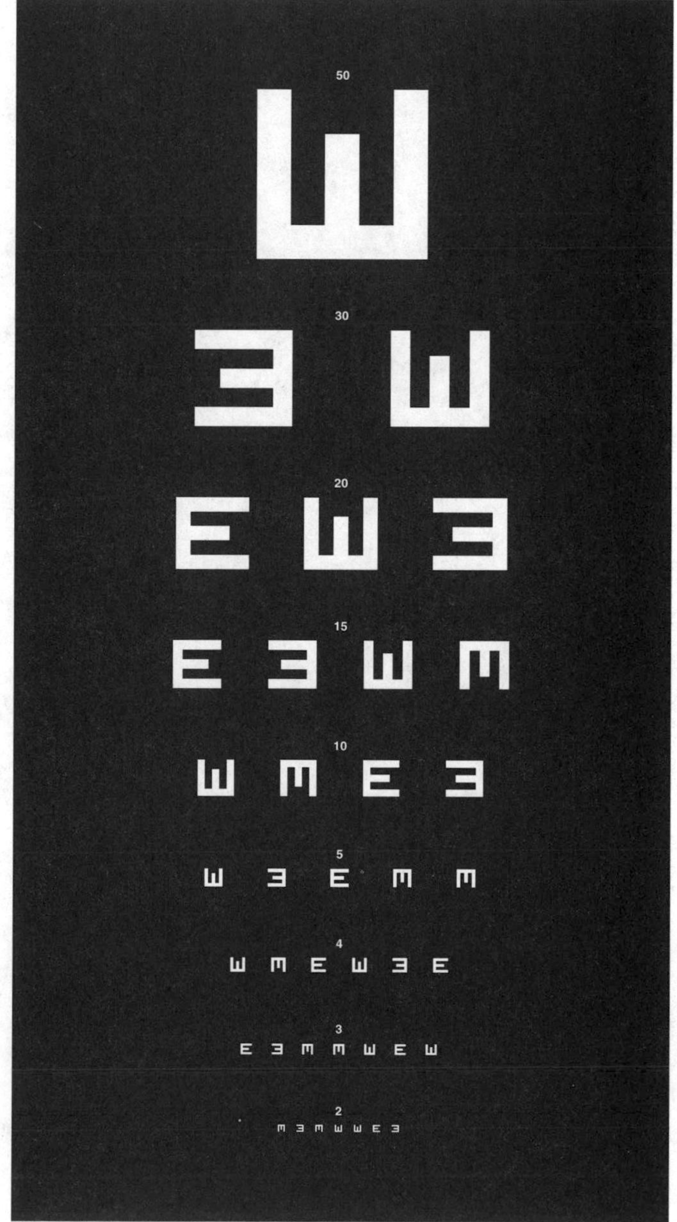

FUNDAMENTALS TEST CARDS

The next page has reversed type cards.

Fundamentals
By
W. H. Bates, M. D.

1. Glasses discarded permanently.

2. Central Fixation is seeing best where you are looking.

3. Favorable conditions: Light may be bright or dim. The distance of the print from the eyes, where seen best, also varies with people.

4. Shifting: With normal sight the eyes are moving all the time.

5. Swinging: When the eyes move slowly or rapidly from side to side, stationary objects appear to move in the opposite direction.

6. Long Swing: Stand with the feet about one foot apart, turn the body to the right—at the same time lifting the heel of the left foot. Do not move the head or eyes or pay any attention to the apparent movement of stationary objects. Now place the left heel on the floor, turn the body to the left, raising the heel of the right foot. Alternate.

7. Drifting Swing: When practicing this swing, one pays no attention to the clearness of stationary objects, which appear to be moving. The eyes wander from point to point slowly, easily, or lazily, so that the stare or strain may be avoided.

8. Variable Swing: Hold the forefinger of one hand six inches from the right eye about the same distance to the right. Look straight ahead and move the head a short distance from side to side. The finger appears to move.

9. Stationary Objects Moving: By moving the head and eyes a short distance from side to side, being sure to blink, one can imagine stationary objects to be moving.

10. Memory: Improving the memory of letters and other objects improves the vision for everything.

11. Imagination: We see only what we think we see, or what we imagine. We can only imagine what we remember.

12. Rest: All cases of imperfect sight are improved by closing the eyes and resting them.

13. Palming: The closed eyes may be covered with the palm of one or both hands.

14. Blinking: The normal eye blinks, or closes and opens very frequently.

15. Mental Pictures: As long as one is awake one has all kinds of memories of mental pictures. If these pictures are remembered easily, perfectly, the vision is benefited.

Fundamentals
By
W. H. Bates, M. D.

1. Glasses discarded permanently.

2. Central Fixation is seeing best where you are looking.

3. Favorable conditions: Light may be bright or dim. The distance of the print from the eyes, where seen best, also varies with people.

4. Shifting: With normal sight the eyes are moving all the time.

5. Swinging: When the eyes move slowly or rapidly from side to side, stationary objects appear to move in the opposite direction.

6. Long Swing: Stand with the feet about one foot apart, turn the body to the right—at the same time lifting the heel of the left foot. Do not move the head or eyes or pay any attention to the apparent movement of stationary objects. Now place the left heel on the floor, turn the body to the left, raising the heel of the right foot. Alternate.

7. Drifting Swing: When practicing this swing, one pays no attention to the clearness of stationary objects, which appear to be moving. The eyes wander from point to point slowly, easily, or lazily, so that the stare or strain may be avoided.

8. Variable Swing: Hold the forefinger of one hand six inches from the right eye about the same distance to the right. Look straight ahead and move the head a short distance from side to side. The finger appears to move.

9. Stationary Objects Moving: By moving the head and eyes a short distance from side to side, being sure to blink, one can imagine stationary objects to be moving.

10. Memory: Improving the memory of letters and other objects improves the vision for everything.

11. Imagination: We see only what we think we see, or what we imagine. We can only imagine what we remember.

12. Rest: All cases of imperfect sight are improved by closing the eyes and resting them.

13. Palming: The closed eyes may be covered with the palm of one or both hands.

14. Blinking: The normal eye blinks, or closes and opens very frequently.

15. Mental Pictures: As long as one is awake one has all kinds of memories of mental pictures. If these pictures are remembered easily, perfectly, the vision is benefited.

Fundamentals

By

W. H. Bates, M. D.

1. Glasses discarded permanently.

2. Central Fixation is seeing best where you are looking.

3. Favorable conditions: Light may be bright or dim. The distance of the print from the eyes, where seen best, also varies with people.

4. Shifting: With normal sight the eyes are moving all the time.

5. Swinging: When the eyes move slowly or rapidly from side to side, stationary objects appear to move in the opposite direction.

6. Long Swing: Stand with the feet about one foot apart, turn the body to the right—at the same time lifting the heel of the left foot. Do not move the head or eyes or pay any attention to the apparent movement of stationary objects. Now place the left heel on the floor, turn the body to the left, raising the heel of the right foot. Alternate.

7. Drifting Swing: When practicing this swing, one pays no attention to the clearness of stationary objects, which appear to be moving. The eyes wander from point to point slowly, easily, or lazily, so that the stare or strain may be avoided.

8. Variable Swing: Hold the forefinger of one hand six inches from the right eye about the same distance to the right. Look straight ahead and move the head a short distance from side to side. The finger appears to move.

9. Stationary Objects Moving: By moving the head and eyes a short distance from side to side, being sure to blink, one can imagine stationary objects to be moving.

10. Memory: Improving the memory of letters and other objects improves the vision for everything.

11. Imagination: We see only what we think we see, or what we imagine. We can only imagine what we remember.

12. Rest: All cases of imperfect sight are improved by closing the eyes and resting them.

13. Palming: The closed eyes may be covered with the palm of one or both hands.

14. Blinking: The normal eye blinks, or closes and opens very frequently.

15. Mental Pictures: As long as one is awake one has all kinds of memories of mental pictures. If these pictures are remembered easily, perfectly, the vision is benefited.

Fundamentals

By

W. H. Bates, M. D.

1. Glasses discarded permanently.

2. Central Fixation is seeing best where you are looking.

3. Favorable conditions: Light may be bright or dim. The distance of the print from the eyes, where seen best, also varies with people.

4. Shifting: With normal sight the eyes are moving all the time.

5. Swinging: When the eyes move slowly or rapidly from side to side, stationary objects appear to move in the opposite direction.

6. Long Swing: Stand with the feet about one foot apart, turn the body to the right—at the same time lifting the heel of the left foot. Do not move the head or eyes or pay any attention to the apparent movement of stationary objects. Now place the left heel on the floor, turn the body to the left, raising the heel of the right foot. Alternate.

7. Drifting Swing: When practicing this swing, one pays no attention to the clearness of stationary objects, which appear to be moving. The eyes wander from point to point slowly, easily, or lazily, so that the stare or strain may be avoided.

8. Variable Swing: Hold the forefinger of one hand six inches from the right eye about the same distance to the right. Look straight ahead and move the head a short distance from side to side. The finger appears to move.

9. Stationary Objects Moving: By moving the head and eyes a short distance from side to side, being sure to blink, one can imagine stationary objects to be moving.

10. Memory: Improving the memory of letters and other objects improves the vision for everything.

11. Imagination: We see only what we think we see, or what we imagine. We can only imagine what we remember.

12. Rest: All cases of imperfect sight are improved by closing the eyes and resting them.

13. Palming: The closed eyes may be covered with the palm of one or both hands.

14. Blinking: The normal eye blinks, or closes and opens very frequently.

15. Mental Pictures: As long as one is awake one has all kinds of memories of mental pictures. If these pictures are remembered easily, perfectly, the vision is benefited.

NEAR EYECHARTS

Hold the Near Eyechart fourteen inches away. The numbers above each line refer to acuity at a distance of fourteen inches. For example, "200" above the letter "S" indicates that this is the 20/200 (equivalent) line; "70" above the letters "T C H" indicates that this is the 20/70 line. The bottom line is 3-point type—20/20 or 14/14 normal near vision.

For more information on reading, see Chapter 22, "Reading—For All Ages," and Chapter 3, "Understanding Lenses and Prescriptions," in *Relearning to See*.

The chart can be cut along the edges and pasted onto cardboard.

The next page has reversed type cards.

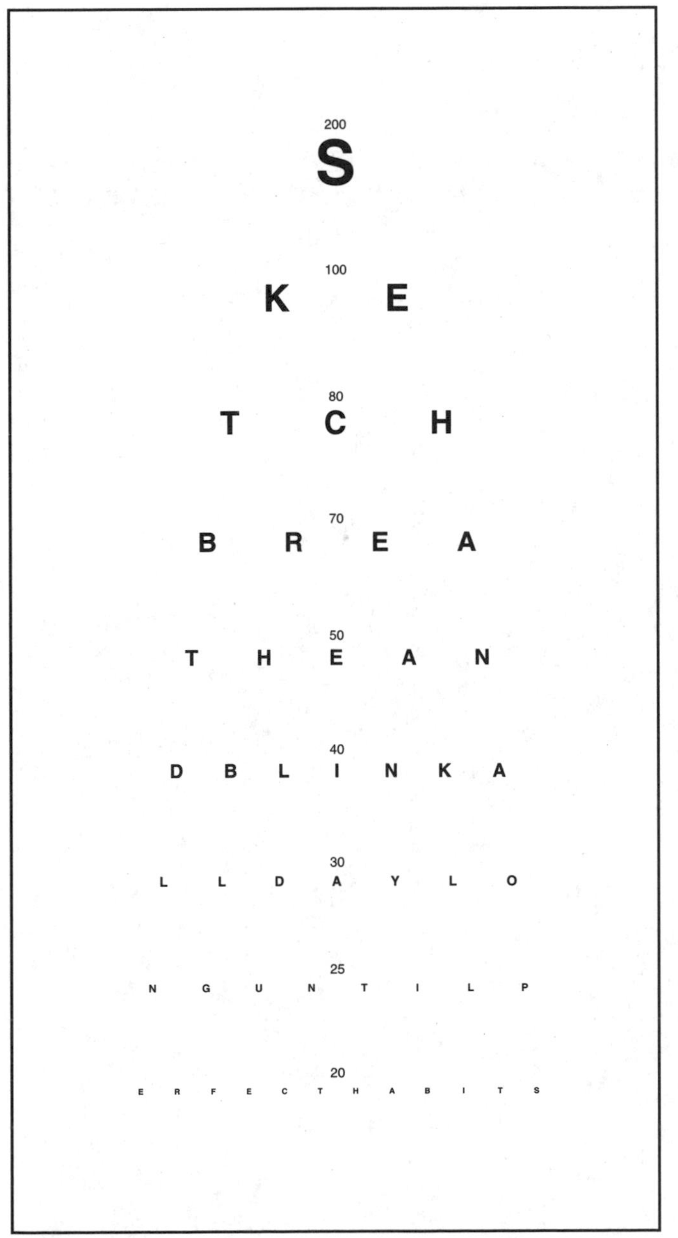

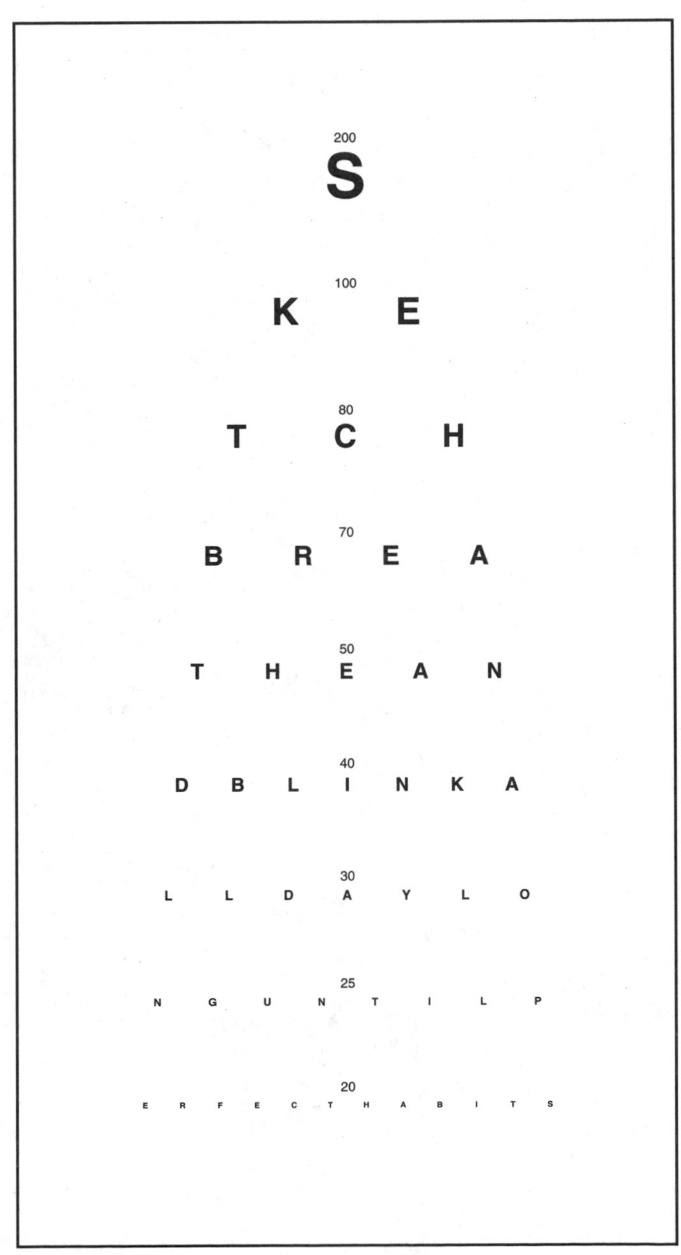

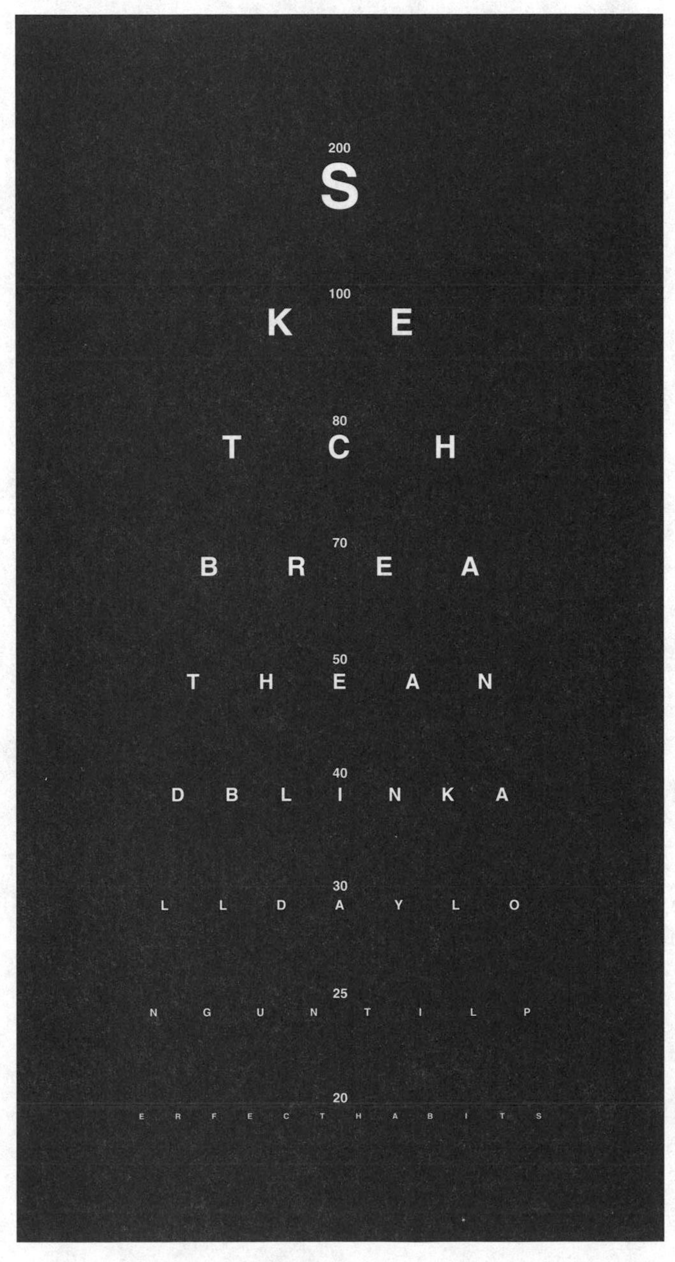
200
S
100
K E
80
T C H
70
B R E A
50
T H E A N
40
D B L I N K A
30
L L D A Y L O
25
N G U N T I L P
20
E R F E C T H A B I T S

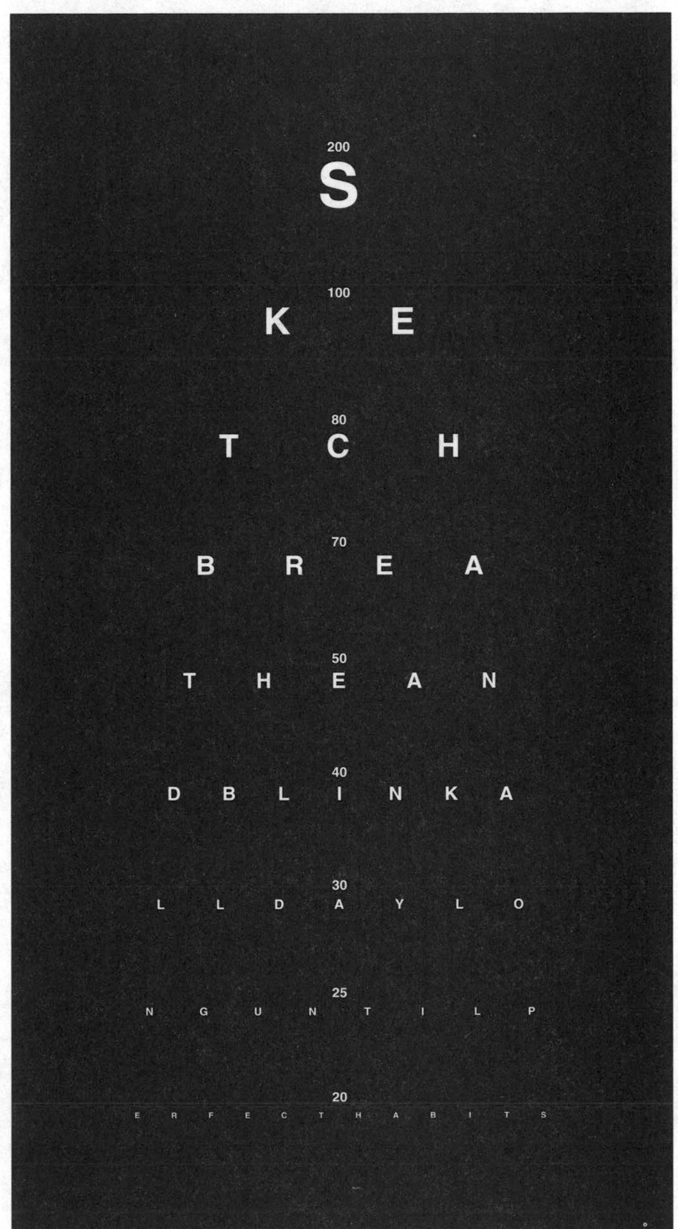
200
S
100
K E
80
T C H
70
B R E A
50
T H E A N
40
D B L I N K A
30
L L D A Y L O
25
N G U N T I L P
20
E R F E C T H A B I T S

INDEX